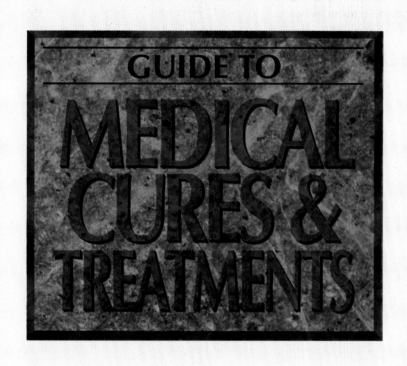

GUIDE TO
MEDICAL
CURES &
TREATMENTS

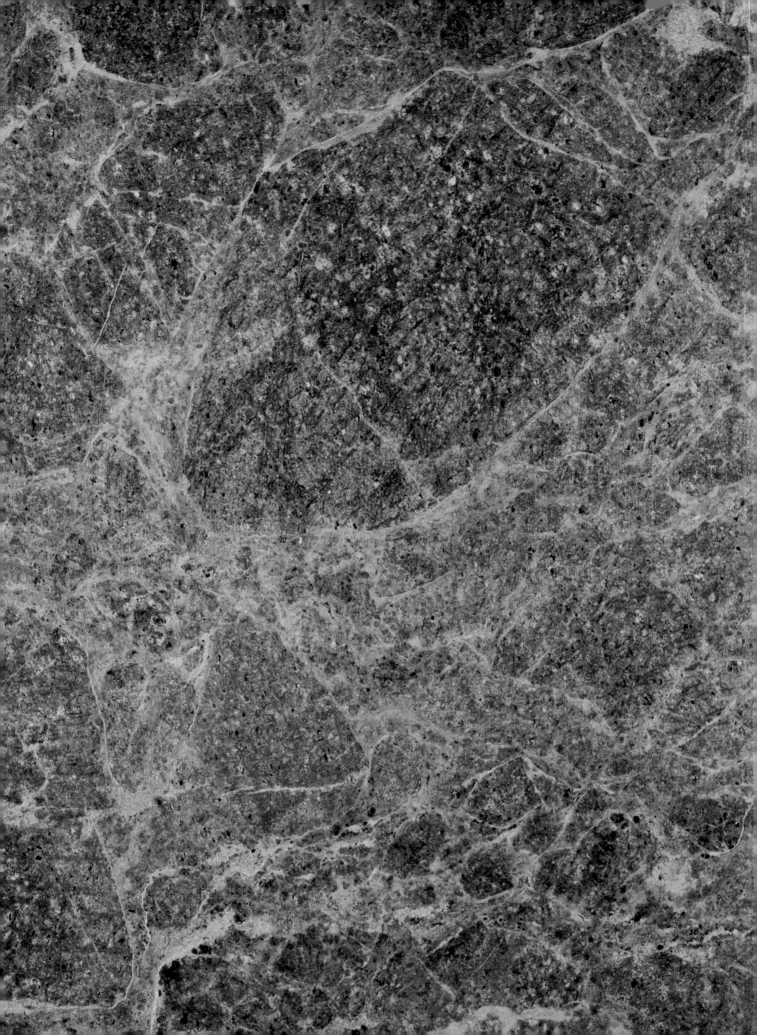

READER'S DIGEST

GUIDE TO
MEDICAL CURES & TREATMENTS

The Reader's Digest Association, Inc.
Pleasantville, New York • Montreal

STAFF

Project Editor
Gayla Visalli

Art Associate
Barbara Lapic

CONTRIBUTORS

Editorial Director
Genell J. Subak-Sharpe

Art Editor
Judy Speicher

Writers and Editors
Diana Benzaia
Susan Carleton
Catherine Caruthers
Mark Deitch
Diane Goetz
Ann Forer
Jennifer Freeman
Helene MacLean
Emily Paulsen
Sharon Pestka
Sarah Subak-Sharpe
Luba Vikhanski

Medical Editors
Morton D. Bogdonoff, M.D.
Valerie Ulene, M.D.

Medical Consultants
Raul Artal, M.D.
Nancy Barone, D.C.
Philip M. Kasofsky, M.D.
Mathew H.M. Lee, M.D.
George D. Roston, D.D.S.

Illustrators
Enid Hatton–Medical
Ray Skibinski–Herbal

Researchers/Technical Support
Arlyn Apollo
Mikola De Roo
Gabby Immerman
Carl Li
Briar Lee Mitchell
Letta Neely
Debra Rabinowitz
Dushan G. Lukic

Photo Research
PhotoSearch, Inc.

Technical Assistant
Christel Henning

READER'S DIGEST GENERAL BOOKS

Editor-in-Chief
Books and Home Entertainment
Barbara J. Morgan

Editor
U.S. General Books
Susan Wernert Lewis

Editorial Director
Jane Polley

Art Director
Evelyn Bauer

Research Director
Laurel A. Gilbride

Affinity Directors
Will Bradbury
Jim Dwyer
Joseph Gonzalez
Kaari Ward

Design Directors
Perri DeFino
Robert M. Grant
Joel Musler

Business Manager
Vidya Tejwani

Copy Chief
Edward W. Atkinson

Picture Editor
Marion Bodine

Senior Research Librarian
Jo Manning

Library of Congress Cataloging in Publication Data

Guide to medical cures & treatments.
    p.   cm.
  Includes index.
  ISBN 0-89577-846-7
  1. Medicine, Popular. I. Reader's Digest Association.
RC81.G885 1996   95-39005
610—dc20

The acknowledgments and credits that appear on page 480 are hereby made a part of this copyright page.

Printed in the United States of America
Third Printing, February 1997

TABLE OF CONTENTS

***Directory of Diseases
Covered in This Book***
*Many diseases have several
names; some are used mostly
by doctors, while others are
part of everyday language. For
example, myocardial infarction,
heart attack, and coronary
thrombosis all refer to the same
disorder. The alphabetical
directory below lists the most
common terms for the diseases
covered in this book. The index
starting on page 470 has an
even more complete listing.*

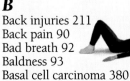

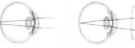

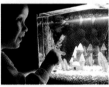

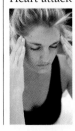

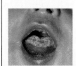

ABOUT THIS BOOK

In today's world, wise people are prepared to make informed decisions regarding their own and their family's health. This means knowing not only about diseases and how they are treated, but also what effect nutritional and lifestyle habits have in preventing illness. Is a particular medical problem something you can handle yourself? If not, how do you decide whom to consult? By using this handy A-to-Z medical reference, you will quickly find the information you need.

But the GUIDE TO MEDICAL CURES & TREATMENTS offers you much more than the usual home medical reference. It begins with an illustrated section on the human body that presents an overview of the various organ systems and how they work together. This is followed by a comprehensive survey of today's health-care system, which describes what to expect from various medical disciplines and provides insight into diagnostic and medical decision-making processes, as well as the domains of various medical specialties and the role of new and experimental treatments. A section on natural medicine covers dozens of alternative therapies—from acupuncture to yoga. You'll learn how these practices evolved, how to distinguish between reputable practitioners and charlatans, and what the advantages and shortcomings are of different alternative approaches.

The heart of the book—the A-to-Z section—is densely filled with information on the symptoms and diagnostic methods of more than 450 common diseases and disorders, how they are treated by both conventional and alternative medical practitioners, and what steps you can take to care for yourself. You'll also find lists of questions that you might want to ask your doctor, plus case histories (included with a number of entries), which are based on real patients; only their names have been changed to protect their privacy.

Following the A-to-Z section is a compendium of the most commonly used prescription and over-the-counter medications. Easy-to-use tables list generic and brand names for each drug, tell what it's used for, and give the major side effects and any precautions you should take while on the medication. Lastly, there is a directory of health resources that lists addresses and phone numbers of nearly 300 organizations, associations, and self-help or support groups.

This book was created by a team of medical educators and practitioners working with skilled medical writers and illustrators to ensure that the text is accurate, up-to-date, and understandable. Throughout, full-color illustrations and photographs are used to make the text even more meaningful.

We believe that no other home medical reference offers so much information on such a range of health problems and their treatments. And no other text allows you to compare conventional treatments, alternative therapies, and self-treatment in such an objective, straightforward presentation. The GUIDE TO MEDICAL CURES & TREATMENTS may well become the most important book in your home health library.

—The Editors

The brain, spinal cord, and peripheral nerves that make up the nervous system function as the body's communications network. The nervous system controls all other organ systems; it also is linked directly with the eyes, ears, and other sensory organs.

The respiratory and circulatory systems work in concert to provide a constant supply of oxygen to every cell in the body.

The endocrine system is made up of various glands that secrete hormones, the chemical messengers that control every bodily process. Hormones are also produced by such other organs as the stomach, lungs, kidneys, and heart.

The renal system filters wastes from the blood, which are then excreted through the urinary tract. The kidneys also produce hormones that are instrumental in controlling blood pressure and the manufacturing of red blood cells.

The organs of the digestive system form a hollow tube that extends from the mouth to the anus. As food passes through this tube, the various organs break it down into molecules that the body can turn into energy and new tissue.

The reproductive organs do more than ensure the survival of the species by producing future generations; they also make the hormones that give males and females their respective physical characteristics.

The adult skeleton contains more than 200 bones, giving the body its form and ability to move. Bones also store calcium and other essential minerals and serve as manufacturing plants for blood cells.

The body's 600 or so voluntary muscles work with the skeletal and nervous systems to make movement possible. Involuntary muscles are instrumental in the smooth functioning of all the other body systems.

The skin acts as a protective barrier against a hostile outside environment. It also manufactures vitamin D, helps regulate body temperature, and is essential to the sense of touch.

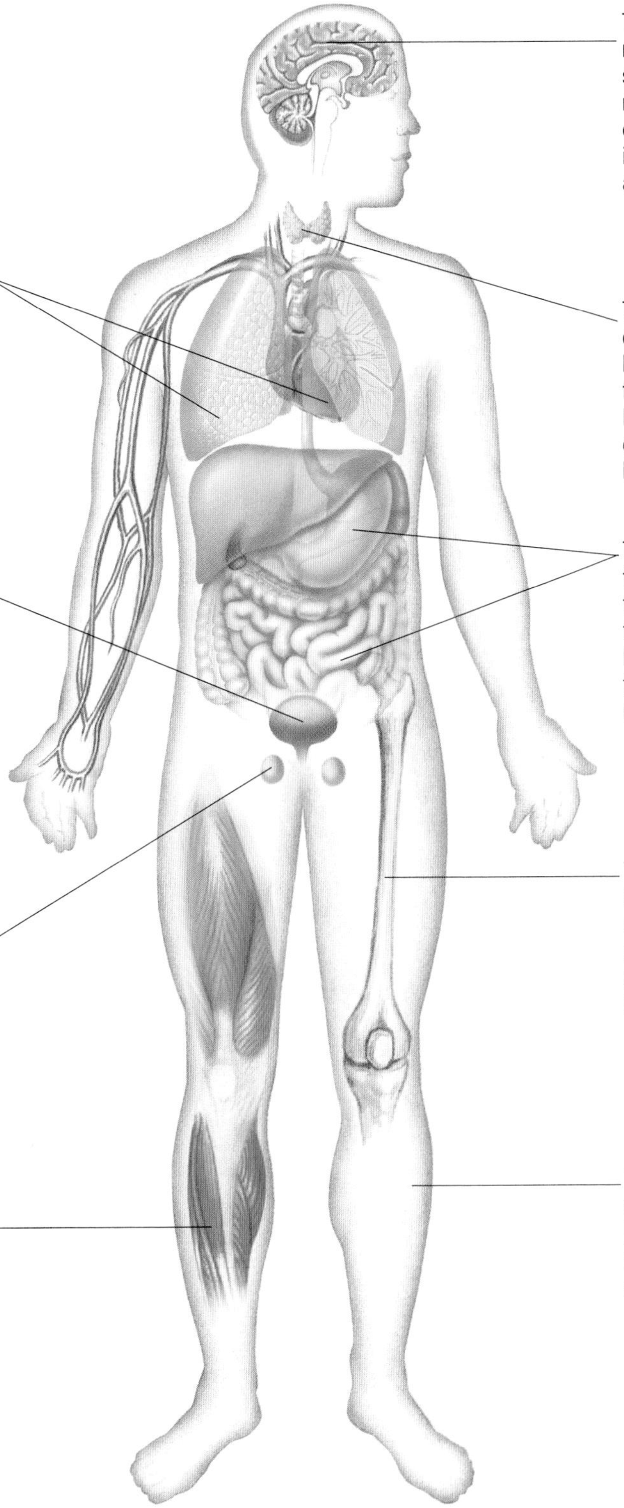

Philosophers and scientists alike have observed that human beings and other forms of animal life are made up of the same elements found in ordinary soil and water. But when these 20 or so basic elements combine in thousands of different ways to form a human body, the result is one of the most complex organisms on the planet and a never-ending source of both wonderment and mystery.

About 75 to 80 percent of an adult's body consists of slightly salty water; the rest is made up of chemical compounds, many of them unique to human beings. These various compounds are arranged to form hundreds of different kinds of cells, the body's smallest, most basic units.

All human life begins with the fusing of two cells, and the subsequent division and multiplication of cells to form a complete body follows the same general blueprint even though no two people are exactly alike. The average body contains 80 to 100 trillion cells, each programmed to grow, carry out a specific function, and even replicate itself. But, with the exception of blood cells, none function independently; instead, similar cells join together to form specific types of tissue—muscle, nerve, bone, and so forth. Each body organ is made up of a collection of related tissues. Finally, organs are organized into the different body systems illustrated above and on the following pages.

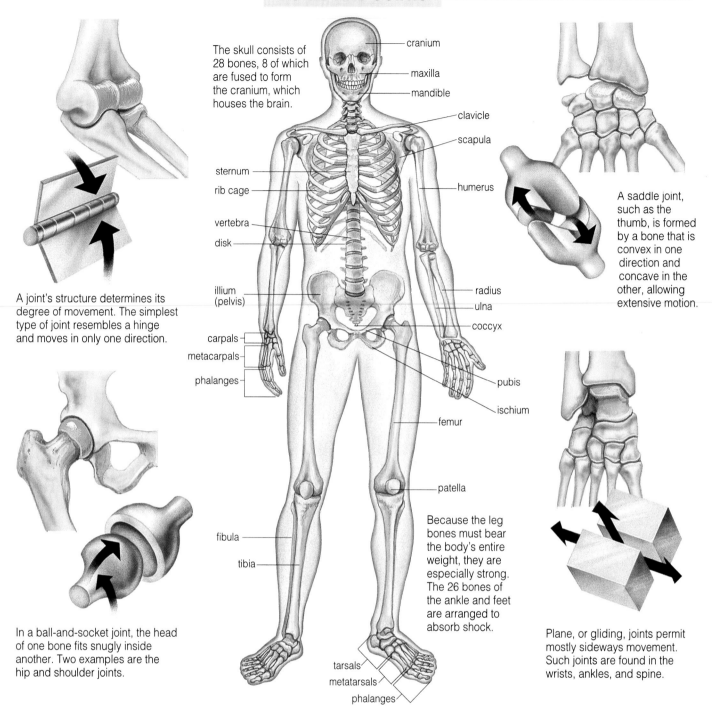

The skull consists of 28 bones, 8 of which are fused to form the cranium, which houses the brain.

cranium
maxilla
mandible
clavicle
scapula
humerus
sternum
rib cage
vertebra
disk
illium (pelvis)
radius
ulna
coccyx
carpals
metacarpals
phalanges
pubis
ischium
femur
patella
fibula
tibia
tarsals
metatarsals
phalanges

A joint's structure determines its degree of movement. The simplest type of joint resembles a hinge and moves in only one direction.

A saddle joint, such as the thumb, is formed by a bone that is convex in one direction and concave in the other, allowing extensive motion.

In a ball-and-socket joint, the head of one bone fits snugly inside another. Two examples are the hip and shoulder joints.

Because the leg bones must bear the body's entire weight, they are especially strong. The 26 bones of the ankle and feet are arranged to absorb shock.

Plane, or gliding, joints permit mostly sideways movement. Such joints are found in the wrists, ankles, and spine.

The human skeleton is an engineering marvel with numerous functions: Not only does it give the body its needed support and a protective framework for vital internal organs, but it also serves as a storehouse for calcium and other essential minerals and is critical in making new blood cells. Although we tend to regard bones as being inert, in reality they are in a constant state of flux and also change dramatically over a lifetime. At birth, a baby has about 350 bones, a number of which are soft and pliable. As the child grows, the bones harden and many, such as those in the skull, fuse together.

The typical adult skeleton has 206 bones and weighs only about 20 pounds. Ounce for ounce, however, compact bone tissue is one of nature's strongest materials. A cubic inch of bone can bear 19,000 pounds, making it four times stronger than reinforced concrete. Bones derive their incredible strength from their honeycombed structure and composition of calcium, phosphorus, and other mineral salts held together by collagen fibers. Nerves and blood vessels permeate the honeycombed structure and calcium and other minerals constantly move in and out of bone tissue. New blood cells are continually being made in the marrow, the spongy interior.

Cartilage, a tough, slippery material, covers the ends of bones, cushioning the joints and reducing friction. Ligaments act as bindings to keep bones in place, and tendons attach muscles to the bones. To permit movement, bones act as levers, the joints are fulcrums, and muscles contract to provide the necessary force (see facing page).

Age takes its toll on bones and joints. The knees and hips are especially vulnerable to degenerative arthritis. And with advancing age, bones begin to lose some of their calcium, making them porous and weak, a condition called osteoporosis (page 320).

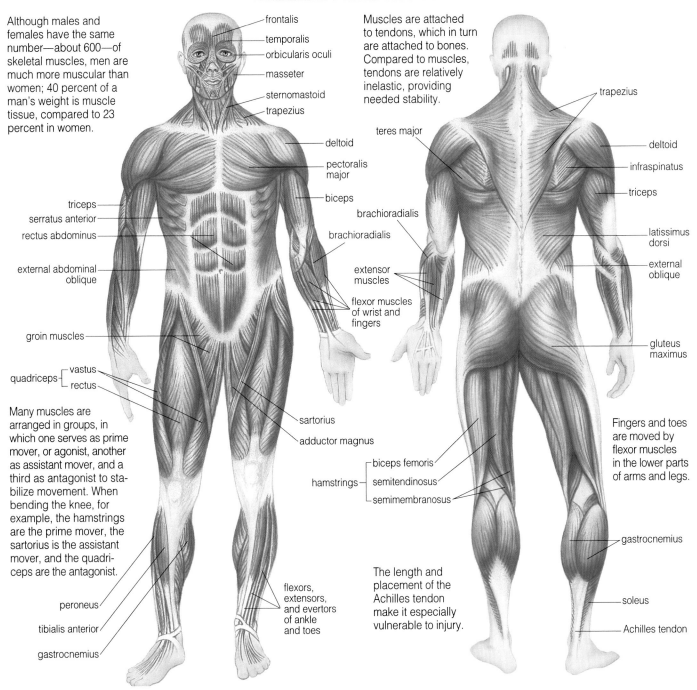

Although males and females have the same number—about 600—of skeletal muscles, men are much more muscular than women; 40 percent of a man's weight is muscle tissue, compared to 23 percent in women.

frontalis
temporalis
orbicularis oculi
masseter
sternomastoid
trapezius
deltoid
pectoralis major
biceps

triceps
serratus anterior
rectus abdominus
external abdominal oblique
groin muscles

quadriceps — vastus
— rectus

Many muscles are arranged in groups, in which one serves as prime mover, or agonist, another as assistant mover, and a third as antagonist to stabilize movement. When bending the knee, for example, the hamstrings are the prime mover, the sartorius is the assistant mover, and the quadriceps are the antagonist.

peroneus
tibialis anterior
gastrocnemius

sartorius
adductor magnus

flexors, extensors, and evertors of ankle and toes

Muscles are attached to tendons, which in turn are attached to bones. Compared to muscles, tendons are relatively inelastic, providing needed stability.

teres major
brachioradialis
brachioradialis
extensor muscles
flexor muscles of wrist and fingers

trapezius
deltoid
infraspinatus
triceps
latissimus dorsi
external oblique
gluteus maximus

hamstrings — biceps femoris
— semitendinosus
— semimembranosus

Fingers and toes are moved by flexor muscles in the lower parts of arms and legs.

The length and placement of the Achilles tendon make it especially vulnerable to injury.

gastrocnemius
soleus
Achilles tendon

The body contains three types of muscle: cardiac, found only in the heart; involuntary smooth muscles, which are part of various organs; and the skeletal muscles, which are attached to bones and make voluntary movement possible.

Skeletal muscles—the body's most abundant tissue—are made up of bundles of long fibers bound together by connective tissue. Each fiber is surrounded by tiny capillaries, which deliver a steady supply of oxygen needed for the muscles to function. The fibers in a particular muscle remain constant in number throughout life, but they enlarge when exercised frequently and shrink, or atrophy, with disuse and age.

Every set of muscles is served by one or more nerves. Movement occurs when nerve signals set off specific chemical reactions that cause certain muscles to contract. Most muscle disorders are actually due to nerve problems. The muscle weakness of multiple sclerosis is one example.

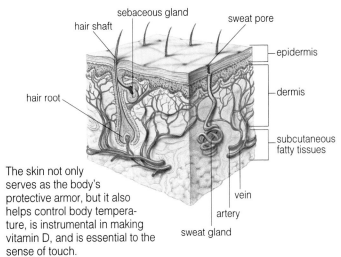

hair shaft
sebaceous gland
sweat pore
epidermis
dermis
hair root
subcutaneous fatty tissues
vein
artery
sweat gland

The skin not only serves as the body's protective armor, but it also helps control body temperature, is instrumental in making vitamin D, and is essential to the sense of touch.

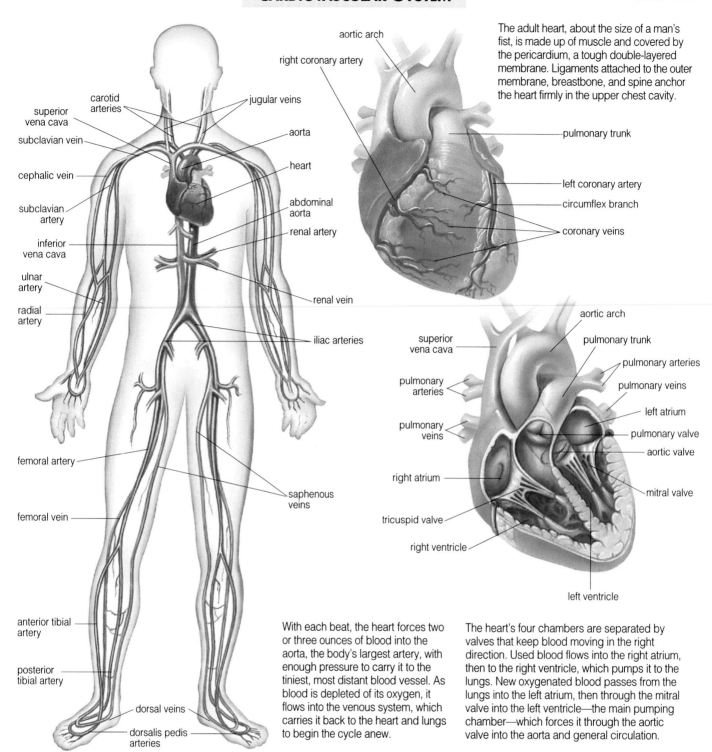

aortic arch

right coronary artery

carotid arteries

jugular veins

superior vena cava

subclavian vein

aorta

cephalic vein

heart

subclavian artery

abdominal aorta

inferior vena cava

renal artery

ulnar artery

radial artery

renal vein

iliac arteries

femoral artery

saphenous veins

femoral vein

anterior tibial artery

posterior tibial artery

dorsal veins

dorsalis pedis arteries

The adult heart, about the size of a man's fist, is made up of muscle and covered by the pericardium, a tough double-layered membrane. Ligaments attached to the outer membrane, breastbone, and spine anchor the heart firmly in the upper chest cavity.

pulmonary trunk

left coronary artery

circumflex branch

coronary veins

aortic arch

superior vena cava

pulmonary trunk

pulmonary arteries

pulmonary veins

pulmonary arteries

left atrium

pulmonary valve

pulmonary veins

aortic valve

right atrium

mitral valve

tricuspid valve

right ventricle

left ventricle

With each beat, the heart forces two or three ounces of blood into the aorta, the body's largest artery, with enough pressure to carry it to the tiniest, most distant blood vessel. As blood is depleted of its oxygen, it flows into the venous system, which carries it back to the heart and lungs to begin the cycle anew.

The heart's four chambers are separated by valves that keep blood moving in the right direction. Used blood flows into the right atrium, then to the right ventricle, which pumps it to the lungs. New oxygenated blood passes from the lungs into the left atrium, then through the mitral valve into the left ventricle—the main pumping chamber—which forces it through the aortic valve into the aorta and general circulation.

The adult body has some 60,000 miles of blood vessels that supply oxygen and other nutrients to every cell and carry away carbon dioxide and other wastes. The heart, one of nature's most durable pumps, constantly circulates 8 to 10 pints of blood through this vast network. On a typical day, the heart beats more than 100,000 times, pumping out 2,600 gallons of blood. This adds up to more than 2.5 billion heartbeats over an average lifetime, with never more than a fraction of a second's rest between each beat.

Although the heart is designed to last a lifetime, cardiovascular disease remains our leading cause of death, claiming more than 900,000 lives a year. Most of these deaths are due to heart attacks, often in the prime of life. The American Heart Association estimates that 56 million Americans suffer from a cardiovascular disorder, with high blood pressure and coronary artery disease the most prevalent. These disorders are epidemic world wide, concentrated mostly in developed nations. They are a relatively modern phenomenon that experts attribute to a combination of lifestyle factors (for example, eating a high-fat diet, smoking, not exercising) and heredity. Increasingly, however, researchers are showing that heart attacks, strokes, and other cardiovascular events can be prevented by adopting a prudent, heart-healthy lifestyle (see Angina, page 79, and Heart Attack, page 216).

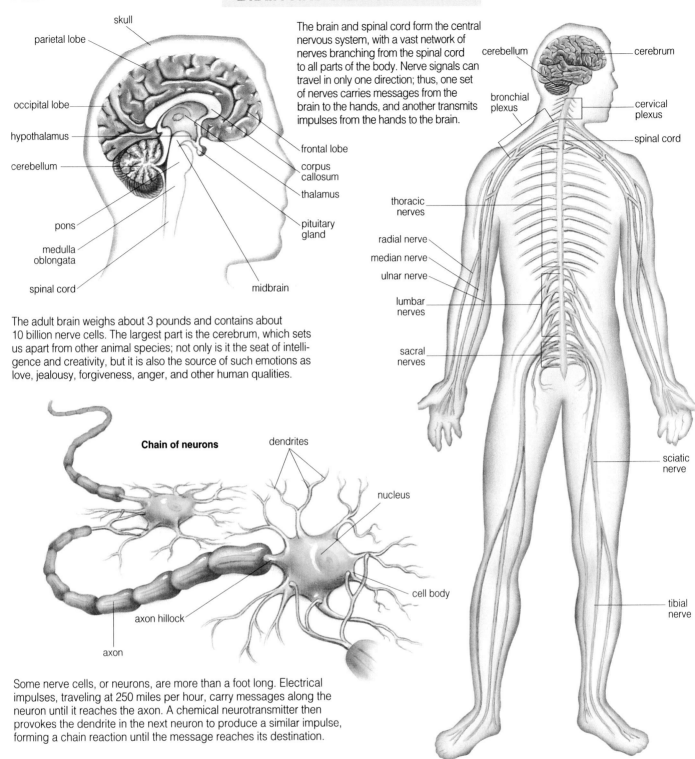

skull
parietal lobe
occipital lobe
hypothalamus
cerebellum
pons
medulla oblongata
spinal cord
midbrain
frontal lobe
corpus callosum
thalamus
pituitary gland

The brain and spinal cord form the central nervous system, with a vast network of nerves branching from the spinal cord to all parts of the body. Nerve signals can travel in only one direction; thus, one set of nerves carries messages from the brain to the hands, and another transmits impulses from the hands to the brain.

cerebellum
cerebrum
bronchial plexus
cervical plexus
spinal cord
thoracic nerves
radial nerve
median nerve
ulnar nerve
lumbar nerves
sacral nerves
sciatic nerve
tibial nerve

The adult brain weighs about 3 pounds and contains about 10 billion nerve cells. The largest part is the cerebrum, which sets us apart from other animal species; not only is it the seat of intelligence and creativity, but it is also the source of such emotions as love, jealousy, forgiveness, anger, and other human qualities.

Chain of neurons
dendrites
nucleus
cell body
axon hillock
axon

Some nerve cells, or neurons, are more than a foot long. Electrical impulses, traveling at 250 miles per hour, carry messages along the neuron until it reaches the axon. A chemical neurotransmitter then provokes the dendrite in the next neuron to produce a similar impulse, forming a chain reaction until the message reaches its destination.

All our movements, thoughts, sensations, and bodily functions are controlled by the brain and nervous system, the most highly evolved among all living creatures and the least understood. Neuroscientists are only beginning to unravel the myriad mysteries of the human brain, and many predict we will never fully understand so many of the things we take for granted: memory, language, creativity, and so forth.

Taken as a whole, the nervous system is actually a complex branching network of systems with many overlapping parts and functions, all controlled by the brain and its spinal cord extension. Such automatic, or involuntary, functions as breathing, circulation, and digestion are directed largely by

the autonomic nervous system, which is divided into the sympathetic and parasympathetic components. In simplified terms, these two systems act as switches to turn organs on and off, thus maintaining a state of balance.

Superficial sensory nerves receive messages from the outside world and transmit them to the brain, where they are interpreted and sent back through the body via the cranial or spinal nerves. All this takes only a split second and often requires little or no thought. However, when something goes awry with the brain or other componets of the nervous system, manifestations can be disastrous, ranging from trivial movement disorders to paralysis and dementia.

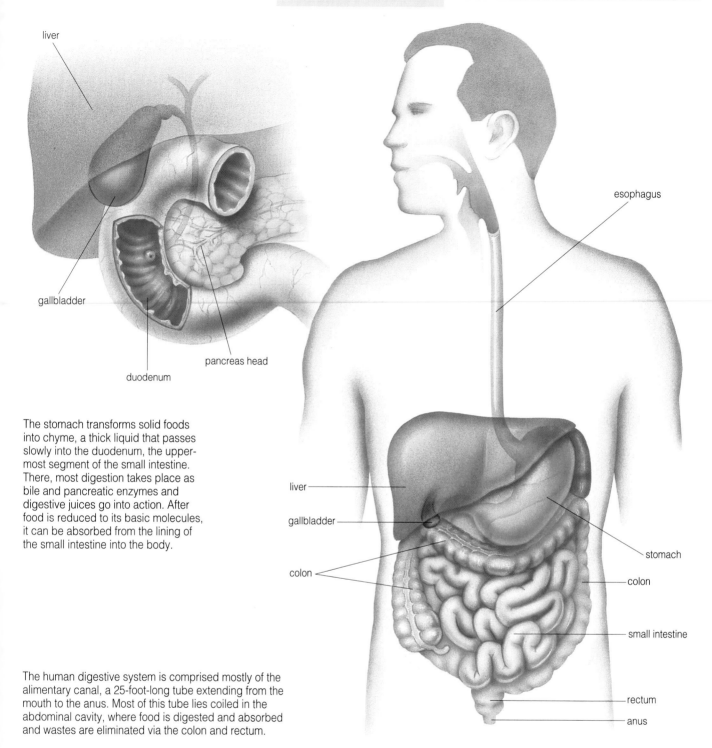

liver

esophagus

gallbladder

pancreas head

duodenum

The stomach transforms solid foods into chyme, a thick liquid that passes slowly into the duodenum, the upper-most segment of the small intestine. There, most digestion takes place as bile and pancreatic enzymes and digestive juices go into action. After food is reduced to its basic molecules, it can be absorbed from the lining of the small intestine into the body.

liver

gallbladder

colon

stomach

colon

small intestine

rectum

anus

The human digestive system is comprised mostly of the alimentary canal, a 25-foot-long tube extending from the mouth to the anus. Most of this tube lies coiled in the abdominal cavity, where food is digested and absorbed and wastes are eliminated via the colon and rectum.

Digestion is a complex chemical and mechanical process that begins when food is chewed and mixed with saliva, which adds moisture and also begins breaking down starch-es. Swallowing forces a bolus of food into the esophagus, a 10-inch muscular tube that transports it to the stomach. Contractions of this muscular organ further pulverize food and mix it with hydrochloric acid and other powerful gastric juices. Little by little, the partially digested food passes from the stomach to the duodenum, the site of even more chemical action. Pancreatic enzymes and juices flow into this upper-most segment of the small intestine, where they break down proteins and carbohydrates. To make fats more soluble, the liver produces bile, which exerts an emulsifying action that transforms globules of fat into minute droplets.

Peristalsis, rhythmic contractions of the intestinal muscles, propels the digested food onward through the small intestine, which is lined with villi, tiny hairlike structures. Molecules can pass through these tiny projections and are then absorbed by the underlying network of blood and lymph vessels. Finally, material that cannot be absorbed from the small intestine passes into the colon. Here, fluid is extracted and returned to the circulation and the remaining fecal material is passed in a bowel movement. The total time required to fully digest a meal varies, but on average, it takes 24 to 36 hours.

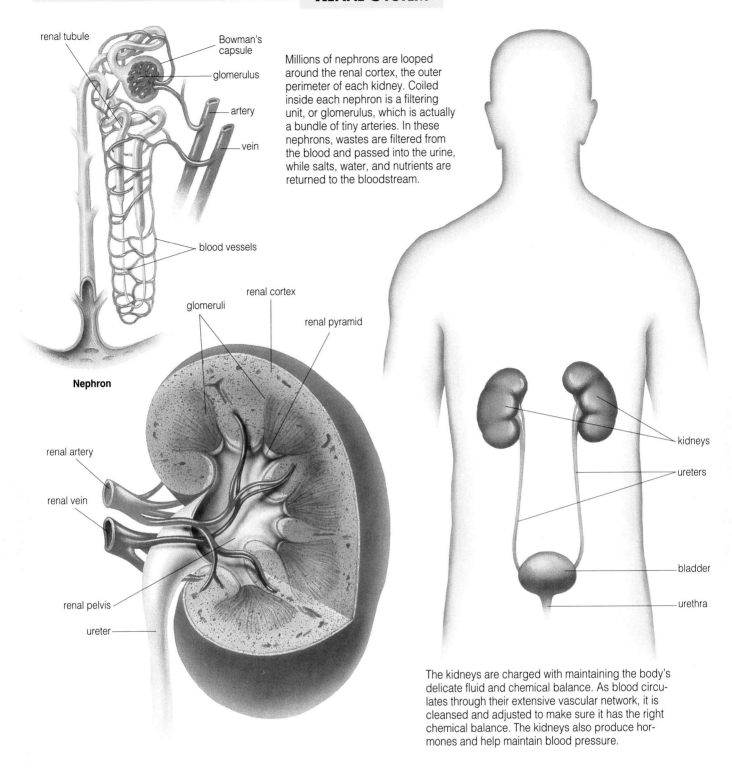

renal tubule

Bowman's capsule

glomerulus

artery

vein

blood vessels

Nephron

Millions of nephrons are looped around the renal cortex, the outer perimeter of each kidney. Coiled inside each nephron is a filtering unit, or glomerulus, which is actually a bundle of tiny arteries. In these nephrons, wastes are filtered from the blood and passed into the urine, while salts, water, and nutrients are returned to the bloodstream.

glomeruli

renal cortex

renal pyramid

renal artery

renal vein

renal pelvis

ureter

kidneys

ureters

bladder

urethra

The kidneys are charged with maintaining the body's delicate fluid and chemical balance. As blood circulates through their extensive vascular network, it is cleansed and adjusted to make sure it has the right chemical balance. The kidneys also produce hormones and help maintain blood pressure.

The body's excretory system is made up of a pair of kidneys and ureters, urinary bladder, and urethra. Kidneys do most of the work; the other structures transport or store urine.

The kidneys are bean-shaped organs, about four inches long and weighing only five ounces. They function as extraordinarily efficient chemical treatment plants, cleansing the blood of urea and other toxic wastes while maintaining the proper balance of fluid, salts, and other blood components. They are also instrumental in maintaining blood pressure.

The renal arteries branch off the abdominal aorta and carry a prodigious amount of blood. Each day, up to 500 quarts of fluid circulate through the kidneys. After it is cleansed, most of this fluid is returned to the bloodstream; only two to four pints are excreted as urine. This waste material collects in the central portion of the kidney—the renal pelvis—and from there it passes into the ureter, a long, narrow tube that carries the urine to the bladder. A normal adult bladder can hold about one pint of liquid, but when it is about half full, it begins to send nerve signals of an urge to urinate. Voluntary muscles in the pelvic floor control bladder function; when these muscles drop, the sphincter that controls the bladder opening relaxes and urine flows into the urethra. The female urethra is about 1.5 inches long and carries only urine; the 8-inch male urethra transports both semen and urine.

The respiratory system is often likened to an upside-down tree, with the trachea serving as the trunk, and the bronchi as the branches. The large bronchi branch out into ever smaller bronchioles, comparable to tree twigs.

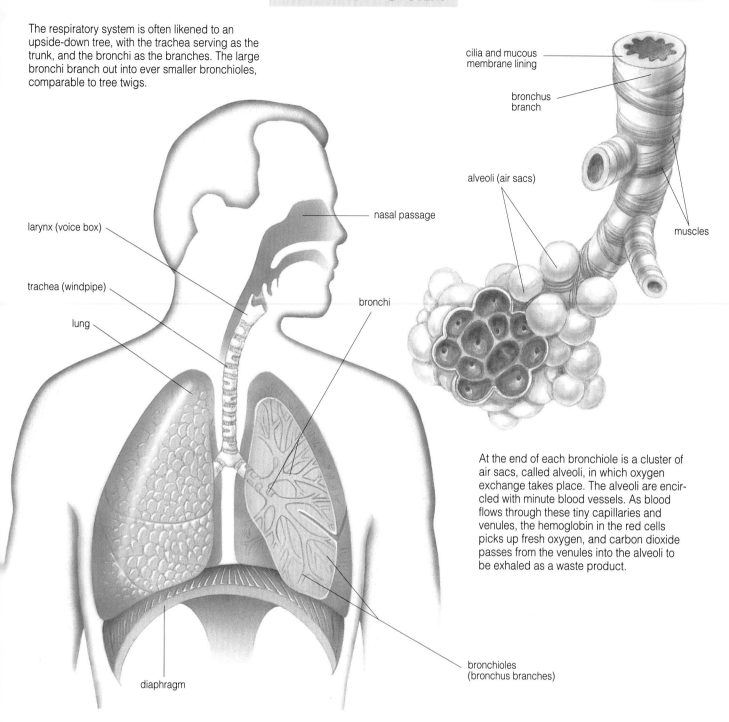

cilia and mucous membrane lining

bronchus branch

alveoli (air sacs)

muscles

nasal passage

larynx (voice box)

trachea (windpipe)

lung

bronchi

diaphragm

bronchioles (bronchus branches)

At the end of each bronchiole is a cluster of air sacs, called alveoli, in which oxygen exchange takes place. The alveoli are encircled with minute blood vessels. As blood flows through these tiny capillaries and venules, the hemoglobin in the red cells picks up fresh oxygen, and carbon dioxide passes from the venules into the alveoli to be exhaled as a waste product.

Of all the substances needed to sustain life, oxygen—an odorless, colorless, and tasteless gas—is perhaps the most critical because it is essential for all stages of metabolism, the various biochemical functions that maintain the body. Without oxygen, cells begin to die within minutes.

With each breath, oxygen is taken into the lungs and carbon dioxide and other wastes are expelled. Although you can deliberately hold your breath for a short period, breathing actually is an automatic process controlled by the brain's respiratory center. When performing quiet activities, a person takes about 14 breaths a minute, but the respiration rate may be slower during sleep or mediation and higher during exercise or other activities that demand extra oxygen.

Air is inhaled through the nose or mouth and passes through the larynx, or voice box, into the trachea, or the windpipe, and then to the bronchi and bronchioles, air tubes that branch off the trachea. These tubes are lined with millions of cilia, hairlike strands that beat rhythmically to keep dust, germs, and other airborne particles out of the lungs. The cilia also help clear the lungs of mucus produced by the mucous cells lining the bronchial tubes.

The bronchioles terminate in clusters of alveoli, tiny, balloon-like air sacs that are responsible for ensuring that the blood has a steady supply of fresh oxygen. Oxygen exchange takes place on the surface of the lungs' 700 million or so alveoli, which, if flattened out, would almost cover a tennis court. The air sacs are elastic, expanding during inhalation and deflating partially as air is exhaled. If alveoli lose their elasticity, as is the case in emphysema (page 175), stale air becomes trapped in the sacs and the body becomes starved for oxygen.

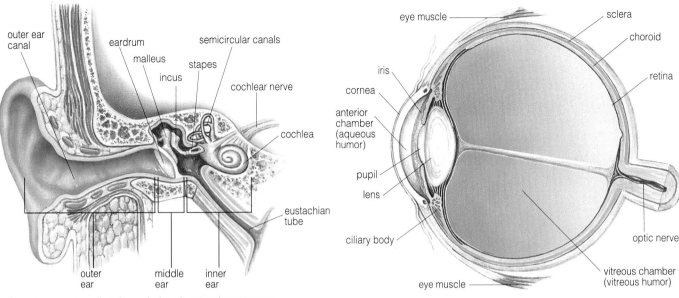

Sound waves traveling through the air enter the outer ear and move through the middle ear into the inner ear, where they are transformed by an arrangement of tiny bones into vibrations. The vibrations then travel through fluid in the inner ear and are converted into electrical nerve impulses to be interpreted by the brain.

Light enters the eye through the lens and is focused on the retina at the back of the eyeball, where light-sensitive cells transform it into electrical impulses. The optic nerve then transmits these impulses to the brain, which interprets the image.

The tongue's surface is covered with millions of projections called papillae, giving it a furry, somewhat irregular surface. There are four types of papillae, three of which contain tastebuds. Although these buds can distinguish only four basic tastes—sour, sweet, salt, and bitter—complex nerve connections and the sense of smell allow us to detect subtle differences.

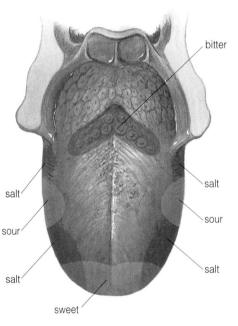

Our sense of smell is centered in the olfactory membrane at the top of the nasal passage. As air passes through the nose, it stimulates cells in this membrane to generate electrical impulses that enable the brain to distinguish specific odors.

Virtually everything that we perceive about our surroundings comes through information collected by the five basic senses—sight, hearing, taste, smell, and touch. Of these, sight and hearing are generally considered the most vital; in fact, however, all work in concert to provide a total picture. This cooperative process is especially apparent when you eat—odor is critical in distinguishing between foods that have a similar taste and texture. This is the reason that food seems to lack taste when you have a cold. However, when you are deprived of one particular sense, others can help compensate; for example, you can use touch and sound to find your way in the dark.

All sensory organs are complex extensions of the central nervous system (page 13), with a direct pathway to the brain, which allows instantaneous processing of information. (The eye's optic nerve is actually an extension of the brain.) The moment you touch an object, you know whether it is soft or hard, hot or cold, smooth or rough. Because information is processed so fast, we give little thought to the complexity of what is involved. Sounds entering the ear or light coming into the eye are immediately broken down and transformed into electrical impulses that are decoded and reassembled in the brain. A similar electrical transformation takes place in identifying an odor, interpreting a touch, and a recognizing a taste.

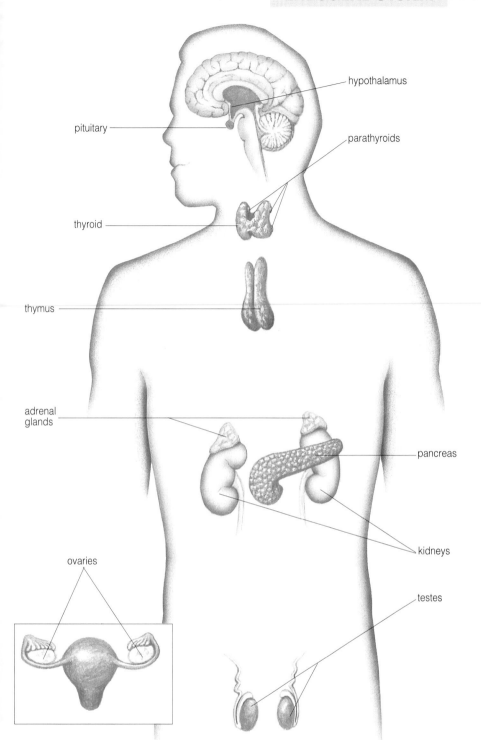

hypothalamus

pituitary

parathyroids

thyroid

thymus

adrenal glands

pancreas

kidneys

ovaries

testes

A finely tuned feedback system, directed by the hypothalamus in the brain, controls hormone levels throughout the body. The hypothalamus senses when levels of a certain hormone are low and passes this information on to the pituitary, which acts as the body's master gland. The pituitary immediately secretes hormones that signal another endocrine gland to pump out the needed hormone(s). When hormone levels are adequate, the hypothalamus switches off the pituitary's action.

Each endocrine gland produces hormones that have specific functions throughout the body. Thyroid hormones, for example, control metabolism and are instrumental in normal growth and development. Calcitonin, also produced by the thyroid, lowers levels of calcium in the blood, while parathyroid hormones raise it. The thymus gland is instrumental in the immune system. Hormones produced by the adrenal glands trigger the body's fight-or-flight response to stress and also control levels of fluids and minerals and glucose metabolism. The pancreas makes insulin and glucagon, hormones that regulate blood levels of glucose. Finally, the gonads produce male and female sex hormones essential to reproduction.

Hormones are chemical messengers that influence virtually every body cell and function. Often working in concert with each other, as well as with the nervous system, hormones control growth, metabolism, digestion, blood pressure, reproduction, and response to stress, among many other functions. Understandably, hormonal imbalances can have profound effects throughout the body.

Although scientists know that hormones are key to almost every body process, much remains to be learned about how they work. For example, we still do not understand how the thymus and pineal glands and their hormones work. And from time to time, yet another hormone is discovered.

In addition to being produced by various endocrine glands, hormones are secreted by other organs, including the lungs, intestines, heart, and kidneys. Regardless of their origin, however, they all travel through the bloodstream in very small amounts, seeking out target organs or cells, which they then stimulate to perform a particular function. Some hormones, such as insulin, are too large to actually enter a cell; instead, they attach themselves to a preprogrammed receptor that triggers the desired response. Other hormones, such as the steroids produced by the adrenal glands, are small enough to penetrate target cells and elicit the desired response from its genetic material.

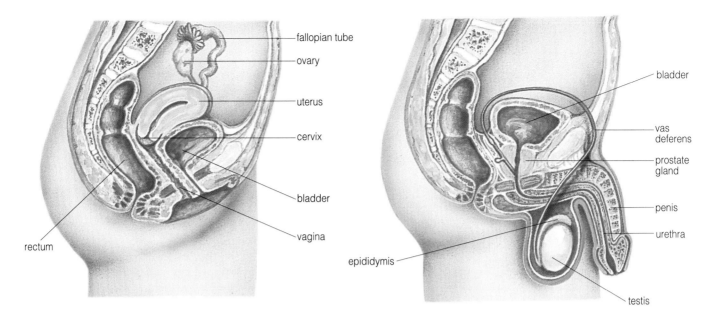

The female reproductive organs lie protected within the pelvic cavity, which can expand to accommodate a growing fetus. At birth, the ovaries harbor their lifetime complement of some 600,000 immature eggs, or oocytes. By puberty, many of these oocytes have disappeared; before menopause, about 400 will develop into mature ova; typically, one or two during a menstrual cycle.

The male reproductive system is designed to manufacture, store, and release sperm, beginning at puberty and continuing throughout life. An individual sperm takes an average of 72 days to mature, but huge numbers of sperm are constantly being made simultaneously; over a typical lifetime, a man produces some 12 trillion sperm.

Each month during a woman's reproductive years, an ovary is stimulated to mature a follicle, which then discharges a mature egg. The egg enters the fallopian tube where, if circumstances are right, fertilization takes place. Within 24 to 30 hours, the merged cell divides and over the next four days, it continues to divide as it travels to the uterus. In six to seven days, the embryo implants itself in the uterus lining, the endometrium, and continues to divide and grow. By the end of the first month, the fetus has begun to take shape, with a heart, budding arms and legs, and rudimentary eyes and central nervous system.

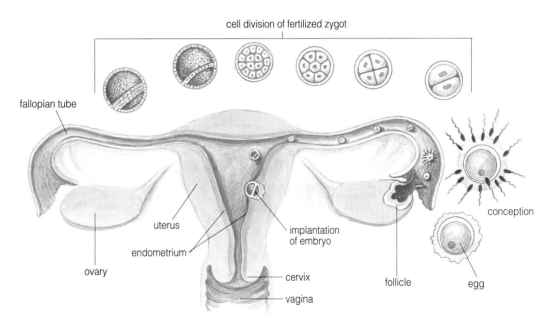

Reproduction remains one of life's most profound wonders. Just the notion that two barely visible cells can merge and form a new human being in just nine months is nothing short of a miracle. Of course, many things can go awry along the way, but most babies are healthy at birth with all the organs needed to grow into a normal adult.

Sex hormones—principally testosterone in men and estrogen in women—directly control reproduction. But many factors influence both the male and female reproductive systems, including overall health, nutrition, and stress. Genetics are also instrumental. Both the mother and father contribute half of the genes needed to make a new human being, and it is this genetic material that determines many of the offspring's characteristics, such as eye and hair color, height, body build, and blood type.

Sex is also determined at the moment of conception and depends upon which sex chromosome is donated by the father. Female cells have two X chromosomes; thus, when an egg divides, it must have an X chromosome. In contrast, males have an X and a Y chromosome, and a sperm can carry either one. So if an egg is fertilized by an X sperm, the baby will be a girl with two female X chromosomes; if the father contributes a Y sperm, the offspring will be a boy with the characteristic male XY chromosomes.

Most lymph nodes are clustered in the neck, armpits, abdomen, and groin. Fluid that drains from body tissues into the lymphatic system filters through at least one lymph node, where layers of tightly packed white blood cells attack and kill any harmful organisms. The swollen lymph nodes that are a sign of disease develop when large numbers of organisms or cancer cells collect in them.

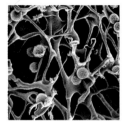

The above enlargement shows the internal filtering structure of a lymph node.

Blood vessels transport white blood cells, antibodies, and other protective substances produced by the immune system. The lymphatic system also returns body fluid to the bloodstream after it has been filtered through lymph nodes.

White blood cells are manufactured in the bone marrow and sent out into the bloodstream and lymphatic system. There are several types of white blood cells: Some are killer cells that destroy invading organisms, cancer cells, and other substances they recognize as foreign to body tissue; others release chemicals that cause inflammation, and still others engulf and digest bacteria.

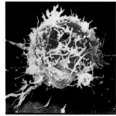

A magnified view of a T lymphocyte, a killer white blood cell.

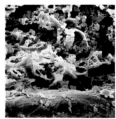

Developing red blood cells are seen as red dots in this enlarged view of bone marrow.

The tonsils are small masses of lymphoid tissue situated at the back of the throat. Along with the adenoids, these glands protect the upper respiratory tract against inhaled organisms. Unlike lymph nodes, the tonsils and adenoids are not enclosed in a capsule. Other clusters of nonencapsulated lymphoid tissue are located in parts of the small intestine.

The thymus is a gland made up of lymphoid tissue. White blood cells that pass through this gland are programmed to become T lymphocytes. The body's most abundant white blood cells, these protect against viruses and other organisms. After puberty, the thymus gradually begins to shrink, although some active tissue remains into old age.

Lymph, a milky substance that contains white blood cells (lymphocytes), proteins, and fats, constantly bathes body tissues as it circulates through the network of lymphatic vessels. The lymphatic system does not have a pump like the heart; instead, lymph is kept moving through the vessels by movement of the body's muscles and a system of one-way valves.

The spleen, a fist-sized organ on the upper left side of the abdomen, is the body's largest lymph node. It has a dual function: As part of the immune system, it produces some antibodies and lymphocytes and helps filter and destroy invading organisms in the bloodstream; it also removes worn-out red blood cells from the bloodstream and breaks them down so that their iron can be reused. Despite its importance, the spleen is not an essential organ; if it must be removed due to injury or disease, its immune system functions are assumed by other lymphatic tissue.

The human body is constantly bombarded by millions of viruses, bacteria, and other disease-causing microorganisms, or pathogens. Fortunately, most of these are thwarted by the body's own protective physical and chemical barriers, such as the skin, saliva, tears, mucus, and stomach acid. The millions of bacteria that live on the skin and the body's mucous membranes also help protect against certain invaders. When a pathogen does manage to evade these defenses and enter the body, it is attacked almost immediately by one or more components of the immune system.

The immune system uses extremely sensitive chemical sensors to recognize a foreign organism or tissue, especially one that can cause disease. Sometimes it overreacts to a harmless substance, such as pollen or a certain food or medication; this can set the stage for an allergic reaction. In other cases, the immune system mistakenly attacks normal body tissue as if it were foreign, resulting in an autoimmune disease such as lupus or rheumatoid arthritis. Most of the time, however, the immune system holds fast as our first line of defense against a host of potentially deadly diseases.

Infectious Agents

Disease-causing organisms vary from tiny viruses to parasites such as the tapeworm, which can grow 20 feet long. Regardless of the size or species of the invading organism, a healthy immune system will mount a vigorous defense against it. The exact nature of that defense varies, however, according to the type and number of invading organisms. The more common types are illustrated below.

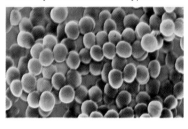

Protozoa are tiny single-celled organisms. Common protozoal infections include giardiasis, an intestinal infection caused by drinking giardia-infected water, and toxoplasmosis, which comes from eating undercooked meat or handling the feces of an infected cat.

Bacteria come in many shapes, including the spheres of various cocci species (staphylococci is shown below), the rods of bacilli, and the spirals of spirochetes like those that cause Lyme disease and syphilis.

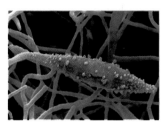

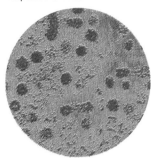

Viruses, the smallest and most prevalent of all life forms, can multiply only after invading the cell of another organism. The enlargement below shows the hepatitis B virus.

Fungi are yeast-like parasites that most commonly grow on the skin or mucous membranes. Ringworm of the scalp is shown above; other common fungal infections include yeast vaginitis and athlete's foot.

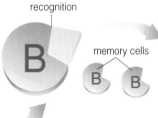

Various worms, or helminths, such as roundworms (left), are parasites that cause diseases.

How the Immune System Fights Infection

Whenever a foreign organism enters the body, chemical signals send the immune system into action. Different types of white blood cells rush to the site of infection to halt the organisms from spreading to other parts of the body.

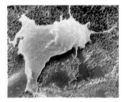

Certain white blood cells, called phagocytes, literally engulf an invading organism.

white blood cells

invading organisms

Organisms that manage to escape the body's first line of defense are met with more concerted and complicated efforts. One calls into action B lymphocytes, white cells that are programmed to recognize a specific organism. In the presence of this organism, the B cells multiply rapidly, producing memory cells that can change into plasma cells; the latter then make antibodies to seek out and destroy the organism. After the infection, remaining memory cells are prepared to go into action if again confronted with the same disease organism.

As part of the immune system's first line of defense, killer lymphocytes release chemicals to destroy invading organisms, while mast cells and eosinophils release substances that produce inflammation. If the invader is a virus, specialized white cells give off interferons, proteins that prevent viruses from reproducing in body cells.

recognition

memory cells

plasma cells

antibodies

organism attacked by antibody

B lymphocytes

disease organisms

killer T cell

invading organism

cell and organism destroyed

infected cell

Another second line of defense involves T lymphocytes, which attack both outside invaders and cancer cells. When a killer T cell recognizes the remains of an organism killed by a phagocyte, it rapidly produces additional T cells to seek out other infected tissue. It then secretes a chemical called lymphokine, which destroys the invader. The killer T cells mount a similar defense against cancer cells. Disease occurs when these natural defenses are weakened by other forces or so overwhelmed that they cannot mount an effective counterattack.

memory T cell

disease organism

lymphokine

New Choices in Healing

Medicine is undergoing a quiet revolution. Only a few years ago, most mainstream physicians and practitioners of alternative therapies tended to view each other with suspicion, if not disdain. Physicians often charged that alternative practitioners were charlatans; in turn, therapists outside of the mainstream claimed that doctors relied too much on potentially dangerous drugs and surgery, and were so overly specialized that they failed to treat the patient as a whole.

Increasingly, both camps are recognizing that each has a place in the healing process—a trend that is being embraced by a growing number of patients. For example, at least one-third of respondents in a 1990 Harvard Medical School survey said that they had been to alternative practitioners. Most patients also saw physicians, but the researchers estimated that visits to alternative practitioners actually exceeded those to primary-care physicians. In keeping with the trend, some insurance policies now cover certain alternative therapies, especially if the treatments are recommended by a physician.

The Historic Perspective

Until the early part of the 20th century, physicians and alternative practitioners competed more or less on equal footing in America, because there were few standards or regulations. Thus, the traveling medicine man could legally call himself a doctor and peddle worthless patent medicines.

This changed dramatically in 1910, when strict standards, based on scientific principles, were adopted for medical schools. Within a few years, only graduates of accredited medical schools could join the American Medical Association, and practitioners of homeopathy, chiropractic, naturopathy, and other "unorthodox" disciplines were shunned by scientific medicine. If the benefits of a therapy could not be documented scientifically, it was discounted as worthless. Some, such as homeopathy, virtually disappeared, and others, such as chiropractic, were relegated to a questionable gray area. Of course, real quackery did not disappear, but government agencies and regulations made life more difficult for charlatans as well as for legitimate alternative practitioners.

Searching for a Common Ground

The pendulum began to swing back with the development of osteopathy and psychiatry as recognized medical specialties, and acceptance of the ancient observation that emotional factors play an important role in health and illness. The 1960s brought renewed interest in Eastern philosophy and healing practices, as well as growing polarization between scientific medicine and alternative therapies. Still, it became increasingly difficult for physicians to discount benefits of certain alternative practices, and conventional medicine started to embrace some of them. In particular, pain clinics began to incorporate such therapies as acupuncture, meditation, and biofeedback training into their therapeutic regimens.

As college graduates of the sixties matured and some entered medical school, a middle ground began to emerge between the two opposing groups. There are still diehards at each extreme, but their numbers are decreasing as more physicians and alternative practitioners recognize that neither has all of the answers but both have things to offer. The basic principles and modalities of conventional medicine are discussed on pages 24–31, while natural, or alternative, therapies are covered on pages 32–61.

A Medical System in Transition

A few decades ago, most families relied upon a general practitioner to look after most of their medical needs. This doctor delivered babies, treated childhood illnesses, set broken bones, performed surgery, and comforted the aged and dying. But lacking vaccines, antibiotics, and other modern medications and daring surgical procedures, these doctors were helpless against many diseases that are now easily cured.

Today, with the growing complexity of conventional medicine, more doctors are specializing in specific parts of the body. Consequently, families are likely to be attended by several doctors, either individual practitioners or members of a prepaid health maintenance organization (HMO).

Faced with a rapidly changing health care system, skyrocketing health-care costs, and so many medical specialists and subspecialists, patients often don't know where to start when they have medical problems. They are baffled by the technology and complexity of modern medicine, and may feel alienated from their physicians, who perhaps don't take the time to explain various procedures.

Experts agree that it's essential in this era of medical specialization and group care for individuals to have a primary physician to oversee and coordinate care. Most primary-care physicians are trained in family practice, internal medicine, pediatrics, or gynecology. If you have a chronic disorder such as heart disease, diabetes, or arthritis, your primary doctor may specialize in that area, and still oversee your care for other problems. Whenever sickness strikes, you should start by seeing your primary doctor, who can, if appropriate, refer you to specialists.

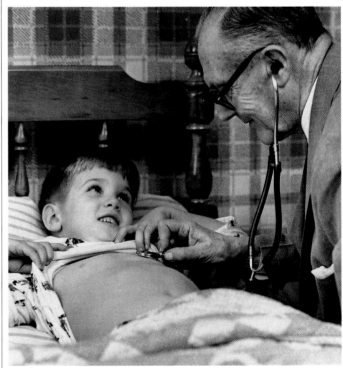

Gone are the days when a family doctor was expected to make routine house calls and treat family members of all ages for a wide range of ailments.

The Diagnostic Process

All medical treatment hinges on an accurate diagnosis, and this begins with a careful medical history. Often, your doctor can zero in on what's ailing you simply by asking the right questions. Of course, you must describe your concerns and symptoms truthfully and accurately. Patients are sometimes afraid to bring up what's really worrying them, and they wait for the doctor to broach the subject. On the other hand, talking about deeply personal matters, even to a doctor, can be embarrassing. It's important to be as forthright as possible.

After taking a medical history, the doctor does a physical examination. Although the emphasis varies according to the symptoms, a typical exam usually includes measuring your height, weight, and blood pressure, and checking your heart and other organs, abdomen, mouth, throat, and eyes for any abnormalities. Routine laboratory tests—blood and urine analyses and perhaps a chest X-ray and an electrocardiogram (ECG)—round out a complete physical. If more information is needed, additional tests may be ordered, or a medical specialist consulted. After gathering as much data as possible, the doctor interprets it and arrives at a diagnosis.

NEW INSIGHTS INTO THE HUMAN BODY

New imaging techniques allow doctors to examine virtually every internal organ without resorting to exploratory surgery. In addition to standard X-rays, these include the following:

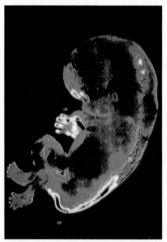

▶ Ultrasound, in which high-frequency sound waves are used in a system similar to sonar for producing images. The waves enter the body painlessly and reflect off internal organs. These reflections can be seen on a video monitor; a computer also records the patterns of reflection and prints out images for later analysis. An audio component can be added to study blood flow through various vessels. Ultrasound is especially useful during pregnancy because it does not expose the fetus to harmful X-rays or drugs.

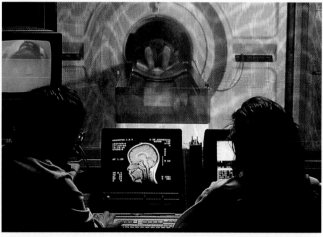

▶ Magnetic resonance imaging, or MRI, in which a powerful magnet instead of the radiation of an X-ray produces three-dimensional views of internal organs. The technique is based on the physics principle that every atom in the body has a nucleus. Radio waves from the MRI machine's magnet, directed into the body, temporarily move the nuclei out of alignment. When the radio waves are stopped, the nuclei move back to their normal alignment, creating signals that are transmitted to a computer and converted into three-dimensional video and film images.

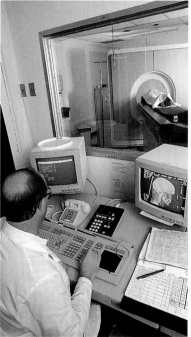

▶ Computed tomography, or CT scans, in which multiple X-rays create a three-dimensional view of a cross-section of the body. The patient is placed inside a scanning machine, while an X-ray unit takes hundreds of films as it revolves around the part of the body under examination. A computer reconstructs the multiple images into a three-dimensional view of a cross section of the body. To make organs stand out, a contrast dye may be used. Color can also be added to the images.

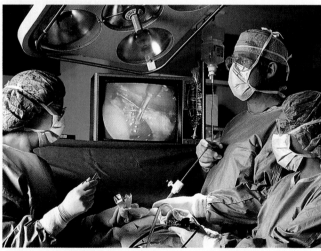

▶ Fiberoptics, in which powerful lights and magnifying devices allow doctors to view internal organs directly. The fiberoptic devices are contained in thin tubes, or catheters, that are inserted into the body through the mouth, anus, or other natural opening, or via a small incision. Common fiberoptic examinations include colonoscopy to study the large intestine, laparoscopy to examine the abdominal cavity, and arthoscopy to view the inside of a joint. During the examination, tissue samples can be collected. Also, many operations, such as removal of colon polyps or repair of a joint, can be performed using fiberoptic technology.

Conventional Medicine

Conventional, or allopathic, medicine focuses mostly on the diagnosis and treatment of disease, although preventive practices as part of this system have gained considerable influence in recent years.

Obviously, treatments vary according to the disorder, but all are aimed at reversing or repairing the underlying condition. If a cure is impossible, the doctor tries to manage or ease the symptoms as much as possible.

Before prescribing a specific course of treatment, a physician weighs the potential benefits against the possible risks. Sometimes the risks or costs of treatment outweigh possible benefits; in other cases, the condition may not warrant immediate treatment but require periodic monitoring. In any event, you as the patient should participate as an informed partner with your doctor in all decision making.

Types of Treatment

All conventional treatments are classified in one of three categories: preventive, noninvasive, or surgery (invasive).

Preventive medicine emphasizes taking specific action to forestall disease. Some aspects are so commonplace that we take them for granted. For example, many killer diseases of the past are now rare or, in the case of smallpox, extinct, thanks to routine immunization. Improved sanitation and other public health measures have rendered cholera, plague, typhoid fever, and tuberculosis rare in industrialized nations, but they are still rampant in undeveloped countries and, given the right circumstances, can spread to developed nations.

Often, preventive medicine calls for a wait-and-see approach in which patients have frequent checkups, but no specific therapy is prescribed. For example, if your family medical history indicates that you have a high risk of developing cancer of the breast or the colon, you will probably be advised to undergo frequent screening examinations to look for any suspicious changes. This allows your doctor to detect cancer in its earliest, most treatable stage.

In other cases, the preventive measures might include drug therapy or even surgery. For instance, low-dose aspirin and other drugs are prescribed routinely now to prevent a heart attack in a high-risk patient. Some people who have a hereditary type of colon polyps that invariably develop into colon cancer may be advised to have a preventive colectomy, an operation in which the entire colon is removed.

Most often, however, preventive medicine emphasizes a healthy lifestyle. Experts now agree that our most common killer diseases can often be prevented by not smoking, by exercising regularly, eating a well-balanced diet, maintaining normal weight, and controlling stress. For many people, certain aspects of alternative medicine, such as meditation, yoga, massage, and biofeedback, have become an important part of their preventive regimens.

Noninvasive therapy usually entails taking drugs, ranging from an occasional nonprescription painkiller to an intensive regimen of chemotherapy for cancer. (Other noninvasive modalities include radiation, sound waves, and psychological counseling.) The introduction of scores of new drugs in the last 50 years has forever changed the practice of medicine. At the turn of the century, infectious diseases were the leading cause of death, and the average life expectancy was about 50 years. Today, not only do vaccines prevent many diseases that formerly killed people in their youth, but antibiotics can also cure most bacterial infections. Consequently, life expectancy in the United States now exceeds 75 years.

Serious incurable diseases such as diabetes and high blood pressure can be controlled by drugs. Similarly, drugs help minimize the crippling effects of arthritis and control many forms of mental illness. But much remains to be done. AIDS and other deadly diseases still defy a cure; researchers hope that these will soon be conquered by drugs or vaccines.

Although drugs can be life-saving, they can also produce adverse side effects that range from minor and annoying to potentially fatal. Medications are not "magic bullets" that attack only the disease; instead, they affect the entire body. Some trigger the immune system to mount an allergic reaction; others damage healthy as well as diseased tissue; and still others produce quite unpredictable reactions. A few of the latter have led to new drug uses and discoveries. For example, the observation that certain allergy medications reduce appetite resulted in the development of new diet pills; the ability of a blood pressure drug to stimulate hair growth produced a somewhat effective treatment for baldness.

Researchers are always seeking to minimize any adverse side effects by devising new ways to deliver medications to their target tissues and bypass organs that would be adversely affected. Some of these are already in use. For example, medicated skin patches effectively deliver small, steady amounts of drugs directly into the bloodstream, thus avoiding the potential problems of having larger doses circulating at any time.

A healthy lifestyle, which includes a nutritious diet, plenty of exercise, and control of weight and stress, is the best preventive medicine.

Enteric coatings that cause a pill to remain intact until it reaches the small intestine protect the stomach from irritation. Cloning techniques that produce special antibodies to carry drugs make it easier to target cancer drugs on tumor cells while sparing normal tissue.

Fetuses, young children, and the elderly are especially vulnerable to adverse drug effects, and in these groups, medications should be used only under a doctor's careful supervision. In general, medicines must always be used cautiously, if at all, during pregnancy, and dosages should be carefully adjusted for children and the elderly.

For anyone, the risk of adverse drug effects increases with the number of medications taken simultaneously because many drugs interact with each other. These dangers can be minimized by always giving a doctor and pharmacist a list of all medications you are taking—including vitamins and non-prescription drugs—before adding more. Many pharmacists now keep computer patient drug profiles, making it easy to spot potentially harmful combinations.

Surgery, an invasive procedure that requires making an incision and using various instruments to enter the body, has also made tremendous advances in recent years. It is an ancient art that was typically practiced in years past by barbers and veterinarians, rather than physicians. Until the 20th century, surgery had a high mortality rate from infection and other complications. Modern anesthesia and antiseptic techniques revolutionized the practice, making most operations painless with greatly reduced risk.

There are now hundreds of different surgical procedures. Operations are performed to repair a damaged structure, to remove a diseased organ, or to alleviate a chronic symptom such as pain. In some instances, surgery may be aimed at preventing a future disease or problem; such a case would be removal of a benign growth to prevent its becoming cancerous. Some operations, especially cosmetic plastic surgery, are intended primarily to enhance self-esteem and a sense of well-being rather than alleviate a medical problem. Doctors may also use surgical procedures, such as biopsies and exploratory surgery, to help in making a diagnosis.

In the 1970s and 1980s, surgery underwent another revolution: Development of powerful surgical microscopes and fiberoptic techniques made it possible to perform delicate operations through tiny puncture incisions. For example, some back surgery that once required a long incision and weeks of recuperation can now be performed using microsurgery methods that necessitate only a brief hospital stay.

Coronary bypass surgery and other heart operations that were impossible a few decades ago are now routine. In fact, critics charge that a large percentage of bypass procedures are unnecessary, and that many patients would do just as well with medication and lifestyle changes. In nonemergency cases many insurance companies and other third-party payers now require a presurgery second opinion to make sure that the operation is really needed. (See box, lower left.)

For some diseases, most notably cancer, surgery is the major treatment. But it is often combined with other approaches, such as radiation and chemotherapy, to produce even better results. Similarly, arthritis treatment may entail a combination of medication and exercise, as well as surgery.

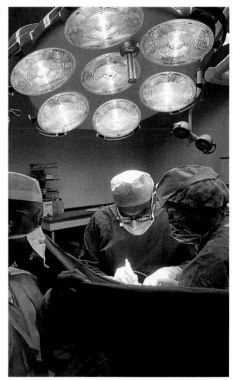

Fiberoptic technology and powerful surgical microscopes now enable surgeons to perform complex procedures through tubes inserted into tiny incisions or natural body openings.

Small amounts of powerful chemotherapy drugs for cancer are often combined to increase their effectiveness and minimize side effects.

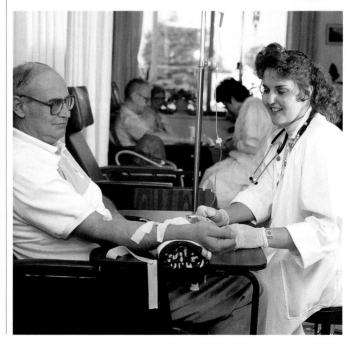

SHOULD YOU SEEK A SECOND OPINION?
Studies show that a large percentage of surgery done in the U.S. each year could be avoided. Because all operations carry a risk, and most are more costly than other treatments, make sure that surgery is the best treatment option. In particular, always seek a second opinion before having any of the following operations:

Cataract removal	Knee surgery
Coronary artery bypass and other heart operations	Prostate surgery
Gallbladder removal	Spinal disk removal and other back operations
Hernia repair	Tonsillectomy
Hysterectomy	

Laboratory Medicine

All doctors rely on laboratory tests in making many of their medical decisions. Some tests may be done on samples of blood, urine, or body tissue. For others, the patient may be sent to a special laboratory for X-rays (page 27), function studies (described below) or scans, imaging, or certain invasive procedures such as colonoscopy (explained on page 23). The following are some of the more common tests that you may encounter as part of a diagnostic process.

Urinalysis. Urine studies are the oldest medical tests. Ancient physicians diagnosed disease by studying the color and smell of urine, and some even tasted it. By this last method, early Greek physicians could discern diabetes, when the urine had a sweet taste because of the presence of blood sugar, or glucose. Today, urine is studied not only for glucose, but also for blood cells, protein, bacteria, hormones, and chemicals. Some urine tests can be done at home. Included

studied, especially if sickle cell disease, anemia, leukemia, or another type of blood disorder is suspected.

Biopsies. These tests require examination of a sample of tissue under a microscope for abnormalities. In some biopsies, a tumor or piece of tissue is removed surgically. In other cases, such as in a bone, liver, or breast biopsy, the sample may be obtained by aspiration with a hollow needle inserted through the skin and overlying tissue.

Pap smear. This test involves scraping cells from the surface of a woman's cervix and then studying them microscopically for abnormalities that indicate possible cancer. Pap smears, which are included as part of most gynecological examinations, should be performed every one to three years.

Function tests. These are diagnostic studies done in special laboratories to assess how well an organ or organ system is functioning. Common examples include hearing and vision tests, spirometry to assess lung function, exercise stress tests to study cardiovascular capability, and nerve and muscle studies. In some cases, such as a fertility workup, function tests are usually combined with other types of laboratory analyses.

The Cost Factor

In recent years, testing has emerged as the fastest growing and most costly aspect of medical care in the United States. Computers and other technological advances are responsible for much of this growth, but changes in medical practice are also a factor. For example, many doctors say they order tests as a protective measure against malpractice suits, even though they may not expect the results to alter treatment. Others perhaps use tests to boost income, because they can charge higher fees (and are more likely to be reimbursed by insurance and other third-party payers) for tests and procedures than for time spent counselling their patients in preventive measures.

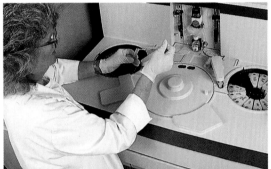

Modern medical laboratories are equipped with a wide array of sophisticated machines that can perform multiple tests using a single blood sample.

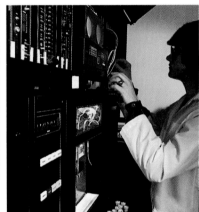

are early pregnancy tests, which can now detect pregnancy as soon as two weeks after conception; and a glucose test, in which chemical strips dipped in a urine sample can detect sugar, a sign that diabetes is out of control. For other analyses, the urine specimen may be collected at home or in a doctor's office, and then sent to a laboratory.

Blood tests. Your blood speaks volumes about your health, and blood tests can detect many conditions long before any symptoms appear. Certain of these tests involve measuring levels of substances carried in the blood, such as cholesterol, hormones, enzymes, drugs, and numerous body chemicals. A biochemical profile, which may involve 40 or more such measurements, can now be done very quickly in a sequential multiple analyzer (SMA) machine with just one or two test tubes of blood. The results are reported on a computer printout that compares your numbers with normal ones.

Although automated blood analysis is fast and relatively inexpensive, errors are common, and you should not be unduly alarmed by an abnormal result. In such cases, a second, less automated, and more precise test will be done to confirm the results of the first one.

Other tests involve looking through a microscope at the blood cells themselves. For a total blood count, the numbers of different blood cells in a specific amount of blood are estimated. The size, shapes, and color of the cells may also be

In some instances, costly screening tests only rarely uncover an abnormality, raising the question of whether they are cost-effective. For example, ultrasound is now performed frequently during pregnancy to screen for certain birth defects and determine fetal age. Some economists question whether this is an appropriate use of medical resources because the large majority of pregnancies are normal. As an alternative, they suggest that ultrasound be reserved for high-risk pregnancies or those in which a problem is already suspected.

Cost is not the only issue—many tests are uncomfortable and some carry a risk of complications. As a patient, you can protect yourself from being given any unnecessary tests by asking the following questions:

▶ Why do I need this test?
▶ Is it painful?
▶ Is there any risk of complications?
▶ How accurate, usually, are the results?
▶ Am I likely to need additional tests?
▶ How will the results be used?
▶ Will the results affect the course of my treatment?
▶ What will happen if I don't have the test?

Nuclear Medicine

Nuclear medicine involves the use of radioactive materials for either diagnosis or treatment. Until the 1950s, the technology was confined to diagnostic X-rays and radiation treatments for cancer and a few other diseases. Today, it is used in the most sophisticated diagnostic studies and surgical procedures, and includes such subspecialties as nuclear cardiology.

For diagnostic X-rays, relatively low doses of ionizing radiation are beamed through soft tissue onto photographic film, where they make denser tissue, such as bone, stand out.

For therapy, radiation is given in larger doses that kill body tissues by destroying the ability of cells to grow and divide normally. It is especially lethal to tissue that grows fast, with a rapid rate of renewal. This is why it is effective in shrinking and eventually eliminating cancerous tumors. Today, half of all cancer patients receive some form of radiation therapy.

Because radiation cannot distinguish between cancerous and normal tissue, it also damages healthy cells, particularly in the skin, the linings of many internal organs, and the bone marrow, where blood cells are made. If the radiation dosage is not too high, most normal tissue will eventually repair itself. Thus, the challenge is to find a dosage that will kill a cancer without rendering permanent damage to the healthy surrounding tissue. Complicating matters is the fact that radiation damage is cumulative. Even low-level environmental, or background, radiation contributes to the buildup.

The Newer Technologies

As medical researchers learn more about the harmful effects of radiation, they are developing ever safer ways to use it. New technology allows doctors to implant tiny radioactive seeds in some types of tumors to shrink or destroy them while sparing healthy tissue. This approach is now being used for prostate cancer and certain inoperable tumors.

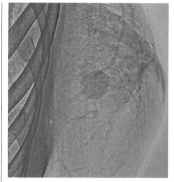
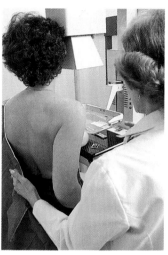

Mammography often can detect breast cancers that are too small to be felt during a physical examination. Above is a mammogram showing a small tumor.

In treating other cancerous growths, computers enable therapists to calculate the precise dosage required and new machines beam radiation directly to the tumor. In still other instances, chemicals carry radiation to an organ without exposing other parts of the body. For example, the use of radioactive iodine often removes the need for surgery in the treatment of an overactive thyroid gland; the thyroid absorbs the iodine, and the radiation destroys part or all of the gland's hormone-making tissue.

New X-ray equipment also delivers less radiation than in the past. The newest mammography machines, for example, require less than one-third of the amount of radiation needed only 20 years ago. In addition, the injection of minute amounts of radioactive particles that can be followed by special gamma cameras allows doctors to study internal organs with less radiation and more accuracy than is possible with X-ray machines alone. For instance, a radioactive material called thallium is used in making heart scans that pinpoint areas where the cardiac muscle is not getting enough blood.

Despite the tremendous advances in nuclear medicine, it is important to realize that there is still a risk involved in exposure to any radiation. Avoid routine diagnostic X-rays unless their benefit clearly outweighs the risk. Hence, the potential risk of an annual chest X-ray is greater than the possible benefits for a healthy person. In contrast, mammography every one or two years for women over the age of 50 is currently recommended because the risk of breast cancer is much higher than any known hazards of this X-ray examination.

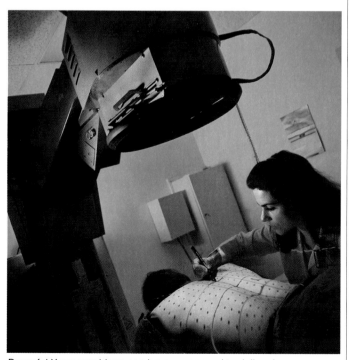

Powerful X-ray machines can be programmed to deliver large amounts of tumor-killing radiation to a very small area, thus sparing as much normal tissue as possible.

RADIATION AND BIRTH DEFECTS

X-rays and other forms of ionizing radiation are especially harmful to a developing fetus; they can cause severe birth defects or even fetal death. Any woman who is pregnant, or who may be pregnant without knowing it, should not be X-rayed. If an X-ray is absolutely necessary, a protective lead shield should be used to cover the fetus.

Even before conception, radiation can cause birth defects by damaging the father's sperm or the mother's eggs. With time, a man's ability to produce healthy sperm usually returns. But a woman does not make new eggs; she is born with her lifetime supply. Fortunately, surgical techniques now allow the ovaries to be moved out of the field of exposure during radiation therapy, and later returned to their normal position.

Psychiatry and Psychotherapy

At some point, one out of every three Americans suffers a mental disorder serious enough to benefit from treatment. Unfortunately, among those who need therapy, only 20 to 25 percent of adults and 60 percent of children undergo it. Why is mental illness so neglected? Experts note that even in this enlightened age, it still carries a social stigma, and large numbers of people who could be helped elect to suffer in silence. Others try to heal themselves, often with little or no success. Still others recognize that they have a problem, but don't know where to go for help, or cannot afford the usually high cost of therapy (see box, below).

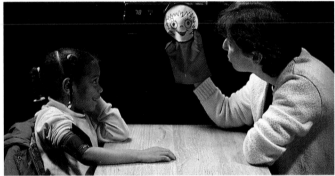

Puppets can allow troubled children to express feelings and concerns they may consider too shameful or frightening to discuss openly.

An Expanding Field

At one time, psychiatry dealt mostly with severe and incapacitating mental illness. Today, psychiatrists and other mental health professionals are called upon to treat a wide range of problems: eating disorders, sexual dysfunction, marital problems, stress-related diseases, personality problems, violent and aggressive behavior, alcoholism and substance abuse, and sleep disorders, among others. As with other medical specialties, mental health professionals tend to concentrate on one or two areas; it might be family therapy, for example, child psychiatry, or treatment of mood disorders.

Psychoactive Drugs

Treatment of mental illness has changed dramatically since the 1950s, when psychoactive drugs were first introduced (see box, opposite page). Before, patients with severe mental illness were institutionalized. Now potent tranquilizers and other drugs enable them to live independently, or at least outside of a mental hospital. Although millions of people have been helped by these new drugs, there are drawbacks. For

LOW-COST ALTERNATIVES

One-on-one psychotherapy is an expensive, long-term undertaking. Some insurance policies cover psychotherapy, but most limit their coverage. Short-term goal-oriented therapy, which is less costly, is covered by most insurance plans. Other low-cost alternatives include group therapy (right), mental health clinics, and counseling provided by psychiatric social workers.

GUIDE TO MENTAL HEALTH PROFESSIONALS

TITLE	WHO THEY ARE AND WHAT THEY DO
Psychiatrists	diagnose and treat mental disorders that are either organic or psychological in origin. Because they are physicians, they can also prescribe drugs.
Clinical psychologists	treat psychological, behavior, and personality disorders. Most have doctorate degrees in psychology and can do psychotherapy, but cannot prescribe drugs or treat any organic illness.
Psychiatric social workers	specialize in counseling patients with mental or emotional problems. They often team up with psychiatrists.
Psychiatric nurses	work in a hospital or mental health clinic, with a psychiatrist, or in private practice. They are registered nurses who have advanced training in treating patients with mental illness.
Counselors	give counsel to distressed persons. In most states, there are no legal definitions or requirements for such personnel. Some have formal training, others are self-styled, and still others are members of the clergy or related professions.

the most part, they do not cure, but instead help to bring the disease under control—a process that usually requires continuing therapy. In treating manic-depression and schizophrenia, for example, life-long drug therapy is necessary, usually in conjunction with counseling.

Persons undergoing this combined approach can often lead productive, relatively normal lives, especially in group homes or similar settings. Too often, however, they are left on their own and may relapse after stopping medication. Mental health experts estimate that up to one-third of the homeless people in U.S. cities are patients who would have been institutionalized in the past.

Side effects of psychoactive drugs pose other hazards, which range from drowsiness and movement disorders to addiction and fatal overdoses. Finding the right dosage or combination of drugs to minimize such effects can be costly and time-consuming. And psychoactive drugs must always be used under close medical supervision.

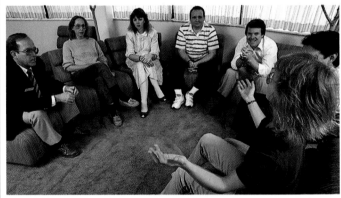

Group psychotherapy is a less expensive alternative to individual therapy. It can also be an adjunct to one-on-one psychotherapy or inpatient treatment, particularly for substance abuse.

Nondrug Therapies

Even if psychoactive drugs are prescribed, nondrug therapy is also recommended. The type of approach varies according to the underlying illness, and may include the following:

Psychodynamic psychotherapy attempts to uncover the source of mental disturbance by having the patient talk freely, especially about childhood experiences and dreams. In its classic Freudian form, it is conducted individually, with the patient talking while the therapist listens. One-on-one psychoanalysis is the most intensive, lengthy, and expensive form of psychotherapy, requiring from one to five sessions a week for three to five years. Variations on this approach include group, couple, or family therapy, in which a therapist treats more than one patient simultaneously.

Short or time-limited psychotherapy has evolved as a popular alternative to classic psychotherapy. In this approach, the patient and therapist agree upon a specific goal and the number of sessions needed to achieve it.

Cognitive therapy, which is also a short-term treatment, seeks to identify and correct distorted thought processes that result in self-defeating behavior. For example, if you are invariably late in meeting assignments because you cannot get started before a deadline looms, the therapist will help pinpoint the attitudes responsible for your poor work habits, and suggest ways to change them. This approach is especially effective in treating depression.

Behavior modification focuses on correcting a faulty habit or behavior without addressing any of the underlying psychological aspects. It is especially helpful in overcoming phobias, bad habits such as smoking, eating disorders, and certain compulsive behavior such as obsessive hand-washing.

ELECTROCONVULSIVE THERAPY

Electroconvulsive therapy (ECT) is a controversial and much misunderstood treatment for severe mental illness. During this process, pulses of electrical current are administered to the brain, producing brief seizures. Doctors do not fully understand how it works, but ECT remains one of the most effective treatments for severe suicidal depression. It is also recommended for psychotic or depressed elderly patients who cannot tolerate any kind of drug therapy.

ECT produces results much faster than antidepressant drugs. There is temporary memory loss, but otherwise, the procedure is relatively safe. And, contrary to popular belief, it is not painful. In fact, the patient does not feel the current and experiences only minor finger or toe movements. Typically, a patient is drowsy or confused for an hour after treatment, although memory loss or difficulty in learning new material may persist for several weeks.

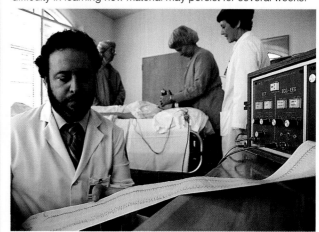

PSYCHOACTIVE DRUGS

CLASS OF DRUG	COMMON EXAMPLES	WHAT IT'S USED FOR	POTENTIAL PROBLEMS
Benzodiazepines (minor tranquilizers)	Librium (chlordiazepoxide); Valium (diazepam); Xanax (alprazolam)	Anxiety; sleep problems	Drowsiness, drug dependency, depressed respiration, especially when combined with alcohol
Neuroleptics (major tranquilizers)	Haldol (haloperidol); Thorazine (chlorpromazine); Serentil (mesoridazine)	Psychotic disorders (schizophrenia, mania, severe paranoia)	Drowsiness, tics, muscle spasms, and other movement abnormalities
Barbiturates	Donnatal (phenobarbital), Seconal (secobarbital)	Sleep problems in people who cannot take benzodiazepines	Same problems as benzodiazepines, only more so; overdose can be fatal
Tricyclic antidepressants	Anafranil (clomipramine); Elavil, Endep (amitriptyline); Surmontil (trimipramine); Tofranil (imipramine)	Clinical depression	Drowsiness, dry mouth, blurred vision, difficulty urinating; overdose can be fatal
Newer antidepressants	Asendin (amoxapine); Ludiomil (maprotiline); Prozac (fluoxetine)	Clinical depression	Same as tricyclics; possible increased risk of suicide during early recovery
MAO inhibitors	Marplan (isocarboxazid); Nardil (phenelzine)	Clinical depression	Severe high blood pressure when taken with foods high in tyramine (e.g.,cheese, meat, red wine)
Lithium	Eskalith, Lithonate, and others	Mania and manic-depression	Lithium toxicity

New or Experimental Treatments

Medical researchers constantly seek new and better treatments, especially for incurable diseases such as AIDS and cancer. Before these can be offered to humans, even on an experimental basis, they must undergo extensive testing, a process during which most are weeded out. Some turn out to be ineffective, others unsafe, and still others are not considered an improvement over existing therapies. Although the list of experimental treatments keeps changing, here are a few that look the most promising in the 1990s:

Immunotherapy

The body's immune system serves as the first line of defense against bacteria, viruses, and other potentially harmful invaders. Immunotherapy manipulates the immune system, either by suppressing or bolstering its natural function of fighting disease. Powerful drugs that suppress the immune system make organ transplantation possible by subduing the body's natural rejection of a foreign tissue.

Sometimes, the immune system goes into action against the body's healthy tissue, resulting in an autoimmune disease. Researchers are working on new immunosuppresive drugs to treat these diseases, which include chronic inflammatory disorders, such as lupus and certain other forms of arthritis.

The opposite approach, bolstering the immune system, is considered one of the most promising new medical frontiers. Several experimental cancer treatments are designed to stimulate the immune system to fight cancer in much the same way that it wards off or rejects any foreign invader. One approach is to develop vaccines against specific cancers. Another involves the use of interferon, interleukin-2, and other natural body chemicals that prompt an immune attack against tumors. Similar immunotherapy approaches are under investigation for the treatment of AIDS.

Yet another experimental cancer treatment, called transfer factor or adoptive therapy, takes a specific antibody from a healthy person and injects it into a patient who has a particular type of cancer, in the hope that it will trigger an immune system attack on the cancer cells.

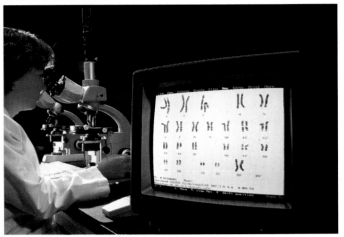

Genetic engineering represents the most hopeful prospect for overcoming hereditary diseases such as cystic fibrosis.

Genetic Engineering

Genes are the individual units of chromosomes, the body's blueprints that make it possible for cells to duplicate themselves in an orderly and consistent fashion. From time to time, genes change, or mutate. Some mutations go unnoticed, but others result in disease. Many genetic diseases, such as cystic fibrosis and muscular dystrophy, are the result of mutations that are inherited, whereas certain cancers develop when the genetic material in cells undergoes mutations during an individual's lifetime.

Environmental factors, such as radiation exposure and tobacco smoking, can prompt genetic mutations that result in disease, but many seem to occur spontaneously, without any obvious promoting factor.

Scientists are just beginning to understand how to manipulate genes to fight disease. Monoclonal antibodies are already used in experimental cancer treatments. Antibodies are the disease-fighting substances produced by the immune system. Genetic engineers can now fuse several types of antibodies—creating super antibodies—and use cloning techniques to produce large quantities of them, which are then injected into cancer patients. Some monoclonal antibodies are engineered to attack cancer cells. Others carry anticancer drugs or radioactive materials directly to the cancer cells, thereby killing them while sparing normal tissue.

Similar genetic engineering holds promise for curing or preventing hereditary diseases. For example, researchers are working on curing cystic fibrosis by getting the body to substitute a normal gene for the one that causes this deadly disease. To accomplish this, the normal gene is attached to a virus that has been rendered harmless, which then carries the gene to the lungs and other target organs. As the gene replicates itself, it replaces the defective one. In time, doctors may be able to replace disease-carrying genes with normal ones during fetal development.

Lasers

A laser, an acronym for light amplification by stimulated emission of radiation, is an extremely intense light beam that produces immense heat and power when it is focused at close range. When a laser beam is directed at any part of the body, the cells absorb its energy and convert it to heat. Almost instantly the tissue becomes charred or evaporates.

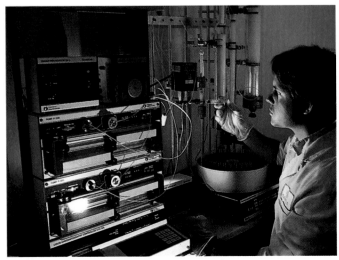

Meticulous laboratory testing is mandatory before new treatments can be offered to humans, even on a voluntary experimental basis.

Lasers have tremendous potential in surgery because they remove tissue with minimal bleeding and scarring. They are now widely used to perform delicate eye surgery, remove birthmarks and other skin blemishes, and burn off small tumors. Lasers have also proved invaluable in the treatment of female infertility due to scarring and closure of the fallopian tubes, which are the passageways between the ovary and the uterus where fertilization takes place.

Researchers believe lasers also have great potential in treating atherosclerosis, the buildup of fatty deposits, or plaque, in arteries. This type of laser surgery already is being performed experimentally to improve circulation in the legs.

Even more exciting are prospects that lasers can be used to unclog coronary arteries, the blood vessels that carry blood to the heart muscle. One approach employs laser surgery in angioplasty, a procedure in which a flexible catheter with a balloon tip is inserted into an artery and the balloon inflated to flatten any fatty deposits. Although angioplasty allows more blood to flow through the artery, it does not remove the plaque and, in time, the arteries renarrow. Researchers are working on ways to manipulate a laser device through the catheter and use its beam to vaporize the plaque. A problem is to control the light beam so it does not puncture the artery walls. But specialists at several major medical centers are now using laser angioplasty on an experimental basis.

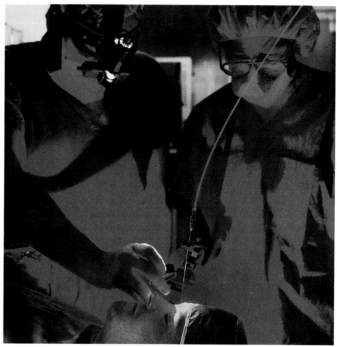

Laser surgery employs powerful light beams that allow surgeons to perform delicate eye operations and other procedures in which bleeding and scarring must be minimized.

THE ROLE OF HUMAN GUINEA PIGS

Before a new drug can be offered to the public, its manufacturer must prove that it is safe and effective, To do this, scientists must test the drug in human beings. As it turns out, this human testing, referred to as clinical trials, is the most costly and time-consuming component of the drug-development process.

Only about 20 percent of the compounds submitted to the Food and Drug Administration (FDA) for clinical trials gain approval for marketing. Critics charge that the testing process is too costly, complicated, and lengthy; they point to other countries where it is much easier to get new drugs approved.

In recent years, the FDA has tried to speed up the procedure, especially for drugs to treat AIDS, but the process still costs an average of $125 million and it takes eight to nine years to bring a new drug to the marketplace.

How Human Testing Works

Contrary to a common public assumption, the FDA itself does not conduct human testing—this is carried out by a pharmaceutical manufacturer, research organization, or a public or private agency. But the FDA reviews and approves the testing procedure, or protocol, as well as the results—often a truckload of volumes.

In the initial, or Phase 1, clinical trials, an experimental drug is given to 20 to 100 healthy volunteers for several months to make sure it is safe. About 70 percent of drugs pass this safety test.

During the next, or Phase 2, testing, several hundred patient volunteers take the drug for a few months to two years to determine whether it is effective as well as safe. For this phase, the volunteers are often divided into two groups, with a number receiving the experimental drug and others getting a placebo. In some instances, a third group may be taking an existing medication in order to find out if the new drug really is superior.

Some 25 to 30 percent of experimental drugs go on to the final Phase 3 testing, which typically involves several thousand patients and lasts for one to four years. During this period, the safety, effectiveness, and dosages are tested. Even if the drug is among the 20 percent that are eventually offered to the public, it must still be monitored for adverse reactions, long-term safety, and efficacy.

How to Volunteer

So-called human guinea pigs are recruited in many ways. Often, a hospital, drug company, or agency simply advertises for participants. Doctors are sometimes enlisted to conduct clinical trials, and may use their own patients or recruit additional volunteers. Teaching hospitals and health agencies, such as the National Cancer Institute, also participate in clinical trials and offer both experimental drugs and treatments to selected patients.

Regardless of who conducts the tests, all participants must be fully informed of any risks involved and then sign an informed consent form. Volunteers are not told whether they are receiving the actual drug or a placebo, because knowing might alter test results.

If it becomes apparent that an experimental drug can save lives or prevent irreversible damage, the study must stop and volunteers receiving a placebo must be offered the new drug. This happened during the human testing of AZT to treat AIDS. After eight months of Phase 2 testing, it was obvious that patients receiving AZT were living longer than those in the placebo group. The test was halted, and a month later the treatment protocol was approved. It took another six months for the FDA to grant final approval. This was in March 1987, some 29 months after the October 1984 start of preclinical tests, a short time compared with the average of 100 months that it usually takes for the entire process.

False Hopes

Desperate patients with incurable diseases often look to experimental treatments as a last resort for a cure. Some clinical studies actually fulfill this hope, and provide excellent medical care during the process. Others fall short of expectations, but still succeed in advancing medical knowledge.

Unfortunately, some people who volunteer for a previously untried treatment become victims of quackery or medical fraud. Always be suspicious if you are asked to pay for an experimental drug; in such cases, ask to see evidence that the FDA has approved the study. Be suspicious too if you learn about the drug from supermarket tabloids or other sensationalized reports. If the source is doubtful, check with your doctor or your nearest FDA office (listed in the U.S. Government section of your phone book) before volunteering.

Natural Medicine

Natural, or alternative, medicine is often thought of as a phenomenon of the so-called New Age; in reality, much of it is older than human history. Every society has herbal cures and folk remedies, many of which have been incorporated into orthodox medicine. In fact, it is estimated that at least half of our modern drugs originated with natural plant sources.

In ancient times, many diseases were attributed to the supernatural—a sick person was thought to be possessed by demons or to have incurred the displeasure of some god. Thus, many treatments were aimed at exorcising demons; priests or shamans often doubled as physicians, because it was felt they could heal by restoring a god's favor.

These beliefs started to change some 3,000 years ago as Indian, Chinese, and Greek philosophers postulated that health signified a balance of internal forces, and that illness occurred when this natural harmony was upset. This idea gave rise to distinct medical systems and practices aimed at maintaining internal harmony. The alternative medicine of today is a direct outgrowth of these millenia-old medical practices, using many of the same techniques.

After the fall of the Roman Empire, a different world view—and with it, different medical practices—took hold in Europe, initiating the rift between Western and Eastern medicine. This rift widened further during the Renaissance, with the rise of scientific inquiry and the beginnings of modern scientific approaches to medicine.

In the 20th century, American physicians embraced scientific medicine wholeheartedly, discarding and even outlawing much of what are now considered alternative therapies. But in other parts of the world, including industrialized European nations, traditional, or natural, therapies continued to coexist with mainstream medicine. Even in India, where the teaching of traditional ayurvedic medicine was banned under British rule, the practice never disappeared, and quickly reemerged when India gained its independence.

In recent years, growing numbers of Americans have come to recognize that achieving and maintaining good health is a personal responsibility, affected by lifestyle. There is increasing emphasis on good nutrition, regular exercise, weight control, and smoking cessation. Many alternative therapies, which were once dismissed as mostly hokum, are now considered complimentary adjuncts to conventional medicine, important in preventing and treating many diseases.

Alternative practitioners and their patients have led the movement toward natural medicine, but several prominent physicians and medical educators, among them Dr. Bernie Segal and Dr. Andrew Weill, have helped to sway both the public and physician colleagues, often with best-selling books. Dr. Weill in particular offers a balanced approach by advocating that patients see mainstream physicians for infections and other acute illnesses, in which they can truly make a difference, and try alternative therapies for chronic problems that conventional medicine is unable to do much about.

Other well-known mainstream physicians, cardiologist Dean Ornish, for instance, advocate a combination of conventional and alternative therapies plus lifestyle changes to treat even serious conditions such as heart disease. The following pages describe some of the more popular alternative therapies and their potential benefits and limitations.

Acupuncture and Other Chinese Remedies

Yin and Yang

Acupuncture is a form of healing based on the concept that all body organs are interconnected by channels, known as meridians, and that illness occurs when the vital energy, or qi (pronounced chee), flowing through these channels is partially blocked. A practitioner of acupuncture attempts to correct this imbalance by inserting thin needles along the meridians at designated points, called acupoints, and in certain cases twirling them, either manually or with an electrical device. He or she may combine the treatment with other traditional practices, such as herbal medicine, diet therapy, and massage.

The most effective acupuncturists are said to contribute their own qi during the procedure. Transmission of energy occurs when the needles are inserted and rotated.

Origins

The Chinese developed the acupuncture system over 2,000 years ago out of a principle of Taoist religious philosophy. As with all traditional Chinese medicine, it is based on the theory that good health depends upon a balance of the forces of yin and yang. These opposites, which exist in nature—as female and male, moon and sun, darkness and light—have their counterparts within the body. Illness occurs when these forces are out of sync, so the goal is to restore balance.

Acupoints were designated according to their assumed clinical function in restoring the balance of yin and yang, thereby improving circulation of both qi and blood. One legend, which attempts to explain how acupoints were determined, says that during wars in ancient times, physicians observed that soldiers who had been struck by arrows in certain parts

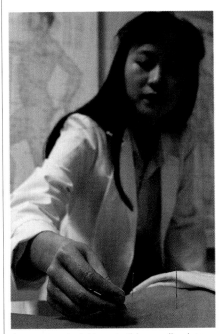

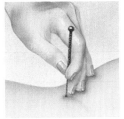

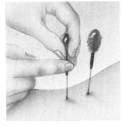

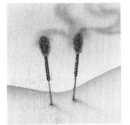

An acupuncturist inserts thin needles into specific acupoints and then twirls the needle (upper right), or applies moxa (center right), an herb that produces penetrating heat when burned (lower right).

of the body were mysteriously cured of specific illnesses.

Western interest in acupuncture has developed sporadically. In the 18th century, when Christian missionaries from Europe were expelled from China, some took acupuncture techniques back home with them. In the 19th century, Chinese workers, who came to America to help build the railroads, brought information about acupuncture, among other remedies, which ultimately caught the attention of some doctors

MOXIBUSTION AND CUPPING
A major method of acupuncture therapy is moxibustion, in which the herb moxa, or mugwort, is applied directly on the skin or indirectly on the needle (see illustration, opposite page) at the acupuncture point. The use of direct moxa is prescribed in specific cases as the prime treatment.

Cupping, shown right, is another traditional Chinese procedure. Glass suction cups, or pulling cups, are placed on the acupoints and the tissues under the cup are pulled upward to stimulate increased blood flow within the cupped area. Cupping is not widely used in the United States. In the past, however, immigrants from Eastern Europe used it to treat a variety of ailments.

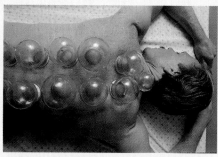

In dry cupping (above) heated cups are placed over the skin to draw tissue into them. In wet cupping, the cups are placed over small skin punctures to produce bleeding.

and healers. More recently, interest in acupuncture has been sparked by two events: the opening of China to the West and the investigation of alternative methods of dealing with pain.

Practitioners
In 14 states, only physicians may perform acupuncture (see page 464 for requirements in your state). These physicians are usually specialists in physical medicine and rehabilitation (physiatrists) or medical doctors trained in China or Korea. Another 21 states require that acupuncturists be licensed, which mandates meeting certain educational and training requirements and passing a test developed by the National Commission for the Certification of Acupuncturists.

When it is used
While many of the claims by acupuncturists are viewed with skepticism by mainstream doctors, there is increasing recognition of their success in alleviating pain, thereby providing an alternative to painkillers, tranquilizers, and sleeping pills. The use of acupuncture for anesthesia in dentistry, childbirth, and some forms of surgery is under study by a number of Western medical practitioners. Researchers are also looking into its usefulness as a way of easing the pain and increasing the range of motion for people who suffer from rheumatoid arthritis and osteoarthritis. Other possible uses of acupuncture include the treatment of allergies, migraine headaches, circulatory disorders, and addictions to nicotine, alcohol, and other drugs.

Interest in acupuncture and other traditional Chinese remedies is increasing in the United States, but their acceptance in Europe is greater. For example, acupuncture is taught in French medical schools and is covered by government health insurance in France and several other European countries.

Precautions
▶ Anyone contemplating acupuncture should be medically assessed before beginning treatment.
▶ Unless your acupuncturist is a licensed M.D. or D.O., or has been recommended by your primary-care doctor, check credentials and training.
▶ Acupuncturists generally sterilize their needles with wet heat (autoclave). Because AIDS, hepatitis B, and other deadly diseases can be transmitted by contaminated needles, however, reuse of needles—even after autoclaving—should be avoided. Disposable needles are available at very low cost.

How it works
There is no parallel in Western medicine for the meridians and acupoints indicated on the traditional acupuncture chart. Within the frame of reference for Western science, it has not been possible to validate the claims of acupuncture as a healing system, nor is there a complete understanding of exactly how it works as an analgesic. Some researchers think its positive effects might result from the release of endorphins, the body's naturally produced analgesics, triggered by the action of the needles. Although the trigger points for pain and for acupuncture have been labeled differently and were discovered independently, recent research into pain has revealed that they represent the same phenomenon and can be explained in terms of how the nervous system functions.

What to expect
Treatment consists of the insertion of hair-thin stainless steel needles a few millimeters below the skin at specifically designated locations. The mystery is that the needles are inserted in one part of the body, yet the sensations of warmth, numbness, or tingling are experienced in another part. The traditional explanation for this phenomenon is that qi is traveling along its proper channel. Western research suggests that the autonomic nervous system is responsible.

In current practice, the needles range in diameter from 10 to 13 mils (thousandths of an inch) and from one to three inches in length. It takes considerable skill and many years of practice to insert the needles perpendicular to the skin without bending them. Their insertion and removal rarely cause pain beyond the sensation of a pin prick. When the patient is relaxed, there is no discomfort at any stage of the procedure.

For treating pain, the length of time that needles are left in place, whether they are twirled manually or hooked up to an electrical rotating device, and whether the acupuncture is combined with heat, depends on the nature of the pain or the desired effect. For example, 5 minutes is said to be sufficient for tooth extraction, while 20 to 30 minutes may be needed for a tonsillectomy, with continuous stimulation by the needles throughout the entire surgical procedure. In the last instance, the analgesic effect lasts about 24 hours.

Most treatments for pain relief take 5 to 15 minutes. Since the effect is presumed to be cumulative, a course of six treatments is usually recommended. Some patients, whose pain has not been alleviated immediately after treatment, report its disappearance days or even weeks later.

Alexander Technique

The Alexander technique is a training process in which a person learns to identify and change faulty posture and movements. The goal is to free the body of muscular tensions that cause stress and fatigue by eliminating common postural problems resulting from such habits as slouching, holding the head in an awkward position when talking on the telephone, or carrying a heavy bag on one shoulder.

A number of poor posture patterns are the result of well-intentioned reminders by parents or teachers to stand or sit up straight. Many people respond by holding their spinal muscles in a constant state of tension instead of aiming for a relaxed balance of head, neck, and torso. Tight or restrictive clothing and high heeled shoes are other common culprits that contribute to incorrect posture and muscle tension.

Origins

The technique was developed in the late 19th century by an Australian actor, F. Mathias Alexander, during a period in his career when he was losing his voice. While examining his movements in a triple mirror, he realized that the tense and artificial postures he habitually assumed with his head, neck, and torso during performances were affecting his vocal chords. By changing his self-defeating habits, he was able to "liberate" his voice.

Encouraged by his success, he began to teach others some of his methods and in 1908, he published one of his earliest pamphlets: "Re-education of the Kinesthetic System (Sensory Appreciation of Muscular Movement) Concerned with the

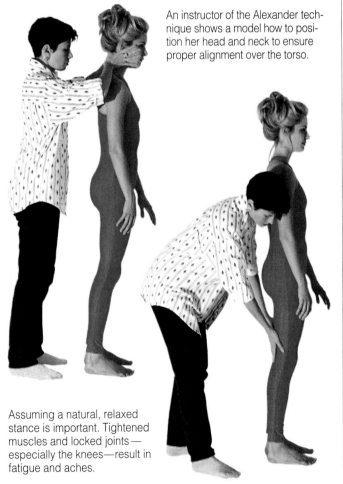

An instructor of the Alexander technique shows a model how to position her head and neck to ensure proper alignment over the torso.

Assuming a natural, relaxed stance is important. Tightened muscles and locked joints—especially the knees—result in fatigue and aches.

Development of Robust Physical Well-Being." In the decades that followed, he attracted many distinguished followers, among them philosopher John Dewey, authors George Bernard Shaw and Aldous Huxley, as well as a number of physicians and scientists. By the time he died in 1955, his technique was being taught worldwide.

Practitioners

Instructors are trained and certified at centers affiliated with the North American Society of Teachers of the Alexander Technique. They may give private lessons and also conduct group classes and workshops.

Some doctors and physical therapists use the method, and many hospitals, rehabilitation centers, and pain clinics now offer instruction to their clients. So do performing arts institutions, including the Juilliard School in New York and the London Academy of Music and Dramatic Arts.

When it is used

The technique is most frequently recommended as a way of dealing with back and neck pain. It is also used to counteract some of the effects of scoliosis (curvature of the spine) and arthritis, to improve respiratory function, and as an adjunct to breathing exercises for asthma patients.

Some performing artists claim that it has helped them to overcome stage fright; many athletes have found that it not only enhances their skills but also helps reduce the likelihood of sports injuries. A growing number of people who work at computers are investigating the Alexander technique as a way of avoiding stress injuries from repetitive movements, which have become a disabling occupational hazard.

How it works

The Alexander technique is based on the assumption that the body can move freely and naturally only when the head, neck, and torso are properly aligned. This requires awareness of faulty muscular movements and correction of them.

What to expect

Teaching sessions usually last from 30 to 45 minutes. Their number is determined by the severity of the problem and how quickly the person learns to correct it. Typically, 10 to 15 classes are sufficient to address most problems.

During one of the first lessons, the student may be told to lie on a padded table while the instructor discusses ways in which the body parts relate to each other. The goal is to help the person achieve a natural rest position that can be practiced at home. Then the student's body is observed as she goes about ordinary tasks—rising from a chair, speaking on the telephone, carrying a pile of books, lifting a heavy carton from the floor. During each of these exercises, the instructor uses a hands-on approach to explore the neck and shoulders of the student for signs of muscle tension. At the same time, the instructor points out faulty movements so that they can be corrected. Critical assessment of posture and movement is often made in front of a mirror so that the client can see the difference between bad habits and better ones.

Aromatherapy

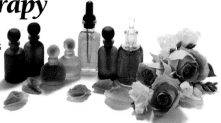

Aromatherapy is the use of oils from herbs and other aromatic plants to achieve relaxation or relief from a disorder. Depending upon the plant, the aromatic, or essential, oil is extracted from the leaves, flowers, roots, seeds, fruit, bark, or resin and then diluted with water or an unscented oil such as jojoba. These solutions may be massaged into skin, inhaled from steam, added to bath water, or used in a compress.

Origins

Aromatic plants, usually applied externally, have been used in many folk remedies since ancient times. Familiar examples include vaporized eucalyptus oil to ease nasal congestion and juniper liniment for the relief of muscle aches.

Modern aromatherapy was born in the 1920s, when a French chemist, Dr. René-Maurice Gattefossé, burned his hand while working in a perfume laboratory. He plunged the injured hand into a container of lavender oil and was amazed by its speedy healing with minimal scarring. He then began to research the healing properties of other aromatic oils.

Practitioners

Aromatherapy is used by trained therapists who often practice other alternative therapies such as massage. Some of the methods can be self-taught and used at home.

When it is used

Practitioners treat a range of medical and emotional problems, including headaches, premenstrual tension, muscle pain, skin disorders, fatigue, insomnia, and stress.

Precautions

▶ Avoid ingesting aromatic oils used for aromatherapy. Many, such as camphor and yellow jasmine, are highly toxic. Make sure that the oils are stored in a safe place out of children's reach.
▶ Many aromatic oils are highly irritating, especially when used in concentrated amounts or on the delicate membranes of the vagina, rectum, or nasal cavities. Follow directions for diluting the oils, and then test the diluted solution on a small patch of skin on the forearm or thigh. Avoid further use if the oil produces redness, itching, or swelling.

How it works

There are two basic mechanisms involved—the sense of smell and the absorptive quality of skin. Practitioners contend that inhalation of a certain scent prompts the brain to release neurochemicals that counter stress and fatigue. They also believe that some oils exert a medicinal effect when absorbed by the skin. Medical benefits of aromatherapy have not been proven, however, and doctors generally discount any therapeutic benefits other than a placebo effect and relaxation.

What to expect

Aromatherapists combine massage and the use of aromatic oils. A session varies according to the problem being treated. The entire body is massaged to relieve stress and general achiness. A facial massage is used to treat headaches and sinus congestion, whereas the back may be massaged to alleviate backache or menstrual cramps.

In addition to massage, an aromatherapist may recommend soaking in a tub of warm water containing a few drops of one or more aromatic oils. Depending upon the oils used, this may induce drowsiness or provide an invigorating lift.

EXAMPLES OF AROMATIC OILS

OIL	SOURCE	WHAT IT'S USED FOR
Chamomile	Dried flowers	Mild, sweet, grain-like aroma. Used in vaporizers, baths, compresses, facial masks, or massages for its soothing effects; also said to speed healing of minor burns, alleviate eczema, and ease muscle pain.
Clary sage	Flowering tops	Strong, pungent aroma. Inhaled or used in vaporizers, baths, compresses, or massages to alleviate anxiety, stress, skin inflammation, and respiratory congestion.
Eucalyptus	Leaves	Strong, invigorating, camphor-like aroma. Used in vaporizers, compresses, baths, and massages to treat nasal and respiratory congestion, alleviate muscle pain, and counter fatigue; applied to the skin as an insect repellant.
Geranium	Leaves	Sharp, spicy fragrance. Used in vaporizers, baths, massages, and (less commonly) mouthwashes and gargles; considered a basic oil to treat stress, acne, eczema, and minor wounds.
Jasmine	Flowers	Subtle floral aroma. Used in facial massages and baths for its relaxing properties.
Juniper berry	Ripe berries	Sharp, peppery fragrance. Used in vaporizers, baths, compresses, and massages for its calming effect; aromatherapists also use it to treat muscle aches and eczema.
Lavender	Flowering tops	Strong, sweet floral fragrance. Used in vaporizers, baths, compresses, and massages to treat stress and skin wounds; said to have antiseptic and anti-inflammatory properties.
Peppermint	Leaves	Fresh, invigorating aroma. Inhaled or used in baths, gargles, and mouthwashes for digestive upsets, sore throat, mouth ulcers, and itchy skin; also used as an insect repellant.
Pine	Resin	Invigorating wood scent. Used in vaporizers, baths, and massages to alleviate muscle aches and treat nasal and chest congestion.
Rose	Flowers	Delicate, persistent floral fragrance. Used in baths and massages for its relaxing qualities. Aromatherapists also use it to treat menstrual problems and other female reproductive disorders.

Art Therapy

Art therapy is the use of visual arts materials to identify and treat emotional trauma and mental disorders. By creating images in drawings, paintings, sculptures, and photographs, patients provide information about suppressed feelings and buried memories that they cannot express with words.

This approach is also an important aspect of rehabilitation programs for people who are recovering from a stroke or an injury affecting hand function. It can help disabled people to improve their self-image and depressed or elderly patients to expand their range of expression.

Origins

The term art therapy was first used in the 1940s to describe the work of psychiatrists and psychologists who were finding that artistic expression provided important insight into the feelings of disturbed children. Independent practitioners eventually established the American Art Therapy Association,

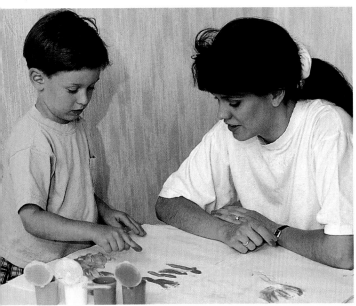

An art therapist encourages a young patient to use finger painting to express feelings that are difficult to put into words.

which issued guidelines for the first formal training program in 1967. An important recent development in the field of art therapy is the formation of Medart International, an organization that investigates and promotes the relationship between established medicine and the visual and performing arts.

Practioners

This method may be used by psychiatrists, psychologists, and psychiatric social workers. To qualify as a professional art therapist, a person must complete a master's degree program that has been approved by the American Art Therapy Association. There are now 122 such programs offered by 16 colleges and universities nationwide.

Practitioners who meet the association's professional standards are given the title of Art Therapist Registered (ATR) and are bound by the same code of patient confidentiality that applies to all psychotherapists. They must also obtain permission from their patients before their artwork can be used for any public display or reproduction.

Precautions
► All art materials used in a therapeutic setting, especially by children, should be nontoxic.
► People with allergies should be especially careful about the contents of paints and solvents.

When it is used

Art therapy is used with patients who cannot or will not employ words to achieve the personal insight that is a cornerstone of traditional psychotherapy. By surmounting language barriers, this therapy can be especially effective with disturbed children and patients who speak a different language from the therapist. It is also helpful in rehabilitating hand/motor skills following a stroke or injury and assessing the progress of a patient by comparing an early attempt at a self-portrait with a similar attempt after physical therapy.

How it works

By providing a patient with a nonverbal means of expressing repressed thoughts and feelings, art therapy can help ease guilt and anger. Sexually abused children often render images whose meaning can eventually be discussed. Through drawings and paintings, a schizophrenic patient may offer the therapist a view into a disordered mind, thus providing some clues for how treatment might proceed.

Art therapy can also enable mentally ill deaf adults to describe early conflicts with family members and to alleviate symptoms of aggression, hostility, and depression. Physically handicapped children, neglected elderly persons, alcoholics, and prison inmates all can be helped to build self-esteem through sculpture, painting, or photography, especially when they see their work exhibited for other people's appreciation.

What to expect

Through supportive discussions with an art therapist, patients become aware of the messages conveyed in their drawings, paintings, or sculptures. When previously unacknowledged frustration, rage, or confusion has been brought to light, the patient can be helped to take positive steps for dealing with it. Practiced in a family setting, art therapy can also resolve interpersonal problems.

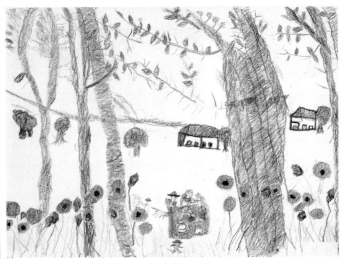

Art therapy can help a stroke patient, such as the creator of this picture, with visual organization, memory, and concentration.

Ayurveda

This ancient healing system from India stresses the mind/body relationship in the maintenance of good health. As in other Asian medical practices, a balance of vital energy, in this case, prana, is considered the key. The system is based on balancing three basic life forces, or doshas—vata, responsible for all movement in the body; pitta, which controls digestion and energy production; and kapha, responsible for the body's structure and stability. Illness occurs when any of the doshas is out of sync; individuals must know their dominant dosha and follow a diet and lifestyle that keeps it balanced with the others.

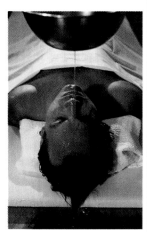

During an ayurvedic session, a warm aromatic oil is poured over the skin, which is then massaged.

Origins

Ayurveda, meaning the "science of life and longevity" in Sanskrit, is believed to be about 5,000 years old, predating all other medical systems. The two classic Ayurveda textbooks are more than 2,000 years old. *Charaka Samhita,* named for the person who was the ayurvedic counterpart of Hippocrates, outlines the principles of health maintenance and treatment of disease, and *Sushruta Samhita* describes elaborate surgical procedures, including reconstructive plastic surgery, gallbladder removal, and other operations that most people consider modern.

Ayurvedic medicine spread with the Hindu culture to Indonesia, Tibet, and eventually to the West, where some of its principles were picked up by the ancient Greek physicians. As Buddhism developed, this healing system was carried to China and other Asian countries.

During the 1800s, the British banned all ayurvedic schools in India, replacing them with Western medical schools. For the next century, ayurvedic medicine was relegated to folk practices in rural areas. When India regained its independence in 1947, ayurvedic schools were again legalized. Today, there are 100 ayurvedic schools in India, equal in number to the Western ones, and many Indian physicians incorporate both styles of medicine into their practices.

In recent years, Ayurveda has spread to the United States. Major clinics have been established in Lancaster, Massachusetts, and Albuquerque, New Mexico.

Practitioners

In India, Ayurveda practitioners must undergo five to six years of training in a traditional ayurvedic medical school before they can treat patients. In the United States, this training is abbreviated into a short course of several months at an ayurvedic institute. Whichever training they have received, ayurvedic physicians are not licensed to practice medicine here, unless they are trained also in another discipline, such as traditional medicine, osteopathy, or chiropractic.

When it is used

Unlike Western medicine, which comes into play when illness strikes, Ayurveda is incorporated into a person's lifestyle. It governs all aspects of life, such as diet, exercise, and sexual practices. An ayurvedic practitioner is consulted only to identify and correct an imbalance among the three life forces. At ayurvedic clinics in the United States, patients are usually treated by both a Western and an ayurvedic physician.

How it works

Ayurvedic philosophy holds that each person is born with a particular ratio of doshas, with one dominating. This dominant dosha determines personality type and also influences one's susceptibility to certain illnesses. For example, pitta people tend to have fiery dispositions and are prone to developing high blood pressure and digestive disorders, so a pitta-related disease may be treated with a bland diet and numerous herbal remedies. Because the mind is seen as an integral force in maintaining health and overcoming illness, meditation or yoga may also be employed.

What to expect

An ayurvedic doctor begins by assessing the patient's dosha pattern. Pulses play a critical role in this assessment—a practitioner feels pulses throughout the body, looking for dosha imbalances as reflected in the nature of a pulse. Seven types of body tissue—plasma, red blood cells, muscle, fat, bone, nerve, and reproductive tissue—are also examined.

Ayurvedic physicians do not focus on a specific disease or an organ system, but instead treat the entire body and mind. Purification to rid the body of toxins is an important part of treatment; methods may include sweat baths, enemas, nasal washes, bloodletting, and oil massages. The practitioner will also recommend a specific diet, meditation or yoga routine, and herbal remedies.

THE SPA EXPERIENCE

For centuries, health enthusiasts have journeyed to special locales such as the Belgian town of Spa to partake of fresh air, healing waters, and a variety of traditional and nontraditional medical treatments. Today, spas remain an integral part of health care in many European countries, where national health plans often pay for a sojourn in a preventive or therapeutic medical facility that may look more like a luxury resort than a clinic.

Spas have gained popularity in the United States as well, although few insurance companies presently pay for their services. Still, those who can afford the fees (which range from $1,000 to $4,000 per week) stand to benefit from a spa visit. Most of the 150 spas in this country provide low-fat meals, exercise and meditation classes, and massage and other body therapies. Popular spas, some relaxed and indulgent and others run with the no-nonsense rigor of an army camp, are typically located in scenic areas; the settings themselves often have a salutary effect.

A growing number of spas address specific medical problems, such as hypertension, obesity, and heart disease. Still others approach health promotion from the perspective of a particular discipline—Ayurveda, for example. In general, though, some of the best spas draw on a variety of disciplines, including traditional Western medicine. As such, they focus less on treating illness than on giving visitors the feeling of healthful living—an experience that they can, ideally, carry forward after returning home.

Precautions

▶ Before agreeing to ayurvedic treatments, ask about costs and cancellation policies. Some clinics ask for advance payment and require two week's notice of cancellation to qualify for a refund.

Biofeedback Training

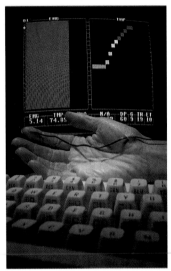

Electronic sensors and signals are utilized to teach a person how to control bodily functions, such as blood flow, that normally are automatic or involuntary.

Biofeedback training allows a person to gain a measure of control over bodily functions that are usually automatic, or involuntary—for example, heartbeat, blood pressure, skin temperature, blood flow to the hands and feet, even brain-wave patterns. Some doctors believe that the results are similar to those of self-hypnosis.

Electronic monitors used to measure these responses produce visible or audible signals. During the training, a person learns how to alter the electronic signals and, in the process, change an involuntary bodily response.

Origins

In the early years of radio, the term "feedback" was created to describe the design principle that enabled electronic systems to self-correct through an information loop. Biofeedback training applies this principle to the correction, or self-regulation, of one's own biological systems.

Experiments in applying biofeedback principles to the body were conducted as part of dream-sleep studies in the late 1950s. The subjects were trained to produce alpha brain-wave patterns, which indicate a mental state of relaxed alertness, on an electroencephalograph screen.

Eventually, scientists at the Menninger Foundation in Kansas were able to teach patients how to alleviate their migraine headaches by redirecting some of the blood flow from constricted blood vessels in the scalp to their hands. To do this, patients were instructed to concentrate on raising their hand temperature by visualizing holding something warm, such as a cup of hot coffee. Since then, biofeedback training has been used to treat numerous ailments.

Practitioners

The training may be done by a physician, psychologist, physical therapist, or laboratory technician, often in a rehabilitation center or a pain clinic.

When it is used

Common uses are to control pain, relieve asthma attacks, rehabilitate muscles damaged by stroke or accident, and treat insomnia, migraine headaches, and other stress-related conditions. Biofeedback training is often combined with visualization and breathing exercises. Researchers in a Duke University heart attack prevention program have used the training to modify Type A personality traits, especially persistent feelings of anger and hostility, which are thought to increase the risk of heart attack.

In some cases, biofeedback can help eliminate the need for medications such as tranquilizers or prescription painkillers. In other instances, such as the control of high blood pressure, it may be combined with medication.

How it works

The goal of biofeedback training is to teach individuals how to become active participants in their own treatment, even though they may be unaware of actually controlling a bodily function. A classic example of how the process works is the experiment, conducted in 1970 at Harvard Medical School, in which male subjects were taught to modify their blood pressure. Success in decreasing their blood pressure and maintaining it at a lower level was indicated by a flashing light; after 20 such flashes, the reward was a glimpse of a nude pinup. Most of the subjects indicated that they had no awareness of actually controlling the flashing lights, nor were they conscious of what response was being measured. However, they were aware of the nude picture.

Some researchers believe that biofeedback contributes to improved physical and mental health because it fosters a feeling of power over bodily functions that were assumed to be beyond one's conscious control. Thus, even if a cure is not achieved, biofeedback training adds an important sense of well-being that may increase the efficacy of medical therapy.

What to expect

Electronic monitors are used to measure specific physical responses; the types of monitors most commonly employed during biofeedback training are:
▶ Electromyograph (EMG), which monitors muscular tension and electrical activity in the muscles.
▶ Electroencephalograph (EEG), which records brain waves.
▶ Skin temperature monitor, which senses minute changes that indicate shifts in blood flow.

The type of disorder over which the patient seeks control determines the kind of monitor used. For example, if a person wants to reduce muscle tension that is causing severe neck pain, EMG electrodes are placed on the muscles in question. These electrodes convert electrical activity of the muscles into a visual image on a screen or into audio signals heard through earphones. The therapist then teaches the patient how to change the signals to reduce the muscle tension. Similarly, by learning to control changes recorded by the EEG, a person can help manage stress, pain, insomnia, and in some cases, epileptic seizures.

Temperature monitors, which sense even slight fluctuations in skin temperature due to changes in blood flow, help patients learn to abort a migraine headache during the early warning stage. They also help people who suffer from circulatory disorders reduce the discomfort of cold hands and feet.

At first, simply seeing the image or hearing the signal is all that is needed to relax muscles or alter blood flow. Eventually, a patient is able to achieve desired results without the presence of a monitor. With practice, people can become increasingly skilled at controlling these involuntary processes.

Precautions
▶ Be wary of mail-order or other sources of biofeedback equipment to use at home because such devices vary in quality. Also, a trained therapist can teach you the most effective techniques, something you do not get with a do-it-yourself approach.
▶ Check with your doctor before undergoing biofeedback training, especially if you have a chronic disorder such as diabetes or high blood pressure. Biofeedback training can alter the need for some medications, and dosages may need to be adjusted.

Chiropractic

Chiropractic is a system of treatment based on the belief that the foundation of good health is the unhampered flow of nerve impulses that originate in the brain and spinal cord and then travel to all parts of the body. Therapy begins with analyzing the patient's spinal column for abnormal alignments of the vertebrae. When such misalignments, called subluxations, are located, they are corrected by manipulation to restore the normal flow of nerve impulses. Many chiropractors also make recommendations about nutrition and exercise, but they do not prescribe drugs or do surgery.

Origins

Energetic hands-on therapy was widely practiced by ancient healers, and manipulation of the backbone is still common in a number of cultures. In an independent movement in the United States, a systematic method of spinal manipulation was developed at the end of the 19th century by a healer in Iowa named Daniel David Palmer. In 1895, he gained local fame by curing a janitor's deafness when he manipulated a displaced vertebra. Following this success, Palmer devoted himself to refining his method of spinal treatments.

One of Palmer's early patients described his technique as "chiropractic," Greek for "accomplished by hand." The word caught on and The Palmer Infirmary and Chiropractic Institute was established in Davenport, Iowa, as a teaching and treatment center. In 1913, the year that Palmer died, Kansas became the first state to license chiropractic healers.

It is only in recent years and as a result of court battles and congressional hearings that this alternative therapy has overcome charges of quackery by the medical establishment. While it is not unusual for physicians such as orthopedists and rehabilitation specialists to refer patients to a chiropractor, there are still many mainstream doctors who feel that this treatment has the potential for doing more harm than good.

Even so, chiropractic seems to be attracting more patients than ever, due to an increase in sports injuries and the recent growth in musculoskeletal problems resulting from working at computers. Visits are now covered by Medicare, Medicaid, and many other health insurance plans. In addition, the American Hospital Association has made some facilities at member hospitals available to qualified practitioners.

Practitioners

Chiropractors are licensed in all 50 states and there are some 20 chiropractic colleges nationwide. Graduates hold a doctor of chiropractic, or D.C. degree. Studies stress the biomedical sciences and provide training in manipulation techniques. Some liberal arts colleges also offer a bachelor's degree in chiropractic, after which graduate study at a chiropractic college is required. Of the approximately 50,000 chiropractors in the United States, about half belong to the American Chiropractic Association, the profession's largest organization.

Years ago, many chiropractors believed spinal manipulation to be the preferred treatment for virtually every ailment. In recent decades, most have come to recognize the limitations of their therapy; they see their work as yet another way to deal with health problems. The majority of chiropractors consider themselves "mixers," who provide a holistic service that includes counseling about nutrition, exercise, and other lifestyle issues in addition to manipulations. A minority are "straights," who follow a strict philosophy of musculoskeletal adjustments.

When it is used

Most people consult a chiropractor because of pain that appears to originate in the musculoskeletal system, usually the neck and/or back. For some patients, the pain has come on suddenly, resulting from an injury on the job, in an automobile accident, or while participating in a sport. For others, the pain may be chronic, perhaps the cumulative effect of years of poor posture, a sedentary lifestyle, and increasing weight. Still others may be suffering from job-related muscle and skeletal problems, such as repetitive stress injuries. Individuals with vague, persistent symptoms such as fatigue and headaches also consult chiropractors for both spinal manipulation and counseling on nutrition and exercise.

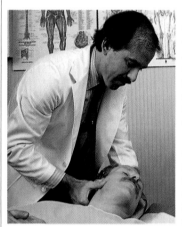

Before attempting adjustments or realignment of vertebrae, a chiropractor rotates the head and neck, feeling for tight muscles and tender points. One manipulative technique involves a rapid motion to increase joint mobility and reduce muscle spasms and pain.

Chiropractic manipulations are said to affect the 31 pairs of nerves that arise from the spinal cord and carry messages between the brain and the rest of the body.

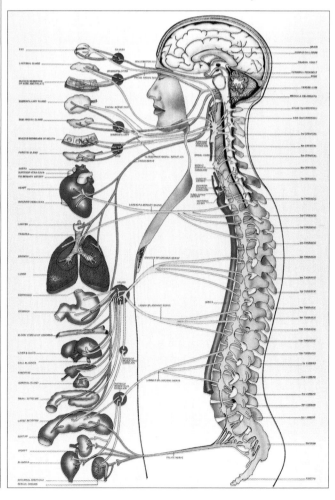

CHIROPRACTIC (CONTINUED)

How it works

The spinal cord gives rise to 31 pairs of spinal nerves, which carry messages to and from the brain and to all parts of the body. These spinal nerves pass through openings in the vertebrae, and when the progress of a nerve is impeded, it is said to be "pinched." The problem may be the result of an injury, a muscle spasm, a slipped (ruptured) vertebral disk, spinal arthritis, or some other structural abnormality.

With X-rays plus a hands-on exploration of the spine, the chiropractor tries to locate the vertebrae that need realignment. The chiropractic method is most successful in cases in which it is possible to restore normal joint movement by improving anatomical relationships. The intimate hands-on approach may also have a positive effect on healing.

Many practitioners believe that chiropractic can be most effective in treating acute pain of recent onset, before it has reached a chronic stage. Some researchers theorize that when pain is allowed to become chronic, the body loses its ability to produce endorphins, body chemicals that act as natural painkillers. This theory is based on the notion that long-term overstimulation of nerves, which occurs in chronic pain, prevents them from triggering production of painkilling chemicals.

What to expect

A visit to a chiropractor involves many of the same steps as a visit to a traditional physician. The evaluation begins with taking the patient's medical history, including questions about symptoms, past illnesses and injuries, and stresses from one's job or other situations. This is followed by a physical examination that includes blood pressure measurement, orthopedic and postural testing, a study of posture and spinal motion, and a series of X-rays. Most of these procedures may take up the entire first visit. Before the second visit, the practitioner has evaluated all this information and is ready to start treatment.

To begin, the patient lies down on a specially designed table. Muscles may be energetically massaged before manipulative techniques are used for spinal adjustment, which often produces a popping sound similar to that of cracking your knuckles. Because certain manipulative techniques involve quick, rapid motion, some transient discomfort may be experienced, especially in acute cases.

Sometimes electrical devices are employed that produce muscle fatigue to alleviate muscle spasms. Moist heat may also be applied, especially if there are muscle spasms. When it's appropriate, a supportive collar, brace, or sling may be recommended for use between treatments. Most sessions last no longer than 45 minutes, and the number of sessions depends on the nature of the problem.

Precautions

▶ Be wary of chiropractors who describe themselves as holistic healers and make extravagant claims for their cures.
▶ Do not substitute chiropractic for traditional medical treatment of heart disease, cancer, diabetes, and other organic disorders.
▶ Before undergoing X-rays in a chiropractor's office, make sure the equipment is up-to-date to minimize radiation exposure.
▶ Chiropractic treatments are generally safe for everyone, but there are exceptions. Patients who have osteoporosis and other disorders characterized by weak or brittle bones should avoid it.

The Special Niche of Osteopathy

Osteopathy is a variation of conventional medicine. Its practitioners are fully qualified doctors, licensed in all 50 states to practice the full range of medicine. In addition, osteopathic training is quite similar to traditional medical school and residency. Even so, this particular practice is often confused with chiropractic because of its focus on manipulation.

Origins

The system was developed in the late 1800s by Andrew Taylor Still, a country doctor, to overcome what he perceived as shortcomings of orthodox medicine at that time. In 1892, he founded the American School of Osteopathy in Kirksville, Missouri, and many of his principles are still followed.

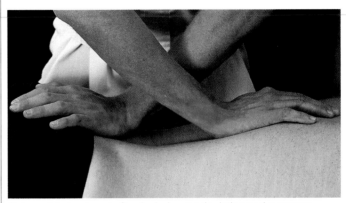

Osteopathic treatment often includes manipulation and massage, especially if the patient has pain.

When it is used

Osteopaths treat the entire spectrum of human disease, and many of their practices are indistinguishable from those of mainstream physicians.

How it works

Osteopathy is based on the premise that all organ systems form an interrelated whole, and that good health reflects a harmonic balance among organs, as well as harmony of mind and body. Any dysfunction of one part is thought to affect the entire organism adversely. Thus, treatment is directed to finding and correcting the underlying cause of the disorder.

What to expect

In making a diagnosis and formulating a treatment plan, an osteopath concentrates on the neuromusculoskeletal system. After taking a detailed medical history, the practitioner typically spends considerable time feeling or palpating the patient's body, looking for areas of inflammation, tenderness, and muscle tightness or spasms. X-rays and laboratory tests may be ordered. A typical treatment often includes manipulation and massage, especially if there is pain.

Like conventional physicians, osteopaths are qualified to prescribe drugs and perform surgery, but they do not rely as much on these modalities as other doctors do. Even when prescribing drugs, an osteopath is likely to perform manipulations as well to increase the effectiveness of the medication. Osteopaths also spend time instructing their patients in self-care, with emphasis on good posture and exercise.

Dance Therapy

Dance therapy, also called dance/movement therapy, employs movement instead of spoken communication to treat the mentally ill. It is also used to enrich the lives of sightless and deaf individuals, especially children, and can be an important aspect of rehabilitation following a stroke or an injury that hinders motion and coordination.

Origins

While dance and movement have long been used for expression, recreation, and religious rituals, the foundation of the present therapy was laid shortly after World War I, when the pioneers in modern dance began to create choreography that expressed inner emotions. At about the same time, new approaches to the treatment of mental illness were developing and therapists increasingly recognized the importance of using body movement as an outlet for emotions that could not be expressed with words.

An early practitioner of dance therapy was Marian Chace, a dance teacher. Having observed that physical movement helped emotionally disturbed children, she began to emphasize their needs for expression rather than their mastery of technique. In the 1940s, a psychiatrist who was impressed with Chace's results invited her to work with mentally ill patients at St. Elizabeth's Hospital in Washington, D.C. In the years that followed, she received national recognition for her accomplishments. She had demonstrated that through dance and movement, patients previously considered hopelessly regressed and withdrawn were able to engage in group activities and take the first steps toward expressing their feelings, even if they were unable to do so verbally.

Other dance therapists appeared on the scene with a variety of techniques, and in 1966, the American Dance Therapy Association was established to set standards for the profession. The association now has about 1,000 members.

Practitioners

Professional dance/movement therapists must undergo training in a graduate level program approved by the American Dance Therapy Association. Those who complete a program are eligible to apply for entry level certification as Dance Therapist Registered (DTR), which indicates that the individual has a master's degree and is qualified to work with a team or under supervision in a professional setting.

After two years of clinical practice, the dance/movement therapist can apply for advanced certification with the association's Academy of Dance Therapists Registered (ADTR). This designation confirms that the holder is fully qualified to teach, provide supervision, and engage in private practice.

When it is used

Dance/movement therapists work with individuals who have social, emotional, cognitive, and/or physical problems. They practice in psychiatric hospitals, community day care and mental health centers, correctional facilities, rehabilitation

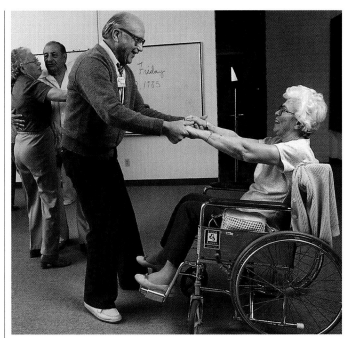

Even a patient confined to a wheelchair can benefit from the social interaction and movement of dance therapy. For others, it can be an important aspect of physical and emotional rehabilitation.

centers, clinics, nursing homes, and geriatric centers. Their work in these last two places is especially important among patients with Alzheimer's disease and others who may be incapable of ordinary social interaction. Some sports coaches also use dance therapy to improve their athletes' agility.

How it works

Participants are encouraged to overcome muscular tensions and to become aware of the way in which their feelings can affect their muscles. With the development of this awareness, they become increasingly capable of the wordless expression of inner feelings in the form of movement, usually accompanied by music. As the therapy progresses, the movements can later be interpreted and discussed.

What to expect

Patients are guided to use their bodies in movements that the therapist is trained to interpret. Through rhythmic body language, for example, an autistic child may achieve a sense of physical order that can have a healing effect on the disordered mind and feelings.

Dance therapy employed to help children with movement disorders, such as cerebral palsy, has multiple goals: to help them gain strength, improve coordination, and experience enjoyable movement free from fear of failure. The same goals apply to an older stroke patient or accident victim as well.

Individuals who are withdrawn can achieve a feeling of connectedness through holding hands in a group and facing other participants. Dance and movement can also have a positive role in the emotional and physical recovery of patients who have survived serious automobile accidents, severe burn injuries, or other mishaps that require lengthy rehabilitation and that could leave a permanent disability.

As therapy progresses, patients may be given an assignment to work on by themselves between sessions, or they may be instructed to prepare a dance improvisation for the therapist and the group to interpret.

Precautions
▶ If you are seeking a dance/movement therapist for personal consultation, remember that only those who have met the requirements for an ADTR (Academy of Dance Therapists Registered) are qualified for private practice.

Herbal Medicine

Herbal medicine is the use of plants—their leaves, stems, bark, flowers, fruits, and seeds—to prevent or cure disease.

Origins

The practice probably originated in prehistoric times when humans discovered, through trial and error, that certain plants had healing powers. During the ancient civilizations of China, Egypt, Persia, and Greece, herbal remedies were codified and, eventually, compiled into books.

With the development of chemistry and the refinement of laboratory methods, herbal medicine gave way to the modern pharmaceutical industry where many drugs are created in test tubes. Still, plant-based ingredients are found in almost half of all prescription and over-the-counter medications used in conventional medicine, including aspirin, digitalis, and atropine, as well as several anticancer medications.

Herbal medicine in China has for centuries been a well-organized system of knowledge based on observations, experiments, and clinical trials, and the effectiveness of a significant number of these remedies has been verified by modern science. Elsewhere, the latest effort in plant codification has been undertaken by a consortium of medical researchers, pharmaceutical companies, and herbalists who are investigating the flora of the rain forests in the hope of discovering new plant sources that might yield cures for heart disease, cancer, AIDS, and other deadly diseases.

Practitioners

Herbal medicine is the specialty of people who call themselves herbalists. It is also part of homeopathy, naturopathy, and aromatherapy, as well as the mainstay of self-styled holistic healers, some with acceptable credentials, many without. Chinese herbal medicine is being popularized in the West by

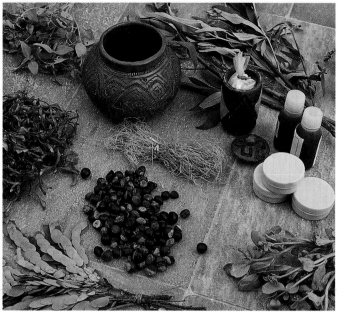

Herbs for medicines are usually dried to preserve their oils and other healing ingredients, then brewed into teas or decoctions (page 45).

acupuncturists and other practitioners of Eastern medicine. Many salespeople in health food stores also consider themselves qualified to recommend the use of herbal extracts. Finally, many home remedies rely upon herbal preparations.

When it is used

For practitioners of herbal medicine, especially Chinese herbalists, there is a plant remedy for almost every disorder. In general, herbs are effective for treating minor ailments such as digestive problems, flu, cough, headache, and rash.

How it works

Herbal medicines that bring about a desired result are found in laboratory analyses to contain substances that trigger specific biochemical responses. For example, the inner bark of a certain type of willow tree chewed by Native Americans to alleviate headaches and other pains contains salicylic acid, the active ingredient of aspirin. Some herbalists still recommend white willow to treat headaches, arthritis, and other painful conditions, contending that it is less likely to produce stomach upset and other adverse effects of aspirin.

Unlike conventional drugs, herbal remedies per se do not have the supervision of the Food and Drug Administration

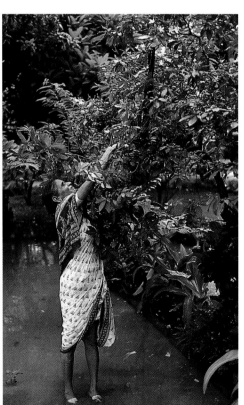

Gathering native herbs is an increasingly important pursuit in many tropical countries where rain forests are rapidly disappearing. Some major pharmaceutical companies are studying these herbs in search of ever more effective drugs.

POISONOUS HERBS

Many herbs are highly toxic, even in small doses. Be cautious of homemade remedies, and if you gather wild herbs, be sure you know what you are picking. The following herbs can be fatal:

Aconite	Lobelia
American and black hellebore	Mayapple (European
Arnica	mandrake)
Autumn crocus	Pokeweed
Belladonna (deadly nightshade)	Rue
Bloodroot	Sassafras
Colts foot	Tansy
Foxglove (digitalis)	Wahoo
Hemlock	Wormwood
Jimsonweed	Yohimbe

THE CHINESE HERBAL PHARMACY

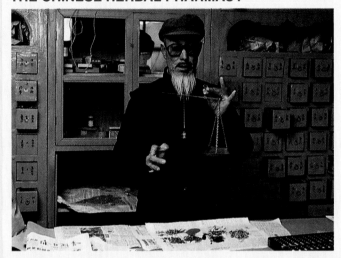

Chinese herbal medicine is thousands of years old, and many of the ideas developed in its infancy are still in use among practitioners throughout the world. For example, the prescriptions shown above, carved on wooden strips, are considered as effective today as when they were first created more than 2,000 years ago.

Throughout the ages, Chinese medical writings have expanded upon past wisdom. Thus, when Chang Chung-ching (A.D. 142-220), who is regarded as the Hippocrates of China, described 287 herbal formulas in his *Treatise on Febrile Diseases and Summaries of Household Remedies,* he drew many of his prescriptions from earlier dynasties. In turn, Chung's followers expanded upon his writings.

During the Ming dynasty (1368-1643), herbal medicine reached new heights—the famed *General Catalog of Herbs* by Li Shih-chen (1518-1593) describes 1,871 herbs and 8,160 herbal prescriptions. In China today, most people continue to rely on ancient herbal remedies, even though they may also see a physician who has been trained in Western medical practices.

Herbal Classification

Chinese herbalists stress that great care is needed to prevent mixing of drugs that are incompatible. Thus, herbal formulas are based upon very specific classifications according to their physical characteristics, and whether they are yin (cool or cold) or yang (warm or hot). More specifically, drugs are classified as follows:

▶ Five flavors: hot, which rid the body of toxins; sour, which are astringents or absorbents; sweet, which are tonics that reinforce warm drugs; bitter, which dry out and purge the body; and salty, which soften and lubricate.
▶ Four directions of action: ascending and floating, which are yang in nature and help expel or purge; and descending and sinking, which are yin in nature and move inward.

While under treatment, patients are also instructed to eat foods that are compatible with the yin or yang nature of their drugs.

Categories of Treatment

Chinese herbal treatments work by inducing one or more of the following physical responses:
▶ Sweating
▶ Vomiting
▶ Purging (promoting elimination via the colon)
▶ Harmonizing (restoring the body's natural homeostasis)
▶ Warming
▶ Removing
▶ Supplementing
▶ Reducing

Specific herbal remedies fall into 17 different categories:
▶ Anthelmintics to kill intestinal parasites.
▶ Antirheumatics, which are taken with sweating agents to treat rheumatism and arthritis.
▶ Antitussives and expectorants to treat coughs, asthma, and excess sputum production.
▶ Astringents to treat rectal prolapse, diarrhea, or sweating.
▶ Blood agents to treat anemia, menstrual problems, ulcers, and other disorders related to bleeding.
▶ Cold agents to treat colds, vomiting, diarrhea, and other symptoms.
▶ Digestive agents to treat abdominal pain and loss of appetite.
▶ Distress agents to treat psychological problems.
▶ Diuretics to treat edema and urinary problems.
▶ Emetics to treat chest congestion, intoxication, or overeating.
▶ External medicines, ointments, and sprays. These preparations are generally toxic if taken internally.
▶ Inhalants to treat fainting, unconsciousness, and high fevers.
▶ Purgatives to treat constipation.
▶ Refreshing agents to detoxify blood during a fever or infection.
▶ Sweating agents to treat such disorders as fevers and chills.
▶ Tonics to treat general weakness.
▶ Tranquilizers to reduce anxiety and treat insomnia and convulsions.

(FDA). Therefore, the consumer has no way of knowing whether an herbal product has been subjected to scientific testing to measure its safety and effectiveness. FDA rules require that herbal products be marketed as foods or food additives and that their labels not make specific medical claims or provide dosage information. Hence, people who use herbal remedies usually turn to books or rely upon the advice of an herbalist or other alternative practitioner.

What to expect

After asking questions about the nature of a problem, an herbalist will prescribe a specific plant and give instructions on how to use it. For medicinal purposes, dried herbs are usually recommended because their increased concentration makes them more potent than the fresh plants.

Leaves and flowers are dried in an airy, shady place; sun bakes out their oils and may also damage other medicinal ingredients. Roots and heavy stems are cleaned, chopped, dried, and then stored in glass jars or other nonmetallic containers in a cool, dry place until they are used.

Medicinal herbs are most often steeped in boiling water and consumed as a tea. These teas, which can be unpleasantly bitter or strong-tasting, should not be confused with the pleasant, commercially available herbal teas, which contain only a small fraction of the herbs used in a medicinal brew.

Precautions
▶ Many plants are poisonous. Make sure that you know exactly what is in an herbal remedy before you take it internally.
▶ Before using any herbal remedy for a child's illness, consult a pediatrician or pediatric nurse.
▶ Take only the recommended dosage. Herbal products that are safe in small amounts can produce severe side effects when taken in larger doses. For example, a plant substance that may be an effective laxative in small quantities can often provoke severe diarrhea when taken in a larger dosage.
▶ Monitor yourself for possible side effects. If you develop a widespread rash, dizziness, difficulty breathing, or other signs of a severe reaction, call a doctor or go to your nearest emergency room because you may be having an anaphylactic reaction.

EXAMPLES OF COMMON HERBAL REMEDIES

Herb	Used for	Precautions
Aloe vera	Skin moisturizer; minor cuts; sunburn	Sometimes promoted as a laxative or for stomach disorders, but internal use is hazardous.
Anise	Cough soother; digestive aid	Generally safe.
Arnica	Anti-inflammatory painkiller for sprains, bruises; muscle aches	For external use only. Causes cardiac toxicity if ingested; stop using if arnica liniment causes dermatitis.
Buckthorn	Laxative; digestive aid; tonic; skin irritations	Generally safe in small doses. Should not be taken during pregnancy.
Chamomile	Tea: sedative; digestive aid; menstrual cramps. Compress: arthritis; skin disorders	Generally safe in small amounts.
Comfrey	Skin wounds, bruises, burns, and boils; reducing swelling of sprains; skin softener	Should not be taken internally because of possible liver toxicity.
Dandelion	Laxative; tonic; diuretic	Generally safe.
Echinacea	Compress: skin sores and stings. Tea: bladder infections; fever; headache	Generally safe in small doses.
Eucalyptus	Nasal and sinus congestion; coughs	Oil irritating to eyes and mucous membranes.
Evening primrose	Painkiller; sedative; autoimmune disorders	Can worsen bleeding disorders.
Fenugreek	Expectorant; digestive tonic; laxative. Poultice: Soothing of boils and skin ulcers	Generally safe.
Fennel	Digestive aid	Generally safe.
Feverfew	Painkiller	Generally safe; may cause mouth sores when chewed.
Garlic	Antiseptic; reducing of high blood pressure and high blood cholesterol	Generally safe, but raw garlic may irritate skin and mucous membranes; should not substitute for prescribed drugs.
Ginseng	General tonic; blood thinner; aphrodisiac	Generally safe, but many claims of its healing power are unproved.
Horehound	Decongestant; expectorant; cough soother; lowering of fever	Generally safe.
Hyssop	Expectorant, sore throat, coughs, digestive aid	Generally safe.
Licorice	Irritated skin and mucous membranes; ulcers; digestive aid	Generally safe; excessive use raises blood pressure.
Marsh mallow	Demulcent to sooth intestinal inflammation and irritation; wound healing	Generally safe; excessive use may cause diarrhea.
Peppermint	Digestive aid	Generally safe.
Sassafras	Skin wounds; relief of poison ivy rash	Should not be taken internally.
Uva-ursi	Diuretic; cystitis; kidney and bladder stones	Generally safe, but should not substitute for antibiotics.
Valerian	Sleep aid; relieving of stress	Generally safe, but should not be used during pregnancy.
Witch hazel	Astringent; skin irritations; hemorrhoids	Should not be taken internally.

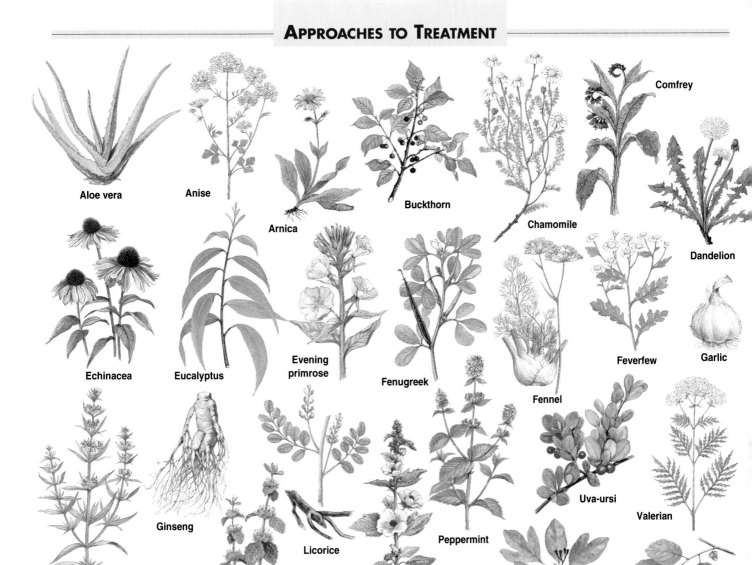

Aloe vera

Anise

Arnica

Buckthorn

Chamomile

Comfrey

Dandelion

Echinacea

Eucalyptus

Evening primrose

Fenugreek

Fennel

Feverfew

Garlic

Ginseng

Licorice

Peppermint

Uva-ursi

Valerian

Hyssop

Horehound

Marsh mallow

Sassafras

Witch hazel

HERBAL RECIPES

Herbal preparations are taken in many forms—alcohol tinctures, fluid extracts, essential oils, syrups, vinegars, capsules, and pills. Lay people are generally advised to obtain these preparations from reliable herbalists or reputable commercial outlets. If you prefer to make your own, herbalists recommend freshly made infusions (teas) or decoctions using the following recipes:

Standard infusion. Place 1 ounce of dried herb or 3 ounces of fresh herb in a teapot or other nonmetalic container, and pour in 1 pint of boiling water. Let it steep for 10 minutes, strain out herbs, and drink while still fresh. (Note: Some remedies may call for stronger or milder teas; adjust recipe according to instructions.)

Decoction. Place 1 ounce of herb in a glass, enamel, or stainless steel pan (not aluminum), add 3 cups of water and bring to a boil; lower heat and simmer for 10 minutes or until the liquid is reduced by one-third. Strain and drink the recommended amount while the liquid is still hot. (Note: decoctions are usually made from roots or woody herbs.)

Compresses. Soak gauze or fine cloth in an infusion or decoction and apply to skin. (Test first on a small area for irritation.)

Poultice. Boil or cook herb (for example, garlic) or other recommended substance (for example, oatmeal), wrap in gauze, press out excess fluid, and apply while still hot.

BACH FLOWER REMEDIES

Of the several variations on herbalism, one of the best known is the system of Dr. Edward Bach, an English bacteriologist and homeopath who created and used flower essences as an alternative to conventional drug remedies. His preparations were made by immersing flowers in water and then exposing this combination to heat or to sunlight. He believed that these essences, individually and in combination, would restore the mental and emotional balance essential for physical well-being.

The best-known of the Bach concoctions is the Rescue Remedy, a combination of five different formulas, which is reserved for especially trying situations such as the death of a loved one. Other Bach remedies include agrimony to relieve anxiety; impatiens to reduce emotional irritability; and a combination of larch, holly, and mustard flower essences for asthma.

Since Bach's death in 1936, several practitioners in the United States have developed comparable remedies. The best-known among these is a group called the 72 Flower Essence Society (FES), whose products are based on flowers native to California.

Flower essences are sold in small bottles with eye droppers from which a drop or two is usually placed under the tongue at specified times. The drops can be found in many health food stores, and are also available from mail order catalogs.

Homeopathy

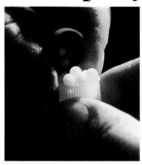

Homeopathic medicines are so diluted that only an undetectable fraction remains.

Homeopathy is based on the theory that the cause of an illness is similar to its cure. Thus, treatment involves giving a small amount of a very diluted natural substance that, if taken in larger doses, would cause the same symptoms as the ailment itself.

Origins

Samuel Hahnemann, a German physician, evolved the principles of homeopathy early in the 19th century, after abandoning what he considered to be the crude practices of his colleagues. He became especially interested in references to "similars" by Paracelsus, a 16th-century Swiss physician and alchemist who had concluded that the same substances which cause illness in large amounts will cure it in small doses. After conducting experiments, Hahnemann announced his findings in 1810, and a list of "proven" remedies appeared in 1821. Hahnemann's principles of homeopathy state that:

▶ Substances that produce symptoms similar or identical to those experienced by the patient will produce the cure; in other words, "like cures like."

▶ Only one medicine is given at a time.

▶ The least possible amount of the curative substance is the most effective for relieving symptoms.

▶ The patient's positive attitude is an essential factor in the success of the healing process.

Homeopathic practice became the rage in Europe and the United States and, in 1844, the American Institute of Homeopathy was established by a group of distinguished doctors. When the American Medical Association was founded a few years later, it took a hostile position against its predecessor. In a short time, homeopathy declined in the United States, but it never went out of style in Europe. Homeopathic pharmacies, hospitals, and clinics abound throughout Europe

Precautions

▶ Beware of extravagant claims by any practitioner who holds out the promise of a cure for a serious condition that is unresponsive to conventional treatment.

▶ If your symptoms haven't been alleviated in one or two homeopathic visits, it's time to see your physician.

▶ A large number of homeopathic guides and remedies can be found in health food stores. Such self-treatment should be confined to minor ailments.

today, and the services are covered by most national health insurance plans. In this country, homeopathy is enjoying a revival, because its adherents consider it a natural approach and its treatments do not cause the side effects of many of the drugs used in conventional medicine.

Practitioners

In three states—Arizona, Nevada, and Connecticut—practitioners of homeopathy must be licensed, and in Connecticut they must also receive board certification. Elsewhere in the United States, health providers already licensed in their own specialty are not required to have a specific license in homeopathy. Thus, some acupuncturists, naturopaths, herbalists, and M.D.s also refer to themselves as homeopaths.

When it is used

Homeopaths claim to treat virtually all conditions, but most concede that their methods work best against chronic disorders such as headaches, allergies, intestinal diseases, and asthma. Remedies are often prescribed as an adjunct to other alternative procedures, such as acupuncture and chiropractic. Most homeopaths recommend that conventional medicine also be used for injuries, infections, and cancer and other serious diseases. In these cases, homeopathy is considered an adjunct to enhance the effect of conventional medicine.

How it works

Even the most enthusiastic proponents of homeopathy are not sure exactly how it works. Practitioners believe that symptoms are an expression of the body's attempt to heal itself. Therefore, they seek the substance that produces in healthy people the symptoms experienced in the illness.

Homeopathic medicines are prepared by a series of dilutions. An extract is mixed with 100 times as much water or water and alcohol, shaken energetically, then diluted again. Shaking between each dilution is essential; substances that are diluted without the shaking do not work. This process is repeated until it is impossible to discover any trace of the original extract. Practitioners claim that the more diluted the remedy, the more effective it will be. They ascribe its effectiveness to the transmission of "vital energy" that resonates within the patient's body. Some assume that confidence in the healer can also improve the patient's condition.

What to expect

In the first encounter, a practitioner will ask many questions and conduct a physical examination. A single remedy is then selected. (Even if this treatment does not produce a cure, it is not likely to do any harm because it is so diluted.) If the wrong remedy is chosen, it is said to have missed the ailment's "center of gravity," and a different one will be tried. The correct remedy may worsen symptoms initially, indicating that the body's defenses are rallying to produce a cure.

THE MATERIA MEDICA OF HOMEOPATHY

Some 2,000 homeopathic remedies are classified according to the symptoms that they are said to counter. Examples include:

▶ Aconite (monkshood). Symptoms, such as a high fever, are intense and come on suddenly. Aconite is normally administered at the onset of an illness.

▶ Apis Mellifica (honey bee venom). Symptoms include acute inflammation marked by stinging, burning, redness, and swelling.

▶ Arsenicum Album (white arsenic or arsenious acid). Symptoms include extreme agitation, fear, weakness, fatigue, chills, and burning pain, all worsening at night.

▶ Belladonna (deadly nightshade). Symptoms come on suddenly and violently, and may include fever, inflammation, and cramps.

▶ Gelsemium (yellow jasmine). Drowsiness, fatigue, mental sluggishness, and physical weakness predominate.

▶ Mercurius Vivus (mercury). Symptoms include marked inflammation of the skin and mucous membranes, pus formation, pain and, in some cases, open sores.

▶ Nux vomica (poison nut tree). Symptoms include headaches, chills, indigestion, muscle spasms, and back pain.

Hydrotherapy

Hydrotherapy is the use of water to treat disease, alleviate pain, induce relaxation, and maintain general good health. For therapeutic purposes, the water may be hot or cold, or in the form of ice or steam. Treatments include immersion baths (usually in cool water), hot tub soaks, sitz baths (a shortened hip bath), mud baths, steam baths, saunas, needle showers, salt rubs, pressure hosing, hot or cold packs, douches, and colonic irrigation (washing of the inner wall of the large intestine). Hydrotherapy may also take the form of drinking water that has special qualities, such as the mineral waters offered by European spas as an aid to digestion.

Origins
Because of the almost universal availability of water, it has been used to promote health and to cure illness by all cultures. The elaborate and efficient public baths built by the ancient Romans are a typical example; they were usually combined with gymnasiums to foster socializing and physical and mental well-being by alternating exercise with relaxation. In Finland, saunas have been a ritual for 2,000 years. Russian and Turkish steam baths, introduced years ago to Americans by immigrant populations, remain popular to this day. In recent years, hydrotherapy has gained an important place in physical therapy and rehabilitation medicine.

Practitioners
In hospitals, hydrotherapy is performed by doctors, nurses, nurses' aides, and physical therapists. At a spa or health club, it may be supervised by a physical therapist, a massage specialist, or an ayurvedic practitioner. However, the most common site for hydrotherapy is the home, where the techniques are used as forms of self-treatment.

When it is used
In rehabilitation facilities and mental hospitals, hydrotherapy is used to relax muscles and joints, soothe anxiety, relieve stress, and enhance mobility. This last may be achieved through swimming and underwater exercise, which can help maintain and extend range of motion for patients who have arthritis and other joint and muscle disorders.

As part of a pain management program, hydrotherapy in the form of warm baths in a darkened room can help patients focus on breathing exercises and other pain-control methods.

Hydrotherapy is also promoted by health clubs and spas as a natural way of treating aching muscles and painful joints, with a combination of showers and steam or whirlpools, after participation in athletic activities.

At home, it is employed as an aid to relaxation, to alleviate minor aches and pains, and to induce sleep.

How it works
The way in which hydrotherapy works depends on its form:
▶ Sitz baths soothe many conditions, including hemorrhoids, anal fissures, and vaginal infections.

Precautions
▶ Pregnant women and people who have diabetes, high blood pressure, or any chronic coronary condition should avoid hot tubs, steam baths, and saunas.
▶ An ice pack should not be placed directly on the skin; instead, it should be wrapped in a towel or cloth.

WATER AEROBICS
An increasingly popular form of hydrotherapy is water aerobics, or modified aerobic dancing done in the shallow end of a swimming pool. Water aerobics offers all the benefits of other forms of aerobic exercise without the joint strain and risk of injury inherent in any weight-bearing activity. It is particularly beneficial for older people, pregnant women, anyone with a sports injury or arthritis, and those who are overweight.

▶ Floating in a pool or special tub permits a person who has arthritis or has suffered a stroke to exercise joints in a way that might otherwise be too difficult or painful.
▶ Medicinal baths in warm to hot water affect metabolism of the body tissues lying just under the skin, or improve circulation by increasing the flow of blood to surface areas.
▶ A steam bath clears nasal congestion and soothes sore muscles and stiff joints.
▶ An ice pack reduces swelling and inflammation following a bruise, sports injury, or tooth extraction.
▶ Medicated vapor relieves chest congestion.
▶ A warm, wet dressing helps to bring a boil to a head so that it can break on its own or be drained.
▶ Cold, wet towels wrapped around an individual suffering from heat exhaustion quickly bring down the person's temperature, and therefore are an effective emergency treatment.

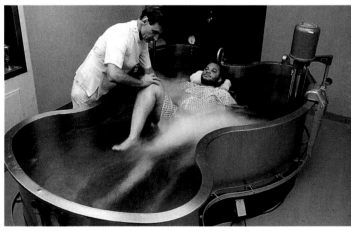

Underwater exercise is an important part of the physical therapy and rehabilitation of patients who have suffered a stroke or whose arthritis makes movement difficult and painful.

What to expect
In rehabilitation centers, hydrotherapy may include immersion baths, needle showers, underwater muscle massage with powerful water jets, douches, and cold or hot wet wrappings of a body part or of the entire body.

In the past, some forms of hydrotherapy were widely used to calm agitated or aggressive patients with mental illnesses. Today, medications have made this use of hydrotherapy largely obsolete. However, some mental institutions may employ a flotation tank to calm severely agitated patients. Use of such a tank induces deep relaxation by allowing the body to float in warm water, often in a darkened room from which all environmental stimuli have been removed.

Hypnosis

Hypnosis is an altered state of consciousness in which a very highly concentrated state of attention is focused on a specific idea or memory. The patient (or subject) is fully awake but responds only to the therapist's suggestions. There is abundant empirical evidence that hypnotherapy produces desired results for many people. Some, however, are incapable of achieving a deep trance state. Others can reach only a light hypnotic state because they are unable or unconsciously unwilling to achieve this form of total concentration.

Origins

From ancient healers to Dr. Franz Mesmer, an 18th-century Viennese physician who cast his subjects into a trance as a theatrical entertainment (hence mesmerizing), hypnosis has had a colorful history. Not until the late 1950s did it begin to

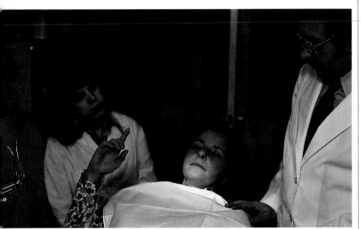

Hypnosis may be a solution for a dental patient who cannot tolerate anesthesia or one who has an intense fear of dental procedures.

overcome its association with charlatans and movie villains. In 1958, the American Medical Association acknowledged for the first time that hypnosis was a useful therapeutic tool.

Practitioners

Hypnotherapy, as the medical use of hypnosis is called, is practiced by physicians (especially psychiatrists), dentists, psychologists, naturopaths, physical therapists, psychiatric social workers, and holistic healers. Legitimate hypnotherapy should not be confused with staged hypnosis, which is sometimes presented as entertainment.

When it is used

A psychotherapist or other health-care professional may use hypnosis in several ways. One is behavior modification; for example, helping a patient to overcome a weight problem or nicotine addiction. Another is the calling up of traumatic events, such as childhood abuse, that may have been denied

Precautions

▶ Be wary of self-styled hypnotherapists who advertise their services in the Yellow Pages or newspaper classified ads. Instead, ask your doctor for a referral or call the psychiatry department of the nearest teaching hospital and ask for names of qualified hypnotherapists in your area.

VISUALIZATION

Visualization entails concentrating fully on a specific image. It may be combined with hypnosis or another therapy to induce relaxation, counteract anxiety, or control pain perception.

Dr. Herbert Benson, a Harvard psychologist and author of *The Relaxation Response,* urges patients to use visualization to overcome stress. For example, he instructs them to visualize a peaceful landscape while tensing and relaxing different muscle groups to achieve more complete relaxation.

or buried as a means of self-protection. Two other uses are the diagnosing of multiple personalities and the treating of phobias, such as fear of flying.

Pain management is another major application of hypnosis. A deep trance state may be induced to serve as anesthesia during surgery; a lighter trance is often employed to ease the pain of childbirth. And for controlling chronic pain, many people are now taught the techniques of self-hypnosis.

How it works

To control pain through hypnosis, patients are taught to become intensely aware of their body sensations, to track their breathing, and to eliminate distracting thoughts and images. Then they are instructed to focus on the pain—its location, intensity, and shape. Through this technique, they become active participants in pain control, learning to modify its features, shift its level, and raise and lower its intensity. Eventually they can learn to transfer the skills developed during hypnosis to control other troublesome problems.

To help a patient remember a blocked out traumatic event or a critical childhood experience, the hypnotist will put him in a hypnotic trance and suggest mentally going back to the time and place in question. This regression is often done in steps; for example, he may be instructed to visit a childhood classroom or former home. Typically, the subject begins to speak in a childlike voice and assume a different posture. If the flashback scene is especially painful, he may cry, but the crying is likely to be that of a child, rather than an adult. After the subject is instructed to end the trance, voice and posture return to normal, and often there is no memory of what happened during hypnosis.

In diagnosing and treating multiple personality disorders, the hypnotist tries to get the other personalities to come forth. Again, there is often a dramatic change in voice and bearing as different personalities emerge.

What to expect

A hypnotic trance is most successfully induced in a subject who is cooperative and who can relax, maintain a state of mental alertness, and concentrate on repeated instructions, which sometimes involve visualization (see box, above). They may be repeated in a low, confident voice as the hypnotherapist leads the subject into a deep trance. As the suggestibility level increases, breathing and pulse rate slow down. At this point, the therapist can instill desired images; for example, having a smoker concentrate on a scenario in which all ashtrays are discarded and all tobacco smoke becomes noxious.

Most patients can learn the techniques of self-hypnosis and visualization, thereby reinforcing and extending the efforts of the therapist. Audio and video tapes that offer instructions in hypnosis and visualization are available for home use.

Light Therapy

Light therapy employs either natural or artificial light to treat various disorders, ranging from psoriasis and other skin diseases to soft bones and seasonal affective disorder (SAD), a type of depression that occurs during the winter.

Origins

Exposure to bright sunlight and to the ultraviolet rays of sun lamps has been used to treat skin diseases for many years. The application of light therapy for treating SAD dates from the late 1980s when doctors first recognized the link between depression and the long, dark days of mid-winter.

Practitioners

Light therapy may be administered by a physician, physical therapist, or psychologist. It is also carried out at home under instructions by a qualified health professional.

When it is used

Light therapy is now the treatment of choice for SAD, largely replacing the use of antidepressants and psychotherapy.

Ultraviolet light has several uses. One is to treat psoriasis, often in conjunction with drugs, as well as other nonspecific skin conditions that cause itching. Another is to treat rickets

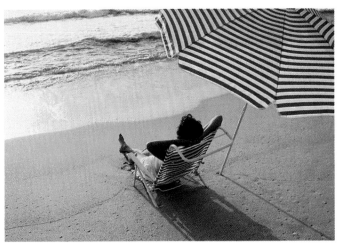

Taking a winter vacation in a warm, sunny clime is a good way to beat the winter blues, but one should be careful not to indulge in too much direct sun exposure, which can damage the skin.

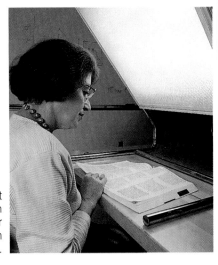

While undergoing light therapy, a patient can read or go about other routine activities that can be done while sitting.

(in children) or osteomalacia (in adults). These disorders, in which the bones become soft, are caused by a lack of vitamin D, which the body makes when the skin is exposed to sunlight. Elderly shut-ins benefit from such treatment in two ways: The light therapy helps strengthen their bones, and at the same time helps them counter depression. Infants born with jaundice are also sometimes exposed to ultraviolet light.

Other potential uses of light therapy include treatment for jet lag, sleep disorders, and the biorhythm problems that are often experienced by people who work at night.

How it works

Exposure to varying levels of light affects the biological clock of all living creatures. In humans, lack of sunshine has a more profound psychological effect than was formerly recognized. (Some researchers estimate that 20 percent of people who live in the northern United States and Canada could benefit from light therapy, with women outnumbering men four to one.) Daylight stimulates the human brain to produce hormones and other brain chemicals that are essential for psychological and emotional well-being.

For most SAD sufferers, daily exposure to a few hours of very bright fluorescent lights relieves their symptoms as effectively as a winter vacation in the sunny tropics. Within four days of beginning treatment, most patients show a marked improvement—much more quickly than with antidepressant medication. Benefits seem to be the same whether therapy takes place during the day or night.

Ultraviolet light also directly affects the skin in several ways: It promotes the manufacture of vitamin D and slows the growth of new skin cells in psoriasis. Its drying effect may help improve acne. In some people, however, sunlight triggers a flare-up of acne; one should proceed with caution.

What to expect

The special fluorescent lights used for treating SAD are housed in boxes containing a reflector and a light-diffusing cover. The treatments, which are simple, painless, inexpensive, and harmless when done properly, usually take two or three hours a day, although some people benefit from as little as half an hour of exposure.

During a treatment, the patient can nap, read, or go about other quiet activities. New types of light therapy devices that would not interfere with a patient's daily routine are being investigated. One of these is a computer-controlled gadget that switches on a bright light early in the morning to simulate the arrival of dawn before the time of the usual winter sunrise. Studies at New York's Columbia-Presbyterian Medical Center, where the device was developed, found that test volunteers woke up feeling alert and vigorous.

Precautions

► Light therapy is effective only with lights specifically designed for this purpose. Other types of bright lights, such as halogen lamps and sunlamps, are not suitable.

► To avoid eye irritation and damage, do not look directly at the light source. Always cover the eyes of babies who are being exposed to bright, direct light.

► Because ultraviolet light increases the risk of skin cancer, its use should be carefully monitored by a doctor.

Macrobiotics

Macrobiotics is a dietary discipline based on the East Asian concept that good health depends on establishing a harmonious balance of the opposing life forces (yang and yin), and that this applies to foods as well as other aspects of life.

Origins

The regimen was developed during the first half of the 20th century by George Ohsawa, a Japanese philosophy student who claimed to have cured his tuberculosis by devising a diet based on the spiritual principles and practices of Oriental medicine. He created the term macrobiotics, which in Greek means "a broad view of life," and described his regimen in a 1920 book, *A New Theory of Nutrition and Its Therapeutic Effect*. The book is now in its 700th edition in Japan.

IS IT YIN OR YANG? The macrobiotic classification of foods as yin or yang weighs at least 15 factors. Plant foods are generally yin, representing the earth's upward force. Thus, they are thought to slow metabolism, have a calming effect, and produce other yin effects, such as reducing body temperature. Animal foods represent the heaven's downward, or yang, force, and have the opposite effect of speeding up metabolism.

Within each classification, however, there are many gradations, ranging from most yin to most yang (see box, below left).

Geography and the season are also taken into consideration. As much as possible, foods should be locally grown. Persons who live in cold, northern (yin) climates should lean toward yang foods and means of preparation, while the opposite applies to those living in warmer (yang) climates. Similarly, yin foods and cooking methods are to be followed during the warm summer months, and yang foods and preparation should dominate in the colder winter months.

By the time of his death in 1966, Ohsawa had written over 300 books and had traveled throughout the world promoting his dietary philosophy. He found a receptive audience in the early 1960s among young Americans, who flocked to macrobiotic restaurants and health food stores.

Practitioners

A number of alternative therapists, including acupuncturists, naturopaths, practitioners of Oriental medicine, and holistic healers, have incorporated macrobiotics into their practices.

When it is used

As a therapy, macrobiotics is used to treat various ailments through a limited diet. It may, for example, be recommended as a treatment for eating disorders or for coping with stress. Many of its proponents also believe that it provides a spiritual or mystical foundation for the way life should be lived.

How it works

Macrobiotics classifies all foods as yang or yin instead of by nutritional content and the designations of carbohydrate, protein, and fat (see box, below). In general, a macrobiotic diet calls for 50 to 60 percent of calories to come from whole cereal grains, the foods that are most balanced in yin and yang; 25 to 30 percent from vegetables; 10 to 15 percent from beans and sea vegetables; 5 to 10 percent from fish, shellfish, seasonal fruits, and nuts; and 5 percent from soups made with vegetables, grains, or miso (fermented soy).

The extreme macrobiotic diets of the early 1960s were sometimes limited to brown rice only, which is balanced in its yin and yang qualities but is not complete nutritionally. Those were soon abandoned when faithful followers developed severe malnutrition. Today's macrobiotic diet is similar to many vegetarian regimens, especially those that eschew milk and eggs but allow inclusion of seafood.

What to expect

Following a diagnosis based on the individual's appearance, symptoms, and current diet, the macrobiotic therapist recommends changes aimed at correcting the imbalance of yang and yin foods. Modifications depend on the availability of local grains, vegetables, and fruit. Brown rice and herbal tea are considered basic. Bananas, mangoes, and other tropical fruits are avoided in temperate climates. Even though fish and some meat may be acceptable, all dairy products are excluded. Processed foods, whether frozen or canned, are also prohibited at all times.

A person may be taught new ways in which to prepare foods. Copper and aluminum pans, for example, are not used because traces of their metals can leach into foods. Instead, stainless steel, enamel, glass, and ceramic cookware, as well as wooden or bamboo spoons, are recommended.

MACROBIOTIC FOOD CLASSIFICATION

Food group	More Yin	More Yang
Grains	Corn, long-grain rice, summer wheat	Millet, buckwheat, short-grain rice, winter wheat
Beans	Soybeans and other oily beans	Chickpeas, lentils, and other nonoily beans
Vegetables	All those grown above ground	Carrots and other root vegetables
Seaweed	Harvested in warm water close to shore	Harvested in deeper, cold water
Nuts	Peanuts, cashews, and other oily nuts	Almonds, chestnuts, and other less oily nuts
Fruits	Citrus, mango, and other tropical fruits	Apples, cherries, and other temperate fruits
Sweeteners	Sugar, honey, and maple syrup	Barley malt and rice honey

Precautions

►A rigorous macrobiotic diet can have dangerous consequences if imposed on children and adolescents. Because it is low in calories and certain nutrients, it can also further jeopardize the health of people with AIDS, cancer, and malabsorption diseases.
► If you devise your own macrobiotic diet as a way of losing weight, ask your doctor or a qualified nutritionist about supplements, especially of vitamin B_{12}.

Massage

In therapeutic massage, touch is used to induce relaxation and promote well-being. Though there are many forms of the practice, all employ systematic stroking, rubbing, pressing, kneading, or thumping of the skin, muscles, and joints. Massage is also combined sometimes with other techniques, especially aroma and water therapies.

Origins

Massage is an instinctive means of communication and giving comfort. Among animals, mothers stroke their young, and the adults of many species rub or groom each other.

Medically, massage is our oldest form of treatment and one that is used by every culture. The earliest Chinese, Egyptian, and Indian medical writings all describe preventive and ther-

medicine, and it was relegated to seedy massage parlors or scorned as a pleasure of the pampered rich. In recent years, the pendulum has begun to swing back, and massage by hand is once again considered a useful therapeutic tool.

Practitioners

Almost everyone can do a simple form of massage on himself or someone else, but special instruction is needed to master the techniques of the therapeutic form. Depending upon the practice, training ranges from a few weeks to a year or more. For membership, the American Massage Therapy Association requires 500 hours of study, including courses in anatomy and physiology. There are also institutes that teach and certify certain specialized forms of massage such as rolfing, a vigorous deep kneading, and reflexology and shiatsu, techniques in which specific pressure points are pressed or massaged to alleviate pain and other symptoms.

Most massage therapists practice independently, although some work in tandem with physical therapists, sports medicine physicians, rehabilitation specialists, osteopaths, chiropractors, and other health professionals. To find a reputable practitioner, call the rehabilitation, or physiatry, department of a hospital.

When it is used

Massage is employed to alleviate stiffness, tension, and soreness in muscles, and to promote comfort and help overcome stress. Many athletic trainers recommend massage to loosen muscles before competition as well as to ease soreness afterwards. Massage can also relieve leg cramps. If you are often awakened by leg cramps or suffer restless leg syndrome, try massaging your legs before going to bed. Back and shoulder massages help some women manage labor pains, and gentle massage is one way to comfort a colicky baby. Migraines and tension headaches can be alleviated by massage; the same is true of lower back pain due to muscle spasms.

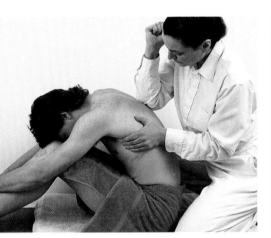
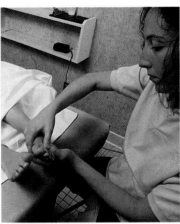
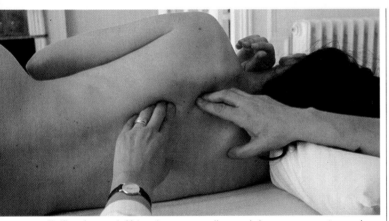

Rolfing (upper left) involves pummeling and deep massage to manipulate connective tissue. In contrast, reflexology (upper right) concentrates on stimulating specific pressure points, usually on the feet. Shiatsu (lower photo) is another form of pressure-point massage.

How it works

In general, massage works by easing muscle and psychological tension and promoting relaxation. The use of aromatic oils during massage—a variation of aromatherapy—can help deepen relaxation. Massage increases blood flow to the area being rubbed, and this may speed healing. Contrary to common claims, however, massage cannot speed the expelling of toxins from the body.

Practitioners of massage techniques that employ pressure points—for example, shiatsu, reflexology, and acupressure—claim benefits similar to those of acupuncture. The idea is to apply pressure to a specific part of the body to elicit a response elsewhere (see next page for more details.)

What to expect

For Swedish, or European, massage, the person receiving treatment undresses and then reclines on a padded table, mattress, or floor pad, and the massager stands or kneels at his side. A towel or sheet is draped over parts of the body that are not being massaged. A warm, often scented oil is applied to the exposed skin, which is then massaged with different strokes. Depending upon the stroke, the fingers, thumbs, palms, or edges of the hand, as well as elbows and forearms, are used. Most strokes are gentle and pleasant. In deep massage, however, the muscles are vigorously prodded

apeutic uses of massage. Galen, a second-century Roman physician, massaged both the emperor and gladiators, and wrote more than a dozen medical books about massage.

The most familiar form in the United States, Swedish, or classic massage, was developed in Sweden in the early 1800s by Per Henrik Ling; before his death in 1838, institutes for it had been established in several countries.

Following World War I, massage by hand was gradually replaced by the electrical devices used in physical therapy. By the 1940s, massage therapy had been eclipsed by modern

MASSAGE (CONTINUED)

and thumped. The effect should be invigorating rather than uncomfortable; let the practitioner know if the massage produces any sharp or radiating pain.

Rolfing, another vigorous form of massage, involves manipulating the deep connective tissue, or fascia, that holds the muscles together. During a session, the rolfer uses his hands, fingers, and elbows to press deeply or pummel different parts of the body. A session can be quite painful, but devotees say they feel wonderful afterwards.

There are a few other therapies that incorporate massage as part of their overall approach. For example, Hellerwork, an outgrowth of rolfing, combines deep-tissue massage with posture exercises. And polarity uses massage to harness and redirect the body's flow of energy. It also employs yoga, exercise, and nutritional and psychological counseling to provide a total approach to health and healing.

Precautions

▶ Refrain from massage during a fever, infectious illness, or bout of phlebitis, because it may worsen the underlying condition.
▶ Avoid rolfing and other deep-tissue massage techniques if you have osteoporosis or similar bone disorders; vigorous pummeling may result in a fracture.
▶ Discontinue back massage immediately if it produces a sharp pain or sends pain radiating to the buttocks or legs.
▶ Avoid massaging directly over a bruise, burn, unhealed wound or incision, varicose vein, or skin infection or rash. Instead, gently massage the adjacent areas to ease discomfort.
▶ Consult your doctor before undergoing massage if you have a chronic disorder such as diabetes or heart disease.
▶ Steer clear of massagers who advertise their services in the personal columns, especially those offering sensuous massages.

PRESSURE-POINT MASSAGE TECHNIQUES

Shiatsu, acupressure, zone therapy, and other pressure-point massage techniques differ from whole-body massage in that they concentrate on specific points, which are comparable to the acupoints of acupuncture. The objective is to maintain or restore the proper flow and balance of vital energy within the body.

Shiatsu. This is a Japanese massage technique that combines aspects of Chinese acupuncture and philosophy with body massage. Pressure points, or tsubos, are situated along 12 pathways, or meridians, extending from head to toe or fingertip. Shiatsu practitioners believe that the life energy, or qi, flows along these meridians; pain and disease occur when this energy flow is blocked or misdirected.

The area between the ribs and pelvis, referred to as the hara, is considered the body's storehouse of qi, and a shiatsu treatment begins and ends with the therapist massaging this section. A proper flow of energy is then restored by massaging and pressing upon the relevant tsubos.

Practitioners also strive to bring the force of yin, which is deep and internal, and yang, which is more active and superficial, into proper harmony. Thus, a patient suffering from yin symptoms such as fatigue and drowsiness would be given a treatment designed to stimulate the more energetic yang forces, whereas a calming yin treatment would be administered to a person complaining of headache or restlessness.

During a typical shiatsu session, the person may be clothed or unclothed and usually lies on a carpeted floor or mat, with the therapist kneeling at her side. Pressure is applied mostly with the fingers, although practitioners may also use the entire hand, elbow, knee, and other body parts. A session lasts generally from 45 to 60 minutes,

and the areas being massaged may vary depending upon whether there is an underlying disorder. Although shiatsu is used to treat certain medical problems, such as back pain or headaches, it is more often considered a preventive therapy to help keep the body functioning properly.

Acupressure. This technique differs from shiatsu in that its goal is to treat specific disorders by pressing upon the acupoints

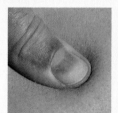

Reflexologists stimulate specific points on the foot or hand to treat disorders of corresponding internal organs. The objective is to redirect the flow of the body's bioelectrical energy.

used by acupuncturists. The appropriate acupoint is identified, and the therapist uses a fingertip or thumb to press upon it. A circular motion may then be used to stimulate deep, constant pressure.

Reflexology. Also referred to as zone therapy, reflexology aims to treat disorders by massaging and stimulating points, usually on the hands and feet, that correspond to specific internal organs. Unlike acupressure and shiatsu, which originated in Asia, reflexology was developed by an American, Dr. William Fitzgerald, an ear, nose, and throat specialist who introduced the technique in 1913.

Fitzgerald divided the body into 10 vertical zones through which he believed bioelectrical energy flowed to specific points in the hands and feet. In the 1940s, Eunice Ingham, a physical therapist, refined Fitzgerald's techniques, concentrating on pressure points in the feet. Today, reflexologists may use points in the feet, hands, ears, and elsewhere on the body, although foot massage remains the primary focus of the discipline. The basic techniques are finger walking, in which fingers are inched over the foot by bending and unbending the first joint; flexing, in which a thumb is pressed into the sole and the foot is then flexed several times; thumb walking, in which the thumb is inched up the sole of the foot toward the toes; and finger rolling, in which the tip of each toe is massaged with the tip of the index finger.

Pressure Points in Reflexology

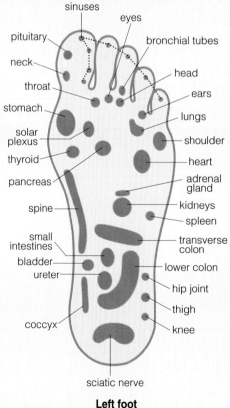

sinuses
eyes
pituitary
bronchial tubes
neck
head
throat
ears
stomach
lungs
solar plexus
shoulder
thyroid
heart
pancreas
adrenal gland
spine
kidneys
spleen
small intestines
transverse colon
bladder
ureter
lower colon
hip joint
thigh
coccyx
knee
sciatic nerve

Left foot

Meditation

Meditation is a mental discipline that is aimed at achieving complete relaxation. It is often promoted as an alternative to tranquilizers and painkillers in the management of emotional stress and physical pain.

Origins

This ancient art has been used for centuries by both healers and spiritual leaders. It is a central practice in many Eastern religions. Buddhist spiritual leaders, for example, believe that meditation frees the mind to release its healing power. In the United States, widespread interest in meditation dates to the 1960s when Maharishi Mahesh Yogi came from India to teach his technique. Called transcendental meditation, it requires no special mental or physical discipline other than the chanting of, or concentration on, a specific sound or thought during two daily half-hour sessions. By the early 1970s, some 90,000 men and women had tried this form of meditation, and many of them volunteered as subjects of medical studies to document its effects. The University of Massachusetts Medical School became the first in this country to establish a clinic whose prime purpose is intensive training in meditative disciplines.

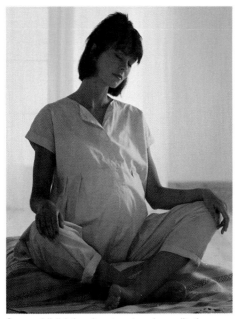

Some childbirth educators teach meditation as a way to overcome fear and manage pain.

Practitioners

Classes in meditation are sometimes conducted by physicians, psychologists, and physical therapists, as well as by yoga instructors, acupuncturists, and other alternative practitioners. Therapists trained in the techniques have been conducting classes in schools of the performing arts, and they are being invited into the corporate world to teach meditation for stress management. Some have also put their instructions on tapes and in books for home use.

When it is used

Meditation is used as a means of managing pain, coping with psychological stress, overcoming insomnia, and dealing with panic and anxiety. It is also an adjunct to conventional medicine in controlling asthma, high blood pressure, angina, and other chronic disorders.

How it works

Research indicates that meditation produces changes in the nervous system that are the opposite of the "fight-or-flight" response to danger. Specifically, meditation appears to reduce the body's production of cortisol, the hormone that triggers the response. Reduced cortisol levels foster relaxation.

Western researchers, who have studied the physical effects of meditation on yogis and Zen Buddhists as they are in the process of using it, have found that it slows metabolism, reduces oxygen consumption, and lowers carbon dioxide production. Brain studies done in the United States and in Japan indicate that there is also an increase in alpha brain waves, which normally occur during relaxation.

What to expect

As the aim of meditation is to achieve a heightened sense of mindfulness through concentration, activities are geared to this goal. For example, Dr. Jon Kabat-Zinn, a psychologist who pioneered the use of meditation in pain management, starts by urging members of a group to concentrate totally on each detail of a raisin: its appearance, feel, smell, taste, texture, and so on. Participants are then asked to transfer this heightened awareness to their breathing. Finally, they are instructed to focus completely on their pain, so they can begin to gain control over it.

The ability to concentrate on breathing to the exclusion of all other activities also has a calming effect, which can help overcome anxiety and relieve panic attacks. By focusing entirely on taking in and letting out one deep breath at a time, a person can control the feelings of panic.

Precautions

▶ If you're experiencing pain or other distressing symptoms, consult a doctor for a diagnosis before you join a meditation group.
▶ Although meditation lowers blood pressure, the effect is usually temporary. Hence, the technique should be used in conjunction with, not as a substitute for, conventional hypertension therapy.

HEALING IMAGES

Guided imagery, also referred to as waking dream therapy, uses mental pictures to fight disease and produce other desired effects. Until recently, imagery was practiced mostly by psychiatrists. A celebrated example was the 14-year-old boy whose tic was permanently cured by Sigmund Freud through imagery—the only complete cure described in all of Freud's case studies, and the only one in which he used this method.

Today, both alternative and conventional health professionals are teaching imagery to patients who have a variety of ailments, everything from stress-related headaches to cancer. In simple terms, imagery attempts to enlist the brain to play an active part in healing. For example, the Simonton Imagery Process encourages cancer patients to imagine the positive effects of radiation on cancer cells, and to enjoy the feeling of control that comes from being in touch with the body. It is thought that this psychological involvement strengthens the patient's immune system.

Dr. Gerald Epstein, a professor of psychiatry at New York's Mount Sinai Medical Center, has outlined dozens of imaging exercises in a book on healing visualizations. He describes one patient who credited her image of a broken bone knitting itself back together with healing her fractured wrist in three weeks instead of the anticipated three months. Epstein concedes that the rapid healing may have been a coincidence, but he believes he has witnessed similar results in too many other patients for coincidence to be the sole explanation.

People who are perfectly well can also benefit from imagery. For example, many athletes, dancers, and musicians resort to imagery to improve their performance; actors sometimes draw upon it to overcome stage fright or help remember their lines.

Music Therapy

In this treatment, music and rhythm are used to improve physical and psychological functioning and provide an alternative means of communication for persons who are unable to put their feelings or thoughts into words.

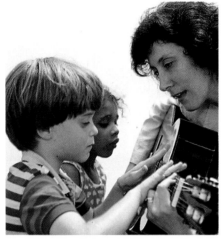
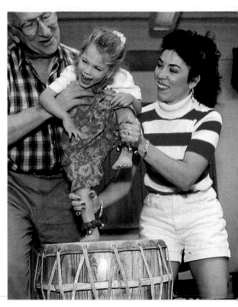

Above, autistic children, who are usually withdrawn, respond to a guitar. At right, a blind, multiply handicapped child learns alternate stepping with the help of rhythmic music.

Origins

Music therapy probably began when the earliest humans stomped or clapped to invoke healing spirits or to exorcise a sick person's demons. Greek myths contain metaphors for the healing power of music, and musical cures were part of many ancient cultures and religions.

More recently, a number of American health professionals have adopted music therapy in their practices. One doctor noted for his work in this field is Oliver Sacks, a neurologist and the author of *Awakenings,* who recognized the healing power of music in 1969 when working with catatonic patients. His 1973 book, later made into a movie, described how music therapy helped many of these patients adjust to the world around them after years of being catatonic. At the Rusk Institute for Rehabilitation Medicine in New York, music therapy has been integrated into programs for patients of all ages who have both physical and/or mental disabilities.

Practitioners

Licensed practitioners have completed an approved course of study and are certified by the American Association for Music Therapy, the National Association for Music Therapy, or the Certification Board for Music Therapy.

When it is used

Music therapy encompasses three major subdivisions:

Medicine: In this practice, music is used to help manage organic disorders, such as pain, and for rehabilitation after a stroke or a serious accident. The aged and patients with Parkinson's disease improve coordination and learn to walk with a steadier gait by exercising to music. Singing or playing certain musical instruments may contribute to improved lung function. Singing is also used to overcome speech disorders.

Psychotherapy: Music, as a universal language, can help psychotherapists to communicate with patients who are unable to verbalize their problems. It is especially beneficial in treating autistic and emotionally disturbed children.

Special education: In this application, music helps improve the coordination of children with neurological disabilities, as well as those who are blind or deaf. When incorporated into group activities, it also contributes to socialization.

How it works

The healing effects of music on all aspects of mind/body function are universally accepted but not scientifically understood. Some researchers believe that music reaches a part of the brain that is not involved with verbal skills. For example, old songs often spark remarkable responses from Alzheimer's patients. Some researchers believe that music activates a flow of stored memory that is otherwise inaccessible.

Research suggests that musical experiences may also trigger the production of endorphins, brain chemicals that are natural painkillers. Studies by anesthesiologists indicate that playing music during surgery reduces the need for anesthesia. Dentists have also observed that their patients don't need as much painkiller when music is being played.

What to expect

Activities may proceed on a one-to-one basis or in a group, depending on the desired result. Participants join in actively or listen passively. For example, a young group may drum rhythmically or exercise to jazz, while geriatric patients may listen to music that was popular during their younger years.

A DRAMATIC ROUTE TO HEALING

To most of us, play acting is little more than a flight of fancy. But to the emotionally disturbed or developmentally handicapped, drama, used as therapy (an outgrowth of music therapy), is a valuable method in the healing process. The goal is to enable a person to experiment with thoughts and emotions in a nonthreatening setting. By assuming a dramatic role, many people can act out emotions they would be unable to express otherwise.

Drama therapy is especially effective in settings where individuals have difficulty relating to each other; for example, in schools for emotionally disturbed children. It is also used in prisons and in programs for those who have difficulty living in society.

In some instances, the patients create their own dramas, but more commonly, a drama therapist draws upon a familiar story, such as a fairy tale, that can be applied to the situation at hand. The therapist then observes how the various players interpret their roles, and in later sessions uses the drama as a basis for discussing their own problems.

In other situations, drama therapy may be used to build a sense of self-worth. For example, schoolchildren from minority groups may be encouraged to put on a play for their classmates that depicts some special event in their history or aspect of their cultural heritage. This exercise can be educational for the audience as well as therapeutic for the actors.

Precautions

▶ Check the qualifications of a music therapist before beginning a course of treatment. The American Association for Music Therapy (see Health Resources, page 465) maintains lists of board-certified music therapists.

Naturopathy and Natural Healing

Naturopathy is based on natural means of healing diseases. Its practitioners often employ the entire spectrum of alternative therapies. Instead of conventional drugs, for example, they may choose from among herbal medicines, homeopathic remedies, nutrition and diet therapy, acupuncture, hydrotherapy, and physical therapy.

Naturopaths describe themselves as holistic practitioners who rely heavily on patient counseling and education. They also include among their treatments some practices of conventional medicine. For instance, they may use diathermy (a form of electrotherapy) for backaches. Many practitioners are also trained in techniques of behavior modification, such as biofeedback and hypnosis; others offer massage and other therapies for stress management.

Origins

Naturopathy originated during the 19th century, when a medical regimen based on hydrotherapy, exercise, fresh air, sunlight, and herbal teas gained a large following in Germany. The system was brought to the United States by a German healer, Benedict Lust, who founded the American School of Naturopathy in New York in 1902.

Lust called for the elimination of "evil" habits such as overeating, the use of alcoholic drinks, tea, coffee, and cocoa, and advocated corrective habits of breathing, exercise, and a wholesome mental outlook. He also recommended good nutrition, periodic fasting, and various forms of hydrotherapy. He took a militant stand against "the drugs, vaccines, and serums employed by superstitious moderns" in favor of "natural forces much more orthodox than the artificial resources of the druggist," which he described as harmful and irritating to the human body.

Naturopathy quickly developed a nationwide following, and in 1909, California became the first state to pass a law regulating natural medicine. But eventually, the practice could not compete successfully with modern medical and surgical techniques, nor could it deal with widespread accusations of quackery. By the 1960s, naturopathy had all but vanished from the scene. Today it is making a comeback.

Practitioners

The designation N.D. stands for Doctor of Naturopathy and indicates that the practitioner has completed studies in one of three naturopathy schools located in Seattle, Washington; Portland, Oregon; or Toronto, Canada. The course of study covers nutrition and various alternative therapies, including herbal medicine, homeopathy, Chinese medicine, massage, and manipulation. Hydrotherapy and other aspects of physical medicine are also studied. Persons with this degree are licensed to practice in seven states: Alaska, Arizona, Connecticut, Hawaii, Montana, Oregon, and Washington.

Some aspects of naturopathy and natural healing are also performed by acupuncturists, herbalists, massage therapists, nutritionists, and chiropractors, as well as by self-proclaimed healers with no formal credentials.

When it is used

While some people prefer a naturopathic practitioner as their primary doctor, others may visit one for specific treatments, such as hydrotherapy for arthritis or herbal preparations as

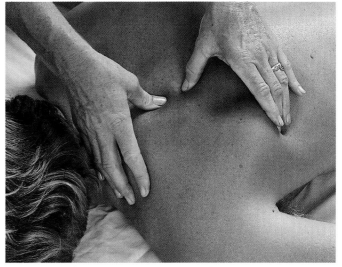

Naturopaths often incorporate massage and other hands-on techniques as part of their natural practices.

alternatives to pharmaceutical medications. Actually, some components of natural healing are used by most people as simple self-care: for example, a high-fiber diet to treat constipation, a warm bath to ease stress, exercise to alleviate depression, or self-massage for muscle aches.

How it works

The major premise of natural healing is that the human organism is capable of resisting disease and healing itself. Therefore the way to achieve wellness is to promote the body's self-healing capabilities. Naturopaths emphasize the responsibility of each individual in eating a sensible diet, exercising, and following a prudent, healthful lifestyle.

What to expect

The first visit is devoted to exploring the patient's medical history and lifestyle. After a diagnosis is made, the patient and practitioner evolve a holistic program. Here, for example, is a summary of the treatment for osteoarthritis as presented in the *Encyclopedia of Natural Medicine* by Michael Murray, N.D. and Joseph Pizzorno, N.D.:

Diet: Avoid all simple carbohydrates (sugars); stress starchy and high-fiber foods, and flavonoid-rich berries such as blueberries and raspberries; keep fats to a minimum; eliminate tomatoes, potatoes, eggplant, and peppers.

Supplements: Take niacinamide, methionine, pantothenic acid, zinc, and copper, and vitamins A, B_6, C, and E.

Botanical medicines: Use yucca leaves and extract and the powdered root of devil's claw.

Physical therapy and exercise: Include isometric exercises and swimming daily. Try short-wave diathermy and other physical therapy treatments that may be helpful.

Precautions

▶ When faced with a serious illness, such as diabetes or cancer, naturopathy should be approached as an adjunct to, not substitute for, conventional medicine.
▶ Be wary of any alternative practitioner who hesitates to refer any patient who has symptoms of serious illness, such as heart disease, diabetes, or cancer, to a medical doctor.

Nutrition Therapy

Nutrition therapy is based on the premise that diet in general or certain vitamins and minerals in particular can prevent or cure disease. Practices range from simply eating a balanced diet to maintain good health to taking megadoses of vitamins and/or minerals to ward off disease or treat mental illness.

A growing body of scientific evidence indicates that nutrition is even more important in preventive medicine than previously thought. But the majority of doctors and nutritionists still stress that for most people, a varied diet—low in fat and sugar, high in fiber and starches, and low enough in calories to maintain ideal weight—will suffice.

Origins

Physicians have been prescribing special diets since the time of the ancient Greeks, and they continue to do so for patients with nutrition-related diseases. The more recent practice of

megavitamin therapy (consuming at least 10 times the Recommended Dietary Allowance, or RDA) originated with Dr. Linus Pauling, a Nobel laureate chemist who coined the term orthomolecular therapy (meaning therapy with the right molecules) in 1968, when he began to advocate very large doses of vitamin C to prevent or treat the common cold. During the 1970s, megavitamin therapy was promoted as an alternative treatment for mental illness. More recently, it has been advocated by food faddists and self-styled healers, as well as some conventional practitioners, as a cure for asthma, allergies, AIDS, and even cancer. Although good nutrition plays a role in treating these problems, there is no scientific proof that it can produce a cure.

Practitioners

Nutrition therapy is practiced by many of the 46,000 registered dietitians (R.D.) who are members of the American Dietetic Association. In addition, more than 500 doctors and

ADULT RDA'S FOR MAJOR VITAMINS AND MINERALS

NUTRIENT	ADULT RANGE*	NEEDED FOR	SOURCES
FAT-SOLUBLE VITAMINS:			
Vitamin A	800-1000 RE**	Vision, reproduction, teeth, bones, hair, immune system	Dairy products, green or yellow vegetables, orange or yellow fruits, organ meats
Vitamin D	10 mcg	Bone growth and calcium absorption	Fish liver oil, liver, vitamin D fortified milk, egg yolks, sun
Vitamin E	8-10 IU‡	Making red blood cells and muscle tissue; preventing oxidation of fatty acids	Cooked greens, whole grains, seafood, poultry, eggs, seeds and nuts, wheat germ
Vitamin K	60-80 mcg	Blood clotting	Leafy green vegetables, potatoes, organ meats, grains
WATER-SOLUBLE VITAMINS:			
Vitamin C	60 mg	Immune system, healing, formation of bones, teeth, and blood vessels	Citrus fruits, tomatoes, green peppers, melons, broccoli, other fruits and vegetables
Thiamin	1.1-1.5 mg	Metabolism and nerve function	Seafood, pork, fortified cereals and breads
Riboflavin	1.3-1.7 mg	Vision and metabolism	Dairy products, organ meats, green leafy vegetables, red meats, dark poultry meat, fortified cereals
Niacin	15-19 mg	Proper nerve function; making digestive enzymes	Poultry, seafood, seeds, nuts, fortified cereals and breads
Vitamin B$_6$	1.6-2 mg	Formation of red blood cells; metabolism and nerve function	Fish, poultry, meats, spinach, bananas, cereals, sweet and white potatoes, prunes
Folate	180-200 mcg	Making DNA; formation of red blood cells	Liver, whole grains, fruits, legumes, dark green leafy vegetables
Vitamin B$_{12}$	2 mcg	Building genetic material; formation of red blood cells	Meats, eggs, seafood, milk, and milk products
MINERALS:			
Calcium	800-1200 mg	Bone and tooth formation; heart, muscle, and nerve function	Milk, milk products, green leafy vegetables, tofu, broccoli, canned salmon and sardines (with bones)
Iron	10-15 mg	Making myoglobin and hemoglobin	Liver, red meat, fish, dried apricots, legumes, soybean flour, raisins
Magnesium	280-350 mg	Making digestive enzymes, DNA, and cells	Beans, oysters, scallops, fortified cereals, green vegetables
Phosphorus	800-1200 mg	Tooth and bone growth; nerve and muscle function	Poultry, meat, dairy products, egg yolks, fish, legumes
Selenium	55-70 mcg	Preventing oxidation of fatty acids in tandem with vitamin E	Seafood, egg yolks, chicken, mushrooms, garlic, onions
Zinc	12-15 mg	Metabolism and the digestive system	Yogurt, beef, wheat germ, liver, fortified cereals

* Lower number is for women; higher for men, except for iron, which women require in the larger amounts.
**Retinol equivalent, the preferred unit of measure for vitamin A. One RE is equal to 3.5 IU from plant sources and 10 IU from animal sources. (Vitamin manufacturers measure vitamin A in IU.)
‡ Alpha tocopherol equivalents, the standard measuring unit of dietary vitamin E.

HIGH-DOSE ANTIOXIDANT VITAMIN THERAPY

NUTRIENT	MEGADOSE	UNPROVED HEALTH CLAIMS	POTENTIAL DANGERS
Vitamin A	15,000-25,000 RE per day	Reduces risk of breast, lung, colon, prostate, and cervical cancer; helps prevent heart disease and stroke; retards macular degeneration.	May cause liver damage, hair loss, blurred vision, headaches, fatigue, diarrhea, irregular periods, dry skin, benign skin yellowing, rashes, joint and bone pain. May lead to birth defects if taken during pregnancy.
Vitamin E	200-400 IU per day	Enhances fertility and improves sexual potency; retards aging process; helps prevent cancer and heart attacks; deters cataracts; relieves premenstrual syndrome and nocturnal leg cramps; protects against radiation damage from sun, air pollutants, and other environmental toxins.	Appears safe in recommended doses; may cause bleeding problems in rare cases of vitamin K deficiency or when taken with aspirin.
Vitamin C	250-1000 mg per day	Helps prevent cancer, heart attacks, and heart disease; bolsters immunity against colds and other infections; lowers blood cholesterol; protects against pollutants and environmental toxins; improves adaptation to stress; retards macular degeneration; deters cataracts; enhances fertility in men.	May cause excessive gas, diarrhea, urinary burning, mouth and intestinal irritation, damage to tooth enamel; can cause hemorrhages in patients with advanced cancer.

other health professionals have passed a qualifying examination given by the American Board of Nutrition, and an equal number of members of the American Nutritionists Association have obtained advanced degrees in this specialty.

Nutritionists may be licensed and/or certified depending on state requirements. There are 29 states in which practitioners must meet certain educational standards and pass an examination before they are legally entitled to call themselves certified dietitians or certified nutritionists. But anyone, regardless of training, can call himself a nutritionist or diet counselor, a situation that has unfortunately left the door open to widespread quackery.

Many chiropractors, naturopaths, herbalists, acupuncturists, and health-food salespeople also double as nutrition counselors, as do some fitness trainers, health-club workers, and diet-center personnel.

When it is used
Nutrition therapists are consulted to treat obesity, eating disorders, and diseases caused by deficiencies of certain vitamins and minerals. Although deficiency diseases are rare in the United States, they still occur, especially among the poor. The elderly and alcoholics are also vulnerable because they often consume very limited types and amounts of food.

Nutrition therapy has become an important component of treating diabetes, heart disease, and intestinal disorders. A nutrition therapist may also be asked to recommend dietary changes for a hyperactive child or for a person with allergies, lactose intolerance, or metabolic disorders. Healthy people, such as athletes and pregnant women, also turn to nutrition therapists for dietary advice to meet their special needs.

High-dose vitamins are used in both conventional and alternative medicine, but for very different purposes. For example, very high doses of niacin (a B vitamin) are sometimes used in conventional medicine to lower blood cholesterol. High-dose vitamin E may be prescribed to treat fibrocystic breasts, and alcoholics may be given large amounts of thiamine. Alternative practitioners, on the other hand, recommend high doses of vitamins—the benefits of which are unproven—for a wider range of illnesses. Research indicates that beta carotene (a precursor of vitamin A) and vitamins A,C, and E (antioxidant

nutrients that offset harmful effects of oxygen metabolism) may help prevent cancer and heart disease and slow the aging process, but new data suggest that eating foods high in these nutrients is more effective than taking supplements.

How it works
Because vitamins and minerals are essential to normal metabolism and other body functions (see chart, opposite page), keeping a proper balance of them in the system is important to good health. However, a vitamin or mineral consumed in amounts greater than your body readily needs takes on the properties of a drug, and as with any drug, it carries a risk of side effects (see chart, above). For example, excesses of vitamins A and D, which are stored in the liver and fatty tissue, can lead to toxicity. High doses of minerals, especially iron, potassium, and lithium, can also be toxic.

What to expect
Nutrition therapy begins with a careful health assessment and a review of the patient's diet. If the person has a chronic health problem such as diabetes, the nutrition therapist should work with the primary-care physician.

In cases that involve obesity or eating disorders, psychotherapy and behavior modification play an important role in long-term success. Some nutritionists ask that clients keep a careful food diary; others inspect the client's kitchen shelves. Occasionally, nutrition therapists even show clients how to make wise choices at supermarkets and restaurants.

Precautions

▶ Never undertake to treat yourself or a family member with megavitamins. Vitamins in large amounts are powerful drugs with a high risk of unpleasant or lethal side effects.

▶ Keep vitamin and mineral pills out of children's reach. Iron overdose is a leading cause of poisoning death in children.

▶ Nutrition fraud is one of the most common forms of medical quackery. Be wary of any nutrition counselor who:

• Diagnoses deficiencies with hair or saliva tests (both worthless).

• Sells a private brand of nutritional supplements.

• Promises a nutritional cure for arthritis, asthma, or any other incurable chronic disease.

Pet Therapy

Pet therapy promotes human well-being through bonding with an animal, most often a cat, dog, or other household pet.

Origins

The domestication of animals and birds probably originated in prehistoric times. By the time the Egyptians exalted the cat to the status of a god about 3,000 B.C., household pets were common. In the late 1800s, the first seeing eye dogs for the blind were trained, utilizing the deep bond that develops between a sightless owner and an animal and inspiring the concept of pet therapy. In recent years, new therapeutic uses have been found for pets. This process began with an investigation of the contribution of pets to mental health. Since then, numerous medical studies have documented physical benefits as well.

Practitioners

Pet therapy may be initiated by a psychotherapist, physician, social worker, or family counselor. More often, it takes place informally, as when a parent gives a disabled child a pet to care for to help in building self-esteem, or an older person acquires a pet in order to cope with a loved one's death.

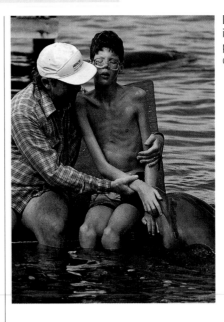

Dolphins are employed in a special education program for disabled children in Florida.

When it is used

Many situations are appropriate. Pet therapists have taken animals into nursing homes to be hugged and stroked by lonely residents who are usually unresponsive to those around them. Mentally disturbed, handicapped, and autistic children have received therapeutic benefits from touching and caring for a variety of animals, including horses and dolphins as well as household

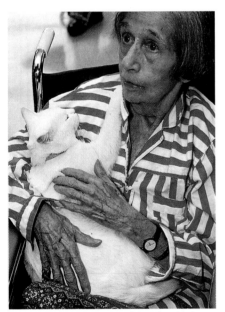

Holding or stroking a trusting animal helps a withdrawn person connect with a living creature, a critical step in establishing or restoring social interaction.

pets. Residential treatment programs for such children often involve some animal care. Also, a study at the Mayo Clinic found that cancer patients who were offered a companion cat while undergoing chemotherapy suffered fewer adverse side effects than patients who did not have an animal.

Prison rehabilitation programs sometimes include one-to-one involvement with an animal, during which participants may recall pleasures of childhood or enjoy for the first time a childhood pleasure they never had. Pediatricians have found that when there's a cat or dog in their office, children find a visit less threatening and are easier to examine. Dentists have noted that the presence of an aquarium in the waiting room eases the tension of anxious patients. Teachers often use animals to foster a sense of responsibility among young children.

How it works

Every pet owner understands the rewards of having an animal that gives unconditional affection. But no one has yet explained why the companionship of a pet reduces heart rate and lowers blood pressure, or why elderly people who own pets make fewer visits to their doctor than those who don't. Numerous scientific studies have shown that pet owners also recover from surgery faster and survive a heart attack longer than those without pets. Some observers have noted that people who love their pets generally take better care of their own health because the animals depend upon them.

What to expect

Pet therapy takes many forms. Physically abused children, given the care of farm animals, may learn to express love for them which they themselves have not received. For a housebound older person, the playful antics of a kitten or the purr of a contented cat might be a comforting distraction from pain. Dog owners can enjoy the health benefits of a daily walk and social interaction with other dog owners.

In a program at an upstate New York center for disturbed children, youngsters are allowed to care for injured wildlife and then release the animals to the wild after they have recovered. Dr. Samuel B. Ross, the initiator of this program, observed that: "It's an especially powerful experience for these kids who are, in a sense, wounded themselves. If you take care of a disabled animal and see that it can survive, then you get the feeling that you can survive yourself."

Precautions

► Don't give anyone an animal without first making sure that it will be welcome, and that the person will be able to care for it.
► If you're embarking on pet ownership for the first time, be sure to choose an animal that is compatible with your lifestyle. If you must work long hours, for example, you may have trouble caring for and training a dog.
► If you or a member of your household suffers from allergies, avoid getting an animal that has fur or feathers. In such cases, consider tropical fish or even an ant farm.

Spiritual Healing

Spiritual healing is the curing of disease through powers outside the limits of medical intervention. It is based on the concept that whatever one truly believes can be made to happen.

Origins

Virtually every ancient culture and religion believed that a specific person in the community was chosen by the spirit(s) to heal both physical and mental illness through supernatural powers. These healers were referred to as medicine men, priests, or shamans, and they were called upon to intercede with the spirits on behalf of their followers. For example, the Bible refers to miracles accomplished through faith and the transfer of positive thoughts from the healer to the sufferer. Whatever its origins, spiritual healing has always involved a belief in a universal healing force.

Practitioners

Spiritual healing is performed by people who claim to be endowed with the gift of thought or energy transference, which gives them a special link to a person in need of healing. One type of spiritual healing is practiced by Christian Scientists, who elect to treat themselves and their loved ones through prayer and faith in God, rather than depend on a physician. Alcoholics Anonymous and other 12-step support groups also rely heavily on spiritualism.

Therapeutic touch, which is practiced by countless conventional doctors and nurses as a routine part of patient care, is closely related to spiritual healing. Many observers believe that when a skilled, compassionate physician or nurse touches or clasps the hand of a trusting patient, an actual transference of healing energy takes place.

When it is used

Spiritual healers attempt to cure various acute and chronic diseases, including arthritis, cancer, diabetes, and even AIDS. Many people who go to spiritual healers for help have already exhausted the capabilities of more orthodox practitioners.

Precautions

▶ Because many people seek out a spiritual healer as an act of desperation, they are vulnerable to charlatans. While trust in the healer is a critical factor in the success of the encounter, financial commitments should be made with extreme caution.

How it works

No one can explain how spiritual healing works. Conventional physicians concede that there are hopelessly ill patients who miraculously recover, and in some of these cases, spiritualism is a factor. Spiritual healers contend that such cures are accomplished when patients become one with God (or with their own concept of a superior power).

Western researchers have studied psychic phenomena, including healing, in the United States and Europe, but they have yet to produce tangible results that are convincing to skeptics. Still, a growing number of conventional physicians, foremost among them cancer surgeon and author Dr. Bernie Siegel, are emphasizing the power of spirituality in the healing process. Most physicians report that patients who have a reservoir of spiritual faith tend to confront serious illness with unusual strength and calmness.

What to expect

Although some spiritual healers claim to have accomplished healing at a distance through the power of their thoughts, most practitioners work at the side of the patient. To prepare themselves for a healing session, they may spend time in prayer and meditation. Deep breathing, chanting, and other relaxation techniques contribute to the trance-like state that many healers enter for their work.

The healers remain passive until they feel they have been overtaken by healing power, which is then transferred to the ailing person. This transfer may be achieved solely through concentration, or it may involve a laying on of hands.

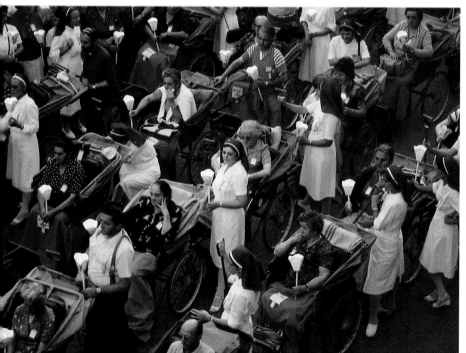

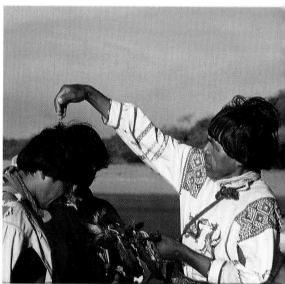

Native American shamans (below) continue to practice spiritual healing using the words and rituals of their predecessors. And each year, thousands of the faithful flock to Lourdes (left) seeking a miracle cure.

Yoga and Other Movement Therapies

Movement therapies employ structured exercise regimens and mental discipline to achieve both physical and emotional health. They range from the gentle approaches of yoga and t'ai chi to the more vigorous movements of aerobics and such martial arts as karate. They also include physical therapy.

Yoga emphasizes meditation, deep breathing, and pre-scribed body positions and movements. The martial arts incorporate meditation and structured movement as well, but the emphasis is more on self-control and self-defense. Despite the military aspects of these disciplines, they are rooted in nonviolence, with the goal of achieving mental and physical health. Aerobic conditioning has the additional aim of improving cardiovascular function, and physical therapy seeks to prevent or treat musculoskeletal problems.

Origins

Movement therapies trace their roots to ancient Eastern philosophy and practice. The term *yoga,* for example, comes from the Sanskrit word yuga meaning "to yoke" or "to join." Yoga practitioners, or yogis, believe that they can achieve cosmic union through movement and meditation.

Some people theorize that martial arts evolved from ancient dance rituals and meditative practices. Another theory, based on legend, holds that they began with Bodhidarma, the Buddhist monk who founded Zen Buddhism. According to this story, he taught young monks and was dismayed by their physical weakness, which he attributed to inactivity; so Bodhidarma developed ritualistic exercises to help increase their strength and stamina.

Practitioners

Yoga is taught in this country by physical therapists, physiatrists (specialists in physical rehabilitation), psychologists, and dance instructors, as well as by yogis and some of their advanced students. Many yogis are interested in transmitting all aspects of their way of life, including, often, pacifism and vegetarianism, through which they believe a spiritual unity with the cosmos can be achieved.

Martial arts are being taught mostly as a means of self-defense and building strength and coordination, but some instructors also emphasize meditation and spiritualism.

When it is used

Movement therapy is used to increase strength, counter stress, and control pain; devotees are all ages and come from every walk of life. Certain movements have been found effective in rehabilitation programs for victims of stroke or injury, and some yoga exercises have been adapted for the elderly and infirm so that they can be done in bed or in a wheelchair.

A number of psychotherapists have their patients learn yoga or t'ai chi to lessen anxiety and reduce panic attacks. Judo is sometimes recommended to help an overly shy child gain confidence and self-esteem.

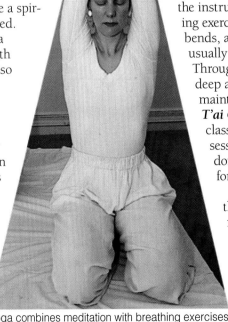

Yoga combines meditation with breathing exercises and controlled movements to achieve well-being.

Precautions
▶ Before you sign up for a series of classes in any movement therapy, ask permission to attend a session as an observer.
▶ Some yoga movements are difficult or impossible to achieve without expert instruction and considerable practice. Go slow, and stop any movement or position that causes pain.

Dancers and other performance artists use yoga and other movement therapies to overcome muscle tension and to limber up their bodies before rehearsals and performances. Dr. Dean Ornish, a California cardiologist, incorporates yoga in his innovative regimen for heart patients. At the Commonweal Cancer Help Program and research center in California, terminally ill cancer patients are taught yoga as a means of achieving serenity. The National Institute on Aging has been studying t'ai chi as an alternative therapy to help the elderly increase their fitness and mobility.

How it works

As currently practiced in the United States, yoga, t'ai chi, and other movement therapies are viewed as a means of achieving mind/body harmony as well as physical strength. Performed regularly, they can help reverse the ill effects of a sedentary lifestyle, promote musculoskeletal strengthening of the body, and increase the suppleness of the spine. People who practice yoga or t'ai chi often describe a feeling of energy flowing through them. The breathing exercises of these therapies stimulate circulation while relaxing the body and mind. They also increase the capacity for focused concentration, and are often combined with meditation.

What to expect

Following is a more detailed description of what you can expect in a yoga or martial arts class. See boxes, opposite page, for aerobics and physical therapy.

Yoga. Instruction may take place one-on-one or in an organized class. Participants wear any attire that allows for freedom of movement. In general, shoes are not worn. During a typical beginning session, the instructor leads the class in a series of breathing exercises to warm up. A routine of stretches, bends, and other movements follows. The pace is usually relaxed and the movements flowing. Throughout the session, strong mental focus and deep abdominal breathing help participants maintain specific postures as long as possible.

T'ai Chi. Instruction is usually given in a class, although some students opt for private sessions. Clothing that allows complete freedom of movement is appropriate, and comfortable, lightweight shoes may be worn.

Serious t'ai chi practitioners perform their routines daily. They execute the movements in a continuous, consistent, and somewhat slow rhythm. During the routine, all mental energy is focused on t'ai chi. The goals are to attain a mental state of complete calm and concentration, and to improve the technique continuously, thereby achieving both physical and emotional fitness.

AEROBIC EXERCISE CONDITIONING

Aerobic exercise is any activity that requires extra oxygen and leads to improved cardiovascular function. Examples include brisk walking, jogging, stair climbing, swimming, and cycling. Such exercise forms the foundation for any well rounded fitness program.

Numerous studies have documented the value of aerobic conditioning: People who exercise vigorously on a regular basis live longer, have fewer heart attacks and other serious diseases, and enjoy a greater sense of well-being than their sedentary peers. Three basics are essential for a conditioning effect:

Frequency—three or four times a week.

Intensity—vigorous enough to increase your heartbeat to its target zone (see how to find it, right).

Duration—at least 15 to 20 minutes per session.

Some exercise physiologists add a fourth basic—*balance*. Excessive exercise can strain joints and supporting structures and increase the risk of sprains, stress fractures, and other injuries.

Designing an Exercise Conditioning Program

▶ Start with a physical checkup, especially if you are over the age of 40 or if you have any cardiovascular risk factors. These include a history of heart disease, diabetes, high blood cholesterol levels, high blood pressure, obesity, and a cigarette habit. A doctor may also recommend an exercise tolerance test to determine your safe level of physical activity.

▶ Next, pick an activity that you enjoy—if exercise is a drudgery, chances are you won't stick with it long enough to get in shape. Also consider what is appropriate for your age and general health. Almost everyone can undertake a walking program, whereas jogging, racketball, and high-impact aerobic dancing require not only stamina but also sturdy joints.

▶ Select the right equipment. Walking requires only well-fitted walking shoes and a safe, comfortable place to walk. If you would rather work out on a stationary cycle or other equipment, try it out before making an investment. If you are considering joining a health club, visit several and then sign up for a short trial period before committing yourself to a long-term membership. After a few sessions, you may decide this particular club is not to your liking.

▶ Start slowly and gradually build endurance. Many people do too much too soon, and end up with aching muscles and joints or more serious injuries. For example, if you are beginning a walking program, start by walking a mile at a comfortable pace. Over the next few weeks, gradually increase your speed and distance; for most people, two miles in 30 to 40 minutes is a reasonable goal.

▶ Include a few minutes of warm-up and cool-down stretching exercises before and after each session. These help to prevent painful muscle tightness and injuries from overuse.

How to Find Your Target Heart Rate

Formula	Example for a 40-year-old
Subtract your age from 220	$220 - 40 = 180$
Multiply the result by 75 percent	$180 \times .75 = 135$

The result is the target number of heartbeats per minute. To find out if your heartbeat is in the target zone, exercise at peak intensity for 10 to 15 minutes; stop, find your pulse, and count the heartbeats for 10 seconds. Multiply by 6 to determine your heart rate.

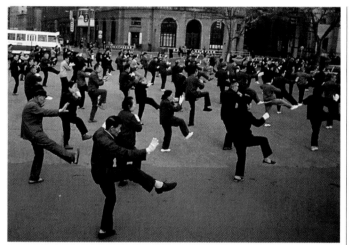

In parks and other public places throughout China, millions gather in the early morning to perform t'ai chi, an exercise ritual that the government has standardized with a routine of 24 movements.

Karate. This martial art is taught in a variety of settings, ranging from community centers to specialized schools. It is practiced barefoot, and traditional, loose-fitting white cotton jacket and trousers are usually worn. In a typical session, students meditate and stretch to warm up, then practice stances, kicks, punches, and blocks, controlling their movements with the help of deep, slow abdominal breathing. Finally, in unison, they perform formal exercises called katas.

Judo. Another hard martial art, judo is taught in most of the same settings as karate. Classes are also conducted in a similar manner, and the same type of clothing is worn. Judo students work on posture, balance, and judgment to perfect throws, falls, holds, and punches intended to disable attackers.

THE GROWING ROLE OF PHYSICAL THERAPY

Physical therapists are the health professionals most concerned with all aspects of movement, from restoring motion to joints that have been stiffened by arthritis to guiding novice athletes in techniques designed to prevent sports injuries.

Until fairly recently, most people consulted physical therapists only for rehabilitation following an injury or a debilitating illness. Now, however, healthy people who want to get the maximum benefit from exercise are consulting them for pointers on designing a program, avoiding injury, and managing minor problems such as muscle soreness. In addition, physical therapy is being employed increasingly in the management of both acute and chronic pain. In a sense, the field is bridging the gap between the medical disciplines of orthopedics, sports medicine, and physical medicine and the movement therapies such as yoga and the martial arts.

Physical therapy can be divided into three main categories:

▶ Preventive, in which a therapist helps develop low-risk fitness programs to prevent chronic diseases and such problems as lower back pain and tennis elbow.

▶ Treatment, in which a therapist designs individual programs for patients with specific injuries such as broken bones, or musculoskeletal problems such as chronic tendinitis.

▶ Rehabilitative, in which a therapist works over a long period with patients who have severe, debilitating conditions such as neuromuscular damage from a stroke or head injury. Rehabilitative personnel sometimes practice in tandem with occupational therapists, health professionals who help people with physical disabilities and movement disorders regain muscular control and find ways to perform the tasks of everyday living.

Physical therapists use several modes of treatment, including specialized exercises, electrical stimulation of nerves, hydrotherapy, heat and cold therapy, and massage. Sessions may take place in the patient's home, in a rehabilitation or physical therapy department of a hospital, or on the premises of an independent practice. Most health insurance policies cover a limited number of therapy sessions if they've been prescribed by a physician.

Introduction

Taking charge of your own health care, deciding when to see a doctor, when an alternative practitioner might be more appropriate, and what you can handle yourself, is an intelligent, perhaps even necessary approach these days. Unfortunately, there are no easy guidelines—many physicians with years of training and experience often find such decisions difficult. Still, the more you know about how diseases can be treated, the more likely you are to make appropriate choices in managing your own and your family's medical care.

When to Call a Doctor

Tens of thousands of Americans die needlessly each year because of denial and delay. Among them are heart attack victims who wait an average of six hours to call a doctor, and other people who ignore for months the common warning signs of cancer.

By contrast, those who run to a medical specialist for every ache, pain, and sniffle not only drive up medical costs, but also increase their risk of adverse reactions from overtreatment. The ideal is to find a middle ground based on common sense and knowledge.

Whom to See

As stressed in the previous section, everyone should have a primary-care physician to oversee and coordinate medical care. This might be a family practitioner, an internist, an osteopath, a pediatrician (for children), or a gyne-

cologist (for women). The doctor may be a private practitioner or a gatekeeper physician with a health-maintenance organization or other managed-care group. The important thing is that she knows your medical history and has a stake in maintaining your health.

When you are injured or acute illness strikes, always turn first to a conventionally trained medical doctor. These practitioners are the best qualified to treat trauma and other emergencies, infections, diabetes, heart disease, cancer, and other serious illnesses.

If you suffer from a chronic pain syndrome or some other condition for which conventional medicine can do little, you might be better off seeing an alternative practitioner. And in many cases, you may be the best person to manage your illness, often under the guidance of a medical professional.

In the box to the right and on the next two pages is a listing of medical signs and symptoms and their possible causes. The remainder of the section describes more than 450 diseases and conditions, both common and rare, and provides information on how they are treated, not only by mainstream physicians but also by alternative practitioners and with self-care. It also details how disorders are diagnosed and lists some important questions you should ask the health professional to whom you entrust your medical care. The goal is to help you make informed decisions about your well-being.

PROBLEMS THAT DEMAND PROMPT MEDICAL ATTENTION

Call your local Emergency Medical Service or get to the nearest emergency room if any of the following develop:

Possible heart attack:
▶ Severe pain, lightheadedness, fainting, sweating, nausea, or shortness of breath
▶ Feeling of pain, pressure, fullness, or squeezing in the center chest that lasts more than two minutes
▶ Pain spreading from the center chest to the shoulders, neck, or arms

Possible stroke or mini-stroke:
▶ Sudden weakness or numbness on one side of the body, usually affecting the face, an arm, or leg
▶ Sudden loss of speech, or difficulty speaking or understanding speech
▶ Loss of vision or dimness, usually in one eye or half of both eyes
▶ Unexplained dizziness, unsteady gait, lack of coordination, or falling
▶ Sudden severe headache unlike any experienced in the past
▶ Abrupt loss of memory or altered mental abilities

Possible shock:
▶ Cold, clammy, and pale skin
▶ Weakness and lightheadedness
▶ Rapid, weak pulse
▶ Rapid, shallow, and irregular breathing
▶ Agitation and feeling of apprehension

Possible anaphylactic reaction:
▶ Severe swelling, especially around the eyes, mouth, and face
▶ Weak, rapid pulse
▶ Difficulty breathing
▶ Possible nausea, vomiting, and abdominal cramps
▶ Bluish tinge to skin and nails
▶ Confusion, dizziness, possible loss of consciousness

Possible internal bleeding:
▶ Coughing or vomiting up blood, which may look like coffee grounds
▶ Blood in the stool or urine
▶ Bleeding from a body opening, such as the ears, nose, or mouth
▶ Abdominal swelling and tenderness
▶ Excessive thirst

Fevers:
See a doctor as soon as possible if:
▶ Body temperature rises to 100.5° F (38° C) in a baby younger than 3 months
▶ Body temperature rises to 103° F (39.4° C) in a child or adult of any age
▶ Body temperature rises to 101° F (38.3° C) and stays there for three days
▶ Low-grade fever recurs or persists for two or more weeks
▶ Fever of any degree is accompanied by severe headache, stiff neck, swelling of the throat, or mental confusion

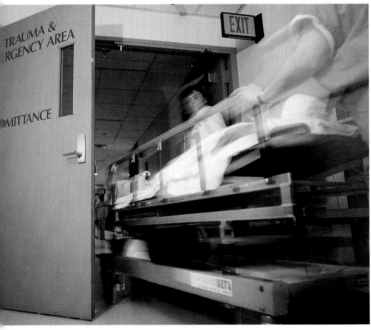

Delays in seeking medical attention for serious problems such as heart attacks are responsible for tens of thousands of deaths each year.

Signs & Symptoms

In medical terms, a sign is any visible indication of disease—bleeding, a rash, or swelling, for example. A symptom is something you can feel, such as pain, fever, or nausea, and it may or may not be accompanied by a physical change. Below are common signs and symptoms and their possible causes.

COMMON SIGNS AND SYMPTOMS

SIGN OR SYMPTOM	POSSIBLE CAUSES
Anxiety	Alcoholism, panic attack, premenstrual syndrome, stress, a thyroid disorder
Belching	Gallbladder disease, indigestion, a malabsorption syndrome
Bleeding and bruises	
Gums	Periodontal disease, leukemia, vitamin deficiency
Eye	Diabetes, high blood pressure, injury
Nose	A clotting disorder, high blood pressure, injury, nasal polyps or tumors
Rectal	Anal fissure, colon cancer or polyps, diverticulitis or other intestinal disorder, hemorrhoids, ulcers
Skin	Allergic reaction, anemia, a blood or clotting disorder, Cushing's syndrome, drug reaction, hemophilia, injury, leukemia
Sputum	Bronchitis, lung cancer, pneumonia, pulmonary embolism, throat infection, tuberculosis
Urine	Bladder infection, urinary tract cancer, kidney stone, prostate disorder
Vagina	Abortion or miscarriage, cancer, a hormonal disorder, infection, menstrual abnormalities, injury, polyps
Vomit	Cirrhosis of the liver, esophageal tear, ulcers
Breathlessness	Anemia, anxiety, asthma, heart disease, hyperventilation, a lung disorder
Confusion	Addiction, alcoholism, Alzheimer's disease or other dementia, drug reaction, head injury, stroke
Constipation	Appendicitis, colon cancer or other bowel disorder, diabetes, diet, drug side effects, inactivity, pregnancy, a thyroid disorder
Coughing	Asthma, bronchitis, common cold, croup, cystic fibrosis, flu, pneumonia
Cyanosis (bluish skin)	A circulatory disorder, congenital heart defect, cystic fibrosis, heart failure, respiratory failure, Raynaud's disease
Delirium	Alcohol or drug abuse, brain tumor or abscess, encephalitis, head injury, heatstroke, meningitis, mountain sickness, poisoning, psychosis, Reye's syndrome
Diarrhea	AIDS, allergies, celiac disease, food poisoning, inflammatory bowel disease, irritable bowel syndome or other colon disorder, infection, a malabsorption syndrome, traveler's diarrhea
Dizziness	Alcohol or drug abuse, anemia, a brain disorder, cardiac arrhythmia, drug reaction, ear infection, Ménière's disease, stroke or mini-stroke, tumor

SIGN OR SYMPTOM	POSSIBLE CAUSES
Fatigue	Anemia, cancer, chronic fatigue syndrome, depression, flu or other infectious disorder, heart disease, hepatitis, mononucleosis, premenstrual syndrome, respiratory disorders
Fever	Abscess, AIDS, appendicitis, cancer, infection (bacterial or viral), medication side effects, rheumatoid arthritis or other autoimmune diseases
Fainting	Anxiety, blood loss, cardiac arrhythmias, heart attack or other heart condition, hyperventilation, hypoglycemia, stroke
Gait changes	Arthritis, a back disorder, multiple sclerosis or other neuromuscular disorder, Parkinson's disease, stroke
Hallucinations	Alcoholism, drug reaction, fever, schizophrenia or other psychotic disorder
Hirsutism	Cancer, Cushing's syndrome, drug side effects, hormonal imbalances, polycystic ovaries or other ovarian disorder
Hoarseness	Anxiety, asthma, bronchitis, cancer, common cold, croup, polyps, smoking, thyroid deficiency
Impotence	Alcoholism, depression, diabetes, drug reaction, multiple sclerosis, hormonal abnormalities, a nerve disorder, surgery for prostate tumors or disease, a thyroid disorder
Insomnia	Alcohol and caffeine use, anxiety or depression, drug side effects, a thyroid disorder
Intestinal gas	Colic, colon cancer or other bowel disorder, diet, indigestion, a malabsorption syndrome
Itching	Allergies, chickenpox or other rash, dry skin, eczema, fungal or other infection, liver disease, stress, vaginitis
Jaundice	Anemia, blocked bile duct, cirrhosis, hepatitis or other liver disorder, gallbladder disease, a pancreatic disorder, infant prematurity
Loss of appetite	AIDS, anemia, cancer, depression, a digestive disorder, drug reaction, an eating disorder, infection, loss of taste
Mood changes	Alcohol or drug abuse, depression or other psychological disorder, drug reaction, a hormonal disorder, menopause, premenstrual syndrome, psychological stress
Nausea and vomiting	Alcohol abuse, appendicitis, brain injury, drug reaction, ear infection, gallbladder disease, food poisoning, gastritis, glaucoma, heart attack, hepatitis, indigestion, infection, intestinal obstruction, Ménière's disease, morning sickness, motion sickness, ulcers, vertigo

SIGN OR SYMPTOM	POSSIBLE CAUSES
Nightmares	Alcohol or drug abuse, anxiety, depression, fever, post-traumatic stress syndrome
Numbness or tingling	Bell's palsy, carpal tunnel syndrome, a circulatory disorder, neuropathy, Raynaud's disease, shingles
Pain:	
Abdomen	Appendicitis, a digestive disorder, gallstones, hepatitis, intestinal disorders, menstrual cramps, pelvic inflammatory disease, tubal pregnancy
Back	Arthritis, muscle spasms or strain, osteoporosis, ruptured disk
Chest	Angina, an esophageal disorder, heart attack, heartburn, pleurisy, pneumonia, pneumothorax
Ear	Infection, foreign body
Eye	Conjunctivitis, glaucoma, foreign body, iritis, sinus infection, injury, sty, tumors
Face	Bell's palsy, dental disease, headache, shingles, sinus infection, temporomandibular joint disorder
Foot	Arthritis, bunions, corns or calluses, gout, neuromas, warts
Generalized aches	Flu, lupus, mononucleosis, rheumatoid arthritis, shingles
Head	Brain tumor, migraine or other type of headache, muscle tension, sinusitis, stroke
Knee	Arthritis, chondromalacia patella, infection, Lyme disease, strain or other injury
Leg	A circulatory disorder, fracture, muscle injury, phlebitis, shin splints
Mouth	Canker sores, cold sores, dental cavities, gum disease, infection
Neck	Arthritis, meningitis, muscle injury, slipped disk, stress
Joint/muscle	Arthritis, lupus, strain or sprain, tendinitis
Throat	Cold, flu, laryngitis, strep infection, tonsillitis, quinsy
Painful intercourse	
In males	Penile warts, prostatic or urethral infection
In females	Menopausal dryness, vaginitis, premenstrual syndrome
Palpitations	Anemia, anxiety, caffeine, heart disease, hypoglycemia, menopause, medications, premenstrual syndrome, a thyroid disorder
Rashes	Allergies, drug reactions, eczema, an infectious disease, lupus, rosacea, toxic shock syndrome
Runny nose	Allergies, common cold, sinus infection
Seizures	Brain tumor, drug side effect, cerebral palsy, epilepsy, fever, head injury, hypoglycemia, toxemia of pregnancy, meningitis, poisoning
Speech problems	Alcohol abuse, Alzheimer's disease, Bell's palsy, multiple sclerosis, stroke, Parkinson's disease

SIGN OR SYMPTOM	POSSIBLE CAUSES
Swallowing problems	Anxiety, diphtheria, an esophageal disorder, pharyngitis, strep throat, throat cancer, tonsillitis, quinsy
Sweating	Anxiety, drug reaction, fever, heart attack, infection, menopause, stress, a thyroid disorder
Swelling and lumps	
Abdominal	Cancer, heart failure, hernias, internal bleeding, intestinal gas, kidney failure, liver disease, pregnancy, uterine tumor
Breast	Cancer, fibrocystic condition, mastitis
Generalized	Anaphylactic reaction, drug reaction, heart failure, kidney disease, phlebitis, a liver disorder, thyroid disease
Joints	Arthritis, sprains
Skin or body surface	Abscess, cysts or other benign growths, cancer, edema, enlarged or obstructed lymph glands, ganglion, hives, infection, moles, warts
Taste changes	Bell's palsy, cancer, drug reaction, gum or dental disease, liver disease, loss of smell, pregnancy, a salivary disorder
Thirst	Diabetes, fever, heat exhaustion
Tinnitus (ringing in the ears)	Brain injury or tumor, cold or flu, drug side effects, ear infection, exposure to loud noise, Ménière's disease, earwax buildup, otosclerosis, vertigo
Tremor	Alcoholism, anxiety, Parkinson's disease, a thyroid disorder
Urinary problems	
Discolored urine	Bladder or kidney infection, kidney stones, liver or gallbladder disease, urinary tract cancer
Incontinence	Aging, Alzheimer's disease, a bladder disorder, nerve deterioration, spinal injury, stroke
Urgency	Bladder infection, bladder tumor, diabetes, interstitial cystitis, drug reaction, pregnancy
Painful urination	Bladder infection, gonorrhea or other sexually transmitted disease, kidney infection, kidney or bladder stones, prostatitis, urethritis, vaginitis
Vaginal discharge	Cancer, cervicitis, gonorrhea, vaginitis, pregnancy, premenstrual syndrome
Vision problems	Cataracts, detached retina, glaucoma, iritis, macular degeneration, mini-stroke, retinopathy
Weakness	Anemia, cancer, Guillain-Barré syndrome, heart disease, infection, liver disease, multiple sclerosis, muscular dystrophy, myasthenia gravis, rheumatoid arthritis
Weight changes	
Unexplained gain	Heart failure, kidney disease, liver disease, medications, toxemia of pregnancy, underactive thyroid
Unexplained loss	AIDS, anemia, cancer, diabetes, an eating disorder, infection, an intestinal disorder, malabsorption syndrome, ulcers
Wheezing	Allergies, asthma, bronchitis, emphysema, heart failure, lung disorders

Acne

(Acne vulgaris)

Acne, our most common skin disorder, is characterized by whiteheads, blackheads, pimples, and cysts. Nearly everyone is afflicted at some time in life, but acne is particularly common in teenagers. The hormonal changes of puberty enlarge the skin's sebaceous glands, increasing their output of an

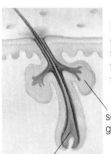

In a normal hair follicle, the sebaceous gland produces sebum, which reaches the skin surface through a pore.

sebaceous gland

hair root

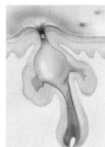

A closed comedone, or whitehead, appears when blockage develops below the surface of the skin Bacteria thrive in this environment, helping to promote acne eruptions.

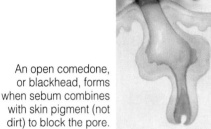

An open comedone, or blackhead, forms when sebum combines with skin pigment (not dirt) to block the pore.

As pressure builds, a large, infected cyst can form, resulting in the most severe type of acne.

oily substance called sebum. A buildup of sebum mixed with bacteria, dead skin cells, and other debris clogs pores, leading to one or more forms of acne (see illustrations above). Birth control pills are sometimes a triggering factor.

Diagnostic Studies and Procedures

Acne is easily diagnosed by its appearance, although a doctor will also ask questions about provoking factors.

Medical Treatments

For mild to moderate acne, treatment typically starts with a 2.5 or 5 percent strength of benzoyl peroxide. This non-prescription medication comes in lotion, gel, and cleanser forms, and in strengths up to 10 percent. Because benzoyl peroxide can irritate the skin, it should be applied only as directed and in the mildest effective strength. Drying agents, such as salicylic acid, alcohol, and sodium thiosulfate, may be combined with it or used alone.

A topical antibiotic, usually erythromycin or clindamycin cream, is prescribed for persistent acne. If one of

these is ineffective, tetracycline or some other oral medication may be used.

Severe, unremitting acne may be treated with tretinoin (Retin-A) or isotretinoin (Accutane), powerful drugs derived from vitamin A. Available in cream, gel, or liquid form, Retin-A is the preferred choice because it has fewer side effects than Accutane, which is taken orally and is generally reserved for the most serious cases.

In more than half of the people who use Accutane, acne never returns. But its many potential side effects include dry, fragile, peeling, or itching skin; hair loss; conjunctivitis, dry eyes, cataracts, and other visual problems; intestinal upsets; and decreased liver function. Accutane can also cause birth defects, and should be discontinued several months before attempting pregnancy. Both Retin-A and Accutane increase the skin's sensitivity to sun, so a sunblock with an SPF of 15 or more should be applied before going outdoors.

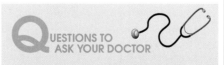

QUESTIONS TO ASK YOUR DOCTOR

▶ When is it safe to attempt a pregnancy after stopping Accutane? Does Retin-A pose a risk to the fetus?
▶ What types of birth control pills are least likely to promote acne?
▶ What can be done about acne scars?

Alternative Therapies

Aromatherapy. Using the aromatic oils of plants or flowers can counter stress, which is sometimes a factor in a flare-up of acne. Aromatherapists recommend massaging the affected areas with essence of juniper in an olive oil base, and then bathing them with lavender water and applying lavender cream. These and any other topical substances should be used cautiously because they can irritate the skin and also may interact adversely with skin medications.

Herbal Medicine. Long-standing herbal remedies for acne include agrimony, burdock root, clover, aloe vera, horsetail, iris, lavender, lemon balm, tansy, and white birch bark. Some of these herbal preparations are applied directly to the skin as a healing lotion or poultice; others are used for cleansing.

Homeopathy. Homeopathic substances recommended for acne include kali bromium, sulphur lotion or ointment, carbo vegetabilis, and thuya.

Self-Treatment

Always refrain from picking or squeezing pimples; this spreads the infection and can cause scarring.

Keep skin clean, but avoid harsh scrubbing and overwashing—acne is not caused by dirty skin and you can't wash it away. Cleanse once or twice a day with a mild, unscented soap. If your skin is very oily, try a drying soap that contains benzoyl peroxide. Use warm water and your fingertips (not a wash cloth or scrub brush). Avoid the use of washing granules or other exfoliates, which can worsen acne by increasing skin irritation.

Periodically apply a facial masque of mud, clay, or oatmeal to help remove oil from the skin. Steer clear of oily moisturizes and hair pomades; shampoo often and wear your hair pulled back from your face. Use non-oily water-based makeup and sunscreen.

Diet does not cause acne, but in some people, certain foods, such as those high in iodine, may make it worse. One at a time, eliminate foods you think affect your acne to see if your skin improves. Stress also does not cause acne but may worsen it; stress reduction techniques such as meditation may be helpful.

Other Causes of Skin Eruptions

Rosacea exhibits acne-like cysts and pustules, as well as flushing, swelling, and reddening of the skin. Allergies can also produce acne-like eruptions.

Addictions

Strictly speaking, an addiction is a compelling physical and psychological need for a habit-forming chemical substance, without regard for destructive consequences. In recent years, this definition has been expanded to include practically any compulsive behavior, ranging from overexercise and compulsive gambling to shoplifting and sex. There are now more than 200 such addictions that are being addressed by 12-step groups modeled on Alcoholics Anonymous (see box, opposite page).

The chemical addictions most prevalent in the United States are nicotine, alcohol, cocaine and crack cocaine, heroin, and amphetamines and other prescription drugs. No one fully understands why use of these substances evolves into abuse or addiction in some people and not others. However, research points to at least three possible explanations: a genetic predisposition, an abnormality in brain chemistry, and a personality disorder. Most likely, it is a combination of these factors that leads to addiction.

Diagnostic Studies and Procedures

Blood and urine tests can detect recent use of alcohol and other chemical substances, but there is no precise test to diagnose addiction. Instead, doctors look for specific patterns of behavior. The American Psychiatric Association's guidelines for a diagnosis of addiction, technically called "psychoactive substance dependence," require at least three of these statements to be true:

▶ The substance is taken in larger amounts or over a longer period than the person intended.
▶ There is persistent desire for the drug or unsuccessful efforts to stop its use.
▶ The person spends a great deal of time trying to get the substance, taking it, or recovering from its effects.
▶ Use of the substance disrupts social obligations or work activities.
▶ The person continues to use the substance despite knowing that it is causing problems; an example would be drinking, even though it makes an ulcer worse or threatens loss of a job.
▶ There is marked tolerance, meaning that increasing amounts are needed to achieve the same results. For example, it now takes an entire bottle of liquor to become intoxicated, compared to three or four drinks in the past.

▶ Attempts to stop using the substance produce withdrawal symptoms.
▶ The substance is taken to avoid the withdrawal symptoms.

Medical Treatments

Treatment, which varies according to the addictive substance, should be tailored to each individual. The chances of success increase if all of those involved—doctor, patient, and family members—recognize that addiction is an illness with complicated physical, psychological, and social components, and not simply a bad habit or sign of weakness. They should also understand that most addictions require a multifaceted approach to treatment.

Nicotine. This powerful stimulant is the addictive substance in tobacco. Within seconds of being inhaled, nicotine reaches the brain, which signals the adrenal glands to pump out adrenaline and other stress hormones. People think that a cigarette is relaxing; in reality, it creates a heightened state of tension. When the effect wears off, the smoker experiences jitteriness and other withdrawal symptoms, which are quelled by another cigarette.

When used properly, nicotine-based drugs make quitting easier by relieving withdrawal symptoms, which—in addition to jitteriness—may include headaches, muscle aches, nausea, irritability, and fatigue. They come in two forms: a gum that is chewed very slowly and a medicated skin patch. (A nicotine nasal spray is in the testing stage.)

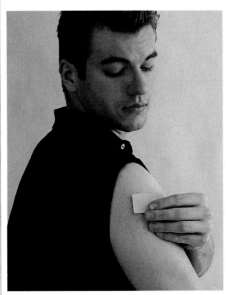

A nicotine patch blocks craving by delivering small amounts of the substance through the skin and into the bloodstream.

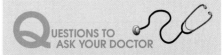
Nicotine from these sources is absorbed into the bloodstream, satisfying the body's craving for it and thus preventing withdrawal symptoms. There are hazards, however, and in an overdose, nicotine is a deadly poison. Nicotine gum and patches must be used exactly as directed, including NOT smoking, to avoid overdosage. After a few weeks, the person should be accustomed to not smoking, and can gradually be weaned off the drug.

To date, the only non-nicotine drug prescribed to aid smoking cessation is Clonidine, a medication originally developed to treat high blood pressure. Some studies suggest that it minimizes nicotine withdrawal symptoms, although it does not block entirely the desire to smoke.

Alcoholism. Medical treatment for alcoholism follows three stages. Stage one involves detoxification, during which alcohol is stopped completely and any nutritional deficiencies and other disorders are treated. Valium or other antianxiety drugs may be given to reduce tremor, hallucinations, and other withdrawal symptoms. Detoxification usually takes place in a clinic, hospital, or residential facility that specializes in drug dependency.

In stage two, the patient begins psychological counseling, which often entails joining the 12-step program of Alcoholics Anonymous or some other support group (see box, opposite page). Long-term abstinence and rehabilitation, which often involve the cooperation of family members, form the focus of stage three. Depending upon the severity of the drinking problem and the patient's overall health, counseling, and rehabilitation may be carried out in a residential program or on an outpatient basis.

In the past, the drug disulfiram (Antabuse) was widely prescribed as a deterrent to drinking. Antabuse produces severe nausea, palpitations, and other very unpleasant physical reactions when combined with even a minute amount of alcohol. But it is not a cure for alcoholism, and most treatment programs have abandoned its use.

Cocaine and Crack Cocaine. Treatment for cocaine abuse usually follows the same three-step program as for alcoholism, with one important difference: Because cocaine withdrawal can result in severe depression, antidepressant drugs are often prescribed for the early stages of detoxification.

Heroin. Substitution of methadone, a comparatively harmless addictive drug, for heroin continues to be the treatment of choice for this addiction. Although methadone itself is addictive, people taking it can hold a job and live a normal life if they are disciplined enough to use the drug exactly as recommended. The major disadvantage is that methadone must be taken daily to prevent withdrawal symptoms.

Prescription Drugs. People who abuse tranquilizers, narcotic painkillers, amphetamines, and other prescription drugs should not stop taking them without medical supervision. Because withdrawal symptoms can pose a serious danger, gradual detoxification is usually necessary.

Alternative Therapies

Although overcoming some addictions requires medical supervision, alternative therapies can ease withdrawal. More importantly, certain alternative therapies provide the tools a person needs for permanently changing behavior patterns that fostered the addiction.

Acupuncture. No one knows how it works, but there's considerable anecdotal evidence that this ancient Chinese procedure helps people overcome drug addictions. Typically, the acupuncturist inserts sterile steel needles in the cartilage of the outer ear, twirling them, and leaving them in place for half an hour. With repeated treatments, many persons have been able to stop smoking, and others have even been able to overcome heroin addiction.

Hypnosis and Visualization. Cigarette smoking is especially amenable to these approaches, perhaps because nicotine withdrawal does not require medical supervision. During hypnosis, a person

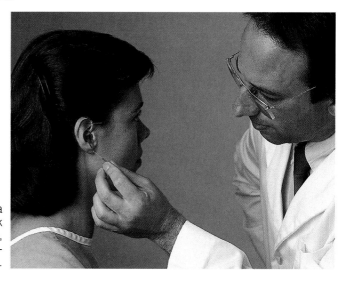

Acupuncturists use a point in the ear to block craving for nicotine, the addictive substance in cigarettes.

is highly receptive to the power of suggestion. Some hypnotists instruct their clients to discard all cigarettes, lighters, and ashtrays at a specific time. They may also plant the notion that smoking is unpleasant; for example, that cigarette smoke has a disgusting odor. Hypnotists often teach visualization or self-hypnosis as additional tools in resisting the urge to smoke.

Meditation and Yoga. Many people turn to cigarettes, alcohol, or other addictive substances as a means of dealing with stress. Meditation, yoga, and other relaxation therapies provide an alternative that is not self-destructive and has other health benefits as well. Relaxation therapy often precedes the actual cessation of smoking; in treating alcoholism and drug addictions, it is usually added during the counseling or rehabilitation stages.

Self-Treatment

Self-treatment remains the most effective way of giving up smoking. About 95 percent of smokers who quit do so on their own, usually abruptly, or cold turkey. Relapses are common, however, and most people make several attempts before quitting for good. To improve your own chances of success, make a systematic plan for stopping, beginning with an analysis of why you continue to smoke and a list of alternatives. For example, many women won't give up smoking because they are afraid of gaining weight. Joining an exercise class can help prevent weight gain and provide other health benefits as well.

Self-treatment is not recommended during the detoxification stage of overcoming substance addictions. After this

initial phase, however, self-treatment is the key to success. The goal of counseling, for instance, is to help strengthen a person's emotional resources so that he can overcome the urge to resume previous behavior. This does not mean, though, that one must go it alone; there are dozens of support and self-help groups ready to help.

THE 12 STEPS

1. Admit we are powerless over [our addiction]—that our lives have become unmanageable.
2. Come to believe that a Power greater than ourselves can restore us to sanity.
3. Make a decision to turn our will and our lives over to the care of God as we understand Him.
4. Make a searching and fearless moral inventory of ourselves.
5. Admit to God, to ourselves, and to another human being the exact nature of our wrongs.
6. Become entirely ready to have God remove all these defects of character.
7. Humbly ask Him to remove our shortcomings.
8. Make a list of all persons we have harmed and become willing to make amends to them all.
9. Make direct amends to such people wherever possible, except when to do so would injure them or others.
10. Continue to take personal inventory and when we are wrong, admit it.
11. Seek through prayer and meditation to improve our conscious contact with God as we understand Him.
12. Having a spiritual awakening as the result of these steps, and trying to carry this message to others and practicing these principles in all our affairs.

Adrenal Disorders

(Addison's disease; adrenal virilism; aldosteronism; Conn's syndrome; Cushing's syndrome; pheochromocytoma)

The adrenal glands produce a number of hormones, complex chemical substances that regulate many vital functions of the body. These include adrenaline, also called epinephrine, and other hormones released during stress; hydrocortisone and other steroids, which help control the immune system as well as regulate blood glucose levels and blood pressure; aldosterone, which maintains proper

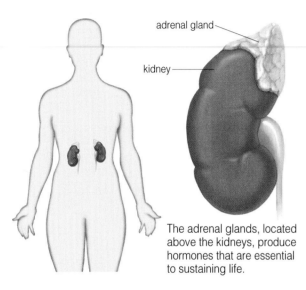

adrenal gland

kidney

The adrenal glands, located above the kidneys, produce hormones that are essential to sustaining life.

fluid and chemical balances; and androgens, progesterone, and estrogen, which are essential for reproduction. Some of these hormones are also produced elsewhere in the body, but the adrenal cortex is the sole source of epinephrine, aldosterone, and hydrocortisone.

Symptoms of adrenal disorders vary. In Addison's disease, the adrenal glands are gradually destroyed, resulting in severe weight loss, darkened skin, fatigue, low blood pressure, and sometimes low glucose levels.

Excessive androgen production is the cause of premature sexual development in boys and masculinization—beard growth, deepening of the voice, acne, and perhaps balding—in women.

In Conn's syndrome, increased aldosterone upsets the body's sodium and potassium balance, leading to muscle weakness, high blood pressure, and excessive thirst and urine production.

Cushing's syndrome, which is often due to the long-term use of steroid drugs, is marked by excessive cortisone,

which causes thinning of the skin and bones, easy bruising, mood changes, high blood pressure, and weight gain, especially on the trunk and upper back.

A pheochromocytoma is a tumor that produces excessive adrenaline and other stress hormones. This overproduction leads to erratic high blood pressure, palpitations, profuse sweating, and extreme anxiety.

Diagnostic Studies and Procedures

Adrenal disorders are diagnosed by characteristic symptoms and blood and urine tests to measure hormone levels. In some instances, all of the patient's urine is collected for a 24-hour period, then analyzed for the presence of potassium, sodium, and hormones.

Medical Treatments

The objective is to restore normal hormonal levels and function. In some disorders, such as Addison's disease, this requires lifelong replacement of hormones.

When Cushing's syndrome is the result of taking steroid medications, it can be reversed by slowly tapering off these drugs. This process must be done under a doctor's supervision, because stopping the medication too abruptly can lead to shock.

Adrenal virilism is treated with medications that suppress overproduction of androgen, or by surgery if a tumor is the source of the excessive hormones.

Conn's syndrome and pheochromocytoma usually are treated surgically to remove the hormone-producing tumors. But drugs may also be used to suppress hormone production.

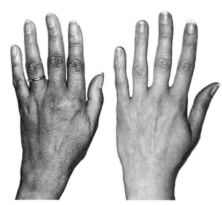

A darkening of the skin, such as the condition on the left, is one of the first obvious signs of Addison's disease.

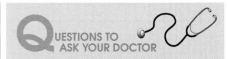
Alternative Therapies

Adrenal disorders are potentially life threatening, so alternative therapies should be used only with the approval of the primary physician and as adjuncts to medical treatment.

Herbal Medicine. An herbalist may recommend licorice, which contains a chemical that increases the output of hormones in patients who have Addison's disease. A physician should be consulted before self-treating with licorice extract, which can send blood pressure soaring if taken in large amounts for any length of time.

Reflexology. Reflexologists believe that adrenal disorders can be alleviated by gently pressing the adrenal point, situated on the narrowest part of the sole, about midway between the heel and toes, and simultaneously rotating the foot. Another adrenal point is on the palm, just below the middle finger.

Self-Treatment

Addison's disease is a lifelong condition, and it is important to recognize symptoms of an impending adrenal crisis—profound weakness, fatigue, dizziness or fainting, and severe pain in the abdomen. Infection, an injury, or other physical stress can precipitate a crisis unless extra cortisone is taken. Patients should wear a Medic-Alert bracelet or pendant and avoid sports in which they risk a fracture or other injury. Swimming, walking, and use of exercise machines are usually safe.

Treatment of adrenal virilism reverses some of the masculine changes such as new beard growth. However, it does not get rid of existing facial hair; this can be removed by electrolysis. Avoid plucking, which irritates skin and worsens the acne that often accompanies adrenal virilization.

Other Causes of Adrenal Symptoms

In diagnosing an adrenal disorder, a doctor should rule out tumors of the pituitary and other hormone-producing glands. He should also investigate the overuse of steroid drugs.

AIDS

(Acquired immune deficiency syndrome)
AIDS, first described in 1981, is not a single disease, but rather, an increasing vulnerability to many disorders, especially infections. These result from the progressive destruction of the immune system by the human immunodeficiency virus (HIV).

The virus is transmitted when a body fluid of an infected individual—blood, semen, vaginal secretions, or breast milk—is absorbed into the bloodstream of a healthy person. The major exception appears to be saliva, which has never been shown to be a carrier.

Worldwide, heterosexual intercourse is the most common mode of HIV transmission. In the United States, most cases result from male homosexual intercourse or the sharing of hypodermic needles. However, heterosexual intercourse is gaining as a source of infection, and about one-third of babies born to HIV-infected women develop AIDS. Before development of an HIV screening test in 1986, the infection was often spread through contaminated blood transfusions and the coagulation factors used to treat hemophilia.

Whenever a virus enters the body, a healthy immune system produces a variety of fighter cells, which include the T-cell lymphocytes. HIV invades T-cells and uses their genetic material to multiply itself. The virus eventually destroys the T-cells, producing many new HIV particles in the process. In time, the immune system is overwhelmed by the infection, and the person becomes increasingly susceptible to the infections and other diseases that make up the AIDS complex.

It takes an average of 10 years from the time of infection to develop full-blown AIDS, and throughout that entire period, contact with body fluids from the person harboring the virus can spread the infection.

Diagnostic Studies and Procedures

There is no direct test to diagnose an HIV infection; the tests currently available detect instead antibodies made in response to the virus. These antibodies are not detectable until at least six weeks after infection; in rare cases, it may take a year or more for them to develop. A negative result, therefore, does not necessarily rule out the existence of an HIV infection.

The most common test for HIV is a blood analysis called ELISA, short for enzyme-linked immunosorbent assay. Because the ELISA test can be falsely positive, however, a firm diagnosis also requires a positive response to another antibody test called the Western blot test, which specifically detects HIV antibodies. Once an HIV infection has been confirmed, frequent blood tests to measure T-cell levels will indicate just how fast the disease is progressing, even in the absence of any symptoms.

Medical Treatments

AIDS remains incurable so far, but there are several drugs that delay the onset of AIDS symptoms, and other drugs and vaccines are in the testing stage. While none of the medications below appear to prolong life, any of them may extend the period of relative health, especially when used early in the infection.

Azidothymidine (AZT). The first AIDS drug, this gained FDA approval in 1987. It works by interfering with replication of the HIV within the T-cells. Contrary to early optimistic expectations, it does not prolong life, but it does delay the onset of AIDS symptoms. Doctors disagree, however, on whether AZT should be initiated as soon as a patient tests HIV positive and risk its side effects (which include anemia and reduced white blood cells), or whether they should wait for symptoms.

Dideoxyinosine (DDI). This drug is similar to AZT, but it has different adverse effects, such as pancreatitis and nerve problems. Thus, DDI may be taken by patients who are unable to tolerate AZT.

Dideoxycytidine (DDC). Used in combination with AZT, this drug helps to prevent the virus from multiplying.

Erythropoietin. This synthetic hormone stimulates bone marrow cells to produce red blood cells and counter anemia caused by AZT.

Interleukin-2. Infusions of this protein appear to increase T-cell production in HIV-positive individuals who do not yet have AIDS. Its use, although promising, is still experimental.

Pentamidine. This is an aerosol drug that is inhaled periodically to prevent *Pneumocystis carinii* pneumonia, a common infection among AIDS patients.

Trimethoprim and sulfamethoxazole. Marketed as Bactrim or Septra, these antibiotics are taken either to prevent or treat pneumocystis pneumonia.

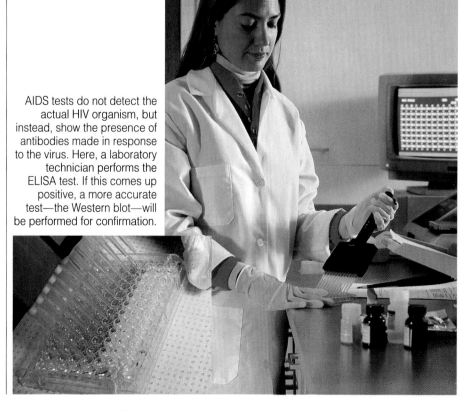

AIDS tests do not detect the actual HIV organism, but instead, show the presence of antibodies made in response to the virus. Here, a laboratory technician performs the ELISA test. If this comes up positive, a more accurate test—the Western blot—will be performed for confirmation.

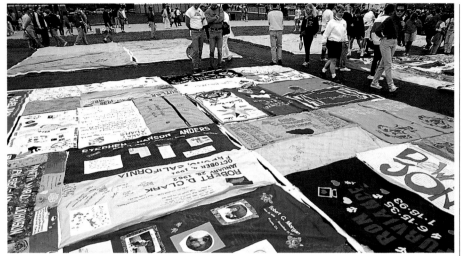

The AIDS Names Project gave rise to the AIDS quilt, with each square a memorial to someone who died of the disease. The quilt now covers several acres when spread out each year near the Washington Memorial in Washington, D.C. Sadly, it continues to grow.

AIDS (CONTINUED)

gp-160. This is an experimental vaccine that may slow the progress of HIV, but like other vaccines that are currently being tested, it does not prevent it.

HIV infection follows an unpredictable course; no two cases are exactly the same. Additional treatments depend upon the AIDS-related diseases or infections involved. For example, AIDS increases the risk of developing cancer, notably lymphoma (page 281), Kaposi's sarcoma (page 260), and cervical cancer (page 127). These are treated by surgery, radiation, and chemotherapy. Pneumocystis pneumonia is treated with drugs, as is toxoplasmosis (page 419), a parasitic infection. Toxoplasmosis cysts may be removed surgically.

The knowledge that one is infected with HIV is also psychologically difficult to deal with. In addition to medical treatment, most doctors also advise that patients seek counseling.

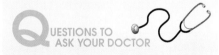

QUESTIONS TO ASK YOUR DOCTOR

▶ Should I be taking supplemental vitamins? Which ones and in what doses?
▶ What should I do to protect others from becoming infected? Specifically, what sexual practices are safe? And what should be avoided?
▶ Should my partner or family members undergo HIV testing?
▶ Is it safe for me to have a cat or other pet? What precautions should I take to avoid toxoplasmosis and other animal-borne infections?

Alternative Therapies

Any alternative therapy should be undertaken as an adjunct to medical treatment and with the full knowledge of the primary-care physician. Some therapies can actually hasten the bodily decline of AIDS, especially if they restrict essential nutrients or exacerbate diarrhea and other digestive problems. People with AIDS should be very suspicious of anyone who promises miracle cures or claims to have the ability to revitalize the immune system.

Aromatherapy and Massage. Massage, alone or combined with aromatic oils, helps overcome stress. Deep muscle massage and acupressure also have a restorative effect on the body's energy. When used with an oil chosen for its appealing scent, the result can be reduction of the negative feelings that are thought to have a detrimental effect on the levels of T-cells.

Meditation and Yoga. These relaxation techniques enhance the immune system and, when combined with guided imagery or visualization, may even slow the progress of HIV infection. Many traditional medical approaches now include instruction in meditation, yoga, and visualization.

Nutrition Therapy. Maintaining a healthful nutritional status is vital to bolstering the immune system, preventing weight loss, and preserving strength. Before making any changes in diet, however, it's best to consult a clinical dietitian, in particular, one who specializes in working with AIDS patients. Some alternative diets can

actually weaken rather than strengthen the immune system. For example, a rigid macrobiotic regimen that restricts calories, protein, and fluids, while relying mostly on brown rice, grains, and vegetables can exacerbate the weight loss, muscle wasting, and diarrhea common with AIDS.

Also be wary of so-called immune-power supplements, such as megadose vitamin C, which can irritate the intestinal tract and promote diarrhea. A high-fat diet may provide vital extra calories, but it can also worsen diarrhea and other digestive problems.

Self-Treatment

Living with AIDS is like living with any progressive, chronic disease in that patients are responsible for most of their day-to-day care. Still, AIDS is a special burden, not only because it is fatal eventually but also because of the stigma, public fear, and extensive misinformation that surround the disease. Most communities now have self-help and support groups where people with HIV infection can discuss their emotional and physical problems in an understanding environment.

As noted earlier, maintaining good nutrition is paramount. But this is only part of a healthful lifestyle. Regular exercise is also important to bolster strength and fitness. Some studies also indicate that aerobic exercise may raise blood levels of certain white cells that fight infections. A typical regimen calls for 30 to 45 minutes of moderate exercise—brisk walking or bicycle riding are good choices—three or four times a week. Don't overdo, however, and get adequate rest between sessions.

MYTHS ABOUT AIDS

From the beginning, myths have persisted regarding ways in which the HIV organism is transmitted. Following are ways in which you CANNOT contract AIDS, despite widespread beliefs to the contrary.

▶ *Casual contact,* such as touching, hand holding, and hugging.
▶ *Donating blood.* A person who receives a blood transfusion from an infected person can contract HIV, but there is no way that you can get the virus by donating blood for the use of others.
▶ *Mosquito and other insect bites.* Numerous scientific studies have failed to find any insect that can carry or transmit the HIV organism.

Allergies

An allergy is an exaggerated response by the body's immune system against a normally harmless substance, or allergen. Almost anything can trigger an allergic reaction. In addition to those pictured to the right, some common allergens are molds, tobacco smoke, certain foods and food additives, insect venom, and chemicals in plants, cosmetics, perfumes, detergents, and soaps.

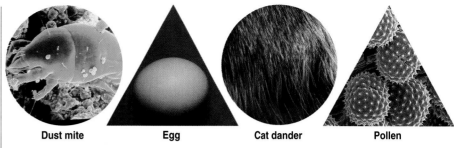

Dust mite **Egg** **Cat dander** **Pollen**

These are among the most common human allergens, which can provoke reactions ranging from hives and hay fever to life-threatening asthma.

The first time an allergen enters the body, the immune system reacts by making a defensive antibody called IgE. This initial exposure does not produce symptoms, but the IgE antibodies become attached to other defending parts of the immune system, either basophils, types of white blood cells, or mast cells, which line the airways, intestines, and skin. On a future exposure to the allergen, the programmed antibodies bind to it and signal the mast cells or basophils to produce a barrage of histamines and other substances that cause allergic symptoms.

Because histamines exert the greatest effect on the skin, mucous membranes, eyes, lungs, and gastrointestinal tract, most allergic reactions involve these organs. Depending on the nature of the allergy, symptoms range from the sneezing, runny nose, and itchy, teary eyes of hay fever, to hives, headaches, diarrhea, and the life-threatening systemic collapse of anaphylactic shock.

Doctors do not fully understand why so many people develop allergies. But because they run in families, an inherited predisposition is likely.

Diagnostic Studies and Procedures

In most cases, symptoms of an allergic reaction are self-evident, but finding just what triggers them often requires considerable detective work. Doctors start by asking a number of questions such as: Are the symptoms seasonal? Do other family members have similar symptoms? What seems to trigger them? Do you own any pets?

A physical examination helps to rule out other conditions that have similar symptoms. Allergy tests may then be ordered to pinpoint specific allergens. The most common are skin tests, in which the skin is exposed to small amounts of suspected allergens and then observed for a reaction.

Alternative studies include provocation tests, in which the patient inhales or ingests suspected allergens, and blood tests to look for IgE antibodies.

Exposure to allergens should always be done in a doctor's office or clinic, so that if a severe reaction should occur, it can be treated immediately.

Medical Treatments

Doctors agree that the best approach is to identify and then avoid the suspected allergen. Unfortunately, avoidance is not always possible. In such cases, treatments vary according to severity of symptoms and the types of allergens.

Allergy Medications. Hay fever and other types of pollen allergies are usually treated with drugs that counteract or inhibit histamines. The antihistamines in many nonprescription allergy medications produce drowsiness. (Such antihistamines should never be taken with alcohol, which increases their sedative effect. Also, they may worsen glaucoma, as well as prostate and urinary tract disorders.) There are prescription antihistamines, which do not enter the brain and are nonsedating; examples include terfenadine (Seldane) and astemizole (Hismanal). An alternative prescription medication, chromolyn sodium (Nasalcrom), is an aerosol nasal spray that inhibits the mast cells from releasing histamine, thus preventing nasal congestion.

In severe cases, steroids may also be prescribed. These work by temporarily blocking the action of white blood cells. They also block prostaglandins, body chemicals that produce inflammation and swelling. Steroids that are used for treating allergies are usually inhaled or applied to the skin.

Other allergy medications work by countering specific symptoms. For example, decongestants relieve nasal stuffiness by constricting the tiny blood vessels in the nose. Topical medications and sprays help to alleviate itching, inflammation, and other skin reactions. Some types, such as calamine, work by soothing and lubricating the surface of the skin; others, such as benzocaine, are local anesthetics that numb the skin.

Allergy Shots. Also called desensitization or immunotherapy, these are usually reserved for severe allergies that can't be controlled adequately with

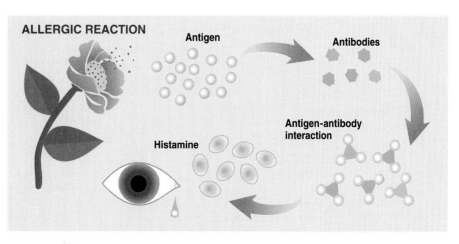

An allergic reaction develops when an antigen (in this case, pollen) enters the body. The immune system responds by producing antibodies that then attack the antigen. This antigen-antibody interaction prompts certain cells to release histamines and other chemicals, which produce symptoms such as runny eyes and nose.

ALLERGIC REACTION

Antigen

Antibodies

Antigen-antibody interaction

Histamine

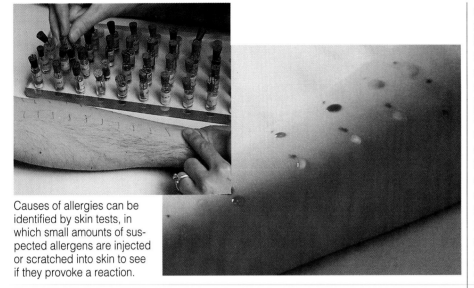

Causes of allergies can be identified by skin tests, in which small amounts of suspected allergens are injected or scratched into skin to see if they provoke a reaction.

ALLERGIES (CONTINUED)

medication. Periodic injections of increasing amounts of the allergenic extract are given over a long period, usually one to three years. The objective is to build up a natural tolerance to the allergens, thereby reducing symptoms and the need for medications.

Anaphylaxis or Anaphylactic Shock. This must always be treated as a life-threatening emergency. Symptoms that indicate anaphylaxis are facial redness and swelling, widespread itching and hives, difficulty breathing and swallowing, cramps, diarrhea, a sudden drop in blood pressure, and possibly unconsciousness. A previous widespread allergic reaction, such as extensive hives and swelling, sets the stage for a more severe response upon future exposure to that allergen. For example, a person who is hypersensitive to bee venom can suffer shock from just one sting (see case on opposite page). Treatment consists of injections of epinephrine (adrenaline), followed by observation until the person has recovered.

Anyone who has suffered a hypersensitive reaction or is allergic to penicillin or another antibiotic should wear a Medic-Alert bracelet containing this information. They should also carry an emergency kit that includes a syringe of adrenaline, plus antihistamines. These kits require a doctor's prescription.

Alternative Therapies

Treatment of severe allergies should be overseen by a physician, preferably an allergist. Some alternative therapies, approached with caution, may help to alleviate symptoms, though it is doubtful that any could produce immunity.

Acupuncture and Acupressure. These treatments are aimed at overcoming specific symptoms, such as skin itchiness or a runny nose. In acupuncture, the needles are inserted into the points related to the affected organs.

Acupressure, which also helps to relieve symptoms at the onset of an allergy attack, can be done as a self-care measure. The point to press is in the web of the hand next to the bone that connects with the index finger. Steady pressure should be applied for at least two minutes on each hand, all the while breathing deeply. The effect is said to be similar to an antihistamine.

Herbal Medicine. Chamomile is an ancient herbal remedy for the itchiness and skin inflammation of hives, and it is widely used in skin ointments and lotions. A compress soaked in chamomile tea may also relieve the itching and skin eruptions from poison ivy.

Inhaling steam that contains cloves, bayberry, or eucalyptus can help to ease nasal and sinus congestion.

A word of caution: Some herbal remedies are chemically related to certain

> QUESTIONS TO
> ASK YOUR DOCTOR
>
> ▶ Are there medications or foods that I should avoid while taking medictions to control allergy symptoms?
> ▶ Will foods I eat during pregnancy have any effect on my child if my family has a tendency to develop food allergies?
> ▶ Am I a candidate for allergy shots?

allergens and can provoke an allergic reaction; always use them with caution.

Homeopathy. Practitioners sometimes treat specific symptoms, such as giving euphrasia or arsenicum for hay fever, or may approach the problem as one component of widespread hypersensitivity.

Meditation. Stress tends to exacerbate allergies and such allergy-related diseases as asthma. Many sufferers find that meditation, yoga, and other relaxation therapies reduce the number and severity of attacks. Although it should not substitute for conventional therapy, meditation may be worth investigating as an additional treatment that can reduce the need for medication.

Naturopathy. Naturopaths have devoted considerable attention to food allergies, and many of their elimination diets are similar to those of more conventional physicians. Their use of dietary supplements to suppress allergies is more questionable, and should be checked with a doctor.

Nutrition Therapy. Counseling by a qualified nutritionist can be very helpful for an individual who has a long list of food allergies. Some allergy diets eliminate entire groups of foods; in such cases, nutrition therapists can suggest supplements or alternatives that will provide a well-balanced diet. They can also pinpoint the potential problems in restaurant dining and teach a patient how to spot the offending ingredients in prepared foods.

Self-Treatment

Anyone who has allergies knows that avoidance is the main line of defense against attacks. For example, seasonal hay fever can be minimized by staying indoors when pollen counts are high and investing in air conditioners for both home and car. If outdoor work is essential, wearing a disposable pollen mask and eye goggles is a good idea.

People with numerous allergies often react to animal dander. If you can't bear to part with a pet, try to keep it outdoors, or at least out of your bedroom. Some animals, such as poodles and rex cats, are said to be less allergenic than others. Recent studies also indicate that female cats are less allergenic than males. Bathing a cat weekly with plain water may reduce its allergy-provoking dander. In any event, before acquiring a pet, you should spend some time with it so you can make sure it does not trigger an allergic reaction.

Martin Bowman vividly remembers all of his encounters with bees. The first occurred when he was a 10-year-old camper and was stung repeatedly after he disturbed a nest of yellow jackets. His next sting occurred when he was in college.

"At that time, I was stung on my hand and my entire arm swelled," he recalls. This should have been a tip-off that he was hypersensitive to bee venom—a fact that was immediately apparent after a third, near-fatal encounter. By then, Bowman was a physician, and was driving with his family to a beach in North Carolina.

"It was a hot day, and we had the car windows open," he relates. "As we approached a small town, a yellow jacket flew in one of the windows and set off a panic among our kids in the backseat." The insect flew forward and stung Bowman on the neck. "Within minutes, my entire face was red and swollen and I was having difficulty breathing."

As a physician, he realized exactly what was happening—he was suffering an anaphylactic reaction to the yellow-jacket sting. "I knew I had to get a shot of adrenaline immediately. My wife was at the wheel and, as luck would have it, we spotted a pharmacy just down the street."

Accompanied by his wife, Bowman rushed into the drugstore. The pharmacist responded to their plea for adrenaline, which Bowman was able to inject himself. A few minutes later, his breathing returned to normal and the swelling started to go down. To be on the safe side, Bowman went to the local emergency room, and a few hours later, the family continued their journey, this time with a supply of antihistamines and adrenaline.

Bowman's experience is typical of those who are hypersensitive to bee venom. His first exposure was severe, prompting his immune system to produce an abundance of bee-venom antibodies. His second encounter indicated hypersensitivity, but fell short of anaphylaxis, which is always a danger in such cases.

Now, Bowman always carries a bee-sting emergency kit if there is any possibility of encountering bees. He also avoids any unnecessary risks.

Following are additional actions that help to reduce exposure to common household allergens:

▶ Use mold-inhibiting paint rather than wallpaper, which promotes mold growth.
▶ Consider discarding rugs, deeply upholstered furniture, and other dust-catching furnishings in favor of wood or tile floors and wood furniture.
▶ Keep the bedroom free of clutter and, if possible, avoid using it as a study or workplace. Objects with crevices or soft, plush surfaces that collect dust should be removed.
▶ Vacuum mattresses regularly and encase them in airtight plastic covers.
▶ Buy pillows and comforters that are filled with synthetic fibers rather than kapok or feathers.
▶ Avoid heavy drapes and venetian blinds—notorious dust catchers. Use window shades instead. If you do use curtains, launder them frequently.
▶ Wear a dust mask when vacuuming or dusting. Better still, have someone else do these tasks for you when you are away from the house.

▶ Keep your bedroom window closed, and use air conditioning, which cleans, cools, and dries the air.
▶ Don't hang laundry (especially sheets) out to dry—allergy-provoking pollens and molds may collect on them.
▶ If your child has allergies, avoid giving him stuffed toys. Many of these contain kapok or other fibers that are highly allergenic.
▶ Make sure that filters on air conditioners and humidifiers are cleaned or changed regularly.
▶ Treat damp areas, such as the basement and garage, with antimildew spray and use space heaters for additional drying.

Other Causes of Allergic Symptoms
Chronic sinus infections can cause nasal congestion and other symptoms similar to those of allergies. Itchiness and chronic hives may be caused by drug reactions. Less commonly, liver disorders or lymphatic cancer can produce unexplained itchiness. The rash and itching of psoriasis may also be mistaken for an allergic reaction.

DEALING WITH POISON IVY, POISON OAK, OR POISON SUMAC

Almost everyone reacts to the oils in these plants, but prompt action often can avert or minimize symptoms.

▶ If you think your hands have been affected, keep them away from your face and other parts of your body.
▶ As soon as possible, wash all exposed skin surfaces with water and either laundry detergent or dishwashing liquid, if available.
▶ Wear rubber gloves to promptly remove all clothing that came in contact with the leaves, and wash it separately in hot, soapy water. If you are very sensitive to these plants, it may be a good idea to discard the clothing.
▶ Avoid handling shovels, rakes, hoes, and other tools that have come in contact with the plants.
▶ Don't burn these plants; inhaling the smoke can cause lung inflammation.
▶ Use calamine lotion, cold compresses, or a paste of baking soda to ease the itching. Try to avoid scratching.
▶ Herbalists recommend rubbing the affected skin with aloe vera leaves, crushed plantain leaves, or juice squeezed from the jewelweed, or impatiens, flower.
▶ If the blisters feel feverish, coat them with vitamin E oil to reduce inflammation.
▶ If an itchy rash develops and interferes with sleep and other normal activities, ask your doctor for a prescription medication to alleviate the itchiness.

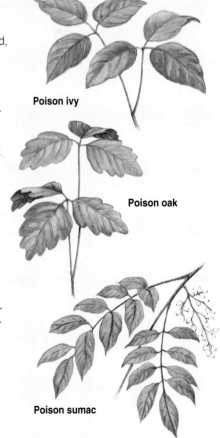

Poison ivy

Poison oak

Poison sumac

Alzheimer's Disease

(Dementia of the Alzheimer type)
Alzheimer's disease is a brain disorder in which memory, thought processes, and behavior become progressively impaired. It is named for Dr. Alois Alzheimer, the German neurologist who first described it in the early 1900s. He discovered during an autopsy of a woman who had died of progressive dementia that her brain was riddled with plaques and tangles of abnormal nerve cells, the hallmarks of the disease.

What causes Alzheimer's disease remains unknown, but studies have revealed the presence of an abnormal substance, called amyloid protein, among the plaques and tangles. Researchers are now trying to determine

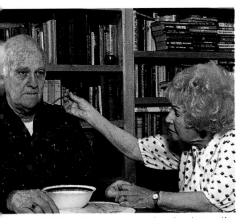

As Alzheimer's progresses, the simplest self-care often requires help, which can place a tremendous burden on family members.

whether these abnormalities stem from an infection, or genetic trait, or perhaps are caused by an environmental toxin.

Diagnostic Studies and Procedures

Only an autopsy can reveal the brain irregularities of Alzheimer's disease. Thus, diagnosis in a living person requires a process of elimination to rule out other possible causes of progressive mental deterioration. Family members and friends may be called upon to fill in the details about previous illnesses, accidents, medications, and personal habits, especially diet, alcohol use, and substance abuse.

The physical examination is usually concentrated on neurological function, although a doctor may also look for circulatory or respiratory disorders.

Special studies might include psychological tests, blood and urine analyses, skull X-rays, electroencephalography, and perhaps a CT brain scan or MRI.

Medical Treatments

Until recently, there was little that doctors could do to treat Alzheimer's disease. This situation is changing with a drug called tacrine (Cognex), which was released in 1993. Long-term effects of the medication are unknown, but about 20 percent of the patients who received it in clinical trials experienced significant improvement in mental functioning. For an additional 20 percent, the disease's progress was slowed down. Patients taking Cognex must undergo frequent blood tests to determine if there is any liver damage, the major adverse effect of the drug.

Some of the more troubling symptoms of Alzheimer's can be treated with older medications. For example, sedatives may be prescribed for sleep problems, antipsychotic drugs to calm psychosis and aggressiveness, and stimulants such as methylphenidate (Ritalin) to combat fatigue and improve mood. These drugs should be used only under regular medical monitoring, however, because they can also impair mental functioning.

Alternative Therapies

As with medical treatments, the goal of any alternative therapy for Alzheimer's disease is to provide comfort.

Hydrotherapy. As an alternative to drugs, some nursing homes use warm baths to soothe agitated or anxious patients. A word of caution, however: To prevent accidental drowning, an elderly person with Alzheimer's should never be left alone in a hot tub or bath.

Music Therapy. There is ample evidence that people with declining mental function can receive a great deal of pleasure from listening to music, both alone and with family members, and from group activities planned around singing. Even when verbal memory fades, the ability to recognize and remember music remains intact. Music therapists find that playing songs popular during a patient's youth, or music associated with a particular time and place, jogs other memories and helps in retrieving past experiences.

Nutrition Therapy. Some proponents of vitamin therapy recommend high doses of antioxidants—vitamins A, C, and E and the mineral selenium—to

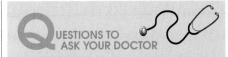

QUESTIONS TO ASK YOUR DOCTOR

▶ Which symptoms might nutritional supplements be likely to relieve?
▶ How often should medications be reviewed for possible adjustment of the dosage?
▶ Are we good candidates for any nearby research programs?

slow the progress of Alzheimer's disease. When consumed in food, these nutrients help counter the damage of unstable molecules called free radicals, which are a by-product of oxygen metabolism. As yet, there is no convincing scientific evidence that antioxidant supplements can benefit Alzheimer's patients or stave off other diseases of aging. A diet that emphasizes fruits, vegetables, legumes, and grains provides ample antioxidants.

Pet Therapy. Nursing homes often provide gentle cats, dogs, or other animals for Alzheimer's patients. Simply making contact with another living creature can be immensely comforting, and may improve human interaction.

Self-Treatment

Following a set routine in a familiar environment helps Alzheimer's patients cope with the early stages of memory loss. Unavoidable changes should be made gradually to avoid disorientation and confusion. For example, many patients suddenly become incontinent when they are hospitalized or moved to a new place. Often, they simply don't know how to find the bathroom, and the problem resolves itself when they return to a familiar setting.

In the early stages of memory loss, some Alzheimer patients write notes to themselves and post them in obvious places. This eases some of the anxiety over forgetting important tasks and appointments. Family members can coax memories by recalling past events, going through old photo albums, or accompanying the patient on an outing to a former neighborhood.

Other Causes of Dementia

During the diagnostic process, disorders that should be ruled out include alcoholism, nutritional deficiencies, depression, overuse of tranquilizers and other drugs affecting mental function, a brain tumor, stroke, Parkinson's disease, and circulatory problems.

Amenorrhea

(Menstrual failure)

Amenorrhea is the medical term for failure to menstruate. It is a normal condition in girls who have not yet reached puberty, and in women who are pregnant, in the early stage of breast-feeding, or postmenopausal. Otherwise, it is considered abnormal, and warrants medical investigation.

The condition may be primary, in which menstruation has not yet started by the age of 16, or secondary, in which menstruation has stopped for at least six months.

Most cases of primary amenorrhea are traced to hormonal imbalances or malnutrition; less commonly, the failure to menstruate is due to genetic or structural abnormalities, such as the absence of a uterus.

Secondary amenorrhea often develops during strenuous dieting for weight loss. It is one of the hallmarks of anorexia nervosa (page 170), a serious eating disorder. Other precipitating factors include stress, overexercising, the use of oral contraceptives and other medications, extreme obesity, hormonal disorders, and tumors.

Diagnostic Studies and Procedures

To diagnose primary amenorrhea, a doctor will take a complete medical history and perform a physical examination. During the exam, he will inspect the breasts, look for secondary sex characteristics, and check the vaginal walls for moistness (this last is an indication of whether the ovaries have begun to secrete estrogen). A teenager should be made aware of these procedures beforehand, when it is the first time she has to undergo a pelvic examination. If the doctor is male, she will probably feel more comfortable having her mother present.

The first step in tracking down the causes of unexplained interruption in menstruation is to rule out pregnancy and menopause—the two most common reasons. Besides undergoing a pelvic examination, the woman will have blood and urine tests to determine if there are hormonal abnormalities. Other studies may include X-rays and various other imaging procedures such as ultrasound, CT scanning, or MRI. These tests can detect tumors or any other abnormalities that could be linked to the amenorrhea.

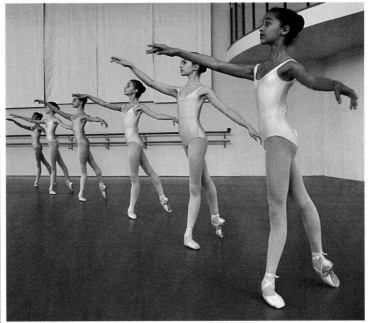

Dancers and gymnasts and other women whose activities demand lots of exercise as well as a lithe, thin body often develop amenorrhea.

Medical Treatments

Hormone therapy is prescribed for amenorrhea due to a thyroid disorder or other endocrine abnormality. If there are no obvious problems to account for either primary or secondary amenorrhea, a doctor may try to initiate menstruation by prescribing estrogen and progesterone, the female sex hormones that control the menstrual cycle.

Estrogen replacement is important for young women whose ovaries have ceased to function. Even if this does not induce menstruation, it can help prevent osteoporosis, a thinning of the bones that usually develops after menopause but can occur earlier due to prolonged ovarian failure. Amenorrhea caused by tumors may require surgery.

Alternative Therapies

Herbal Medicine. Tincture of American hellebore is recommended by both herbalists and homeopaths for amenorrhea. The highly diluted doses of homeopathy are safe; but even a small amount of the tincture is toxic and should not be in-

gested. A safer choice is tincture of calendula flowers. In the past, a number of other herbs including angelica, juniper, mayapple, pennyroyal, and tansy were used to induce menstruation or to terminate pregnancy because they caused abdominal cramps. These herbs are now considered toxic and should not be ingested.

Nutrition Therapy. This is the preferred treatment for amenorrhea that is related to excessive thinness or obesity. A sports nutritionist can help an athlete or dancer plan a diet that provides enough nutrition for proper ovarian function and menstruation without jeopardizing athletic performance.

Meditation and Yoga. Amenorrhea related to stress can often be cured by meditation, yoga, or other relaxation techniques. These may also be useful adjuncts to psychotherapy for women whose amenorrhea is related to overexercise or anorexia nervosa.

Self-Treatment

Moderation is the key to successful self-treatment of amenorrhea resulting from overexercise, crash dieting, or stress. It is important for young women athletes to recognize the long-term consequences of amenorrhea related to lack of estrogen, which can lead to infertility and premature bone loss.

Other Causes of Amenorrhea

Chronic diseases such as diabetes, thyroid disease, and some types of cancer can also lead to secondary amenorrhea, and should be ruled out in the process of making a diagnosis.

QUESTIONS TO ASK YOUR DOCTOR

▶ Should I be taking calcium to prevent bone loss?
▶ Is the failure of my ovaries likely to be permanent?
▶ Does my failure to menstruate mean I don't need to worry about pregnancy?

Anal Disorders

(Anal fissure; anorectal abscess; anorectal fistula; pruritus ani)

Anal disorders typically cause pain and itching, especially during or after bowel movements. Most often, the problem is due to an infection, an injury, pinworms, or simply poor hygiene. In some cases, anal discomfort is caused by a more serious problem. This might be a fissure, an ulcerated tear in the anal wall; a fistula, an abnormal opening from the rectum to the skin's surface or a nearby organ; or an abscess.

Diagnostic Studies and Procedures

A doctor can diagnose most anal disorders simply by examining the area. Identifying the size and location of a fistula, however, may require an internal examination with a sigmoidoscope, a tube with magnifying and lighting devices. Additional tests may be needed to identify its cause.

Medical Treatments

Treatment of anal disorders varies according to the underlying problem.
Anal Fissures. A medicated cream may be prescribed to alleviate irritation of the area. Severe cases may require surgery to remove the ulceration. This is a last-resort treatment because it can result in fecal incontinence.
Anorectal Abscesses. These usually require lancing with a sharp instrument, and then draining of the pus. If the abscess is large, a wick impregnated with antibiotics may be inserted temporarily into the pocket.
Anorectal Fistulas. Because fistulas don't disappear on their own, surgical repair is invariably necessary. The operation, which will be performed under general or local anesthesia, involves either opening or excising the fistula tract. The underlying cause of the fistula should also be treated.
Anal Itching. When this problem, known medically as pruritus ani, is due to pinworms, a prescription medicine quickly eliminates them. Pinworms are most common in children, but a doctor may advocate treating an entire family to prevent the spread and reinfection of the worms (page 441).

Alternative Therapies

Herbal Medicine. To promote healing of an anal fissure, herbalists recommend compresses soaked in warm echinacea tea or witch hazel; this last also alleviates itching.

Naturopathy and Nutrition Therapy.
Most anal fissures are due to chronic constipation, a condition that usually can be remedied by a high-fiber diet, increased exercise, and adequate fluid intake. Many naturopaths advocate adding 1 tablespoon of blackstrap molasses to a cup of warm water and drinking the mixture. Some suggest applying vitamin E oil to a fissure to hasten healing.

To relieve anal itching, naturopaths recommend soaking a cotton pad in apple cider vinegar and placing it on the affected area. This may burn at first, especially if the area is raw. Leave the pad on overnight, holding it in place with a sanitary napkin.

Self-Treatment

With the exception of fistulas and some abscesses, most anal disorders can be controlled with proper self-care. First and foremost, avoid straining during bowel movements. If necessary, use a stool softener or suppository. Some people find that squatting makes bowel movements easier, but it's a difficult position to achieve on an ordinary toilet. Try placing your feet on a stool and drawing your knees upward.

Most anal itching is due to poor hygiene or a reaction to chemicals in soap or toilet paper. Wipe carefully after bowel movements, but avoid excessive rubbing. A moistened wipe is gentler than toilet paper. Pat the area dry after cleaning and apply unscented talcum powder.

Soaking in a warm sitz bath relieves itching and irritation. To increase the effectiveness, add a half-cup of baking soda to the water. Avoid scratching; this only makes matters worse.

Nonprescription medications that contain mild anesthetics, such as benzocaine or pramoxine hydrochloride,

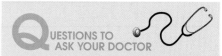

QUESTIONS TO ASK YOUR DOCTOR

▶ Do you recommend a laxative? If so, what kind should I use?
▶ What is the risk of bowel incontinence after surgical repair of a fistula or fissure?
▶ What can I do to avoid a recurrence of an abscess, fissure, fistula, or other anal disorder?

can relieve irritation and itching, as can hydrocortisone creams and ointments in 0.5 percent strength. Make sure that these topical medications are applied only to the external skin and not to the inside of the rectum itself.

A small abscess can sometimes be healed by applying warm compresses. Don't attempt to lance it yourself, as this can lead to a serious infection.

Caffeine, alcohol, high doses of vitamin C, and certain spicy foods may cause anal irritation. Try eliminating all such culprits from your diet for a few days and see if this helps. Return each suspect one by one. If symptoms return, you will know what foods to avoid in the future.

Anal itching caused by an allergic response to a personal product can be alleviated by using plain, unscented, or hypoallergenic products and wearing loose-fitting cotton underwear.

Anyone with an anal fissure, fistula, or abscess should avoid anal intercourse. Similarly, forego enemas or the insertion of any object in the anal canal.

Other Causes of Anal Discomfort

Hemorrhoids often cause anal itching and irritation; so do fungal infections and certain digestive disorders, as well as some medications.

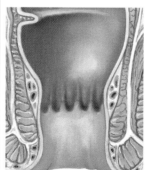

Even a normal anal area is sensitive to pain because of its rich nerve supply.

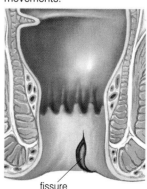

A fissure can produce intense pain during bowel movements.

fissure

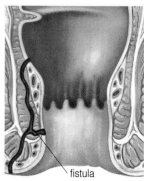

fistula

A fistula is usually a consequence of inflammatory bowel disease or other disorders.

Anemia

(Aplastic, hemolytic, iron deficiency, and pernicious anemias)

There are many forms of anemia, the most common blood disorder. All are marked by abnormalities in the number or function of red blood cells, or erythrocytes. These blood cells get their red color from hemoglobin, an iron-rich substance that carries oxygen.

The prevalent causes of anemia are malnutrition, metabolic defects, certain drugs, environmental toxins, excessive blood loss, and cancer and various other diseases.

Diagnostic Studies and Procedures

All types of anemia produce weakness and fatigue, skin pallor, shortness of breath, and palpitations. But accurate diagnosis requires blood analyses, starting with a complete blood count, or CBC, in which the various cells in a specific amount of blood are counted with the aid of a microscope. While counting the cells, a lab technician will also look for abnormalities in their shape, size, color, and distribution.

For some anemias, diagnosis also requires analysis of bone marrow, which is obtained by aspiration with a hollow needle. In the United States, the common types of anemia are:

Iron deficiency anemia, the most prevalent, results when the body lacks enough iron to make hemoglobin. This can be caused by inadequate diet, an intestinal disorder, or excessive blood loss, usually through heavy menstrual periods or other chronic bleeding.

Aplastic anemia occurs when the bone marrow cannot make enough of certain blood cells—red, white, or platelets—even though the ones produced are generally normal. Possible causes of aplastic anemia are a hereditary defect or a thymus gland tumor. Exposure to radiation and certain chemicals, including arsenic, benzene, and some pesticides, may be implicated, as well as anticancer drugs and some antibiotics.The condition may also develop following infections with a number of viruses. In about half of all cases, however, a cause cannot be found.

Folic acid deficiency anemia almost always results from a deficiency of this B vitamin, which is needed to make hemoglobin. This anemia is especially common in alcoholics; less often, it is due to an intestinal disorder.

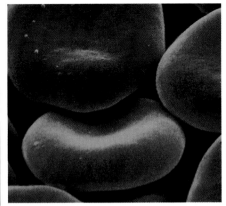

Normal red blood cells live about 120 days. Their iron is then recycled through the liver and bone marrow to make new cells.

Hemolytic anemia occurs when red blood cells are destroyed faster than the body can produce new ones. Sometimes this is due to an autoimmune disease in which the immune system attacks the red blood cells.

Pernicious anemia is caused by a deficiency of vitamin B_{12}, usually when the stomach fails to produce intrinsic factor, a substance needed to absorb the vitamin into the bloodstream.

Medical Treatments

Iron deficiency anemia responds generally to iron pills and an increased intake of iron-rich foods, especially liver and lean red meats. Other good sources of iron are whole grains, dark green vegetables, and legumes. Because chemicals in certain foods inhibit iron absorption, they should not be taken at the same meal with iron-rich foods. Included are dairy products, nuts, tea, and coffee. Citrus fruits, on the other hand, enhance iron absorption.

In severe cases of iron deficiency anemia, involving major blood loss, a transfusion may be necessary.

Aplastic anemia caused by radiation, drugs, or industrial chemicals is treated with transfusions until the bone mar-

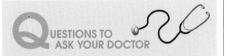

QUESTIONS TO ASK YOUR DOCTOR

▶ How much extra iron do I need to meet my own and my baby's requirements during pregnancy?
▶ Do any of my medications carry a risk of causing anemia?
▶ How can I determine if chemicals in my workplace cause anemia? How can I safeguard myself when working with them?

row can resume its normal function. In recent years, bone marrow transplantation, in which the patient's marrow is destroyed and replaced with healthy marrow from a donor, has cured some cases, especially in patients under age 30. Another relatively new treatment consists of injections of equine antithymocyte globulin (ATG), a substance obtained from horse serum. This approach has helped about 60 percent of patients. Alternatively, cyclosporine—a drug that suppresses the immune system—may be used.

Folic acid deficiency anemia is treated with vitamin supplements and an increased intake of organ meats, raw fruits, and vegetables. If intestinal absorption is the problem, folic acid must be given by injection.

Hemolytic anemia caused by medication can be treated by withdrawing it. If an autoimmune disorder is at fault, corticosteroids or other drugs to suppress the immune system are prescribed. In some cases, removal of the spleen, which destroys red blood cells, cures the problem. Transfusions are sometimes necessary.

Pernicious anemia is treated with vitamin B_{12} injections. Initially, the shots are given at least weekly. As the body's vitamin B_{12} stores are replenished, monthly injections suffice.

Alternative Therapies

Anemia is a serious condition that does not lend itself to alternative therapies. In some cases, however, they may be useful adjuncts to medical treatment.

Herbal Medicine. Dandelion tea and wine are ancient herbal remedies for anemia, especially if it's due to iron deficiency. Brewing the tea or wine in a cast-iron pot increases the iron content. Using cast iron cookware to prepare acidic foods such as tomato sauce also adds significant iron to the diet.

Self-Treatment

Self-diagnosis and treatment of anemia are potentially dangerous. By all means, consume a healthful, balanced diet, but don't resort to taking iron pills and other supplements without consulting a doctor first. Too much iron damages the liver, heart, and other organs.

Other Causes of Anemia

Genetic disorders such as sickle cell disease and Cooley's anemia can cause abnormal red cells. A severe infestation of hookworms or other intestinal parasites can lead to anemia.

Aneurysms

(Abdominal, aortic, and dissecting aneurysms)

An aneurysm is a bulging in the wall of a weakened segment of a blood vessel. The aorta, the body's largest artery, is most often affected, although aneurysms develop also in arteries at the base of the brain and in some of the smaller vessels within the brain.

Aneurysms usually do not produce symptoms until they are large enough to press on nearby organs. For example, an aortic aneurysm that occurs near the heart can cause chest pain and other symptoms that mimic angina or a heart attack. In this type of aneurysm, the artery's inner and outer walls may divide, allowing blood to seep between the layers and reducing blood flow to other parts of the body. This is called a dissecting aortic aneurysm and it is especially dangerous.

An abdominal aortic aneurysm can sometimes be felt as a throbbing, tender mass just under the skin, below the ribcage in the center of the abdomen. If it leaks blood, it can cause pain that radiates to the back and groin. In a carotid aneurysm, the throbbing is felt in the neck, and there may also be a visible bulging under the skin.

Arteriosclerosis, a hardening of the arteries, promotes aneurysms, as does high blood pressure. Other causes are congenital defects and inherited disorders. For instance, coarctation of the aorta, a congenital defect in which a segment of the artery is stiff and narrowed, can lead to an aortic aneurysm in the normal portion. Anyone with Marfan's syndrome, a hereditary disorder characterized by eye, skeletal, and cardiovascular abnormalities, is also prone to aneurysms.

As an aneurysm enlarges, the danger increases that it might suddenly rupture. A burst aneurysm is usually fatal within minutes, especially if the aorta or carotid arteries are involved, although immediate surgery to halt bleeding and repair the break is sometimes life-saving.

Diagnostic Studies and Procedures

During a physical examination, a doctor can often feel and hear the abnormal throbbing of an aneurysm. As blood flows through the weakened segment of the vessel, it may also make a distinctive sound that can be heard through a stethoscope. A doctor may suspect coarctation of the aorta if blood pressure is elevated in the arms and upper body, and normal or low in the trunk and legs. This is confirmed by measuring blood pressure separately in the arms and the legs.

Imaging studies, ranging from ordinary X-rays to a CT scan or MRI and ultrasound, confirm the presence of an aneurysm. Asymptomatic aneurysms sometimes show up on X-rays or scans taken for some other purpose.

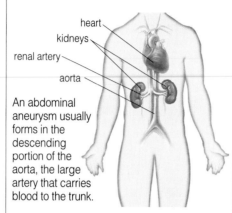

heart
kidneys
renal artery
aorta

An abdominal aneurysm usually forms in the descending portion of the aorta, the large artery that carries blood to the trunk.

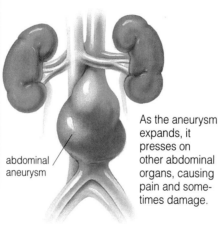

abdominal aneurysm

As the aneurysm expands, it presses on other abdominal organs, causing pain and sometimes damage.

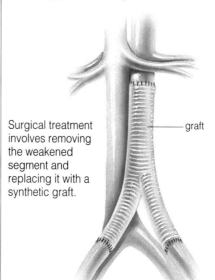

graft

Surgical treatment involves removing the weakened segment and replacing it with a synthetic graft.

Medical Treatments

A small aneurysm that is neither enlarging nor producing symptoms usually requires only regular monitoring with X-rays or other tests to detect any enlargement.

Surgery, sometimes on an emergency basis, is required if the aneurysm is growing or in danger of rupture. A promising experimental treatment for an expanding aneurysm entails lining the weakened artery with a thin tube.

Coarctation of the aorta also requires surgical repair, although some cases can be resolved by balloon angioplasty. In this procedure, a balloon-tipped catheter is inserted into the aorta, and the balloon is inflated at the narrowed site to stretch the artery, thereby allowing normal blood flow.

Alternative Therapies

There are no safe alternative approaches for an aneurysm, although meditation and other relaxation techniques are useful adjunctive therapies if high blood pressure is a contributing factor. In such cases, salt restriction, weight loss, and other nutritional therapies may also be beneficial.

Self-Treatment

An aneurysm does not lend itself to self-treatment. However, preventive measures may be recommended in certain situations. For example, patients with Marfan's syndrome are advised to avoid competitive or endurance sports. Some athletes with undiagnosed Marfan's syndrome have died suddenly during a strenuous competitive event. Flo Hyman, a member of the U.S. Olympic volleyball team in 1984, is a notable example of sudden death due to Marfan's syndrome.

Because atherosclerosis increases the risk of an aneurysm, a diet low in saturated fat and high in fiber, which will help reduce blood cholesterol levels, is advisable. Smoking and excess weight can also contribute to conditions that provoke aneurysms, so stopping smoking and controlling weight are important aspects of preventive self-care. Moderate exercise, approved by a physician, may also be beneficial.

Other Causes of Aneurysm Symptoms

The pain of an abdominal aneurysm, which may be felt in the back or sides, sometimes leads a doctor to suspect a ruptured spinal disk, kidney disease, or intestinal disorder.

Angina

(Angina pectoris; chest pain; coronary artery disease)

Angina is recurrent chest pain that originates under the breastbone (sternum), often spreading to the neck, jaw, arms, and upper back. The nature of the pain varies, but it is usually described as a sensation of pressure, tightness, heaviness, or choking, and

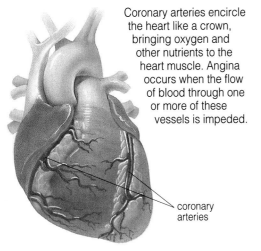

Coronary arteries encircle the heart like a crown, bringing oxygen and other nutrients to the heart muscle. Angina occurs when the flow of blood through one or more of these vessels is impeded.

coronary arteries

it is often accompanied by shortness of breath. Severe angina may feel like a heart attack, but it is a temporary condition that does not cause permanent damage. It does, however, signal an increased risk of a heart attack.

Angina occurs when the heart muscle is not getting enough oxygen. The most common cause is atherosclerosis, a narrowing of the coronary arteries due to deposits of fatty plaque. The narrowed arteries may be able to deliver enough oxygen-rich blood to the heart muscle to carry on normal activities. But when the heart must work harder, such as during unaccustomed physical exertion or periods of stress, the heart muscle becomes starved for oxygen, a condition called ischemia.

A heavy meal or exposure to cold may also precipitate angina because blood flow is diverted from the coronary arteries to other parts of the body.

Some people experience angina while resting or even sleeping. This unprovoked, or variant, angina is sometimes caused by a spasm in the coronary artery, usually at the site of fatty deposits. More often, it is classified as unstable angina, and is a warning sign of impending heart attack.

Diagnostic Studies and Procedures

There is no specific test for angina, but a doctor can usually tell whether or not the pain arises from the heart by asking three key questions: What provokes the discomfort? What is it like? And what alleviates it? Angina is suspected when there are other cardiovascular risk factors, such as cigarette use, a family history of early heart attacks, elevated blood pressure and cholesterol levels,

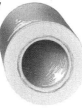

In a normal coronary artery, tiny muscles that surround the vessel cause it to widen or narrow, thereby controlling the amount of blood flowing through it.

Angina occurs when a buildup of fatty deposits (left) reduces blood flow and deprives the heart muscle of needed oxygen.

diabetes, and so forth. During a physical examination, the doctor listens carefully to the heart for any abnormal sounds or beats.

Routine tests include an electrocardiogram (ECG), blood pressure measurement, blood and urine tests, and a chest X-ray. If a doctor suspects angina, additional tests may be ordered to assess any underlying heart disease.

An exercise stress test can usually confirm that physical exertion brings on ischemia. This test is sometimes combined with echocardiography, an examination using high-frequency sound waves, or nuclear scanning, in which thallium or another radioactive substance is injected into the bloodstream and then tracked by special gamma cameras. These last two tests can often pinpoint the areas of heart muscle that are deprived of blood.

A more invasive procedure, cardiac catheterization, is needed to make a precise diagnosis of coronary artery disease. In this examination, a thin, flexible tube is inserted into an artery in the leg (or less commonly, the arm) and threaded to the heart. A dye is then injected into the coronary arteries to make them visible on X-rays.

Medical Treatments

There are numerous effective treatments for angina, ranging from exercise conditioning and medication to surgery. Depending upon the severity of symptoms and the degree of coronary disease, lifestyle changes and drugs are usually tried first, with surgery reserved for cases that cannot be controlled by more moderate approaches.

Exercise Conditioning. After an exercise stress test, a doctor prescribes a regimen of physical activity designed to increase endurance without provoking angina. Patients are taught to monitor their heart rate, and to increase their exercise gradually. This conditioning prompts the coronary arteries to build collateral circulation, increasing blood flow to segments of the heart muscle receiving inadequate blood.

Drug Therapy. There are numerous drugs that control or prevent angina. The choice depends on the circumstances and whether or not there are other contributing disorders, such as high blood pressure.

Two classes of drugs—nitrates and calcium channel blockers—open, or dilate, the arteries, allowing more blood to flow through them. This action lowers blood pressure, reduces the heart's workload, and increases blood flow to the heart muscle.

A third class of drugs, beta blockers, alleviates angina by reducing the action of norepinephrine, a neurotransmitter that carries signals from the sympathetic nervous system. Blocking these signals also reduces the heart's workload by allowing it to beat slower and less forcefully than usual.

Calcium channel blockers and beta blockers are taken daily to prevent angina; nitroglycerin—the most commonly prescribed nitrate—is used both to stop and prevent angina. During an attack, a nitroglycerin pill placed under the tongue or in the cheek pocket is absorbed rapidly into the bloodstream, usually providing relief within five minutes. The effect wears off quickly, however; for more sustained or preventive action, nitroglycerin is available as a skin patch or ointment. In these forms, the drug is slowly absorbed through the skin, thus providing protection from attacks.

A note of caution: Nitroglycerin can cause flushing, dizziness, and headache. Doctors advise sitting down when

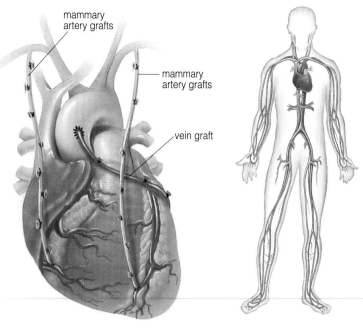
mammary artery grafts
mammary artery grafts
vein graft

During coronary bypass surgery, segments of healthy blood vessels are transplanted to the heart to carry blood around the areas of blockage. Some grafts are made with veins, usually taken from the legs. For others, portions of the mammary artery in the chest are moved to the heart.

ANGINA (CONTINUED)

taking the medication: This reduces dizziness and prevents fainting from a sudden drop in blood pressure.

Angioplasty. This is an invasive procedure designed to alleviate angina by physically opening up narrowed blood vessels. It is similar to cardiac catheterization, except that a catheter with a balloon tip is inserted into the coronary arteries while being followed on a fluoroscope monitor, a special type of moving X-ray. When the catheter reaches a narrowed segment, the balloon is inflated to flatten the plaque. In a new variation, a rotating blade similar to a tiny roto-rooter shaves the plaque into tiny particles, rather than simply flattening it out. In another, still experimental variation, a laser beam is used to vaporize the plaque.

Coronary Bypass Surgery. This operation is reserved for severe coronary disease that cannot be adequately controlled with drugs and is not amenable to angioplasty. Segments of healthy blood vessels, from either an artery in the chest wall or a vein in the leg, are used to bypass severely narrowed parts of the coronary arteries. Up to seven or even eight bypass grafts may be done in a single operation, greatly increasing blood flow to the heart muscle and reducing the incidence of angina and the risk of a heart attack.

The operation usually takes 3 or 4 hours, although some complicated cases require 8 to 10 hours. The patient then spends two or three days in an intensive care unit, and another five to seven days in the hospital. Even though the operation is relatively safe, it is not risk-free, and the potential dangers must be weighed against the benefits that are expected.

Alternative Therapies

Angina is always a serious warning sign, and any alternative therapy should be considered an adjunct to, not a substitute for, conventional medical treatments. A number of prominent researchers and cardiologists have been trying out combinations of conventional and alternative therapies, especially in preventive cardiology. Alternative approaches include:

Exercise Conditioning. This involves following a specific exercise regimen to improve cardiovascular function. The objective is to increase physical activity without provoking an attack of angina. After undergoing an exercise stress test to determine his maximum safe exercise level, the patient is given an exercise program calling for gradual increases in activity. With conditioning, the heart pumps more efficiently, and the body also uses oxygen more efficiently, reducing the heart's workload. Exercise also helps build collateral coronary arteries to increase blood flow to heart muscle.

Herbal Medicine. To treat angina, herbalists recommend hawthorn, sweet woodruff, and a number of other herbs that increase blood flow. They also advocate garlic to prevent angina by attacking its underlying causes, high blood cholesterol as well as high blood pressure. (An odorless garlic pill is available; whether or not it has the same benefits as fresh garlic has not yet been determined.)

A note of caution: Some highly toxic plants such as foxglove (digitalis) are used to make prescription heart medicines, but brewing your own drugs from them can be fatal.

Meditation and Yoga. These are among the relaxation techniques being used by researchers who are studying their potential in treating angina and coronary heart disease. The initial results indicate that for some patients, these alternative therapies reduce their need for drugs and surgery.

Nutrition Therapy. Its role in coronary disease is well established. Both alternative and conventional practitioners now advocate low-fat, high-fiber diets. The late Nathan Pritikin developed a very low-fat, mostly vegetarian diet for angina patients that has since been adopted by many mainstream physicians and nutritionists. Nutrition therapists may also recommend high doses of vitamin E, an antioxidant that is believed to lower levels of the harmful

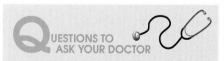

QUESTIONS TO ASK YOUR DOCTOR

▶ Is it safe for me to take a daily aspirin?
▶ What exercise guidelines should I follow? What warning signs indicate that I should stop?
▶ How can I tell the difference between angina and a heart attack?

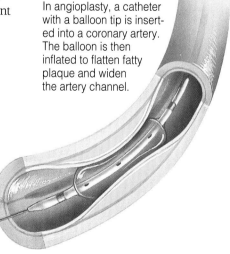
In angioplasty, a catheter with a balloon tip is inserted into a coronary artery. The balloon is then inflated to flatten fatty plaque and widen the artery channel.

Josh Sanford's angina began as an uncomfortable shortness of breath during strenuous exercise. At first, the 54-year-old college soccer coach attributed the difficulty in breathing to his age and the fact that he was trying to keep up with much younger players. Then during a practice session, he suddenly developed sharp chest pains that spread to his jaw.

"At first, I thought I was having a heart attack," he remembers. "But after I sat down for a few minutes, the pain went away. By the time practice was over, I felt fine again." Two days later, however, he suffered a similar bout of pain while running up a flight of stairs. Sanford decided it was time to see his doctor.

"I told him about my episodes of chest pain and he asked if I had other symptoms, such as shortness of breath. I hadn't connected the two until he explained that angina often takes the form of breathlessness."

Blood tests revealed that Sanford had very high cholesterol levels, and an exercise stress test confirmed that his symptoms were, indeed, due to angina. Next came coronary angiography, which showed marked blockages in two arteries.

"I had to make some hard decisions," Sanford recalls. "A cardiologist recommended balloon angioplasty, but I knew that its benefits were often temporary." He had been reading about Dr. Dean Ornish's program to treat heart disease with diet, exercise, and meditation. "I decided to give it a try, and it changed my life."

Sanford had always been active, so the exercise regimen was easy, not however, the low-fat vegetarian diet. "I was a meat and potatoes man," he says. "Now it's no meat, but lots of vegetables, grains, pasta, and fruit. I also learned the value of meditation. Instead of getting uptight and yelling during a match, I close my eyes, do some deep breathing, and stay calm."

Sanford has now gone for six months without an angina attack; and at his last checkup, his cholesterol levels were in the desirable range. "I carry nitroglycerin tablets just in case," he says, "but I don't expect ever to need them."

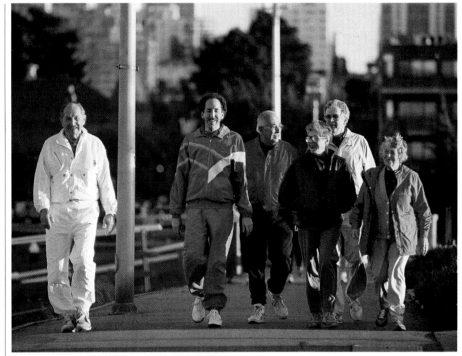

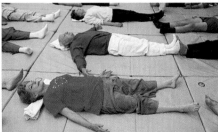

Dr. Dean Ornish (in turquoise in photo above) has developed an innovative heart disease treatment and prevention program in Sausalito, California, that combines a very low-fat diet, exercise, and relaxation therapies, such as meditation and yoga (left). He has demonstrated that patients who follow this regimen have been able to reduce their medication dosage, and some have also shown regression in the fatty deposits in their coronary arteries.

LDL cholesterol. Lecithin is also advocated, but its benefits are not as well documented as those of vitamin E.

Shiatsu. Practitioners of this Japanese massage therapy believe that pressing upon points in the inner forearm can alleviate an angina attack.

Self-Treatment

It is increasingly clear that a prudent lifestyle is central in both preventing and treating the underlying coronary disease that causes angina. Especially critical factors are not smoking, getting enough exercise, controlling stress, and eating a balanced low-fat diet that is also high in fiber and complex carbohydrates. Many doctors also recommend a daily aspirin to prevent a heart attack, but check with your doctor first — even low-dose aspirin is hazardous for people with uncontrolled high blood pressure, ulcers, and certain bleeding disorders.

The following are some specific self-help strategies for preventing angina:

▶ Eat four or five small meals, evenly spread throughout the day, rather than two or three large ones. After a heavy meal, blood is diverted to the digestive system, reducing flow to the heart and other muscles. Avoid exercise for at least one hour after eating.

▶ Go easy on alcohol. An occasional drink or two probably is not harmful, but excessive alcohol can damage the heart muscle.

▶ Avoid going out on cold, windy days. The cold constricts blood vessels and increases the chance of suffering an attack of angina.

Other Causes of Chest Pain

Indigestion, esophageal spasms, heartburn, and panic attacks are among the many noncardiac causes of chest pains. An overactive thyroid, or hyperthyroidism, can also cause irregular heartbeats and chest pain. Pericarditis, an inflammation of the sac surrounding the heart, should be ruled out, as should structural problems, such as a broken rib. Asthma, a collapsed lung, and other pulmonary disorders can also produce shortness of breath similar to that of angina.

Anxiety

(Generalized anxiety; hyperventilation; panic attacks)

Anxiety, often referred to as excessive nervousness, is a pervasive sense of apprehension. Sometimes the feeling is prompted by worry over an impending event, such as a school examination or medical test. This type of anxiety is a normal response to a specific circumstance. In contrast, generalized anxiety produces feelings of foreboding that stem from almost any uncertainty or even no apparent provocation. When carried to extremes, this type of anxiety leads to emotional exhaustion, sleeplessness, and an increased risk of stress-related illnesses.

Acute anxiety sometimes takes the form of a panic attack. This is an episode of intense fear accompanied by physical symptoms, such as chest pain, difficulty breathing, and a feeling of impending doom. Recent studies have indicated that panic attacks are likely to run in families, and they may begin in early adolescence.

Hyperventilation, or overbreathing, is common during a panic attack, and this rapid, shallow breathing upsets the balance of oxygen and carbon dioxide in the blood. This in turn leads to dizziness, palpitations, chest pain, and other unpleasant physical symptoms that are so distressing, they themselves engender fear and anxiety, resulting in a vicious cycle of increasingly frequent panic attacks. People with anxiety go to great lengths to avoid what they think are triggers. Many even fear venturing from the safety of their homes, a condition called agoraphobia (see Fears and Phobias, page 184).

Diagnostic Studies and Procedures

Some people who experience chronic anxiety fail to relate their physical symptoms to their emotional apprehensions. These people may go from doctor to doctor trying to find causes for troubling symptoms—back pain, frequent headaches, muscle and joint aches, indigestion, and diarrhea. Typically, a physical examination and medical tests fail to find an organic cause for all the problems. At this point, a physician may suspect anxiety as the underlying cause and suggest that the patient consult a psychiatrist or other mental health professional for diagnosis and treatment.

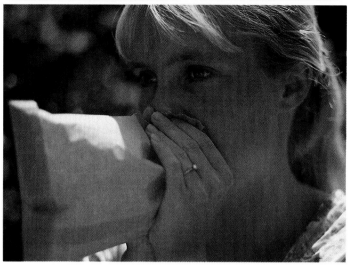

Overbreathing during a panic attack decreases the carbon dioxide content of the blood, causing palpitations, dizziness, and other frightening symptoms. Breathing into a paper bag helps restore the normal balance of oxygen and carbon dioxide, thus alleviating the symptoms.

Panic attacks are easier to diagnose than generalized anxiety. Typically, they are sudden and unprovoked and last for only 5 to 10 minutes, although they may seem much longer to the sufferer. According to the diagnostic guidelines of the American Psychiatric Association, a panic attack is characterized by the presence of at least four of the following signs and symptoms:

▸ Shortness of breath.
▸ Dizziness, unsteadiness, or faintness.
▸ Palpitations.
▸ Trembling and shaking.
▸ Profuse sweating.
▸ Chest pains or discomfort.
▸ Nausea and abdominal distress.
▸ Gagging or a choking sensation.
▸ Hot and cold flashes.
▸ Numbness or tingling sensations in the hands or feet.
▸ Dizziness or vertigo.
▸ Fear of losing control.
▸ Intense fear of dying.

Medical Treatments

The two approaches to treatment, medication and psychological counseling, are often combined.

Drug Therapy. Antianxiety drugs, or tranquilizers, are the major medical treatments for both generalized anxiety and panic attacks. A class of drugs,

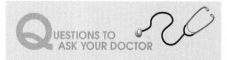

QUESTIONS TO ASK YOUR DOCTOR

▸ Do any of the drugs I'm taking produce symptoms of anxiety?
▸ How long can I take antianxiety drugs without becoming addicted?

known as benzodiazepines and marketed as Librium, Valium, Ativan, and Xanax, are the most widely prescribed antianxiety medications. These drugs appear to work by increasing the action of a brain chemical that blocks the transmission of nerve impulses in the brain, thus reducing the feelings of jittery nerves and restlessness. In the process, they can cause drowsiness and lethargy. They also heighten the effects of alcohol, sometimes dangerously so, because the combination can lead to respiratory arrest and death.

After three months of benzodiazepine treatment, 90 percent of panic-attack patients show marked improvement and 50 percent are entirely free of them.

Although tranquilizers are highly effective in easing anxiety and overcoming panic attacks, they should not be used for an extended period of time—usually defined as more than 12 consecutive weeks—because continued use can lead to psychological dependence and addiction. However, anyone who has been taking tranquilizers regularly for several months should not stop them abruptly. Instead a doctor's guidance should be sought for gradually dispensing with them.

Less addictive drugs are sometimes prescribed instead of tranquilizers. Among them, beta blockers—normally used to treat high blood pressure and angina—are effective against specific kinds of anxiety, especially stage fright. These medications ease feelings of anxiety by blocking the action of norepinephrine, or noradrenaline, a neurotransmitter that the body produces in response to stress.

A CASE IN POINT

Mindy Markowitz, a 25-year-old art director, started suffering panic attacks at the age of 17. At the time, she was editor of her high school yearbook, applying to college, and breaking up with her boyfriend. The attacks would begin with a sudden, intense wave of "horrible fear" that came out of nowhere, sometimes during the day, sometimes waking her from sleep at night.

She also experienced palpitations, nausea, trembling, a sensation of choking, and profuse sweating, but because she felt perfectly healthy when she was not having an attack, she did not seek medical treatment. Instead, she dealt with the occurrences by "just sitting quietly" until the symptoms subsided.

Over the next few years, she sometimes went for several months without any attacks, only to have them return as severe as ever. But she refused to let them interfere with her school or work, even though they sometimes left her feeling exhausted. After she took a new job, however, the attacks came with increasing frequency, sometimes two or three times a day. She finally sought medical help after reading about a clinic for victims of panic attacks.

Markowitz's physical symptoms indicated that her attacks were originating in the autonomic nervous system and were probably triggered by a surge in adrenal hormones, which are released in response to stress. The clinic psychiatrist prescribed a short course of Valium to interrupt the frequency of attacks. He also urged Markowitz to enter group therapy with several other people who were suffering from similar episodes.

At one of the sessions, a fellow patient described how biofeedback training had helped him control his attacks without having to take medication. Markowitz decided to give it a try, and enrolled in the clinic's biofeedback training program. Within six weeks, she, too, was off medication and enjoying freedom from panic attacks.

"Now if I feel a rush of fear," she explains, "I put my biofeedback training to work to slow down my heartbeat and regain a sense of calmness."

In the past, meprobamate (Equanil or Miltown), a tranquilizer, and phenobarbital, a barbiturate, were used to treat anxiety. They are rarely prescribed for this purpose today because of their addictiveness and potential for abuse.

Psychotherapy. Psychiatrists and other mental health professionals usually recommend some form of psychotherapy in addition to tranquilizers. Treatment may range from long-term one-on-one psychotherapy to short-term cognitive therapy. During the latter, patients are helped to correct distorted ways of thinking about themselves and their fears. Through cognitive therapy, for example, a person can control panic attacks by learning to interpret and calmly handle the alarming symptoms rather than overreacting to them, which usually intensifies the problem.

Another approach is to enter group therapy, in which patients share common fears and seek workable ways of dealing with them.

Alternative Therapies

Alternative therapies that emphasize relaxation techniques are often incorporated into conventional medical treatment for anxiety and panic attacks. The breathing exercises of relaxation methods are especially helpful in preventing or stopping hyperventilation. Specific therapies may include:

Biofeedback. Patients learn how to control overbreathing and other physical responses that trigger or worsen panic attacks. Certain techniques can then be applied in situations that are likely to provoke an episode.

Herbal Medicine. Caffeine-free herbal teas can help calm jittery nerves. In addition, some herbs contain chemicals that can offset the common effects of anxiety. For example, betony can lower blood pressure, and lemon balm, mint, and valerian can counter insomnia.

Hypnosis and Visualization. These are especially useful in controlling panic attacks. During a few sessions with a hypnotist, a person can learn to quell anxious feelings by combining deep breathing exercises with meditation or visualization of a particular setting or situation. Methods of self-hypnosis can also be learned by using an audio tape or home course.

Massage. Few activities are more conducive to releasing stress than a massage, either from a professional therapist or someone close to you.

The use of aromatic oils or lotions makes this therapy even more relaxing.

Music Therapy. Listening to music is a time-honored method of relaxation. To alleviate anxiety, music therapists recommend soothing classical music rather than loud, percussive types. Music associated with a happy event or time period can also be beneficial.

Yoga and T'ai Chi. These movement therapies are directed to achieving emotional well-being by balancing mental and physical energies. Yoga is especially helpful in developing the ability to breathe deeply and slowly and thus avoid hyperventilation. Consult a professional instructor to learn specific postures or techniques that are particularly suited to overcoming anxiety.

Self-Treatment

Setting aside at least 30 minutes each day for quiet, private time does wonders in dissipating anxiety. Try using this time to meditate, do yoga or t'ai chi, or listen to music. Or simply clear your mind of pressing obligations by reading, exercising, or engaging in some other pleasurable activity. Additional self-help measures include:

Breathing Exercises. Hyperventilation can be controlled by breathing into and out of a paper or plastic bag. This forces you to reinhale some of the carbon dioxide that is exhaled during rapid, shallow breathing. At other times, practice slow, deep breathing, inhaling through your nose and slowly exhaling through your mouth.

Exercise. Daily aerobic exercise contributes to both physical and emotional health. Choose a noncompetitive activity such as swimming, biking, or walking.

Stimulants. Overuse of caffeine, nicotine, and other stimulants contributes to feelings of anxiety. Switch to decaffeinated beverages and, if you smoke, make every effort to stop.

Diet. Some people find that certain foods promote feelings of anxiety. This may be an allergic reaction or an exaggerated response to a food additive. Keep a food diary, and try to eliminate items that provoke symptoms.

Other Causes of Anxiety

Alcohol abuse, excessive caffeine, or the use of diet pills, steroids, and certain other medications can produce feelings of anxiety. For many women, anxiety is part of the premenstrual syndrome. An overactive thyroid gland can also provoke jitteriness.

Appendicitis

The appendix is a small, pouch-shaped organ located in the lower right side of the abdomen, where the small intestine empties into the colon. In humans, the appendix has no known function, and generally does not cause problems unless it becomes inflamed, enlarged, and filled with pus—a condition referred to as appendicitis.

Although appendicitis can occur at any age, it is most common between the years of 10 and 30, and is rare before the age of 2. Appendicitis begins usually with a feeling of general malaise and pain near the navel. This pain quickly intensifies and becomes con-

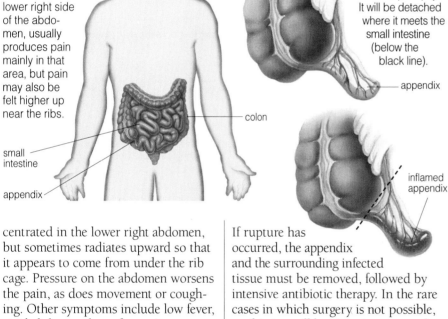

Inflammation in the appendix, situated on the lower right side of the abdomen, usually produces pain mainly in that area, but pain may also be felt higher up near the ribs.

small intestine

appendix

colon

When an appendix is inflamed, it must be removed promptly. It will be detached where it meets the small intestine (below the black line).

appendix

inflamed appendix

centrated in the lower right abdomen, but sometimes radiates upward so that it appears to come from under the rib cage. Pressure on the abdomen worsens the pain, as does movement or coughing. Other symptoms include low fever, rigid abdomen, loss of appetite, nausea, vomiting, constipation, or, more rarely, diarrhea. Lying on the left side with the legs drawn up in a fetal position often brings some temporary relief.

Diagnostic Studies and Procedures

A doctor will press, or palpate, the abdomen, feeling for the rigidity that is typical. Blood tests showing an elevated white cell count, a common indication of any infection, coupled with the other characteristic symptoms will raise a suspicion of appendicitis.

There are no specific diagnostic tests for the problem but an ultrasound examination often shows that the appendix is enlarged. If the diagnosis is still uncertain after a physical exami-

nation and ultrasound, laparotomy may be ordered, particularly in women, because the symptoms may indicate an ovarian cyst or other gynecologic disorder. In this procedure, a viewing tube is inserted into a small incision near the navel, allowing a doctor to examine the abdominal organs.

Medical Treatments

An operation to remove the appendix, called an appendectomy, will be done immediately; it is the only treatment for acute appendicitis. Prompt surgery is important to prevent rupture and spreading of the infection.

A ruptured appendix invariably leads to peritonitis, a serious infection of the lining around the abdominal cavity.

If rupture has occurred, the appendix and the surrounding infected tissue must be removed, followed by intensive antibiotic therapy. In the rare cases in which surgery is not possible, antibiotics will be given intravenously.

An uncomplicated appendectomy takes about an hour to perform. Most patients are released from the hospital in 5 or 6 days, and recover fully within a week to 10 days.

Alternative Therapies

While there is no substitute for surgical treatment, such relaxation techniques as meditation, visualization, and self-hypnosis can reduce postoperative pain. Other approaches include:

Acupuncture. In China, acupuncture substitutes for painkillers following an appendectomy and some other types of surgery. When James Reston, a New York Times columnist, developed appendicitis during a trip to China,

local anesthesia was used for the operation and acupuncture to alleviate postoperative pain. His subsequent reports on the effectiveness of this approach spurred interest in the United States for using this technique to alleviate pain.

Music Therapy. Listening to music dulls the perception of pain, perhaps by increasing the brain's production of endorphins—the body's natural painkillers. Studies show that surgery patients who listen to music often can reduce their need for painkillers.

Nutrition Therapy. Some nutritionists and doctors believe that eating high-fiber foods, such as whole-grain cereals and breads, fresh fruit, and vegetables, may help prevent appendicitis.

Self-Treatment

There is no self-treatment for acute appendicitis; your best course is to seek medical treatment as quickly as you can. Go to the nearest emergency room if you are unable to reach your own doctor. If you cannot get to a hospital immediately, apply ice packs and stay as quiet as possible.

Constipation is common with this condition, but you should never take a laxative if the symptoms suggest the possibility of appendicitis because it can cause the appendix to rupture.

While recovering from an appendectomy, an ice pack applied to the area of the incision numbs the pain. After the stitches or surgical staples have been removed, application of vitamin E oil or cream to the incision may promote healing and help to reduce scarring. Generally, physicians advise against lifting any heavy objects for at least six weeks, as such activity can put undue stress on the incision and slow the healing process.

Other Causes of Abdominal Pain

Other disorders that produce pain like that of appendicitis include pelvic inflammatory disease, tubal pregnancy, a ruptured ovarian cyst, Crohn's disease, and other intestinal disorders.

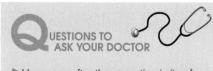

QUESTIONS TO ASK YOUR DOCTOR

▶ How soon after the operation is it safe to resume my exercise routine?
▶ When can I return to work?
▶ When can I drive?

Arthritis

(Rheumatic diseases)

Arthritis is the medical term for any disease that produces inflammation, pain, and stiffness in one or more joints. There are more than 100 different types, all of which are classified as rheumatic diseases.

Arthritis develops when cartilage, the tough, slippery material covering the ends of bones, is destroyed faster than the body can repair it. Aging, excessive wear and tear, infection, and inflammation contribute to the process. As the cartilage roughens and wears down, the ends of the bones become increasingly exposed and eventually damaged.

Osteoarthritis, also called degenerative joint disease, is the most common type. It is caused by natural deterioration from aging, as well as injuries to and overuse of joints in sports or work. Other contributing factors include an inherited predisposition, excessive weight, and skeletal abnormalities.

Rheumatoid arthritis is one of the most serious forms. It is systemic and can affect the blood vessels, heart, and other organs in addition to joints. Though the cause is unknown, most researchers consider it an autoimmune disorder, in which the immune system attacks the body. Its course is unpredictable, but most people experience remissions in which the disease is quiescent, interrupted by flare-ups that cause progressive, irreversible damage.

Some types of arthritis are caused by infection, including such sexually transmitted diseases as gonorrhea and Reiter's syndrome. Auto-immune diseases such as lupus (page 278) often involve an immune-system attack on joints. Still other types, such as gout, are due to metabolic defects, which are often hereditary.

Diagnostic Studies and Procedures

A diagnosis of osteoarthritis is based on symptoms, X-ray results, and the extent of pain and loss of mobility found in studies of joint movements. Rheumatoid arthritis is confirmed by an additional finding of the rheumatoid factor, an abnormal antibody, in the blood and joint (synovial) fluid. Rheumatoid factor shows up in about 80 percent of patients with this condition, although several tests, taken at different times,

may be needed to detect it. Infectious forms of arthritis usually can be diagnosed by the presence of bacteria or other organisms in joint fluid.

Medical Treatments

An approach that combines medication, exercise, and rest is basic to treating most forms of arthritis, with physical or rehabilitative medicine and alternative therapies as important adjuncts. For more serious types, such as rheumatoid arthritis and lupus, treatment should be coordinated by a rheumatologist, a specialist in these disorders.

Drug Therapy. Arthritis medications suppress inflammation and alleviate pain, but several drugs and dosages may have to be tried to achieve the best results with the least adverse side effects. The two main categories are nonsteroidal anti-inflammatory drugs (known as NSAIDs) and corticosteroids. Of the NSAIDs, aspirin remains the drug of choice for those who can tolerate it in large therapeutic doses of 16 or more tablets a day. Other NSAIDs include: ibuprofen, which is sold in both non-prescription and prescription dosages; and stronger prescription drugs, such as indomethacin (Indocin), ketoprofen (Orudis), naproxen (Naprosyn), piroxicam (Feldene), and sulindac (Clinoril).

Osteoarthritis that is free of inflammation can be treated with the nonprescription painkiller acetaminophen. Otherwise, the NSAIDs used for rheumatoid arthritis are prescribed.

The corticosteroids are synthetic versions of cortisone, one of the adrenal hormones. These are powerful drugs

intended for short-term use and are reserved for cases that cannot be controlled adequately by NSAIDs. Cortisone injected directly into the affected joints reduces adverse reactions, but even so, overuse can reduce resistance to infections, weaken bones, and cause other serious side effects.

Drugs prescribed for severe rheumatoid arthritis that is not helped by other medications include chloroquine (Aralen), usually employed for malaria, and cyclophosphamide (Cytoxan) and methotrexate, agents that suppress the immune system. Penicillamine (Cuprimine and Depen), a chelating agent normally used to remove copper and other metals from the body, appears to remove rheumatoid factor also; the possible result is a remission of arthritis.

Compounds of gold salts, usually injected, can produce remission of rheumatoid arthritis also, but how or why they work is unknown. Patients receiving all such medications must be closely monitored for adverse effects.

Pain-Control Devices. The use of TENS, short for transcutaneous electrical nerve stimulation, sometimes reduces the need for painkillers. TENS electrodes are placed on the skin at specific trigger points, where they stimulate nerves that block pain signals. TENS battery operated devices are available at surgical or medical supply stores, but a doctor or physical therapist should provide instruction on using them properly.

Surgical Treatments. With surgical advances in arthroplasty—the repair or replacement of joints—mobility can

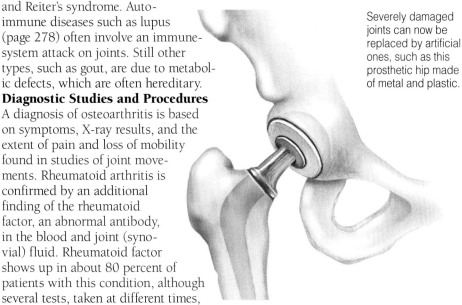

Severely damaged joints can now be replaced by artificial ones, such as this prosthetic hip made of metal and plastic.

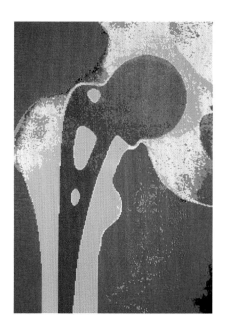

ARTHRITIS (CONTINUED)

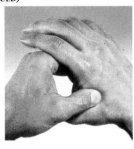

To alleviate pain in finger joints, press into the webbing between the fore-finger and thumb. Keep hand relaxed and maintain the pressure for 1 to 2 minutes. Repeat as needed.

now be restored to many severely disabled arthritis patients. It is possible to restructure certain joints, such as those in the feet and wrists, using grafted cartilage and other tissue, and to replace badly diseased hips, knees, shoulders, and fingers with artificial ones made of metal and plastic.

Microsurgery employing arthroscopy, a tube with fiberoptic magnifying devices, has further revolutionized joint surgery. An arthroscope is inserted into the joint through a small incision, and a magnified view of interior tissues is projected on a television screen. While viewing the screen, the surgeon manipulates tiny instruments inside the arthroscope to repair the joint.

Other surgical procedures include osteotomy, in which a bone is cut and then reset to improve alignment, and synovectomy, in which portions of the diseased synovial membrane—the sac surrounding the joint—are removed.

Alternative Therapies

Many alternatives, included as part of arthritis treatment, can help to relieve pain. A word of caution, however: Most forms of arthritis are incurable and arthritis quackery is common. Be wary of any healers who promise a cure.

Acupuncture. Pain relief is the major benefit of acupuncture, although some practitioners claim that their treatments reduce inflammation and induce remissions of rheumatoid arthritis. Since spontaneous remissions are common in this disease, it is impossible to attribute them to any particular therapy.

Chiropractic. Spinal manipulation and massage temporarily alleviate the stiffness and pain of some types of arthritis, but a chiropractor should not be considered a substitute for a rheumatologist.

Herbal Medicine. To promote bone repair and cartilage elasticity, herbalists recommend comfrey. As natural anti-inflammatories, they advocate devil's claw, licorice, wild yam, willow bark, and yucca. Because tension and stress can trigger an arthritis flare-up, herbal teas are advised as substitutes for beverages that contain caffeine.

Hydrotherapy. Water therapies, including underwater exercise, hot and cold wet packs, and powerful directional showers, can improve circulation, help retain joint mobility, and possibly slow tissue deterioration and fusing of joints.

Massage Therapy. Massage can relax stiff joints but it cannot restore lost function and mobility.

Nutrition Therapy and Megavitamins. There is renewed medical interest in the effects of high-dose vitamin supplements and trace minerals on rheumatic diseases. Even so, there still are no nutritional cures for arthritis. Before taking high-dose vitamins, consult a doctor or qualified nutritionist; some supplements interact with arthritis medications and others, such as high-dose vitamin A, are potentially toxic.

Yoga and T'ai Chi. These and other gentle routines such as dance therapy utilize body movements and postures that reduce physical stress. Combined

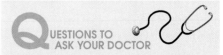

with meditation and breathing exercises, these movement therapies also help to strengthen muscles around joints, promote flexibility, and manage pain.

Self-Treatment

Self-care plays a critical role. Only an individual can judge the best balance of rest and exercise, heat and cold, and medication adjustments.

Rest. Fatigue exacerbates arthritis; even mild tiredness is an important warning that your body needs rest. Rest individual joints as needed by using a cane, for example, to relieve stress on hips and knees, orthotic devices in footwear to ease stress on ankles and feet, and splints to support wrists and hands. Strive for a balance when using splints, however, because excessive immobilization can result in a frozen joint.

Exercise. Putting all arthritic joints through a daily range-of-motion routine minimizes stiffness and retains joint function. Special resistance exercises promote muscle strength, and also help maintain mobility. A physical therapist or rehabilitative specialist can recommend the best exercises.

Special Accommodations. Review your daily routine and rearrange access to key elements, such as clothing and kitchen supplies, to minimize uncomfortable or difficult movements. There are also numerous aids, such as special eating utensils, jar openers, raised toilet seats, combs and toothbrushes, among others, to make routine tasks easier.

Weight Control. Excessive weight increases stress on joints, and speeds up the destructive course of arthritis. Consult a nutritionist to work out a sensible weight-loss diet.

Other Causes of Joint Disease

Infections, including Lyme disease, rheumatic fever, and gonorrhea, should be ruled out when diagnosing arthritis.

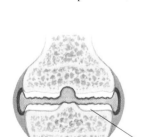

In a normal joint, cartilage cushions the ends of the bones.

cartilage

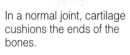

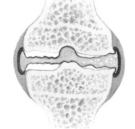

When inflammation develops around a joint, the cartilage begins to erode. Researchers don't fully understood the destructive process, but they do know that antibodies trigger the inflammation.

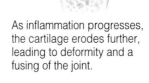

As inflammation progresses, the cartilage erodes further, leading to deformity and a fusing of the joint.

Asthma

(Bronchial asthma; reversible hyperreactive lung disease)

Asthma is a chronic disease in which the air passages, or bronchi, overact to normally harmless substances or circumstances. When these triggering

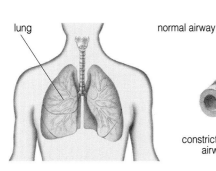

An asthma attack occurs when muscles controlling the small airways in the lungs constrict, making it more difficult for air to flow in and out of the airsacs. The airways then become inflamed and clogged with mucus.

factors enter the bronchi, the airways constrict to hinder the flow of air in and out of the lungs. Very soon, the bronchi become inflamed, and the membranes lining them secrete a sticky mucus. The result is wheezing, coughing, and difficulty in breathing. A severe attack can be life-threatening.

Asthma triggers vary from person to person; some of the most common are allergens such as pollen, animal dander, and house dust; irritants such as air pollution, tobacco smoke, perfumes, and chemicals; cold air; certain foods and food additives; aspirin and related medications; anxiety and stress; and vigorous exercise.

No one knows why some people develop hyperreactive lungs, although an inherited predisposition appears to play a role. Many people think that emotional problems are a major cause, but researchers have discounted this. Asthma is a difficult disease that may lead to emotional problems, and stress can sometimes provoke a flare-up, but it is not itself a psychological disorder. Although asthma differs from an allergic reaction, allergies are often involved and can also trigger attacks.

Most common in children, asthma often subsides during adolescence, but never fully disappears. It is not unusual for adults to suffer a recurrence after

going years without a flare-up. This return often as not comes on the heels of a respiratory infection.

Diagnostic Studies and Procedures

Wheezing and other symptoms may point to asthma, but lung function tests will still be necessary to distinguish it from other disorders. Testing begins with spirometry to measure the amount of air that is breathed in and out of lungs under different circumstances. Spirometry is sometimes combined with challenge testing to identify the specific asthma triggers and to measure the effectiveness of medications. In a challenge test, the patient is exposed to a suspected trigger and its effect is then measured by spirometry.

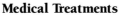

Medical Treatments

Doctors approach asthma treatment with two major goals: to prevent attacks and to reverse any flare-up as quickly as possible. Prevention entails teaching patients how to control their disorder with drugs, lifestyle changes, and, increasingly, alternative therapies.

Asthma patients are also taught to use a peak-flow meter, a simple handheld device that measures the amount of air that can be exhaled after taking a deep breath. A drop in the normal peak-flow reading points to an imminent attack; an increase indicates that therapy is working. Prompt treatment with bronchodilator drugs to open the airways during an asthma attack can usually stop it before it becomes an emergency. The most common prescription medications for asthma are:

Beta-2 Agonists. These drugs, most of which both prevent and stop attacks, are the most widely used asthma medications in the United States. Included are albuterol (Proventil and Ventolin), isoetharine (Bronkometer), metaproterenol (Alupent and Metaprel), and terbutaline (Brethine). Available in pill, liquid, and aerosol forms, they work by relaxing the muscles that control the airways. They also reduce the flow of

mucus by inhibiting histamine production, and help to clear mucus from the lungs. Their side effects include shakiness, tremor, and an increased heart rate; long-term use can cause anxiety and restlessness.

Another drug in this class, epinephrine (Adrenalin), is inhaled or injected, and works faster and more forcefully than other beta-2 agonists. It is usually reserved for severe attacks that are not controlled by the other medications.

Xanthines. This category includes aminophylline (Mudrane), oxtriphylline (Choledyl), theophylline (Slo-Bid, Theo-Dur, and others), and dyphylline (Dilor and Lufyllin). These drugs, which are chemically related to caffeine, relax and open the airways, allowing more air to flow. They also make the heart beat faster and stimulate breathing. Difficulty in finding the right dosage is their major drawback, because the margin between a safe, effective blood level and a dangerously high one is very narrow. Theophyllines work best when they are taken daily, thereby maintaining a constant level of the drug in the bloodstream.

Adverse reactions to a small overdose include agitation, headache, nausea, abdominal cramps, and palpitations. A larger overdose can cause serious irregular heartbeats and convulsions. Once a safe dosage is found, however, the drugs are highly effective.

Adrenocorticoids. These drugs are related to steroid hormones produced by the adrenal glands. Aerosol steroids include beclomethasone (Vanceril and Beclovent), flunisolide (AeroBid), and triamcinolone (Azmacort); the most common oral and injected form is prednisone. Steroids are potent anti-inflammatory medications that are highly effective in treating severe asthma. Experts recommend that they be used in high doses for a short period of time to stop a sustained flare-up. Their long-term use is limited by their side effects, which include lowered immunity, bone loss, weight gain, and mood swings and other mental changes.

Because they can cause growth problems and other long-term adverse side effects, their use in children is limited to severe asthma that cannot be controlled by other medications.

Cromolyn Sodium. This inhaled antihistamine, marketed as Intal, is highly effective in preventing asthma, but it

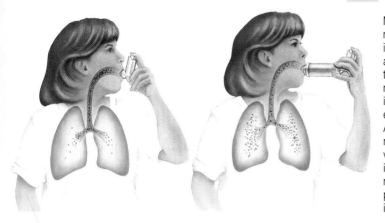

Most asthma medications come in aerosol form, administered through a metered-dose inhaler (left) or extender (right). An extender, or nebulizer, converts liquid medication to a fine mist, allowing it to penetrate deeper into the lungs.

ASTHMA (CONTINUED)

does not help during an actual attack. It is especially beneficial in preventing asthma that is triggered by allergens, exercise, and environmental chemicals or pollutants. It may be taken just before exercising or, if appropriate, used several times a day. Because some people briefly experience coughing or breathlessness immediately after inhaling cromolyn sodium, it can worsen an asthma attack. Otherwise, it is a safe drug with minimal side effects.

Alternative Therapies

Despite favorable anecdotal accounts, it has not been proven that acupuncture, chiropractic, reflexology, and other manipulative techniques are of much help against asthma. Also, the Bach flower remedies and other forms of aromatherapy may actually trigger an attack in asthmatics who are sensitive to perfumes. In contrast, alternative approaches that emphasize breathing exercises and relaxation, or that help to increase physical endurance are important adjuncts to medical treatment, especially if they reduce the need for steroids and other powerful drugs.

Alexander Technique. By using this training to improve posture and learn proper breathing methods, asthma patients are often able to increase their control over the disease.

Biofeedback, Hypnosis, and Visualization. These techniques help asthmatics gain a measure of control over breathing and other normally involuntary functions. When practiced during the early, or prodrome, stages of an attack, they may even abort it.

Homeopathy. Practitioners recommend a number of substances, including aconite, arsenicum album, and phosphorus. If a flare-up does not improve within a few minutes, however, a conventional drug should be used.

Hydrotherapy. Swimming is one of the best exercises for asthma because it improves endurance and increases lung capacity in an environment free of dust and other asthma triggers. Taking a hot shower or relaxing in a warm tub of water are also beneficial; the warmth eases tensions and the moist air helps clear the lungs of mucus.

Massage. This provides an excellent means of countering stress. Massage combined with postural drainage— a percussive tapping of the back while the head is lower than chest (see page 151)—clears mucus from the lungs.

Meditation and Yoga. These and other relaxation therapies are useful in overcoming the stress that often precipitates an asthma flare-up. They can also lessen the stress and panicky feeling that can exacerbate an attack.

Nutrition Therapy. Many foods and food additives, especially sulfites, will trigger asthma in susceptible people. A nutrition therapist can help identify such foods, and structure a balanced diet that eliminates them. One should avoid, however, an overly restricted diet that does not provide adequate nutrition. Some high-dose supplements,

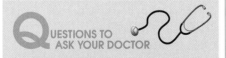

Q**UESTIONS TO ASK YOUR DOCTOR**

▶ Should I use a nebulizer to take inhaled medications?
▶ What are the possible side effects of my asthma drugs? Do they interact with any other drugs or foods?
▶ How does pregnancy affect asthma? What are the chances that my child will also have asthma?
▶ Would changing jobs or moving to a new locale help?

especially beta carotene, vitamins C and E, and magnesium, are touted as being beneficial for asthma sufferers, but they should not be taken without the guidance of a doctor or nutritionist.

Self-Treatment

Careful self-treatment is the key to keeping asthma under control. First and foremost, identify what sets off an attack and then make every effort to avoid it. If a triggering factor cannot be avoided, take a preventive drug such as cromolyn sodium. Other important self-care measures include:

▶ Take asthma medications correctly. To allow inhaled drugs to penetrate to the smallest airways, thereby increasing their effectiveness, use a nebulizer, or extender, instead of a metered-dose inhaler, or whiffer. Check with your doctor if you are uncertain as to how or when to take medication.
▶ Practice daily postural drainage to help loosen and remove mucus from your breathing passages.
▶ Contact your doctor immediately if you catch a cold or other respiratory infection. Increasing preventive medication at this time can help ward off a severe flare-up.
▶ Do not smoke, and don't allow anyone to smoke in your home, office, car, or other surroundings.
▶ Keep a diary of symptoms that signal an impending attack (for example, unproductive coughing, apprehension, rapid breathing). When you sense one coming on, do breathing exercises, perhaps combined with meditation or visualization, to overcome it. Also drink a glass of water; this keeps mucus thin and flowing, rather than thick and sticky. If necessary, take a preventive dose of medication.
▶ Avoid inhaling cold air. If you have to go out when it's cold, cover your face and inhale through your nose.
▶ Stay indoors when air pollution or pollen counts are high. If you must go outdoors, wear a protective face mask.

Other Causes of Difficult Breathing

Panic attacks may produce wheezing and a choking sensation similar to those of asthma. In children, chronic adenoid and sinus infections can be mistaken for asthma, as can cystic fibrosis. Among adults, congestive heart failure and a number of chronic lung disorders, such as emphysema, chronic bronchitis, and bronchiectasis should also be ruled out.

Autism

(Infantile autism; pervasive developmental disorder)

Autism is a complex syndrome of childhood in which intellectual growth is uneven and social development is impaired. Common characteristics include unresponsiveness, inability to speak or communicate and understand, refusal to seek or accept physical comforting, and an unusual insistence upon routines. For example, autistic children often make repetitive body movements, and even the most trivial change in their physical environment or routine can provoke rage or extreme anxiety. Some autistic children mimic sounds or develop intelligible speech patterns, and some are mute. About 20 to 40 percent have seizures.

The cause of autism is unknown, but it is classified as a neurophysiologic disorder. Parental behavior has no bearing on it, though some cases have been linked to rubella contracted before birth, hereditary metabolic disorders, encephalitis, and meningitis. Sometimes autism develops in children who have appeared to be normal, but then inexplicably regress. Autistic boys outnumber girls at least two to one.

A number of autistic children appear to have low IQs, others are normal, and a few are extremely intelligent but cannot adjust socially. Occasionally, an autistic child will have unusual talent in math or art.

Diagnostic Studies and Procedures

Although babies may demonstrate some symptoms of autism, the problem usually is not diagnosed until about age three when it becomes clear that the child's speech is delayed or abnormal. Diagnosis requires a careful physical and neurologic examination to rule out other causes. A specialist in childhood developmental disorders may administer psychological tests, but testing is difficult if the child does not yet speak or is intellectually impaired.

Medical Treatments

Because there is no cure for autism, treatment focuses on trying to help a child develop language and social skills. This usually entails a combination of speech and behavioral therapy, special education, and in some cases, medication. Antipsychotic drugs are sometimes prescribed for children who are aggressive or self-destructive.

Anticonvulsant medications such as carbamazepine (Tegretol) or phenobarbital (Bellatal, Donnatal, and others) are given to children who suffer seizures.

Since autism involves so many variables, each child must be evaluated individually to develop the most appropriate treatment program. Children with near-normal or normal IQs are often helped by psychotherapy, with emphasis on behavior modification designed to foster social skills. Some autistic children do well living at home; others improve while living in a closely supervised treatment facility with other learning disabled children.

Alternative Therapies

In recent years, a few alternative therapies have been used experimentally with autistic children, often producing marked improvement. These include:

Art Therapy. Therapists working with autistic children encourage them to use a variety of materials—clay, crayons, paints, and cutouts, for example. The goal is to help them express themselves while overcoming ritualistic behavior.

Dance and Music Therapy. These modalities are used separately or in combination. Group dance and music therapy fosters social interaction while breaking ritualistic patterns. Music may also be used to calm agitated or aggressive behavior; in some cases, it also provides a means of self-expression.

Pet Therapy. This is a relatively new approach that has met with considerable success. In an experimental program in Florida, autistic and other developmentally impaired children have been learning to swim and interact with dolphins. Another program on Long Island in New York has been using cats to encourage autistic children to connect with other living creatures. Researchers report that such approaches seem to take many children out of their solitude, boost their learning skills, and increase their interrelationships with people.

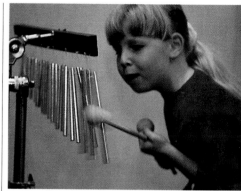

Music therapy has become an important component in the quest to help autistic children find a means of self-expression.

Self-Treatment

About 15 percent of autistic children eventually become self-sufficient, although most continue to require a sheltered environment. Otherwise, autism demands life-long care, a task that is trying, even under the best circumstances. Because the strain often leads to depression, anger, and guilt among parents and siblings, it's important for them to work with qualified mental health professionals. Recommended home treatment includes:

Teaching Verbal Skills. This should be done in brief, one-on-one sessions in which the child is encouraged to communicate verbally. Because autistic children learn by rote, a single word or concept must be repeated many times in the same way. Children who cannot speak are taught to communicate through body language, art, or other creative therapies. Special education programs that use computers to foster communication skills also appear to be promising.

Teaching Social Skills. Parents can apply many of the tactics used by professionals to encourage an autistic child to break out of self-imposed isolation. Plan activities that are simple and unthreatening, such as listening to music or dancing together. In all activities, go slowly, breaking each task or skill into small steps.

Other Causes of Autistic Symptoms

Before diagnosing autism, doctors should rule out a thyroid hormone deficiency, deafness, an organic brain disease such as encephalitis, and such metabolic disorders as phenylketonuria, or PKU. Sometimes child abuse and post-traumatic stress syndrome can also produce symptoms similar to those of autism.

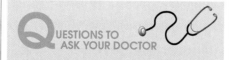

QUESTIONS TO ASK YOUR DOCTOR

▶ Would my child do better in a residential care facility?
▶ If medication has been prescribed, what are the side effects? Will these drugs affect normal growth?

Back Pain

(Backache; back strain; piriformis syndrome; sciatica)

At least 80 percent of all Americans suffer an occasional backache, and for 15 percent, the problem is chronic. The majority of backaches originate in the lumbar spine, between the waist and tailbone; the cervical spine (neck) is the second most common source of pain. Depending upon the cause, the pain may be constant, dull, and centered in one area; or it may be acute or stabbing, and spread from the lower back to the buttocks and legs or from the neck to the jaw and arms.

Most back pain is due to muscle strains and spasms, often the result of improper lifting or abrupt twisting.

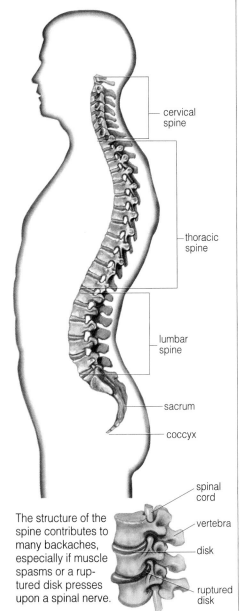

The structure of the spine contributes to many backaches, especially if muscle spasms or a ruptured disk presses upon a spinal nerve.

cervical spine

thoracic spine

lumbar spine

sacrum

coccyx

spinal cord

vertebra

disk

ruptured disk

Poor posture, obesity, and pregnancy are common contributing factors, as is a sedentary lifestyle.

A slipped (prolapsed) or ruptured disk, the spongy cushion that lies between each pair of vertebrae, can also cause back pain, especially if the disk pinches a nerve in the neck or lower back. So can a structural abnormality, such as a curved spine (scoliosis). You should see a doctor if back pain persists for more than two weeks despite rest, or if it recurs. Don't delay if the pain is accompanied by other symptoms, such as numbness in the arms or legs, or loss of bowel or bladder control.

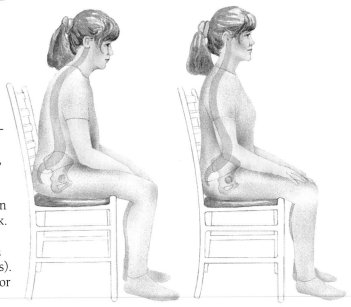

A practitioner of the Alexander technique analyzes poor posture habits (left), then teaches how to achieve proper alignment (right).

Diagnostic Studies and Procedures

After examining your back and testing nerve reflexes, the doctor will probably order X-rays of the back. If a ruptured disk is suspected, imaging studies such as computed tomography (CT) scans or magnetic resonance imaging (MRI) can pinpoint the problem. Other tests may include bone density studies and nerve and muscle evaluations.

Medical Treatments

Most simple backaches can be managed with aspirin (or stronger nonsteroidal anti-inflammatory drugs) and rest (see Self-Treatment). If this conservative course proves inadequate, a muscle relaxant and perhaps a cortisone injection may be tried.

Sometimes immobilizing the back with a brace, neck collar, or traction is needed, especially if the problem stems from a back injury. Persistent back pain caused by a ruptured disk may require surgery to remove the disk.

Back pain due to a structural abnormality or disease requires treatment of the underlying condition.

Alternative Therapies

Back pain is one area in which alternative therapies are widely used and often highly effective. Included are:

Acupuncture or Acupressure. These techniques, the cornerstones of traditional Chinese medicine, are widely used to overcome chronic back pain.

Treatments involve inserting needles into or pressing on the meridians (body points) related to back pain. Some patients report relief after the first treatment; more commonly, however, a series of six or more sessions is needed to produce results.

Alexander Technique. Many chronic back problems are due to poor posture, which often can be remedied by training in the Alexander technique. After carefully analyzing a person's posture and body movement, the practitioner will teach exercises and movements designed to bring the back bones into proper alignment and to strengthen the supporting muscles.

Chiropractic. This alternative therapy, which involves manipulating the spine to correct faulty alignment, is one of the most widely used treatments for back pain. Even physicians who are critical of other aspects of chiropractic often recommend it for back patients, but to be sure that there is no underlying medical problem, a physician should be consulted first.

Massage. Because so many backaches are caused by muscle spasms, massage designed to relax the tensed muscles is a natural remedy. Techniques may range from the relatively gentle Swedish (classic) massage to rolfing, a deep massage that calls for considerable pummeling. (A word of caution: Rolfing can be dangerous for people with osteoporosis, spinal arthritis, and other degenerative bone disorders.)

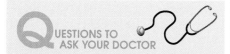

QUESTIONS TO ASK YOUR DOCTOR

▶ Is it safe for me to exercise? If so, what exercises do your recommend?
▶ Would surgery help my particular back problem?

Osteopathy and Physical Therapy. These approaches include such methods as massage, electrical stimulation, ultrasound, and manipulation to relax tensed muscles and alleviate pain.

Yoga and T'ai Chi. These and other movement therapies can strengthen supporting muscles, improve posture, and reduce stress—all important elements in controlling back pain.

Self-Treatment

Appropriate self-care is the key to overcoming and preventing back pain. Although most simple backaches are easily self-treated, you should consult a doctor to rule out a serious underlying problem before embarking on a self-treatment regimen for back pain.

During an acute flare-up, back pain due to muscle strain or an injury requires rest in order to heal. Lie on a firm surface, such as a hard mattress or floor mat. Don't lie on your stomach (even though this may be the most comfortable position); instead, position yourself on your back with your knees slightly bent and supported by a pillow, or on your side with the knees bent. For extra relief, try using a heating pad, an ice pack, or alternating applications of heat and ice.

As soon as the pain eases, start exercises designed to strengthen your back (see illustrations). A word of warning, however: If an exercise produces pain, STOP it immediately. Pain is a warning that something is wrong. Other preventive measures include:

▶ Use the correct techniques for lifting and carrying (see illustrations).
▶ If you work at a desk or computer display terminal, make sure that your chair provides proper back support, and that the desk and chair are comfortable heights for you (see page 123 for illustrations of correct positions).
▶ Avoid prolonged periods of sitting; they put undue stress on the back muscles. Whether at work,

or in a car, theater, or airplane, take a break to stretch and walk around at least once every hour or so.
▶ If your job requires long periods of standing, rest one foot on a low stool to ease back strain. Try to move about every few minutes.
▶ Work to improve posture through such exercises as yoga, dance, and the Alexander technique.
▶ Sleep on a firm mattress, or put a bed board under it.

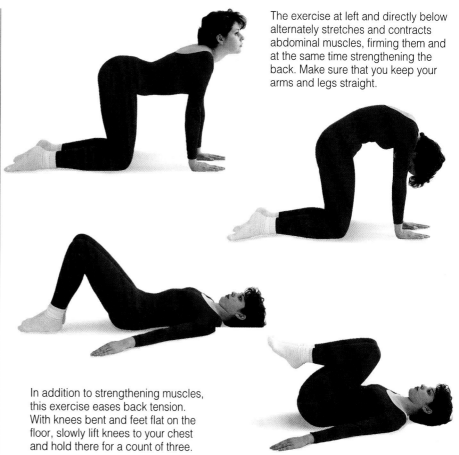

The exercise at left and directly below alternately stretches and contracts abdominal muscles, firming them and at the same time strengthening the back. Make sure that you keep your arms and legs straight.

In addition to strengthening muscles, this exercise eases back tension. With knees bent and feet flat on the floor, slowly lift knees to your chest and hold there for a count of three.

Other Causes of Back Pain

Severe osteoporosis, or thinning of the bones, often results in compression of the spinal column, spontaneous fractures of the vertebrae, and chronic back pain. Arthritis can also cause chronic back pain. A less common cause is cancer that has spread to the bones.

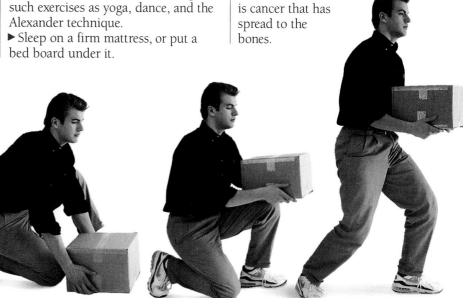

To lift heavy objects from the floor or ground, use your thigh muscles rather than arms and back. Keep the back straight, lifting the weight by straightening your legs.

Bad Breath

(*Fetor oris, halitosis*)
Most people cannot smell their
own bad breath, but it is all
too apparent to others.
Among the many
causes of unpleasant
breath odor, smoking,
eating certain foods,
and poor dental hygiene
are the most common.

Foods and drinks affect the
breath either directly or indirectly
through the lungs and digestive system.
Wine, beer, and other alcoholic beverages leave a residue in the mouth that
alters breath odor, and the digestive
process produces a somewhat different,
sour smell. Foods with relatively high
sulfur content—garlic, onions, fish,
and meat, for example—can create a
lingering breath odor because, as they
are digested, sulfur compounds enter
the bloodstream, travel to the lungs,
and are exhaled. As the body metabolizes these compounds (in about 12 to
24 hours) the odor disappears.

Anything that dries the mouth also
promotes bad breath. A steady flow of
saliva controls the oral bacteria. When
saliva production falls, such as during
sleep, the bacteria quickly multiply,
feeding on particles of food in the
mouth and forming a sticky film called
plaque on the teeth. This process produces so-called morning breath.

Drugs that reduce the flow of saliva,
including antihistamines, antidepressants, and diuretics, as well as disorders of the salivary glands, are other
causes of unpleasant breath from a dry
mouth. Also, saliva production naturally
declines with age, which explains why
many older people have bad breath.

Diagnostic Studies and Procedures

The above causes of bad breath are easy
to determine, but tracking down others
may require considerable detective
work. A thorough dental checkup is
a logical first step. If the problem lies
elsewhere, a doctor may find the cause
during a physical examination of the
mouth, throat, and lungs. Sometimes
the nature of the odor provides important clues. For example, breath that
smells fruity or like nail polish indicates possible diabetes.

Blood and urine tests are done to
look for diabetes and liver or kidney
disorders. A chest X-ray and analysis of

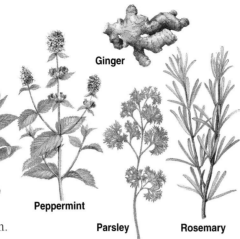

Many herbs, especially the ones above, are
natural breath-fresheners. The leaves can
be eaten fresh, or their extracts can be incorporated into mouthwashes.

a sputum sample can pinpoint a common lung disorder such as pneumonia,
which may cause stale breath. In some
cases, however, extensive medical testing fails to find an underlying cause.

Medical Treatments

Treatment obviously depends on the
cause. Bad breath that stems from poor
oral hygiene can be remedied by filling
any cavities, scaling and cleaning the
teeth, and treating gum disease. Special
mouthwashes or artificial saliva may
remedy a chronic dry mouth. Antibiotics might be prescribed to treat an
underlying infection, such as chronic
bronchitis. Other treatments will be
tailored to the specific problem.

Alternative Therapies

Herbal Medicine. Parsley, which is
packed with chlorophyll, is a popular
herbal breath-freshener. Eating a sprig
of fresh parsley after having onions and
other odorous foods often prevents the
bad breath associated with them.

Alfalfa, which is also high in chlor-
phyll, is another herbal remedy for bad
breath. Herbalists recommend one
tablespoon of alfalfa juice (sold in
health food stores) twice daily. Alternatively, alfalfa tablets may be taken.

Other herbs recommended to counter
bad breath are cloves, ginger (root),
peppermint, fennel, anise seeds, sage,
and rosemary. The leaves of some of
these are chewed; extracts of others are
mixed at a ratio of three parts water to
one part extract to make a mouthwash.
Naturopathy. Practitioners often advise
a cleansing three-day fast, which they
believe rids the body of toxins and

reduces the causes of bad breath. One
regimen calls for eating only raw foods
for two days before and after fasting.

Self-Treatment

In the majority of cases, bad breath is
easily eliminated by diligent self-care,
starting with a look at your diet. Often,
simply avoiding raw onions, garlic, and
similar foods is all that is needed to
freshen breath.

Careful dental hygiene is crucial. See
a dentist or dental hygienist every six
months (more often if necessary) for a
checkup and cleaning. Floss daily and
brush your teeth every morning and
evening as well as after eating. If
brushing after every meal is impractical, at least rinse your mouth with
water or a mouthwash.

Unfortunately, most mouthwashes
just mask breath odor, rather than
eliminate its cause. Those that contain
zinc and sodium benzoate, however,
help to neutralize the odor-causing
waste products from bacteria. Rinsing
and gargling with warm salt water or
1 teaspoon of a 3-percent solution of
hydrogen peroxide in ½ cup of water
also helps control oral bacteria and
eliminate bad breath.

The tongue can contribute to bad
breath; clean it with a soft brush or
rinse your mouth with warm water and
salt, baking soda, or a 3-percent solution of hydrogen peroxide.

To help prevent dry mouth, drink
at least eight glasses of water or other
fluids throughout the day. Fruit juice
stimulates saliva secretion, as does
chewing sugarless gum.

Other Causes of Bad Breath

A number of diseases affect breath
odor, including diabetes, chronic bronchitis and other lung infections, tonsillitis, gastritis, hepatitis, cirrhosis of the
liver, and some types of cancer. With
kidney failure, the breath has a urine-
like odor. Illnesses that cause vomiting
produce temporary bad breath, as does
prolonged fasting.

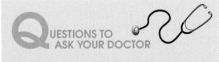

QUESTIONS TO ASK YOUR DOCTOR

▶ Am I using the proper flossing and brushing techniques?
▶ Do any of the medications I am taking cause dry mouth? Will changing the dosage or switching drugs help?

Baldness

(Alopecia)

Baldness involves the complete or partial loss of hair, usually on the scalp, but sometimes other places as well.

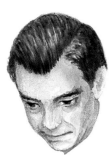

Normally, we shed 50 to 100 hairs every day as part of a natural growth, resting, and renewal process. When a hair is in the resting stage, it loosens gradually from its root and is shed. A few months later, a new hair begins to grow in its place.

With aging, it is normal for hair to thin in women and men. But many men experience more extensive hair loss due to a hereditary condition called male pattern baldness, or androgenic alopecia, which can occur any time after the teen years. Typically, it begins with a slow thinning of all scalp hair; then the hair gradually recedes from the forehead and thins at the crown, eventually leaving just a fringe around the back of the head and over the ears.

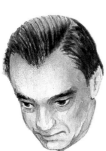

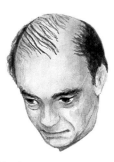

The illustrations above show the typical development of male pattern baldness, which is usually inherited from the mother's side of a man's family.

Hair follicles in balding areas metabolize androgens, male sex hormones, in a different way than those on other parts of the scalp and body, causing some hair follicles to shrink. Hair growth slows, and eventually the hair dies, resulting in permanent baldness.

Women may experience temporary hair loss from hormonal changes during pregnancy, menopause, or postmenopausal hormone therapy. When a woman has female pattern baldness at about the time of menopause, this is due to major shifts in androgen levels, and like male pattern baldness, it tends to be hereditary. Excessive perming, straightening, or hair coloring can also cause excessive hair loss in women, as can wearing a tight pony tail.

A temporary type of hair loss called alopecia areata produces patchy baldness in both men and women. Some researchers believe that this is an autoimmune reaction in which the body's immune system attacks healthy hair follicles. In many cases, the hair grows back within 6 to 24 months.

Fungal infections of the scalp, such as ringworm, also cause hair loss that is generally reversible with treatment.

Diagnostic Studies and Procedures

The cause of most baldness is easily diagnosed on the basis of appearance and medical history, such as recent illness or drug use. A fungal infection can be detected by examining the skin with a special light.

Medical Treatments

Drug Therapy. Hair loss due to male pattern baldness may be treated with minoxidil (Rogaine), a reformulation of a blood pressure medication that causes excessive growth of scalp and body hair as a side effect. It is now prescribed as a topical lotion that is applied daily to the scalp. It takes several months to show results, and only about one-third of men experience significant hair regrowth. The new hair is finer and thinner than normal, and the drug must be used continuously to maintain the new hair growth.

Alopecia areata can sometimes be halted by applying a topical steroid or injecting it into the scalp to lower the immune system's attack on the hair follicles.

Plastic Surgery. Two procedures are now available. The oldest is hair transplantation, in which small circles, or plugs, of skin containing healthy hair follicles are transplanted from the back and sides of the head to the balding site. If the plugs take, they continue to grow hair. Surgery is usually done in stages, but sometimes entire strips of skin with hair can be moved. Transplantation is expensive; each plug costs $30 to $35, and an average procedure requires from 50 to 200 plugs.

The second surgical approach is scalp reduction, in which a surgeon removes an oval-shaped piece of scalp from the top of the head, then pulls the part of

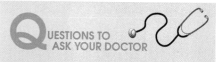
the scalp that still contains hair upward to fill in the missing piece.

Experimental Treatments. Some physicians have successfully stimulated hair growth by rubbing a chemical irritant onto the scalp. The resulting inflammation sometimes produces hair growth. In another experimental approach, allergen sensitizers are applied to the scalp. These procedures must be done by a professional, and they work for only a few people.

Alternative Therapies

There are numerous claims of alternative cures for baldness, but there's no proof that any really help.

Herbal Medicine. An ancient remedy calls for rubbing onion juice on the scalp and then exposing it to the sun. Some herbalists today recommend a rosemary hair tonic. There is no evidence that either works.

Self-Treatment

Although self-care cannot halt male pattern baldness, gentle treatment may slow its progression. Never brush wet hair, as this action can weaken and break it. Instead, comb gently with a large-tooth comb. Use mild shampoo and warm, not hot water, rinse with cool water, and gently towel dry. Both men and women concerned with hair loss should avoid perming and the use of hot hair dryers and hair coloring.

Another option is a hair piece. Some new types are quite natural looking and can be attached with glue or by anchoring the piece to other hair with fine wires. These hair pieces do not shift or fall off even while the wearer is swimming and showering. They are made with either human or artificial hair and range in price from a few hundred to a few thousand dollars.

Other Causes of Hair Loss

Diseases that often produce hair loss include lupus, thyroid insufficiency, and scleroderma, a hardening of the skin. A high fever, radiation exposure, and certain drugs, especially cancer chemotherapy, also produce hair loss.

Bedsores

(Decubitus ulcers; pressure sores; trophic ulcers)

These painful ulcers are a potentially serious problem for anyone who is bedridden, confined to a wheelchair, or lacks sensation because of paralysis or some other condition. If a person does not change position every few hours, either independently or with help, blood flow is reduced wherever there is unrelieved pressure. The result is cell death, skin deterioration, and eventually, the development of pressure sores. Places where bone is close to the skin, such as the heels, hips, and base of the spine, are particularly vulnerable.

Diagnostic Studies and Procedures

A bedsore is usually diagnosed by observation. The first warning sign is an area of redness over a pressure point. The skin there gradually thickens and swells, leading to blisters and open sores. Finally, skin ulcerations develop, sometimes becoming progressively deeper until the bone is exposed. At this stage, osteomyelitis, a serious bone inflammation, is likely to develop.

Medical Treatments

If the source of pressure is identified and corrected at an early stage, bedsores can be treated with special gels, creams, and antibiotics.

More advanced bedsores require debridement to remove the dead tissue. Special gels or 1.5-percent hydrogen peroxide may be applied to speed sloughing, so that the diseased tissue can be lifted away with forceps. Deeper sores require surgical removal of damaged tissue and bone. Skin grafts may be needed to cover large areas.

Alternative Therapies

Severe bedsores always require medical treatment. For milder cases, certain homemade remedies can be used, but special care must be taken to avoid infecting open wounds.

Herbal Medicine. Many herbalists recommend myrrh for bedsores because of its astringent and antiseptic properties. Before use, however, it should be tested on a small area of skin to make sure that it does not cause further irritation, and it should never be applied to an open sore.

Hydrotherapy. Wet dressings and special whirlpool baths promote the sloughing of dead tissue. Whirlpool baths also facilitate healing by increasing blood flow to the skin.

Naturopathy. Poultices of certain natural substances are recommended for the treatment of weeping sores, but if a wound is deep or infected, a health professional should be consulted. A poultice made of raw, unprocessed honey is said to promote healing. So too is a dressing of papaya pulp or a poultice of grated raw or mashed cooked carrots placed on the sore and changed every two to three hours.

Self-Treatment

To prevent bedsores from developing or from progressing past the initial stages, self-care is fundamental.

If you are the patient, shift positions frequently and be alert to any red or sore spots. If feasible, exercise in bed to maintain muscle tone and good circulation. This helps to prevent not only bedsores but also the formation of clots that can lead to phlebitis, a pulmonary embolism, or other serious complications. Periodically lift each foot, one at

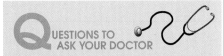

a time, move it in a circle, and flex it up and down. Then lift each leg in turn, without bending your knee, and hold it up for a count of 10 seconds. As strength increases, hold the legs up for longer periods.

Knee bends can also be performed while lying in bed, by lifting each leg in turn and flexing and straightening the knee joint. Try to do all of the above exercises four or five times a day, gradually increasing the number of repetitions during each session.

In a wheelchair, use a foam rubber cushion covered with sheepskin and raise your buttocks off the seat periodically. Do not sit for extended periods in the same position.

If you are caring for someone who is unable to move himself, shift the patient every few hours. Keep the skin clean and dry by washing it thoroughly at least once a day, or more often if the patient is incontinent. Avoid rubbing harshly; gentle sponging with a small amount of soap is best. Pat the skin dry with a soft towel and apply talcum powder where needed. Use a moisturizing lotion to prevent dryness.

Change sheets every day or two, or whenever they are soiled or damp. If the patient eats in bed, make sure that all crumbs and food particles are carefully removed after each meal.

An egg-carton-type of foam rubber pad under the bottom sheet can help relieve pressure. A water bed also can help distribute the body's weight more evenly. Consider using a bed cradle that will keep the covers away from the knees, toes, and heels. For extra protection, sheepskin pads can be used to cushion the heels and elbows, and a larger sheepskin mat can be placed under the buttocks to cushion the hip.

Other Causes of Skin Ulcers

Bacterial infections can lead to skin ulcers, as can varicose veins and other circulatory problems in the legs.

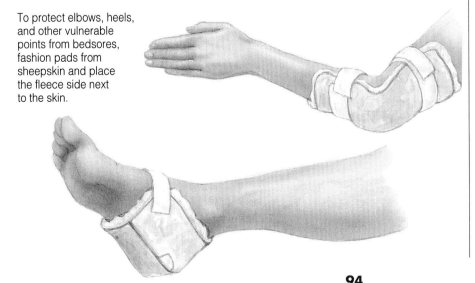

To protect elbows, heels, and other vulnerable points from bedsores, fashion pads from sheepskin and place the fleece side next to the skin.

Bell's Palsy

(Facial palsy)

Bell's palsy is a paralysis of the facial muscles that control movement and expression. Each year, about 40,000 Americans develop the condition; most are over 40, although the disorder can occur at any age.

Paralysis, which occurs on one side of the face, is usually temporary. The symptoms include an inability to close one eye plus weakness and lack of muscle tone on the affected side. The face may feel as if it is twisted, and speaking and eating may become difficult. In some cases, one side of the mouth droops and the senses of taste and hearing are impaired. The eye may also become abnormally dry.

Bell's palsy usually develops rapidly, often coming on overnight, but some patients recall a warning pain behind the ear a few hours to a few days before the onset. The paralysis is thought to be caused by a swelling of the facial nerve that runs from the brain to the face. As the nerve swells, it becomes compressed within the surrounding bony enclosure.

The underlying cause is unknown, but because Bell's palsy often follows an earache, cold, or other viral infection, some doctors believe that a virus may be involved. Injuries to the head and pregnancy have also been implicated.

In 80 to 90 percent of cases, Bell's palsy is a temporary condition. If paralysis begins to reverse by the end of the second week, the prognosis for a full recovery is good.

Diagnostic Studies and Procedures

Most occurrences can be diagnosed by the characteristic symptoms and their rapid onset. If there is any doubt, a doctor will order X-rays and perhaps a CT scan or MRI of the skull to rule out a tumor, fracture, or bone erosion. Blood tests can help detect a possible underlying infection.

If facial paralysis persists, nerve conduction tests or electromyography (EMG) may be ordered to assess the extent of nerve activity and damage.

Medical Treatments

Treatment for this condition is somewhat controversial. Because most cases resolve themselves without therapy, some doctors advise a wait-and-see policy. Others advocate prompt medical intervention in the hope of shortening the course of the paralysis.

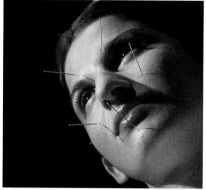

Acupuncture can be helpful for many conditions, including Bell's palsy, in which the facial nerve swells and is compressed within its bony channel in the mastoid bone.

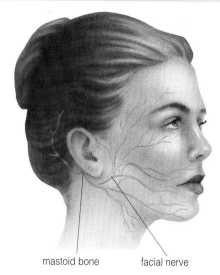

mastoid bone   facial nerve

If improvement fails to occur within two weeks, treatment is advisable. There are two approaches: The most common entails taking corticosteroid drugs such as prednisone to reduce nerve swelling and inflammation. Typically, the drug is given in high doses for five days, and then tapered off and stopped over the next five days.

Sometimes surgery is performed to widen the bony canal that surrounds the facial nerve. But this operation is done only as a last resort.

Alternative Therapies

Alternative therapies for Bell's palsy are even more controversial than those of conventional medicine, because their efficacy is doubtful. Those that are sometimes suggested include:

Acupuncture. Stimulation of meridians controlling nerves in the head and face is said to reduce swelling and reverse paralysis, provided the nerve has not been permanently damaged.

Aromatherapy. Facial massage using aromatic oils can prevent muscle spasms and may speed recovery.

Herbal Medicine. Traditional Chinese herbalists recommend the Pueraria combination, which is made up of kudzu root, ma-huang, ginger, jujube

fruit, cinnamon, peony root, and licorice for acute numbness of facial nerves, and a combination of cinnamon, atractylodes, and aconite for chronic disorders of these nerves.

Self-Treatment

Self-care is directed to preventing long-term eye damage and alleviating symptoms while awaiting recovery. Because you probably will not be able to blink or close your eye, it should be protected with an eye patch, especially while sleeping. Artificial tears or medicated eyedrops help to alleviate eye dryness.

Special facial exercises and self-massage can prevent long-term contracture and damage to the facial muscles. A physical therapist can prescribe exercises to do at home.

Wearing a splint helps to prevent drooping of the lower part of the face. A doctor or physical therapist can supply an appropriate one, or you can fashion your own from a long strip of cotton or linen.

Chewing and swallowing may be difficult, so avoid foods that can cause choking. In fact, you may want to switch to a liquid diet until the paralysis disappears.

Other Causes of Facial Paralysis

Infection, Guillain-Barré syndrome, Lyme disease, shingles, stroke, or a tumor are among the many other causes of facial paralysis. Spasms of the facial muscles, called hemifacial spasm, can cause symptoms similar to those of Bell's palsy. In rare cases, women develop a condition called facial hemiatrophy of Romberg, which entails loss of fatty tissue just under the skin. This disorder progresses slowly, resulting in facial atrophy and distortion.

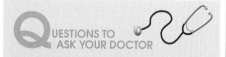

QUESTIONS TO ASK YOUR DOCTOR

▶ Am I likely to suffer permanent nerve damage?
▶ How can I best protect my eye until the paralysis disappears?
▶ How can I avoid choking and other problems with eating?

Bites and Stings

(Insect, marine, and snake)
Consequences of venom from poisonous insects, spiders, marine life, and snakes range from minor to life threatening; anyone who spends time outdoors should be aware of the hazards.
Bee stings. Most stings from flying insects in the *Hymenoptera* family—bees, wasps, hornets, and yellow jackets—are more of a nuisance than a health hazard. However, certain proteins excreted in their venom can cause potentially fatal allergic reactions in people who are hypersensitive to them.
Spiders and scorpions. Spiders to be concerned about are the black widow and brown recluse. Only the female black widow bites. Be especially wary if she is guarding an egg mass. Brown recluse, or violin, spiders hide in dark, out-of-the-way places, including the folds of blankets or clothing, and will bite if disturbed. There are about 70 species of scorpions in North America. Their stings are painful, but not especially dangerous, unlike those of their cousins in tropical countries.
Sea creatures. Although bites and stings from marine life in coastal waters can be very painful, most are not poisonous. The primary exceptions are stingrays, the Portuguese man-of-war, and some types of jellyfish.
Snakes. About 45,000 Americans are bitten by snakes every year. Of this number, about 9,000 experience snake venom poisoning, but only about 15 deaths occur as a result.

Two types of poisonous snakes are indigenous to the United States: pit vipers and coral snakes. A pit viper, which includes the rattlesnake, copperhead, and cottonmouth (also called water moccasin), has a triangular head with a pit between the eyes and slit-like pupils. The coral snake, a variety of cobra, has a rounded head and black rings bordered at both ends by bands of yellow (see illustrations, opposite page).

All other U.S. snakes, which also have round heads, are not poisonous. Their bites, however, can cause a painful infection if they go untreated.

Diagnostic Studies and Procedures

Diagnostic studies are not required to assess bites and stings. Instead, knowledge of what caused the bite and development of these symptoms indicate whether or not a bite is serious.

FIRST AID FOR INSECT BITES OR STINGS

1. If stung by a bee or other flying insect, remove the stinger by gently scraping the skin with a knife blade, fingernail, credit card, or similar object. Do not remove it with tweezers, because squeezing may force more venom into the body.
2. If the bite was from a spider or scorpion, keep the victim lying down with the area of the bite lower than the heart.
3. Wash the wound with soap and water, if available, and apply ice or cold compresses to the sting or bite area to slow the spread of the venom.
4. If the person has a known sensitivity to bee venom, find out if she is carrying a syringe of injectable adrenaline (epinephrine); if so, use it immediately, and then go to a hospital emergency room.
5. If adrenaline is not available and signs of a severe allergic reaction develop, apply a constriction band as described under first aid for snake bites and get to a hospital emergency room right away.

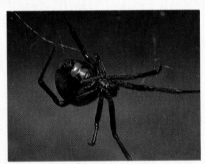
Black widow spider

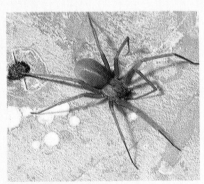
Brown recluse spider

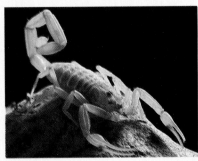
Scorpion

After a bee sting. Signs of a hypersensitive reaction include severe swelling beyond the site of the bite, hives or other rash, severe itching, wheezing or other breathing problems, weakness or dizziness, stomach cramps, nausea and vomiting, severe anxiety, and possible loss of consciousness.
After a bite by a crawling insect.
General signs of poisoning include a painful stinging or burning sensation when bitten, redness and swelling at the site of the bite, and worsening pain over the course of several hours. At the spot where a brown recluse spider has bitten, a blister develops and, within a day or two, chills, fever, nausea, vomiting, and weakness may occur, possibly followed by tissue death advancing over a wider area.

A bite by a black widow spider causes profuse sweating, stomach cramps, nausea, vomiting, tightness in the chest, and difficulty in breathing.

The area around a scorpion sting becomes numb and tingly; nausea, vomiting, muscle spasms (especially around the site of the bite) follow, and sometimes convulsions and shock.
After a marine bite or sting. Stingray venom produces immediate pain, which spreads rapidly over the next 90 minutes; this is followed by dizziness, weakness, nausea and vomiting, diarrhea, cramps, sweating, anxiety, lymph node pain and, in the worst cases, difficulty in breathing and arrhythmias.

Jellyfish or Portuguese man-of-war venom causes pain, itching, and long, red wheals on the skin, followed by weakness, nausea, headache, muscle pain and spasms, sweating, tearing, difficulty breathing, and chest pain. In some cases, shock may develop.
After a poisonous snake bite. If venom has been injected, there is usually pain and swelling, followed by skin discoloration. Severe poisoning is marked by general weakness or drowsiness, rapid pulse, increased salivation and sweating, breathing difficulty, blurred or dimming vision, swollen eyelids, slurred speech, nausea and vomiting, convulsions, and shock, possibly advancing to coma and death.

Medical Treatments

If the person is hypersensitive to bee venom, a sting requires an immediate injection with adrenaline, or epinephrine, which can prevent anaphylactic shock. An antihistamine also may be given. If avoiding bees is difficult, desensitization may be recommended. This involves weekly injections of diluted bee venom for a year or more to permit the body to build up resistance.

Treatment for poisonous spider or scorpion bites depends on the creature involved and the severity of symptoms. Sometimes local therapy to ease discomfort is all that is needed. In other cases, treatment may require antivenin injections, hospitalization, and even life support until the crisis is past. Steroid injections may be given if the wound from a brown recluse continues to expand after the first 12 to 24 hours.

A sting from a marine animal may require a tetanus shot, antibiotic

therapy, and, depending on the wound, removal of the stinger and surgical closure. Painkillers and topical lotions containing an antihistamine, anesthetic, and corticosteroids also may be prescribed. In more serious cases, especially if shock occurs, hospitalization for intravenous therapy and oxygen support may be necessary.

Immediate treatment for a poisonous snake bite usually involves extracting the venom by suction (see box, below). Some doctors also cut open the wound and excise a block of tissue around the bite. If symptoms are severe, antivenin may be given intravenously for several hours or, less commonly, by intramuscular injection. However, antivenin

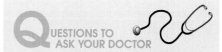

QUESTIONS TO ASK YOUR DOCTOR

▶ Should I carry a syringe of epinephrine to deal with bee stings?
▶ How long does it usually take for a snake (or poisonous spider) bite to heal?

itself could cause an anaphylactic reaction, so sensitivity must be tested first by exposure to a diluted solution of it. Even so, careful monitoring is essential after giving snake antivenin. A tetanus shot, antibiotics, and a painkilling medication will also be administered when indicated.

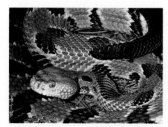

Besides the rattles on its tail, a rattlesnake has a triangular head and a pit between its eyes.

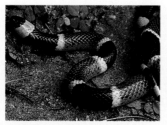

Distinctive bands of red, black, and yellow markings make the colorful coral snake easy to spot.

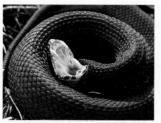

The cottonmouth, or water moccasin, is so named because the inside of its mouth is white.

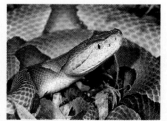

A copperhead is distinguished by its copper-colored head and reddish brown hourglass markings.

FIRST AID FOR SNAKE BITES

Start first aid immediately if you will not be able to reach a hospital emergency room within 30 minutes. Even after applying first aid, obtain medical help as soon as possible.

1. Keep the victim from walking or otherwise moving around, because motion speeds distribution of the snake venom throughout the body. Have the person recline, preferably with the bitten part at or below heart level.

2. Use a tie, belt, or rope to apply a light constriction band to a bite on the arm or leg, about four to six inches above the wound (A). Make it snug but loose enough to slip a finger underneath. Move the band a few inches higher if the area around it begins to swell. If moving the person is necessary, immobilize the limb with a splint, made from a blanket, towel, or rolled newspaper.

3. If a snake-bite kit is available, use the extractor in it to remove as much venom as possible (B), following the kit's directions care-

fully. Prompt action is a must—up to 35 percent of the venom can be removed if an extractor is used within the first five minutes after the bite has occurred.

4. If a snake-bite kit is not available, try to squeeze out as much venom as possible. The venom also may be sucked from the wound with the mouth because the digestive system neutralizes venom as long as the person sucking does not have any open sores or cuts in or around the mouth. While sucking out venom, be sure to spit out the venom and rinse the mouth periodically. In the past, first aid manuals gave instructions to make shallow cuts over the fang marks. Experts now feel that this action increases the chance of infection, so they discourage it. In fact, these incisions actually decrease the amount of venom that can be removed with an extractor.

5. After removing as much venom as possible, wash the wound area thoroughly if soap and warm water are available, Alternatively, cleanse it with an antiseptic pad or wipe (C).

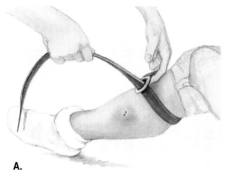

A.
A constriction band should be applied loosely enough to slip a finger underneath.

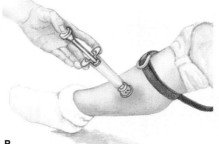

B.
Snake-bite kits contain an extractor that can remove up to a third of the venom.

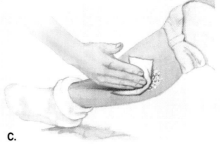

C.
Use an antiseptic wipe or a clean cloth with soap and warm water to wash the area.

FIRST AID FOR MARINE BITES OR STINGS

1. Remove any stingers or tentacles left in the skin with tweezers or fingers covered by a cloth to prevent further injury.
2. Wash the area with sea water, rubbing alcohol, or ammonia, but do not rub it.
3. If possible, immerse a stingray injury in very hot water for 30 to 90 minutes.
4. After an injury from a Portuguese man-of-war or jellyfish, soak the area in a 50/50 solution of vinegar and water for 30 minutes, and then apply a paste of meat tenderizer (papain) and sea water. If meat tenderizer is unavailable, use baking soda.
5. If nausea, vomiting, or breathing problems develop, seek immediate emergency care.

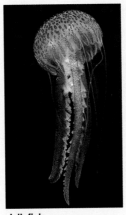

Jellyfish

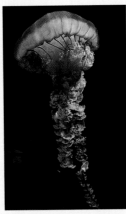

Portuguese man-of-war

A jellyfish has a translucent body and tentacles studded with stinging cells. A Portuguese man-of-war is actually a colony of organisms with long tentacles that bear multiple stinging cells.

BITES AND STINGS (CONTINUED)

If shock develops following any type of bite or sting, treatment will probably include blood transfusions, intravenous fluids, and possibly oxygen and respirator support. During recuperation, a large wound will be cleaned of dead tissue. The wound may also be enclosed in a plastic bag and exposed to high concentrations of oxygen (oxygen therapy) to help speed healing.

Alternative Therapies

If you are bitten by a venomous creature, immediate medical attention is called for. Alternative therapies may provide relief, however, for lesser bites and stings. These can also speed healing of severe bites and stings when used as a supplement to medical treatment.

Herbal Medicine. Herbalists praise slippery elm, extracted from the inner bark of the red elm tree, for its healing properties. Some recommend mixing the powder with water and making a poultice to treat uncomplicated bites.

For more extensive wounds, an herbalist may use a poultice made with ground comfrey root or crushed burdock root, place it over the wound, and cover it with a bandage. A poultice should be changed daily and before it is reapplied, the wound should be cleansed thoroughly with soap and sterile water, or with hydrogen peroxide to help prevent an infection.

Chamomile or witch hazel extracts can be applied directly to minor bites and stings to promote healing.

Native Americans use the leaves and roots of the echinacea plant to treat snake and insect bites and a poultice of yarrow flowers to treat wounds.

There is some evidence that eating raw garlic may help prevent infection.

Naturopathy. Application of a fresh-cut slice of raw onion to a bee sting is one of several natural methods to alleviate the swelling and pain. Another is to smear it with honey and then apply an ice pack. The juice squeezed from plantain leaves that have been bruised and heated until they wilt is said to relieve many bee and insect stings. Also, the leaves from a lesser known member of the plantain family, the psyllium plant, have long been used to soothe minor bites and stings.

Self-Treatment

Most insect bites are not harmful; they produce only minor pain and irritation, which often abates when you apply ice followed by calamine lotion. You can also ease the itching of mosquito and other bites by applying a poultice of cornstarch or baking soda and fresh lemon juice. If itching persists, try a cool compress soaked in Burow's solution, which is available without a prescription at most pharmacies.

Immediate first aid (see box on page 96) is important for more serious bites and stings, especially if there are any symptoms of anaphylactic shock or venom poisoning.

Do not use ice on a snake bite. Wash the wound with soap and water and apply a simple bandage. If you are bitten on an arm or leg, remove rings, shoes, or other items that may become constrictive if swelling occurs. Call your doctor for advice on whether a tetanus shot and antibiotics are advisable.

If there is the slightest possibility that a snake bite is poisonous, head for a hospital emergency room immediately if you will be able to reach it within 30 minutes. If transportation will take longer, start first aid immediately (see box, page 97). Try to identify the type of snake involved so you can report it to health-care personnel.

Other Types of Bites

Bite wounds from both humans and animals are among the most common injuries seen in hospital emergency rooms. Cat bites occur more often than dog bites—and, according to the American Red Cross, are more likely to cause infection, because cats' mouths harbor a greater variety of bacteria. A severe dog bite, however, causes more extensive tissue damage.

Human bites are as serious as those of most animals because they, too, commonly cause infection. Therefore, even a bite that seems minor should receive medical attention and antibiotics to prevent complications.

For both human and animal bites, first aid consists of cleaning the wound with soap and warm water and then applying an antiseptic such as hydrogen peroxide. See a doctor for any deep puncture wound.

THE THREAT OF RABIES

Rabies is a major concern with all animal bites. This usually fatal disease is contracted by direct contact with the saliva of an infected animal, which can be either domestic or wild.

To protect against rabies, have all pets vaccinated yearly, and never approach a stray cat or dog. Also stay away from wild animals, raccoons in particular. Any wild animal that allows a human to come close is probably ill. If you see such an animal, report it to your local animal control office or warden.

Bladder Cancer

(Bladder carcinoma)

Bladder cancer is any malignancy of the urinary bladder. Each year, more than 50,000 Americans are diagnosed with the disease, which causes about 11,000 deaths. Men outnumber women three to one, and the incidence is higher among whites than other races.

Certain environmental factors seem to increase the risk of bladder cancer. Included are cigarette smoking and exposure to naphthaline, benzidine, aniline dyes, and chemicals used in rubber and leather processing. Research has also implicated cyclamates, a type of artifical sweetner, but these have been banned in the United States.

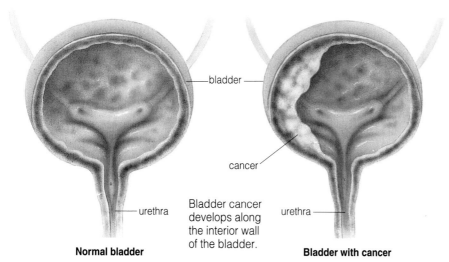

Normal bladder

bladder

cancer

urethra

Bladder cancer develops along the interior wall of the bladder.

urethra

Bladder with cancer

Blood in the urine, or hematuria, is the most common warning sign. There may also be burning or pain during urination. Advanced bladder cancer may cause fatigue, weight loss, and abdominal, pelvic, or back pain.

Diagnostic Studies and Procedures

A urinalysis can detect even invisible blood in urine. If malignancy is suspected, imaging such as ultrasound, CT scans, or MRI, or an intravenous pyelogram (IVP, a special X-ray of the urinary tract) can usually locate the tumor.

A cystoscope, a flexible viewing tube with magnifying devices, allows a doctor to inspect the urethra and bladder and collect tissue samples. If cancer is confirmed, additional tests will be performed to determine its extent.

Medical Treatments

If diagnosed early, bladder cancer is highly curable. Superficial tumors are treated with a procedure called trans-

JOB RELATED RISKS

Occupations linked to an increased risk of bladder cancer include:

Asbestos handlers	Metal workers
Chemical workers	Petroleum workers
Hairdressers and manicurists	Printers
Leather tanners	Rubber workers
Machinists	Textile workers
	Truck drivers

urethral electroresection, in which an instrument similar to a cystoscope is passed through the urethra to the bladder and an electrical current or laser beam destroys the cancer. Anticancer drugs may also be instilled directly into the bladder weekly for about six weeks.

Because bladder cancer often recurs, follow-up visits are recommended every two or three months during the first two years, and then every four months thereafter.

About 12 percent of patients with superficial bladder cancer eventually develop more invasive cancers that require surgery. The operation may be followed by radiation or chemotherapy.

In the most advanced cases, the bladder must be removed and a new exit for urine created through the lower abdomen. Most commonly, a pouch to collect urine is created from a segment of the small intestine. Then an opening, or stoma, is made in the abdominal wall, and this allows the urine to flow to an external collection bag, which has to be emptied periodically. Sometimes, the ureters, tubes that carry urine from the kidneys to the bladder, will be attached to a segment of the lower

colon, thus allowing urine to pass from the kidneys into the rectum instead.

Alternative Therapies

To improve their quality of life, some cancer patients adopt the following alternative approaches:

Nutrition Therapy. Although diet cannot cure cancer, some researchers believe it is important in preventing it. For example, a low intake of vitamin A is associated with an increased risk of bladder cancer. To increase vitamin A in your diet, eat more yellow or orange fruits and vegetables, plus broccoli and dark green leafy vegetables.

Yoga and Meditation. These and other relaxation therapies, such as massage and visualization, can help patients cope with cancer pain and the side effects of treatments. There is also some evidence that visualization may bolster the body's ability to fight cancer.

Self-Treatment

If you smoke, quit immediately. Also minimize exposure to possible cancer-causing agents. Use protective equipment if your job requires exposure to harmful chemicals (see box, above).

Some studies have linked heavy consumption of coffee (more than four cups a day) with an increased risk of bladder cancer. Chemical caffeine removers have also been linked to the disease. If you drink caffeine-free coffee, try to find water-decaffeinated brands to avoid this possible risk.

Recent results of two long-term studies did not find a link between hair dyes and bladder cancer—a fear raised by earlier research. Still, some experts advise using semipermanent, light-colored dyes that wash out in a few weeks.

If treatment results in a urinary stoma, consider joining a support group of fellow patients. Such groups offer emotional support and helpful advice.

Other Causes of Bladder Symptoms

An enlarged prostate, cystitis, a bladder infection or obstruction, urethritis, and bladder stones all can cause symptoms similar to those of bladder cancer.

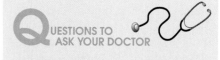

QUESTIONS TO ASK YOUR DOCTOR

▶ What can I do to reduce my risk of bladder cancer?
▶ Will I maintain normal urinary function after treatment for bladder cancer?

Bladder Disorders

The urinary bladder is a muscular pouch that can expand to hold about a pint of urine. When almost half full, the bladder begins signaling a feeling of fullness. During urination, the bladder muscle contracts to release urine in such a way that it cannot flow back into the ureters, the tubes linking the kidneys and bladder.

Bladder disorders may occur as a result of an injury, disease, or an inherited condition. Anatomical differences between men and women predispose them to different bladder problems. Women are much more prone than men to bladder and urethral infections, because their urethra is very short and located close to the anus and the vagina, sites that often harbor bacteria that can invade the bladder. Prostate gland disorders account for many of the male bladder problems.

The most common bladder disorder, cystitis, is discussed on page 152. Below are some of the other problems that are frequently encountered.

Bladder stones, or urinary bladder calculi, are comprised of calcium oxalate or calcium phosphate crystals or, in a small percentage of cases, uric acid or cystine crystals. They vary in size from microscopic to several centimeters in diameter.

Some bladder stones appear spontaneously, without any apparent cause. Others may be precipitated by over-excretion of calcium or uric acid, reduced excretion of urine due to an enlarged prostate or some other structural abnormality, or a urinary tract infection.

Sometimes, no reason can be discovered for the production of bladder stones. Small ones may be passed without symptoms, but a large stone can cause excruciating pain in the lower back, abdomen, or pubic area, as well as blood in the urine and a sudden interruption in urinary flow. There may also be fever and chills, especially if the urinary tract is infected.

Urethritis is an inflammation of the urethra, the narrow tube in which urine and, in men, semen passes out of the body. Women are especially susceptible to urethritis that is caused by a bacterial infection. The disorder in men is more often due to an enlarged or inflamed prostate gland or a sexually transmitted disease, such as chlamydia

or gonorrhea. Symptoms include pain or a burning sensation during urination or ejaculation, a feeling of urgency when urinating, and, in males, an abnormal discharge from the penis.

Urinary fistulas are abnormal passages that link the bladder or urethra to another organ. In women, a fistula sometimes develops between the bladder and vagina. The most common symptom is a flow of urine from the vagina. Trauma during childbirth is the most frequent cause, although a urinary fistula may also develop as a result of radiation therapy and tumors.

Urethral stricture in men is caused by a narrowing or blockage of the urethra within the penis; in women, it may be secondary to repeated bouts of cystitis. Urinary tract injuries or infections can produce scar tissue that obstructs the urethral passage. Symptoms include pain and difficulty in urinating.

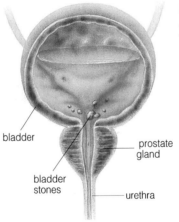

bladder

bladder stones

prostate gland

urethra

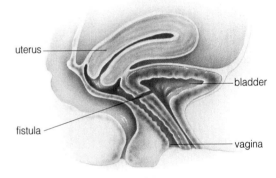

Bladder stones (left) can block the urethra, causing pain and a backup of urine. A fistula between bladder and vagina (below) is signaled by urine flow from the vagina.

uterus

bladder

fistula

vagina

Vesicoureteral reflux (VR) is a back-up of urine into the ureters caused by a malfunction of the one-way valve that leads from the ureter into the bladder. The backup occurs when the bladder contracts to release urine. Then, as the bladder relaxes, the urine flows back into it. The result is a buildup of stagnant urine, which increases the risk of infection and inflammation.

The most common urinary tract problem among children, VR is usually caused by congenital structural anomalies, although it may be due also to an obstruction of the bladder outlet, a urinary tract infection, or other disorders. VR is often asymptomatic; when symptoms do occur, they are usually the result of a secondary infection and may include painful urination, pain in the

abdomen or side, increased urinary frequency and urgency, blood in the urine, and fever.

Diagnostic Studies and Procedures

If bladder stones are suspected, a physician or urologist will perform a complete physical examination and seek confirmation of the diagnosis through urinalysis, a special X-ray procedure called intravenous urography, and possibly a bladder ultrasound evaluation that employs sound waves to identify the site and size of stones.

Urethritis is diagnosed by analyses of urine and vaginal or penile discharge to determine whether an infection is present and, if so, what type.

To diagnose a urethral stricture or a urinary fistula both the urethra and bladder will be examined with a cystoscope, a narrow, flexible viewing tube, inserted into the urethra. If a fistula is confirmed, its opening can be tracked

by inspecting the vagina after infusing the bladder with an opaque dye.

If VR is suspected, the urologist may order intravenous urography and a filling and voiding cystourethrogram, an X-ray study to determine whether urine stays in the bladder or flows back toward the kidney. If reflux is found, a kidney ultrasound evaluation or intravenous pyelogram (X-rays taken after a dye is injected into the renal circulation) may be done to detect possible kidney damage. Cystoscopy also can confirm certain structural problems that may be causing VR.

Medical Treatment

Bladder stones. If the bladder stones are small, they do not require medical therapy other than monitoring to make sure that they are expelled during

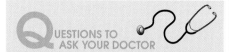
urination. Depending upon the cause and symptoms, antibiotics and pain-killers may be prescribed.

If stones are large and obstructing the flow of urine, immediate treatment is necessary. Depending on their size, composition, and location in the urinary tract, stones may be removed by one of several methods: extraction through a flexible tube or cystoscope; crushing with sound waves in a process called extracorporeal shock-wave lithotripsy; or medication to promote dissolution. In severe cases, surgical removal may be needed.

If the composition of the stones or their cause can be determined, further steps may be taken to reduce the risk of recurrence. Procedures might include alleviating prostate enlargement, prescribing diuretics, modifying the diet, or treating an underlying disease.

Urethritis. If the underlying cause is chlamydia, it is generally treated with 10 days of tetracycline or erythromycin; gonorrhea is treated with a cephalosporin plus doxycycline; other bacterial infections may require sulfa drugs. If a sexually transmitted disease is involved, partners should also be tested and treated.

Urethral stricture. A physician may try to widen the narrowed area by inserting a thin instrument into the urethra after giving a local anesthetic. If this does not work, the stricture can be widened surgically, through a cystoscope or an open incision.

Urinary fistula. Surgical closure of the fistula is the first-choice treatment. If this is not possible, the flow of urine may be diverted to bypass the fistula.

Vesicoureteral reflux. Mild reflux often improves or disappears as a child grows. In the meantime, prophylactic antibiotics may be given to keep the urine, bladder, and kidneys free of infection. Urine samples should be checked periodically to make sure that the urine is bacteria-free. For children with moderate or severe reflux, surgery may be recommended because of the risk of kidney damage.

Alternative Therapies
Some alternative approaches may help promote the natural passage of small bladder stones and also prevent their recurrences (large, obstructive stones require prompt medical attention). Otherwise, alternative therapies are useful primarily for symptomatic relief.
Acupuncture. Stimulation of points along the urinary bladder, kidney, and stomach meridians may ease pain and facilitate the passage of stones. Similarly, acupuncture needles placed along the bladder, liver, kidney, and spleen meridians are said to help relieve pain.
Herbal Medicine. Herbalists recommend a tea made from uva-ursi (bearberry) leaves to treat bladder stones and other urinary disorders. Other herbal remedies include teas made from goldenrod, watermelon seeds, or marsh mallow root.
Nutrition Therapy and Naturopathy. For bladder stones, a therapist may advise taking daily supplements of 10 milligrams of magnesium and 10 milligrams of vitamin B_6 to reduce calcium oxalate, a substance found in some stones. To reduce the formation of oxalate stones, she might suggest adopting a low-salt diet and not taking vitamin C supplements. Limiting such oxalate-rich foods as spinach, chard, beet greens, and rhubarb, as well as tea and chocolate, also may help.

To help prevent urethritis, naturopaths suggest a regular intake of citrus fruits and juices to acidify the urine, which may help stop bacterial growth. Blueberry and cranberry juices also contain a compound that inhibits the growth of bladder bacteria.

Self-Treatment
Self-care can play a significant role in both the treatment and prevention of bladder disorders. It's a good idea to increase consumption of water and other nonalcoholic fluids to at least 10 glasses a day. Extra fluids dilute the urine, helping to prevent urethritis as well as bladder stones, and also to pass those that may have formed.

If you have high levels of uric acid, talk to your doctor about dietary changes that may reduce its formation. Avoiding legumes, organ meats, and other foods high in purine may help.

If bladder stones contain calcium, lowering calcium intake may be a good idea, but this should be done only under a doctor's supervision, because too little calcium can contribute to osteoporosis. In any event, avoid high-dose calcium supplements and calcium-based antacids. Inactivity can also increase calcium in the urine. Walking and other physical activity that exercises the back, legs, and other weight-bearing bones enables the body to absorb and store calcium rather than excrete it, possibly lowering the risk of recurrent bladder stones.

Other measures to alleviate bladder problems include the following:
► Try heat to soothe the pain of urethritis; sitting in a warm bath or using a heating pad may help.
► Don't delay urination. Holding urine increases bladder irritation.
► Bathe daily, but avoid perfumed soaps, bubble baths, genital deodorants, and feminine hygiene products, which can irritate the genital area and set the stage for urethritis. Scented toilet paper may also be irritating.
► Empty the bladder before sex. Afterwards, drink a glass of water and wait an hour to urinate again. This allows the bladder to fill enough to flush out bacteria. Using a mild, unscented, and water-soluble lubricant or contraceptive foam or jelly (which is bactericidal) during intercourse can make penetration easier and lessen trauma to the urethra and bladder.

Other Causes of Bladder Problems
Cystitis, caused by infection and/or inflammation of the bladder, produces symptoms similar to those of urethritis; frequently, the two conditions coexist.

Interstitial cystitis, marked by inflammation of the bladder wall without an active infection, can also cause chronic, debilitating bladder pain, especially in women. In men, an enlarged or inflamed prostate (prostatitis) may cause similar problems. Stress, too, can manifest itself in urinary tract problems, especially an irritable bladder.

Following menopause, many women experience increased urinary urgency, even when the bladder is relatively empty. This is caused by thinning of tissues in the lower urinary tract due to lack of estrogen. Incontinence, the inability to control urination, may be caused by these and other bladder problems, as well as nerve disorders.

Bleeding Emergencies

(Hemorrhaging)

A bleeding emergency, or hemorrhage, is a crisis in which steps must be taken promptly to stop loss of blood before it becomes life threatening. On average, an adult has about 10.5 pints of blood; the loss of even two pints can be fatal.

After a serious accident, injury, or rupture of a major artery, a bleeding emergency may come on rapidly. It develops more slowly when blood loss is associated with an ulcer or other chronic condition, but diagnosis and treatment are still mandatory. For example, many disorders involving internal organs, especially the kidneys, stomach, colon, uterus, and lungs, may lead to a bleeding emergency. Manifestations range from bleeding in an eye or ear, to vomiting or coughing up large amounts of blood, to severe bleeding from the vagina or rectum.

Excessive blood loss is also one of the risks of major surgery. In anticipation of this possibility, a patient might consider providing a quantity of his own blood beforehand so that it will be available if needed. If this is not feasible, the lost blood can be replaced with donor transfusions.

Any unexpected bleeding, even though not severe enough to be considered an emergency, also warrants prompt diagnosis. Examples include profuse rectal bleeding; vaginal bleeding not associated with menstruation; blood in the urine; or unexplained bruises. In such cases, tests are usually needed to detect the underlying cause.

Diagnostic Studies and Procedures

Heavy blood loss from an open wound requires immediate first aid. If you are the only person available to do this at the time of an accident, start first aid right after calling the emergency medical service (see box, opposite page).

In assessing a bleeding emergency, a doctor tries to determine the source of the bleeding, the volume of blood lost, and whether the patient is in shock. Finding the source of internal bleeding is sometimes difficult; a physician will look for unusual swelling, tenderness, bruises, and bleeding from body openings. Vital signs—blood pressure, heart and respiration rate, and consciousness—will also be noted.

ASSEMBLING A FIRST AID KIT

Arrange the following items in a tool box or divided make-up kit.
► Adhesive strip bandages
► Analgesic tablets such as aspirin, acetaminophen, or ibuprofen (Add liquid acetaminophen for children.)
► Angle-edged tweezers to pluck out glass and splinters
► Antibiotic ointment for minor cuts
► Antihistamine cream for insect bites and itching
► Antiseptics such as betadine, isopropyl alcohol, or antiseptic towelettes to clean and disinfect wounds
► Calamine lotion
► Cotton tip applicators and cotton balls
► Disposable latex gloves
► Elastic bandage for sprains
► A firm piece of plastic, such as an expired credit card, to scrape away the stinger after a bee sting
► Flashlight and batteries
► Fragrance-free soap
► Instant ice compress
► Ipecac syrup and activated charcoal for poisoning accidents
► Oral thermometer
► Scissors
► Sterile four-inch gauze pads, long gauze roll, and tape
► Telephone numbers for the family's primary-care physician, emergency medical service, fire department, and poison control center

Bright red blood spurting from a wound indicates that an artery has been severed; it demands attention before the slower, steady bleeding of an injured vein. Other factors to consider include:
► Bleeding that persists despite all efforts to control it.

► Any deep puncture or laceration.
► Severed or crushed nerve, tendon, bone, or muscle.
► Skin broken by a bite.
► Heavy contamination of a wound by soil or organic matter.
► Foreign object(s) imbedded deep in the tissue.

As soon as a patient has been stabilized, X-rays and other studies may be ordered to find sites of internal bleeding. A CT scan or MRI should be done if there is a possibility of a head injury and bleeding inside the skull.

Medical Treatments

The first priority is to stop the bleeding. If this cannot be accomplished by applying pressure to the related artery, emergency surgery may be performed to repair the damaged blood vessels and close the wound.

Follow-up treatment for a severe open wound depends on its origin. In most cases, antibiotics are given to guard against infection. The wound is cleansed, foreign matter is removed, topical antibacterial salve is applied if needed, and a new dressing is put on.

If the wound is the result of an animal bite, the local health department must be contacted and, if appropriate, rabies immunization carried out. A tetanus shot may also be administered.

Treatment for closed wounds is based on evidence of internal damage as revealed by diagnostic studies. If a significant amount of blood has been lost, transfusions may be necessary. Bleeding associated with anticoagulant drugs such as warfarin (Coumadin) is treated with an injection of vitamin K.

HOW TO STOP A NOSEBLEED

Most minor nosebleeds stop after a few minutes of gentle pressure against the bony cartilage that forms the midline of the nose. If bleeding is profuse, bright red, and continues for more than 10 to 15 minutes, the following first aid should be applied :

1. Sit with the upper body tilted forward, allowing blood to drain out of the nose rather than flow back into the throat where it may cause choking.
2. Apply pressure to both nostrils by squeezing the upper part of the nose firmly between your thumb and index finger.
3. Apply ice or a cold compress to the forehead, upper part of the nose, and the upper back of the neck.
4. If packing is necessary, use gauze or a strip of a clean handkerchief or other woven

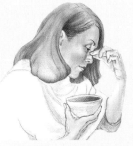

To stop a nosebleed, lean slightly forward and pinch the bridge of your nose.

material. Do not insert either tissue or cotton balls into the nostrils. Avoid removing the packing for several hours. If it is taken out too soon, clots may be disturbed and the bleeding will start again.
5. Seek medical attention if the bleeding persists, if it was caused by a head or nose injury, or if the patient has high blood pressure or a bleeding disorder.

FIRST AID FOR HEMORRHAGING

Follow these steps to stop blood flow, protect the wound from infection, and when necessary, to treat the injured person for shock.

1. Apply direct pressure by placing the palm of your hand on the wound—over a dressing—to compress injured blood vessels against the more firm underlying muscle or bone (top illustration, far right); this will halt bleeding without interfering with normal circulation. If heavy gauze pads are not available, use any folded cloth, such as a clean handkerchief or section torn from a garment. If nothing is available to use as a compress, apply your bare hand.

2. Maintain pressure until the bleeding stops. If the improvised dressing is soaked through, add several more layers (do not remove the original compress) and continue the hand pressure as firmly as possible.

3. Do not disturb the clotting process after bleeding stops. Leave the wound undisturbed, even though the dressing may be blood-soaked. Hold it in place with a pressure bandage, if possible. Otherwise, use a strip of cloth, wind it around the dressing, and tie it with the knot over the wound (lower illustration, far right).

4. If a wound has been sustained in the arm or leg, raise the limb above the level of the heart so that the force of gravity can slow the flow of blood to the injured area.

5. Watch for any signs of shock—pale or bluish skin that feels moist or clammy; weakness; a rapid faint pulse; rapid, shallow breathing; and possible loss of consciousness. Begin first aid for shock immediately:

    a. Have the person lie down, face up, with the legs propped up so that they are at a higher level than the heart.

    b. Remove or loosen all constricting clothing.

    c. Cover the person with a blanket or with whatever outer garments are available.

    d. Reassure the person. Do not provide anything, not even water, to drink. If vomiting occurs, turn the person's head to one side to prevent choking.

6. Transfer the injured person to the nearest hospital for further treatment. If you suspect internal bleeding, minimize movement and call for an ambulance.

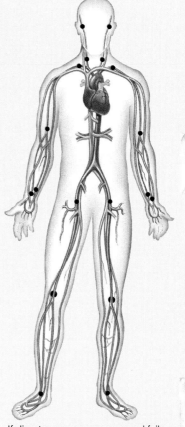

If direct pressure over a wound fails to halt bleeding, press upon the artery feeding the wound at one of the points illustrated above. (Small dots indicate points located on the front of the body, large dots, on the back.)

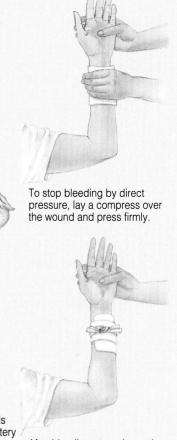

To stop bleeding by direct pressure, lay a compress over the wound and press firmly.

After bleeding stops, leave the compress in place and bind snugly with a clean cloth, tying the knot over the wound.

Alternative Therapies

Alternative therapies have a limited role to play in the handling of a bleeding emergency. But both the injured person and the one administering first aid can benefit from a knowledge of deep-breathing exercises to maintain calm. These and other relaxation techniques can also be helpful during recovery from a major hemorrhage or in managing pain during recuperation.

Alternative therapies recommended for less serious bleeding include:

Herbal Medicine. Chinese herbalists advocate agrimony for treating heavy menstrual periods. Indian herbalists prescribe garlic as a remedy for heavy periods. Gel from a freshly cut aloe stem is said to stop bleeding and speed healing of minor cuts.

Nutrition Therapy. Any significant blood loss can lead to iron deficiency anemia. Iron supplements may be prescribed as well as iron-rich food (red meat, liver, egg yolks, and iron-fortified cereal products) to help build new red blood cells. Extra protein is also needed for the repair of tissue. To promote clotting, foods that are rich in vitamin K—green leafy vegetables, milk, and liver—are recommended.

Self-Treatment

A knowledge of first aid can make the difference between life and death in any emergency. The American Red Cross offers first aid courses that take just one day, and many community hospitals have similar programs.

A first aid kit (see box, opposite page, top) should be in the medicine cabinet of every home, the trunk of every car, and the backpack of every hiker. Someone should check it periodically and replenish any supplies as needed.

If a painkiller is needed, do not take aspirin, ibuprofen, or other non-steroidal anti-inflammatory drugs, because these medications interfere with the normal clotting of blood. Acetaminophen is a safe alternative.

Other Causes of Bleeding

Abnormal bleeding is a warning sign of many cancers and should never be ignored. Fortunately, most bleeding has easily treated causes. For example, a small amount of blood when brushing the teeth is usually caused by gum disease. Blood in the urine may indicate cystitis or bladder or kidney stones. In athletes, blood in the urine sometimes results from excessive running. Rectal bleeding or blood in the stools usually is due to hemorrhoids, polyps, or inflammation of the colon.

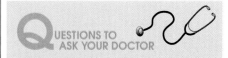

QUESTIONS TO ASK YOUR DOCTOR

▶ Could any of the medications that I take be responsible for an increased tendency to bleed?

▶ What's the best antibacterial solution to use on a cut before bandaging it?

Body Odor

The body exudes many odors, some of them tolerable, perhaps even agreeable, and others unpleasant. For example, the smell of fresh perspiration usually is not offensive. (That of stale perspiration is, however, because bacteria that live on the skin create malodorous substances in sweat.) Menstrual blood develops a disagreeable odor when exposed to air, and certain foods, especially onions and garlic, as well as alcoholic beverages, can produce a strong and distinctive body odor.

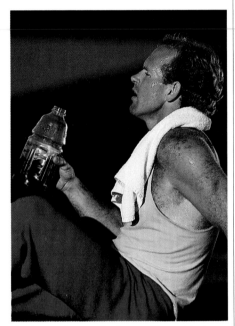

Fresh sweat normally does not have an unpleasant odor, but bacteria and fungi can make it malodorous as it dries and ages.

Body odor generally originates in the underarms, genital area, and feet because perspiration cannot readily evaporate from these areas and bacterial and fungal action are encouraged.

Diagnostic Studies and Procedures
An unpleasant body odor is rarely of mysterious origin and usually vanishes with bathing; if it does not, these are some possibilities to consider.

An untreated infection can be the source of the problem. Athlete's foot, a fungal infection, is the most common cause of foot odor. Vaginal yeast infections have a fishy smell. And any skin infection that is allowed to fester under an airtight dressing will produce a bad odor. Also, gangrene, which denotes tissue death, smells like rotting meat.

Certain medications may also be the source. Frequent application of a topical over-the-counter acne preparation that contains benzoyl peroxide may produce an unwanted smell. Other medications used topically or taken internally should be reviewed with your doctor to find out whether they might be causing body odors.

An offensive smell can also originate in the faulty metabolism of a particular food or food group. If body odor is a persistent problem, a doctor will investigate the diet to try to track down the cause. There is some evidence, for example, that foods high in the chemical choline—found in eggs, liver, and legumes—may produce a distinctive odor in perspiration; eliminating them from the diet may help.

Medical Treatments
In practically all cases, body odor does not require medical treatment. The exceptions are problems due to an infection or underlying disease. Topical antifungal creams or powders will clear up most cases of athlete's foot, and antiyeast preparations can cure the majority of vaginal yeast infections.

Exposing skin ulcers to the air, removing diseased tissue, and applying appropriate antibiotics can heal most skin ulcers and infections. However, gangrenous tissue must be surgically removed. If poor circulation is contributing to the infection, it must be treated as well.

Alternative Therapies
Natural deodorants, many of which are available in health food stores, are recommended to counter body odor. Other alternative approaches include:
Herbal Medicine. Extracts of astringent herbs such as witch hazel, sage, and betony have mild antiperspirant properties when applied to the skin. A few drops of mint oil added to bathwater acts as a natural deodorant.
Nutrition Therapy. In addition to exploring the possibility that a change in diet might be the solution to offensive body odor, a nutritionist may also suggest such dietary supplements as zinc or magnesium, which are said to counteract unpleasant smells carried in the perspiration of some people.

Self-Treatment
In the vast majority of cases, simple self-treatment is all that is needed. To control most unpleasant odors, bathe daily and refrain from using perfumes,

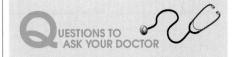
deodorants, and antiperspirants as an alternative to bathing. (Also heed warnings not to use these products on broken skin and discontinue their use if a rash appears.) Roll-on or cream deodorants are preferable to aerosols, which may contain propellants harmful to the lungs or the environment.

Genital areas can be kept free of unpleasant odors by daily washing with mild soap and water. Women should avoid overuse of douches and feminine hygiene products, because they can irritate sensitive tissues.

Even after odor has been eliminated from the body, it may linger on some clothing. If washing with detergent does not remove it, try soaking the garments for at least an hour in warm salt water, using about 3 tablespoons of salt per quart of water.

To prevent the bad odors that may develop because of bacterial decomposition on sweaty feet, podiatrists make the following recommendations:
▶ Wear shoes made of natural materials, such as leather and cotton canvas, that allow air to circulate.
▶ Don't wear the same shoes, especially sneakers, everyday; give them a chance to air out. It also helps to dust them with a deodorant foot powder.
▶ In hot weather, choose open footwear that permits air to circulate.
▶ Wear white cotton socks with sneakers. After exercising, bathe feet with warm water and soap, dry them thoroughly, and change into dry socks and different shoes.

If athlete's foot does not respond within a week to self-treatment with a nonprescription drug, see a dermatologist for a prescription medication. Sometimes the infection spreads to the nails and can be especially difficult to cure, even with professional treatment.

Other Causes of Body Odor
In unusual cases, a serious underlying disease such as diabetes or cancer can cause an unpleasant body odor.

Boils

(Furuncles)

A boil is a painful swelling of the skin caused by a bacterial infection in a hair follicle. Technically called furuncles, boils usually develop in hairy parts of the body that are exposed to friction and pressure. They appear most often on the face, scalp, back of the neck, armpits, and buttocks, and are more common in men than in women.

Possible causes of boils are poor personal hygiene or an immune system compromised by diabetes or other chronic illness. Nutritional deficiencies and exposure to certain industrial chemicals may also be implicated.

A boil can be as small as a green pea or larger than a marble. In larger ones, the infection involves both the hair follicle and surrounding tissue.

Boils that form in a cluster are called carbuncles. When they appear simultaneously in different parts of the body, the condition is called furunculosis. This occurs when the bacteria are spread from the original site to other parts of the body by contaminated objects such as towels, unwashed hands, or shaving implements.

Diagnostic Studies and Procedures

Boils are easily diagnosed by their characteristic appearance. As a boil begins to form, it is accompanied by mild pain and itching. When pus collects and the boil increases in size, it becomes more painful and tender to the touch.

Typically, within two weeks or less, it will come to a head and have a white or yellow center; if there are no complications, it will burst spontaneously, then drain, and heal.

RESISTANT GERMS

In recent years, an alarming number of bacteria have developed resistance to our most widely prescribed antibiotics. Researchers are especially worried about *Staphylococcus aureus,* the microorganism responsible for most boils.

S. aureus, which normally resides in the throat and nose, can cause toxic shock syndrome and other deadly types of blood poisoning if it invades the bloodstream. This bacterium has developed resistance to all antibiotics except vancomycin, and researchers warn that it is only a matter of time until *S. aureus* can also elude this drug, raising the specter of a rise in fatal staph infections.

The bacterial agent responsible for most boils is *Staphylococcus aureus.* Staph infections are not dangerous when they are strictly local and promptly eliminated, but when the organisim invades the bloodstream, the resulting illness can be life threatening (see box, lower left).

Medical Treatments

A boil or carbuncle that resists self-treatment and becomes more painful and red should be seen by a doctor, especially if it is accompanied by a feeling of malaise and a fever. In such cases, oral antibiotics are given (usually one of the newer penicillin variants), and if necessary, the boil is lanced surgically and drained. A topical antibiotic is applied and the area is covered with sterile gauze. The doctor usually provides instructions to follow until the area is completely healed.

If the boil is large and deep, the doctor may, after lancing and draining it, leave it uncovered and insert an antibiotic-impregnated wick of gauze into the incision to kill any remaining bacteria. The wick is pulled out a bit each day, and finally removed completely when the infection is cleared up. This procedure may leave a hairline scar.

Many people develop boils when their resistance to infection is low, or when they are in crowded unsanitary surroundings. Recurrent boils or carbuncles, however, should be brought to a doctor's attention to find the underlying cause. This is especially important when boils occur in or around the nose, providing a route for the infection to travel to the brain.

Alternative Therapies

Herbal Medicine. Herbalists advocate the application of poultices soaked in a strong infusion of comfrey and linseed oil. Such applications are said to soften the boil and make it easier to drain. Also recommended for poultices are dried burdock and echinacea. Some herbal books suggest applying a paste made from the powdered root of goldenseal. Caution is needed, however, because goldenseal may cause skin ulcers (see box, page 339).

Nutrition Therapy. A nutritionist may review the diet and suggest the elimination of sugar, food allergens, and other components that might suppress the immune system. There is some evidence that dietary zinc supplements are effective in preventing recurrent boils.

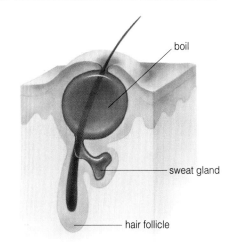

A boil forms in a hair follicle and may also infect surrounding tissue.

Other supplements that are thought to be helpful are vitamins A, C, and E and beta carotene.

Self-Treatment

Prompt self-treatment clears up most boils. Hot compresses applied several times a day bring the boil to a head more quickly so that it can be drained. You can use tap water that has been boiled and cooled to a tolerable temperature, or make Epsom salt packs by dissolving two tablespoons of the salts in a cup of hot water.

Never squeeze a boil to break it open, as this can force the bacteria inward into the bloodstream. Use the compresses to encourage a spontaneous opening, clean the area carefully with hydrogen peroxide, alcohol, or Betadine, and cover it with sterile gauze. Do not make an airtight dressing, however; exposure to oxygen promotes healing. Antibacterial soaps can help to prevent boils but are not an effective treatment for existing ones.

Other Causes of Skin Infections

Impetigo, a bacterial skin infection, can produce abscesses that resemble boils. See a doctor promptly if a sore persists or recurs or if several boil-like lesions appear in a cluster.

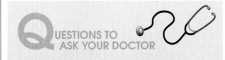

QUESTIONS TO ASK YOUR DOCTOR

▶ What can I do to prevent spreading the infection that causes boils to others?
▶ Could my recurrent boils be due to a nutritional deficiency? If so, what supplements should I take?

Bone Cancer

(Ewing's and other sarcomas)

Bone cancer is a relatively rare malignancy that can occur at any age, but more often it seems to strike during childhood or adolescence.

There are several different types:

Osteogenic sarcoma and *Ewing's sarcoma* are the most common in children.

Parosteal sarcoma, a slow-growing tumor, affects adults.

Chondrosarcoma, also an adult disease, develops in cartilage, most often in the knee, trunk, shoulders, or upper thighs, where it may cause tender masses.

Giant cell tumors of the bone often begin in the knee and affect women more often than men.

Adamantinoma of the long bones usually involves the shinbone.

Chordoma arises in the vertebrae of the lower back, and can also involve the skull and affect vision.

Most childhood bone cancers develop during periods of rapid growth, but the cause is unknown. Excessive radiation exposure through repeated X-rays is linked to some cancers. Paget's disease, which causes bone overgrowth, is sometimes implicated.

A hallmark of bone cancer is increasing pain that cannot be relieved with painkillers. Other symptoms include unexplained fractures, fatigue, loss of

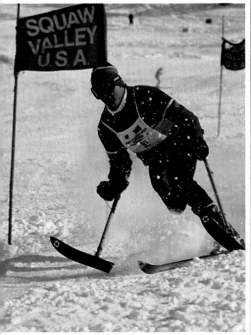

An amputation due to bone cancer has not kept Senator Edward Kennedy's son, Edward, Jr., from skiing and other sports.

appetite and weight, and a persistent low-grade fever. Depending on the tumor site, there may also be swelling.

Diagnostic Studies and Procedures

Characteristic symptoms usually alert a doctor to the possibility of bone cancer. After a physical examination, he will probably order X-rays of the affected bones and perhaps scans of the entire skeleton and the lungs.

Special bone scans to show where new bone is forming may be ordered. One imaging technique, called scintigraphy, involves injecting a radioactive substance into a vein and then scanning the skeleton with a special camera, which will reveal areas of increased blood flow characteristic of a tumor.

A definitive diagnosis requires a biopsy of tissue removed from the tumor. Blood studies can help determine whether the tumor originated in the bone or has metastasized from a cancer elsewhere in the body.

Medical Treatments

Treatment should be carried out by a team of specialists at a comprehensive cancer center, because these cancers are uncommon and therapy is constantly being refined. Surgery is usually called for, but not necessarily amputation. Sometimes the tumor can be removed along with a margin of healthy tissue, followed by radiation treatments and chemotherapy to eradicate any remaining cancer cells.

When amputation is necessary, surgeons can sometimes replace the diseased bone with either a metal substitute or with bone from some other part of the person's body.

A few bone cancers, especially Ewing's sarcoma, are sometimes cured with radiation and chemotherapy, either alone or following surgery.

Alternative Therapies

Potentially useful adjuncts to conventional treatments include:

Acupuncture. This technique is helpful in alleviating the pain, which can be severe with bone cancer.

Herbal Medicine. Some traditional Chinese herbal combinations may help to reduce the nausea and other side effects of radiation and chemotherapy.

T'ai Chi and Other Movement Therapies. Gentle exercise is instrumental in regeneration of healthy bone after radiation treatments, which destroy both healthy and cancerous bone tissue. Before embarking on any

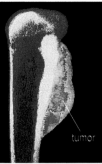

A bone tumor is often evident on special X-rays, but a biopsy is necessary to tell whether or not it is cancerous.

exercise regimen, check with your doctor. Too much weight placed on the weakened bones can result in fractures.

Self-Treatment

Maintaining a healthy diet can be very difficult for bone cancer patients. Both the disease and its treatments suppress appetite. Emphasize foods that are high in protein, calcium, and the nutrients needed to boost the immune system—zinc and vitamins A, B_6, and C. Fruit milkshakes and creamed vegetable soups are examples. (Talk to your doctor about supplements and enriched foods.) Frequent, nutritious snacks may be easier to cope with than three regular meals. Foods served cold or at room temperature are less likely to provoke nausea than hot dishes.

Recovery often demands extensive physical therapy and rehabilitation, especially after an amputation. The rehabilitation should be part of the overall treatment plan, and some aspects may begin before or during the active treatment phase.

Consider joining a support group of patients with similar problems. New bioengineering technology has produced truly amazing artificial limbs, but learning to use them often requires determination, patience, and support.

Other Causes of Bone Tumors

Cancers that arise elsewhere and spread to the bones are actually much more common than primary bone cancer. Malignancies of the breast, lung, thyroid, prostate, and kidneys are most likely to spread to the skeleton.

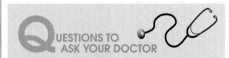

QUESTIONS TO ASK YOUR DOCTOR

▶ What kind of bone cancer do I have?
▶ Is an amputation necessary or can the cancer be treated with less radical methods?
▶ What kind of rehabilitation will be needed following treatment?

Bowlegs

(Genu varum)

At birth, all babies are somewhat bow-legged because, within the cramped space in the uterus, the legs are likely to fold over each other. This condition is referred to as *genu varum* in medical parlance. (In Latin, *genu* means knees and *varum* means inwardly curved.) In the simplest terms, legs are defined as bowed if, when the ankles touch each other, the unbent knees do not.

In practically all cases, mildly bowed legs correct themselves, even if the condition persists until the child is three years old. When only one leg is bowed, however, the cause may be a turning in of the leg bone resulting from a birth injury or an inherited degenerative disease of the knee.

Diagnostic Studies and Procedures

A pediatrician normally checks a baby's legs during routine examinations. If the bowing is less than 20 degrees, chances are that the problem will correct itself. However, a bowing of more 20 degrees after the age of 18 months, or one that is progressing or causing pain when walking, should be investigated by a pediatric orthopedist. Mildly bowed legs that fail to straighten out spontaneously by the time the child is four years old also warrant an evaluation by an orthopedist.

In arriving at a diagnosis, the doctor will ask about family medical history, nutrition, and any birth injuries. An

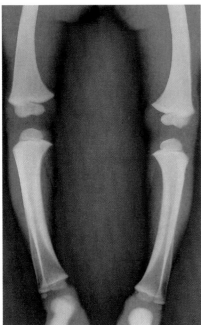

Even markedly bowed legs, such as the ones shown in this X-ray, may correct themselves as the child grows. If not, braces or other treatment may be necessary.

X-ray may show bone deformities or injuries. If there is a family history of bowlegs and knock-knees, a genetic disorder is likely. Other possibilities include Blount's disease, or *tibial osteochondrosis,* in which the shin bone curves inward because the growth plate ceases to function normally. This abnormality may develop in children who walk early, or who are very short or obese. It may appear also during the adolescent growth spurt.

Bowlegs may indicate rickets, a disease caused by vitamin D deficiency due either to an inadequate amount in the diet, a lack of exposure to sunlight, or a genetic inability to absorb the vitamin. Without sufficient vitamin D, the body cannot utilize calcium, and the result is soft and deformed bones. Nutritional rickets is very rare in the United States, thanks to fortified milk and other basic foods that are enriched with vitamin D. Laboratory tests can detect the genetic form.

Medical Treatments

If the bowing is severe or worsening, braces and surgery are the first options to be considered. Correction should be undertaken as early as possible, first with braces, and if this treatment shows no positive results, with surgery to correct the faulty knee structure.

Blount's disease usually requires surgery to rotate the shin bone to its proper position. Otherwise the condition may eventually result in disabling problems of the knee joints.

Nutritional rickets is treated with large doses of vitamin D. The treatment of rickets that is caused by a genetic metabolic defect will vary depending on the nature of the disorder.

Alternative Therapies

Responsible practitioners of acupuncture, chiropractic, and most other alternative therapies would not undertake the basic treatment of bowlegs. Some alternative therapies, however, may improve the underlying causes.

Light Therapy.

Exposure to sunlight or an ultraviolet lamp stimulates the skin's production of vitamin D. Be careful when exposing a baby to the sun, however, because of the danger of sunburn. A few minutes in the early morning or late afternoon two or three times a week is all that is usually needed.

Massage Therapies.

Massage, using gentle manipulative exercises by a practitioner trained in pediatric care, may be helpful. Physical therapists on the staffs of orthopedic clinics are also knowledgeable about these techniques, and can show you how to exercise the child's legs yourself.

Nutrition Therapy.

If a physician has determined that a dietary deficiency or a metabolic abnormality is the cause of bowlegs, she may suggest that a nutrition therapist be consulted to prescribe the appropriate amounts of such supplements as calcium and vitamin D. Careful monitoring is necessary when giving a young child supplements of these nutrients because they are stored in the body and excessive amounts can result in severe liver damage, metabolic abnormalities, and kidney disorders.

Self-Treatment

When a baby appears to be bowlegged, parents should not encourage early walking, which can exacerbate the problem. They should also avoid bulky diapers, which can push the development of bowlegs, especially when a baby starts standing and attempting to walk. If your baby is overweight, consult a pediatrician about a change in diet.

Other Causes of Bowlegs

In rare cases, an inherited metabolic disorder called neurofibromatosis may produce leg bowing and other neuromuscular abnormalities. Sometimes bowing occurs as a result of a fracture in the growth plate, or metaphyses, the part of a long bone that abuts the cartilage and covers the end of the bone. This condition usually corrects itself as the bone heals.

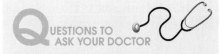

▶ Is there any value in putting special wedges in my baby's walking shoes ?
▶ Can extra amounts of vitamin D harm my bowlegged toddler? What is the safe dosage?
▶ Are night braces or splints advisable?

Brain Tumors

(Meningioma; acoustic neuroma; acoustic schwannoma; pinealoma; glioma)

A brain tumor is any abnormal growth or mass that develops in the skull space usually occupied exclusively by the brain. It may be noncancerous or malignant; both types of growths are potentially life threatening because they encroach on normal brain tissue, which, because of the surrounding skull, becomes compressed.

Symptoms include severe or persistent headaches, personality changes, increased irritability and moodiness, unusual sleepiness, unexplained nausea and vomiting, paralysis, and balance problems. There may also be some deficits of the senses, including hearing, vision, speech, taste, and smell.

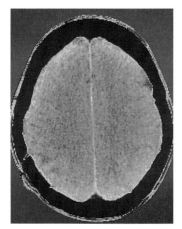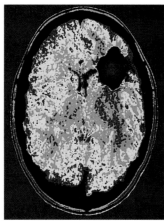

A brain tumor can often be found with a CT scan. On the left is a scan showing a normal brain. The one on the right reveals a glioma.

The most common noncancerous type of brain tumor is called a meningioma, because it arises from the meninges, the thin membranes that cover the brain and the spinal cord.

Of the primary brain cancers, gliomas are the most prevalent, accounting for about 45 percent of cases. Gliomas and other primary brain cancers seldom metastasize. Their rate of growth varies greatly; some may be present for years without causing any problems, while others are rapidly fatal.

There has been a baffling increase in primary brain cancers in recent years, especially among children and young adults. The causes remain largely unknown, although some evidence points to environmental factors. The increase may be linked to a viral infection or possibly exposure to radiation or certain chemicals.

Diagnostic Studies and Procedures

Characteristic symptoms raise a suspicion of a brain tumor. The presence of one is confirmed by various imaging techniques—usually X-rays of the skull and CT scans or MRI. A biopsy of the tumor cells is necessary, however, to learn whether or not it is malignant.

Medical Treatments

Brain tumors are most often treated with radiation, surgery, or a combination of the two. In some cases, a surgeon can remove the entire tumor and effect a complete cure. Developments in computer-assisted surgery, which now make it possible for surgeons to remove tumors deep within the brain, have increased the chances of surgical cure for some types of brain tumors.

If a tumor is inoperable, if it recurs or metastizes, or if only part of it can be removed, radiation is used. With a technique known as radiosurgery, high-dose radiation can be beamed directly into the tumor to shrink it.

In recent years, cancer specialists have also developed methods for using chemotherapy to treat brain cancer. A protective barrier prevents most drugs from penetrating the brain. But doctors can now administer doses directly into the brain via a small, implanted tube.

Another promising experimental treatment involves implanting one or more polymer wafers about the size of a nickel into the brain. The wafer peels away like the skin of an onion over a period of a month, dispensing a powerful drug called BCNU. This system targets the drug directly to the brain over an extended period of time, without exposing other parts of the body to the toxic side effects.

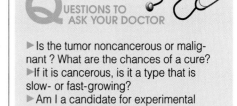

QUESTIONS TO ASK YOUR DOCTOR

► Is the tumor noncancerous or malignant? What are the chances of a cure?
► If it is cancerous, is it a type that is slow- or fast-growing?
► Am I a candidate for experimental treatments? If so, how do I go about enlisting in such programs?

Alternative Therapies

Alternative therapies are unlikely to cure a brain tumor, but they can help relieve some of the symptoms.

Acupuncture. This is often used to lessen cancer pain. It may be combined with chemotherapy and radiation as part of the overall treatment program.

Hypnosis and Imagery. These techniques also help cancer patients to control pain, as well as nausea and other unpleasant symptoms. Self-hypnosis is now being taught to patients at many pain and cancer centers.

The goal of guided imagery goes beyond pain control. While the patient relaxes in a trancelike state, a therapist or a tape recording instructs him to visualize the condition mentally and then to imagine ways of helping the immune system eradicate it. This technique requires patients to study and understand the body's immune system, and then to visualize how it can overcome the tumor. The efficacy of guided imagery has not been proven scientifically, but some researchers theorize that it may bolster the immune system by reducing stress and its effects.

Self-Treatment

Although self-treatment of a brain tumor is not possible, working with speech and physical therapists during the recovery period after surgery can help to overcome some or all of the residual disability.

Other Causes of Brain Tumors

Most malignant brain tumors arise elsewhere in the body and then spread to the brain. Sometimes, a metastatic brain tumor is found before the primary cancer has been diagnosed. Thus, the discovery of a brain malignancy usually prompts a search for cancer in other parts of the body, especially the lungs, breasts, and bones, using imaging techniques similar to those employed in detecting a brain tumor.

Breast Cancer

(Mammary carcinoma)

Breast cancer is the most common malignancy in women, and second only to lung cancer in female cancer mortality. Presently, about one in nine American women develops this disease at some time in her life, compared to one in 17 in 1950. Experts are uncertain whether this represents a true rise in the incidence of breast cancer or improved detection of it due to mammography and better public awareness.

The risk of breast cancer increases with age, especially after menopause. Risk is also higher among women who had their first child after age 30 or never had children; already have had cancer in one breast; had an early first menstrual period or a late menopause; or have a close relative, such as a sister or mother, who was diagnosed with breast cancer before menopause.

Some studies have linked a high-fat diet to an increased risk of breast cancer, but others have shown otherwise. Cancer specialists emphasize that about 70 percent of all cases of breast cancer arise in women with none of the above risk factors. In rare instances, men also develop breast cancer, accounting for less than five percent of occurrences.

Diagnostic Studies and Procedures

Early detection is the single most important factor in surviving breast cancer, because early, localized malignancies are more than 90 percent curable. The American Cancer Society (ACS) recommends that all women age 20 or older perform a monthly self-examination of their breasts (see box, page 113). Although more than 80 percent of the lumps found by women during self-examination are benign, women initially discover more than 85 percent of all breast cancers.

Breast examination by a physician is recommended every three years between the ages of 20 and 40 and annually thereafter. The age at which a woman should begin regular screening with mammography remains controversial. Present guidelines from the National Cancer Institute recommend starting annual mammography at age 50, but many cancer experts advocate beginning at age 40. There is no doubt, however, that mammography is the most effective means of early breast cancer detection in women over 50 because it can locate suspicious areas of calcification, a common sign of cancer, long before a tumor is large enough to be felt by a woman or her doctors. Mammography is not as effective in younger women because they have denser, lumpier breasts, making it harder to discern normal from abnormal tissue.

Mammography should be scheduled for the week after menstruation, when breasts are unlikely to be swollen and painful. To help assure an accurate mammogram and avoid repeats, no deodorant, powder, cream, or other substance should be applied to breasts or the underarm area that day because they can cause misleading results.

If any suspicious areas are found by mammography or physical examination, a biopsy is necessary to rule out cancer. In most cases, a doctor will attempt to obtain a tissue sample by aspiration, a procedure in which a hollow needle is inserted into the lump. If fluid can be withdrawn, it will be analyzed for malignant cells, but such

WARNING SIGNS OF BREAST CANCER

Any of the following warrant a prompt doctor's evaluation.
► A lump that persists throughout the menstrual cycle.
► Any change in breast shape, symmetry, or contour.
► Persistent pain or tenderness.
► Thickening or hardening of the breast tissue in one region.
► Redness, pitting, dimpling, or inflammation of the skin.
► Clear or bloody nipple discharge.
► Nipple retraction or indentation.

lumps, especially those that disappear after aspiration, are usually harmless cysts. If a lump returns rapidly, no fluid can be withdrawn, or malignant cells are detected in the fluid, another biopsy is necessary. Again, this may be done by needle. With a new procedure called stereotaxic needle aspiration, a special X-ray scanning technique is used during aspiration to locate suspicious areas too small to be felt.

In some cases, a surgical biopsy is necessary. This may be excisional, in which the entire mass is removed, or incisional, in which only part of the lump is taken out. A pathologist will then determine whether the tissue is cancerous, and if so, what kind of cancer it is. Cells from a cancerous lump will also be tested to determine if they are stimulated by estrogen or progesterone, a finding that may influence the choice of anticancer drugs.

If breast cancer is diagnosed, additional tests are needed to find out if it has metastasized to other parts of the body. These may include a bone scan, X-rays, and sampling of lymph nodes.

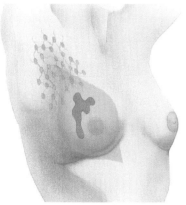

With a modified radical mastectomy the breast, lymph nodes, and perhaps some chest muscle are removed.

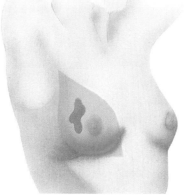

With a total, or simple, mastectomy all breast tissue is removed but not the nodes or underlying chest muscle.

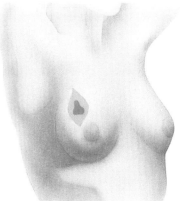

With a partial mastectomy, or lumpectomy, the tumor, a margin of normal breast tissue, and perhaps a few nodes are taken out.

Medical Treatments

Surgery. Treatment varies according to the type and stage of cancer, but surgery remains the first choice for most tumors. The majority of operations now are less disfiguring than the radical mastectomy that was standard until the 1970s. Operations for breast cancer are:

Extended radical mastectomy involves removal of the breast, underarm lymph nodes, and underlying chest muscles. This procedure, rarely performed today, is reserved for women with large tumors that are attached to or have invaded the chest muscle and its connective tissues. If the mammary lymph nodes deep in the chest are involved, they will also be removed.

Modified radical mastectomy is the removal of the breast, underarm lymph nodes, and sometimes part of the chest muscle. The amount of tissue removed from the underarm depends on the spread of the tumor. This remains the most common operation for women with invasive breast cancer.

Total, or simple, mastectomy is the removal of the entire breast, including its extensions to the armpit and sometimes near the collarbone. Because the lymph nodes are left intact, radiation therapy usually follows the operation.

Subcutaneous mastectomy involves removing the breast tissue but leaving the skin and nipple intact. A prosthesis is then slipped under the skin to restore normal appearance. This procedure is rarely performed, because it may miss cancer cells and the cosmetic results are often poor.

Lumpectomy or partial mastectomy involves removal of the cancerous lump and a surrounding margin of normal tissue. Some of the armpit lymph nodes are also taken out and examined for spread, and the operation is followed by radiation therapy.

Preventative, or prophylactic, mastectomy is the removal of a breast to prevent the development of cancer. This operation is done only if a woman has a very high risk of breast cancer and is so worried by the prospect that she cannot live a normal life.

Breast reconstruction by a plastic surgeon can sometimes be performed immediately following a mastectomy, but more often it is done after the original incision has healed. If the opposite breast is larger, it may be reduced in size to match the reconstructed one, either at the same time as the reconstruction or in a later operation.

In the past, a prosthetic implant filled with silicone gel was the first choice for reconstruction. Because questions have arisen about the long-term safety of silicone, many women are now opting for implants filled with a saline solution, or a more extensive procedure in which fatty tissue from the woman's own buttocks or elsewhere is used to reconstruct a breast.

Radiation Therapy. The purpose of this treatment is to destroy any cancer cells that may have escaped surgical removal. Radiation is routinely administered after a simple mastectomy and a lumpectomy, or if numerous lymph nodes have been affected. It is also prescribed for recurring or inoperable cancer, and to alleviate the pain of advanced cancer.

Typically, radiation treatments are begun two or three weeks after the surgery, or after the scar has healed and the woman has regained the use of her arm. Immediate side effects include blistering of the skin and fatigue. Later, the skin exposed to the radiation may darken, thicken, and lack sensitivity if any nerve endings have been damaged. Long-term complications may include

Exercises that involve raising the arms can help prevent arm swelling after a mastectomy.

impaired lung function due to scar tissue, an increased risk of heart disease, and easy fracturing of the ribs.

Chemotherapy. Studies indicate that adjuvant chemotherapy greatly increases long-term survival, even for women with localized stage I cancer (see box, below). Chemotherapy may begin before surgery; however, it is usually started a few weeks afterwards. This treatment is also prescribed for recurrent or inoperable cancers.

Chemotherapy appears to be most effective in preventing a recurrence among younger women who have not gone through menopause. The side effects—loss of hair, nausea, reduced immunity to infections, mouth sores, fatigue, and bleeding problems—are temporary, but still very trying. For this reason, chemotherapy may not be recommended for an older woman, especially if her cancer is localized.

Hormone Therapy. Cancer specialists now believe that almost all breast cancer patients can benefit from hormone therapy, even if their tumors are not the type stimulated by estrogen or progesterone. Tamoxifen (Nolvadex), a drug that blocks estrogen, is the treatment of choice. It has fewer side effects than anticancer drugs, although it may cause hot flashes and other menopausal symptoms in younger women.

Other, more radical approaches to hormone manipulation include *ovarian ablation*, a procedure in which the ovaries are either surgically removed or destroyed by chemicals or radiation, and perhaps the removal of other hormone-producing glands.

STAGES OF BREAST CANCER

Based on a combination of parameters, five stages of breast cancer have been designated:

▶ **Stage 0** is noninvasive cancer, or carcinoma in situ, with no metastases.
▶ **Stage I** refers to small (2 centimeters or less) invasive tumors without metastases.
▶ **Stage IIA** refers to small tumors (2 centimeters or less) with metastases to regional lymph nodes and larger (2 to 5 centimeters) tumors without metastases. Stage IIB includes large tumors (more than 5 centimeters) without metastases.

▶ **Stage IIIA** includes tumors of any size associated with spread to fixed adjacent lymph nodes, and large (more than 5 centimeters) tumors associated with metastases to adjacent nodes. Stage IIIB cancer includes locally advanced tumors and those with spread to internal mammary lymph nodes.
▶ **Stage IV** encompasses all tumors with distant metastases.

Experimental Treatments. Women with advanced breast cancer may be candidates for experimental therapies such as *hyperthermia*, in which very high fevers are induced to kill cancer cells; *photodynamic therapy*, which uses a light-sensitive anticancer drug; and *bone marrow transplantation*, in which the woman's bone marrow is destroyed by drugs and then replaced with healthy marrow to bolster the body's ability to fight the cancer.

Alternative Therapies

Cancer requires scrupulous medical and surgical treatment. Nonetheless, certain alternative therapies may play an adjunctive role in its care.

Herbal Medicine. Herbalists have long recommended tropical periwinkle to treat breast cancer and other malignancies. Indeed, a periwinkle alkaloid is used to make vincristine, a very potent chemotherapy agent. Oncologists stress, however, that this drug should be used only under careful medical supervision rather than to resort to herbal periwinkle extracts, which can be highly toxic.

Meditation, Self-Hypnosis, and Visualization. Studies indicate that women with advanced breast cancer who participate in group support sessions that include these techniques have significantly longer survival rates than those who do not. Scientists have not yet been able to explain this effect, but some theorize that the methods mobilize the immune system to fight the further spread of cancer.

Nutrition Therapy. Some nutritionists recommend daily supplements of beta carotene (precursor to vitamin A) and vitamins C and E, both to help prevent cancer and to slow its growth. However, studies suggest that foods high in these antioxidants are more effective. Good sources of beta carotene are orange and dark green vegetables and yellow and orange fruits; of vitamin C, many fruits and vegetables, especially citrus fruits and bell peppers; of vitamin E, wheat germ, legumes, seafood, and poultry.

Although the role of other dietary components remains controversial, some studies suggest that a low-fat diet may cut the risk of breast cancer and its recurrence. Such a regimen requires limiting the intake of all fats, especially those from animals, as well as animal protein, while increasing foods high in fiber, such as whole-grain products and fresh fruits and vegetables.

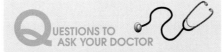

QUESTIONS TO ASK YOUR DOCTOR

▶ Is your mammography equipment used only for breast examinations? (The answer should always be yes.) How many rads does it deliver? (It should be less than one rad for a two-film examination.)
▶ What type of cancer do I have and is it localized?
▶ Can breast reconstruction be performed at the time of mastectomy? What are the risks of reconstruction?
▶ How often should I schedule follow-up doctor visits?

Other nutrition therapists and some naturopaths may recommend extreme macrobiotic and other restricted, low-calorie diets for breast cancer patients. Oncologists warn that these diets should be avoided because they do not provide adequate calories, protein, and other nutrients that the body needs for recovery or to prevent the wasting that occurs in advanced cancer.

Yoga. Regular practice of yoga, meditation, and other relaxation techniques can help alleviate the stress and anxiety caused by cancer, which in turn may boost immune system function.

Self-Treatment

Increasingly, women are expected to play a decision-making role in their overall treatment. This demands being well-informed and not hesitating to question your doctor and voice your concerns. Under the best of circumstances, a diagnosis of breast cancer is psychologically devastating. Joining a support group such as the American Cancer Society's Reach to Recovery program, or simply talking to women who have recovered from breast cancer, can be reassuring.

Concerns about physical appearance following a mastectomy are normal. However, women who do not undergo immediate breast reconstruction are usually relieved to find that, with a well-fit prosthesis, they can wear most of their clothing without anyone being able to tell they have had this surgery.

Initially, use a temporary prosthesis such as cotton fluff inserted into your regular bra, or one that is slightly larger to accommodate bandages. Take this to the hospital with you to avoid the stress of finding something to wear for

the trip home. After healing is complete, plan to shop for a permanent prosthesis. Some regular lingerie departments sell breast prostheses, but you may feel more comfortable and find a wider selection at a specialty shop. Make sure that you try on several different types. Prices vary, but many insurance policies and Medicare cover at least part of the cost. If you cannot find a ready-made prosthesis that looks and feels right, consider investing in a customized one made to match exactly the contour of your other breast.

A prosthesis usually is not necessary after a lumpectomy, but a bra should be worn day and night for several days following surgery to prevent traction of the wound and to help the breast regain its previous shape.

Self-help measures can help to minimize common complications affecting the arm and hand on the mastectomy side. To minimize swelling, exercise your arm as soon as your surgeon says it is okay. Lift it as high as you comfortably can several times a day to promote the flow of lymph. Also, "walk" your fingers up a wall as high as possible and do isometric, or pumping, exercises for the hand such as squeezing a rubber ball. If arm swelling still occurs, talk to your doctor about wearing an elastic sleeve to reduce swelling and improve lymph flow.

If lymph nodes have been removed, the arm and hand on that side are more vulnerable to infection. It is best to avoid anything that constricts or burdens them. Wear loose fitting clothing and switch your watch and purse to the opposite arm. Also have blood drawn or blood pressure measured on the opposite arm. Try to minimize cuts or injuries; for example, use an electric razor if you shave underarm hair; wear protective gloves for gardening and other tasks; and use special care when trimming nails and cuticles.

If you do get a cut or burn, wash it immediately with soap and water and apply an antiseptic plus an antibiotic cream. Consult your doctor promptly if an infection develops.

Other Causes of Breast Symptoms

Many women experience swelling and tenderness of the breasts as part of premenstrual syndrome. Benign fibrocystic breast lumps are also exceedingly common. Nursing mothers often develop mastitis, a bacterial breast infection.

Breast Lumps

(Cystic mastitis; fibrocystic breast syndrome; fibroadenoma; lipoma)

Although women often react with alarm to any change in their breasts, especially the appearance of a lump, most breast problems are benign disorders. Indeed, more than 80 percent of all breast lumps that appear before menopause are not cancerous.

Fibrocystic breast syndrome is the most common cause of breast lumps. Some doctors refer to it as a disease, but most now consider it a normal variation of breast tissue that makes it appear lumpy. The condition seems to be an exaggeration of changes that normally occur in the breast each month, due to fluctuations in the female hormones. These changing hormone levels prepare the breasts for milk production by increasing fluid and blood flow. When conception does not occur, the excess fluid should be reabsorbed by the body, but often some of it accumulates in small sacs called cysts. With time, the sacs may fill with fibrous tissue, leading to permanent lumps.

For unknown reasons, the breast lumpiness is often accompanied by swelling, tenderness, or pain, especially during the premenstrual week. This discomfort, which is referred to as

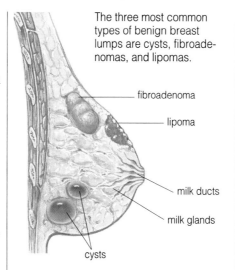

The three most common types of benign breast lumps are cysts, fibroadenomas, and lipomas.

fibroadenoma
lipoma
milk ducts
milk glands
cysts

cystic mastalgia, commonly begins when a woman is in her twenties and often continues until menopause. Some women have fibrocystic symptoms throughout their menstruating years; others find that they come and go.

During pregnancy and breast-feeding, fibrocystic breast discomfort stops, as a rule. Many women find that their monthly discomfort is reduced even after they discontinue breast-feeding.

After menopause, fibrocystic problems usually disappear, but they may in fact worsen in the months leading up to the last menstrual cycle. Contrary to popular belief, fibrocystic breasts

do not increase the risk of breast cancer, but their lumpiness can make it more difficult to detect any tumors that do develop.

Fibroadenoma is the most common benign breast tumor. Although its cause is unknown, female hormones may be a factor. Most develop as a single, firm, round lump that moves freely and painlessly under the skin.

These tumors normally grow very slowly, but in rare cases, they may enlarge rapidly during pregnancy. It is not uncommon for women who have had one fibroadenoma to develop a second one months or years later. These benign breast tumors do not increase the risk of breast cancer.

Lipomas are benign tumors composed of fat cells. They usually lie just below the skin, and may cause dimpling similar to that of breast cancer.

Diagnostic Studies and Procedures

Any unusual or new breast lump should be examined by a doctor. Even if you have fibrocystic breasts, you should be alert to any changes in them. The first step in diagnosis usually involves inserting a hollow needle into the lump. If fluid is easily removed, the likely diagnosis is a cyst. If no fluid can be removed and the lump is solid, mammography and perhaps a biopsy should be done.

A CASE IN POINT

Martha Stockwell, a schoolteacher and mother of two, discovered her first benign breast lump at age 28, during her monthly breast self-examination. Stockwell often developed breast cysts during her premenstrual period, but unlike this hard lump, the cysts were soft and they usually disappeared after menstruation. Her gynecologist advised her to wait and see if it went away after her next period, but she was so worried, she insisted on scheduling an immediate doctor's appointment.

As the doctor examined Stockwell's breast, he assured her he didn't think the lump was a cause for concern. He was unable to draw any fluid from it, however, indicating that it was not a typical cyst. So he instructed Stockwell to get a mammogram. Ordinarily, mammography is recommended for women under age 40 only if there is a suspicious lump.

The mammogram showed a round, solid tumor without the calcification that is typical of breast cancer. Again, the doctor was reassuring. "It looks like a benign fibroma," he said, "but the only way we can rule out cancer is to do a biopsy."

Stockwell found the lump's presence worrisome, and asked that it be removed. This was done in an excisional biopsy performed on an outpatient basis. The next day, her doctor called with the good news that the lump had been a benign fibroadenoma.

The scenario was repeated some 20 years later. This time, her doctor was more concerned because Stockwell was at an age when the risk of breast cancer rises sharply and the lump appeared to be growing rapidly. However, the news was again good—an excisional biopsy confirmed another fibroadenoma. Over the next three years, she developed four

more lumps, but these turned out to be fluid-filled cysts that disappeared after needle drainage. Her breasts seemed more tender than usual, even though she was entering menopause.

"In most women, fibrocystic conditions taper off during menopause," her doctor explained, "but there are exceptions. We think hormonal changes are to blame. Eventually, the tenderness and the appearance of new benign lumps subside." At the same time, he warned Stockwell that she must be extra diligent about annual mammography and seeing a doctor promptly for new lumps.

"We know that cysts and fibroadenomas don't increase the risk of cancer," he said, "but age does. What feels like a fibroadenoma or a cyst may turn out to be a malignant tumor, so every new breast lump must be assumed to be cancerous until proven otherwise."

Medical Treatments

In severe cases of persistent breast pain that is not alleviated by self-care, your doctor may prescribe a diuretic to prevent fluid retention. She may also have you try certain hormonal agents, such as tamoxifen (an estrogen blocker), bromocriptine (a prolactin blocker), or danazol (a synthetic androgen). These drugs are used only as a last resort because of their significant side effects, which range from cessation of menstruation and weight gain to growth of facial and body hair, elevation of blood pressure, headache, fatigue, depression, and blood clots.

A fibroadenoma that is not growing or causing symptoms does not require treatment, although many doctors advocate that it be biopsied to be on the safe side. If the tumor is growing or causing other problems, it can be surgically removed under local anesthesia, usually as an outpatient procedure.

Lipomas are removed as a rule because of the difficulty of distinguishing these benign tumors from cancer. This procedure, too, can be performed under local anesthesia on an outpatient basis. The removal of small tumors usually does not affect appearance.

Alternative Therapies

Herbal Medicine. A comfrey poultice has been reported to ease breast tenderness. Some herbalists also recommend taking two to four grams of evening primrose oil each day. Avoid herbal remedies that contain ginseng, which can have steroidal effects similar to estrogen; they may exacerbate fibrocystic syndrome and cystic mastitis.

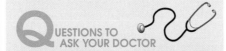

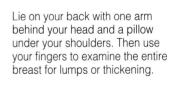

QUESTIONS TO ASK YOUR DOCTOR

▶ What type of breast changes should warrant a visit to a doctor?
▶ How often should I have a breast checkup?
▶ Is it necessary to have fluid removed from recurrent cysts?

Nutrition Therapy. For fibrocystic syndrome, a nutrition therapist might prescribe daily supplements of 400 to 1,000 International Units of vitamin E, which may alter blood fats and indirectly influence hormone levels. In addition, 100 to 200 milligrams of vitamin B_6 may help.

Intake of salt should be reduced, especially in the second half of the menstrual cycle, to help reduce fluid retention and swelling.

Studies indicate that reducing fat intake to less than 15 percent of total calories alleviates symptoms in many women. Accompanying this change should be an increased intake of complex carbohydrates and high-fiber foods, such as fresh vegetables and fruits, plus whole grains.

Self-Treatment

A painkiller such as aspirin, ibuprofen, or acetaminophen may be all that is needed to reduce breast discomfort.

The role of methylxanthines, a substance in coffee, chocolate, tea, colas, and other caffeine-containing beverages, is debatable, but some women report relief when they restrict these

substances. Also, it's wise to avoid over-the-counter medications such as wake-up pills, cold remedies, and aspirin combinations that contain caffeine.

You can ease anxiety about benign breast disorders by examining your breasts regularly and learning to recognize your own pattern of breast lumpiness. For several months, practice daily breast self-examination (see illustrations, below). Make a chart for each breast, noting any lumps or discomfort. Keep track of your menstrual cycle on the same chart. Identifying patterns allows you to discern variations that could signal a new breast problem, which might warrant medical attention. Also note any effects of self-care, such as reduction of caffeine, salt, or fat.

A few modest changes in lifestyle can help alleviate the discomfort of fibrocystic breasts.

▶ Wear a bra that fits well and gives your breasts good support. When your breasts are swollen, you may be more comfortable in a brassiere one cup size larger than normal.
▶ Try to sleep on your back and wear a brassiere to bed when your breasts are swollen and tender.
▶ Alternate applications of warm and cool compresses on the painful breasts.
▶ During painful times, avoid activities that jar the breasts, such as jogging and high-impact aerobics. Always wear a support bra during such activities.

Other Causes of Breast Symptoms

Breast cancer produces lumps that are sometimes difficult to distinguish from benign changes. Pregnancy also causes breast swelling and tenderness.

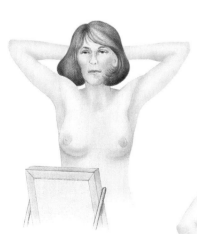

To do a thorough breast exam, stand before a mirror, clasp your hands behind your head, tighten chest muscles, and check the breast contours for symmetry.

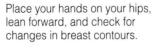

Place your hands on your hips, lean forward, and check for changes in breast contours.

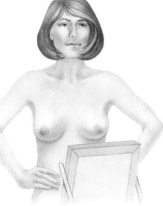

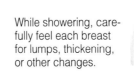

While showering, carefully feel each breast for lumps, thickening, or other changes.

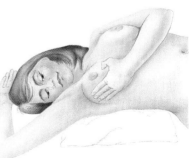

Lie on your back with one arm behind your head and a pillow under your shoulders. Then use your fingers to examine the entire breast for lumps or thickening.

Bronchitis

(Acute infectious bronchitis; chronic bronchitis)

Bronchitis refers to inflammation of the bronchi, the tubes that connect the windpipe, or trachea, with the lungs. When the bronchi become inflamed, breathing is more difficult and the membranes lining the airways produce large amounts of thick mucus, which trigger coughing spells.

Acute bronchitis typically develops in cold weather, when a cold or flu virus attacks the airways; it's often accompanied by a secondary bacterial infection.

Chronic bronchitis is characterized by a mucus-producing cough that lasts for three or more months and recurs yearly, normally in the winter. Smoking is the usual cause, and asthma, emphysema, and other chronic lung problems may increase vulnerability to the disorder. Less frequently, the condition is caused by breathing air that is polluted with hazardous dust, chemicals, or other environmental irritants.

Diagnostic Studies and Procedures

The patient's description of symptoms is important in diagnosing both the acute and chronic forms. A doctor will want to know about recent respiratory infections and any exposure to possible airway irritants. She will also order a sputum culture to identify a causative bacterium, and possibly a chest X-ray. For chronic bronchitis, pulmonary function tests should also be done to detect possible emphysema.

Medical Treatments

Antibiotics are usually prescribed to eradicate bacterial infections. Expectorants, which make the mucus easier to cough up, may also be recommended.

Long-term antibiotic therapy may be needed for chronic bronchitis, or the drugs may be given prophylactically during a cold or flu. Bronchodilators might be prescribed to open the bronchial tubes, and an inhaled steroid given to reduce inflammation.

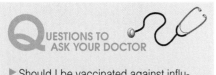

QUESTIONS TO ASK YOUR DOCTOR

▶ Should I be vaccinated against influenza and pneumococcal pneumonia?
▶ What should I do if I have difficulty breathing or I have chest pain?

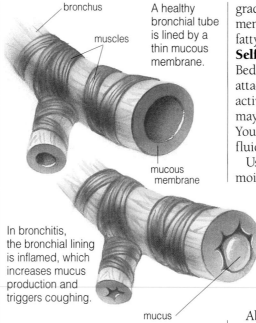

bronchus

muscles

A healthy bronchial tube is lined by a thin mucous membrane.

mucous membrane

In bronchitis, the bronchial lining is inflamed, which increases mucus production and triggers coughing.

mucus

Alternative Therapies

Although alternative therapies do not rid the body of the bacteria that causes most bronchitis, some may alleviate coughing and other symptoms.

Aromatherapy. Massaging the upper body with oil of basil essence is recommended for chronic colds and coughs.

Herbal Medicine. Herbalists often advocate garlic to cure bronchitis. Patients are instructed to keep a garlic clove in the mouth at all times except when sleeping, using new cloves twice a day. They also recommend eucalyptus tea as an expectorant, and capsules containing garlic, parsley, and echinacea. Some advise drinking coltsfoot or angelica root tea, but these herbs should not be ingested because they are linked to an increased risk of cancer.

Chinese herbalists use three different formulas: The Blue Dragon combination is given when there is a cough accompanied by watery sputum and chest congestion; the Minor Bupleurum when there is both fever and a cough that produces sticky yellow mucus; and the Ophiopogon combination for a harsh, dry cough.

Homeopathy. Practitioners urge that aconitum be taken as soon as the symptoms appear. Alternatively, a combination of aconitum, bryonia, and chamomile may be advocated.

Naturopathy and Nutrition Therapy. For acute bronchitis, some naturopaths recommend three days of fasting, followed by a rejuvenating diet that gradually reintroduces food. This regimen eschews dairy products, poultry, fatty meats, and all fried foods.

Self-Treatment

Bed rest is advisable during an acute attack, with a gradual return to normal activities as symptoms disappear. It may take a week or two to recover fully. You should drink at least 10 glasses of fluids a day to thin the mucus.

Use a cool-mist humidifier to keep air moist. Hot showers also help alleviate congestion. Take aspirin or acetaminophen to relieve a low-grade fever. However, do not give aspirin to anyone under the age of 18 during the course of a cold, flu, or other viral infection, because it increases the risk of Reye's syndrome (see page 437). Abstaining from smoking is especially important. Smoking not only delays recovery but also sets the stage for chronic bronchitis, emphysema, and other serious lung disorders. In addi-

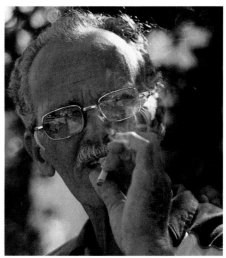

Cigarette smoking is the most common cause of chronic bronchitis.

tion, don't allow anyone to smoke in your presence; secondhand smoke is also highly irritating to the bronchi.

If you have chronic bronchitis, stay away from people who have colds, and try to remain indoors during periods of high air pollution. If your work environment contains irritating dust or chemicals, wear a filtration mask.

Other Causes of Bronchial Coughs

Pneumonia, emphysema, and asthma can produce symptoms similar to those of chronic bronchitis and should be ruled out in the diagnostic process.

Bruises

(Contusion; hematoma)

A bruise develops when blood escapes from damaged blood vessels into the surrounding tissues under the skin, usually as the result of a blow directly to the injured area. The exception is a black eye, which may result from a hit at the temple or forehead, as well as on the eye itself. This happens because the blood follows a gravitational path. Bruised tissues under and around the eye are likely to swell, in some cases causing the eye to shut.

Although the skin over a bruise remains unbroken, it quickly becomes discolored, turning reddish initially, then "black and blue" or purple, and finally yellow or pale green, as damaged blood cells die and are reabsorbed into the blood stream.

The extent of a bruise is self-limiting, because nearby undamaged vessels contract and restrict any further blood flow to that area. Meanwhile, blood platelets collect and activate the clotting mechanism that closes off the break. Unless more serious injuries are present, most bruises will heal themselves in a week to 10 days.

Diagnostic Studies and Procedures

Bruises, also called contusions and hematomas, are usually obvious by their appearance, particularly if they develop as a result of a blow, fall, or dislocation. If they form uneven blotches or remain painful over a long period, medical investigation is warranted, which may include blood tests to measure platelets, clotting factors, and clotting time.

Medical Treatments

There are no medical treatments for bruises as such. Simple bruises are self-healing, and even more extensive ones respond well to self-treatment. Some doctors suggest substituting other pain-killers for aspirin as a treatment for bruising, because aspirin is known to disrupt the blood's clotting mechanism. However, there is little evidence that this approach will make any difference.

An ophthalmologist should be consulted promptly if an injury to the eye causes blurred vision or severe pain or if there is bleeding in the eye.

Alternative Therapies

Herbal Medicine. Herbalists recommend applications of a poultice made from the leaves of comfrey steeped in boiling water. This mix should be

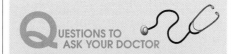

cooled and applied between gauze layers to the bruised areas (see illustrations, below). Avoid skin irritation by applying lanolin first. The active chemical agent in comfrey is allantoin, which has a healing effect on skin tissue.

Tincture of arnica, or an arnica cream derived from the dried flowers of the plant *Arnica montana,* is also said to be effective in treating bruises, especially if applied soon after being injured.

Self-Treatment

Although bruises will heal themselves, prompt self-treatment can sometimes reduce their size and tenderness. During the first 24 hours following the injury, frequent application of an ice pack or cold water compress to the bruised area slows down the bleeding and reduces swelling and pain. After ice treatment, healing through the reabsorbtion of blood cells is promoted by the use of warm compresses or the application of a heating pad.

If a bruise forms on an arm or a leg, swelling can be reduced by keeping the affected limb elevated.

Bruises that develop in conjunction with a pulled muscle or a sprain in the wrist or ankle should be treated with the standard RICE approach: rest, ice, compression, and elevation.

The bruise of a black eye calls for somewhat different self-treatment. To

reduce swelling, apply an ice pack or cold compress as soon as possible after being injured; follow with warm wet compresses the next day. There is no value to the folk remedy of applying raw steak to the bruise. Any benefit comes from the coolness of the meat and a compress is more convenient.

Other Causes of Bruises

Sometimes spontaneous bruises occur when there is a serious underlying disease, possibly a bleeding disorder such as hemophilia, or a serious blood disease such as leukemia or aplastic anemia. Long-term use of corticosteroid medications can also cause easy bruising, as can vitamin C deficiency.

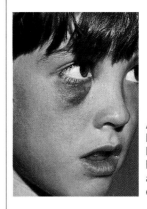

A black eye may be caused by a blow to the forehead or temple, as well as to the eye area itself.

A condition called purpura simplex, which usually occurs in women, is characterized by the spontaneous appearance of bruises on the upper arms, thighs, and buttocks. In most cases, there are no other blood abnormalities and clotting mechanisms are normal. The cause of this easy bleeding is unknown; unless symptoms of an underlying disorder become apparent, it is not a cause for concern, and it requires no special attention.

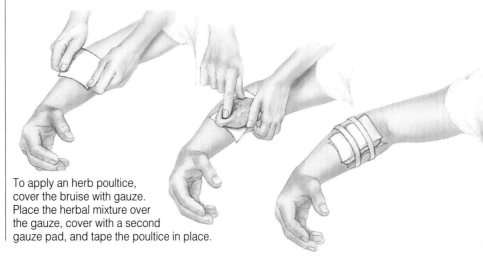

To apply an herb poultice, cover the bruise with gauze. Place the herbal mixture over the gauze, cover with a second gauze pad, and tape the poultice in place.

Bunions

(Hallux valgus)

A bunion is a deformity, or protrusion, of the joint at the base of the big toe, in which there is usually pain, inflammation, and swelling. The big toe appears to be turned inward and may overlap the second toe, and sometimes the third toe as well. The condition is almost always accompanied by inflammation of the nearby bursa, the fluid-filled sac that acts as a cushion between the tendons and bones.

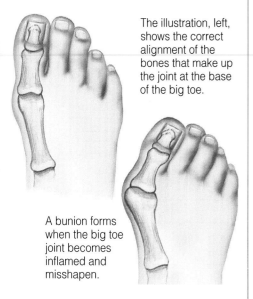

The illustration, left, shows the correct alignment of the bones that make up the joint at the base of the big toe.

A bunion forms when the big toe joint becomes inflamed and misshapen.

Much more common in women than in men, bunions are usually due to a combination of factors, typically starting with an inherited weakness of the joint. Pressure from improperly fitted shoes, particularly those with high heels and narrow toes, forces the toes together in an abnormal position. In time this leads to a permanently deformed joint.

Diagnostic Studies and Procedures

A physical examination is usually all that is necessary to ascertain that a bunion is present. However, a doctor may order foot X-rays to determine the extent of the deformity and decide upon a course of treatment.

Medical Treatments

Aspirin, ibuprofen, or stronger prescription nonsteroidal anti-inflammatory drugs can usually alleviate the pain and inflammation of a bunion.

Surgery to remove the bunion and realign the toe joint may be necessary in severe cases, especially when the bunion causes difficulty in walking and puts abnormal stress on the foot, hip,

and spine. This operation, called a bunionectomy, involves opening the joint capsule and cutting tendons attached to the base of the metatarsal and the toe bones to permit the bones to straighten as they heal. The section of the metatarsal bone that is protruding may be removed, along with the sesamoid bone, another small bone that is attached to a tendon.

The operation is most often done on an outpatient basis under local or spinal anesthesia. About six weeks are required for complete recovery. To permit healing during that time, excessive weight should not be put on the foot. The foot is wrapped firmly with an elastic bandage, and special shoes are worn during the healing period.

Most people are able to return to work and other daily activities within a few days after the operation, but vigorous exercise should be avoided until healing is complete. Any sign of infection and inflammation should be reported promptly to the doctor.

Alternative Therapies

Alternative treatments cannot cure a bunion, but they can be helpful in reducing the pain and inflammation.

Acupuncture. Stimulation of certain points may alleviate pain and inflammation of the metatarsophalangeal joint, where bunions form.

Hydrotherapy. Soaking the painful joint in a whirlpool footbath, or simply applying a wet compress can relieve pain, especially after standing up for a long period. Experiment with water temperature; some people find hot or warm water is the most effective, while others prefer tepid or cold water.

Massage. An inflamed joint should not be massaged directly, but the area around it can be soothed with gentle massaging. To alleviate pain, some therapists press upon a point on the side of the foot just below the second toe and parallel to the bunion. Other pain points are located just below the ankle bone, near the tip of the thumb, and in the space adjacent to the first joint of the thumb.

Physical Therapy. Special foot exercises sometimes help prevent bunions by strengthening foot muscles. Three that physical therapists and podiatrists often recommend are:

▶ *Marble pick-up.* Place a marble or similar object on the floor and practice picking it up with your toes.

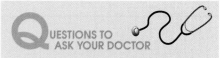
▶ *Bottle roll.* Place a soda or other round bottle on the floor and, while seated, roll your entire foot over it 10 times. Repeat with the other foot.

▶ *Foot and toe stretches.* While seated, lift one bare foot five or six inches off the floor. Make six small circles in both directions with the entire foot, then stretch your toes out and upward as far as you can. Repeat with the other foot.

Self-Treatment

The key to treating a bunion is to select the proper shoes. Most mild bunions can be controlled by wearing properly fitted, low-heeled shoes with a toe box that is wide enough to accommodate the deformed toe. Women should not wear heels higher than one inch or shoes with pointed or narrow toes. It should be possible to wiggle the toes freely inside the shoes.

When trying on a pair of new shoes, be sure to try the one for the foot with the bunion. You may need to increase your shoe size, or even cut out a piece of the shoe around the bump. Certain styles of sandals with adjustable straps often provide the greatest comfort; tennis shoes or other athletic shoes are also a popular choice. In addition, make sure that socks or stockings are neither too tight nor too big.

Pharmacies and some shoe repair shops carry special devices for adapting shoes to accommodate bunions. Experiment with these to see what helps the most. An arch support can alleviate pressure on the bunion, and ring-shaped adhesive pads can be worn around and over it. Make certain that these devices fit comfortably inside your shoes, or they will do more harm than good. To help keep your big toe properly aligned, try placing a foam rubber pad between it and your second toe at bedtime.

Other Causes of Bunions

Rheumatoid arthritis can cause a deformity similar to a bunion, as can chronic gout and other rheumatic disorders.

Burns

About 2 million Americans are burned seriously enough each year to require medical attention, almost half of them children. Although in most people's minds, burns are associated with fire or flames, they can also be caused by chemicals, steam, and electricity.

The resulting injuries range from mild to fatal. Minor burns simply make the outer layer of skin red and painful, but severe burns penetrate more deeply and can damage nerves, blood vessels, glands, and even muscle and bone. They can also cause life-threatening metabolic abnormalities and disrupt the immune system.

Diagnostic Studies and Procedures

A physical examination is the only means of diagnosis that is necessary for simple burns. Severe, extensive burns require blood and urine analyses, as well as studies of kidney and liver function. In addition, any assessment of a burn patient requires classifying the injury by degree and extent of body involvement. This task can be difficult, because the depth of a burn is often hard to measure. In general, burns are classified as follows:

First-degree, which causes both pain and redness but no blisters, and the damage is confined to the epidermis, the skin's tough outer layer.

Second-degree, which produces blisters and damages both the epidermis and the dermis, the inner layer of the skin. These can be quite painful but usually are not serious unless they cover a large part of the body or the blisters become infected.

Third-degree, which looks charred, white, or blackened, and extends to the tissue below the skin. Such burns usually are not painful at first, because the nerve endings are damaged. But all third-degree burns are considered a medical emergency; they can be fatal if they cover more than 30 percent of the body's surface, or if they impair any of the vital functions.

Medical Treatments

First-degree burns generally do not require a doctor's care. Any second-degree burn with blisters more than one inch across or that affects the hands, face, feet, or genitals, should be seen by a doctor. In the past, blisters were often opened, but now, most burn specialists advocate letting them drain naturally to reduce the risk of infection. If a blister is opened, it must be done under sterile conditions to avoid infection. The doctor may prescribe antibiotics to prevent infection and recommend immunization against tetanus.

If the burn involves a joint, manipulation and perhaps splinting will be needed to prevent a permanent shortening of the skin, which may develop when scar tissue formation takes place. Depending on the severity of the burn, the doctor may arrange for physical or occupational therapy.

Third-degree burns need immediate attention by medical professionals, preferably in a burn center or hospital critical care unit. Shock often follows serious burns, and blood or plasma transfusions may be given to combat it. Oxygen is usually administered, and if the lungs or airways have been damaged, a breathing tube may be inserted. Antibiotics will be prescribed to prevent an infection.

Fluid replacement to make up for what is lost through the damaged skin is also critical. For extensive burns, the fluids are given intravenously.

Deep burn wounds also demand special care. The damaged tissue must be excised and the remaining tissue covered with a sterile dressing or artificial skin. Skin regenerates itself after first- and second-degree burns, but not third-degree. The margins may heal but

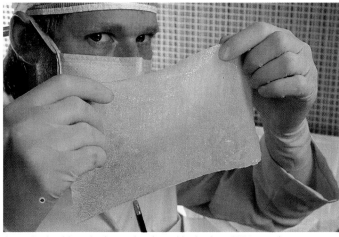

A synthetic skin substitute, developed in the late 1980s, makes skin grafting easier and less painful.

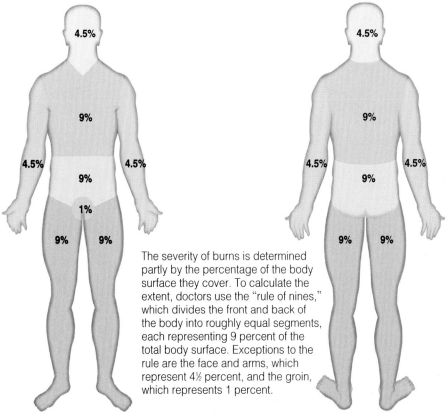

The severity of burns is determined partly by the percentage of the body surface they cover. To calculate the extent, doctors use the "rule of nines," which divides the front and back of the body into roughly equal segments, each representing 9 percent of the total body surface. Exceptions to the rule are the face and arms, which represent 4½ percent, and the groin, which represents 1 percent.

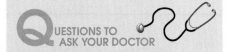

BURNS (CONTINUED)

the destroyed skin will be replaced by thick scar tissue. Skin grafting is often necessary in the treatment of these deep burns. The development of artificial skin has made the procedure simpler and less painful than it once was.

Alternative Therapies

Alternative therapies can be helpful in treating first- and second-degree burns, particularly if they are not extensive. Alternative approaches used for any third-degree burn should supplement conventional medical care.

Herbal Medicine. Aloe vera is recommended to treat minor burns because of its anesthetic and healing properties. The natural way to use it is from the plant, which can be grown in a pot indoors. When needed, break off a leaf and squeeze it out over the burned area. Or make a poultice by wrapping a freshly cut leaf in gauze. If you don't have a plant, use aloe vera gel or cream, available in pharmacies and health food stores. The higher the percentage of aloe vera, the more effective it will be. However, aloe should not be applied to open blisters or third-degree burns.

Other herbs that may be used also to treat minor burns include comfrey, calendula, and witch hazel. Typically, they are applied as compresses that have been soaked in decoctions.

Hypnosis and Meditation. These and other relaxation techniques may help

burn victims cope with the pain of wound care, which involves removal of dressings and dead tissue. The methods may also be used as part of rehabilitation following a severe burn.

Nutrition Therapy. A diet that is high in both calories for energy and protein for tissue repair is important for recovery from burns, particularly if they are extensive. Fluid intake should be kept high, and the diet supplemented with vitamin C for wound healing, B vitamins to meet the body's increased metabolic demands, and vitamin A and potassium to promote skin health. When applied to the skin, vitamin E may speed healing.

Self-Treatment

For first- and second-degree burns, immerse the burned part in cool water if possible. Apply cold packs to reduce the pain and swelling, but do not apply ice directly to the skin. Leave a cold pack on for 20 minutes, remove it for 10 minutes, and then reapply it.

Take aspirin or ibuprofen for pain and inflammation. If you are pregnant or have a history of ulcers, be sure to ask your doctor if these medications are safe for you to take.

Should blisters develop, do not puncture them—this increases the risk of infection. If a blister opens on its own, wash the area gently with soap and water, apply an antibiotic ointment, and cover with a sterile bandage. Change the dressings at least once a day, and call your doctor if you see any signs of infection or inflammation.

If a burn was caused by a corrosive chemical, as in a product for unclogging household drains, remove all contaminated clothing and jewelry and immediately flush the

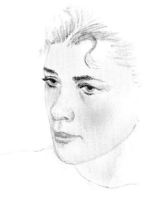

If a chemical splashes in your eye, flush it with water, leaning your head to one side to avoid washing the substance into the other eye.

burned area with cool water for 15 to 30 minutes. Be sure to read the first aid instructions on the product's label.

If your eye has been burned by chemicals, flush it with water at once, being careful not to get the chemical into the other eye. Cover your eye with a cool compress and go directly to the nearest hospital emergency room.

If you receive an electrical burn, call your doctor right away. These burns are often more severe than they look, sometimes causing greater damage within the body than on its surface.

If you have been seriously burned, don't try to remove burned clothing or attempt any self-treatment. Instead, call an ambulance or have someone take you to the nearest emergency room as fast as possible.

Other Causes of Burns

Excessive sun exposure can result in an extensive first- or second-degree burn that requires medical attention.

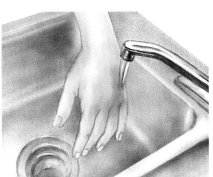

If you receive a first- or second-degree burn, first immerse it in cool water.

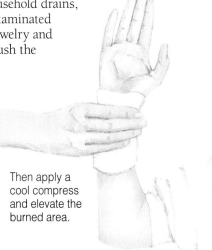

Then apply a cool compress and elevate the burned area.

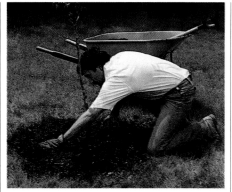

Bursitis

(Inflammation of a bursa)

Bursitis is a rheumatic condition that occurs when a bursa becomes inflamed and painful. The bursae are small sacs or pouches at the ends of bones that act as cushions between the bones and muscles, tendons, or skin. They contain a lubricating fluid to eliminate joint friction and maintain smooth movement of muscles over the bones.

Inflamed bursae produce tenderness and swelling near the affected joint. This ranges from minor discomfort to severe and virtually disabling pain that makes it almost impossible to move the joint. The condition can result from a sudden and extreme traumatic pressure or, more often, from continuous strain. Some occupations and sports that require constant, repetitious motion can lead to either acute or chronic bursitis; so-called housemaid's knee, which is caused by frequent kneeling, is one of the most familiar examples. The joints most commonly affected are the shoulders, knees, elbows, and hips.

Diagnostic Studies and Procedures

Bursitis is easily diagnosed on the basis of symptoms and a physical examination. Your account of recent activities helps a doctor determine the cause of the flare-up and also provides clues to whether or not the problem might be a sign of a more general condition.

During the physical examination, a doctor manipulates the joint to identify the most painful area and to determine the degree of joint mobility. An X-ray, blood studies, and other tests may be ordered to rule out conditions that cause similar symptoms.

Medical Treatments

Aspirin, ibuprofen, and stronger non-steroidal anti-inflammatory drugs are the mainstays to relieve both pain and inflammation of bursitis. In acute

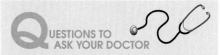

▶ When is it safe to start exercising? What kinds of exercise should I do and what should I avoid?
▶ Could my weight be a factor?
▶ How can I prevent future episodes, especially if my job demands the movements that caused it?

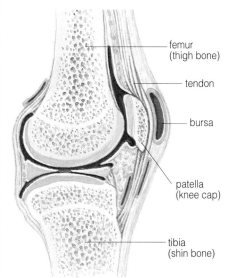

Gardeners are especially vulnerable to knee bursitis because of the pressure they exert on the joint by kneeling.

cases, a corticosteroid such as cortisone, a powerful anti-inflammatory drug, may be injected into the inflamed area. When given by this type of injection, steroids are less likely to produce serious side effects than when taken orally.

Excess fluid in the bursa may be drawn off with a hollow needle and syringe to reduce swelling, then the joint wrapped with an elastic bandage. If a shoulder or elbow is involved, the doctor may recommend an arm sling to rest and protect the joint.

Alternative Therapies

Chiropractic. Manipulation may ease pain caused by bursitis, particularly if misalignment is involved. A patient who has any form of arthritis should bring this to the chiropractor's attention before beginning treatment, however, because manipulation can be harmful in certain cases.

Herbal Medicine. Some herbal remedies may ease the swelling and pain of bursitis, although none are a substitute for medical treatment. Many herbalists recommend rubbing fresh garlic on the painful area, as well as taking garlic pills twice a day.

A poultice made with 3 tablespoons of horseradish stirred into ½ of boiled milk is also said to alleviate pain. It should be applied hot, using a piece of cheesecloth or a gauze pad, and removed when it has cooled. A note of caution: Both garlic and horseradish may irritate mucous membranes and skin. Test the substance first on a small area of skin, and avoid using it if it produces blistering, reddening, or a rash.

Hydrotherapy. Ice is used first in an acute attack of bursitis to alleviate pain and reduce swelling. After the first two days, switch to heat treatment. You can

apply heat with hot packs, a heating pad, an infrared lamp, or by taking hot showers or baths.

Self-Treatment

Most cases of bursitis will clear up within a week or two with attentive self-care. (See a doctor, however, if the pain and swelling are severe enough to prevent joint movement, if the condition worsens, or if there is no improvement after four or five days.)

Rest the affected area as much as possible and wrap it firmly, but not too tightly, in an elastic bandage. Take aspirin or ibuprofen to alleviate the pain and inflammation, ingesting them with milk or food to prevent stomach irritation. Use heat or cold treatments for additional pain relief.

As the bursitis disappears, you can begin gentle and gradual exercising to gain muscle strength. A physical therapist at a sports medicine center or an athletic trainer can provide guidance as to which exercises are beneficial and which ones should be avoided.

The most important aspect of self-treatment is determining what activity triggered the bursitis. Once you know what it is, you can avoid overdoing it or learn better techniques for performing that particular motion.

Other Causes of Bursitis Symptoms

Some forms of arthritis, including gout, can cause inflammation of the bursae. Tendinitis, an inflammation of the thick tissue that connects muscles and bones, may also mimic bursitis.

femur (thigh bone)

tendon

bursa

patella (knee cap)

tibia (shin bone)

Bursae are fluid-filled sacs that act as cushions between bones and tendons or skin, as shown in this illustration of a knee joint.

Canker Sores

(Aphthous stomatitis)

Canker sores are small, painful mouth ulcers that develop most often in the soft fold of tissue where the inner cheeks meet the gums. Other common sites include the soft palate, tongue, and floor of the mouth; it is not unusual for two or three to appear at a time, even 10 or more in some cases.

They start as small red areas and within a day or two, each center forms a yellow or white crater. Ranging in size from an one-eighth inch to one-half inch or more across, they can be painful enough to interfere with speaking and eating the first two or three days. Some people also develop a low-grade fever, swollen lymph nodes, and feelings of general malaise.

Their specific cause is unknown, but canker sores are frequently linked to fatigue, stress, poor diet, or debilitated physical condition due to another illness. People with AIDS or certain types of cancer often develop the sores, possibly due to a weakened immune system. In contrast, some researchers believe that the sores are more likely to develop when the body's immune system attacks healthy tissue.

Another possible cause is irritation from overly vigorous brushing of the teeth, eating certain foods, dental fillings that scrape the mouth, and poorly fitted dentures. In women, canker sores often appear just prior to menstruation. Recurring attacks are common, but most canker sores heal within two weeks and leave no scars.

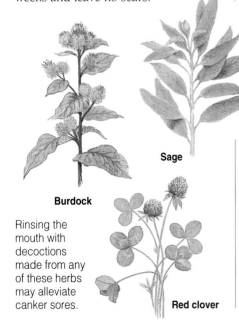

Sage

Burdock

Red clover

Rinsing the mouth with decoctions made from any of these herbs may alleviate canker sores.

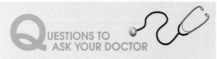

QUESTIONS TO ASK YOUR DOCTOR

▶ Could stress be behind my recurrent canker sores?
▶ Can irritation from spicy foods or smoking trigger canker sores?
▶ Do you think an antibiotic mouthwash might be helpful in my case?

Diagnostic Studies and Procedures

The sores are readily diagnosed by a visual examination. In some cases, a laboratory culture may be needed to distinguish them from those of herpes, and to rule out the presence of a secondary bacterial infection.

Medical Treatments

Medical care is not usually necessary unless the condition persists or recurs frequently. In such cases, a mouthwash with tetracycline may be prescribed to relieve pain, especially if a secondary infection is present. In severe cases, a doctor may prescribe steroid medication to be used both as a mouthwash and in tablet form. Other prescription products are anesthetic mouthwashes to make eating more comfortable, and a paste that is applied to the ulcer to relieve pain and promote healing.

Alternative Therapies

Aromatherapy. Lemon oil applied during a facial massage is recommended for treating canker sores.

Herbal Medicine. The tannic acid in tea is astringent, helping to dry up canker sores and bring relief from pain. Dip a regular teabag into boiling water, squeeze out most of the water, allow it to cool, then apply it to the canker sore for three minutes. Repeat as needed until the sore disappears. Herbalists also suggest rinsing the mouth with a rose water decoction, made by simmering rose petals in a pint of water. Other popular herbal remedies include rinses made from raspberry leaf, burdock, sage, or red clover decoctions. Tincture of myrrh may be applied directly to the sore, but caution is recommended, because it can damage delicate mouth tissue.

Naturopathy and Nutrition Therapy. Until the sores heal, it's best to eat soothing, cool foods. Milk, gelatin, ice cream, puddings, and custard usually are well tolerated. Yogurt with active lactobacillus acidophilus cultures is both soothing and reportedly speeds healing. In fact, many naturopaths advocate acidophilus pills, starting with two tablets per meal, decreasing the dosage as the condition clears up.

Onions, either raw or cooked, are recommended for their high sulfur content. Avoid chocolate, citrus fruits, acidic foods, and salty or spicy foods, which are likely to irritate the ulcers.

If you suffer from recurrent sores, have a nutritionist analyze your diet to make sure it provides adequate folic acid, iron, zinc, and vitamin B$_{12}$. A limited number of studies have shown a link between canker sores and deficiencies of these nutrients.

Yoga and Meditation. Because canker sores at times appear to be related to stress, these and other relaxation techniques, including breathing exercises, can be a helpful aspect of both treatment and prevention.

Self-Treatment

Most canker sores will clear up within 7 to 10 days. In the meantime, to relieve pain, try an over-the-counter anesthetic gel or liquid, applying it directly to the ulcer. A styptic pencil, such as those used by barbers to stop bleeding from minor nicks, numbs the nerve endings and provides temporary relief. Aspirin, acetaminophen, or ibuprofen can also help with pain.

Rinse your mouth several times a day with a mild solution of salt water (½ teaspoon of salt in 1 cup of warm water), and clean the sores frequently with a cotton swab dipped in a solution of one part 3-percent hydrogen peroxide to four parts water.

To clean teeth, use a soft toothbrush and baking soda, which is less irritating than toothpaste. See your dentist if you think the sores are being caused by braces, dentures, or a rough tooth.

Other Causes of Mouth Ulcers

A herpes simplex infection causes fever blisters or cold sores that resemble canker sores. If you have previously had a herpes infection, the sores may recur at the same time canker sores appear because they seem to share precipitating factors. Also, oral thrush, a yeast infection, shows up as white patches in the mouth, which can result in small painful ulcers. Smoking promotes mouth sores in some people, but it more commonly causes leukoplakia, thick whitish patches that often evolve into cancer.

Cardiac Arrhythmias

(Bradycardia; fibrillation; palpitations; and tachycardia)

Cardiac arrhythmias are characterized by an abnormal series of heartbeats, classified as bradycardia (too slow), tachycardia (too fast), or irregular (erratic). During bradycardia, fainting may occur because the brain does not get enough oxygen. In some forms of tachycardia, such as fibrillation, the rhythm is lost entirely, dissolving into quivering of the heart muscle.

Arrhythmias are usually caused by damage to the heart muscle or the sinus node, the heart's natural pacemaker. Such damage may be due to a heart attack, congenital defect, damaged heart valve, or a heart infection such as bacterial endocarditis (page 178).

Diagnostic Studies and Procedures

Diagnosis begins with an electrocardiogram, or ECG, to measure the heart's electrical activity with electrodes placed on the patient's chest, preferably during a period of arrhythmia. If the problem is episodic, a portable ECG machine, called a Holter monitor, may be worn for 24 to 48 hours.

When computers are used to enhance the ECG, a process called signal averaging, it becomes possible to predict, in some cases, whether or not the patient is likely to experience ventricular arrhythmias. Transesophageal echocardiography, which produces ultrasound images of the heart through a tube inserted into the esophagus, makes it

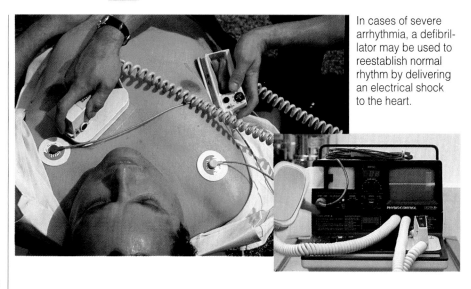

In cases of severe arrhythmia, a defibrillator may be used to reestablish normal rhythm by delivering an electrical shock to the heart.

possible to evaluate the atria, the heart's two upper chambers, and look for potential causes of arrhythmias arising from this area of the heart.

A new diagnostic approach, called electrophysiology testing, is used in special circumstances, such as for patients who have experienced sudden, unexplained cardiac arrest. Electrodes are guided into the heart through a catheter, then drugs are administered to provoke an arrhythmia.

Medical Treatments

Most arrhythmias can be controlled with beta blockers and other drugs that stabilize heart rate. Some cases, however, require implantation of an artificial pacemaker, a tiny, battery-operated device placed under the skin with electrodes attached to the heart.

Fibrillation and certain other serious arrhythmias are usually treated by the administration of an electrical shock (defibrillation) to the heart in order to reestablish a normal heart rhythm.

Alternative Therapies

Any alternative therapies that help to prevent heart disease can also prevent cardiac arrhythmias.

Herbal Medicine. Chinese herbalists recommend several herbal combinations: bupleurum, cinnamon, and ginger or bupleurum and dragon bone formulas for the treatment of palpitations; pinellia and magnolia for tachycardia; and the atratylodes and hoelen herbal combination for treating bradycardia.

Shiatsu. Pressing upon certain points along the inner forearm is said to help slow down palpitations that are precipitated by anxiety.

Yoga and Meditation. The breathing exercises of these relaxation therapies help some people control palpitations related to stress.

Self-Treatment

All cardiac arrhythmias that are persistent or serious require medical treatment. During an attack of tachycardia, however, it is sometimes possible to slow the heart rate by rubbing your neck or bearing down as though you're having a bowel movement. Dizziness due to bradycardia can be temporarily overcome by resting with the head lower than the heart. On a long-term basis, the best approach is to reduce stress, abstain from using alcohol and tobacco, and limit daily caffeine intake.

Other Causes of Arrhythmias

Certain drugs, including allergy medications and diet pills, can cause irregular heartbeats. In some people, exercise can trigger arrhythmias.

The heart's rhythmic beating is coordinated by the sinus node through a series of electrical impulses that travel along specific pathways.

sinus node

atrioventricular node

electrical pathway

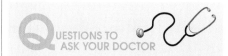

QUESTIONS TO ASK YOUR DOCTOR

▶ Is it safe to engage in vigorous or sustained exercise? If not, what can I substitute as a means of staying fit?
▶ If I am at risk of sudden death from arrhythmia, should I consider having a defibrillator implanted?
▶ Are there any safe nonprescription allergy medications that will not provoke a fast heartbeat?

Carpal Tunnel Syndrome

(Repetitive stress injury)

Carpal tunnel syndrome, which encompasses a range of symptoms affecting the hands and wrists, is now the most common hand problem that primary-care physicians see. It has been estimated that millions of Americans presently have the syndrome, due primarily to their occupations.

Typical symptoms are persistent numbness, burning, and tingling of the hands, as if they had fallen asleep. These conditions are likely to worsen at night, and may even wake you up. Many people also experience stiff, swollen wrist joints and loss of hand strength and dexterity, especially when performing fine movements such as picking up a button or sewing.

The direct cause is pressure on the median nerve, which carries messages between the hand and brain. The carpal tunnel itself is a narrow opening in the wrist, made up of eight bones that form three sides of the tunnel, and the transverse carpal ligament, a tough band of tissue that forms the fourth side. The tunnel is situated on the palm side of the wrist, and nine tendons as well as the median nerve pass through it. If any of these tendons swells, or if an injury causes the space inside the tunnel to decrease, the median nerve may become irritated or pinched, leading to inflammation, swelling, and the characteristic symptoms.

Anyone whose job or hobby calls for repeating the same motions over and over, especially if the wrists are hyper-

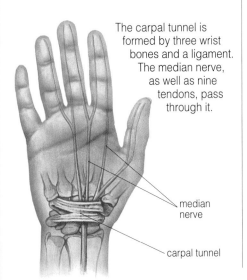

The carpal tunnel is formed by three wrist bones and a ligament. The median nerve, as well as nine tendons, pass through it.

median nerve

carpal tunnel

flexed or hyperextended, are vulnerable to the syndrome, which is also referred to as repetitive stress injury. Computer operators, pianists, meat packers, and jackhammer operators are among those who have a high risk of carpal tunnel syndrome. Pregnant women are also vulnerable to the disorder because of general tissue swelling and fluid retention, especially in the hands and feet.

Diagnostic Studies and Procedures

Two simple office tests point to a diagnosis of carpal tunnel syndrome. In one, called Phalen's test, you put the backs of your hands against each other with the wrists completely flexed. If you feel numbness, tingling, or pain within 60 seconds, the median nerve is probably compressed. In the second, called Tinel's test, the doctor will tap the palm area over the median nerve. Again, any tingling or numbness indicates median nerve compression.

The definitive diagnostic test, however, is electromyography (EMG). In this nerve conduction study, performed by a neurologist, electrical stimulation is used to detect any abnormal electrical activity when nerves and muscles are at rest and during contraction.

Medical Treatments

Treatment usually starts with rest and immobilization of the affected hand and wrist. Special splints may be used to hold the wrist in a straight, unflexed position. Some patients wear the splint only at night, while others require it all the time until symptoms abate.

Anti-inflammatory medications such as aspirin and ibuprofen may be prescribed, as well as muscle relaxants and stronger prescription pain relievers if needed. In more severe cases, cortisone injections directly into the wrist can provide dramatic relief of pain and inflammation, but will not permanently cure the condition.

Progression of the syndrome, marked by increasing pain, a weakening of grip strength, and shrinking of the muscles at the base of the thumb, calls for more intensive treatment. A removable cast, worn at all times except when showering or bathing, may be tried. If this does not produce improvement, surgery by a hand specialist may be necessary to release the trapped nerve. The surgery involves cutting and releasing the transverse ligament, which relieves pressure on the median nerve. Many people report that their symp-

toms completely disappear right after surgery. The problems may return, however, with the resumption of the activities that produced them.

Alternative Therapies

Many doctors recommend a trial of these therapies before resorting to surgery. They can also be used as adjuncts to conventional treatment.

Acupuncture. Meridians affecting the neck, back, and shoulders as well as the hands, wrists, and arms are stimulated in an attempt to heal the entire length of the injured nerve.

Alexander Technique. A practitioner will assess your posture and movements and suggest changes that are likely to correct faulty habits that contribute to the syndrome.

Chiropractic. Practitioners manipulate misaligned or fixated joints to relieve nerve pressure, and are likely to adjust not only the wrist, but also the areas where the median nerve is connected to the rest of the nervous system, including the arm, shoulder, and neck. Adjusting the neck, or cervical spine, is considered particularly important.

Many chiropractors, as well as some acupuncturists, use transcutaneous nerve stimulation, or TENS, a method of relieving pain by delivering mild electrical pulses to the skin that cause the body to produce endorphins, its own natural painkillers.

Some chiropractors also use ultrasound and may recommend other alternative approaches.

Nutrition Therapy and Naturopathy. Deficiencies of vitamins B_6 and B_{12} appear to play a role in some cases of carpal tunnel syndrome. A nutritionist can assess your diet and suggest taking supplements or eating foods rich in these vitamins, including meat, fish, and other animal products for both, plus whole grains, spinach, potatoes, and bananas for B_6. Caution is needed, however, because excessive B_6 also produces hand numbness and tingling.

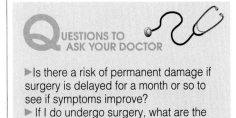

QUESTIONS TO ASK YOUR DOCTOR

▶ Is there a risk of permanent damage if surgery is delayed for a month or so to see if symptoms improve?
▶ If I do undergo surgery, what are the chances that the problem will recur?

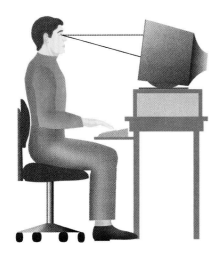

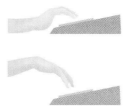

When working at a video display terminal, your back should be straight, your feet flat on the floor, and your lower arm and wrist straight, not flexed, as shown above.

Osteopathy. Osteopaths combine the medical training of a traditional physician with manipulation techniques. They are likely to emphasize exercising and stretching to increase range of motion and may also prescribe medication and perform surgery, if needed.

Physical Therapy. Doctors, chiropractors, and osteopaths often refer patients to a physical therapist as an important aspect of treatment. These therapists can teach proper work habits and correct posture, and also design a therapeutic exercise program tailored to specific needs. In addition, they may use hydrotherapy, electrotherapy, ultrasound, massage, and a new type of electrical treatment called interferential current therapy to restore function and alleviate pain.

Self-Treatment

The most fundamental aspect of self-treatment is keeping your wrists in proper alignment, neither overflexed nor overextended. Pay attention to the position of your hands and wrists, both when working and at ease. They should be comfortably straight.

Make sure your work environment is designed to minimize stress on your joints. If you work at a computer or desk, adjust your chair to a comfortable height that allows you to place your feet flat on the floor and sit up straight, with good support for the lower back. If your chair lacks support, place a cushion or a rolled-up towel in the small of your back.

A computer monitor should be at or a little below eye level, and documents should be placed in a holder that keeps you from craning or bending your neck. Use a wrist rest if you spend a

good part of your day at the keyboard; these are sold in most computer stores, or you can fashion one from a folded towel. Don't angle your head forward, but keep it aligned straight above your spine. Try to avoid slouching.

Stand up and walk around whenever possible, for example, while talking on the phone or reading mail. In any event, take brief breaks at least once every hour, and perform the following simple exercises in a sitting position.

▶ Cross your arms over your head and take your right elbow in your left hand. Pull the elbow toward your opposite arm and hold it for a few seconds. Repeat with the other elbow.

▶ Raise one arm over your head, then reach around to the opposite ear. Pull your head toward your shoulder for 10 seconds, reverse position and repeat with the other arm.

▶ Clasp your hands behind your head. Without letting your shoulders come up, gently try to move your elbows backward for five seconds or more.

▶ With your hands in your lap, make circles with your shoulders, rolling them forward, upward, and back while maintaining your head and neck in straight alignment. Do this five times, then reverse the circle and roll your shoulders from back to front five times.

▶ Limber up your hands by massaging and stretching your fingers, bending your wrist back and forth, and clenching and unclenching your fist.

Other Causes of Hand and Wrist Symptoms

Some systemic diseases, such as rheumatoid arthritis, diabetes, and thyroid disease, are associated with carpal tunnel syndrome. Certain nerve and circulatory disorders, such as Raynaud's syndrome, can cause hand numbness and tingling. A fractured or dislocated wrist that is not properly set or a herniated disc in the cervical spine can also trigger the symptoms of carpal tunnel syndrome.

A CASE IN POINT

Amy Greene, a 29-year-old reporter, was delighted when her newspaper put in a computer network to replace its old typewriters. Six months later, with her hands crippled by carpal tunnel syndrome, she rued the day.

Greene's problems started three months after switching to the computer. "I do all my writing at the keyboard," she explained. "Because a computer keyboard does not require as much effort as a typewriter, I thought it was actually easier on my hands." What she didn't realize was that typing with her wrists in a flexed position was puting extra stress on the nerves to her fingers. Consequently, she was often awakened at night by shooting pains in her arms and tingling sensations in her hands.

"My fingers were so swollen I couldn't wear my rings," she recalls, "and my hands were too weak in the morning to hold a cup of coffee."

At first, aspirin, soaking her hands in cool water, and gently exercising her fingers provided temporary relief, but after an hour or so at her keyboard, the swelling and pain would return. "My boss suggested I use a wrist support," she said. "It helped some, but only temporarily."

Fearing that her job was at stake, she consulted an orthopedist, who quickly diagnosed carpal tunnel syndrome. After injecting cortisone into both wrists to ease the inflammation, he referred Greene to a physical therapist. "He told me I had to rest my wrists completely to allow the inflamed nerves to heal." She was fitted with a special splint to hold her wrists in a fixed position, and told to forego typing for at least a month.

"Unfortunately, I simply couldn't do that. Even though I wore the splints while typing, my symptoms were getting worse."

Finally, she took a three-month disability leave to undergo wrist surgery, followed by occupational therapy to learn the proper typing technique. She had her computer workstation adjusted to a proper height, and her traditional keyboard replaced with one that puts less stress on her wrists. Greene's condition has improved, but she still wears wrist splints at night and when typing.

Cataracts

A cataract is a progressive eye disorder in which the lens becomes increasingly cloudy and stiff. This clouding blocks the passage of light to the back of the eyeball, causing a painless deterioration of vision. Cataracts are a normal—but not inevitable—part of aging, affecting more than half of all Americans over the age of 65. In rare cases, babies are born with congenital cataracts.

A number of environmental factors increase the risk of developing this disorder, including exposure to X-rays, infrared radiation, and the sun's ultraviolet rays. Smoking is implicated in 20 percent of all cataract cases in the United States. Research indicates that the damage is caused by a substance inhaled in tobacco smoke that is transported to the eye through the bloodstream, rather than the exposure of the eye to airborne smoke.

Diagnostic Studies and Procedures

Blurred, dimmed, or double vision and a frequent need for a new eyeglass prescription usually raise a suspicion of cataracts. The individual may also be aware of seeing a scattering of light beams in the glare from a spotlight, headlights, or the sun.

An ophthalmologist or optometrist can easily detect an incipient cataract during a routine eye examination. The diagnosis is confirmed by dilating the pupil with eye drops and then directing an intense, narrowly focused light ray onto various parts of the retina. The extent of a cataract's effect on vision depends on its size and location.

Medical Treatments

There is no medicine that can cure or dissolve cataracts; instead, they are treated surgically. However, cataract surgery has become so routine today, it is often done on an outpatient basis.

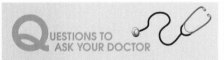

In general, the operation is not performed until the cataracts are interfering with normal activities such as reading, driving, and working. Any person whose job requires keen eyesight may undergo their removal sooner than one whose lifestyle or work demands less of the eyes. If a person has cataracts in both eyes, the eye that has less vision will be corrected first, and when healing is complete, the second one will be dealt with.

There are three major methods for removing cataracts:
▶ *Extracapsular surgery,* in which the lens is removed except for the back half of its outer covering, or capsule.
▶ *Phacoemulsification,* a variation of extracapsular surgery in which only the core of the lens is removed after breaking it up with ultrasound.
▶ *Intracapsular,* in which the entire lens and its capsule are removed. (This is a rare operation.)

In most cases, the lens is replaced by a plastic disc, or intraocular lens, inserted into the capsule. The artificial lens is a permanent implant, though occasionally it becomes clouded and has to be replaced. Other alternatives include a removable contact lens, or special eyeglasses created for this purpose.

Recovery from the operation itself takes no more than a day or so, but becoming used to the new lens requires more time. Some people adjust in only a few weeks, while others may need as much as several months.

Alternative Therapies

Alternative therapies cannot cure cataracts, but some may help resolve their underlying causes. For example, behavior modification therapies, such as hypnosis, biofeedback training, and even acupuncture, are often helpful to smokers who want to quit. More direct alternative approaches may include:
Herbal Medicine. A traditional Chinese formula known as hachimijiogan is said to contain ingredients that protect the eye against the formation of cataracts and to slow their progress

surgical instrument

lens

Cataracts look like opaque or cloudy areas in the pupil.

In one type of cataract removal, an incision is made at the edge of the iris, and a special instrument (upper left) is used to force the lens out.

when they begin to appear. The preparation, which is used mostly in China and Japan, is taken in daily oral doses.
Naturopathy and Nutrition Therapy. Practitioners may recommend supplements of selenium, vitamin E, and beta carotene (precursor to vitamin A), antioxidants that prevent tissue damage from oxygen metabolism—a factor in the development of cataracts. Studies indicate that supplements are of limited benefit, but increasing intake of food sources—yellow, orange, and dark green vegetables, whole-grain cereals and breads, and legumes—may help.

Self-Treatment

In the early stages of a cataract's development, simple measures such as improved lighting and new prescription glasses permit many patients to perform most everyday tasks. Other self-help measures include:
▶ Wearing sunglasses whenever there is enough sunlight to cause a sunburn. When choosing nonprescription sunglasses, look for a label indicating that the lenses block out 100 percent of the sun's ultraviolet rays.
▶ Wearing protective goggles or eyewear to prevent eye injuries, especially if your job is risky, such as arc-welding or sand-blasting.
▶ Wearing protective glasses if you are a health-care professional exposed either to laser beams or infrared radiation.
▶ Stopping smoking, whatever your age; you will protect not only your eyes but also your general health.

Other Causes of Cataracts

Uveitis, a chronic eye inflammation, can cause cataracts at a young age; so too can diabetes and the long-term use of corticosteroid medications.

Cavities

(Dental caries)

A cavity is an area of decay in a tooth, resulting from the interaction between oral bacteria and sugar and other carbohydrates in the mouth. In the course of metabolizing the sugars (and starches transformed into sugar by saliva), the bacteria create an acid that becomes part of a sticky substance known as dental plaque. Plaque clings to the tooth and begins to erode the enamel, producing holes, or cavities. Tooth enamel is the strongest material in the body, but it does not renew itself. As bacteria and the acids they form further penetrate the damaged tooth surface, a cavity enlarges to the point where it invades the dentin—the bony material inside a tooth (see illustration).

Diagnostic Studies and Procedures

During a routine checkup, a dentist examines each tooth with an angled mirror and metal probe to make sure that surfaces are intact. Where doubt exists, an X-ray may be taken. In addition, a complete set of dental X-rays is routinely taken every three or four years to detect any hidden problems.

Medical Treatments

If the work is expected to be extensive and painful, the dentist gives the patient the option of having an anesthetic such as Novocain injected into the gum. To prepare a tooth for filling, the dentist cleans out the cavity with a high-speed water-cooled drill, sterilizes the interior, and dries it.

A filling that matches the tooth is then chosen from a wide range of long-lasting compounds. Unless there are unexpected complications, a simple cavity can be filled in one visit.

If the cavity has extended to the dentin, the area may be injected with

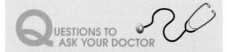

a calcium phosphate solution to stimulate new dentin growth. A temporary filling will be placed in the cavity, then later removed and replaced with a permanent filling.

When a cavity has reached into the pulp of the tooth, the patient may be referred to a specialist, an endodontist, for root-canal work. This procedure kills the nerve, eliminating pain and usually saving the tooth, which can then be cleaned out and filled as usual.

If only the base of the tooth remains after extensive decay or root-canal work, the dentist fills the socket of the tooth with cement and covers it with a crown. This usually takes three or four sessions because it involves laboratory work and precision fitting.

Alternative Therapies

Herbal Medicine. The compounds in green tea are reported to kill the bacteria responsible for causing tooth decay. The same compounds occur in sage, coriander, and thyme.

A traditional temporary remedy for a toothache has been oil of cloves, but this is not recommended today because it can damage delicate gum tissue.

Nutrition Therapy. A diet that provides adequate calcium and other minerals is essential to building strong teeth. For this purpose, babies and young children may also be given fluoride drops with their food, especially if the local water does not contain added

fluoride. Reducing sugar intake, especially sticky sweets that adhere to the teeth, helps to prevent cavities.

Relaxation Techniques. Hypnosis, biofeedback, and similar techniques can help people to overcome a fear of dentists. Hypnosis is also used as an alternative for patients who cannot tolerate Novocain and other anesthetics.

Self-Treatment

Good oral hygiene is the key to preventing cavities. Visiting your dentist regularly and flossing and brushing properly can prevent most decay.

Toothpastes with added fluoride also help prevent cavities. However, be careful about allowing children to use extra-strength fluoridated types. Eating the toothpaste can lead to fluoride toxicity. Also, pregnant women should not take fluoride supplements because it can cause tooth mottling in the child.

Never allow a baby to fall asleep with a bottle of milk, juice, or other sweetened liquid because this can cause "baby-bottle caries." If a bottle is essential at bedtime, fill it with water.

The application of a dental sealant on the chewing and grinding surfaces of a child's back teeth is the best way to protect them from cavities. The procedure is usually scheduled when the permanent molars begin to appear—typically between ages 6 and 8, and again at age 12.

Other Causes of Cavities

Long-term use of drugs that reduce the flow of saliva, such as antihistamines, tranquilizers, and antidepressants, increase the risk of cavities. Radiation therapy of the head and neck and diseases affecting the salivary glands also contribute to tooth decay by reducing the output of saliva. Accidents that chip or break tooth enamel make the surface more vulnerable to decay.

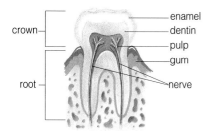

Tooth decay progresses from the surface of the tooth, or enamel (A), to the dentin, a bony substance inside the tooth (B). When decay extends through the dentin into the pulp (C), it can reach a nerve and cause a toothache. An abscess may also form below the root.

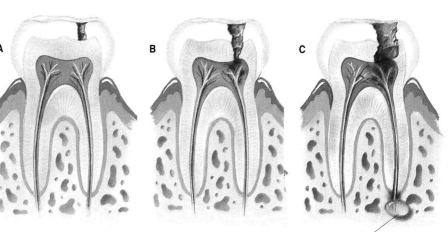

Cerebral Palsy

(CP)

Cerebral palsy is a neurological disorder that affects basic functions, including movement, speech, and posture. Between 500,000 and 700,000 Americans have it in varying degrees. There are several types including: *spastic,* in which movement is stiff and difficult; *athetoid,* in which movement is involuntary or uncontrolled; *ataxic,* in which balance and depth perception are abnormal; and *mixed,* a combination of types.

Cerebral palsy is caused by brain and nervous system damage sustained before birth, during labor, or shortly after birth. Depending upon the area and extent of the damage, symptoms may include spasms, tics, gait abnormalities, seizures, and poor muscle tone. Sight, hearing, speech, and intellect also may be affected.

Diagnostic Studies and Procedures

The disorder may be obvious at birth, or it may not become apparent for several months. Early diagnosis is important, however, so that therapy can begin as soon as possible.

If cerebral palsy is suspected, a pediatric neurologist should be consulted for diagnostic tests to determine the extent and location of brain damage and to rule out other disorders. Tests are likely to include electroencephalography to measure the brain's electrical activity; electromyography, or EMG,

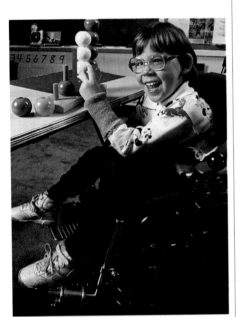

Many children afflicted with cerebral palsy can develop skills in self-care with the help of physical and occupational therapy.

to measure electrical activity in the muscles during movement; and a CT scan to look for brain abnormalities. Blood and urine samples will also be studied to rule out other disorders that produce similar symptoms.

Medical Treatments

Planning of treatment should involve a team of health professionals, including physical, speech, and occupational therapists; a psychologist; a neurologist; and an orthopedist. Beacause there is no cure for cerebral palsy, the goal is to help the child achieve as much independence as possible.

Seizures can often be controlled with anticonvulsant medications. Orthopedic treatment may include braces, splints, and casts to prevent contractures and other deformities of the arms and legs. Some children need orthopedic surgery to cut contracted muscles and tendons, thus allowing them to stretch, or to fuse together certain bones to stabilize joints. Such surgery can enable a child to walk or to maintain balance better.

Alternative Therapies

Several allied health professions and alternative practices play an important role in helping children with cerebral palsy to develop their full potential.

Dance and Music Therapies. These approaches can help children to improve their coordination, build muscle tone and strength, and gain self-confidence. It is important, however, that the instructor be specially trained to work with handicapped children.

Massage Therapy. This is beneficial in alleviating spasms and reducing muscle contractions. The therapist should consult the child's primary care doctor in planning the therapy.

Physical, Occupational, and Speech Therapy. Professionals in these fields specialize in teaching living skills. Physical therapists use exercise and relaxation techniques to teach children how to walk with the aid of braces, crutches, and other devices, or how to transfer from a wheelchair to a bed and chair. They also show parents how to incorporate therapy into the child's daily routine. Occupational therapists help a child develop useful skills such as typing or mastery of special devices to perform routine tasks. Speech therapists teach communication skills, including sign language for children who are unable to speak.

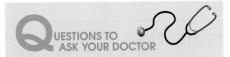

Self-Treatment

Cerebral palsy is a life-long condition that usually demands adaptation and training in order to achieve self-sufficiency. The earlier a diagnosis is made, the sooner a child can receive special education services.

Many children with cerebral palsy attend regular public schools, but others require special classes, and the more disabled may need developmental day-care programs that are geared especially to their needs.

Parents can do a great deal to provide a home environment that stimulates the child to learn and to explore. Regular exercise, beginning in infancy, is critical to achieving as much movement control as possible. Initially, passive exercises performed by parents or other caregivers are used, but at an early age, the child should be encouraged to participate in and eventually perform appropriate exercises.

Toilet training is usually delayed and difficult to achieve if the nerves that affect bowel and bladder control are damaged. Talking to other parents who have been through this stage may yield helpful tips. Special large-handled eating utensils, toothbrushes, and dressing aids, such as those used by people with severe arthritis, are valuable in learning to perform basic self-care.

A large number of cerebral palsy cases could be prevented by improved prenatal care. Several types of infections, including toxoplasmosis, genital herpes, rubella, and cytomegalovirus, increase the risk of cerebral palsy. A woman with any of these diseases should consult an obstetrician who specializes in high-risk pregnancies. Some studies indicate smoking and alcohol use during pregnancy also increase the risk.

Other Causes of Palsy

A head injury, brain tumor, stroke, and brain infection are among the possible causes of palsy.

Cervical Cancer

(Cervical carcinoma)

After decades of decline, the incidence of cervical cancer is again on the rise, especially in women under age 50. According to the American Cancer Society, about 80,000 women are now diagnosed with cervical cancer each year, but the malignancy is invasive in only 16,000 of these cases. (Invasive cancer may cause unusual vaginal bleeding, a watery discharge, and dull pelvic pain.) The remaining 65,000 have carcinoma in situ, an asymptomatic preinvasive condition.

Cervical cancer most commonly develops between the ages of 40 and 55. Its precise cause is unknown, but factors linked to an increased risk include beginning sexual intercourse before the age of 18 and having multiple sex partners; contracting genital warts; and tobacco use. Some studies also suggest that use of oral contraceptives increases risk; others implicate a deficiency of folic acid.

Diagnostic Studies and Procedures

The best means of early detection is a pap smear, which all women should have at least every three years, and more often if they have any of the high-risk factors listed above.

In a pap test, a sample of cells is collected from the cervix and sent to a laboratory for evaluation. If abnormal cells are detected, colposcopy will usually be

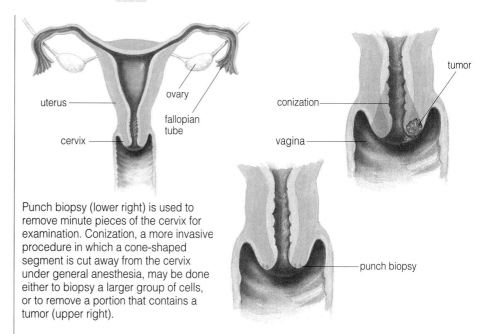

Punch biopsy (lower right) is used to remove minute pieces of the cervix for examination. Conization, a more invasive procedure in which a cone-shaped segment is cut away from the cervix under general anesthesia, may be done either to biopsy a larger group of cells, or to remove a portion that contains a tumor (upper right).

THE FOUR STAGES OF CERVICAL CANCER

Stage 0. Preinvasive carcinoma in situ (100 percent five-year survival).
Stage I. Cancer confined to the cervix (85 percent five-year survival).
Stage II. Cancer extends to the upper third of the vagina or the tissue around the uterus (the parametrium), but not the pelvic wall (50 to 60 percent five-year survival).
Stage III. Cancer involves the vagina (but not the lower third) and/or the pelvic side wall, and possibly the kidneys (30 percent five-year survival).
Stage IV. Cancer extends beyond the pelvic organs, involving the bladder or rectum, or metastases to distant organs, most often the lung, liver, and sometimes the bone (10 percent five-year survival).

In stages III and IV, the cancer also involves the lymph nodes in 50 percent or more of the patients, increasing the chance of distant spread.

done to locate the site of the abnormal cells and biopsy them. This is achieved with the aid of a colposcope, a slender optical instrument with a light at the end to magnify the surface of the cervix and vagina. Fragments of cervix will be removed and studied by a pathologist (punch biopsy) to determine whether the cells show dysplasia, a change in tissue that may develop into carcinoma in situ or more invasive cancer.

Medical Treatments

In some cases of mild dysplasia, no treatment is given, but frequent pap smears and physical examinations are performed. More often, the abnormal tissue is destroyed using one of three methods: a freezing technique called cryosurgery; hot cauterization with an electrical probe; or laser surgery.

Treatment of cancer depends upon its stage (see box, left). Carcinoma in situ is sometimes treated with conization (illustrated above), which usually preserves a woman's ability to have a baby. In other cases, radiation therapy or a hysterectomy may be advised, especially if a woman has completed her family or is past menopause.

More extensive cervical cancer almost always requires surgery, often a radical hysterectomy. This operation may be followed up with radiation therapy. Occasionally, radiation precedes or substitutes for surgery.

Radiation can be administered externally in the form of low-dose X-rays, or internally as radioactive rods inserted into the vagina and uterus.

Alternative Therapies

While there is no substitute for medical care of cervical cancer, acupuncture, meditation, and other relaxation therapies may be employed to control pain. More controversial is the use of garlic inserted into the vagina. Though it is said to have anticancer properties, it is highly irritating to mucous membranes.

Self-Treatment

After cryosurgery, use sanitary napkins, not tampons, to absorb discharge. Plan on at least six weeks to recover fully from a hysterectomy. In the meantime, avoid lifting heavy objects and any other activity that will put a strain on the incision. If constipation is a problem, use a stool softener. Following treatment for cervical cancer, check with your doctor before resuming sexual intercourse, although it is usually safe when healing is complete.

Other Causes of Cervical Symptoms

Polyps, infections, and chronic pelvic inflammatory disease can produce bleeding, pain, and other symptoms similar to those of cervical cancer.

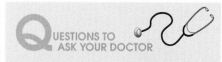

QUESTIONS TO ASK YOUR DOCTOR

► How often should I have a pap smear?
► What happens if mild dysplasia or cervical overgrowth is not treated?
► Does estrogen replacement therapy increase the risk of cervical cancer?

Chickenpox

(Varicella)
Chickenpox is a highly contagious childhood disease. About 95 percent of all children have been infected with it before adolescence, most commonly between ages three and nine.

The disease is caused by the varicella zoster virus, which is transmitted by direct contact with an infected person. It is contagious a day or two before its characteristic itchy rash appears, so a child may catch it from another before signs of infection are apparent. Clusters of small red bumps progress to blisters and scabs within 24 hours, but new clusters continue forming for four or five days. The disease remains conta-

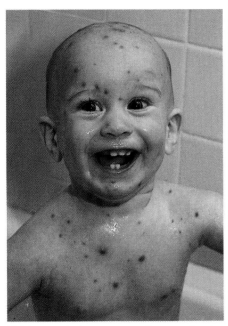

Chickenpox lesions progress from small red bumps to blisters that eventually break and form scabs within 24 hours.

gious until the final crop of blisters forms scabs. The virus then becomes dormant in the body, but may reappear years later as shingles. A person who lacks immunity to the varicella virus can contract chickenpox if exposed to someone with a shingles rash.

Diagnostic Studies and Procedures
Pediatricians usually diagnose chickenpox over the phone, to avoid having infected children in the office where they may give it to others. The parent's description of symptoms is the essential diagnostic tool. A fever and the typical rash are the key signs.

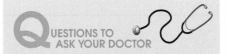

QUESTIONS TO ASK YOUR DOCTOR

▶ If I've never had chickenpox, is it risky for me to take care of a child who has it? What should I do if my child gets chickenpox while I'm pregnant?
▶ Do you favor immunizing children against chickenpox? And what about adults who have not had the disease?

Medical Treatments
A pediatrician's care is not usually required, unless the patient has a weakened immune system or develops severe complications. In such cases, acyclovir, an antiviral drug, may be administered intravenously.

Common complications of chickenpox are skin infections from scratching the blisters. These are usually treated with antibiotics. If itching is intense and the child cannot be prevented from scratching, the doctor may prescribe an antihistamine pill or ointment.

The disease is much more serious in adults than in children; complications may include pneumonia (page 338), hepatitis (page 225), and even encephalitis (page 177), a brain inflammation. Any adult who contracts chickenpox should seek prompt medical care.

Alternative Therapies
Herbal Medicine. Some practitioners recommend adding essences of ginger or elecampane to bath water to alleviate itchy skin. Others advocate drinking mild catnip tea to reduce fever and promote sleep. Some herbal books suggest drinking an infusion of yarrow leaves and flower tops to reduce fever, but this may cause an upset stomach. Also, yarrow contains derivatives of salicylic acid, the major ingredient in aspirin, which is contraindicated for children with chickenpox.
Hydrotherapy. Soothing baths often relieve itching, at least temporarily. Use lukewarm water and add to it 4 to 8 ounces of baking soda, or 1 to 2 cups of finely ground oatmeal. You can grind the oatmeal in a coffee grinder or blender, or purchase preground colloidal oatmeal at a pharmacy.
Nutrition Therapy. No special diet is required, but the child should be encouraged to drink plenty of fluids, especially if there is fever. Some natur-

opaths advise giving soy or almond milk instead of cow's milk until the infection clears up. Drinking diluted grape juice and eating grapes is sometimes suggested to reduce fever, but no evidence exists to support this advice.
Self-Treatment
Scratching the blisters can lead to infection and scarring. Cut the child's nails short and wash his hands often with antibacterial soap. Put a pair of light mittens or socks on a baby's hands.

Give the sick child a lukewarm sponge bath with mild soap several times a day. Do not rub the skin, but pat it dry instead, to reduce the chances of infection. Apply calamine lotion or a mild antihistamine lotion to alleviate itching and dry the blisters. For blisters in the mouth, have the child gargle with salt water.

Give acetaminophen for fever and general achiness, but never give aspirin to a child or adolescent with chickenpox. When taken during a viral infection, aspirin increases the risk of Reye's syndrome, a potentially fatal illness (see page 437 for more details).
Other Causes of Childhood Rashes
In a young child, herpes, heat rash, or impetigo may look like chickenpox. Also, some children develop very mild cases, with little or no rash, and their chickenpox may be mistaken for a cold or other mild viral infection.

CHICKENPOX IMMUNIZATION
Chickenpox can be prevented or modified by an injection of zoster immune globulin (ZIG), provided it is given within 96 hours of exposure to the disease. This is usually done if a child has leukemia or some other disorder that lowers the body's resistance. It is also sometimes given to newborn babies whose mothers developed chickenpox within five days of giving birth or two days after delivery.

There is a also a new vaccine that was approved by the Food and Drug Administration in 1995 despite controversy over its use. Some officials argue that because chickenpox is usually harmless, albeit uncomfortable for the child and inconvenient for the parents, a vaccine is not worth the cost. However, supporters of chickenpox immunization argue that about 100 children die from the disease each year, and that adults who contract it can suffer severe complications. Childhood immunization may also prevent shingles (see page 376 for more on this adult form of chickenpox).

Chlamydia

(Chlamydia trachomatis)
Chlamydia are tiny parasitic microorganisms, closely related to bacteria. They are usually transferred from one person to another through sexual contact. In fact, chlamydial infection is now the most common sexually transmitted disease in the United States. The infection also can be passed from a woman to her infant during a vaginal delivery, causing infections of the lungs, ears, and eyes, and, in rare cases, even death in the newborn.

Chlamydia can infect the male or female genital tract, the urinary tract, and the anus. The most common symptoms in women are vaginal itching and a smelly, yellowish discharge. Without treatment, the infection can worsen and spread, causing abdominal pain, bleeding between menstrual periods, painful intercourse, painful or frequent urination, nausea, and fever.

The usual symptoms in men are a discharge from the penis and itching or burning around the penis opening, particularly during urination. If untreated, the infection may worsen, causing fever and pain in the groin.

In many cases, especially in women, chlamydial infections do not produce symptoms until they progress to pelvic inflammatory disease (page 331). Even without treatment, initial symptoms in both males and females may subside within a month while the infection continues to spread throughout the reproductive tracts, causing chronic bladder and urethral problems, as well as infertility in both women and men.

Diagnostic Studies and Procedures
If chlamydial infection is suspected, a sample of secretions from the woman's vagina and vulva or the man's penis is taken. In addition, a urine specimen may be requested, and men may be asked to provide a specimen of seminal fluid. These samples are then cultured and analyzed. When chlamydia is found, it is not uncommon for the bacteria that cause gonorrhea also to be detected, because these two infections often occur together.

Medical Treatments
In adults, chlamydial infection is treated with antibiotics, which usually cures the disease in the early stages. Tetra-

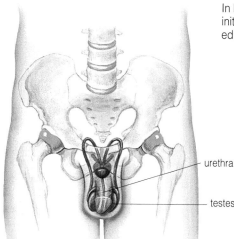
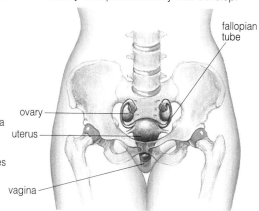

In both men and women, reproductive organs are the initial targets of chlamydia, but if the disease is untreated, chronic urinary tract problems may also develop.

fallopian tube — ovary — uterus — vagina — urethra — testes

cycline is the antibiotic of choice, although erythromycin is an effective alternative for pregnant women, who should avoid tetracycline because it can damage the baby's teeth.

Antibiotic therapy lasts from 10 to 14 days. The entire course of treatment must be completed, even though the symptoms are likely to disappear somewhat sooner. To prevent reinfection, sexual partners must also be treated.

Because antibiotics do not distinguish between chlamydia and beneficial bacteria, such as lactobacilli, organisms that help control the growth of yeast (*Candida albicans*) in the reproductive and gastrointestinal tracts, some doctors suggest that a woman also use a vaginal antifungal medication while taking antibiotics for other problems. Several preparations are available as over-the-counter creams and suppositories. Look for products that contain clotrimazole, miconazole, or nystatin.

In certain advanced cases of chlamydia, the infected glands may have to be drained or, in rare cases, surgically removed. Even after the appropriate therapy, relapses may occur. Therefore, many doctors recommend having a retest one month after the initial round of therapy is completed.

Alternative Therapies
Only a full course of antibiotics can eradicate chlamydia, but some alternative therapies may augment their effectiveness and reduce side effects.
Herbal Medicine. Garlic is promoted for its natural antibiotic properties. It may be taken fresh or in odorless pill form. Other herbal remedies that may augment antibiotic therapy include echinacea, horsetail, pau d'arco, and

saw palmetto. Some herbalists also recommend chaparral, but this herb has been linked to liver toxicity and should be avoided.
Nutrition Therapy. To prevent yeast overgrowth while patients are on antibiotics, nutrition therapists suggest taking acidophilus pills or eating yogurt made with active lactobacillus or acidophilus cultures. It's also advisable to increase fluid intake, especially if the bladder and urethra are infected.

Self-Treatment
You can reduce your risk of contracting chlamydia by limiting your number of sexual partners and by always using a condom. Some studies have shown that spermicides containing nonoxynol-9 kill bacteria and chlamydia.

Anyone with a chlamydial infection should abstain from all sexual intercourse until antibiotic treatment is completed and follow-up tests show that the infection has cleared up.

Other Causes of Genital Discharges
Genital discharges and discomfort also may be caused by other sexually transmitted diseases, such as gonorrhea and syphilis, as well as by yeast infections and cervical cancer in women or by urethritis in men.

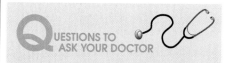

QUESTIONS TO ASK YOUR DOCTOR

► When will it be safe to resume sexual relations?
► Should I be tested for a chlamydial infection before my baby is born? If chlamydia is present, would a cesarean delivery be advisable?

Cholera

Cholera is an acute intestinal illness caused by a particular strain of the *Vibrio cholerae* bacterium. Usually, the disorder is mild, but in approximately one case in 10, cholera produces profuse watery diarrhea, vomiting, and leg cramps. These, in turn, cause a rapid

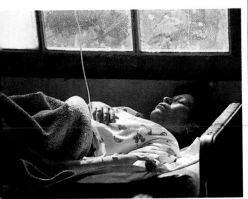

In addition to being debilitating, the diarrhea and vomiting of cholera can lead to severe dehydration and even death.

loss of body fluids and salts and result in dehydration and shock that, if left untreated, can be fatal.

A person may contract cholera by eating food or drinking water that has been contaminated by body wastes or vomit from infected individuals, as well as by eating raw shellfish from waters infested with cholera bacteria. However, it is not spread through casual contact with an infected person.

Epidemics are likely to occur in areas where there is inadequate sewage and water sanitation. In recent years, cholera epidemics have been occurring continuously in parts of Africa, Asia, and South and Central America. (Even where sanitation is normally adequate, cholera is likely to follow after a disaster such an an earthquake or flood.) However, Americans who visit these places are at very low risk of getting the disease if they observe simple dietary precautions (see Self-Treatment).

Diagnostic Studies and Procedures
Diagnosis is based on laboratory identification of the cholera organism in a fresh sample of the patient's stool.

Medical Treatments
Emergency treatment consists of immediate rehydration therapy to replace fluids and salts lost through diarrhea. When patients are severely dehydrated,

they will be given intravenous fluids in rapid succession until the body's fluid volume, blood pressure, and pulse return to normal.

Persons who are only moderately affected usually respond well to an oral rehydration solution. The standard formula calls for 20 grams of glucose, 3.5 grams of sodium chloride, 1.5 grams of potassium, and 2.9 grams of trisodium citrate or 2.5 grams of sodium bicarbonate per liter of sterile water.

Although most cholera patients will recover completely with rehydration alone, the addition of antibiotic treatment reduces the volume and duration of diarrhea. Tetracycline, taken orally every 6 hours for 72 hours, kills the bacteria and usually ends diarrhea within 48 hours. An alternative is a single dose of doxycycline, considered almost as effective as tetracycline.

Immunization is sometimes recommended for people traveling to areas where cholera is widespread, but public health officials generally advise against it. Only 50 percent of those who receive cholera vaccine develop immunity against the disease, and even then, it lasts only a few months. Still, some local authorities in countries where cholera is endemic may require that travelers present proof of having been vaccinated. In such cases, a single dose of vaccine is sufficient to satisfy the requirements. In any event, cholera vaccination should definitely be avoided during pregnancy.

Alternative Therapies
There are no alternative treatments for cholera, although some may alleviate symptoms. For example, relaxation exercises can be helpful in overcoming

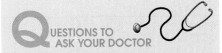

exhaustion from fluid loss. Some herbs that contain tannins, such as tormentil root and witch hazel, taken as teas, are also helpful in controlling diarrhea.

Self-Treatment
Prevention is the best self-treatment for cholera. A simple rule to follow is: "Boil it, cook it, peel it, or forget it." The Centers for Disease Control and Prevention (CDC) makes the following recommendations for travelers to places where cholera is endemic:

▶ Drink only water that has been boiled or treated with chlorine or iodine. Other safe beverages include tea or coffee made with boiled water, and carbonated bottled beverages served without ice unless the water to make it has been boiled.
▶ Eat only vegetables and other foods that have been thoroughly cooked and are still hot, or fruit that you have peeled yourself. Avoid fresh salads.
▶ Avoid undercooked or raw fish or shellfish, including ceviche.

Other Causes of Cholera-like Symptoms
Diarrhea is a symptom of most types of food poisoning, including salmonella and *Escherichia coli* infection (a common cause of traveler's diarrhea).

COUNTRIES WITH CHOLERA OUTBREAKS IN 1994

Africa		Southeast Asia	Nepal	Central America
Angola	Mauritania	Cambodia	Sri Lanka	Belize
Benin	Mozambique	China	**South America**	Costa Rica
Burkina Faso	Niger	Indonesia	Argentina	El Salvaador
Burundi	Nigeria	Laos	Bolivia	Guatemala
Cameroon	Rwanda	Malaysia	Brazil	Honduras
Chad	Sao Tome and Principe	Vietnam	Chile	Mexico
Cote d'Ivoire	Somalia	**Indian Subcontinent**	Columbia	Nicaragua
Djibouti	Swaziland	Afganistan	Ecuador	Panama
Ghana	Tanzania	Bhutan	French Guiana	**Eastern Europe**
Guinea	Togo	India	Guyana	Ukraine
Kenya	Uganda	Iraq	Peru	**South Pacific**
Liberia	Zaire	Iran	Suriname	Tuvalu
Malawi	Zambia		Venezuela	
Mali	Zimbabwe			

Cholesterol Disorders

(Hypercholesterolemia; hyperlipidemia; familial hypercholesterolemia)
Cholesterol is a lipid (fatty substance) that circulates in blood and is essential to many vital functions, such as the making of cell walls and certain hormones. When cholesterol levels are too high, atherosclerosis—the buildup of fatty deposits in artery walls—may develop, impeding blood flow and raising the risk of heart disease and stroke.

As cholesterol and other lipids circulate, they are attached to proteins in

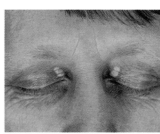

Xanthomas, small fat deposits beneath the skin, develop in many people who have a hereditary form of hypercholesterolemia. Otherwise, high-cholesterol levels are not readily apparent.

complexes called lipoproteins, which are classified according to how efficiently they carry cholesterol. Low density lipoproteins (LDLs) tend to deposit cholesterol on arterial walls. Thus, LDL is often referred to as the "bad" cholesterol. In comparison, high density lipoprotein (HDL) is known as the "good" lipid because it carries cholesterol back to the liver. Very low density lipoproteins (VLDLs) largely carry triglycerides, but convert to LDLs after depositing their triglycerides.

The liver makes all the cholesterol that the body needs. Why

some people have levels elevated well beyond these needs is not understood, but we do know some contributing factors. A diet high in saturated fat is one. It seems to encourage the liver to manufacture more cholesterol. High-cholesterol foods, such as liver and egg yolks, can also raise levels. In some people, there is a hereditary link. Their condition, known as familial hypercholesterolemia, can show up even in childhood. Diabetes, liver and kidney disorders, obesity, alcoholism, smoking, and stress are also related to high cholesterol.

Diagnostic Studies and Procedures

Lipid levels are measured by blood tests. For accuracy, they should be performed after an overnight fast. A total serum cholesterol level of less than 200 mg/dl is considered desirable for adults, with the LDLs under 130 mg/dl and HDLs over 35 mg/dl. Cholesterol levels may be expressed as an HDL ratio, or the result when total cholesterol is divided by HDL cholesterol. A ratio of 4.5 or less is considered desirable. If HDL levels are particularly high, and LDL levels correspondingly low, a total serum cholesterol level over 200 mg/dl may not be harmful.

Medical Treatments

The first step in treating hypercholesterolemia is adopting a lifestyle that includes a diet low in calories, cholesterol, and saturated fat, as well as weight reduction and increased exercise.

It is relatively easy to get the fat out of favorite foods, as illustrated by these two meals. The one at the left is fried and served with a butter-flavored gravy. The equally tasty meal, above, contains a fraction of the fat, thanks to baking instead of frying and using herbs and lemon for flavoring.

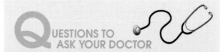
QUESTIONS TO ASK YOUR DOCTOR

▶ What is my total serum cholesterol level; also my HDL and LDL levels and my HDL ratio?
▶ How often should I have my cholesterol level checked?
▶ What are the side effects of my medication? How often should I be tested for hidden adverse reactions?

If such measures do not provide sufficient benefit, drug therapy, with one or more of the following medications, might be necessary:

Bile-acid sequestrants. Cholestyramine (Questran) and colestipol (Colestid) work in the intestines to bind bile acids, thus preventing them from being absorbed. As a result, the liver takes more LDL cholesterol from the blood to make bile, thereby lowering cholesterol levels 15 to 25 percent. Several of these products are formulated as powders or granules to be dissolved in water or fruit juice. Because they are not absorbed into the bloodstream, their side effects are limited to the intestinal tract, and may include bloating, gas, diarrhea, or constipation.

Fibric acids. These drugs include clofibrate (Atromid-S) and gemfibrozil (Lopid), which are usually taken as capsules or tablets twice a day. It is not clearly understood how these drugs work, but it is thought that they slow the production of VLDLs and thereby lead to a reduction of serum LDLs and triglycerides. Some also increase levels of protective HDLs. In general, fibric acids are not as effective as several other cholesterol-lowering agents.

Statins. These are the newest and most powerful cholesterol-lowering drugs, achieving an average 25 percent reduction by interfering with the liver's manufacturing of cholesterol. Included in this category are lovastatin (Mevacor), pravastatin (Pravachol), and simvastatin (Zocor). Although these drugs are safe for most people, regular checkups are necessary to look for signs of possible liver or kidney problems. They also may cause muscle weakness.

Nicotinic Acid or Niacin. High doses of this inexpensive and highly effective B vitamin are often recommended to start. It works by reducing the liver's

A CASE IN POINT

A routine insurance examination in 1964 alerted Bob Bailey, a 42-year-old university professor, to the fact that he had dangerously high cholesterol. At that time, doctors were not as concerned with cholesterol as they are today, but Bailey's reading of 420 was clearly alarming.

"My doctor told me to cut out eggs and other high-cholesterol foods, but that was about all," Bailey recalls. "So I decided to do some research myself."

At his university library, Bailey ran across an article describing the cholesterol-lowering properties of high-dose niacin, and another crediting vegetarianism with the low incidence of heart attacks among Seventh Day Adventists. An herbal textbook advocated garlic and evening primrose oil, and a book on

natural medicine recommended lecithin. "I decided to do my own controlled clinical study," Bailey says. He started by switching to a mostly vegetarian diet, and six months later, his cholesterol had dropped to 340.

"My doctor seemed pleased, but my research told me that 340 was still far too high." So, he added 3 tablespoons of lecithin to his daily regimen. At his next checkup, his cholesterol was 325.

"I talked to my doctor about niacin, and he warned me that I'd probably suffer hot flashes and other side effects," Bailey recalls. Another trip to the library unearthed what seemed a reasonable approach—start with 200 milligrams morning and evening, and then gradually increase the dosage by 100 milligrams

every two or three weeks until reaching 2,000 to 3,000 milligrams a day.

At Bailey's next checkup, his cholesterol was down to 220, and he decided to see if substituting primrose oil for lecithin would make a difference. At his next checkup, the cholesterol was unchanged, leading him to conclude that, for him, neither made much difference.

In the intervening years, Bailey has cut his niacin dosage from 3,000 to 2,000 milligrams a day. Periodic liver function tests indicate that he continues to tolerate the drug without organ damage, and his total cholesterol ranges between 180 and 200. He credits an exercise program that he started when he retired at 67 with the further improvement. At the age of 72, he still has no sign of heart disease.

CHOLESTEROL DISORDERS (CONTINUED)

production of VLDLs, which in turn decreases LDL levels. Unfortunately, high doses can cause intense flushes of the skin, similar to menopausal hot flashes. This adverse side effect can sometimes be avoided by starting with a low dose and gradually increasing it, or by taking time-released forms.

Probucol. This drug, marketed as Lorelco, is taken in tablet form twice a day. It is believed to alter the makeup of LDL, causing cells to remove it more quickly from the bloodstream.

A few patients with familial hypercholesterolemia have received heart and liver transplants; the new liver appears to handle cholesterol properly.

Alternative Therapies

The following alternative therapies can help lower blood cholesterol levels:

Herbal Medicine. Capsaicin (a component of hot red pepper, or cayenne), hawthorn berries, black currants, primrose oil, and kelp have all been reported to help lower cholesterol. Better documented are the benefits of garlic, taken raw or in capsule form.

Nutrition Therapy. Doctors and alternative practitioners alike recognize that diet plays a key role in cholesterol reduction. Cutting saturated fat intake to 10 percent of total calories and increasing dietary fiber is widely recommended. Dietary cholesterol should not exceed 300 milligrams a day; fats should be mostly polyunsaturated and monounsaturated (see box, right).

Soluble fiber, found in vegetables, fruits, oat bran, and psyllium products, can help lower serum cholesterol. Good food sources are dry beans, brown rice, oatmeal, barley, apples, broccoli, carrots, bananas, and peaches.

Vitamin E supplements have been shown to elevate levels of HDL. Often advocated for lowering cholesterol is a tablespoon of lecithin before meals.

Some nutritionists also recommend taking fish oil supplements to lower cholesterol. These are high in omega-3 fatty acids, but caution is advised because they have blood-thinning properties that can cause bleeding. It is better to have a serving of a cold-water fish such as halibut, tuna, or salmon once or twice a week.

TYPES OF FATS ACCORDING TO SATURATION

Mostly Polyunsaturated

Corn oil	Soybean oil
Cotton seed oil	Sunflower oil
Safflower oil	

Mostly Monounsaturated

Canola oil	Peanut oil
Olive oil	Sesame oil

Mostly Saturated

Animal fats	Coconut oil
Butter	Palm and palm
Cocoa butter	kernel oils

Yoga and Meditation. Studies have linked stress with elevated cholesterol. Meditation, yoga, and other relaxation therapies are now advocated as part of a program to reduce heart disease risk.

Self-Treatment

Self-care emphasizes a healthy lifestyle for both prevention and management of cholesterol disorders. Strategies include:

Not smoking. A component in tobacco smoke may be instrumental in initiating the blood vessel damage that leads to atherosclerosis.

Exercising regularly. At least 30 minutes of sustained physical activity three or four times a week can improve the balance of HDL/LDL cholesterol.

Maintaining ideal weight. Obesity increases cholesterol levels, adds to the heart's workload, and raises the risk of hypertension and diabetes. Losing even 10 or 15 pounds can lower levels.

Practicing moderation. Limit alcohol to one or two drinks a day. At this level, alcohol may even raise levels of HDL cholesterol, but a higher intake offsets any gain by damaging the liver and other organs. Limit caffeine to the equivalent of three of four cups of coffee a day. A higher intake has been linked to a rise in serum cholesterol.

Other Causes of High Cholesterol

Diabetes can raise cholesterol levels, as can certain drugs such as isotretinoin (Accutane), a medication for severe acne, and anabolic steroids, which are sometimes misused by athletes.

Chronic Fatigue Syndrome

Chronic fatigue syndrome, commonly referred to as CFS, is a condition of unknown origin whose main symptom is unremitting and disabling exhaustion. In some cases, the syndrome follows an infectious illness. In others, the symptoms appear during a time of unusual stress, or they may start gradually, with no apparent cause, at any time from adolescence through middle age. At least two-thirds of sufferers are white middle-class women.

Although the cause of chronic fatigue syndrome is unknown, under investigation as possible causes are hormone deficiencies, allergies, the reactivation of a dormant virus, and neurological damage sustained in a previous illness.

Recent studies have discounted a number of earlier suspects, including infection with the Epstein-Barr virus, cytomegalovirus, herpes virus, and viruses similar to HIV, the organism that causes AIDS.

Experts disagree on what role, if any, psychological factors play. About half the individuals diagnosed as having CFS seem to have had a pre-existing psychiatric disorder. Other patients develop depression and anxiety only after the syndrome has taken hold.

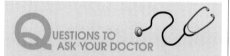

Q UESTIONS TO ASK YOUR DOCTOR

► Am I a good candidate for a CFS research project? If so, how can I enroll?
► Does CFS increase my susceptibility to other diseases related to reduced immunity, such as lupus, arthritis, or cancer?

Diagnostic Studies and Procedure

There is no specific test for chronic fatigue syndrome; instead, the government's Centers for Disease Control and Prevention (CDC) has compiled the following list of conditions that must be present to make a diagnosis:
► Debilitating fatigue lasting for at least six months.
► The exclusion, by examination and testing, of other disorders that may cause fatigue.
► A combination of eight or more

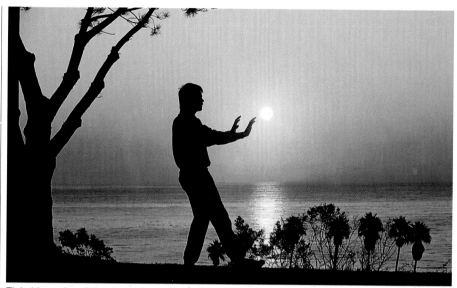

T'ai chi requires little physical energy, and the slow, focused movements are thought to relieve fatigue. To obtain the full benefits, the mind should be concentrated fully on each movement.

symptoms that develop over the course of a few days and persist for six months or more. These include:
  Mild fever
  Sore throat
  Painful lymph nodes
  Generalized muscle weakness
  Muscle aches
  Headache
  Joint pains
  Prolonged fatigue after exercise
  Inability to concentrate and other
    nervous system complaints
  Altered sleep habits

Medical Treatments

Because there is no single treatment for the syndrome, symptoms are treated as they present themselves. Aspirin and other nonsteroidal anti-inflammatory medications are helpful in alleviating fever, headaches, and muscle and joint pains. Antidepressants or other psychotropic drugs may be prescribed for depression and anxiety.

Alternative Therapies

A number of the drugs prescribed for chronic fatigue syndrome can cause side effects that add to the debilitating nature of the disorder, thus many patients turn to alternative therapies before traditional medicine.

Herbal Medicine. Among the herbs that are commonly recommended are: purple coneflower, or echinacea, extract or capsules, which is said to stimulate the immune system; licorice root capsules and dried or fresh shitake mushrooms, which are used in Chinese medicine to increase resistance to dis-

ease; and suma, a South American herb similar to ginseng that is taken as capsules or tablets or as a tonic to fight fatigue. Also suggested are teas, extracts, or tablets of rosemary, ginseng root (both American and Siberian), peppermint, and rose hips.

Naturopathy. Practitioners recommend several dietary supplements intended to strengthen the immune system: a multivitamin and mineral supplement with a high content of all the B vitamins; also, beta carotene (precursor to vitamin A), extra vitamin C, and zinc. (If megadoses are advised, consult your doctor.)

T'ai Chi. These gentle exercises are said to refresh the fatigued body. Although they require relatively little physical energy, the exercises do help to tone muscles. Doing them in a group can also boost morale.

Self-Treatment

To cope with chronic fatigue syndrome, follow a regimen of good nutrition, adequate rest, and moderate exercise. Keep your life balanced; avoid stressful circumstances and overexertion. Join a support group, which can provide comfort and understanding as well as referrals and treatment suggestions.

Other Causes of Chronic Fatigue

Among the many diseases that should be ruled out when diagnosing chronic fatigue syndrome are depression, lupus, leukemia and other cancers, hepatitis, AIDS, anemia, and heart, lung, liver, and kidney diseases. Also, side effects of certain drugs produce symptoms of chronic fatigue syndrome.

Cirrhosis

(Alcoholic, hepatic, and other forms of cirrhosis)

Cirrhosis refers to progressive scarring of the liver, in which fibrous bands and hard nodules replace healthy tissue and reduce normal liver function. This organ, which filters toxic substances

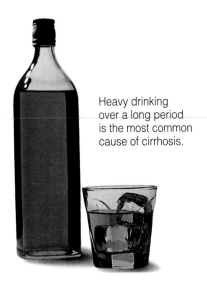

Heavy drinking over a long period is the most common cause of cirrhosis.

from the blood and performs numerous other chemical and metabolic tasks, can function even when a large number of its cells are destroyed, but unchecked cirrhosis is eventually fatal.

The usual symptoms of cirrhosis are loss of weight and appetite, jaundice, nausea and vomiting, weakness, and abdominal pain. Generalized itching and intestinal bleeding may also occur.

Excessive alcohol intake is the most common cause of cirrhosis; a liver infection, chronic hepatitis, and a congenital defect are other possible causes. A variant called biliary cirrhosis, which affects the ducts that transport bile

from the liver to the intestines, can be due to disease of the bile ducts.

Diagnostic Studies and Procedures

A physical examination is the first step in diagnosis. The abdomen is palpated, or pressed, to determine if the liver feels hard and the spleen is enlarged. Such findings generally suggest the presence of cirrhosis.

Diagnostic studies include blood and urine tests, X-rays, and ultrasound scans. A definitive diagnosis may require a biopsy, in which a needle is used to take a sample of liver tissue.

Medical Treatments

Medical treatment depends upon the underlying cause. Alcoholic cirrhosis is treated mainly by nonmedical means, such as cessation of drinking and dietary changes. Biliary cirrhosis may involve surgery if a bile duct is obstructed. Sometimes, congenital cirrhosis can be controlled, but because scarring is irreversible, a liver transplant is the only cure in many cases.

Alternative Therapies

These therapies cannot cure cirrhosis, but some may be useful in minimizing symptoms and preventing any further deterioration of liver tissues.

Herbal Medicine. Many herbal preparations are said to improve liver function and promote regeneration of liver cells. These include milk thistle extract, available as silymarin pills, and cynarin, a substance in artichokes that is believed to reduce liver inflammation. Garlic capsules are promoted to detoxify the liver. Other herbal remedies include barberry, black radish, dandelion, and echinacea.

Naturopathy and Nutrition Therapy. A clinical nutritionist or dietitian can provide dietary guidance, especially in cases of alcoholism where malnutrition often contributes to deterioration of the

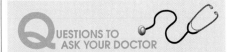

QUESTIONS TO ASK YOUR DOCTOR

▶ What foods should I avoid?
▶ Should I receive immunization against hepatitis B?

liver. Anyone with cirrhosis must consume precisely the correct amount of protein, since too much can lead to a buildup of ammonia and the risk of a coma, while too little prevents the liver from manufacturing new cells.

Some naturopaths and nutritionists recommend that protein be derived mostly from vegetable sources, such as beans and nuts, rather than from meat. Sufficient carbohydrates and fat must be consumed to provide for the body's energy needs, so that protein can go toward repairing the liver. Vitamin B complex and other supplements are usually needed too.

Self-Treatment

Total abstention from alcohol is critical, but abstaining can be very difficult. Detoxification should be carried out under careful medical supervision. After that, a support group such as Alcoholics Anonymous provides the best chance of long-term success in overcoming alcoholism.

People vary regarding how much alcohol it takes to induce cirrhosis, but it's usually in the range of a pint or more of whiskey or other spirits a day (or the equivalent in beer or wine) over several years. Limiting alcohol consumption to one or two drinks at a time on an occasional basis is probably safe. Other self-care measures include:
▶ Take only those medications, including over-the-counter preparations, that your doctor feels are necessary. Most drugs are metabolized by the liver, and unneeded ones increase its workload.
▶ Avoid working with chemicals that give off fumes toxic to the liver.
▶ Minimize the danger of hepatitis by avoiding raw shellfish and other potentially contaminated foods.

Other Causes of Cirrhosis

Cirrhosis can be inborn. It can also be the result of Wilson's disease, a hereditary disorder in which copper accumulates in the liver; hemochromatosis, a genetic tendency to conserve iron; and cystic fibrosis.

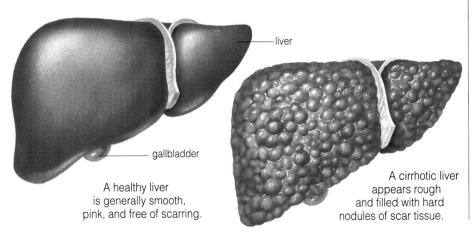

A healthy liver is generally smooth, pink, and free of scarring.

liver

gallbladder

A cirrhotic liver appears rough and filled with hard nodules of scar tissue.

Clubfoot

(Equinovarus congenita)

A clubfoot is a deformity of the lower leg and foot that occurs during fetal development. Twice as common in males as in females, the abnormality may affect one or both feet. In most cases, the front of the foot turns down and in, and the heel also turns inward. The arch is abnormally high, the ankle joint may be rigid or stiff, and the calf is abnormally small.

Most club feet are thought to be a congenital defect in the prenatal development of ankle bones and surrounding muscles. Usually, no cause for the malformation can be identified. However, some medications such as methotrexate, used to treat severe arthritis and psoriasis, have been linked to fetal abnormalities, including clubfoot.

There are cases in which the feet appear deformed immediately after birth because of a cramped fetal position in the womb, and they soon assume a normal shape on their own. These are not true clubfeet.

Diagnostic Studies and Procedures

Sometimes what appears to be a deformed limb may show up on a fetal sonogram, but this is not a reliable test. Diagnosis is usually made when the baby is examined immediately after birth, at which time a clubfoot is easily recognized on the basis of its appearance. X-rays confirm the diagnosis and provide precise information about the placement of the foot and ankle bones.

Medical Treatments

A pediatric orthopedist should be consulted as soon as possible following the baby's birth, because clubfoot is not a condition that can be expected to correct itself with time or exercises and it is more difficult to correct if allowed to go untreated.

Ideally, the foot is manipulated toward a normal position when the baby is a few days old, and the new

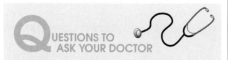

Q UESTIONS TO ASK YOUR DOCTOR

▶ How long must my child wear special orthopedic shoes?
▶ If surgical correction is needed, can it be done in a single operation?
▶ Will massage and exercise help?

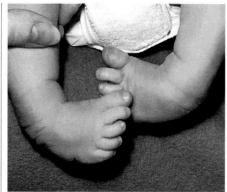

Clubfoot develops during gestation, when foot bones form in abnormal positions, causing the heel and front of the foot to turn down and inward.

position is maintained by a cast or a splint covered with an adhesive bandage. During the first few weeks, manipulation and compression are repeated every few days, along with a change of cast or splinting designed to move the foot to a more normal position.

By the time the baby is about two months old, the casts are changed at one- to two-week intervals. When normal positioning of the foot has been achieved, corrective shoes are worn for a time to maintain it.

If a deformed foot cannot be coaxed into a normal position by manipulation and casts, surgical correction is necessary. This is done usually when the baby is 6 to 12 months old.

With prompt and complete treatment, a child born with a clubfoot can eventually have a normal foot, engage in sports, and wear the same shoes as his peers. But the foot should be evaluated periodically by a pediatric orthopedist to be sure it is still growing normally.

Although orthotic devices—special shoe inserts—are not used for treatment, they may be recommended later on to help maintain proper alignment of the foot and ankle bones following either type of correction.

In some cases, an abnormality in foot development does not become obvious until a baby is a few months old. At that point, the problem is also treated with progressive casting or splinting, corrective footwear, and eventual surgery, if necessary. Even an adult whose deformity was not corrected during childhood can achieve some measure of foot normalcy through operations in which the foot bones are resectioned and then fused.

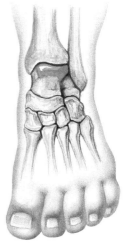

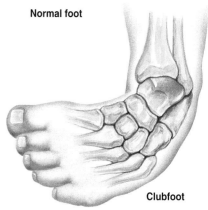

To straighten a clubfoot in a newborn, an orthopedic surgeon manipulates the bones toward the normal position and holds them in place with a splint or cast. This procedure is repeated at regular intervals until the bone alignment is normal.

Normal foot

Clubfoot

Alternative Therapies

Although not recommended as a substitute for conventional treatment of clubfoot in infancy, massage therapies may hasten the correction in certain cases. Such treatments should not be undertaken, however, without the approval of the orthopedist who is overseeing the correction.

Self-Treatment

Children who are handicapped by their deformity can profit from exercises that are designed to stabilize their gait and prevent fatigue. A physical therapist can demonstrate the routines for parent and child, so that the exercises can be supervised at home.

Parents should avoid overprotection of a child with a clubfoot, because it can have a crippling effect on psychological and emotional development.

Other Causes of Foot Deformities

A birth injury or an accident during infancy can result in deformities similar to those of clubfoot, as can neuromuscular disorders, such as cerebral palsy and muscular dystrophy. A clubfoot-like deformity may also be one of the manifestations of genetic dwarfism.

Cluster Headaches

(Horton's headache)

Cluster headaches are caused by abnormalities in the blood vessels of the head. Nicknamed "suicide headaches" because of their severity, they appear in clusters just as their name implies. These headaches generally occur daily, sometimes several times a day, for weeks or months at a time and then suddenly disappear, only to recur weeks, months, or even years later.

The excruciating pain is usually localized to one side of the head, commonly around the eye. During an attack, the eye on the affected side often tears and may become quite red, the nostril may become congested or runny, and the face may flush. The headaches start and end abruptly, usually without warning, often beginning during sleep. Most last for less than an hour.

While the causes of cluster headaches are not well understood, a few potential triggers have been identified. Alcohol and tobacco both appear to precipitate attacks in some people, as do certain foods. Stress and other psychological factors sometimes trigger cluster headaches, but not to the same extent as in other types. For many people, cluster attacks are seasonal and occur at the same time each year, indicating that an individual's underlying biologic rhythm may play a role.

Men with cluster headaches outnumber women four to one. Many sufferers seem to fit a certain personality profile; that is, they are hard-driving, so-called Type A individuals.

Diagnostic Studies and Procedures

The physician's most important tool is a thorough history of the occurrences. By studying the patterns and characteristics of a patient's headaches, the doctor can usually differentiate cluster headaches from migraines or headaches that

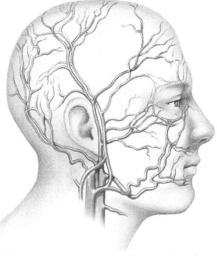

Although the exact causes of cluster headaches are unknown, abnormalities in the blood vessels of the head seem to play a role in their development.

arise from tumors and other potentially dangerous medical conditions.

When consulting a doctor, be prepared to describe the frequency and duration of the headaches, possible precipitating factors, and the nature of the pain and what alleviates it. To identify triggers and accurately report the frequency and duration of symptoms, it may help to keep a log or journal for a few months (see Self-Treatment).

A complete physical examination, including a neurologic workup, should be performed, along with blood tests to exclude other diagnoses. In some cases, imaging studies such as a CT brain scan or MRI may be necessary.

Medical Treatments

There are several drugs that can prevent cluster headaches, but they must be taken regularly and are ineffective if taken once an attack begins. Lithium carbonate, more commonly prescribed to treat manic-depression, provides relief in up to 90 percent of patients.

Other possible medications include corticosteroids; methysergide (Sansert), a migraine drug; cyproheptadine (Periactin), an antihistimine; indomethacin (Indocin), a common arthritis drug; and calcium-channel blockers such as verapamil (Calan and others). The last are vasodilators normally used to lower blood pressure.

The drugs containing ergot that are frequently used to treat migraines are also useful in preventing cluster headaches but caution must be exercised to avoid ergot toxicity.

During an acute attack, the two most effective treatments appear to be ergot drugs and inhaled oxygen, which seem to work by constricting the blood vessels in the head.

Alternative Therapies

There are few alternatives to medical therapy that are effective in relieving cluster headaches; approaches that focus on preventing them are generally the most successful.

Acupressure. Pressing the webbed area between the thumb and forefinger is said to relieve headaches.

Biofeedback. Some patients are helped by biofeedback training to learn how to divert blood flow from the scalp vessels to other parts of the body.

Herbal Medicine. Herbalists recommend one to three capsules of feverfew daily to prevent migraines, and some also advocate taking this herb to prevent cluster headaches.

Meditation and Visualization. Patients whose headaches are triggered by stress may benefit from these relaxation techniques. Meditation can also help with pain management during an attack.

Self-Treatment

Self-treatment starts with prevention. Identify those things that set off your headaches and try to avoid them. Document your headaches in a journal, making note of anything that could possibly have caused them. See if any patterns emerge and, if they do, try to eliminate the potential trigger.

When a cluster does develop, using a portable oxygen inhaler helps about 80 percent of patients. Talk to your physician about obtaining one.

Individuals who suffer from cluster headaches usually have their own coping routines. For example, some people sit quietly in a darkened room, while others feel better if they stand or pace. Some even bang their heads against a padded surface, but it is doubtful that this can alleviate the pain.

Other Causes of Headaches

Cluster headaches can be confused with other forms of headache, particularly vascular types such as migraines. Conditions that may mimic cluster headaches include sinusitis, congestion or infection of the sinus cavities in the forehead and cheekbones; trigeminal neuralgia, a disorder affecting one of the facial nerves; aneurysms, abnormalities of the blood vessels in the head or neck; and brain tumors.

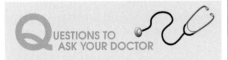

QUESTIONS TO ASK YOUR DOCTOR

▶ What kind of portable oxygen sources are available that I might use when I get a headache?
▶ Should I try preventive medications? If so, what precautions should I follow?

Cold Sores

(Fever blisters; herpes simplex)

Cold sores appear as small, painful blisters around the mouth. They occur usually in groups, with a red ring surrounding each blister, and last for one to three weeks. During this period, the sores fill with fluid, and then crust over, dry up, and disappear.

The Type 1 herpes simplex virus causes most cold sores, although some cases are due to the Type 2 virus that is usually responsible for genital herpes. The herpes virus is highly contagious and, once acquired, it may lie dormant in the body for years. Some people experience recurrent outbreaks throughout their lives. For most persons, though, recurrences stop within a few years of the first outbreak.

A fever, exposure to the sun, or physical or emotional stress can bring on an attack from a dormant virus. Even such

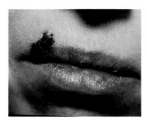

Most cold sores develop on the lips or under the nose.

minor demands on the immune system as fighting a cold or an intestinal infection can result in a flare-up of cold sores. Women have a higher risk of developing them during their menstrual periods and in the premenstrual phase.

Diagnostic Studies and Procedures

Cold sores almost always are diagnosed on the basis of symptoms and the characteristic appearance of the blisters. If a secondary bacterial infection develops, a laboratory culture may be ordered.

Medical Treatments

In most instances, cold sores heal themselves without any medical treatment. An exception would be an eruption that occurs in someone who has a compromised immune system or an infection near or in the eyes. In the latter case, prompt treatment with antiviral eyedrops or ointment, usually vidarabine (Vira-A), trifluridine (Viroptic), or idoxuridine (Herplex Liquifilm and Stoxil) is needed to prevent eye damage. The medication should be applied to the eyes several times a day.

Extensive cold sores in the mouth area may be treated with acyclovir (Zovirax), an antiviral agent. An antibiotic ointment may also be prescribed if a bacterial infection develops.

Alternative Therapies

Herbal Medicine. Herbalists may prescribe echinacea tea, tablets, or tincture in order to stimulate the immune system against viral infections. A few drops of lavender oil applied to the sore may promote healing.

Homeopathy. To speed healing, practitioners suggest applying a solution made with one part calendula tincture and three parts water to the sores after they have opened. Other homeopathic remedies include rhustoxicodendron, a general anti-infective, and sepia. Oozing blisters may be treated with topical natrum muriaticum or graphites.

Naturopathy and Nutrition Therapy. High doses of vitamin C are said to be effective against cold sores, although there is no definitive scientific proof for this belief. An amino acid called L-lysine is also used sometimes by persons who have recurrent attacks of cold sores. It comes in pills or in a cream to be applied to the sores.

Other natural or nutritional remedies are supplements of vitamin B complex, lozenges of zinc gluconate, acidophilus pills or yogurt containing acidophilus cultures, and garlic capsules.

Self-Treatment

Minor pain can be relieved with acetaminophen, aspirin, or ibuprofen. Remember, however, that aspirin should not be given to anyone under the age of 18 years during a viral infection because of an increased risk of Reye's syndrome, a potentially life-threatening disorder (see page 437).

Applying an ice cube to the lesion for an hour or so when it first appears can help speed healing. Dipping a cotton ball in cold milk and applying it to the sore has the same effect. Even better, use one of these techniques at the first sign of a cold sore, which may be a stinging, tingling, or itching sensation on a part of the mouth where outbreaks are likely to occur.

Once a blister develops, soothe it by drinking cool liquids, sucking frozen juice bars, or applying petroleum salve or over-the-counter anesthetics. Salves are particularly helpful for softening scabs that form as cold sores heal. Avoid irritating salty and acidic foods

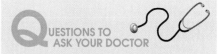

QUESTIONS TO ASK YOUR DOCTOR

▶ What precautions are necessary to keep the virus from spreading within the household?
▶ If I get cold sores, am I more likely to get shingles, which is also caused by a type of herpes virus?

until the lesion heals completely. Don't try to mask a cold sore with makeup, as this action can make it worse.

Because cold sores are very contagious, you should avoid kissing and other skin contact with a person who has one. Be particularly careful about sexual contact with anyone who has a cold sore; the herpes virus can be transmitted through oral-genital contact, resulting in genital herpes.

Also, wash your hands frequently to avoid spreading the virus to others, and avoid sharing glasses, cups, eating utensils, towels, and washcloths.

Other Causes of Skin Blisters

Cold sores are sometimes confused with impetigo, a skin infection caused by a bacterium that produces a red rash with many small blisters. A canker sore on the lips may feel like a cold sore, but it has a different appearance. Chickenpox and shingles, which are also caused by a virus in the herpes family, produce tiny, blister-like lesions that may appear on the face.

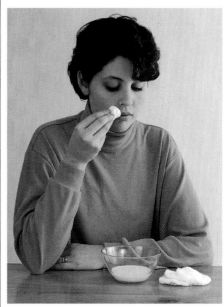

When a cold sore first appears, apply a cotton ball soaked in cold milk to speed healing.

Colic

(Infantile colic syndrome)

Colic is a self-limiting condition in which an otherwise healthy baby cries inconsolably for several hours at a time. No one can say with certainty what causes colic, but about 10 percent of all infants develop it. The prolonged crying usually begins a few days after birth, tapers off at two months, and comes to an end at about three months. Crying episodes occur most commonly in the early evening, but they may also take place at other times of the day.

Between periods of crying, a colicky baby is completely normal. One current theory is that colicky babies have immature nervous systems that are

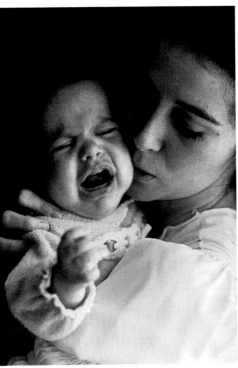

Body contact, rocking, and soothing sounds can sometimes quiet a colicky baby.

incapable of tuning out the stimuli that overwhelm them. This supersensitivity seems to be corrected as their physiological development catches up and can process the environmental overload.

Diagnostic Studies and Procedures

Before deciding that a baby is colicky, other causes for the crying should be ruled out. An allergic reaction to milk in any form—whether breast milk or formula—should be investigated, especially if the crying is accompanied by diarrhea or excessive gassiness.

A doctor should be consulted if the crying turns into screams of pain; if it goes on for more than three hours; and especially if the crying occurs after a fall or other injury.

Extended periods of fussy crying that begin after the baby is four weeks old do not represent colic, and a doctor should be consulted to find the cause.

Medical Treatments

After physical causes for the crying are ruled out, medical treatment of colic is not needed. In the past, sedating colicky babies with phenobarbital and similar drugs was sometimes recommended, but these drugs are no longer used for this purpose because they are constipating and potentially addictive. However, tranquilizers and/or sleeping pills may be prescribed for a mother who has become emotionally and physically exhausted.

A doctor may also recommend counseling for mothers and other family members, especially when the colicky infant is a first-born child. Older siblings who feel neglected and angry should also be encouraged to talk honestly to a professional counselor about their mixed emotions. Counseling can be especially important for a parent who is increasingly enraged by the demands of a colicky baby because these circumstances can lead to child abuse, often with tragic consequences.

Alternative Therapies

Acupressure. For a colicky infant, applying pressure to the web of skin between the thumb and forefinger may bring relief, as may a gentle massage to the center of the abdomen about two inches above the navel.

Herbal medicine. Grippe water, which is infused with dill seed, is commonly used to treat colicky infants in Europe and Canada. Chamomile and fennel may also be helpful. Check with a pediatrician, though, before giving an infant any herbal remedy.

Meditation and Yoga. An overburdened mother may benefit from these relaxation techniques, which can help her to achieve a state of calmness and emotional stability. Breathing exercises to overcome anxiety and tension can be practiced even while rocking the baby.

Nutrition Therapy. A mother who is breast-feeding should try to eliminate caffeine and such gas-producing foods as onions, cucumbers, cabbage, and legumes from her diet.

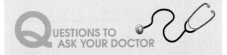

Self-Treatment

Caring for a colicky baby is a stressful responsibility. One of the best things a mother can do to help herself cope with the situation is to set aside a little time, even if it's only a few minutes each day, for a relaxing or pleasurable activity.

Above all, be patient. All babies outgrow colic eventually, usually by their second or third month. In the meantime, here are some ways to comfort a colicky baby:

▶ Rock the baby in a cradle or your arms or sit with her in a rocking chair.
▶ Keep the baby next to you in an infant sling or carrier whenever possible.
▶ Whisper loving words, hum softly, or sing soothing lullabies.
▶ Try an outing in the stroller or automobile. Often the motion of a brief ride in the car does the trick. In fact, there is a new FDA-approved gadget called SleepTight, which can be attached under a crib, that simulates the sound and motion of a car.
▶ Ease the baby into sleep. After a warm bath and a gentle massage, put the baby in the crib, reduce all stimuli to a minimum, and turn off the light.
▶ Promote sleep at night by interrupting a daytime nap that lasts for more than three hours. Wake and feed the baby, and then amuse him for a while before the bedtime feeding.
▶ Swaddling often helps; try wrapping the baby firmly in a light blanket.
▶ Set up orderly rituals for feeding, bathing, outing, and bedtime, and try not to vary them. Keep excitement, visitors, noise, and disorder at a minimum, especially during the late afternoon and evening.

Other Causes of Crying

Although colic is the most common cause of prolonged infant crying, other possible causes include a mother's drug or alcohol dependency during her pregnancy, allergy to formula or breast milk, malabsorption and other intestinal problems, and autism.

Collapsed Lung

(Pneumothorax)

A lung collapses when air enters the pleural space, which lies between the membranes (pleura) that line the chest cavity and the lungs. Although this can occur without a person having any symptoms, usually there is sudden, sharp chest pain, shortness of breath, and occasionally, a dry, hacking cough.

With an open pneumothorax, outside air enters the space through a wound that penetrates the chest.

With a closed pneumothorax, air may leak from the lungs or airways, either because of an injury or a spontaneous rupture. The latter, referred to as a simple spontaneous pneumothorax, sometimes occurs in a normal, healthy person who has a congenital weakness in part of a lung. This condition is most common among otherwise healthy young men, but it can occur at any age in both sexes.

A complicated pneumothorax also involves a spontaneous rupture, but the condition is worsened by the presence of other lung diseases, such as emphysema or cystic fibrosis. It occurs mostly in middle-aged and older people.

Diagnostic Studies and Procedures

If a pneumothorax is suspected, a doctor first listens to the chest sounds with a stethoscope, and then orders chest X-rays. In some cases, more invasive procedures such as thoracoscopy may be performed. For this examination a catheter with lighting devices is inserted into the chest cavity so that the doctor can view the pleural membranes and the space between them.

Medical Treatments

A small, simple, spontaneous pneumothorax that is confined to a limited portion of the lung often does not require any treatment other than repeated X-rays to make sure that it is healing on its own.

A larger rupture is treated by inserting a tube into the chest cavity to allow air to escape from the pleural space. If the rupture is extensive, it may be necessary to insert a needle into the chest to remove the air. Needle insertion may also be required if the pneumothorax is increasing in size. As a last resort, surgery may be performed to correct an underlying problem.

Some patients have repeated occurrences of pneumothorax; in such cases,

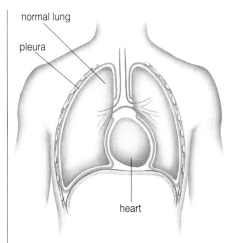

normal lung

pleura

heart

Normally, there is no air in the space between the pleural membranes lining the chest cavity and a lung itself.

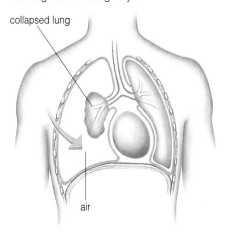

With a collapsed lung, air leaking from the lung into the pleural space prevents the lung from inflating fully.

collapsed lung

air

surgery may be necessary to remove the weakened segments of the lung. This procedure effectively prevents any future ruptures from occurring.

Alternative Therapies

A collapsed lung should always be treated immediately by a doctor. Alternative therapies can be applied as an adjunct approach during convalescence. These measures are also effective in treating some of the respiratory problems that increase the risk of a collapsed lung.

Herbal Medicine. Hyssop and lungwort teas or decoctions are advocated for treating mild lung problems and promoting respiratory health. Herbalists also suggest garlic because of its ability to fight off infection, build immunity, and generally strengthen the respiratory tract.

Nutrition Therapy. Vitamins A and C are said to strengthen the immune system and heal inflamed lung tissue. Some practitioners also believe that magnesium is beneficial to the muscles used in breathing. In general, maintaining a balanced diet with plenty of fresh fruits and vegetables will help promote healthy respiratory function.

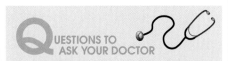

QUESTIONS TO ASK YOUR DOCTOR

▶ What precautions should be taken after recovery from a collapsed lung?
▶ Is it safe to jog or engage in other endurance activities?
▶ Does coughing or sneezing increase the chance of a recurrence?

Reflexology. In this form of massage, application of pressure to certain points on the feet and hands relieves tension in specific areas of the body. Lung disorders are treated by pushing the knuckles of the fist against the base of the patient's toes and the ball of the foot. Pressing on the tips of the fingers and the middle of the palm is believed to improve breathing.

Self-Treatment

There is no self-treatment for a collapsed lung, because the situation may deteriorate very rapidly into a medical emergency. If you think you have this condition, go immediately to the nearest hospital emergency room.

As a follow-up to medical treatment, good self-care may help prevent a recurrence, especially if bronchitis, emphysema, or another chronic lung disorder is present. If you are a smoker, make every effort to stop, and avoid smoke-filled environments. If your job involves exposure to toxic substances or fumes, protect your lungs with the proper safety equipment. People with chronic lung disorders should also avoid going outdoors on days when the air pollution index is high.

Other Causes of Chest Symptoms

Chest pain accompanied by shortness of breath may be caused by angina or a heart attack. Breathing problems may also signal heart failure. Pneumonia and pleurisy, inflammation of the pleural membranes, may cause chest pain that feels similar to the pain of pneumothorax. Anxiety and panic attacks can also produce similar symptoms, particularly pressure in the chest.

Colon Polyps

(Benign colon tumors)

Colon polyps are small benign tumors that grow on the inside walls of the large intestine, usually in or near the rectum. They range in size from a tiny grape to a small plum. Some, known as familial polyposis, are inherited, but the cause of most colon polyps is unknown. They become more common after age 40; most adults eventually develop them.

The majority of colon polyps remain small and cause no symptoms. Sometimes, however, they grow large enough to interfere with normal bowel function, causing a change in the size and shape of the stools, possible constipation or diarrhea, bleeding (which may or not be visible in the stool), and abdominal pain.

A more serious concern is that some colon polyps contain cells that are or may become cancerous. This almost always happens in familial polyposis and is common if there are many or recurrent polyps. Thus, early detection and removal of colon polyps can help prevent colon cancer.

Diagnostic Studies and Procedures

Even in the absence of symptoms, anyone over age 40 should be screened annually with a digital rectal examination to check for growths in the lower rectum. Everyone over age 50 should have sigmoidoscopy every three to five years. For this procedure, a hollow viewing tube is inserted into the rectum and lower sigmoid part of the bowel. If abnormalities are detected, or there is a history of familial polyposis, a more extensive diagnostic procedure called colonoscopy is done. The instrument used is similar to the sigmoidoscope but has a much longer flexible tube that enables the physician to examine the entire colon. If any polyps or other suspicious areas are observed, a small tool can be inserted through the scope to take a biopsy sample.

Diagnostic studies may also include a barium enema, in which a chalky substance is inserted into the colon to make it more visible on X-rays. A CT scan or MRI may be ordered if a suspicious growth is found.

Medical Treatments

Small, benign polyps that are causing no problems do not necessarily require surgery, although most doctors will

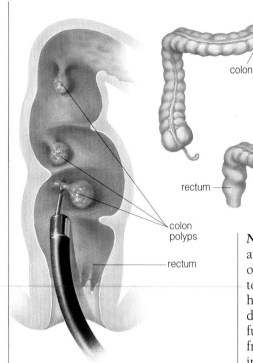

Polyps may develop anywhere along the length of the colon (above right), but they appear most frequently in or just above the rectum. Most of these growths can be removed with the aid of a colonoscope or sigmoidoscope (above).

recommend their removal because they may harbor cancer cells. Small polyps can be taken out usually with the sigmoidoscope or colonoscope, a procedure called polypectomy. Larger polyps may be removed by laparotomy, which involves making a small incision in the abdomen and inserting a special surgical scope through which a section of the colon can be removed.

When confronted with a case of familial polyposis, many doctors recommend a colectomy, or removal of the entire colon, because these polyps almost always develop into a particularly lethal form of colon cancer. This surgery is major and often requires the

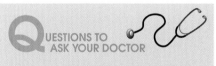

creation of a stoma, an opening in the abdomen to provide a new exit for fecal waste. However, a portion of the small intestine is sometimes used to take over normal bowel function (see Medical Treatments, opposite page, and page 248).

Alternative Therapies

There is no substitute for polyp removal, but alternative therapies may help to reduce their recurrences.

Nutrition Therapy. Many physicians and naturopaths believe that the development of colon polyps that may lead to colon cancer can be limited by a high-fiber, low-fat, and low-protein diet, which promotes healthy bowel function. Such a diet emphasizes fresh fruits and vegetables and whole grains instead of meat, and promotes rapid movement of food through the digestive system, thus reducing the growth of bacteria and chemical compounds that may enhance polyp or cancer growth. Of particular value may be oat and rice bran, as well as foods high in vitamins A and C. Some nutritionists also recommend supplements, particularly of beta carotene (precursor to vitamin A), calcium, and vitamins C and E.

Self-Treatment

Colon polyps cannot be self-treated, but you should pay attention to any changes in your bowel functions that might indicate a problem. In addition, the American Cancer Society (ACS) recommends that everyone over 40 have an annual stool test for hidden blood. This can be done at home, using a kit available at pharmacies or from some ACS chapters. A small sample of stool is smeared on a guaiac-impregnated card to detect enzymes found in hemoglobin, a major component of blood. Unfortunately, dietary factors, such as the recent consumption of red meat or iron supplements, often produce false test results, so be sure to follow instructions carefully. If the test is positive, a colonoscopy should be performed.

Other Causes of Rectal Bleeding

Many conditions produce rectal bleeding, including infection, hemorrhoids, colon cancer, Crohn's disease, diverticulosis, ulcerative colitis, and certain intestinal parasites.

Colon/Rectal Cancer

(Colorectal carcinoma)

Cancer of the colon and rectum is the second most common malignancy in the United States (surpassed only by lung cancer), with about 138,000 new cases and 55,000 deaths a year. Even so, death rates from colorectal cancer have fallen by 29 percent in men and 7 percent in women over the past 30 years, and recent progress promises further reductions in mortality.

It is now known that a single gene is responsible for about one in every seven colon cancers. Other risk factors include the presence of colon polyps, inflammatory bowel disease, and certain other kinds of cancer, especially of the breast, uterus, and ovaries.

Diagnostic Studies and Procedures

Since the gene responsible for colon cancer was found by scientists, it has been possible to identify many high-risk people for special preventive care. But procedures are still too complicated and expensive for widespread use. This situation is expected to change soon; researchers are working on a blood test that will identify people with the trait.

In the meantime, the first step in detecting colon or rectal cancer remains an analysis of a stool sample for hidden, or occult, blood, which can come from a polyp or tumor. (See Self-Treatment, on next page.)

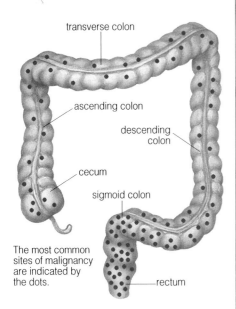

The most common sites of malignancy are indicated by the dots.

Colon cancer most often develops in the rectum and the sigmoid segment.

Two other screening tests are a digital rectal examination, which should be done every year after age 40, and sigmoidoscopy, in which the rectum and lower sigmoid part of the colon are examined with an optical viewing tube. This test, which should be done every three to five years after age 50, is mildly uncomfortable but not truly painful, especially if a flexible rather than rigid instrument is used; most doctors now use flexible versions of the sigmoidoscope.

If colon or rectal cancer is suspected on the basis of these routine screenings, other laboratory tests and diagnostic procedures will be performed. These usually start with a lower GI series, X-rays in which the intestines are viewed after an infusion of barium, a chalky contrast material. These X-rays will be followed by colonoscopy, a more extensive version of sigmoidoscopy that involves the entire colon. At this time, samples of tissue can be collected for microscopic examination, and small growths can be removed.

If cancer is detected, further studies such as MRI and CT and bone scans may be ordered to see if the disease has spread to other parts of the body.

Medical Treatments

Surgery remains the primary treatment for colorectal cancer. In most cases, the operation involves removal of the cancerous segment plus margins of healthy intestine on both ends. The two ends are then stitched together, allowing normal bowel function after healing. The operation may be followed by a course of chemotherapy and/or radiation treatments, especially if the disease is in an advanced stage.

If cancer involves the lower rectum or anus, an artificial opening, or stoma, may have to be created in the abdominal wall to allow fecal waste to exit the body into a special collection bag.

A colectomy—surgery to remove the entire colon—is often recommended for patients who have familial polyposis, because these polyps inevitably develop into an especially lethal form of cancer. Similarly, a colectomy may be necessary for patients with severe inflammatory bowel disease (page 248).

In many such cases, a stoma can be avoided with a procedure known as ileoanal anastomosis. In this operation, the rectum is left in place and a segment of small intestine is attached to

the rectum just above the anal opening, to assume bowel function.

Even when the entire colon and rectum must be removed, it is sometimes possible to avoid wearing and caring for an external pouch by having a continent ileostomy. This approach involves making an internal collection pouch from the lowermost segment of the small intestine, and creating an opening on the lower abdomen. The pouch can be emptied through a nipple valve with a small tube.

COLON/RECTAL CANCER (CONTINUED)

Alternative Therapies

Any form of cancer or precancerous condition needs prompt medical treatment, although alternative therapies can play a supportive role.

Acupuncture. Both acupuncture and acupressure are accepted as useful means of controlling cancer pain.

Nutrition Therapy. No responsible practitioner claims that diet can cure cancer. However, the risk of cancer may be reduced by adhering to a diet that is low in animal fat and high in fiber. Dietary fiber helps prevent constipation by producing soft, bulky stools that pass easily and quickly through the colon. Some studies indicate that this process may also protect against colon cancer. However, if you add more fiber to your diet, do so gradually. A sudden increase may lead to digestive problems.

Recent research suggests that vitamins A, C, and E, as well as calcium, may lower the risk of developing colon cancer, but you should consult a doctor before taking any high-dose supplements, especially if you are undergoing therapy for cancer. In particular, you should avoid taking iron pills, unless they've been prescribed to meet a specific need, because excessive iron is thought to hinder the immune system's defense against cancer.

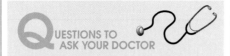

QUESTIONS TO ASK YOUR DOCTOR

▶ Is the new diagnostic test for people with a family history of colorectal cancer available yet?
▶ Am I likely to need a stoma to eliminate wastes? If so, will it be permanent? Where will it be and how does it work?
▶ Will I have radiation therapy or chemotherapy after surgery? If so, for how long will these treatments go on?

Yoga and Meditation. These and other relaxation therapies such as visualization and biofeedback can help with reducing the stress, handling the emotions, and managing the pain of cancer.

Self-Treatment

As in all types of cancers, the goal of self-treatment is to maintain a healthful nutritional status and to cooperate as much as possible with medical therapists. The National Cancer Institute recommends the following guidelines to prevent colon cancer:
▶ Eat fresh or dried fruits for desserts and snacks.
▶ Make beans, lentils, peas, and other legumes a regular part of your diet by including them in soups, stews, casseroles, and salads.

▶ Eat cereals and breads that are made with whole-grain flours.
▶ Leave the skins on potatoes, fruits, and vegetables to increase fiber intake. Similarly, use brown rice, cracked wheat, and buckwheat instead of white rice and refined grains.
▶ Consider low-dose aspirin therapy; recent studies indicate that as little as one pill every other day can significantly reduce an individual's risk of developing colon cancer.

During cancer treatment, have frequent small meals that emphasize nutrient-rich foods. Following surgery, a clinical dietitian can help plan menus that minimize demands on the colon until healing is complete.

If a stoma is necessary, an ostomy therapist will provide instruction in its use (see box, page 141). Joining an ostomy support group such as those affiliated with the American Cancer Society can be helpful. Ostomy patients find they can lead relatively normal lives, including a return to work and resumption of sexual relations, once they have mastered caring for a stoma.

Other Causes of Blood in the Stool

The presence of blood in the stool is not necessarily an indication of cancer. A positive test result is often due to hemorrhoids, ulcers, polyps, diverticulosis, or other noncancerous conditions.

A CASE IN POINT

Margaret Ellis's doctor describes her as a classic colon cancer patient: She had a family history of the disease, as well as a past history of breast and uterine cancers, putting her in a high-risk category. Then blood in her stool alerted her to have colonoscopy, during which two small malignant growths were found in her lower (sigmoid) colon.

"Like most of my patients, Margaret was terrified that she would end up with a colostomy and a stoma," her surgeon recounts. Ellis's fears were bolstered by the fact that her father had had a stoma, and despite her doctor's reassurances that it was highly unlikely she would follow suit, she remained unconvinced.

Two days before her scheduled operation, Ellis was sent for bone scans and an abdominal MRI study to search for signs of possible spread to either the liver or skeleton—two common sites of the

metastases of colon cancer. The MRI showed a small, indistinct spot on her liver—a cause of concern to her surgeon.

On the morning of her operation, Ellis was given a sedative to ease her anxiety. When she woke up several hours later, her first question was: "Do I have a pouch?" Happily, the recovery room nurse assured her that she did not.

Later that day, her surgeon filled in more of the details. The cancer was found to be confined to the inner wall of the colon—a good sign. The suspected liver spot had turned out to be nothing. The rest of her colon was healthy, and yes, she would resume normal bowel function within a week or so!

With her spirits buoyed by so much good news, Ellis set about to make as fast a recovery as possible. Within two days, she was walking up and down the hospital corridors, and complaining to her

husband about her liquid diet. By the end of the first week, her colon had recovered enough to begin the introduction of solid foods.

Nine days after her operation, Ellis was sent home to recuperate. All seemed to be going well until five weeks later when she developed severe abdominal pain. Her doctor told her to come immediately to the emergency room, where he quickly determined that she had an obstructed colon at the surgical site—a complication that required an immediate operation.

"This sometimes happens when scars and adhesions form," the doctor explained afterwards. Ellis took the setback in stride, and two weeks later, she was again at home, able to eat a regular diet and enjoy normal bowel function. Colonoscopy performed six months later showed that the colon was fully healed with no further adhesions.

Common Cold

(Acute coryza; upper respiratory infection)
The common cold is our most ubiquitous illness. On average, adults have two to four colds a year, and some children have 8 to 12. People who work in schools or health care settings, or who have small children, are more likely to catch multiple colds each year.

Symptoms may vary, but the typical cold starts with a sore throat, sneezing, nasal congestion, and a runny nose, frequently followed by a cough that can linger for a week to 10 days.

More than 200 different viruses can cause cold symptoms, but the most common are in the rhinovirus family and are highly contagious. They are often transmitted through the air when someone who has a cold expels them by sneezing or coughing and someone else inhales them. They can also travel from one person to another by direct contact with fingers, tissues, or other objects that can harbor a virus.

Even though so many different viruses are involved, they all produce similar symptoms, which is why all are classified as a single illness.

Colds can occur at any time of the year, but are most common in the late fall, winter, and early spring.

Diagnostic Studies and Procedures
Diagnosis is usually based on the presence of characteristic symptoms. In some cases, a laboratory throat culture may be ordered to rule out strep throat and other bacterial infections.

Medical Treatments
There are no cures for the common cold, and prescription drugs are no more effective than those you can purchase over the counter. A doctor's care is usually not necessary unless complications develop, or you have a chronic disease such as asthma, emphysema, cystic fibrosis, or diabetes that can be made worse by a cold.

The most common complication is a secondary bacterial infection of the ears, throat, sinuses, or lungs. If this should occur, antibiotics may be necessary. Generally, you should see a doctor if symptoms do not improve in 7 to 10 days. Go sooner if your breathing is difficult or painful or you have a persistent fever and chills, an earache, a severe headache, enlarged and tender lymph nodes in the neck, or other severe or unusual symptoms.

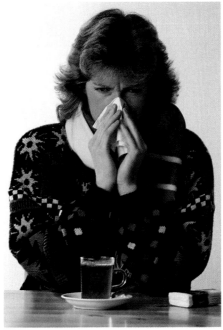

Hot, steamy liquids can decrease congestion, but nothing can cure a cold, except time to allow the body to rid itself of the virus.

Alternative Therapies
There are numerous alternative and folk remedies to alleviate cold symptoms.
Aromatherapy. Massaging the face with diluted eucalyptus oil can ease nasal congestion. Adding a few drops of pine or eucalyptus oil to a tub of hot water and soaking in it can help alleviate chest congestion and muscle aches.
Herbal Medicine. Teas or capsules of echinacea, ginger, horehound, lungwort, and mullein are recommended for general cold symptoms. Gargling with fenugreek tea or sucking lozenges of slippery elm bark may help alleviate a sore throat.

Cayenne tea, or foods flavored with it, stops chills and helps to clear sinuses and lung congestion, as does munching a clove of fresh garlic.

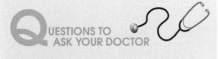

QUESTIONS TO ASK YOUR DOCTOR

▶ Do infants or young children require any special precautions or care when they have colds?
▶ Does smoking or exposure to second-hand smoke increase one's susceptibility to colds?
▶ What precautions should a person with a chronic lung disorder such as asthma or emphysema take during a cold?

Homeopathy. The specific remedy is determined by the type of cold. For example, aconite or belladonna is recommended during the early stage of a cold that comes on suddenly after a chill. Allium cepa, or raw onion, is said to counter colds that produce an irritating nasal discharge, while euphrasia is advised for those with a nonirritating nasal discharge and runny eyes. Arsenicum is the preferred remedy for colds with coughs; bryonia and phosphorus are also recommended.
Hydrotherapy. Hot baths or alternating warm and cool showers help alleviate general achiness. Soaking the feet in hot water is thought to relieve congestion and promote sleep.
Naturopathy and Nutrition Therapy. Hot, steamy liquids such as chicken soup help to thin mucus and clear congestion. In fact, medical studies have confirmed that chicken soup really does ease cold symptoms.

More controversial are high doses of vitamin C. Firm scientific proof is lacking, yet millions of people insist that two to six grams of vitamin C each day has helped prevent colds and shorten the course of those that do develop. (A word of caution: If high doses cause diarrhea, reduce the amount. Also, do not take high-dose vitamin C if you have kidney or bladder problems.)
Yoga. Deep breathing techniques can promote rest and relaxation, which aid healing, and counter nasal congestion.

Self-Treatment
Most colds run their course in seven days regardless of what you do. In the meantime, get plenty of rest and drink extra fluids to thin mucus. A cool-mist humidifier to increase air moisture can relieve nasal symptoms.

Exposure to irritants such as cigarette smoke may prolong cold symptoms. Abstain from smoking at the first sign of a cold, and stay away from smoky or otherwise polluted environments.

If you take cold medications, look for those with ingredients to treat your particular symptoms instead of broad-spectrum combinations to combat 10 or 12 complaints. Remember, ingredients such as antihistamines and decongestants increase the risk of drowsiness and other unwanted side effects.

Other Causes of Cold Symptoms
Many of the symptoms of a cold also accompany the flu, bronchitis, pneumonia, mononucleosis, and allergies.

Conjunctivitis

(Pink eye)

Conjunctivitis is an inflammation of the conjunctiva, the thin membranes that line the inner surface of the eyelid and cover part of the eyeball. It is commonly known as pink eye, because the most obvious symptom is reddening of the affected eye. In addition, the eye usually feels gritty and has a runny discharge. During sleep, the discharge may make the eyelids stick together. Some people also experience intense itching or sensitivity to bright light.

The most common cause of conjunctivitis is a viral infection; occasionally it is due to a bacterium. In rare cases, a sexually transmitted disease such as gonorrhea or chlamydia can be responsible for the inflammation. Genital herpes, contracted from an infected mother during birth, can cause a severe type of conjunctivitis in a newborn. Other possible causes include chemical irritation, air pollution, the sun's ultraviolet rays, exposure to intense light, and an allergic reaction to cosmetics, pollen, or other substances.

A cold or a sore throat may accompany viral conjunctivitis, while middle ear infections are often present with the bacterial form, especially in children.

Diagnostic Studies and Procedures

The patient's own observation of the symptoms, plus a medical history and physical examination by an eye specialist, are the mainstays of diagnosis. In some cases, however, a laboratory culture of the eye discharge may be required to determine if the cause is a virus or a bacterium.

Medical Treatments

Simple viral conjunctivitis almost always clears up on its own in about a week, but since it is sometimes impossible to distinguish from the bacterial form, the doctor will probably prescribe antibiotic eye drops or ointment.

If a herpes virus is involved, antiviral eyedrops or medication will be used. Steroid eye drops, prescribed to treat iritis and certain other eye inflammations, should not be used during a herpes infection because they can cause the infection to spread to the cornea, resulting in permanent eye damage.

Allergic conjunctivitis usually clears up when the source of the allergen is removed. In some cases, prescription antihistamines may be needed.

Alternative Therapies

When using an alternative therapy for self-treatment of the eyes, make sure that any applied substance is sterile.

Herbal Medicine. Herbalists recommend washing the eyes twice a day with weak chamomile tea that is made with boiled water and allowed to cool.

Homeopathy. Belladonna, a natural source of atropine, is sometimes used to treat red, teary eyes in the initial stages of conjunctivitis. For light sensitivity and burning sensations, homeopaths recommend eyebright, an herbal remedy. However, ophthalmologists warn that this herb, which is also known as deadly nightshade, is highly toxic, and should be used only under medical supervision.

Hydrotherapy. Warm water soaks are often effective in relieving symptoms and softening and dissolving crusts on the lashes. Use a disposable gauze pad

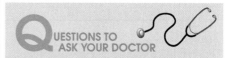

QUESTIONS TO ASK YOUR DOCTOR

▶ How can I tell if my red eyes are due to an allergic reaction? Should I see an allergy specialist?
▶ Can I pick up conjunctivitis by swimming in a public pool? If so, will eye goggles provide adequate protection?

on each eye, wetting it thoroughly with warm, sterile water. To promote healing, add 1 teaspoon of salt to 1 cup of boiled water, and use this solution to saturate the compresses.

Naturopathy. Practitioners make up a poultice of grated apple or grated raw red-skinned potato which they place over the (closed) eye once a day for about half an hour. This is said to reduce eyelid swelling and clear up simple conjunctivitis within two or three days. They may also advocate high doses of vitamin C.

Self-Treatment

Conjunctivitis is highly contagious and is usually transmitted by finger contact. To avoid spreading it or reinfecting yourself, wash your hands often with an antiseptic soap, and use disposable paper towels rather than a cloth towel. Avoid touching your eyes; if you have a discharge, you can use a disposable tissue to gently wipe it away. Do not share washcloths, towels, and other such items, and make sure to launder all bath linens in hot water, with bleach added as a disinfectant.

Discard old eye makeup, and avoid using replacements until the infection is cleared up. Try hypoallergenic brands, if makeup is suspected of causing allergic conjunctivitis. Never share eye makeup with others.

Most conjunctivitis that is environmentally caused can be prevented by taking common-sense precautions. Always use a protective face mask when welding, and wear sunglasses that screen out ultraviolet rays when outdoors in bright sunlight.

Other Causes of Red Eyes

Eye redness and irritation may be caused by a sty, an infected hair follicle on the eyelid. An eyelid disorder called entropion, in which a portion of the eyelid turns inward, causes eye pain and redness. A blocked tear duct or a lack of tears also causes red eyes.

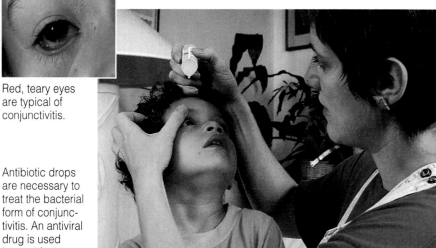

Red, teary eyes are typical of conjunctivitis.

Antibiotic drops are necessary to treat the bacterial form of conjunctivitis. An antiviral drug is used instead for herpes eye infections.

Constipation

Constipation is a condition marked by infrequent bowel movements of hard feces that are difficult to pass. Straining, rectal bleeding, and a sensation of fullness are common.

In some cases, the constipation alternates with diarrhea and it may be accompanied by abdominal cramps, bloating, and gassiness. Chronic constipation often leads to hemorrhoids (page 225) and other rectal problems.

Almost everyone experiences periodic bouts of constipation. However, some people mistakenly correlate the condition with a failure to have a daily bowel movement. In reality, colon function varies considerably, and bowel movements as often as three times a day and as infrequently as twice a week fall within the normal range, so long as the stools are easy to pass.

Most constipation is due to insufficient fiber in the diet (25 to 30 grams per day are recommended) and inadequate intake of fluid. Aging, a sedentary lifestyle, depression, emotional stress, the side effects of certain drugs, and overuse of laxatives and enemas can also be responsible. Occasionally, constipation is a symptom of a serious underlying disorder such as colon cancer or a digestive disease.

Diagnostic Studies and Procedures
Constipation is not usually considered significant medically, unless there is a major change in bowel habits that persists for more than one week. In such cases, a doctor will ask about recent dietary changes, drug use, and other possible contributing factors, and then perform a physical examination.

Laboratory tests of blood and stool samples may be ordered; additional diagnostic tests will depend upon results from these initial procedures. For example, a direct examination of the colon with a sigmoidoscope or a colonoscope—a thin, flexible tube with magnifying and lighting devices—will be ordered if a colon tumor or other disorder is suspected.

Medical Treatments
Medical treatment is not necessary for simple constipation. In some cases, a short course of a fiber-based stool softener may be recommended, but in general, the use of laxatives and enemas is discouraged because they can disrupt normal bowel function.

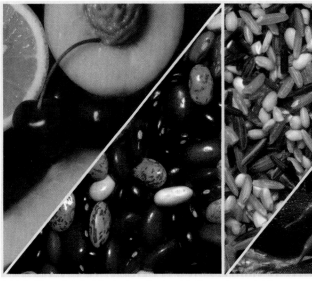

A high-fiber diet that includes plenty of fruits and vegetables, as well as whole grains and dried beans, peas, and other legumes, can prevent constipation.

If constipation is due to a medication such as codeine or an antidepressant, an alternative drug may be prescribed. In cases of severe obstruction, surgery may be necessary, but this is rare.

Alternative Therapies
Eliminating constipation is a major aspect of many alternative therapies, which include:
Ayurveda. Enemas, herbal emetics, and purgatives are central to panchakarma therapy, the ayurveda program of five cleansings designed to restore the body's natural balance.
Herbal Medicine. A number of herbs have a laxative effect, including cascara sagrada, chicory, dandelion, flaxseed, elderberry, goldenrod, licorice, and psyllium seed. Castor oil is another long-recommended remedy. Though it is not toxic (like other parts of the castor bean), it sometimes causes nausea and vomiting and should be used in small amounts, if at all.
Nutrition Therapy. The vast majority of constipation cases can be treated by increasing the amount of fiber in the

diet. One simple remedy is to soak six to eight dried figs or prunes in a glass of water overnight, and drink the water and eat the fruit in the morning.

Nutritionists recommend eating fresh fruits, vegetables, and whole-grain products at every meal and as snacks. Raisins and other dried fruits, brown rice, broccoli, beans, popcorn, and whole-wheat or bran cereals, breads, and crackers are examples of high-fiber foods. Increase fiber intake gradually to avoid bloating, abdominal cramps, and gassiness. Coffee and tea also act as laxatives for some people.

Self-Treatment
Most constipation can be eliminated by adopting a high-fiber diet, drinking 8 to 10 glasses of fluid each day, and establishing a regular exercise program.

When you first get up in the morning, drink a glass of warm water with a teaspoon of lemon juice or blackstrap molasses stirred in. This tonic, followed by food entering an empty stomach, helps to stimulate muscle contractions and push residue out of the bowel.

Set aside a specific time each day to devote at least 10 minutes to an unhurried attempt at a bowel movement. If possible, try to do this about an hour after eating breakfast.

Other Causes of Constipation
An underactive thyroid, or hypothyroidism, can cause constipation. Chronic constipation and recurrent pain in the lower abdomen could be a sign of diverticular disease, irritable bowel syndrome, or intestinal cancer.

QUESTIONS TO ASK YOUR DOCTOR

▶ Do any of the medications I take produce constipation as a side effect? If so, what can I do to counteract or manage this problem?
▶ What tests are indicated if there is blood in the stool?

Corns and Calluses

(Heloma; tyloma)
Corns are small, round mounds of firm, dead skin that usually form over bony areas of the toes. Calluses are thickened areas that most often develop on the balls and heels of the feet and on the hands. Both are caused by friction or pressure against the skin, commonly the result of wearing shoes or socks that do not fit properly or engaging in work or sports activities that involve

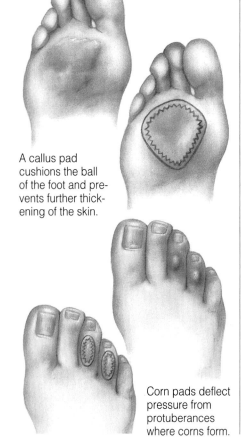

Calluses most commonly form on the balls of the feet, and on the heels as well.

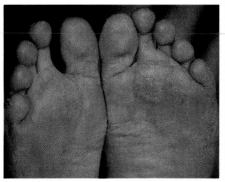

A callus pad cushions the ball of the foot and prevents further thickening of the skin.

Corn pads deflect pressure from protuberances where corns form.

constant rubbing and pressure. In some cases, they are caused by arthritis or deformities in the structure of bones.

Hard corns form over bony protuberances; those between the toes are soft corns. Most corns are yellow, but they may become red when irritated and inflamed. They have a hard, waxy core that forms in the epidermis, or outer layer of the skin, and then bores down into underlying tissue and nerves in the dermis. They cause extreme pain when subjected to pressure.

Calluses vary in size and shape. They are generally painless, but some grow so thick that the skin becomes inflexible and cracks, which can cause discomfort. People with diabetes or reduced circulation may develop a potentially serious infection under a callus.

Diagnostic Studies and Procedures
Corns and calluses are easily diagnosed by sight. To pinpoint the cause, a doctor or podiatrist (foot specialist) will ask about routine recreation and work activities and inspect footwear.

Medical Treatments
In most cases, a doctor's care is not required for these conditions, unless they are severe and persistent or if they become infected and require antibiotics. If they are troublesome, a podiatrist commonly will cut away thickened tissue after injecting a local anesthetic.

Alternative Therapies
Folk remedies abound for treating corns; some are helpful if used in addition to standard self-care methods.

Rubbing castor oil on a corn twice a day is recommended as a way to make it gradually peel off.

Placing a fresh lemon peel on a corn at night, with the inside of the peel against the corn, is said to make the corn disappear within a few days. A strip of fresh pineapple can be used in the same way. The enzymes and acids in these fruits act on the corn.

Taping a moist teabag on the corn for half an hour every day is also said to remove a corn within a week or two.

Poulticing is another popular remedy. One poultice mixture consists of a crumbled piece of bread soaked in ¼ cup of vinegar for half an hour. This is then wrapped in gauze, squeezed to remove excess fluid, taped over the corn, and left in place overnight. Most corns will peel off the next morning, but stubborn ones may require treatment for several nights in succession.

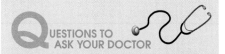

QUESTIONS TO ASK YOUR DOCTOR
► Can flat feet contribute to corns and calluses? If so, what can be done to prevent their formation?
► What precautions should I follow when using nonprescription corn removers?

Soaking the feet in oatmeal water often helps to ease the pain caused by corns. To prepare the soak, boil 2 cups of finely ground oatmeal with 5 quarts of water until the mixture cooks down to about 4 quarts. Strain it, put it in a large basin, and soak your feet in it for at least 20 minutes.

Self-Treatment
The best self-treatment for both corns and calluses is to remove the source of the pressure that has been causing them. This means discarding shoes that do not fit properly and padding the callused areas.

Nonprescription corn and callus pads reduce pressure. Medications, also available without a prescription, soften the skin layers and make them easier to remove, but some can damage skin and should be used with care.

You can usually peel a corn by first softening it and then rubbing it with a pumice stone. One way to soften stubborn corns is to soak the foot in Epsom salts and water for about 15 minutes and then apply a moisturizing cream. Or cover the corn with a moist gauze pad and wrap the foot in plastic for 15 minutes. Remove the plastic and rub the area with a pumice stone.

After peeling, apply a 5 or 10 percent salicylic ointment and cover it with an adhesive bandage. Repeat the treatment daily until the corn disappears.

A word of caution: If you have diabetes or any other medical condition that causes poor circulation, do not attempt self-treatment of calluses and corns. Some methods can increase the risk of infections and other complications. Instead, see a doctor or a podiatrist for professional foot care.

Other Causes of Thickened Skin
Plantar warts, virus-caused benign growths that form on the soles, are sometimes confused with calluses. Morton's neuroma, a growth on a plantar nerve, can cause pressure pain.

Coughs

(Tussis)

A cough is the forcible expulsion of air from the airways to rid them of any obstructions. It is often triggered by excessive fluids in the bronchial passages; but it may also be an attempt to get rid of dust, pollen, and other pollutants in the lungs.

A fit of coughing may have been set off by food or fluid entering the windpipe. A regular intermittent cough could be a nervous tic or simply a manifestation of boredom.

Coughing of limited duration is associated with a cold (page 143), the flu (page 189), or bronchitis (page 114), while chronic coughing usually indicates an underlying condition such as asthma, an allergy, or a lung tumor. A chronic cough is also an inevitable consequence of smoking.

Diagnostic Studies and Procedures

In general, a doctor should be consulted about a nagging cough if:
▶ It is accompanied by chest pains, severe earache, or swollen neck glands.
▶ It lasts for more than three weeks.
▶ It is accompanied by a temperature above 102°F (39°C).
▶ It produces blood or a thick and yellowish-green sputum.
▶ It is accompanied by wheezing and a feeling of breathlessness.

In such circumstances, a doctor will ask about other symptoms, smoking and drinking habits, and occupation, and follow up with a physical examination and chest X-rays.

If a patient does not cough spontaneously, the doctor may try to induce a coughing spell. Any sputum will be examined and cultured for bacteria. Additional tests might include lung scans, pulmonary function tests, and bronchoscopy, a viewing of bronchial passages through special devices.

Medical Treatments

Treatment of any cough depends on the underlying condition. Those associated with colds or flu can be managed with self-care. If coughing interferes with sleep, a suppressant containing codeine may be prescribed for nighttime use.

Alternative Therapies

Aromatherapy. Inhaling the steam from a strong tea made with 1 tablespoon of dried thyme, eucalyptus, chamomile, or peppermint leaves and 1 cup of boiling water helps to ease congestion.

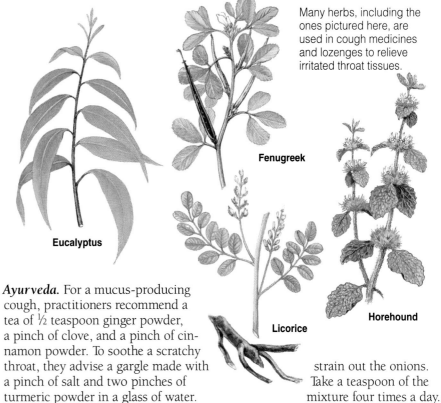

Many herbs, including the ones pictured here, are used in cough medicines and lozenges to relieve irritated throat tissues.

Fenugreek

Eucalyptus

Licorice

Horehound

Ayurveda. For a mucus-producing cough, practitioners recommend a tea of ½ teaspoon ginger powder, a pinch of clove, and a pinch of cinnamon powder. To soothe a scratchy throat, they advise a gargle made with a pinch of salt and two pinches of turmeric powder in a glass of water.

Herbal Medicine. Eucalyptus, horehound, wild cherry, and licorice are among the many herbal remedies that have been incorporated into standard cough medicines and lozenges to soothe a sore, scratchy throat.

Herbalists generally discourage using substances that suppress coughing; for a productive cough, they suggest taking an expectorant such as fenugreek tea, because it thins the secretions and makes them easier to expel. Mullein tea is recommended for a dry, hacking cough; it soothes irritated mucous membranes that line the airways.

Naturopathy. An onion-honey mixture is a time-honored cough remedy. To prepare it, slice an onion into a deep bowl, cover the slices with honey, let the mixture steep overnight, and then

strain out the onions. Take a teaspoon of the mixture four times a day.

Relaxation Therapies. Coughing produced by stress or by a nervous tic can eventually be eliminated by practicing yoga breathing exercises and meditation.

Self-Treatment

The only cure for a smoker's cough is to break the tobacco habit. A cough from a mild respiratory infection will disappear as the body rids itself of the virus.

A doctor may advise a nonprescription expectorant to thin mucus and make it easier to cough up. Be aware, however, that many cough medicines contain ingredients that may interact with other drugs, especially those prescribed for high blood pressure, heart disease, and other chronic illnesses.

Other self-help measures include:
▶ Transform the bathroom into a home steamroom by closing the door, turning on the hot water in the shower, and inhaling the steamy air until the coughing stops.
▶ Drink plenty of hot liquids during the day and use a vaporizer at night.
▶ Suck on herbal or zinc lozenges to get rid of the tickle in your throat.

Other Causes of Coughs

Coughing is a symptom of allergies, asthma, chronic bronchitis, cystic fibrosis, emphysema, lung cancer, and occupational lung disorders. Coughs also occur in croup, laryngitis, pneumonia, pleurisy, and tuberculosis.

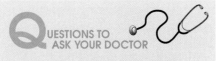

QUESTIONS TO ASK YOUR DOCTOR

▶ If I have bronchitis, will an antibiotic help stop a cough?
▶ How long does it take smoker's cough to disappear after giving up cigarettes?
▶ What tests are needed if a cough produces blood-streaked phlegm?
▶ Will any of the medications I'm taking interact with the ingredients in an over-the-counter cough preparation?

Cradle Cap

(Infantile seborrheic eczema)

Cradle cap is a common condition of infancy in which patches of greasy, yellow flakes and small, pimple-like bumps appear on the scalp and, less often, on eyebrows and lashes. Crusts also may develop behind the ears and on the face, neck, chest, buttocks, and other places where sebaceous glands are located. These glands, which produce sebum, a fatty wax-like skin lubricant, are at the heart of the problem.

Cradle cap is most likely to appear during the first few weeks of life, and it usually clears up by the sixth month.

The cause is unknown, but some dermatologists think that high levels of maternal hormones, which may be transmitted to the baby during the final weeks of pregnancy, trigger the production of excess sebum. This excess not only overstimulates the growth of new cells but also binds the discarded cells together into flakes and crusts.

Dermatologists do not believe that cradle cap is related to the adult form of dandruff, nor has it anything to do with infrequent bathing or any other aspect of hygiene or infant care. Contrary to some media reports, there is no evidence either that cradle cap is a sign of a nutritional deficiency.

Diagnostic Studies and Procedures

The yellow patches of cradle cap are clearly visible, and the condition is readily diagnosed during a regular

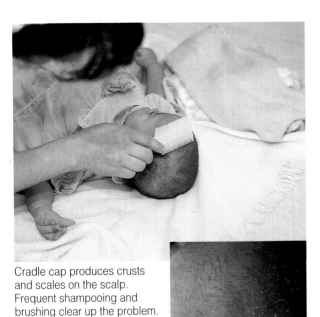

Cradle cap produces crusts and scales on the scalp. Frequent shampooing and brushing clear up the problem.

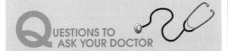
checkup. It is not unusual even for a doctor to make the diagnosis over the telephone, based on the mother's description of the baby's scalp.

Medical Treatments

If cradle cap is not cleared up with simple home care (see Self-Treatment), a doctor may advise the use of a non-prescription cream containing 0.5 percent hydrocortisone. (Although this product is available over the counter, it should not be used on a baby unless a doctor specifically recommends it.) For a severe or very stubborn case of cradle cap, a doctor may also recommend a stronger shampoo that is specially formulated to remove scaly crusts. (Strong shampoo, too, should be used only at the suggestion of a physician.)

In rare cases, a yeast infection may complicate cradle cap, particularly if the crusts and bumps are under the arms and in the neck creases as well as on the scalp. A superimposed yeast infection will make the affected skin bright red and cause severe itching. Should such an infection develop, a doctor will prescribe an antifungal cream.

Alternative Therapies

Aromatherapy. Massaging the baby's scalp with olive oil that contains a few drops of 2 percent sage essence will help loosen the crusts. The olive oil should be shampooed out after each treatment, however, to prevent an oily buildup. If the oil is permitted to build up, the condition may actually become worse.

Herbal Medicine. Herbalists recommend preparing a mixture as follows: Steep ¼ cup of dried nettles in 1 cup of boiling water. When

the solution cools, strain and add ¼ cup of cider vinegar. Before you massage the mixture all over the baby's scalp, try a small sample first to make sure that it doesn't cause any irritation. Be especially careful not to get any of it in the baby's eyes.

Self-Treatment

Because cradle cap is likely to get worse with sweating, the baby should be kept cool and dry. A healthy infant does not need to wear a hat outdoors except in cold weather, and the hat should be removed in a heated car, train, or bus.

When you try out a treatment, give it at least three days to work. Then, if you see no improvement, consider abandoning it for a different one.

You can shampoo the baby as often as once a day. While shampooing, you needn't be fearful about rubbing the fontanel, the soft spot that lies between the bones of the skull at the top of the head. Ordinary rubbing will not injure the underlying brain tissue.

Here are a few other home-care measures that should be helpful:
▶ When bathing the baby, lather the scalp lightly with an ordinary baby shampoo and brush the shampoo into the scalp with a soft hairbrush. Let it stay for a minute or so, and rinse off with warm water or wipe off gently with a washcloth.
▶ Massage baby oil, mineral oil, or petroleum jelly into the baby's scalp to loosen the flakes, and then shampoo. Rub in the lather with a soft brush, then rinse the scalp thoroughly with warm water. Repeat this treatment three or four times a week.
▶ Instead of bathing the baby with soap, consider trying one of the soapless products such as Lowilla cake or Moisturel soap. These are also suitable for use on the scalp.
▶ Gently comb away loose crusts with a baby comb. However, resist the temptation to remove crusts and scales with the tip of a fingernail. When the scales are ready to come off, they don't have to be picked at or peeled.

Other Causes of Crusting Skin

Eczema may produce skin flaking and crusts. Food allergies have also been linked to cradle cap; if the baby is breast-fed, the mother's allergies should also be considered. In some cases, ringworm or another fungal infection might be the cause of skin crusting and hair loss, especially on the scalp.

Crossed Eyes

(Strabismus)

Crossed eyes, or strabismus, involves a misalignment of the eyes. It is one of the most common eye problems in children, but it also occurs in adults (see Other Causes of Crossed Eyes).

Strabismus develops when the eye muscles fail to work together or to function in a parallel manner; one eye or both may turn or wander in or out, up or down. The condition can result from neurological problems, a tumor, or an injury, but most often it is due to imbalance of the eye muscles.

The deviation may be constant or come and go. Sometimes it is obvious from birth; in other cases it doesn't appear until later in a child or adult. Childhood strabismus is often associated with a "lazy eye," or amblyopia, in which just one eye assumes the task of relaying visual messages to the brain.

A newborn baby's eyes tend to wander, but by three or four months, an infant should be able to focus on small objects, and the eyes should be parallel. By six months, he should be able to focus on both distant and near objects. If crossed eyes or excessive squinting persists past four months, the baby should have an eye examination. Even if their eyes appear normal, all children should have them examined by a pediatrician by age six months.

Diagnostic Studies and Procedures

Even when crossed eyes are apparent, a doctor will perform basic vision tests. Adults and older children will be asked to read numbers or letters on a wall chart, and children who cannot read will be tested with a picture chart. In very young children, the doctor estimates the vision of each eye by observing how it follows a small toy or some other brightly colored object.

Next, the external eye muscles will be tested by examining how each eye moves. The doctor may hold a pencil or a flashlight in front of the eyes and ask the patient to focus on this object as it is moved in and out of the visual field. The angle of crossed eyes can be determined with special optical instruments. Drops are then put in the eyes to dilate the pupils for examination with an ophthalmoscope.

Additional tests may include blood and urine studies, X-rays, a CT scan, and other imaging studies.

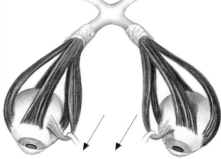

Normal eyes (above) function in a parallel way, both turning at precisely the same angle in unison.

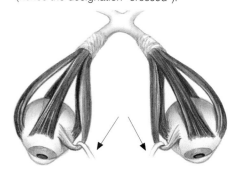

With crossed eyes (below), they move in different directions, at times facing away from each other, as shown, or toward each other (hence the designation "crossed").

Medical Treatments

If there is any underlying medical condition, it will be treated first. Glasses may also be prescribed to improve the wandering eye's ability to focus, and to redirect the line of sight to synchronize and straighten the eyes.

If amblyopia is present, an eye patch may be placed over the normal eye to force the weak eye to focus. Or, eye drops or ointment may be used to blur the vision in the normal eye.

If these approaches do not work, surgery may be performed to straighten the eye muscles. The type of operation varies according to the underlying cause of the problem. In the most common procedure, an eye surgeon makes a small incision in the covering of the eye to adjust the tension exerted by the outer muscles on one or both eyes.

Another operation, called resection surgery, can be done to shorten the muscles and improve alignment. This involves removing a section of muscle, reconnecting the ends, and sewing the muscle back into place.

Recession surgery is performed if a muscle needs to be lengthened. In this operation, the muscles are moved further back, and the incision is closed with absorbable sutures.

Alternative Therapies

Any alternative treatment should be cleared first with an ophthalmologist, who should assume the role of the primary physician in correcting a problem. *Orthoptics.* Eye exercises, or orthoptics, often have a place in treating crossed eyes. Orthoptists are eye-care professionals who undergo special training and are licensed; optometrists may also prescribe or teach orthoptics. Six or eight treatment sessions over the course of several months are usually involved; during this time, the patient learns special exercises to practice at home, and these are modified as needed during periodic evaluations.
Vision Training. Its practitioners seek to teach the eye and brain to work together through a series of exercises that strengthen eye muscles. They also believe that eye problems are often related to emotional stress, nutrition, and other lifestyle factors. The method usually requires more frequent visits to a practitioner than orthoptics, and treatment may continue for months or even years. Most eye-care professionals consider it of questionable value.

Self-Treatment

Exercises you do on your own should be designed by a qualified eye-care professional. Adults with crossed eyes often have double vision and wearing a patch over one eye may help correct this. However, patching should not be attempted without seeking the advice of a medical professional.

Other Causes of Crossed Eyes

Nerve damage can paralyze the eye muscles and result in crossed eyes. Diseases that can cause crossed eyes in adults include thyroid disorders, brain tumors, diabetes, stroke, multiple sclerosis, muscular dystrophy, myasthenia gravis, and temporal arteritis, in which the scalp arteries become inflamed.

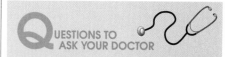

QUESTIONS TO ASK YOUR DOCTOR

▶ How often should a child have an eye examination?
▶ What happens if crossed eyes are not corrected?
▶ Can crossed eyes develop from working long hours at a computer terminal or reading in a dim light?

Croup

(Acute laryngotracheobronchitis)

Croup is an acute illness of early child-hood that affects the upper and lower respiratory passages. Caused by a virus, it frequently follows a cold or the flu. The disorder occurs in the late fall and winter as a rule, and generally lasts no more than a week.

Typically, croup is characterized by hoarseness, wheezing, a tight barking cough, and difficulty in breathing—all consequences of an infection of the lar-ynx and swelling of the vocal chords. A low-pitched, harsh, raspy noise, called stridor, occurs when air passes through the swollen windpipe and over the inflamed vocal cords. Coughing attacks range from mild to severe and tend to be worse at night. Prolonged coughing can continue for half an hour and may end with vomiting.

Diagnostic Studies and Procedures

Croup can usually be diagnosed over the telephone simply by describing the symptoms and cough. In a doctor's office, it is easily identified by listening to the child's breathing and coughing.

Medical Treatments

Medicines are not given for croup unless there is a secondary bacterial infection. In such a case, an antibiotic will be prescribed. Children who develop severe complications, such as threatened airway blockage or pneu-monia, require hospitalization. Inhaled epinephrine may be administered to reduce swelling of the air passage.

Alternative Therapies

Caring for a child with croup requires calmness to quell the anxiety of the youngster—a task that can be difficult if parents themselves are anxious. Relaxation techniques are useful in helping parents overcome their own alarm. Other approaches include:

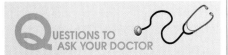

QUESTIONS TO ASK YOUR DOCTOR

▶ Should older children in the family avoid contact with a sibling who has developed croup?
▶ Should my child receive HIB vaccine to protect against croup caused by *Haemophilus influenzae* type B?
▶ Do infected tonsils increase a child's risk of developing croup?

IMPORTANT
Take the child to the nearest emergency room if:
▶ Coughing continues for more than an hour in moist air.
▶ Fever reaches 103°F (39.5°C).
▶ The child begins to turn blue, drool, have difficulty swallowing, or arch the neck back to breathe. These are signs of life-threatening epiglottitis.

Aromatherapy. Add a few drops of gin-ger extract to a warm bath to loosen mucus. After bathing, wrap the child in a heavy towel or light blanket, and put her to bed.

Herbal Medicine. Herbalists suggest drinking diluted echinacea extract, or gargling with fenugreek tea. Another remedy is a hot onion pack on the back or chest. To prepare one, wrap sliced onions with flannel or other cotton cloth and top with a heating pad or hot water bottle. Make sure that the heat source is not so hot as to cause a burn.

Self-Treatment

Croup is almost always treated at home by using a cool-mist humidifier or a steam vaporizer in the child's room around the clock. In fact, this practice during a cold or flu can often prevent the onset of croup. Do not add menthol or aromatic camphor oils to the vapor-izer because they can irritate already inflamed tissues.

During a coughing attack, increase the air moisture by transforming a bathroom into a steamroom. Turn on hot water in the shower and close the bathroom door until the room is dense with steam. Do this as soon as an attack begins, and stay in the bathroom with the child until the attack is over. A frightened child can be comforted by assurances that the steam will make breathing much easier.

Another approach is to pour hot water into a pitcher or bowl and have the child lean over it with a towel draped on the head to make a kind of tent. Never hold a child over hot steam coming from a kettle on the stove; this can result in serious scalding.

A child with croup can breathe more easily sitting up than lying down; use extra pillows or a bolster at night.

Reduce milk and milk products to a minimum during the illness, and offer large amounts of broth and other warm, clear fluids to loosen mucus

---

trapped in the airways. Apple juice and tea with honey and lemon are also helpful for loosening mucus.

Because crying can trigger an attack, even an older child will benefit from being held and cuddled. Use distrac-tions such as storytelling and singing. Also, a few minutes of fresh air can sometimes end an episode.

The effect of passive tobacco smoke can transform croup from a manageable illness into a medical emergency. There-fore, no one should be permitted to smoke indoors when a child has croup. If this rule is unenforceable, keep

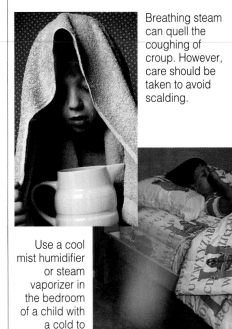

Breathing steam can quell the coughing of croup. However, care should be taken to avoid scalding.

Use a cool mist humidifier or steam vaporizer in the bedroom of a child with a cold to prevent the development of croup.

smoking confined to one designated room, keep the door closed, open the windows from time to time, and make this room off-limits to the child.

Other Causes of Croup-like Symptoms

Asthma can sometimes produce cough-ing and a choking sensation, as can tonsillitis and other respiratory infec-tions. In unusual cases, a foreign object lodged in a child's throat may create a barking cough and difficult breathing. This circumstance can be confirmed by an X-ray. Pertussis, or whooping cough, also causes severe, harsh bouts of coughing that often end in vomiting. These coughing attacks can occur periodically for several months.

Cystic Fibrosis

(CF; mucoviscidosis)

Cystic fibrosis, or CF, is an incurable genetic disease characterized by abnormalities of the exocrine and eccrine glands, which secrete sweat, mucus, digestive juices, and other substances. The abnormal glands produce large amounts of thick, sticky mucus that can clog airways, intestines, and other passageways. Progressive blockage of the bronchial tubes often leads to infection, respiratory failure, and death.

Intestinal blockage usually affects the pancreas, causing poor digestion and impaired absorption resulting in slow growth and undernutrition. The sweat glands are also affected, so that abnormal amounts of sodium, chloride, and potassium are excreted in perspiration.

In 1989, scientists identified the gene that causes the disease, which was a major breakthrough for developing future treatments. Cystic fibrosis develops only if a child inherits the CF gene from each parent. In the United States, it is most common among whites, affecting one baby in 2,000.

Diagnostic Studies and Procedures

Although cystic fibrosis is present at birth, symptoms may not appear right away; most cases are diagnosed by the time a child is three. Common symptoms include recurrent wheezing, a persistent cough that produces large amounts of mucus, repeated bouts of pneumonia, and frequent bowel movements of bulky, greasy, and foul-smelling stools. The child may fail to grow, despite having a healthy appetite.

Parents often notice that the baby's skin has a salty taste. A doctor may find small fleshy growths, or polyps, inside the nose and enlargement of the fingertips and toes. Diagnosis is confirmed by a test to measure the salt content in the child's sweat. In newborns, the immunoreactive trypsinogen test (IRT) is used instead.

Medical Treatments

Isolation of the cystic fibrosis gene has enabled scientists to develop a method for replacing the faulty gene. This treatment, first tried on a patient in April, 1993, involves introducing a harmless virus that has been altered to carry a normal gene that will replace the one causing the disease. Although this approach appears promising, much more study is needed.

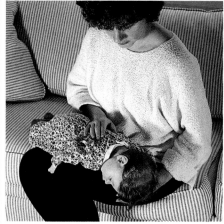

An integral part of self-care for cystic fibrosis is regular postural drainage, in which the child lies with the head and chest tilted downward and a parent or therapist taps or percusses the back to loosen mucus.

Routine care, coordinated by a specialist in pediatric pulmonary diseases, should begin as soon as the diagnosis is made. Treatments vary, depending on the organs involved and the severity of the disease. Digestive problems are controlled usually with pancreatic enzyme supplements, nutritional supplements, and dietary changes.

Treatment of lung problems is aimed at clearing the airways and preventing infection. Prophylactic antibiotics and other drugs, including inhaled medications, may be prescribed. As the disease progresses, oxygen support is often necessary. Bronchial washes may help unclog the airways.

As a last resort, a heart-lung transplant (the transplanting of heart and lungs as a unit) may be tried; if the patient's heart is undamaged, it can then be used as a donor organ for someone who needs only a heart.

Alternative Therapies

Alternative therapies play an important role in maintaining a patient's strength and warding off infection.

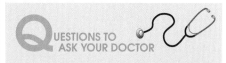

QUESTIONS TO ASK YOUR DOCTOR

▶ Is there a way to enroll in experimental trials of gene therapy for cystic fibrosis? If so, what are the risks of trying it?
▶ If I have one child with this disease, what are my chances of having another?
▶ How reliable are prenatal tests for detecting the disease?

Herbal Medicine. Echinacea, ginger, marsh mallow, and hyssop teas are recommended for thinning mucus to make it easier to cough up.

Naturopathy. Practitioners suggest high doses of vitamin C to strengthen the immune system, vitamins K and the B_6 complex to aid digestion, and pancreatin and other pancreatic enzymes to regulate metabolism. Be sure to check with the child's doctor before giving any nutritional supplement.

Nutrition Therapy. A child with cystic fibrosis usually needs more calories than a healthy one. Certain foods may have to be avoided if they cause intestinal cramps, diarrhea, or constipation. Extra salt may be needed to maintain the body's proper balance of fluids and chemicals, especially during warm weather or a fever.

Acidophilus pills may help restore normal intestinal bacteria when antibiotics are being taken, thereby preventing diarrhea. A clinical dietitian experienced in dealing with cystic fibrosis can provide expert guidance on structuring an appropriate diet.

Physical Therapy. A physical therapist can design an activity program that will help a child with CF maintain strength and fitness without overtaxing his level of endurance.

Self-Treatment

Parents administer day-to-day care, which includes regular bronchial drainage or postural drainage (see illustration, above). As soon as a child is old enough, she should be taught how to perform the routine herself.

Coughing is useful because it helps loosen mucus and remove it from air passages; therefore, cough suppressants should not be taken.

Although it is important to avoid unnecessary contact with people who have a contagious illness, children with CF should be encouraged to lead normal lives. Parents might want to consider joining a CF support group, so they can share insights with other parents who are facing similar problems.

Other Causes of CF Symptoms

The main symptoms of cystic fibrosis are seen in many other conditions. Coughing, wheezing, and spitting up mucus are common to asthma, bronchitis, pneumonia, and other diseases of the lung. Similar digestive problems may be caused by celiac disease and other malabsorption disorders.

Cystitis

(Bladder infections; urinary tract infections; UTI)

Cystitis is an inflammation of the urinary bladder, most often due to a bacterial infection. The irritation of cystitis prompts the bladder nerves to signal a sudden and urgent need to urinate, even though the bladder may be relatively empty. Urination is accompanied often by pain or a burning sensation, and if the infection is severe, only small amounts of urine may pass, usually containing blood. Other possible symptoms include a low-grade fever and pain in the pubic area.

Most bladder infections are caused by *Escherichia coli*, bacteria that normally live in the intestines. Chlamydia, a sexually transmitted organism, also causes cystitis. These can invade the bladder through the urethra—the tube through which urine leaves the body.

Women are especially vulnerable to cystitis because the female urethra is short—about two inches compared with 8 to 10 inches in men—and is located near the vagina and anus where bacteria can flourish. Also, sexual activity can cause bacteria to be introduced into the urethra, resulting in "honeymoon cystitis." An oversized diaphragm, which may apply pressure to the urethra and bladder, also promotes cystitis. Other contributing factors include the hormonal changes of menopause and allergic reactions to tampons, spermicides, and lubricants.

Diagnostic Studies and Procedures

Diagnosis is based on a physical examination and analysis of a urine sample to identify the causative bacteria. A nonprescription home kit, available at most pharmacies, contains urine dipsticks that can confirm a bacterial

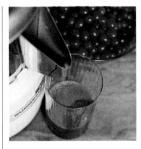

Cranberry juice can help prevent recurrent cystitis, because it acidifies the urine, creating an environment that is inhospitable for bacteria.

infection. A doctor's visit will still be necessary, however, because home tests do not indicate the causative organism.

Medical Treatments

Ideally, therapy should not begin until after a culture has identified the organism, enabling a doctor to prescribe the best antibiotic to eradicate it. In some cases, however, a broad spectrum antibiotic such as sulfamethoxazole with trimethoprim (Bactrim or Septra) or nitrofurantoin (Macrodantin and others) may be prescribed to quickly alleviate symptoms while awaiting results of the urine studies; lab tests may be repeated several days later to make sure that the drug has worked.

The duration of antibiotic therapy varies. Some doctors prescribe a single large dose; others favor a 7- to 10-day course, or an even longer regimen for recurring infections. It is important to take the full course, even though symptoms may disappear within a few days. Some doctors recommend that women who have recurrent cystitis take a low-dose antibiotic on a continuing basis as a preventive measure.

Urinary pain usually abates within a few hours of starting antibiotic therapy. If not, a bladder analgesic such as phenazopyridine (Pyridium) may help.

Alternative Therapies

Alternative therapies will not cure the infection but may relieve symptoms.

Acupuncture. Needles along the bladder, liver, kidney, and spleen meridians are usually helpful in relieving the pain of cystitis.

Herbal Medicine. Alfalfa, which is reputed to be a natural diuretic, is often used to treat urinary tract infections.

Homeopathy. Either sarsaparilla or cantharis may be advocated for painful urination.

Hydrotherapy. Warm sitz baths can help soothe urinary burning sensations as well as ease pain.

Nutrition Therapy. Antibiotics that are prescribed to treat cystitis often kill beneficial bacteria as well, resulting in a vaginal yeast infection and diarrhea. Nutrition therapists advise taking acidophilus capsules three times a day or eating yogurt with active acidophilus cultures. Some also recommend drinking cranberry juice because it appears to contain a bacteria-killing compound; it also acidifies the urine. However, it may cause bladder irritation.

Self-Treatment

The following self-care measures can alleviate cystitis pain, hasten healing, and prevent recurrent infections:

▶ Drink at least 8 to 10 glasses of fluids daily to help flush out the bladder. However, avoid alcohol and caffeine, which cause bladder irritation.

▶ Women should urinate and then drink a full glass of water before sexual intercourse. Wait for an hour afterward and then urinate again; this allows the bladder to fill and wash out bacteria.

▶ Do not use vaginal deodorants or other potentially irritating substances.

▶ Wear cotton underwear and avoid tight garments to allow the genital area to remain dry. Avoid sitting around in a wet bathing suit.

▶ If you use a diaphragm, make sure you are fitted correctly or consider some other birth control method. Also, use sanitary pads instead of tampons.

▶ After a bowel movement, always wipe from front to back; this reduces the spread of bacteria from the rectum to the urethra.

Other Causes of Urinary Problems

Painful urination may be caused also by a bladder disorder called interstitial cystitis, by a sexually transmitted disease such as gonorrhea or, in men, by prostate enlargement. Blood in the urine may be triggered by a stone in the urinary tract, or cancer of the bladder, kidney, or prostate.

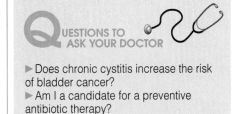

QUESTIONS TO ASK YOUR DOCTOR

▶ Does chronic cystitis increase the risk of bladder cancer?
▶ Am I a candidate for a preventive antibiotic therapy?

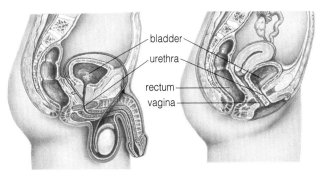

bladder
urethra
rectum
vagina

Cystitis, or bladder infection, is common in women because the urethra, vagina, and rectum are so close together that bacteria from the rectum and vagina can easily enter the urethra.

Dandruff

(Pityriasis simplex)

Dandruff is a form of seborrheic dermatitis, an inflammatory condition in which dead scalp cells flake off, leaving telltale signs on the shoulders and clothing. More severe cases also affect the skin around the nose, behind the ears, or in the armpits or genital area.

The flaking is thought to be caused by scalp cells that are aging too rapidly. Normally, dead skin cells are shed from the scalp during routine hair care. But when the normal growth pattern is altered, and excessive dead cells reach the scalp's surface simultaneously, they stick together and fall off in flakes. However, some researchers dispute this

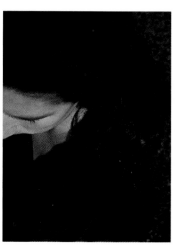
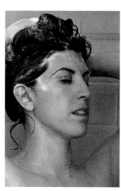

Rapid loss of scalp cells results in dandruff, which can be treated with special shampoos.

view and argue that a yeast called *Pityrosporum ovale* is responsible. Whatever the cause, dandruff does not lead to permanent hair loss or baldness.

Both dry and oily scalps develop dandruff. With an oily scalp, excessive fatty acids irritate the cells around the hair follicles, prompting an even more rapid cell turnover that leads to dandruff. In contrast, the flaking of a dry scalp is due to lack of moisture. Dandruff from a normal scalp is probably the result of poor hair care.

During periods of stress, fatigue, or illness, dandruff may increase. Hair coloring, waving, or straightening may also produce extra flaking.

Diagnostic Studies and Procedures

Dandruff is usually obvious and rarely requires a medical diagnosis. When it is persistent and does not respond to treatment, however, a doctor should rule out other skin disorders. If there is still doubt about the underlying cause, a biopsy may be taken from affected areas for laboratory study.

Medical Treatments

Ordinary dandruff does not need medical treatment, but severe cases may require a medicated shampoo. Some dermatologists prescribe an antifungal shampoo, such as ketoconazole (Nizoral). Although dandruff is not a fungal disease, fungi that normally live on the scalp can increase flaking.

Alternative Therapies

Aromatherapy. Practitioners recommend bathing the affected areas three times a week with a 2 percent essence of geranium in a distilled water base. Another remedy calls for massaging a 10 percent sage essence in an olive oil base into the affected areas, then waiting two hours before washing out the mixture. This procedure should be followed twice a week.

Herbal Medicine. Aloe vera has skin softening properties that can help alleviate dandruff. It is most effective when a freshly cut leaf is rubbed directly onto the affected area. Applying eucalyptus oil to the scalp is advocated by some herbalists.

Massage. Although this therapy cannot cure dandruff, it is a time-honored method for reducing the stress that may be an underlying cause. Reflexology, or foot massage, is also said to be effective.

Relaxation Therapies. All forms of meditation, including yoga, may help relieve a dandruff condition that is related to excessive stress. An increase in exercise may have a similar effect.

Self-Treatment

If your hair is oily, treat dandruff by brushing thoroughly and then washing with a shampoo for oily hair. Follow this with a dandruff shampoo that contains sulfur, such as Sebulex, Sebutone, or Selsun, to remove dead scalp cells and reduce the output of oil glands. Next, apply a lemon rinse, made with the strained juice of one lemon in a cup of lukewarm water. Pour this on, work it through the scalp, and rinse with cool water. Do not use a commercial conditioner, which may actually compound the oil problem. Treat your hair

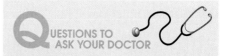

QUESTIONS TO ASK YOUR DOCTOR

▶ At what point should I try using an antifungal shampoo?
▶ What steps can I take to alleviate the itchiness of dandruff?

with this program twice a week until the condition is under control. If you shampoo more frequently, use a standard shampoo for oily hair followed by the lemon rinse. Blow-dry using a cool or warm setting, but avoid letting the hair dry naturally, because lying against the scalp allows wet hair to pick up oil more quickly. If possible, avoid hair spray as it is a magnet for dirt and oil.

Treat dry hair and dandruff first with a thorough brushing, then spread about ¼ cup of hand and body lotion on the hair and work it into the scalp. Wrap the head with a towel that has been soaked in very hot water and wrung out, and leave it in place for about 20 minutes. Next, wash the hair with a mild dandruff shampoo, such as Head & Shoulders or Zincon, that contains zinc pyrithione. If the dandruff persists, try a coal tar shampoo such as Denorex or Polytar. After shampooing, always rinse the scalp thoroughly with lukewarm water.

If you have normal hair, treat dandruff by brushing, washing with plain shampoo, and then applying an aspirin rinse, made by dissolving six aspirin tablets in a cup of warm water. The rinse should be poured over the hair, worked into the scalp, and left on for 15 minutes before rinsing. Once the dandruff disappears, you can return to a normal program of hair care.

For hair that has been bleached or permed, dandruff should be treated by first brushing, then shampooing with a protein, acid-balanced shampoo. Follow this with a mild dandruff shampoo that contains zinc pyrithione, and then rinse and apply a low-pH conditioner with protein.

Other Causes of Dandruff

The silvery scales of psoriasis are sometimes confused with dandruff. Eczema may also be responsible for dandruff. Babies often develop infantile seborrheic eczema, commonly referred to as cradle cap, which appears as thick and yellow crusted patches on the scalp.

Depression

(Disthymic disorder; major depressive episode; manic-depressive disorder)
Many people mistakenly equate sadness with depression. From time to time, everyone feels sad, often for a good reason such as a setback at work or the death of a loved one. Most people cope with such feelings, called reactive depression, and over time, shake off the sadness.

In contrast, clinical depression appears without an apparent reason and increasingly interferes with a person's ability to function.

Psychiatrists categorize the different types of depression according to the following characteristics:
Major depressive episode, in which symptoms (see Diagnostic Criteria, right) have no identifiable cause and prevent the person from performing normal daily activities. The episode may be isolated or recurrent.
Manic episode, in which abnormal euphoria or irritability dominate.
Mixed episode, in which mood alternates between mania and depression for at least one week. (This is also referred to as manic/depression or bipolar disorder.)
Dysthymic disorder, in which a depressed mood prevails, but some normal activities can be performed.

The cause of these disorders is unknown, although some researchers believe that biochemical changes in the brain may be responsible. Because depression tends to run in families, there may be a hereditary link too. Sometimes depression develops as a response—perhaps biochemical—to an infectious disease such as hepatitis. In addition, alcohol and other drugs can induce depression.

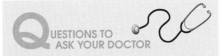

QUESTIONS TO ASK YOUR DOCTOR

▶ How can I tell if I have a normal reactive depression or a more serious form that requires medical treatment?
▶ If alcohol is a depressant, then why does having a drink or two lift my spirits? And what's wrong with doing that?
▶ What action is called for when a person threatens suicide? Should I broach the subject of suicide, or will that simply make matters worse?

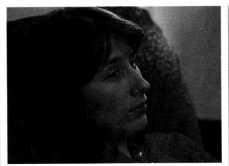

Depressed patients often feel lethargic and withdrawn, and they have lost the capacity for enjoyment.

Diagnostic Studies and Procedures

Diagnosis is based on symptoms and a medical history. If a doctor suspects clinical depression, she will probably refer the patient to a psychiatrist or clinical psychologist for testing.

Medical Treatments

Depression responds to medical treatment better than many other mental disorders. Approaches fall into three categories—medication, psychological therapy, and electroconvulsive therapy.
Drug Therapy. Antidepressant medications include tricyclic drugs, monoamine oxidase (MAO) inhibitors, and serotonin uptake inhibitors, all of which alleviate symptoms, and lithium, a drug that is used on a long-term basis to control the euphoric phase of manic-depressive illness.

Tricyclics, which include amitriptyline (Elavil,Endep, and others), amoxapine (Asendin), and imipramine (Tofranil and others), work by blocking the reabsorption of brain chemicals called neurotransmitters, thereby increasing their levels in the brain. MAO inhibitors, such as isocarboxazid (Marplan) and phenelzine (Nardil), block an enzyme that breaks down neurotransmitters. Fluoxetine (Prozac), the prototype of the newest class of antidepressants, works by blocking the absorption of serotonin; this is a potent brain chemical that seems to have mood-regulating properties.

As responses to antidepressants vary, trial and error is often necessary to find the best medication or combination.

Tricyclic drugs are useful in alleviating such symptoms as loss of appetite and weight, decreased capacity to feel pleasure, lethargy, suicidal thoughts, hopelessness, and excessive guilt. Some of the newer tricyclics take effect within a few days, while older ones require

several weeks. Side effects, such as dry mouth, drowsiness, and constipation, tend to subside with time.

MAO inhibitors are more often prescribed for depression characterized by increased appetite and excessive fatigue and sleepiness. Patients taking them must follow dietary restrictions because tyramine, a substance in cured meat, aged cheese, and red wine, for example, can react with the drug to precipitate a dangerous rise in blood pressure.

The serotonin blocker Prozac works faster than most other antidepressants, and is especially effective in combatting lethargy, drowsiness, and overeating. Among its side effects are nervousness, insomnia, anxiety, and loss of appetite.

Lithium can be highly effective in reducing the frequency and severity of

DIAGNOSTIC CRITERIA

The American Psychiatric Association uses the following symptoms to distinguish among the different types of depression:

Major depressive episode:
Five or more of these symptoms must persist most of the time for two weeks:
1. Overall depressed mood.
2. Diminished interest in or pleasure from most activities.
3. Significant weight loss or gain.
4. Insomnia or excessive sleepiness.
5. Hyperactivity or lethargy.
6. Persistent fatigue.
7. Feelings or worthlessness or guilt.
8. Inability to concentrate or make decisions.
9. Recurrent thoughts of suicide or preoccupation with death.

Manic episode:
Three or more of the following must prevail for at least one week:
1. Inflated self-esteem or grandiosity.
2. Decreased need for sleep.
3. Excessive talkativeness.
4. Racing thoughts and ideas.
5. Easily distracted.
6. Hyperactivity, especially in achieving goals, which may be unrealistic.
7. Excessive pursuit of risky activities, such as sexual indiscretions or gambling.

Dysthymic disorder:
Two or more of the following prevail for at least two years in an adult or one year in a child or adolescent:
1. Poor appetite or overeating.
2. Insomnia or excessive sleepiness.
3. Low energy or fatigue.
4. Low self-esteem.
5. Poor concentration or difficulty in making decisions.
6. Feelings of hopelessness.

manic-depressive cycles, although some patients do better with other drugs such as carbamazepine (Tegretol).

Psychotherapies. These "talking" treatments focus on helping patients resolve emotional problems by gaining insight into their own psychological makeup. Traditional psychotherapy looks for a childhood source of the problem, while other approaches address current conflicts and interpersonal problems.

Behavioral and cognitive forms of psychotherapy teach patients new ways to view the world. Depressed people tend to expect failure and often make false assumptions about the behavior and motives of others. Cognitive therapists strive to help these patients correct their negative beliefs.

Interpersonal therapy is based on the concept that depression occurs when personal relationships are disturbed, and that these relationships perpetuate symptoms, which worsen the interpersonal problems; the end result is a dysfunctional cycle. By focusing on issues, interpersonal therapists help patients understand their illness and feelings, and find ways to improve relationships.

Electroconvulsive Therapy. Although this method, often referred to as ECT or shock treatment, is not used as often as in the past, it is still highly effective in treating suicidal patients. The patient is given a general anesthetic, eliminating pain and memory of the procedure. Electrodes are placed on one or both sides of the scalp and a mild electric shock is administered to the brain, resulting in a minor seizure. There is temporary loss of memory for events of the past 6 to 12 months.

Alternative Therapies

Major or recurrent depression requires medical treatment. Alternative therapies are useful adjuncts that may be adequate for overcoming the milder forms.

Ayurveda. This ancient method of healing from India promotes emotional and physical well being with a regimen of diet, exercise, and herbal remedies designed to correct individual imbalances.

Creative Therapies. Art, music, dance, and other forms of artistic expression are especially beneficial during recovery from depression, because they help a patient to build self-esteem.

Light Therapy. People who repeatedly suffer depression only during the winter have seasonal affective disorder, or SAD, associated with insufficient

---

To her friends and coworkers, 30-year-old Lynda Stevens seemed to have all the ingredients of a happy life: A successful career, a loving marriage, and a healthy baby. About three months after her baby's birth, however, Stevens was overwhelmed with feelings of sadness and insecurity. She worked only part-time, yet she worried constantly that she was not meeting her baby's needs. Most of the time, she felt tired and irritable, and activities she had formerly enjoyed lost all their appeal. She was also increasingly sensitive: Minor frustrations and disputes with her husband and coworkers frequently reduced her to tears.

"I really wasn't myself," Stevens recalls. "My mood was taking a toll on my work and relationships." At her husband's urging, she saw a clinical social worker for help in coping with her problems. The social worker agreed that psychotherapy would be helpful, but also recommended that she see a psychiatrist as her symptoms suggested depression.

At first, Stevens was reluctant to call the doctor. "I thought psychiatrists were only for crazy people," she says. "But when I finally saw the doctor, she explained that depression is a medical illness, just like diabetes or high blood pressure. Correcting my brain chemistry with medication would improve my mood and help me find better ways to cope with day to day problems."

The psychiatrist prescribed desipramine (Norpramin), a tricyclic antidepressant. For the first few weeks on the drug, Stevens noticed little improvement, although she was somewhat less tired. After six weeks, however, she was almost back to normal.

For the next year, Stevens continued both the medication and therapy, which helped her become less self-critical and more relaxed with motherhood. "I know now that I am vulnerable to depression," she notes. "If my mood begins to fall again the way it did before, I'll definitely get help sooner."

---

exposure to daylight. Typical treatment involves sitting under special lights for several hours a day (see page 49).

Naturopathy and Nutrition Therapy. Diet plays a major role in brain function, but there is considerable disagreement over nutritional treatment of any mental disorder. Many nutrition therapists advise a sugar-free, low-fat diet that is high in complex carbohydrates and protein. Some also recommend supplements of B-complex vitamins.

Self-Treatment

Exercise can work as well as antidepressant drugs for mild depression or dysthemia. Aerobic exercise is especially effective, because it stimulates a release of endorphins, the body's own pain-relieving and mood-lifting chemicals.

It's best to stick to normal routines, particularly if you are experiencing reactive depression. Daily chores anchor you in reality; they may also prevent deeper depression.

Never overlook the power of laughter. A funny movie or an amusing book can often improve your mood.

Other Causes of Depression

Chronic fatigue syndrome has many of the hallmarks of depression. Among the elderly, symptoms of depression

are often confused with dementia. An underactive thyroid can cause symptoms similar to those of depression, as can many serious illnesses; for example, depression is common following a heart attack. Medications, such as those used to lower blood pressure, frequently cause transient depression.

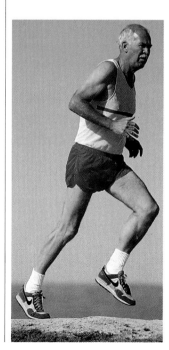

Exercise is a powerful weapon against depression, particularly mild cases.

Dermatitis

Dermatitis is the general term for any inflammation of the skin. Typical symptoms include scaling, itching, flaking, thickening, and changing coloration. Among the many causes are various types of allergic responses, bacterial and viral infections, chemical damage, insect bites, poor circulation, vitamin deficiencies, and stress.

Common forms of the condition include contact dermatitis (poison ivy and similar reactions) and atopic dermatitis or eczema, which is associated with allergies such as asthma and hay fever.

Diagnostic Studies and Procedures

Before making a diagnosis of dermatitis, a doctor takes a complete history and asks questions about known allergies, diet, medications, lifestyle, recent travel, work conditions, and sources of stress. All preparations routinely used on the skin, including cosmetics, antiperspirants, after-shave lotions, and colognes, are also reviewed.

The skin over the entire body, as well as the scalp, fingernails, and toenails are then examined. In uncertain cases, some tests may be done. These could include bacterial cultures, a skin biopsy, and patch tests for allergies. Some skin surfaces may also be examined under ultraviolet light in a darkened room to look for possible fungal infections. If symptoms of dermatitis are severe, referral to a dermatologist (a skin specialist) may be necessary.

Medical Treatments

Treatments vary depending on the diagnosis. For the relief of itching and pain, a cortisone ointment may be needed; in especially severe cases, a short course of corticosteroids may be prescribed.

Nonprescription medicated powders, soaps, and ointments are available to alleviate itching and chapping. Many doctors recommend calamine lotion for mild dermatitis outbreaks. Secondary infections caused by scratching may require either oral or topical antibiotics.

Alternative Therapies

Aromatherapy. Full-body massages using soothing aromatic oils such as rose, clary sage, or peppermint may prove helpful in alleviating itchiness and promoting relaxation to counter stress-related dermatitis.

Herbal Medicine. Aloe vera juice is a soothing treatment for some rashes and skin inflammations. Chickweed, used

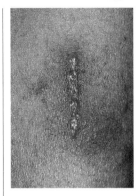

Redness, itching, and scaling are hallmarks of dermatitis. Clear borders suggest that the cause was contact with a specific irritant.

as an ointment, cream, or oil added to bathwater, eases itching and promotes healing. Other herbal remedies for dermatitis include lotions or ointments of comfrey, pau d'arco, stinging nettles, red clover, witch hazel, and elder.

Hydrotherapy. Baking soda or colloidal oatmeal added to bath water can help alleviate itching. To relieve both inflammation and itching, a compress dipped in a mixture of 1 quart cool water and 1 cup Burow's solution (a nonprescription skin product) is suggested. It should be kept on the affected area for 10 to 15 minutes several times a day.

Nutrition Therapy. Some therapists recommend kelp tablets, as well as supplements of vitamin B complex, vitamin E, and zinc. Dietary deficiencies and food allergies that cause dermatitis can often be identified by a nutritionist. Gluten is often a culprit. To determine if it is causing allergy problems for you, eliminate foods that contain wheat, rye, oats, and barley for six weeks and see if the condition improves.

Relaxation Techniques. Many forms of dermatitis, especially eczema and hives, are triggered by stress and further aggravated by repressed feelings. Training in biofeedback skills, breathing exercises, and meditation, as well as counseling in behavior modification, can be effective ways to overcome many skin problems that are often exacerbated by emotional factors.

Self-Treatment

Dermatitis frequently responds well to an over-the-counter anti-itch cream, an application of a nonprescription cortisone ointment, or home remedies, such as the ones described below. If a skin disorder, particularly a rash, fails to improve in several weeks or if it gets worse, consult a dermatologist.

▶ Try to determine the cause and avoid it whenever possible. Certain foods,

jewelry, cosmetics, soaps, and detergents are common culprits. In any event, protect the skin from chemicals that may aggravate existing dermatitis or trigger new outbreaks.

▶ Try not to scratch. It can cause the inflammation to become worse.

▶ Use a mild, nonmedicated soap and warm water to maintain enough surface oil to prevent drying.

▶ Bathe or shower every other day instead of daily, especially during the winter. Use tepid rather than hot water, and apply a nonirritating moisturizer while your skin is still damp.

▶ Protect your skin from the sun, especially if you are taking medications that increase sun sensitivity. Experiment with different sunscreens. Some people are sensitive to PABA or other ingredients in sunscreen products.

▶ To protect hands that are frequently immersed in water, coat them often with a moisturizer containing lanolin. For housework, wear latex gloves to protect hands from dish detergents and household cleaners.

▶ To counteract the drying effects of air-conditioning and central heating, install a humidifier in the bedroom.

▶ Consider clothing fibers as a possible trigger of dermatitis. Common offenders include wool and some synthetics. Certain fabric finishes can also trigger dermatitis. If possible, wash new clothes before wearing them.

▶ Avoid exposing skin to irritating chemicals, especially if you are an artist, artisan, hairdresser, chemical worker, gardener, or hobbyist. When you use such chemicals, wear cotton-lined gloves and sprinkle the interior with talc or cornstarch after each wearing to provide added protection.

Other Causes of Skin Inflammation

Such ailments as herpes, chickenpox, shingles, impetigo, psoriasis, and scabies produce skin eruptions.

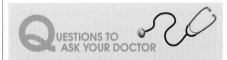

QUESTIONS TO ASK YOUR DOCTOR

▶ Should a cortisone ointment be used for only a limited time? Is it absorbed through the skin in quantities large enough to cause side effects?
▶ Can I safely take antihistamines or other medications to alleviate skin itchiness and dryness?

Detached Retina

If a retina becomes detached from the tissue at the back of the eyeball, it is deprived of its blood supply that is carrying essential oxygen and nutrients. It must be reattached as soon as possible to prevent irreversible loss of sight. Fortunately, advances in repairing minor retinal tears have been preventing the more serious eventuality of complete retinal detachment.

A retina may become detached as the result of a cyst or tumor, a hemorrhage, acute infection, extreme nearsightedness, the aging of eye tissues, or a severe blow to the eye. (Athletes, especially boxers, are particularly vulnerable to retinal detachment.)

Retinal detachment can sometimes be a complication of diabetes, high blood pressure, and cataract surgery. Extremely high stress may also be a factor. A California study of 33 people who had suffered detached retinas concluded that the problem can be precipitated by highly stressful situations that cause a sudden surge in blood pressure.

to shrink. As the gel liquifies, it peels away from the retina and forms the threadlike "floaters" familiar to millions of people as harmless phenomena that come and go without any consequence and for no clear reasons.

When vitreous gel begins to peel away to a greater extent, it pulls on the retina and dazzling flashes of light, or "stars," appear. If the pull leads to a small tear in the retina, blood from damaged blood vessels will enter the vitreous gel through this slight opening. The result of this seepage is a clouding of vision. Prompt diagnosis and treatment of these symptoms by a specialist can prevent an eventual emergency.

Diagnostic Studies and Procedures

Diagnosis is based on an examination of the eye with an ophthalmoscope, which gives the doctor a close-up view of the retina. A technique known as indirect ophthalmoscopy, invented in the 19th century, is used to get a panoramic view of the retina, including the outer periphery. With this procedure, a doctor is able to detect tiny tears at the edge of the retina.

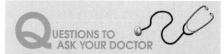

the torn tissue receive laser burns. When the scar forms, it prevents any further leaking of vitreous humor from behind the retina.

Freezing. This outpatient procedure, technically called *cryoretinopexy*, is also performed under a local anesthetic. It has the same purpose as the laser treatment. The ophthalmologist uses a small frozen probe above the retinal tear to produce inflammation that eventually creates scar tissue.

Surgical Repair. An emergency operation is required to reattach a detached retina to the wall of the eye. Various methods may be used depending on how much fluid has seeped behind the retina and for how long the retina itself has been deprived of nourishment. Surgery is performed under general anesthesia in a hospital. Although the hospital stay may be brief, physical activities may have to be severely restricted and only after several weeks is it possible to assess how much sight has been restored.

Alternative Therapies

There are no alternative therapies for a detached retina, although relaxation techniques such as breathing exercises and meditation can be helpful in managing stress that might lead to retinal detachment. These techniques are especially effective during the postsurgical period when physical movement must be kept to a minimum.

Self-Treatment

To prevent injuries that might lead to retinal detachment, it's a good idea to wear protective glasses when engaged in contact and racquet sports. Wraparound goggles should always be worn when working with such hazardous equipment as a blowtorch.

Other Causes of Retinal Detachment

Iritis, a serious eye inflammation, increases the possibility of developing a detached retina.

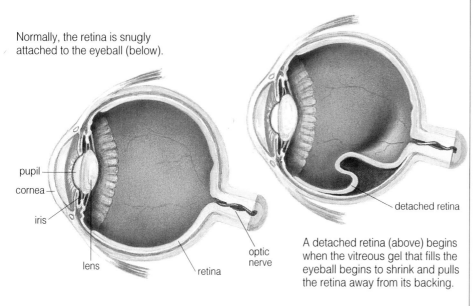

Normally, the retina is snugly attached to the eyeball (below).

pupil
cornea
iris
lens
retina
optic nerve
detached retina

A detached retina (above) begins when the vitreous gel that fills the eyeball begins to shrink and pulls the retina away from its backing.

As pressure increases, fluid is forced from the capillaries behind the retina, causing blisters to form on the retina's surface. When individuals are under chronic stress, the capillaries may become increasingly weakened, making the possibility of detachment an ever-present danger.

The first stage in retinal detachment may be a hole or tear in the retina. This damage can occur if the vitreous gel, or humor, in the center of the eye begins

Medical Treatments

There are no drug treatments for detached retina. Depending on the extent of the retinal damage, several surgical treatments can be considered.

Laser Treatment. To repair a tear in the retina before it becomes detached, photocoagulation may be performed under a local anesthetic in the doctor's office. A mirrored contact lens is placed in the patient's eye, enabling the doctor to see where the retina is torn. The edges of

Diabetes

(Diabetes mellitus; Type I and Type II diabetes)

Diabetes is a chronic metabolic disease in which the body either does not produce or does not fully utilize insulin. As a result, it cannot properly metabolize carbohydrates and, to a lesser extent, protein and fat. Glucose (sugar) builds up in the blood; to rid the body of the excess, the kidneys begin to excrete it in the urine.

Although excessive glucose is circulating, the brain and other tissues that need it for fuel are unable to use it. The body begins to break down fat and protein in an attempt to provide an alternate source of fuel, resulting in serious biochemical imbalances. In the meantime, the high levels of glucose are damaging structures throughout the body, increasing the risk of complications such as heart attack, blindness, kidney failure, stroke, and painful nerve problems. Despite effective treatments, diabetes is one of the leading causes of death in the United States.

There are two major forms: Type I, in which the body stops making insulin completely, and Type II, in which the body produces inadequate insulin or is unable to use it fully. The first type, also called insulin-dependent or juvenile diabetes, usually develops during the first 20 years of life when islet cells in the pancreas are destroyed and can no longer make insulin. Symptoms are frequent urination, weight loss, unusual thirst, weakness, fatigue, and hunger.

Type II, also called non-insulin dependent or adult-onset diabetes, is most common among overweight older people, although it can occur in persons of normal weight. It develops more slowly than Type I; indeed, many individuals have the disease for years

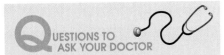

QUESTIONS TO
ASK YOUR DOCTOR

▶ Am I a good candidate for use of an insulin pump?
▶ How often should I have a medical checkup? See an ophthalmologist? Cardiologist? Other specialist?
▶ How does my diabetes affect my prospects of having a child? Are my children likely to have diabetes?

SIGNS OF AN INSULIN OVERDOSE
▶ A tingling sensation in the mouth, the fingers, or other parts of the body
▶ A cold clammy feeling
▶ Paleness
▶ A buzzing in the ears
▶ Excessive sweating
▶ A feeling of weakness or faintness
▶ Headache
▶ Hunger
▶ Abdominal pain
▶ Irritability and a change in mood
▶ Impaired vision
▶ Rapid heartbeat and trembling
▶ Sudden drowsiness
▶ Sudden awakening from sleep, especially if it is accompanied by any of the above symptoms

without knowing it. In addition to symptoms experienced in Type I diabetes, signs may include frequent infections, cramps and tingling sensations, slow healing, impotence in men, and chronic vaginitis in women.

The cause of diabetes is unknown, but researchers believe that Type I develops when the immune system destroys the islet cells. The disease tends to run in families, so there may be a genetic component.

Diagnostic Studies and Procedures

Diagnosis is based on a blood test that measures blood glucose levels. Elevated blood glucose doesn't necessarily indicate diabetes, but it does call for more extensive testing. In general, a diagnosis is established if two separate blood tests, done after fasting for eight hours, show glucose levels of 140 milligrams of glucose per deciliter of blood (mg/dl). In borderline cases, a glucose challenge test may be ordered. This involves measuring glucose after fasting, and again after drinking sugar water.

Medical Treatments

There is no cure for either type of diabetes, but the disease can be controlled with a combination of therapies. People with Type I need regular insulin injections and a special diet and exercise regimen. They must also measure their own blood sugar (see Self-Treatment).

Most people with Type II diabetes can control it with just diet and exercise, especially if they lose weight. In fact, studies show that weight loss alone can produce normal blood glucose levels in more than 80 percent of overweight Type II patients. Others may need oral

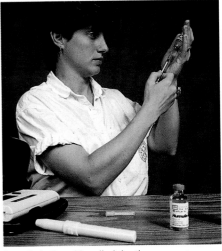

Regularly timed insulin injections are an integral part of managing Type I diabetes.

hypoglycemics to increase insulin production and its effectiveness. These drugs include chlorpropamide (Diabinese), glipizide (Glucotrol), glyburide (Diaßeta and Micronase), tolbutamide (Orinase), and tolazamide (Tolinase).

Patients with both types of diabetes require extra medical care and should establish a close working relationship with a specialist, usually an internist or endocrinologist. Because diabetes affects especially the heart, blood vessels, kidneys, nerves, and eyes, other specialists may be needed. For example, an ophthalmologist should be seen at least every 6 to 12 months to check for diabetic retinopathy, a disorder in which blood vessels in the retina overgrow and rupture. If unchecked, this bleeding can lead to blindness.

Cardiovascular complications, such as high blood pressure and coronary artery disease, are particularly common in diabetes. A significant number of patients develop kidney failure, and require dialysis or a kidney transplant. Reduced circulation to the legs and feet may lead to the need for vascular surgery or even amputation.

There is, however, good news for the 13 million Americans who have diabetes. A 10-year study showed that maintaining normal blood sugar levels dramatically slows the progression of complications. More doctors are now encouraging diabetic patients to follow a regimen that maintains blood glucose levels as near to normal as possible. This involves frequent glucose monitoring (at least four times a day), adjustment of insulin or other medication dosages, changes in exercise patterns, and alteration of the timing, frequency, and content of meals and snacks.

To make insulin injections easier, there is now an insulin pump, which is carried in a pocket or worn on a belt. It can be programmed to administer small amounts of insulin at specific times through a syringe left in place in the abdomen or other convenient site.

Alternative Therapies
Alternative therapies are helpful as adjuncts to medical treatment.

Exercise Conditioning. This improves the body's ability to use insulin. Type I patients who exercise regularly can usually lower their insulin dosage, and Type II patients can often eliminate the need for oral hypoglycemics. Exercise also improves circulation, and may help prevent leg and foot problems.

Homeopathy. Practitioners may prescribe phosphorous to help stabilize blood sugar levels.

Meditation, Self-Hypnosis, and Yoga. These and other relaxation techniques can help lower the levels of stress that may elevate blood glucose.

Nutrition Therapy. The basic diabetic diet is described under Self-Treatment. In addition, many dietitians urge eating beans regularly, as they can help blunt the post-meal rise in glucose levels.

Self-Treatment
All patients must learn to test their blood sugar levels at home and adjust their food-exercise-medication regimens on a daily basis. Parents should

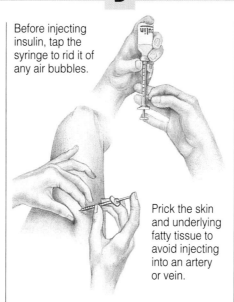

Before injecting insulin, tap the syringe to rid it of any air bubbles.

Prick the skin and underlying fatty tissue to avoid injecting into an artery or vein.

assume this responsibility for young children; by age 9 or 10, most youngsters can use a self-monitoring device.

People with diabetes, especially children and teenagers, need emotional support and continual education to accept responsibility for their own care. Joining a group for diabetic patients or sending a child to a diabetes camp can make it easier to cope with the disease.

A diabetes diet is similar to the healthful diets now recommended for all Americans: Obtain most of your calories from complex carbohydrates, such as vegetables, legumes, fruits, and whole grains, and rely less on animal foods for protein. Avoid refined sugars and restrict fat and cholesterol intake to help reduce the risk of heart disease.

When diabetes is first diagnosed, you should consult with a registered dietitian to develop meal plans compatible with your tastes and lifestyle, and learn to follow the exchange lists developed by the American Diabetes Association. These lists provide simple formulas to assure that you get an appropriate number of calories and other nutrients each day. Eventually, you will not need to rely as heavily on them. In fact, with careful self-testing, you can learn to increase or decrease your insulin dosage to accommodate an occasional departure from your usual diet.

People with diabetes often have poor circulation and are susceptible to skin ulcers, especially on the legs and feet. Fit shoes carefully to avoid corns and other foot problems that can develop into a serious infection. Also keep toenails trimmed. If you have difficulty caring for your feet, see a podiatrist.

Carry in your wallet identification indicating that you have diabetes so that you can receive prompt medical care if you are in an accident or have a high or low blood sugar reaction. Also, be alert for signs of an insulin overdose (see box, opposite page), and carry a source of sugar to use if one occurs.

Other Causes of High Blood Sugar
Certain medications can raise blood sugar. So too can diseases affecting the pancreas. Pregnant women sometimes develop gestational diabetes, which can be detected with a blood glucose test, usually in the second trimester.

A CASE IN POINT

When Ron Harrison developed Type I diabetes in 1961 at the age of 12, he was put on the standard regimen for that time—a strict diet and daily shot of lente insulin, a form that works for 18 to 24 hours. He was also instructed to test his urine for glucose each morning.

Over the next few years, Harrison was hospitalized several times when his diabetes went out of control. "I tried to follow my doctor's instructions," he recalls, "but my regimen just wasn't keeping my blood sugar under control." And the unstable diabetes was reflected in damage to his eyes and kidneys.

Then came a revolutionary innovation in diabetes self-care—the development of a home test to measure blood glucose

instantaneously. Heretofore, Harrison had relied on urine tests, but by the time glucose shows up in the urine, blood levels may have been dangerously high for hours or even days. Results of a blood test done by a doctor often were not available until the next day. The automated test allows patients to measure their glucose and adjust their insulin dosage to avoid dangerous fluctuations.

Referred to a diabetes self-care program, Harrison was at first skeptical. "I had been taught that one shot at the same time every day was the gold standard of treatment," he said. "If that didn't work, you were one of the unlucky ones whose diabetes couldn't be controlled." He learned to measure his blood glucose

several times a day, and to keep a careful diary of test results, food intake, exercise, and other factors affecting insulin needs. He also learned to adjust his insulin dosage by calculating how much would be needed to metabolize a specific amount of food, and how to make further adjustments for exercise. He shifted to a combination of insulins divided into three or more daily doses, which permitted further fine-tuning and adjustments to maintain normal blood glucose levels.

After nearly a decade, Harrison's diabetes remains in check. His kidney function has actually improved and there has been no further damage to his eyes. "Before, I was being controlled by my diabetes; now I'm controlling it," he says.

Diaper Rash

(Diaper dermatitis)

At some time, almost all babies develop diaper rash, which is confined to the skin covered by a diaper. The affected area is dotted with small, pimple-like bumps that may become scaly or crusty. Sometimes the sores ooze and have an unpleasant odor.

Most diaper rash is caused by a yeast or bacterial infection. These organisms thrive in a moist, warm environment, which is enhanced by infrequent changing and/or wearing rubber pants or plastic-coated diapers.

Diaper rash is most common between the ages of six and nine months. Some babies seem to be more vulnerable than others, but those who are breast-fed are less prone to the condition. Diarrhea and the administering of antibiotics increase susceptibility. Other contributing factors include friction, introduction of new foods, and skin contact with stale urine, detergent residue in cloth diapers, and chemicals used in some disposable products.

Diagnostic Studies and Procedures

Most parents can readily recognize a diaper rash by its characteristic appearance and its confinement to the buttocks and genital area; there is usually little or none in the skin creases. In some cases, however, the rash may develop into a more severe infection; the baby should be taken to a doctor if the area is unusually red and inflamed, if pus-filled sores develop, or if there are other symptoms, such as a fever, diarrhea, and listlessness.

Medical Treatments

Ordinary diaper rash does not require medical treatment. If it does not clear up in two or three days of home care, however, a doctor may prescribe a medicated ointment.

Alternative Therapies

Herbal Medicine. Aloe gel applied to the diaper area is said to speed healing, especially if crusty sores develop. Herbalists also suggest comfrey ointment. In stubborn cases, applying a poultice made of powdered comfrey root might help. Using arrowroot powder instead of ordinary baby powder may promote healing of skin sores.

Self-Treatment

Frequent changing is the first step in treating diaper rash and preventing recurrences. However, there is no clear

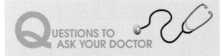

agreement on whether cloth or disposable diapers are better when it comes to preventing the condition. At least two medical studies have found that super absorbent disposable diapers, which contain a gelling material, keep the skin drier and afford greater protection against rash than cloth and regular disposable diapers. On the other hand, between cloth and conventional disposable diapers, cloth keeps the baby drier, especially if it contains an inner layer of nonwoven fabric. If your baby often develops diaper rash, despite frequent changing, experiment with different types of diapers.

If you do use cloth diapers, make sure that they are properly washed and sterilized. Commercial diaper services can usually be trusted to do this adequately. If you wash your own, use hot water and a mild laundry soap. Rinse the diapers, then put them through another wash cycle with a half-cup of chlorine bleach to sterilize them. Add an ounce of white vinegar per gallon of water to the final rinse cycle. This rinse will help later to neutralize the ammonia in the baby's urine.

Home care clears up most diaper rash in two or three days. Here are tactics that usually help.
▶ Leave off the diaper as much as possible. Exposing the skin to the air and preventing contact with urine and feces speeds healing. To minimize mess, place the baby on a rubber mat that is covered with a sheet or towel.
▶ Change the baby as soon as possible after bowel movements; any prolonged skin contact with feces worsens diaper rash, and can cause blistering and infection.
▶ When changing the baby, wash the area with plain water and a mild soap. Don't use commercial diaper wipes; these contain alcohol and other chemi-

cals that may irritate the baby's skin. After washing, pat the skin dry before diapering. Alternatively, use a hair drier set on low.
▶ Before putting on a fresh diaper, you may, as some dermatologists suggest, apply a mild vinegar solution to the baby's bottom. Use one part vinegar to eight parts water, and gently wipe it on the skin after washing. To avoid moisture buildup, allow the skin to dry thoroughly before diapering.
▶ To make the baby more comfortable, apply cornstarch or a commercial baby powder containing cornstarch. Pour a little into your hand and then spread it on the baby's bottom; you and your baby will inhale less of the powder when it is applied this way, than if it is sprinkled directly onto the skin. Avoid talcum powders; they can cause lung damage if inhaled.
▶ To speed healing, try applying vitamin E oil directly to the skin. Skin creams or ointments should not be used until the rash clears up, however, because these can slow healing. When the rash is gone, products that contain zinc oxide or petroleum jelly can be used to protect the skin from a recurrence. These ointments tend to adhere to the skin; to remove them, use a cotton ball dipped in baby oil.
▶ Don't use plastic pants, which keep moisture in. Also avoid the use of thick, bulky diapers or wrapping the material too tightly. The diaper should be loose enough to let in some air.

Other Causes of Infant Rashes

In unusual cases, a rash in the diaper area may be a manifestation of a more general skin disease, such as infantile psoriasis or seborrheic eczema. In such cases, the baby is likely to have rashes on other parts of the body.

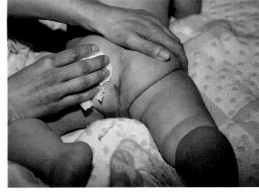

Wiping the baby's bottom with a mild vinegar solution helps prevent diaper rash by neutralizing ammonia.

Diarrhea

Diarrhea, the frequent passage of very loose or watery bowel movements, is a symptom of an underlying disorder, which may have been caused by stress, dietary indiscretion, traveler's diarrhea, flu, food poisoning, or any one of numerous conditions. Although most episodes are minor and temporary, a prolonged bout can lead to dehydration and an upset in body chemistry that could be life threatening, especially in children and the elderly.

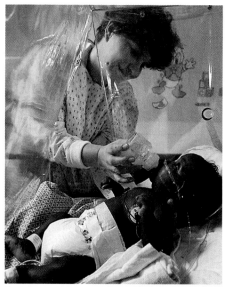

An infant with severe diarrhea may need hospital care to treat dehydration.

You should call a doctor if diarrhea lasts for more than one day in a child under the age of two or two days in an older child or an adult. Consult him even sooner if the diarrhea worsens or is accompanied by other symptoms such as severe abdominal pain, vomiting, fever, or the appearance of blood, mucus, or worms in the stool. Persistent or intermittent mild diarrhea also warrants medical investigation.

Diagnostic Studies and Procedures

The nature of the diarrhea is an important factor in the process of diagnosis. For example, diarrhea that alternates with constipation and periods of normal bowel function may be caused either by irritable bowel syndrome or stress. Blood in the stool can point to the possibility of an infection, cancer, polyps, or an inflamed colon.

After a physical examination, certain tests may be called for, including a stool analysis, X-rays, and colonoscopy, an examination of the entire colon with a special fiberoptic instrument.

Medical Treatments

The choice of antidiarrheal medication depends upon the underlying cause. Most diarrhea resolves itself in a day or two of self-treatment with nonprescription drugs. Diarrhea accompanied by intestinal cramps and spasms may be treated with phenobarbital, paregoric, opium, or other prescription substances to reduce intestinal motility. Antibiotics will be prescribed if a bacterial infection is present. Other drugs called anthelmintics are given if there are intestinal worms.

Even mild diarrhea in a baby or young child poses a danger of dehydration, especially if there is also vomiting, which makes it more difficult to replace fluids and body salts. In severe cases, hospitalization may be necessary to administer intravenous replacement of water and salts. Giving a special rehydration formula such as Pedialyte, which is available at pharmacies, usually can prevent dehydration and the need for intravenous therapy.

Alternative Therapies

Depending on the cause of the diarrhea, alternative therapies may be your sole remedy or may supplement medical or self-treatment.

Acupressure. A shiatsu technique for relieving diarrhea involves applying pressure to the index finger a fraction of an inch from the corner of the nail, on the side facing your thumb (see photograph, below). Use the thumb of the opposite hand to apply pressure for five to seven seconds several times an hour until diarrhea subsides.

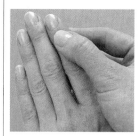

The acupressure point for relieving diarrhea is on the index finger, a little below the nail.

Herbal Medicine. Herbalists often recommend blackberry root bark. Prepared tinctures are available in health food stores, or the bark can be boiled in water for 20 minutes and then strained and taken as a tea. Other

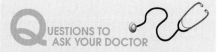

QUESTIONS TO ASK YOUR DOCTOR

▶ Do you recommend medication for mild diarrhea? If so, what kind?
▶ When should I consider taking a fluid replacement for diarrhea, and what kind should I use?

herbal remedies include chamomile tea, raspberry leaf tea, and cayenne capsules. Ginger tea may alleviate any accompanying abdominal cramps and nausea; slippery elm bark capsules may also be recommended.

Nutrition Therapy. Sometimes taking antibiotics leads to diarrhea because they kill certain bacteria that live in the intestines and help maintain normal functioning. Eating yogurt with live acidophilus cultures helps repopulate the colon with these beneficial bacteria.

Self-Treatment

When stress brings on a bout of diarrhea, relaxation can help prevent it. If it is caused by an excess of certain fibrous foods such as bran, dietary modification may be necessary.

Occasional mild diarrhea can be self-treated with an over-the-counter medication that contains bismuth (Pepto-Bismol), attapulgite (Kaopectate), or loperamide (Imodium A-D), although doctors disagree about their value. Do not use such products for more than a day or two without consulting a physician.

During an attack of diarrhea, avoid all solid foods, coffee, milk products, and spices. Take frequent sips of fluids such as flat sodas (ginger ale or cola allowed to fizz out at room temperature), tea, or clear soup. You can also try rice water, made by boiling ½ cup of brown rice in 3 cups of water for 30 to 45 minutes, then straining out the rice; drink about ½ cup of this liquid every hour.

As the diarrhea subsides, add bland foods; for example, the BRAT diet of bananas, rice, applesauce, and toast. Avoid other fruits and raw vegetables until normal bowel function returns.

Other Causes of Diarrhea

Diarrhea also can be caused by serious digestive problems, including colorectal cancer, Crohn's disease, diverticulitis, and ulcerative colitis.

Diphtheria

This acute, highly contagious infection is characterized by a grayish membrane that coats the throat. In the disease's early stages, other symptoms usually include a sore throat, low fever, and swollen glands in the neck. During later stages, the patient may experience difficulty in swallowing or breathing; he may also have a profuse discharge from the nose plus a rapid heartbeat. Although many people think of diphtheria as a children's disease, it can actually strike at any age.

The organism that causes diphtheria is *Corynebacterium diphtheriae*, which spreads by way of droplets expelled

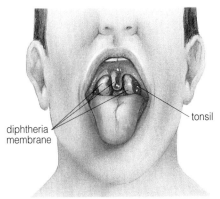

diphtheria membrane — tonsil

A grayish membrane coating the throat is a hallmark of diphtheria.

during coughing, sneezing, or simply breathing. Some strains of the bacterium produce a poisonous exotoxin that travels through the bloodstream and attacks the nerves, heart, kidneys, and reproductive organs. The results can be nerve and heart inflammation, heart failure, shock, and even death.

Diagnostic Studies and Procedures

Because diphtheria is rare in the United States and other industrialized countries, most doctors in these areas have never encountered it and so may not recognize it. Once the classic gray membrane appears, however, a physician will probably suspect diphtheria. A culture for the bacterium, obtained from a sample of throat secretions, can confirm a diagnosis.

Medical Treatments

This disease is so contagious that anyone who has it must be isolated, usually in a hospital intensive-care unit. The diphtheria antitoxin should be given immediately. This will neutralize the

exotoxin, but only that which has not yet attacked body cells; it's less effective, therefore, if given later in the course of the disease. An antibiotic—usually penicillin or erythromycin—is also needed to kill the bacteria.

Depending on the severity of the disease and the presence of complications, supplemental oxygen may be given, and the lungs, heart, and nervous system might be monitored for further signs of complications. If the throat has swollen, artificial respiration may be needed to prevent the patient from suffocating.

Recuperation can be lengthy, particularly if there are heart complications. Bed rest is essential, sometimes for two or three months in severe cases.

Anyone exposed to diphtheria should find out when they were last immunized against the disease, and receive, if necessary, a booster shot or a complete course of immunizations.

Alternative Therapies

Diphtheria is a medical emergency requiring prompt treatment with the diphtheria antitoxin. Any alternative therapies must be used strictly as an adjunct to this medical care.

Aromatherapy. During convalescence, soothing scents may help relax an irritable or restless patient; place a bowl of steaming water containing aromatic oils at the person's bedside. Bach flower remedies may also be used to foster emotional well-being.

Massage. Swedish or other therapeutic massages can help to relax the convalescent. Massage may also tone muscles in preparation for a gradual return to normal physical activity.

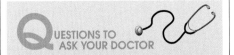

QUESTIONS TO ASK YOUR DOCTOR

▶ What should I do if someone in the family has been exposed to diphtheria?
▶ Is there any way to tell if my child will have an adverse reaction to the DPT shot? How dangerous is such a reaction?
▶ If I have been exposed to diphtheria, do I need a booster shot even though I was recently immunized?

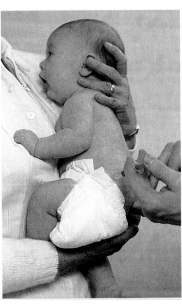

Diphtheria can be prevented by giving the DPT series of immunization. For a baby, these are begun at two months of age.

Self-Treatment

Diphtheria requires medical treatment, but you can take measures to prevent the disease. Keep your immunizations up-to-date; an adult should have a diphtheria booster shot at least every 10 years. If it has been longer since your last one, you need a complete three-dose series of immunizations. This is especially important if you plan to travel to any country that has had recent outbreaks of the disease.

Make sure that children receive the diphtheria vaccine at 2, 4, 6, and 18 months of age. They also need a booster shot when they begin school (usually between the ages of 4 and 6 years) and every 5 to 10 years after that.

For young children, the diphtheria vaccine is usually combined with pertussis and tetanus immunizations in what is called the DPT shot. Although some youngsters do suffer adverse reactions to this injection, they are generally responding to the pertussis component and not the diphtheria vaccine. A child who has previously had an adverse reaction to the DPT shot or who has ever had a seizure or convulsion, should not receive the pertussis vaccine but should be given the diphtheria and tetanus vaccines, which can still be combined in a single shot.

Other Causes of Throat Symptoms

The early symptoms of diphtheria are similar to those of flu, a cold, strep throat, or other upper respiratory infections. Mononucleosis or scarlet fever may cause a very sore throat with no other cold symptoms.

Diverticulosis

(Diverticular disease)

Diverticulosis is a condition in which small pouches, or diverticula, protrude from a weakened segment of the colon wall. Many people have no symptoms. Others experience occasional mild pain or diarrhea or blood in the stools. But if waste material clogs one or more of the pouches, diverticulitis, an inflammation characterized by fever, bleeding, intense pain, and general malaise, may develop. If diverticulitis goes untreated, serious complications can arise, such as perforation of the intestine, which may lead to peritonitis, a life-threatening inflammation of the membrane that lines the abdominal cavity.

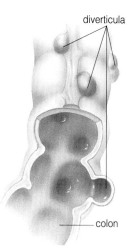

diverticula

colon

Outpouches along the colon may become impacted and inflamed.

Diagnostic Studies and Procedures

When a doctor suspects diverticulitis, he may order a colonoscopy, inspection of the lining of the colon with a flexible tube that has special viewing devices. He may also have a stool sample tested for hidden, or occult, blood.

Medical Treatments

Uncomplicated diverticulosis is usually treated conservatively. A high-fiber diet is generally recommended, as well as laxatives if constipation is part of the problem. Antibiotics will be prescribed to treat any infection. When the infection is severe or heavy bleeding occurs,

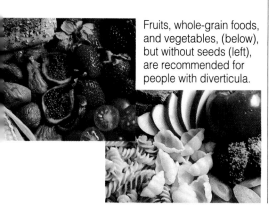

Fruits, whole-grain foods, and vegetables, (below), but without seeds (left), are recommended for people with diverticula.

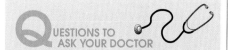

QUESTIONS TO ASK YOUR DOCTOR

▶ What kind of diet should I follow? Are there foods I should avoid?
▶ Do I need an annual colonoscopy because of the risk of colon cancer?

surgery may be necessary to remove the diseased part of the colon. In especially severe cases, the entire colon may have to be removed, but this can usually be done in such a way that normal bowel function will be retained.

Alternative Therapies

Alternative therapies should be used only as adjunctive treatments.

Ayurveda. A series of cleansing enemas may be given to clear the colon. The diet is then adjusted to prevent constipation, which promotes diverticulitis.

Herbal Medicine. Chamomile, papaya, and red clover—consumed either as teas or extract capsules—are among the herbs recommended for diverticulitis. Some herbalists advocate two cups of pau d'arco tea daily to alleviate intestinal inflammation and abdominal cramps. Psyllium seeds, included in many stool softeners, may also be prescribed, but a doctor should be consulted before taking these.

Nutrition Therapy. Diet plays an important role in prevention and treatment of diverticular disease. A low-fiber, high-fat diet increases the risk of diverticulitis, and research indicates that increased fiber intake helps prevent its symptoms in those who have diverticulosis. Spicy or seedy foods should be avoided. Supplements of vitamins A, E, and C, as well as garlic capsules, are sometimes suggested.

A flare-up of diverticulitis calls for a bland, puréed diet devoid of raw fruits and vegetables, alcohol, and caffeine. A psyllium seed laxative may be recommended to prevent constipation. A high-fiber diet can be resumed a month after all symptoms subside.

Self-Treatment

Once diverticula form, they cannot be eliminated, but diligent self-care can prevent acute diverticulitis. In addition to following dietary recommendations, drink at least eight glasses of fluids a day to keep stools soft. Allow yourself a minimum of 10 minutes for a bowel movement at about the same time each

day, but do not strain. (See a doctor if your stool is black, or if you have fever or severe pain.) Exercise helps prevent constipation; make it part of your daily routine. There also appears to be a relationship between diverticulitis, a sedentary lifestyle, and obesity.

Other Causes of Abdominal Pain

Appendicitis causes acute abdominal pain and cramping. Colon polyps, colon or rectal cancer, and inflammatory bowel disorders can bring about bloody stools and altered bowel habits.

A CASE IN POINT

Al Freeman, a 63-year-old businessman, had a long history of intermittent stomach problems—constipation alternating with diarrhea, intestinal gas, and abdominal cramps—all of which he attributed to stress. Then during one siege, which included a low-grade fever, Freeman noticed blood and mucus in his stool.

A gastroenterologist ordered a colonoscopy, which showed that the lower third of the colon was inflamed and there was evidence of more than a dozen outpouches. The doctor advised hospital treatment because of the danger that one or more of the impacted pouches would rupture—an event that could lead to peritonitis.

While in the hospital, Freeman received intensive antibiotic therapy for the inflammation. To quiet his colon, they gave him anticholinergic drugs; he was also put on a low-residue liquid diet.

After a week, he was discharged with instructions to continue the low-residue diet for two more weeks and then to increase his fiber intake gradually. "I was told to eat high-fiber foods, such as oatmeal, whole-grain bread, and beans," he recounts, "and to avoid anything with seeds, hulls, or strings, which could become trapped in one of the pouches." He was also advised to drink at least 10 glasses of water or juice a day and to abstain from alcohol and caffeine. Finally, he was given a fiber stool softener in case of constipation.

Freeman's doctor urged him to have a colonoscopy annually, because colon cancer and diverticulitis produce similar symptoms and it's essential not to confuse one with the other.

Dizziness

(Vertigo; disequilibrium; lightheadedness)
Vision, touch, hearing, the vestibular system in the inner ear, and multiple areas of the brain all contribute to helping maintain balance and orientation in space. Damage to any of these senses or areas can cause dizziness.

When dizziness occurs, it's important to identify the sensation clearly. For example, with true vertigo, an illusion of motion, you feel as if you are spinning or that the room is spinning around you; it often provokes nausea and vomiting. Vertigo is most likely to arise from the vestibular portion of the inner ear, the nerve connecting the inner ear to the brain, or the brain itself. It may result from motion sickness, an inner ear infection, allergic rhinitis, high doses of certain drugs, Ménière's disease (page 288), a blow to the head, tumors, or, less commonly, multiple sclerosis.

Disequilibrium, often referred to as dizziness of the feet, is an unsteady feeling, as though you might fall. If you wear reading glasses, you may have experienced a comparable sensation after removing them quickly. The problem often stems from a neurologic abnormality, such as a degenerative nerve disorder, but use of alcohol or certain medications may also be factors.

The sensation of lightheadedness is difficult to describe precisely; most people say simply that they feel dizzy. Lightheadedness often derives from anxiety or another psychological cause. It may happen in conjunction with hyperventilation, or overbreathing; this occurs when a person breathes too rapidly or deeply, taking in more than the usual amount of oxygen and thereby upsetting the body's balance of oxygen and carbon dioxide.

Diagnostic Studies and Procedures

The extent of a diagnostic evaluation depends upon the suspected cause of the dizziness. Tests range from an ear

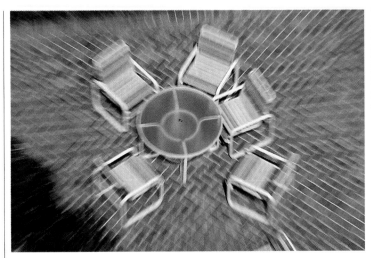

The most uncomfortable form of dizziness is vertigo, an illusion of motion that often causes nausea and vomiting.

examination, if the vestibular system of the inner ear is involved, to CT scans or MRI and other procedures, if a brain disorder is suspected.

Medical Treatments

Therapy for dizziness depends upon the underlying cause.

Nonprescription drugs such as dimenhydrinate and meclizine or prescription drugs such as scopolamine (Transderm Scōp), which is administered through a skin patch usually worn behind the ear, may prevent dizziness from motion sickness.

Antibiotics generally take care of dizziness when it is caused by an inner ear infection.

A change in medication or dosage usually alleviates any dizziness from medication; aspirin, tranquilizers, antimalarial drugs, certain antibiotics and anticonvulsants, and antihypertensive drugs are common offenders. (Ringing in the ears frequently precedes such an episode of dizziness.)

In the case of Ménière's disease, prescription diuretics may reduce fluids in the labyrinth section of the ear. During an attack, prescription antinausea drugs may be helpful.

Surgery can sometimes cure dizziness caused by a tumor along the nerve leading from the inner ear to the brain.

Alternative Therapies

Acupressure. There are two methods used to alleviate dizziness: Apply pressure with a thumb and index finger against the inside of the eye sockets between the eyebrows. Or use a thumb to press between the first and second metatarsal bones of your foot, located about two inches in from the angle where your big and second toes meet.

Herbal Medicine. Ginger is reputed to prevent and alleviate dizziness related to motion sickness, although scientific studies have not documented this. The herb can be taken as fresh ginger tea, two to four capsules of powdered ginger, or slices of candied ginger.

Meditation and Self-Hypnosis. These and other relaxation therapies, such as visualization, can ease anxiety and the lightheadedness it may cause.

Nutrition Therapy. A very low-fat diet has helped some people with inner ear problems and Ménière's disease. Improvement has been noted within two to three weeks of reducing fat to less than 10 percent of calories and increasing intake of fruits, vegetables, and whole-grain products.

Self-Treatment

If you are prone to dizziness, avoid abrupt movements that can bring it on. Get out of bed in stages, sitting for a minute or so before standing up.

Don't become overly hungry—eat several small meals a day. Abstain from alcohol and reduce your intake of caffeine, which can promote hyperventilation. If you do hyperventilate, you can restore a normal balance of oxygen and carbon dioxide by breathing in and out of a small paper bag.

Other Causes of Dizziness

Sometimes dizziness or lightheadedness that leads to fainting is a sign of a heart rhythm disturbance, a heart valve disease, or orthostatic hypotension, a sudden drop in blood pressure when one abruptly changes positions. Vasovagal syndrome, a condition characterized by extreme sensitivity of the vagus nerve in the chest and abdomen, can also cause dizziness and fainting.

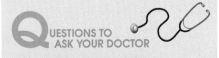

QUESTIONS TO ASK YOUR DOCTOR

▶ Could my dizziness be caused by medication? If so, can I change drugs or take a lower dosage?

Dry Mouth

(Xerostomia)

Dry mouth describes any condition in which reduced secretion of the salivary glands results in inadequate saliva, and the saliva that is produced is thicker than normal. Depending on the severity of the problem, a person may have not only dryness in the mouth, but also increased thirst, dry lips, or, in the worst cases, difficulty chewing and swallowing. Taste and smell may be impaired. Because mouth dryness permits more rapid bacterial growth, tooth decay and gum disease are more likely to occur.

Commonly, dry mouth is a consequence of smoking or a side effect of certain drugs, especially decongestants, antihistamines, antidepressants, atropine, and some heart and ulcer

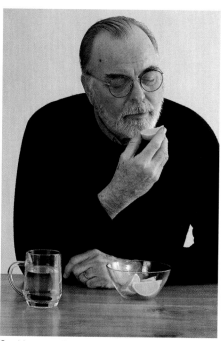

Sucking on a lemon to stimulate saliva flow and taking frequent sips of water or other fluids can alleviate a dry mouth.

medications. Cancer chemotherapy and radiation therapy to the mouth and throat also cause dry mouth. To some degree, all older people experience this condition, because saliva production naturally declines with age.

Diagnostic Studies and Procedures

A doctor or dentist can often diagnose a salivary gland disorder simply by feeling the glands and noting the reduced moisture in the mouth. However,

if the cause is not readily apparent, the physician may order blood tests to check for autoantibodies (antibodies that attack the body) and X-rays to check for structural abnormalities.

Medical Treatments

If an autoimmune disorder, such as lupus (page 278) or Sjögren's syndrome (see section on other causes), is responsible for the dry mouth, treatment is directed to controlling the underlying disease and alleviating the dryness. In severe cases, immunosuppressive drugs are given to halt the immune-system attack on healthy tissue.

If salivary glands suddenly become enlarged and painful, a painkiller with anti-inflammatory action, such as ibuprofen or aspirin, may be advised.

Anyone with dry mouth should see a dentist every three months for cleaning and periodontal treatments to help prevent a potentially dramatic increase in dental cavities and gum disease. The dentist may recommend special preventive fluoride treatments that can be performed at home.

Alternative Therapies

Herbal Medicine. Herbalists recommend sour or bitter herbs to stimulate the flow of saliva. Chinese green tea is a popular remedy. Teas made of ginger, cayenne, lemon balm, or chamomile may help. A mouthwash made of 5 to 10 drops of myrrh in a cup of warm water helps control mouth bacteria. Chewing mint leaves will freshen the mouth and help prevent bad breath—a common consequence of dry mouth.

Homeopathy. If gum disease accompanies dry mouth, practitioners may prescribe staphysagaria, mercurius solubilis, or a folic acid solution.

Nutrition Therapy. Vitamin C and beta carotene, found in such foods as carrots and sweet potatoes, may help prevent gum disease.

Self-Treatment

Self-care can alleviate the discomfort of dry mouth and help prevent dental disease. If you smoke, make every effort to stop; smoking aggravates dry mouth, and greatly increases the risk of serious dental problems. Avoid drugs, such as antihistamines and decongestants, that further decrease salivary secretion. Sip water or other sugar-free fluids throughout the day. To stimulate saliva production, try sucking on a lemon or sugarless lemon drops, nibbling a sour pickle, or chewing sugarless gum.

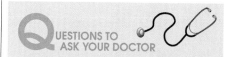

QUESTIONS TO ASK YOUR DOCTOR

▶ What is causing my dry mouth?
▶ If my dry mouth is caused by a drug, can I substitute another medication that doesn't have this side effect?
▶ What other drugs, besides antihistamines and decongestants, should I avoid to prevent worsening of the condition?

If dry mouth makes chewing and swallowing difficult, mash or purée food and moisten it with broth or other low-fat liquids. You may also want to try nonprescription saliva substitutes, available at most pharmacies. Some of the available products are liquid mouth sprays; others are gels that are placed along the gum line and then moved around the mouth to protect mucous membranes. Experiment with different types and tastes, and read product labels carefully to avoid those that contain sugar, which will increase the risk of tooth decay.

To reduce bacteria and freshen your breath, rinse your mouth often with an antiseptic mouthwash. To further protect your teeth, practice scrupulous dental hygiene, brushing your teeth at least twice a day and flossing every evening. Consider using an antibacterial toothpaste made especially for persons with dry mouth problems. Or mix baking soda and a few drops of 3 percent hydrogen peroxide into a paste and use this to brush your teeth, paying special attention to the gum line. To increase the antibacterial effect, let the paste remain in your mouth for a few minutes before rinsing it out.

Other Causes of Dry Mouth

Dry mouth may also accompany facial nerve paralysis (Bell's palsy), mumps, and infection of the mouth, throat, or salivary glands.

An extremely dry mouth is a primary symptom of Sjögren's syndrome, a chronic inflammatory disorder in which the immune system attacks the salivary glands. It may occur alone or in conjunction with other autoimmune diseases, such as systemic lupus erythematosus, rheumatoid arthritis, and scleroderma. Other mucous membranes—the eyes, nasal passages, throat, larynx, bronchi, vagina, and vulva—may also be abnormally dry.

Dry Skin

(Xeroderma)

When skin becomes very dry, it loses its softness, flexibility, moisture, and youthful look. It is rough and itchy and may appear wrinkled, shiny, or scaly.

New skin cells are constantly forming in the junction between the epidermis and dermis. These cells slowly rise to

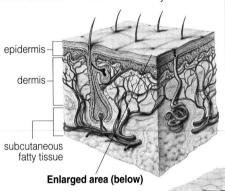

epidermis

dermis

subcutaneous fatty tissue

Enlarged area (below)

The skin constantly renews itself with new cells pushing their way upward from the dermis to the outer epidermis, bringing moisture and oily sebum to make the skin moist and supple.

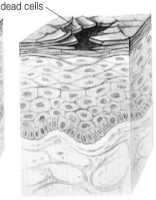

dead cells

epidermis

dermis

Normal skin   **Dry skin**

the outer skin layer, carrying with them moisture from the underlying dermis. They die and are shed as new cells emerge to take their place. This renewal process continues throughout life, but the skin's ability to retain moisture diminishes with age. Skin becomes dry when the moisture evaporates faster than it can be replenished. One reason is that the production of sebum, which contains oils that inhibit evaporation, diminishes as skin ages.

Other factors that promote dry skin include overheated rooms, exposure to soap and other harsh cleansers, frequent bathing in overly hot water, overexposure to the sun, and dry, windy climates. Hormonal changes, especially the drop in estrogen that follows menopause, can also cause skin dryness.

Diagnostic Studies and Procedures

A dermatologist can identify dry skin by its appearance. If the skin is severely dry or if a young person has suddenly developed dry, itchy skin, a physician may order blood tests to determine whether there is an underlying disease. She will also review the patient's medications and relevant lifestyle factors, such as spending time in the sun.

Medical Treatments

Dry skin rarely requires a doctor's care, but a dermatologist can help to design a self-treatment program. If nonprescription products are not effective, a doctor may recommend using Lac-Hydrin, a prescription drug that acts on skin-cell metabolism to help remoisturize overly dry skin.

Alternative Therapies

Aromatherapy. Massages that include the use of eucalyptus or other aromatic oils can help prevent excessive evaporation of moisture; massage also increases blood flow to the skin. Masks and cleansing creams containing essential aromatic oils may be beneficial as well.

Herbal Medicine. Herbalists recommend taking gamma linoleic acid (GLA)—a fatty acid found in evening primrose, black currant, and borage oils—to promote the healthy growth of skin, hair, and nails. The usual dosage consists of two to four "pearls" ingested daily. Lotions containing aloe vera help restore skin moisture.

Nutrition Therapy. Beta carotene (precursor to vitamin A) and vitamins C, D, and E contribute to healthy skin. Besides including foods rich in these nutrients in your diet, apply a thin film of vitamin E or wheat germ oil to the skin as a moisturizer.

Self-Treatment

Diligent self-care is the key to overcoming dry skin.

▶ When in the sun, apply a sunscreen with a SPF of at least 15. If the sunscreen irritates your skin, you may be sensitive to its ingredients. Ask a dermatologist to recommend a product.

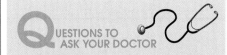

QUESTIONS TO ASK YOUR DOCTOR

▶ Are there special skin care products that might restore moisture to my skin?
▶ Could a medical disorder be causing my dry skin?

▶ Use moisturizers containing urea on your face and body after each washing.
▶ Exercise regularly to improve blood flow to the skin.
▶ If you smoke, stop. Smoking can reduce the flow of blood to the skin and may lower a woman's estrogen levels, thereby speeding the skin's aging.
▶ Take shorter showers, or better still, switch to tub baths. Use warm, not hot, water and oilated or superfatted soaps. If your skin is extremely dry, try a soap substitute. After bathing, pat the skin only semi-dry, then moisturize it.
▶ Avoid astringents and skin toners, unless they are specially formulated for dry skin. Gel masks, rather than paste masks, are appropriate when made for dry skin. Use oil-based makeup, and avoid cosmetics containing alcohol.
▶ In winter, set the thermostat at 68 or 70°F (20 or 21°C), and use a humidifier. In summer, avoid air conditioning, which dries the air, whenever possible.

Other Causes of Dry Skin

Patches of dry, itchy skin may indicate eczema, or, when scaly, psoriasis. Contact dermatitis produces dry, cracked, and scaly skin as a reaction to specific substances.

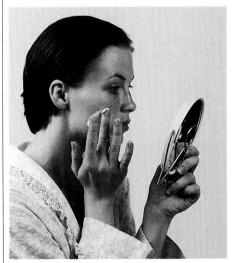

The best time to apply a moisturizer is right after washing, while skin is still moist. Use one that contains urea.

Earaches and Ear Infections

(External otitis; otitis media; labyrinthitis)
At some time, virtually everyone experiences an earache, with children being particularly susceptible. By the age of six, 90 percent of all children have had at least one middle ear infection.

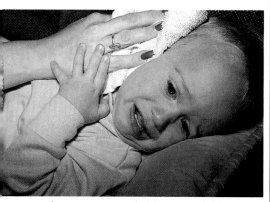

A warm compress held over a painful ear can help alleviate a child's earache.

An earache may be constant or intermittent, with pain that is dull, sharp, burning, or throbbing. Most earaches stem from infections, which are classified according to the part of the ear in which they occur.

Otitis media. This is an infection of the middle ear, the central portion made up of the eardrum (a hollow chamber) and an arrangement of tiny bones that are instrumental in hearing (see illustration, below right).

The middle ear of a child is especially vulnerable to infection because of the position and small size of the eustachian tube, the short, narrow tube that links nasal passages with the middle ear. The infection-causing organism can easily travel from the nasal passages into the middle ear during a cold or other illness in the upper respiratory tract (and nose-blowing during such an illness often forces fluid and mucus into the ear as well). In addition, swelling caused by tonsillitis, an allergy, or enlarged adenoids can block the eustachian tube, thus leading to an infection.

Otitis media can cause a perforated eardrum. In rare cases, mastoiditis, inflammation of the bone behind the ear, may develop.

External otitis. This refers to an infection in the external ear canal, which extends from the ear opening to the eardrum. Also called swimmer's ear, external otitis usually develops when water becomes trapped in the canal, creating prime conditions for a fungal or bacterial infection. Other causes include allergies and a foreign object or chemical irritant in the ear canal.

Inner ear infections. Though uncommon, infections of the innermost part of the ear can be quite serious. An infection of the labyrinth, the semicircular canals of the inner ear, can cause complete loss of hearing.

Barotitis. This ear pain develops during rapid changes in barometric pressure, such as when an airplane takes off or lands. It is usually harmless.

Diagnostic Studies and Procedures

A doctor will ask about recent symptoms such as a runny nose, sore throat, headache, fever, or nasal obstruction. He will then examine the ear with an otoscope, a lighted instrument that provides a magnified view of the inside of the ears. If he suspects a bacterial infection, he may also have a sample of pus or ear discharge cultured.

Medical Treatments

Treatment varies according to the cause and site of the earache. For a bacterial infection, a doctor will give antibiotics, either as ear drops or oral medication. It is critical to complete the entire course of therapy—usually 10 days— even if the symptoms disappear before all medication is used up; otherwise, the infection may recur. Blocked eustachian tubes may be opened with medicated nose drops.

Severe or chronic otitis media may require insertion of a small plastic drainage tube into the eardrum to prevent a buildup of pus and fluid. If a ruptured eardrum does not heal on its own, it will require surgical repair, a procedure called a tympanoplasty.

Depending upon the cause, swimmer's ear is usually treated with antibiotic, antifungal, or corticosteroid ear drops. A wicking device may be placed in the ear canal to carry the drops the length of the canal. Oral antibiotics may also be prescribed.

Inner ear infections are treated by draining accumulated fluid and then administering antibiotics. Surgery may be required to remove infected tissue.

Alternative Therapies

Numerous alternative remedies help alleviate earaches, but these are not substitutes for antibiotics.

Aromatherapy. An aromatherapist may recommend essence of basil in a vegetable oil to be applied around the ear twice daily for about three weeks.

Herbal Medicine. To relieve an earache, some herbalists suggest diluting the oil of one garlic capsule with four parts of a vegetable oil and slowly dripping this mixture into the affected ear and then inserting a puff of cotton in the outer ear to prevent the oil from draining out. Mullein oil is also used as eardrops to alleviate pain. However, eardrops should never be used if there is any chance that the eardrum has ruptured.

The structure of the middle ear makes it especially vulnerable to infection, particularly in young children. A drainage tube (below, right) may be inserted to prevent a ruptured eardrum.

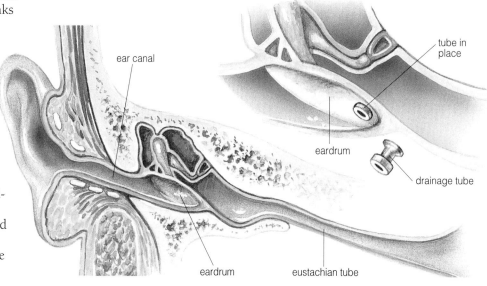

ear canal

tube in place

eardrum

drainage tube

eardrum

eustachian tube

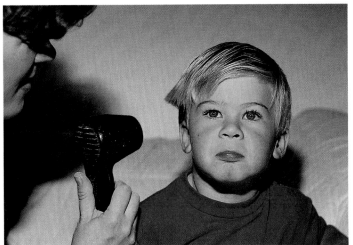

Keeping the ear canal dry is a key to preventing and treating swimmer's ear (external otitis). A hair dryer, set on warm, can be used when the ear has been exposed to water.

EARACHES AND EAR INFECTIONS (CONTINUED)

To fight an ear infection, herbalists suggest echinacea, or purple cone flower. This can be taken three times a day as a tea made from one to two grams of dried roots, a teaspoon of 1:5 tincture, ¼ to ½ teaspoon of 1:1 fluid extract, or 250 to 500 milligrams of 4:1 powdered solid extract.

Chinese herbalists use the pueraria combination (Ko-Ken-Tang) as the formula of choice. It consists of a combination of pueraria, ma-huang, ginger, jujube fruit, cinnamon twigs, and peony and licorice root.

Homeopathy. Ear pain may be treated with aconite, belladonna, ferrum phosphate, pulsatilla, sulphur, mercurius, chamomilla, hepar sulphite, alium cepa, lycopodium, or lachesis.

Naturopathy. Naturopaths often advocate thymus extract and supplements of beta carotene (precursor to vitamin A), vitamin C, zinc, and bioflavonoids as part of a preventive regimen. Zinc lozenges may also be recommended.

A dietary strategy during treatment calls for abstaining from solid foods for three days while drinking juices and other fluids. The regular diet is then resumed in stages: one-half of normal food intake on the first post-fast day; three-fourths on the second day, and then a complete diet.

Heated poultices may alleviate ear pain. One suggested mixture consists of ½ cup of unprocessed bran and ½ cup of kosher salt, wrapped in cheesecloth, heated until warm, and placed on the painful ear for an hour.

Osteopathy. A special technique called cranial osteopathy may be used to adjust the skull bones and to improve the flow of cerebrospinal fluid.

Reflexology. Hand points related to the ears are at the base of the ring finger and the middle portion of the little finger. Pressing or massaging these points for three minutes each hour is said to alleviate pain within a few hours. After the pain has passed, the points should be stimulated every four hours for four days, and then twice a day for two additional weeks.

Self-Treatment

Self-care may help to ease pain and prevent recurrences.

Aspirin or acetaminophen not only relieves pain but also reduces fever. Alternating warm and cold compresses may also help—apply a hot, wet towel to the painful ear for two minutes, then a cold towel for a few seconds. Repeat four or five times an hour until the pain eases. Lying on a heating pad set on low or medium may also help.

About ¼ teaspoon of warm castor oil or olive oil dropped into the ear canal is an old home remedy for earaches.

A ruptured eardrum often heals without treatment in a week or two. During this time, keep the ear clean and dry, and cover it with a plastic patch. Do not insert cotton or any other object.

To relieve barotitis, try swallowing, yawning, or chewing gum to restore normal air pressure in the ears. If discomfort persists, hold your nose, close your mouth, and exhale gently.

Many childhood ear infections can be prevented. Ask your doctor about using decongestant nose drops to prevent swelling and blockage of the eustachian tube. Feed a baby in a sitting position to prevent milk from entering the eustachian tube. Antihistamines may help if allergies are involved.

Use special care when blowing your nose; blow gently, one nostril at a time. Also, avoid sniffing, which can force mucus into the eustachian tube.

Keep the ear canal dry. After showering or shampooing, tilt the head to one side to allow any water to run out of the ear, then hold a hair dryer a few inches from the ear and direct warm (not hot) air into it.

If you are prone to swimmer's ear, always use protective ear plugs and wear a bathing cap while swimming. After swimming, place a few drops of a solution made with equal parts of white vinegar and rubbing (isopropyl) alcohol in each ear canal.

Members of swim teams sometimes use prescription eardrops that alter the acid/alkali balance in the ear canal. A nonprescription solution of boric acid and alcohol, which may produce the same effect, is also available. Again, never use eardrops or rinses if the eardrum has ruptured or ear drainage tubes have been inserted.

When you have swimmer's ear, place cotton in the infected ear when bathing or showering. Cover the cotton with petroleum jelly to make a watertight seal, and pull a shower cap down over the ear. Treat the infection overnight by placing in the ear a cotton ball soaked in Burow's solution or alcohol. In the morning, rinse the ear with 1 tablespoon of 3 percent hydrogen peroxide and ¼ cup of warm water. Consult a doctor if the pain and itching still persist after five days.

Other Causes of Earache

Excessive earwax and any foreign object that injure the external canal or lodge there can cause an earache. Other possible causes are an abscessed tooth, a gum infection, sinusitis, and temperomandibular joint problems.

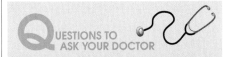

QUESTIONS TO ASK YOUR DOCTOR

▶ Do repeated ear infections carry a risk of permanent hearing loss?
▶ Is my child likely to outgrow recurrent ear infections? In the meantime, should drainage tubes be inserted?
▶ Does swimming in a public pool increase the risk of swimmer's ear?
▶ Can flying when I have a cold or earache cause a ruptured eardrum?

Earwax Buildup

(Cerumen impaction)

Earwax, or cerumen, normally lines the ear canal, a narrow tunnel about one inch long that extends from the outer ear to the eardrum. (This tunnel contains many nerve endings, so that even the slightest touch or pressure can cause discomfort.) Earwax, which is produced by glands in the canal, protects the inside of the ear, especially against water. When too much wax accumulates, however, it can cause pain, itching, ringing in the ears (tinnitus), and temporary loss of hearing.

Diagnostic Studies and Procedures

A doctor can easily detect a buildup of earwax by looking into the ear with an otoscope, a hand-held magnifying device with special lights. Physical examination of the ear canal also allows her to rule out other possible causes of the symptoms, such as an ear infection.

Medical Treatments

Earwax buildup is treated by removing the excess wax. Unless there is also an infection or a foreign body in the ear canal, no medication is needed. The wax may be removed by irrigation, but most ear specialists prefer to roll it out with an instrument shaped like a loop, or to extract it with a small vacuum device that is connected to a thin, flexible tube. These two approaches are more comfortable and less messy than the irrigation method.

Alternative Therapies

Reflexology. If you still have some loss of hearing, reflexologists suggest pressing the tips of your middle finger and ring fingers of one hand with the thumb and first finger of the other; do this for several minutes, four times daily. Other reflex points said to affect hearing are in the spaces behind the last wisdom teeth. Try biting down on a firm object placed between these gums, for five minutes, several times a day.

Homeopathy. To remove earwax, practitioners suggest placing two or three drops of pure olive oil in the ear for two or three nights in a row, and then clearing the ear with irrigation (see illustration below). Alternatively, you can try tincture of plantago or verbascum and thapsus to remove wax.

Self-Treatment

You can usually remove earwax by first softening it and then either allowing it to drain naturally from the ear or irrigating the ear. Do not attempt removal of earwax yourself if you have a perforated eardrum; seek medical treatment.

One approach for softening the wax involves using nonprescription ear drops. To insert the drops, lie down with the ear to be cleaned facing toward the ceiling. With one hand, pull the top of the ear gently up and toward the back of the head. Following the directions on the ear drops package, put the recommended amount into the ear canal. If possible, remain in the same position for 20 minutes; otherwise, gently plug the ear with cotton.

To irrigate the ear canal, sit up, leaning away from the affected side. Fill a soft rubber-bulb syringe with plain warm water or equal parts of warm water and 3-percent hydrogen peroxide, and insert the tip of the syringe into the ear canal. Gently squeeze the bulb to express the water, then leave the head tilted for a few seconds. Next, hold a small bowl beneath the ear and tilt the head the other way to allow the canal to drain. Repeat until the ear feels clear. You should see one or more plugs of earwax in the liquid that drains out.

Another method is to warm a tablespoonful of 3 percent hydrogen peroxide, place 10 drops of it in the ear canal, and allow it to remain for three minutes. Then tilt the head until the liquid runs out onto a tissue. Repeat two or three times. This should soften the wax, which will come out of the ear with the peroxide. If not, remove it by irrigating the ear with warm water.

Do not try to remove the wax with a stick or cotton swab, as this will only push the wax further into the ear canal and possibly cause an infection or damage to the eardrum.

Other Causes of Ear Symptoms

An ear infection, a tooth or gum abscess, or temporomandibular joint problems can bring about ear pain. Excessive use of aspirin or certain antibiotics and other medications sometimes produces ringing in the ears (tinnitus) and perhaps hearing loss. A foreign body in the ear canal, exposure to excessive noise, or trauma can cause ear pain and hearing loss.

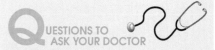

QUESTIONS TO ASK YOUR DOCTOR

▶ Is it safe to remove wax from a small child's ear myself?
▶ Does my excessive earwax suggest a vulnerability to any diseases? What actions should I take? (Some studies have linked excessive earwax to an increased risk of breast cancer.)

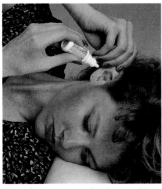

To soften earwax, lie down with the affected ear facing upward. Pulling the ear gently toward the back of the head, insert the prescribed amount of drops into it.

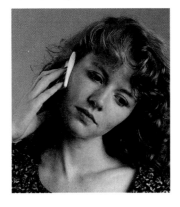

Remain in this position for 20 minutes; otherwise, use a soft cotton plug to prevent the drops from running out.

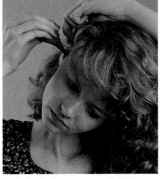

To irrigate the ear canal, fill it with warm water or equal parts warm water and 3 percent hydrogen peroxide, using a soft rubber ball syringe.

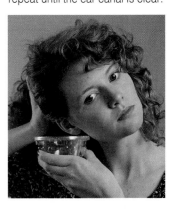

After a few seconds, tilt head in the oposite direction, allowing the water to flow into a small bowl; repeat until the ear canal is clear.

Eating Disorders

(Anorexia nervosa; bulimia)

Two of the most serious eating disorders are anorexia nervosa, a complex disease characterized by a distorted body image and self-starvation, and bulimia, which involves eating huge quantities of food followed by purging, usually through self-induced vomiting and/or laxative abuse.

More than 90 percent of those with either of these conditions are adolescent girls or young women; boys are affected only occasionally. Some persons have features of both disorders.

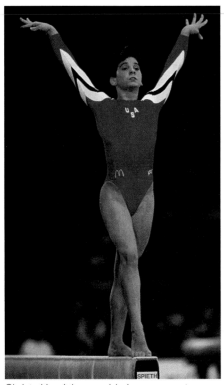

Christy Henrich, a world-class gymnast, was an anorectic who ultimately died of starvation.

Anorexia nervosa typically begins during early adolescence when a young girl becomes convinced that her maturing body is fat. Anorectics tend to be high achievers and are often described as obedient, ideal daughters. Some psychiatrists theorize that their eating behavior represents one aspect of life they feel they can control.

A person with anorexia chronically undereats, becoming thinner and thinner and, in extreme cases, literally starving to death, while remaining firmly convinced that she is over-weight. Many anorectics expend a great

deal of time and energy in preparing food, which they serve to others while eating only tiny amounts themselves. In addition, some of them have ritualistic eating habits, such as cutting food up into tiny pieces or arranging it very precisely on the plate.

The bulimic goes on periodic food binges, gorging on a large quantity of food in a short period of time. These binges are followed by purges, in which the individual forces vomiting and/or uses drugs to stimulate vomiting and bowel movements. Some bulimics also abuse diuretics, drugs that increase excretion of body fluids; others abuse amphetamines to prevent weight gain.

Bulimics and anorectics are secretive about their eating habits and typically deny that they have a problem. They tend to be obsessive about exercising. Many have low self-esteem, and some bulimics also exhibit other addictive behavior, such as alcohol abuse and compulsive shoplifting.

What causes these eating disorders is unknown, but some experts blame problematic family relationships. However, research suggests that eating disorders stem in part from brain chemical and hormonal imbalances.

Anorexia and bulimia are potentially fatal diseases. Anorectics can literally starve themselves to death, while bulimics have a high suicide rate. Metabolic and other changes brought about by their erratic eating behavior increases their risk of heart disease.

Diagnostic Studies and Procedures

Even if an eating disorder is suspected, the first step is a complete physical examination to rule out other illnesses, such as cancer or a chronic infection, particularly if extreme weight loss has occurred. While conducting the examination, the doctor will look for signs of anorexia and bulimia.

Indicators of anorexia include dry skin, thinning and brittle hair, low blood pressure, and a slow heart rate—all signs that the body is responding to starvation by shutting off or slowing down functions that are not vital to sustaining life. Some anorectics complain of constipation and intolerance to cold, and may even develop a soft body hair called lanugo as a response to the lower body temperature that occurs when body fat is lost. Another major symptom of anorexia is the absence of menstruation, due to the loss of body

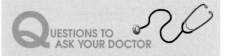

fat and the resulting hormonal changes. Mild anemia, lightheadedness, and sleep problems also suggest anorexia.

In diagnosing bulimia, the physical examination and medical history are also highly important. The doctor will look for damage to the teeth and gums caused by repeated exposure to the stomach acids in vomit. The esophagus may be inflamed due to vomiting, and glands near the cheeks might also be swollen. One or more fingers could be scarred as a result of pushing them down the throat to induce vomiting. And menstrual periods are likely to be irregular. The doctor will ask about dieting and exercise habits, as bulimics frequently diet and exercise incessantly without losing weight and generally regain weight if they do lose it.

Medical Treatments

Treatment of an eating disorder requires both psychological and medical care. Some form of psychotherapy is necessary, as well as medications if the person is severely depressed.

Anorectics often require hospitalization to treat malnutrition and other medical complications of starvation. Even then, calorie intake must be monitored closely to be sure the patient is eating, rather than hiding or disposing of food. (Anorectics have many strategies for misleading others into thinking they have eaten when they have not.)

Intravenous, or tube, feeding, bed rest, and intensive nursing care will probably be needed in order to restore the lost weight. At the same time, behavioral therapy is almost always called for to help change compulsive eating habits and obsessions concerning staying thin.

In many cases, psychological counseling is also recommended for the parents and other family members. Often, the mother also has a history of an eating disorder. She may be overweight or put undue emphasis on being thin. Some psychiatrists theorize that an anorectic daughter may be fulfilling her parents' unconscious desire that she remain a child.

Hospitalization for bulimics is rare, except for some patients who are very depressed. Group therapy works well for many bulimics, who tend to be ashamed of their binging and so feel relieved to find they are not alone in this behavior. Once they are able to discuss the problem in a therapeutic setting, treatment is more likely to work for them. An antidepressant drug may be prescribed in conjunction with dietary and behavioral therapy. Such drugs help control mood by increasing levels of serotonin (a brain chemical with a calming effect) in the circulation.

Alternative Therapies
Biofeedback and Visualization. These two techniques can be combined to reduce stress and help the person create new thought patterns to control compulsive eating habits. During biofeedback training, she becomes aware of the body's responses to compulsive behavior, which enables her to control them. Visualization involves "seeing" a desired response. The bulimic, for example, might learn to see herself eating a normal amount of food and then leaving the table feeling satisfied rather than guilty for overeating.

Hypnosis. Combined with other psychotherapeutic approaches, hypnosis and self-hypnosis can help the bulimic to control the impulse to binge and purge, and the anorectic to overcome the perception of being too fat.

Meditation. Yoga and other forms of meditation can help a person with an eating disorder to control stress, which is essential if treatment is to succeed.

Nutrition Therapy. This is the key to overcoming any eating disorder. A nutrition counselor can provide an understanding of the body's needs for well balanced meals and point out the health hazards of overly restrictive diets. The binge eater and the anorectic both need to learn how to plan menus and set reasonable goals for eating and weight control. The anorectic must also learn to accept more normal concepts of what constitutes ideal weight, overweight, and underweight, and to understand what the consequences of extreme thinness can be. Frequent sessions with a nutritionist may be necessary over a period of time, so that eating habits and weight can be monitored.

Self-Treatment
Because people with eating disorders typically deny their problem, ignoring symptoms and constructing elaborate strategies for deceiving others about their eating habits, self-treatment is usually not effective unless supported by some form of therapy. In general,

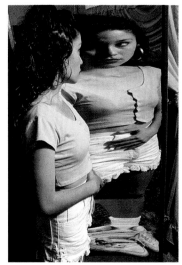

An anorectic perceives of herself as being overweight even though she may be painfully thin.

people with eating disorders are unlikely to seek treatment on their own. Yet the earlier treatment begins, the more likely it is to be successful.

During psychotherapy, anorectics and bulimics gradually learn to stop denying that they have a problem and to set goals for maintaining normal eating habits. Family members may need counseling to understand how they can be helpful and how to avoid being misled or making the problem worse.

Other Causes of Weight Loss
Many serious illnesses can cause severe weight loss and an emaciated appearance; these include cancer, heart disease, thyroid disorders, and AIDS.

A CASE IN POINT

Alice, a tall, slightly chubby 17-year-old student, began dieting when she was 10. By the age of 12, she had graduated to binging and vomiting—a pattern that soon dominated her life. At the time, she was a competitive swimmer, and she had to be thin to remain on the team.

Before a swim meet, Alice would go without eating for several days to get her weight down. But then, an uncontrollable urge to eat would send her to the kitchen—usually late at night when her family was asleep—where she would raid the cupboards and refrigerator for sweets. She later recalled that at a single sitting she might consume an entire pie, a quart of ice cream, and whatever else she could find, stopping only when she was so full that her stomach was painfully distended. By then, she would feel over-

come with remorse, and would spend an hour or more forcing herself to vomit.

The adolescent started taking her mother's diet pills, even though they made her feel jumpy. Occasionally, she took a handful of laxatives as well.

By the time she was 15, Alice was binging and purging at least four times a week. Even so, she slowly gained weight; at 16, she weighed 180 pounds, while standing 5 feet 9 inches tall.

By then, almost every waking thought was centered on food and her weight. Through crash dieting, she managed to lose 30 pounds. She then dropped out of school for five months, staying at home and going through several binge-vomit cycles a day. In desperation, her parents admitted her to a hospital-based program for treatment of eating disorders. But

while there, she became depressed and attempted suicide by cutting her wrists.

Psychiatrists working with Alice generally described her as neatly dressed, well oriented, and rational. After an interview with her, one doctor wrote: "She realizes she has a serious problem with binge eating, but feels rather hopeless about getting the behavior under control."

Summarizing Alice's eating problems, the psychiatrists called it a classic case of bulimia, and recommended both individual psychotherapy and group therapy with other bulimics, to help her achieve a normal eating pattern and to become more comfortable with her body. Her success is reflected in the fact that her average weight now ranges between 150 and 160 pounds—only slightly above her ideal weight of 145 pounds.

Eczema

(Atopic, nummular, or steatotic eczema)
Eczema refers to a wide variety of skin conditions. In general, lesions that are red, blistering, oozing, scaly, brownish, thickened, and itchy may all be considered eczema. The term is often used interchangeably with dermatitis, which causes similar lesions, but unlike eczema, dermatitis usually has an identifiable external cause.

Eczema afflicts people of all ages, but certain forms of the disorder are more prevalent during specific life stages. For example, atopic eczema, sometimes referred to as infantile eczema, occurs mostly in babies, children, and young adults. Nummular, or discoid, eczema occurs mostly in adults. Its red, coin-shaped patches—which may become swollen, blistered, or crusty—sometimes itch and often ooze or thicken.

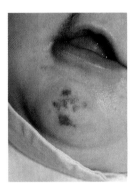

Atopic, or infantile, eczema typically develops early in life and is characterized by itchy blisters.

Some elderly people develop a condition called steatotic eczema, in which the skin becomes dry and scaly. Doctors think this is due to the loss of skin lipids that occurs with aging.

Allergies and eczema appear to be related, and both conditions tend to run in families. Stress can trigger a flare-up.

Diagnostic Studies and Procedures

The appearance of the skin patches usually forms the basis of a diagnosis. To distinguish eczema from allergic, or contact, dermatitis, a doctor will ask about substances to which the skin has been exposed; he may then order skin tests to identify possible allergens. Skin scrapings may also be studied under a microscope to rule out bacterial or fungal skin infections.

Medical Treatments

Anti-inflammatory medications are often prescribed to be taken by mouth or applied to the skin lesions. The most commonly prescribed topical medications are coal tar and cortisone cream. Mild eczema may respond to hydrocortisone in a nonprescription strength of 0.5 or 1 percent, but the prescription strength of 2.5 percent is usually needed. In certain cases, a doctor will recommend applying a liberal coating of hydrocortisone to affected areas at night and then covering them with plastic wrap or other occlusive dressing.

Oral antihistamines are often used to reduce itching and thus break the itch-scratch-itch cycle. If bacterial infection has already developed as a result of scratching, antibiotics may be prescribed. Oral cortisone, sedatives, or tranquilizers can help severe itching.

Alternative Therapies

Herbal Medicine. Creams or ointments containing chickweed, stinging nettle, or heartsease (tricolored sweet violets) are herbal remedies said to alleviate the itchiness and oozing lesions of eczema. For adults, some herbalists also recommend systemic treatments with various teas or tinctures, especially burdock or stinging nettle.

Naturopathy and Nutrition Therapy. A naturopath may recommend taking supplements of zinc, bioflavonoids, and vitamins A, E, and C, as well as two to four capsules of evening primrose oil three times a day, and 1 teaspoon of flaxseed oil once a day.

A food allergy can trigger eczema, especially in a young child. To identify the allergy, nutrition therapists often recommend eliminating such foods as milk products, eggs, tomatoes, and citrus fruits. If the eczema improves, the foods are then reintroduced one at a time; a flare-up may indicate an allergy and avoiding that food in the future should solve the problem.

Relaxation Techniques. Excessive stress frequently aggravates eczema. Meditation, yoga, self-hypnosis, or visualization can improve one's ability to cope with periods of stress.

Self-Treatment

Many of the remedies used for dry skin (page 166) can alleviate eczema too. It is also a good idea to use hypoallergenic skin products that are formulated especially for dry skin.

Adding 1 cup of Aveeno powder or other colloidal oatmeal product, or ½ cup of baking soda, to a tepid bath may help to reduce itching. An over-the-counter antihistamine taken at bedtime can reduce itching and promote sleep.

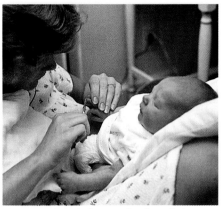

Keeping a baby's fingernails clipped short helps minimize the effects of scratching, which can make a skin condition feel worse.

After bathing or showering, apply a moisturizing cream, gel, or skin medication recommended by a doctor. As much as possible, wear soft cotton clothing next to your skin.

If you live in a dry climate, you may benefit from a central humidifier; conversely, if heat and humidity seem to intensify itching, try using a dehumidifier and air conditioning. And avoid rapid changes of temperature, which can also aggravate eczema.

Brief exposure to the sun's ultraviolet rays can help heal eczema, but it is important not to get sunburned—this can worsen the disorder, in addition to damaging skin and increasing the risk of developing skin cancer later.

If you have severe eczema, you should eschew activities that provoke sweating. Instead of jogging or doing aerobics, for example, try swimming.

Other Causes of Itchy Skin Rashes

Many conditions can cause rashes and itching similar to those of eczema. These include an adverse reaction to medication, hives, prickly heat, diaper rash, scabies, insect bites, and skin infections, especially impetigo, a bacterial infection, and ringworm, caused by a fungal infection.

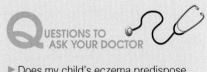

QUESTIONS TO ASK YOUR DOCTOR

▶ Does my child's eczema predispose him to other skin problems?
▶ Are there drugs I should avoid taking because they worsen eczema?
▶ Would moving to a different climate lessen the severity of my eczema?

Edema

(Angioedema; lymphedema)

An abnormal accumulation of fluid in body tissues causes a type of swelling called edema. This swelling may be localized, as with ascites (the distended abdomen that develops in cases of liver disease and some types of cancer), or generalized, occurring throughout the body, as with progressive kidney failure. In the early stages of generalized edema, the swelling may not be obvious, but a rapid, seemingly mysterious weight gain may take place.

Hormonal factors can produce edema. Two examples are the swelling that occurs during pregnancy and the premenstrual phase of a woman's monthly cycle. Heart failure, advanced kidney disease, malnutrition, and thyroid disorders are among the other causes.

Diagnostic Studies and Procedures

Since edema is a symptom of a wide range of disorders, the diagnostic goal is to find the underlying cause. In addition to taking a medical history and conducting a physical examination, a doctor will pay special attention to the location and nature of the swelling. For example, facial puffiness and generalized swelling point to possible kidney failure. Swelling of the lower legs, accompanied by difficult breathing, indicates congestive heart failure. Marked swelling of one leg or arm suggests blockage of that limb's lymph channels. After observing such signs, a doctor will order tests, which may include X-rays and scans, to verify or rule out probable causes.

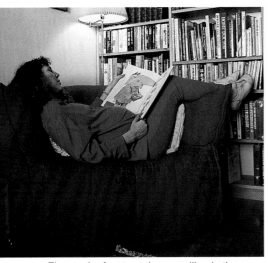

Elevate the feet to reduce swelling in the ankles and lower legs.

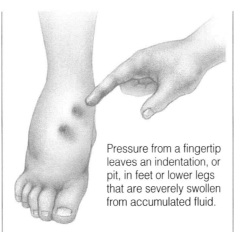

Pressure from a fingertip leaves an indentation, or pit, in feet or lower legs that are severely swollen from accumulated fluid.

Medical Treatments

The medical approach varies according to the underlying cause, but the use of diuretics, commonly referred to as water pills, are a mainstay in the treatment of many forms of edema. For example, diuretics combined with digitalis, a medication that slows and strengthens the heartbeat, may help edema caused by heart failure; however, the digitalis dose must be carefully adjusted to make sure that it is large enough to be effective but not so large as to cause toxicity. Diuretics alone are usually sufficient during the early stages of edema from kidney failure, but this condition may require dialysis eventually. A kidney transplant may also be considered in severe cases.

An antihistamine such as diphenhydramine may counter edema when it is part of an allergic response. Anaphylactic shock—which includes marked, generalized swelling that threatens to block the airway—may necessitate an injection of adrenaline (epinephrine), in addition to antihistamine.

Sometimes excess fluid, as from abdominal swelling related to liver disease or ovarian cancer, can be drained away with a hollow needle.

Alternative Therapies

Edema often has a serious underlying cause that requires conventional medical treatment. Alternative therapies should be considered only after checking with your doctor.

Herbal Medicine. Dr. William Withering, an 18th-century English physician, observed that the leaves of the foxglove, or digitalis, plant reduced edema. Thus, digitalis became the first effective heart medication, and a synthesized form of the herb remains one of the most effective treatments for heart failure. You should never attempt to prepare your own drug, however, because digitalis made from foxglove can be lethal if too much is consumed. Herbalists recommend uva-ursi as a much safer diuretic. The usual dosage is one to three capsules a day or a tea made from one tablespoon of the dried herb in a cup of water.

Nutrition Therapy. Salt restriction is an important aspect of reducing edema. Other dietary limitations may also apply, depending upon the cause of the edema. For example, edema related to kidney disease may require a low-fat, low-protein diet. In such cases, a qualified nutritionist should be consulted in structuring a balanced diet.

T'ai Chi and Yoga. The gentle exercises of these movement therapies can help minimize arm and leg swelling from obstructed lymph vessels.

Self-Treatments

In addition to restricting your intake of salt, you can do the following:

▶ Strive to maintain weight that is ideal for your age and height.

▶ For leg swelling, rest several times a day with your legs elevated. Also, try wearing elastic or surgical stockings.

▶ To prevent arm swelling that results from a mastectomy, do the exercises shown on page 110.

▶ To alleviate nighttime pulmonary edema, sleep in a semi-sitting position; use extra pillows or elevate the head of your bed a few inches.

▶ Abstain from alcohol, or use it in moderation, especially if the edema is related to liver disease.

▶ If your eyelids swell, you may be allergic to your makeup. Try a hypoallergenic brand. Treat lid puffiness with cold compresses or with compresses made from used tea bags.

Other Causes of Fluid Buildup

In addition to the diseases already mentioned, alcoholism, the use of oral contraceptives and other hormonal preparations, injuries, and certain infections may result in edema.

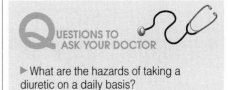

QUESTIONS TO ASK YOUR DOCTOR

▶ What are the hazards of taking a diuretic on a daily basis?
▶ Should I reduce my intake of fluids?
▶ Do I need a special diet?

Electric Shock

Electric shock results when an electric current passes through the body, either from lightning or an artificially generated source. The impact ranges from a slight tingling to electrocution. Between these extremes, electricity may cause minor to major burns and temporary to irreversible tissue damage. A strong electric jolt may also produce traumatic shock, in which the body's vital processes are profoundly disturbed.

In other instances, a brief electrical shock can be therapeutic—for example, one that is administered through a defibrillator can restore a normal heartbeat, thus preventing death from an abnormal heart rhythm.

Factors that determine the severity of an electric shock include:

Type and magnitude of the current. For both AC and DC, damage increases with a higher voltage and amperage.
Resistance of the body at the point where the electrical contact is made. Moist, thin skin is 40 times less resistant than dry, unbroken skin.
Path along which the current travels. If skin resistance is high, the electricity is dissipated along the surface and does not penetrate. If the skin resistance is low, the current enters the body, burning internal tissues. The most dangerous pathway is one that reaches the heart or brain.
Duration of current flow. Internal injuries are directly related to the length of exposure time. For example, when lightning strikes, the voltage is high, but the duration of current flow is extremely brief. A lightning strike rarely causes burns, but it may disrupt the body's internal electrical impulses that control the brain and the heart.

Diagnostic Studies and Procedures

An electric shock does not always produce obvious burns. A careful examination is necessary to detect internal injuries. This starts with assessing vital signs—blood pressure, heart rate, and consciousness—to rule out traumatic shock. The doctor then looks for fractures and other injuries.

Medical Treatments

Treatment will depend on the effects of the electric shock.

Extensive burns may necessitate a tetanus shot, as well as antibiotics and other medications.

DURING A THUNDERSTORM

▶ Seek appropriate shelter at the first sounds of thunder. Thunderclouds discharge the most electricity just before the rain begins to fall.
▶ If you're in a car, stay there, but don't play the radio.
▶ If you're in the water, get to shore as quickly as possible.
▶ If you're in an open area, such as a golf course or camping ground, drop whatever you're holding that might conduct electricity (golf club, metal bat) and lie on your side or squat down on the lowest ground, such as a dry hollow, with your head between your knees. Don't seek refuge under a tall tree or other high structure—lightning strikes the tallest available object.
▶ Do not use the telephone during a thunder and lightning storm. A surge of electricity can travel through the phone line and deliver a fatal shock into the ear.

After a severe shock from lightning, fluids may be restricted to help prevent brain swelling. Sedatives or tranquilizers may also be prescribed. During hospitalization, heart rhythm and kidney function will be closely monitored, and a CT scan or MRI may be ordered to rule out a brain injury or swelling.

Alternative Therapies

Possible alternative treatments are similar to those for burns (page 117).

Self-Treatment

A victim of electric shock needs medical care, but you can prevent such injuries to yourself and family at home.
▶ Unplug all appliances, such as food processors, toasters, and microwave ovens, when they are not in use.
▶ Replace damaged cords and plugs.
▶ Make sure that sockets and outlets are not overloaded.
▶ Cover all unused outlets and extension cord receptacles with safety caps.
▶ Never use a hair drier or other electrical appliance in the tub or shower.

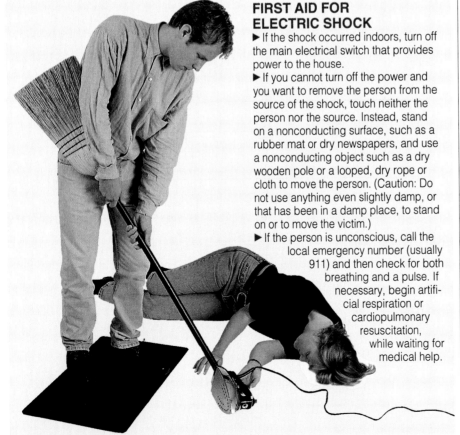

FIRST AID FOR ELECTRIC SHOCK

▶ If the shock occurred indoors, turn off the main electrical switch that provides power to the house.
▶ If you cannot turn off the power and you want to remove the person from the source of the shock, touch neither the person nor the source. Instead, stand on a nonconducting surface, such as a rubber mat or dry newspapers, and use a nonconducting object such as a dry wooden pole or a looped, dry rope or cloth to move the person. (Caution: Do not use anything even slightly damp, or that has been in a damp place, to stand on or to move the victim.)
▶ If the person is unconscious, call the local emergency number (usually 911) and then check for both breathing and a pulse. If necessary, begin artificial respiration or cardiopulmonary resuscitation, while waiting for medical help.

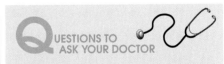

QUESTIONS TO ASK YOUR DOCTOR

▶ If I wear a pacemaker, what special precautions should I take around electrical equipment? Can lightning interfere with its programming?
▶ How should a mild electrical burn be treated?

Emphysema

(Chronic obstructive pulmonary disease; COPD)

Emphysema is a chronic condition in which the alveoli, or air sacs, of the lungs have lost their elasticity and become stretched out and filled with stale air. As a result, the tiny blood vessels in the sacs cannot perform their normal function of picking up a fresh supply of oxygen while getting rid of carbon dioxide and other waste products; thus the breathing process is labored and inefficient.

As the alveoli become more diseased, the body is increasingly starved for oxygen, and the slightest exertion produces shortness of breath and fatigue. A person with emphysema eventually develops a barrel-shaped chest because the lungs are expanded with stale air that cannot be exhaled.

The primary cause of emphysema is smoking, although air pollution, occupational exposure to toxic chemicals and gases, chronic bronchitis and other lung disorders, and an inherited tendency to develop the condition may also be responsible.

Diagnostic Studies and Procedures

Diagnosis begins with gathering background information. A doctor will want to know whether you ever smoked and if you have recurring bronchitis or asthma. This is followed by a physical examination with particular attention to lung function. A definitive diagnosis requires a simple test called spirometry,

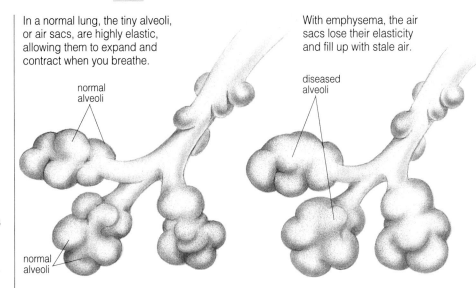

In a normal lung, the tiny alveoli, or air sacs, are highly elastic, allowing them to expand and contract when you breathe.

normal alveoli

normal alveoli

With emphysema, the air sacs lose their elasticity and fill up with stale air.

diseased alveoli

in which you take a deep breath and then exhale as much air as you can as quickly as possible. This test indicates whether you can empty your lungs normally. Other diagnostic studies include lung X-rays, lung scans, and blood studies to check for signs of infection and measure levels of oxygen and carbon dioxide reaching the body's tissues.

Medical Treatments

Emphysema has no cure, but medical treatments can relieve its symptoms, slow the progression of the disease, and help to delay disability.

Drug therapy usually includes the use of bronchodilators, medications that relax the airway and facilitate the flow of air in and out of the lungs. These drugs are usually taken at regular intervals several times a day, rather than only when symptoms appear.

Corticosteroid drugs, in either oral or inhaled form, may be prescribed to counter lung inflammation, and antibiotics may be given, not only to treat airway infections but also to prevent them. For example, a doctor may advise a patient to take antibiotics at the first sign of a cold to stave off a secondary infection—even though the drugs will have no effect against the cold itself. Annual flu shots are a particularly important preventive measure, as is immunization against pneumococcal pneumonia, because these illnesses can be life threatening for any person who has emphysema.

Severe cases may require supplemental oxygen, administered through tubes in the nostrils. This can be given at home, although hospitalization is sometimes necessary.

An experimental operation in which 20 to 30 percent of the damaged lung tissue is removed has brought dramatic improvement to some patients with advanced emphysema. Reducing the size of the distended lungs allows more room for the remaining tissue to inflate when inhaling. The operation does not halt progression of the disease, however; in severe cases, a lung transplant may be considered.

Alternative Therapies

Aromatherapy. Thyme oil, which is extracted from the flowering tops of the plant, is said to have therapeutic qualities useful in alleviating emphysema. Aromatherapists also use the oils from hyssop plants and eucalyptus trees to treat respiratory ailments. These oils may be inhaled by placing a few drops in a bath or a basin of hot water and breathing the vapor, or by putting the drops on a handkerchief and placing it on your pillow at night.

Herbal Medicine. To clear the lungs of phlegm, herbalists recommend adding 1 teaspoon of powdered elecampane root to 1 cup of cold water, letting it stand for 9 to 10 hours, and then heating the water and drinking the solution while it is hot. This remedy should be taken two or three times daily.

Chinese herbalists use the ma-huang combination, which consists of cinnamon, licorice root, apricot seeds, and ma-huang, to treat emphysema and other pulmonary disorders.

T'ai Chi. This gentle exercise is recommended to help emphysema sufferers maintain their muscle tone and fitness without excessive exertion. It also fosters a sense of well-being.

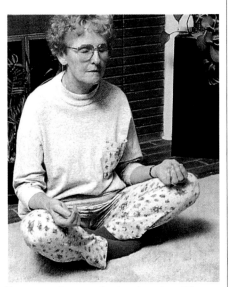

Yoga exercises emphasize deep breathing utilizing the diaphragm. They may help a person with emphysema breathe more efficiently.

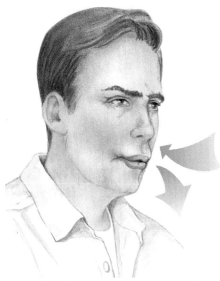

A technique for helping to rid the lungs of stale air is to exhale slowly through lips pursed as if your were going to whistle.

EMPHYSEMA (CONTINUED)

Yoga. Abdominal yoga exercises that emphasize deep diaphragmatic breathing are said to increase oxygen flow.

Self-Treatment

The most important aspect of self-treatment is to quit smoking and to avoid exposure to secondhand smoke and other lung irritants. Because emphy-sema begins years before symptoms appear, stopping smoking while you are still healthy can halt the progression of lung damage before it becomes disabling. Some of the early changes in lung function from smoking may even be reversed after you give up the habit.

Living with emphysema involves pacing yourself and allowing for rest periods whenever you feel short of breath. If you set priorities for daily activities, you won't become overly tired. Regular exercise such as walking can help prevent disability, but you should avoid overly strenuous activities that stress the heart and lungs.

Learn pursed-lip breathing methods to minimize exhaustion during physical activity: Inhale deeply through your nose, and exhale slowly and steadily through a small opening between pursed lips. Exhale for twice as long as you inhale. This technique slows down your breathing and helps expel stale air from your lungs.

If you are overweight, make every effort to lose the extra pounds. Reduce salt intake, especially if you suffer from fluid retention and swelling of the feet and lower legs, a complication that may

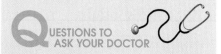

result from cor pulmonale, a form of heart failure that is associated with advanced emphysema.

Other Causes of Breathing Difficulties

Chronic and progressive breathing difficulties can be the result of any lung infection or inflammation, including AIDS-related pneumonia, tuberculosis, chronic bronchitis, and such occupational lung disorders as black lung disease. Bronchiectasis, a condition in which bronchial tubes become dilated and blocked with thick secretions, also hampers breathing, as does congestive heart failure, a condition in which the lungs become congested with fluid that the heart is unable to pump out.

A CASE IN POINT

Robert Warren, a retired professor of public health, prided himself in keeping active. Although no longer teaching at his university, he worked three days a week as a health-policy consultant. He also enjoyed outdoor work, especially gardening and landscaping.

Warren readily admits that his health problems were largely self-induced. Despite a long history of lung disorders, he continued to smoke two packs of cigarettes a day. Over the last few years, he had suffered at least one attack of bronchitis in the winter, with each bout lasting longer than the one before. But after a midwinter vacation in Arizona or some other warm, sunny place, his lungs would clear and he could return to his usual routine. Nevertheless, the cumulative damage to his lungs eventually became impossible to deny.

"Fatigue was my first symptom," Warren recalls. "Climbing stairs was especially trying. By the time I'd get to the top, I was out of breath and each leg felt like it weighed a ton."

At that point, he went to his doctor. After a careful examination of Warren's heart and lungs, the doctor referred him to a testing laboratory for a complete set of pulmonary function tests. These tests confirmed that Warren had chronic obstructive lung disease (COPD), with emphysema the predominant feature.

"I wasn't surprised at the diagnosis," Warren admits. He knew that emphysema was an irreversible, progressive disease, but there were some optimistic findings: Although he had suffered frequent bouts of bronchitis, the ailment was not yet chronic—a good sign. COPD in which bronchitis predominates is especially lethal, because the inflammation and increased mucus in the bronchi further clog the airway.

Warren anticipated the treatment regimen that would be proposed by a team of lung specialists—stop smoking immediately. "I had tried in the past, but now it was a matter of life and death," he says. He quit cold turkey and has not smoked since.

Although Warren was already physically active, his doctor recommended a structured exercise conditioning program that called for walking two miles a day, four or five times a week. Warren also went to a pulmonary therapist to learn diaphragmatic and pursed-lip breathing techniques, which help force stale air out of the lungs.

To avoid future bouts of bronchitis, Warren now spends the entire winter in a warm climate. As an added precaution, he takes antibiotics at the first sign of a cold. He also has prescription bronchodilator medication to help open his airways if he feels short of breath.

It has now been three years since Warren's emphysema was first diagnosed. At his last checkup, his doctor was surprised—and pleased—to note a modest improvement in Warren's pulmonary function test. "This does not mean that the previous damage has been reversed," the doctor explained, "but it does indicate increased capacity of the unaffected lung tissue."

Encephalitis

Any inflammation of the brain is referred to as encephalitis. The most common type, viral encephalitis, may be primary or secondary. Organisms that cause primary encephalitis include the polio, Coxsackie, and Type 1 herpes simplex viruses, as well as tick- or mosquito-borne arboviruses, which sometimes cause outbreaks of equine encephalitis in the summer.

Secondary viral encephalitis can occur as a complication of a disease such as measles, mumps, rubella, or chickenpox. Such bacterial diseases as syphilis, streptococcus pneumonia, and tuberculosis can also be the cause of encephalitis. Sometimes meningitis, an inflammation of the membranes that cover the brain and spinal cord, also involves the brain itself.

Diagnostic Studies and Procedures

Mild viral encephalitis often goes undiagnosed, because the symptoms—fever, headache, and malaise—are short-lived and attributed to flu or another minor illness. However, in its more severe form, encephalitis causes dizziness, confusion, vomiting, and a high fever. As the disease progresses, symptoms may include weakness or paralysis, impaired speech and hearing, delirium, excessive drowsiness, and coma.

If such symptoms develop after a bout of a disease known to cause secondary encephalitis, a doctor should immediately suspect the disorder. But if the symptoms appear abruptly, other possibilities will be considered first.

In addition to studies of blood and spinal-fluid samples, tests may include a CT scan or MRI to rule out a brain abscess or tumor. After encephalitis is confirmed, further tests may be needed to identify the precise cause, so that treatment can be directed to eradicating it.

Medical Treatments

Mild encephalitis usually does not require treatment other than rest. If the the herpes simplex virus is causing the

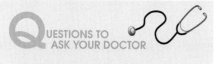

Q UESTIONS TO
ASK YOUR DOCTOR

▶ Aside from the usual immunizations, what steps can I take to protect my child from encephalitis?
▶ Is permanent brain damage likely?

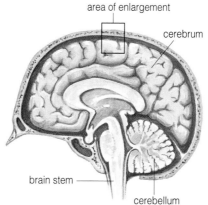

area of enlargement

cerebrum

brain stem

cerebellum

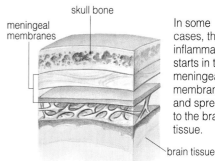

Encephalitis is an inflammation and swelling in any part of the brain; there may also be small hemorrhages scattered throughout.

skull bone

meningeal membranes

brain tissue

In some cases, the inflammation starts in the meningeal membranes and spreads to the brain tissue.

inflammation, intravenous treatment with acyclovir (Zovirax) or vidarabine (Vira-A) is begun as soon as possible and continued for at least 10 days.

When encephalitis is secondary to another infection, the underlying disease is treated. For example, antibiotics are used when the cause is a bacterial infection. Rest, replacement of fluids, and fever control are necessary to speed recovery. Adults can take either aspirin or acetaminophen to reduce a fever. Children can be given acetaminophen (important for preventing a seizure if temperature reaches 103°F), but not aspirin, because it increases the risk of Reye's syndrome (see box, page 437).

If excess fluid accumulates in the brain, mannitol, a diuretic, may be administered intravenously. Alternatively, the fluid may be removed by aspiration or by insertion of a shunt that carries it away from the brain.

The long-term outlook varies considerably and is not necessarily related to the severity of the disease. A person who is extremely ill may make a full recovery, while someone with a seemingly mild case may suffer permanent neurological damage.

Alternative Therapies

The severe symptoms of encephalitis require prompt medical treatment. Alternative therapies should be considered only after checking with the primary-care doctor.

Hydrotherapy. Feverish patients may benefit from cool compresses and sponge baths with cool or tepid water.

Herbal Remedies. To lower fever, some herbalists recommend 10 to 40 drops of boneset extract in a cup of warm water. Others advocate 1 to 3 capsules of feverfew a day, or 2 capsules of white willow bark every three hours. This last should not be given to a child, however,

because it contains salicylate, an ingredient chemically similar to aspirin.

Physical Therapy. Services of physical and occupational therapists may be necessary, especially if the encephalitis results in permanent neurological problems. Some patients also may benefit from speech therapy if that function has been affected.

Self-Treatment

Stay in bed until symptoms abate. Eat light, nourishing meals and drink lots of fluids. During recovery, regularly do moderate exercise, such as walking, to regain your strength.

To avoid encephalitis spread by mosquitoes or ticks, use an insect repellent when outdoors and make sure window screens are in good repair. Place some mosquito netting over cribs and beds if equine encephalitis occurs in your area. When traveling to or camping in mosquito-infested areas, take along fine-mesh netting to sleep under.

Other Causes of Brain Inflammation

Brain inflammation may also be due to toxoplasmosis, a parasitic infection, or aspergillosis, a fungal infection. Lead poisoning can also cause an inflammation of the brain. People with AIDS, patients taking drugs that suppress the immune system, and others with lowered immunity are at a high risk of developing unusual brain infections.

To protect an infant or toddler from equine encephalitis, use mosquito netting over the crib, carriage, or stroller.

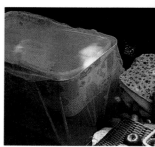

Endocarditis

(Acute and subacute bacterial endocarditis; nonbacterial thrombotic endocarditis)
Endocarditis is an inflammation or infection of the endocardium, the inner lining of the heart valves and chambers, and most often occurs in the valves.

In the past, this condition was often a consequence of rheumatic fever, a childhood infection that commonly attacks the heart, but this is no longer true because strep throat—an infection that can lead to rheumatic fever—is now quickly detected and treated.

Although anyone can develop endocarditis under certain circumstances, today it is most prevalent among intravenous drug abusers and people who have valvular heart disease, especially those with artificial heart valves or certain types of congenital heart defects.

The infection develops when bacteria have an opportunity to invade the bloodstream, for example, during dental procedures or surgery, especially colon, urologic, or gynecologic operations. Skin infections also increase the risk.

Symptoms suggesting endocarditis include a persistent low-grade fever, shortness of breath, increasing weakness, night sweats, joint pain, general malaise, and the appearance of tiny purple spots, or petechia, on the chest, fingers, toes, or in the mouth.

Diagnostic Studies and Procedures
The initial diagnosis is generally made on the basis of medical history and symptoms, and by listening to the

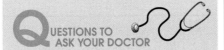

sounds of the heart. Subacute endcarditis, which causes only mild symptoms, can be difficult to detect, but development of a new heart murmur raises suspicion of the disorder. The eyes may also show small hemorrhages in the mucous membranes.

To confirm the diagnosis, a blood sample will be cultured to look for the presence of bacteria. An echocardiogram, or ultrasound imaging of the heart, may also reveal clumps of bacteria on the heart valves.

Medical Treatments
The mainstay of treatment is intensive antibiotic therapy, which is usually given intravenously in a hospital. After the initial crisis is past, oral antibiotics can be substituted for the intravenous drugs, but the therapy is usually continued for at least a month or longer.

In a few cases, surgery may be necessary to remove infected areas or repair or replace a damaged heart valve. The one that most often needs replacing is the mitral valve (see illustration, below), which regulates the flow of

newly oxygenated blood from the left atrium to the left ventricle, the heart's main pumping chamber.

Alternative Therapies
There are no alternative therapies that can substitute for antibiotic treatment in clearing up endocarditis, although some can serve as adjuncts to regular medical treatment.

Exercise. Even while bedridden, you can do certain exercises to prevent clot formation. Ask your doctor about a safe regimen that will help maintain good circulation and muscle tone without straining your heart.

Herbal Medicine. Two garlic capsules daily are recommended to protect the heart against infection.

Massage. During recovery, massage of the legs can be helpful in preventing blood clots from forming.

Naturopathy and Nutrition Therapy. Extra vitamin C is recommended by some nutritionists to strengthen the immune system and protect against infection. Naturopaths also suggest a daily helping of onions to help prevent all forms of heart disease.

Self-Treatment
If you are at risk for developing endocarditis, you should make sure that all health professionals whom you see know that you have this underlying heart problem. They can then prescribe preventive antibiotics before any procedure that increases your chances for infection. For example, a dentist might give you a high dose of penicillin or similar antibiotic before an extraction or cleaning your teeth, to kill any bacteria that may enter the bloodstream through cuts around your gums. People who have had rheumatic fever or who have an artificial heart valve in place may be advised to take antibiotics daily for life, especially if they have had a prior episode of endocarditis.

Anyone addicted to illegal intravenous drugs such as heroin should enter a drug treatment program.

Other Causes of Endocarditis Symptoms
Many of the symptoms of endocarditis are sometimes confused initially with heart-valve disease or flu and other infectious diseases.

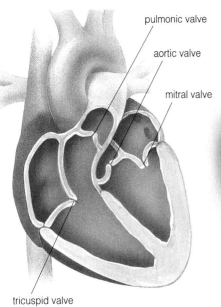

pulmonic valve
aortic valve
mitral valve
tricuspid valve
Normal heart

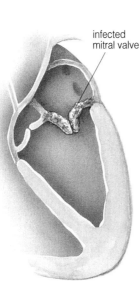

infected mitral valve

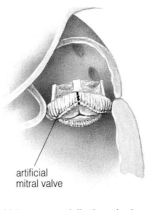

artificial mitral valve

Valves, especially the mitral, are the parts of the heart most susceptible to endocarditis. If a valve has been greatly damaged by the infection, it is possible to surgically implant an artificial one in its place.

Endometriosis

Endometriosis is a disorder of the female reproductive system, in which the endometrial tissue that normally lines the uterus grows in other parts of the body. The most likely locations are on the ovaries, fallopian tubes, colon, outer surface of the uterus, and other pelvic structures. Less commonly, the tissue may migrate to the lungs and other internal organs.

The misplaced tissue responds to the hormonal changes that occur during the menstrual cycle in a manner similar to that of the endometrium itself. When low hormone levels prompt the uterus to shed its endometrial lining as a menstrual period, the endometrial tissue growing outside the uterus also breaks apart and bleeds, but the misplaced blood has no place to go. The tissue becomes swollen and inflamed, often resulting in cramps that become more intense during the latter days of a menstrual period.

When menstruation ends, the abnormal bleeding also stops, but scar tissue forms as the endometrial clumps heal. If this pattern recurs each month, adhesions may develop and cause organs to become twisted or bound together. The condition may gradually worsen, even though symptoms may come and go.

In addition to producing menstrual pain, endometriosis sometimes causes pain throughout the month. It can also lead to infertility, especially if adhesions alter the normal alignment of organs.

Diagnostic Studies and Procedures

Endometriosis can be difficult to diagnose, especially in the approximately 25 percent of cases in which there are no symptoms. When a doctor suspects endometriosis, she may perform a pelvic examination both during and between the woman's menstrual periods.

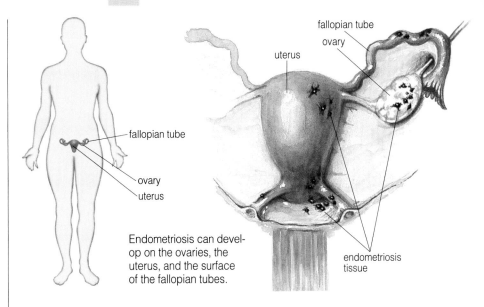

Endometriosis can develop on the ovaries, the uterus, and the surface of the fallopian tubes.

A definite diagnosis requires laparoscopy, in which a viewing instrument is inserted into the abdominal cavity through a small incision near the navel. This procedure, which is usually done under general anesthesia, allows a doctor to examine the pelvic and abdominal organs for signs of endometriosis.

Medical Treatments

There is no cure for endometriosis, but hormonal treatments can slow its growth by temporarily changing the normal patterns of female hormones. One tactic is to mimic the hormone levels of pregnancy by giving high-estrogen oral contraceptives. Endometriosis disappears when a woman is not ovulating, such as during pregnancy. Another is to produce an artificial menopause by giving drugs that halt ovulation temporarily. Without the monthly hormonal stimulation of a menstrual cycle, endometriosis tissue shrinks and eventually disappears. During such therapy, pregnancy cannot occur, although the long-term treatment goal may be to restore fertility.

Surgery may be performed to remove the endometrial tissue growing in abnormal locations. In severe cases, a hysterectomy may be recommended to alleviate symptoms. However, this course is reserved for women with incapacitating menstrual pain who do not plan a future pregnancy.

Alternative Therapies

Alternative therapies cannot cure endometriosis, but some may relieve cramps and other symptoms.

Acupuncture and Acupressure. The methods that relieve menstrual pain can also be helpful for endometriosis.

Some women report success using a rubber stimulating device that, when strapped around an ankle, presses upon an acupressure point used in treating urinary and genital problems.

Aromatherapy. Massages or baths that incorporate juniper, peppermint, or marjoram oil are advocated to relieve menstrual pain. These oils may also be ingested as a tea, or added to a glass of honey and water. The usual dosage is 1 to 3 drops of the oil in a cup of water taken two or three times a day.

Herbal Medicine. Valerian extract, tea, or capsules are recommended for relieving menstrual cramps, and may also help endometriosis. The herbal section of many health food stores carries special preparations for menstrual pain that contain dong quai, pennyroyal, and vitex. Also recommended are white willow capsules; these contain salicylic acid, a painkiller similar to aspirin, but they are not as likely to cause stomach upset and other adverse side effects.

Yoga. The knee to chest position (page 188), deep breathing, and other relaxation methods may be helpful in relieving pain associated with endometriosis.

Self-Treatment

Heat, in the form of a hot bath or a heating pad, often eases the pain of endometriosis. Massaging the area may also help. Some women benefit from over-the-counter pain relievers, such as aspirin, acetaminophen, and ibuprofen.

Other Causes of Pelvic Pain

Chronic pelvic pain can also be due to the presence of fibroid tumors in the uterus, pelvic inflammatory disease, or other disorders that affect the female reproductive organs.

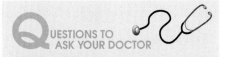

QUESTIONS TO ASK YOUR DOCTOR

▶ Is the endometriosis likely to return after a pregnancy?
▶ Would taking birth control pills be a beneficial course of action?
▶ What are my chances of achieving pregnancy after surgical treatment?
▶ Will my endometriosis go away when I reach menopause?

Esophageal and Swallowing Disorders

(Dysphagia; esophageal diverticula, spasm, stricture, varices, and webs)
The esophagus, or gullet, is a muscular tube, approximately 10 inches long, that extends from the mouth to the stomach. (It is sometimes called the food pipe to distinguish it from the nearby windpipe, or trachea.) Valve mechanisms at both the upper and lower ends, as well as gravity and a wavelike muscular motion called peristalsis, keep food moving through the esophagus in the right direction.

Before it reaches the stomach, the esophagus passes through an opening in the diaphragm called the hiatus. Disorders of the esophagus may occur at any point along the way. Some involve the swallowing mechanism, which may be affected by a congenital malformation or injury to the head or neck, and interfere with the normal passage of food into the stomach. More commonly, the esophagus itself becomes diseased. Esophageal disorders or conditions that may lead to difficulty in swallowing include the following:

Diverticula, which are outpouches that form in the esophagus wall.
Infections, which may spread from the mouth and upper throat or result from an overgrowth of fungi such as candidiasis in the esophagus. Esophageal infections are most common among people taking antibiotics and those with weakened immune systems from immunosuppressive medications or such diseases as cancer and AIDS.
Spasms, or achalasia, in which the muscles controlling the esophageal sphincter contract abnormally.
Stricture, in which abnormal muscle or mucosal tissue, erosion, or tumors narrow the lower esophagus, interfering with the passage of food.
Tumors, whether benign or cancerous, which may develop anywhere along the length of the esophagus.
Ulcerations, which may result from a backflow of digestive acids from the stomach or the accidental swallowing of a caustic substance.
Varices, masses of varicosed veins in the esophagus that are often associated with liver cirrhosis.
Webs, bands of tissue in the esophagus that are sometimes present at birth or that may develop during middle age, usually in association with an iron-deficiency anemia called Plummer-Vinson syndrome.

In addition to difficulty in swallowing, symptoms pointing to an esophageal disorder include chest pain, a burning sensation in the chest and throat, bad breath, frequent choking, and spitting up of undigested food.

Diagnostic Studies and Procedures

A detailed medical history, a careful description of symptoms, and a physical examination tell a doctor a great deal about the nature of esophageal and swallowing disorders, but additional tests are usually needed. An infection necessitates laboratory cultures to identify the bacterium or fungus. Otherwise, tests usually start with

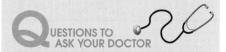

QUESTIONS TO ASK YOUR DOCTOR

► Can very hot or spicy foods interfere with normal swallowing?
► Could the sensation of a lump in my throat be related to stress or other psychological factors?

an upper GI series—X-rays taken after the patient swallows barium, an opaque substance that makes the esophagus visible on film.

Depending upon what the X-rays show, additional tests may include endoscopy (to look at the inside of the esophagus), a CT scan or MRI, ultrasonography, and manometry, which measures the pressures on the upper and lower esophageal sphincters. These tests not only make it possible to determine exactly how long it takes for food to travel from the mouth to the stomach, but they also allow doctors to watch the entire process on a screen.

If endoscopy reveals a tumor or other suspicious area, biopsy samples will be taken during the procedure.

Medical Treatments
Some disorders, such as small pouches (diverticula) in the upper esophagus, do not need medical treatment; more often, however, medication and/or surgery are necessary.
Drug Therapy. The choice of medication depends upon the underlying problem. Mild candidiasis will be treated with nystatin, an antifungal medication that is used as a mouthwash and then swallowed. If this fails to clear up the infection, a stronger antifungal medicine, such as amphotericin B, may be prescribed.

Impacted and inflamed esophageal outpouches will be treated with antibiotics, although it is usually essential to remove the foreign material first. This can be done during endoscopy.

Medications that will relax smooth muscles, such as the calcium-channel blocker nifedipine (Procardia), usually alleviate esophageal spasms.
Surgical Treatments. Extensive webs are generally removed surgically, as are large outpouches in the lower part of the esophagus that interfere with normal eating. Numerous esophageal ulcers or erosions may require removal

esophageal outpouch

muscle stricture

refluxed acid — stomach

esophagus —

stomach —

Anything that narrows the esophagus can cause swallowing problems. Examples include a diverticular outpouch (top), muscle stricture (middle), and ulcerations due to a reflux of stomach acid (bottom).

of part of the esophagus. If a large segment or all of the esophagus must be removed, a section of intestine may be used as a graft to link the throat and stomach. This procedure will restore the ability to eat normally. Alternatively, a portion of stomach may be narrowed to form a tube, which will then be moved higher into the chest cavity to assume the function of the esophagus.

Severe strictures can be widened surgically; in other cases, a doctor may insert a rubber dilator into the esophagus to stretch the narrowed segment or break the stricture.

If medication does not control esophageal spasms, an operation called a myotomy can reduce muscular action.

Variceal sclerotherapy is used to treat esophageal varices that rupture and cause severe bleeding. In this procedure, a varicosed vein is injected with a sclerosing solution that stops the bleeding; the scar tissue that subsequently forms ultimately destroys the diseased vein, thereby preventing future episodes of esophageal bleeding.

Alternative Therapies

Alternative therapies are of the most value in treating those esophageal problems that are related to stress rather than a physical abnormality.

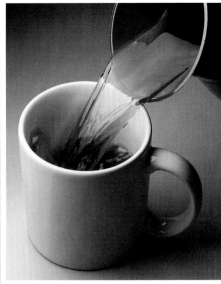

If you have difficulty swallowing, avoid coffee and other hot drinks. Instead, drink beverages served at room temperature.

Nutrition Therapy. A person with a narrowed esophagus or swallowing problems may need a liquid diet. A nutrition therapist can help structure a balanced diet for someone unable to eat solid foods. Naturopaths advise patients who suffer from esophageal spasms to abstain from spicy foods as well as caffeine and alcohol.

Yoga and Meditation. These and other relaxation therapies that call for deep breathing can help overcome stress-related swallowing problems.

Self-Treatment

If you have difficulty swallowing, try eating your food at room temperature, rather than when it is very hot or cold. Chew your food well, and flush it down with fluids. You may need to switch to puréed or liquid foods.

If you have dry mouth, use artificial saliva, and moisten food well before attempting to swallow it.

Do not smoke, and abstain from alcohol or use it in moderation. The combination of smoking and heavy alcohol consumption greatly increases the risk of esophageal cancer. Alcoholism can also lead to cirrhosis of the liver, which is the major cause of esophageal varices and bleeding.

Other Causes of Swallowing Problems

Strokes, myasthenia gravis and other neuromuscular disorders, and tongue, larynx, and throat cancers may create swallowing difficulties. Anxiety can aggravate the problem. Dry mouth, often caused by a medication or disease that reduces saliva production, also affects the swallowing mechanism.

A CASE IN POINT

When Harry Adams, a 46-year-old lawyer, experienced his first episode of an esophageal spasm, he thought he was having a heart attack. The incident took place at a business luncheon during intense contract negotiations.

Adams had skipped breakfast and so was feeling ravenously hungry. He ordered a steak, but before his meal arrived, he joined his colleagues in a couple of drinks. After taking a few hurried bites of his steak, he suddenly experienced severe pains just behind his breastbone that spread to his jaw and mouth. His alarmed companions called for an ambulance, and he was rushed to a nearby hospital.

Even before Adams arrived at the hospital, the emergency medical team had performed an ECG, which appeared normal, and had reassured their patient that they didn't think he was having a heart attack—an opinion later confirmed by an emergency room physician. The episode

was attributed to stress, and Adams was advised to take a much-needed vacation.

A few weeks after returning to work, Adams experienced a second attack—this time during dinner with his family. He had had a hard day at work and things weren't much better at home, with his two teenage sons bringing a quarrel to the table. Again, Adams was rushed to the emergency room, and again, doctors could find no physical explanation for his chest pains. He was advised to see his doctor for a complete checkup.

His doctor found no evidence of heart disease, but the symptoms pointed to a possible esophageal problem. The doctor ordered an upper GI series with fluoroscopy—still and moving X-rays taken after the patient swallows barium to coat the esophagus. The X-rays showed an abnormal narrowing and reduced motility in the lower esophagus, findings that pointed to esophageal spasms. A more definitive test—manometry—then was

used to measure pressure on the upper and lower openings of the esophagus. This test confirmed that Adams's symptoms were, indeed, caused by esophageal spasms. Endoscopy failed to find any physical abnormality, such as esophageal diverticula or obstructions, and other tests ruled out a neuromuscular cause.

The doctor explained that failure to identify a cause was not uncommon. He also assured Adams that the spasms were not a serious health threat.

"Episodes usually can be prevented by eating small, frequent meals," Adams's doctor told him. "When you have difficulty swallowing, switch to bland, puréed foods. Above all, strive to make meals a pleasant, relaxed time."

He also advised his patient to try deep breathing exercises or to consider biofeedback training, if the spasms continued to be a problem. For Adams, peaceful meals and the breathing exercises have so far prevented another attack.

Failure to Thrive

Failure to thrive refers to abnormally slow growth in infants and young children. In general, it describes a child under two years of age who weighs less than 80 percent of the average for children with the same birth weight. The child may also lag in other aspects of development, including speech and motor control. The cause might be organic or nonorganic, but more often it is a mixture of the two.

The most obvious and common organic cause is severe malnutrition; however, failure to thrive may afflict an adequately fed child who has a congenital defect or a disease that interferes with eating and metabolism.

The condition is considered nonorganic when no physical abnormality can be found to account for it. An example would be a baby who is healthy at birth and perhaps even does well initially, but then regresses.

The mother (or primary caregiver) and the family environment play a critical role in nonorganic failure to thrive. Often, poor parenting skills are at fault. A depressed mother may fail to bond with her baby, or parents may fear spoiling a child by responding to crying. Social and economic circumstances also play a role; there simply may not be enough time or money to provide for a baby's needs.

Regardless of the cause, the consequences can be serious if the child continues not to gain weight. Without adequate nutrition, intellectual development may be stunted, and the child may even die.

Diagnostic Studies and Procedures
The first step involves trying to identify organic causes. The physician will ask the parents about any symptoms, previous illnesses, and family history of genetic diseases, also the baby's feeding habits. She might inquire about some

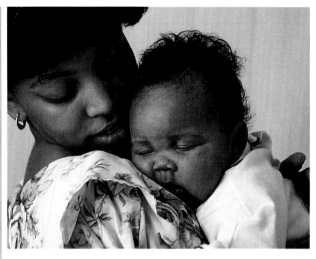
Nurturing and love are as important as good nutrition in helping an infant grow.

aspects of the mother's pregnancy—her diet and whether she smoked or used drugs or alcohol. The baby will then be examined.

In diagnosing failure to thrive, a doctor uses established medical standards for weight, height, head circumference, hand size, and skeletal development. He may test the child's hearing and vision and also order blood, urine, and X-ray studies.

If there appear to be no organic abnormalities, the doctor usually concentrates on identifying psychological factors that could be contributing to the baby's delayed development. He asks the parents to describe the home environment and observes the interaction between the mother and her baby. Looking for signs of emotional deprivation or inadequate attachment, the physician notes whether or not the baby makes eye contact with the mother, responds to being held and spoken to, and takes any interest in the surroundings.

Typically, a child who fails to thrive is listless and withdrawn, and does not respond to cuddling and other stimuli. The youngster may engage in repetitive motions, such as banging its head or rocking back and forth.

Medical Treatments
Any underlying medical problem—an illness or congenital defect—must be treated. A severely malnourished child may be hospitalized for special feeding, possibly including intravenous fluids and nutrients.

Alternative Therapies
Successful treatment often necessitates a team effort by health professionals and alternative practitioners.

Family Counseling. Parents who need to improve their relationship with an unusually demanding baby may require special therapy. A social worker or family therapist might make a home visit to study family dynamics and suggest ways to improve the relationships between the parents and between each parent and the child.

Nutrition Therapy. A diet that provides the protein and calories needed for proper growth and development is critical in overcoming failure to thrive. Consulting a nutritionist experienced in treating infant feeding problems may be necessary to make sure that the baby's diet is sufficient. Often, a listless, malnourished child lacks appetite and must be encouraged to eat frequent, calorie-enriched meals. If finances are a factor, the nutritionist can help the parents to enroll in assistance programs and can instruct them in how to provide nourishing foods at low cost.

Physical and Occupational Therapy. Professionals in these specialties can guide parents in setting up stimulating activities to foster the child's emotional and intellectual development.

Self-Treatment
If failure to thrive is rooted in the parent-child relationship, joining a self-help group composed of parents with similar problems can be a source of support and understanding.

Other Causes of Retarded Growth
Cystic fibrosis, malabsorption disorders, esophageal disorders, anemia, thyroid disorders, congenital heart defects and other anomalies, and HIV and other infections are among the many organic conditions that may account for a baby's failure to thrive.

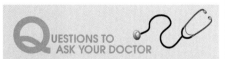

QUESTIONS TO ASK YOUR DOCTOR

▶ Could inadequate breast milk account for my baby's failure to gain weight?
▶ How can I tell if my baby is getting enough to eat at a feeding?
▶ Should I pick up my baby every time she cries?

Fainting

(Syncope)

Fainting is a sudden loss of consciousness, usually brief and preceded by a sense of lightheadedness or dizziness. It represents the body's way of protecting the brain's oxygen supply. When you faint, you involuntarily fall, allowing more blood to flow to the brain.

A classic cause of fainting is orthostatic hypotension, a sudden drop in blood pressure upon standing up. This condition sometimes occurs in younger people who have been confined to bed for a few days, but it is more common in older persons who have circulatory disorders or who are taking medication for high blood pressure or, less frequently, depression.

Some people are susceptible to a type of fainting called vasovagal syndrome. Given the right circumstances, the vagus nerve, which passes through the neck and chest and controls many involuntary processes, suddenly shunts blood to one part of the body, causing it to pool there and decrease the supply to the brain. Unusual stress or fright, the sight of blood, or exposure to certain odors or sounds can bring on this kind of fainting spell. People with this syndrome know they have a tendency to faint and usually feel warning signs, such as sweating or dizziness, so they can take preventive action.

Diabetic patients may feel lightheaded and possibly faint when their blood sugar becomes low from too much insulin. People with certain heart conditions, such as arrythmias, can also be prone to fainting. A person suffering from heat exhaustion (page 222), or anyone who has become dehydrated from heavy physical activity or prolonged diarrhea might also faint.

Diagnostic Studies and Procedures

Because serious underlying disorders can bring about loss of consciousness, a person who has fainted without ostensible cause needs a full medical checkup. This includes an electrocardiogram to evaluate heart function and blood tests to check for anemia.

Medical Treatments

Even though the underlying cause should be investigated, in most cases fainting is a transient reaction that does not call for treatment. If fainting results from orthostatic hypotension brought on by the use of antihypertensive drugs

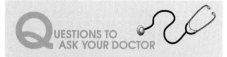

QUESTIONS TO ASK YOUR DOCTOR

► Could medication be responsible for my fainting spells? If so, should I try a lower dosage?
► How can I avoid fainting when I see blood (or some other unpleasant sight)?

or other medications, a lower dosage or an alternative drug will usually prevent future episodes.

If you have diabetes and are prone to developing hypoglycemia, ask your physician to prescribe a glucagon gel, a hormone that raises blood glucose levels rapidly. Always carry the medication with you; when you squeeze a small amount into your mouth, it quickly reverses hypoglycemia.

Fainting related to a heart disorder requires taking care of that problem. Depending upon the specific condition, the treatments may range from lifestyle changes to medication and possibly even surgery.

Alternative Therapies

Nutrition Therapy. Some persons feel lightheaded and may faint when they become overly hungry. For them, eating four to six small meals a day and emphasizing low-sugar foods can help. Some nutritionists also recommend a daily supplement of 200 micrograms of the picolinate form of chromium to help stabilize blood sugar. It takes at least two months to see any improvement with this therapy.

Visualization. This technique may be useful to someone who is prone to an extreme vasovagal response and who invariably faints upon seeing blood or experiencing some similar psychological trauma. Such a person might visualize a scenario in which he gains mastery over the automatic reaction by marshalling inner resources.

Self-Treatment

You can usually prevent fainting by lying down with your head lower than the rest of your body, allowing blood to flow rapidly to the brain. If you cannot lie down, sit with your head lower than your heart, but don't put it between your knees—if you do faint in this position, you might fall on your head and sustain a serious injury.

If you have bouts of orthostatic hypotension, always get out of bed gradually to avoid faintness. Sit on the side of the bed for a minute or two before slowly standing up.

If you have been fasting and feel faint, drink a glass of orange juice or a soda with sugar in it.

Some people require extra salt and fluids, especially during hot weather or a lengthy workout. If this applies to you, drink at least 8 to 10 glasses of water, juice, broth, or other clear fluids daily. You might try a sports drink that replaces the salt lost in perspiration; you may also need to add extra salt when you prepare food.

Other Causes of Fainting

Fainting can be a warning sign of a heart valve problem, a cardiac arrhythmia, or an impending stroke. All of these disorders warrant immediate medical attention. Sometimes, too, fainting episodes occur in the early stages of pregnancy.

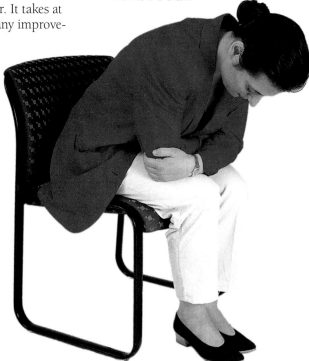

If you feel that you might faint and are unable to lie down, sit down with your head lowered to promote increased blood flow to the brain.

Fears And Phobias

Fear is a strong emotional response to danger, real or imagined. A phobia—the Greek word for fear—is a persistent, irrational fear that is out of all proportion to its cause. People with phobias recognize that their fears are excessive and constraining, but they feel powerless to confront them and often go to great lengths to avoid the dreaded object or situation.

According to the American Psychiatric Association, up to 24 million Americans suffer from one or more phobias, making this the country's most common psychological disorder. Psychiatrists classify phobias according to the following categories:

Specific phobia: fear of a specific object, situation, or event. Common examples include fears of animals, insects, the dark, germs, storms, heights, illness, and death. From 5 to 12 percent of the population suffers from such phobias at some point in life; women are more likely than men to be affected.

Specific phobias often arise during childhood. Although most disappear as a child matures, a few may persist for life. Some feared situations are easy enough to avoid, but others, such as a fear of flying (aerophobia) or of enclosed spaces (claustrophobia), can interfere with an individual's lifestyle and work.

Social phobia: a compelling desire to avoid situations in which it's necessary to face the scrutiny of others. People with this disorder fear being embarrassed or humiliated. For example, some persons are terrified of engaging in casual conversation; others cannot tolerate eating in a public place, using public restrooms, or interacting with a member of the opposite sex. Typically, a social phobia begins in adolescence and often lasts for life. About 3 to 5 percent of the population suffers from some type of a social phobia. Men and women have the disorder in roughly equal numbers.

Agoraphobia: an intense fear of being alone or trapped in a public place. (Agoraphobia is the Greek term for fear of a marketplace.) This is the most limiting of all phobias, causing some people literally to become prisoners in their own homes.

About 0.6 percent of Americans have agoraphobia, with women outnumbering men. Some two-thirds of people

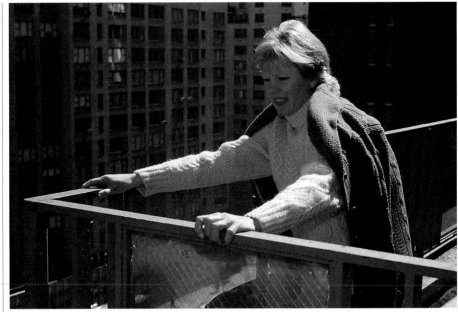

Acrophobia, an intense fear of heights, can sometimes be overcome by deliberately going to a high, yet safe, place and then practicing deep breathing or self-hypnosis.

with agoraphobia experience panic attacks—periods of intense anxiety characterized by chest pains, a rapid heartbeat, sweating, difficulty in breathing, and other symptoms easily mistaken for a heart attack.

Diagnostic Studies and Procedures

The most important diagnostic criterion is a person's instant feeling of extreme anxiety when encountering the feared object or circumstance. A doctor or mental-health professional can easily diagnose a specific phobia simply by having the person describe the fears. The patient usually takes great pains to avoid the dreaded object or situation, even while admitting that the fear is unreasonable and seeking professional help to overcome it.

Some people, however, engage in what is called counterphobic behavior in an attempt to counteract their fears. They deliberately, and often irrationally, seek out the object of their phobia. Thus, a person afraid of heights may take up parachute jumping or rock climbing. Such individuals are unlikely to seek help for their phobias.

People with social phobias often go to great lengths to conceal their fears, although the resulting isolation may prompt them to consult a psychotherapist. Friends and family members should suspect social phobia in a loved one who consistently finds excuses to avoid specific social activities. For example, someone who fears eating

in public may invariably develop a stomachache or plead loss of appetite when invited out for a meal. In reality, the person is afraid of spilling food or committing some other embarrassing act. The anxiety may perpetuate a vicious cycle; for instance, nervousness may prompt the person to spill some food, thus reinforcing the fear.

When a physician or family member suspects agoraphobia, a review of recent behavior usually reveals a typical pattern of increasing constriction of activities. Eventually, the avoidance behavior takes on a life of its own. In severe cases, the agoraphobic may venture away from home only in the company of a friend or family member. Even then, the person will probably check constantly for an escape route and may make a sudden exit, especially if symptoms of a panic attack develop. Some people with severe agoraphobia actually remain in one room at all times. (See Anxiety, page 82.)

Medical Treatments

Drug Therapy. Most phobia sufferers are able to cope with their fears without medication. The exceptions are people with severe agoraphobia accompanied by panic attacks; they may require a prescription medication. Possible medications include antidepressant drugs, especially MAO inhibitors such as phenelzine (Nardil) and isocarboxazid (Marplan), or tricyclic antidepressants, such as imipramine (Tofranil) and desipramine (Norpramin). Other potential drugs are beta blockers, usually propranolol (Inderal), or antianxiety agents such as alprazolam (Xanax).

Psychological Treatments. For most phobias, various forms of psychotherapy can help alleviate the fear. Even in severe cases that require drugs, a doctor will still recommend psychotherapy to get at the root of the problem. The specific approach will depend on the phobia and the degree to which it is limiting the person's life. One-to-one cognitive therapy often helps an agoraphobic. Group therapy is also beneficial in most cases, because it provides mutual support from others who have similar problems.

Alternative Therapies

Alternative therapies that emphasize stress management through relaxation skills are the most helpful in overcoming phobic reactions.

Behavior Modification. This is a key therapy employed by both psychiatrists and alternative therapists in treating phobias. The person gradually learns to overcome the fears through a process called desensitization. For example, a homebound agoraphobic might be instructed to start by opening the front door and spending several minutes looking outside. When the person can do this without anxiety or panic, he goes on to the next assignment, which might be to walk to the end of the

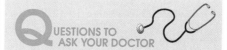

driveway. The eventual goal is to enter a public place without experiencing fear. Practitioners also use similar desensitization exercises in treating simple and social phobias.

Biofeedback Training. With guidance from a qualified therapist, an individual can learn to normalize certain physical responses—for instance, a racing heartbeat and elevated blood pressure—of a phobic reaction.

Hypnosis. This alternative therapy can be especially effective in overcoming simple phobias, such as a fear of flying or heights. While hypnotized, the patient is given instructions on how to respond when confronting the fear. For example, a person who fears flying may be told to imagine himself in the pilot's seat with complete control over the situation. He may also be taught self-hypnosis techniques to practice when in such fearful situations.

Meditation and Visualization. These techniques allow people with phobias to become detached observers rather than victims, permitting them to face their fears instead of trying to avoid them. Slow breathing exercises during meditation or visualization are an important part of these disciplines.

Self-Treatment

Although some of the therapies just described require initial guidance from a professional, once mastered, they can be applied on your own. Also, communicating your fears to close friends and family members—instead of hiding them—can elicit the support you need for dealing with them. Other self-help strategies include:

Breathing Exercises. You can learn to control hyperventilation and the onset of a panic attack by focusing all your attention on taking slow, deep breaths, inhaling through your nose, and exhaling slowly through your mouth. For best results, make this part of a 10-minute daily stress-reduction program.

Self-desensitization. Desensitization is a part of behavior modification, but you can also try it on your own. For example, if family members are eager to adopt a cat but you are terrified of these animals, start by learning more about them from a distance. Look at cat picture books and visit a zoo to watch the lions and other big cats. Then observe a friend stroking her cat, listen to it purr, and imagine yourself stroking it. When you feel comfortable with your visual images of yourself with a cat, try petting a kitten that someone else is holding. Eventually, you may be able to overcome your fear.

Support Groups. There are many organizations—YMCAs, YWCAs, mental-health clinics, and churches, among others—that sponsor support groups to help people overcome their fears. These include groups for people with specific phobias, such as agoraphobia.

Other Causes of Fears

The use of alcohol, crack cocaine, and hallucinogenic drugs can give rise to intense fear. Also, fears may be part of other psychiatric disorders, especially schizophrenia, depression, and post-traumatic stress syndrome, which follows a particularly disturbing event or experience. In unusual cases, the development of fears may be traced to a brain tumor or exposure to LSD and other toxic substances.

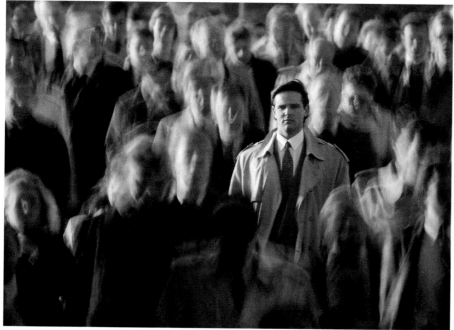

A fear of crowds, a common aspect of agoraphobia, can manifest itself as a panic attack or a strong desire to flee when surrounded by people.

Fever And Chills

(Ague)

Fever, an abnormal rise in body temperature, is sometimes accompanied by chills. With flu, malaria, and certain other diseases, fever may concur or alternate with sweating and chills.

The hypothalamus, which is part of the brain, controls the body's thermostat. It sets the body's temperature normally at about 98.6°F (37°C) when taken orally or about 99.6°F (37.5°C) when taken rectally. Your temperature is slightly lower when you first awake in the morning; this is referred to as the body's basal temperature.

Body temperature rises for a number of reasons, but the most common is the invasion of infectious organisms, which induce the blood's disease-fighting white cells to release pyrogen, a chemical that travels to the brain and prompts the hypothalamus to reset the body's thermostat at a higher level.

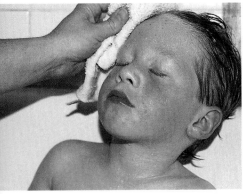

A sponge bath with cool or tepid water often reduces a young child's fever.

The reaction is part of the body's effort to kill the organisms, which often cannot survive a high body temperature.

Diagnostic Studies and Procedures

Because fever is a symptom of a wide range of disorders and not an illness in itself, diagnosis focuses on finding the cause. Diagnostic studies may consist

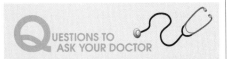

QUESTIONS TO ASK YOUR DOCTOR

▶ How soon after taking aspirin or acetaminophen should my fever go down?
▶ Will lowering a fever prolong a bout of flu or other viral infection?

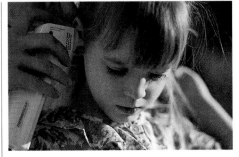

Ear thermometers (left) and oral, rectal, and digital devices (top to bottom below) measure body temperature to the nearest tenth of a degree.

of blood tests, various cultures, X-rays, and possibly a biopsy.

Medical Treatments

The cause of a fever determines whether or not treatment is necessary. Many doctors feel that if a fever does not exceed 102°F (39°C), it is best to leave it alone. However, a prolonged high fever or one above 103°F (39.5°C) can bring on dehydration, headache, nausea, and convulsions, especially in young children. In the frail elderly, an extremely high fever may be life threatening.

In such cases, aspirin and acetaminophen are the most effective drugs for lowering a fever. For very young children—and for anyone with a swallowing problem—pills can be pulverized and mixed with mashed banana or applesauce. Be sure to consult a doctor before giving aspirin to anyone under age 18. In this age group, aspirin given during a viral infection increases the risk of Reye's syndrome, a potentially fatal disorder (see box on page 437).

Alternative Therapies

Several alternative therapies can lower a fever. Such approaches may be useful adjuncts to medical treatment.

Aromatherapy. Aromatic oils, said to reduce a fever when massaged into the skin or converted to vapor for inhalation, include camphor, eucalyptus, lemon, and hyssop.

Herbal Medicine. Tea made with the dried bupleurum root can be effective, as can tea made from boneset, or agueweed, a remedy favored by Native Americans to treat high fevers.

Homeopathy. Numerous remedies are recommended, including aconite, arnica, arsenicum, pulsatilla, pyrogen, and hyoscyamus. The cause and nature of the fever determines what to use.

Hydrotherapy. Applying a cold compress to the forehead and sponging the body with cool or tepid water can

quickly reduce a high fever. Do not sponge a baby with alcohol, however; the fumes can be dangerous.

Self-Treatment

Drink extra fluids to replace those lost through sweating. Good choices are water, fruit juice, lemonade, herbal teas, and clear broth. Avoid alcohol and beverages containing caffeine, which have a diuretic effect that can cause additional fluid loss.

Extra sleep is also important. Stay in bed as much as possible. If chills accompany the fever, use a light blanket that can be removed during periods of fever and sweating.

Other Causes of Fever

A continuing low-grade fever may be a warning sign of tuberculosis and of some types of cancer, especially leukemia and Hodgkin's disease. Fever is also a symptom of mononucleosis, rheumatoid arthritis, and lupus. A sudden high temperature may indicate an acute infection, such as appendicitis. In women, pelvic inflammatory disease or toxic shock syndrome can bring on a high fever, while in children, middle ear infections are a common cause.

WHEN TO SEE A DOCTOR

Consult a doctor if the temperature is:
▶ 100°F (38°C) in a baby under three months of age.
▶ 103°F (39.5°C) in a child or adult under 60; 102°F (39°C) in an adult over 60.
▶ 101°F for more than three days.
Also, see a doctor if a low-grade (less than 101°F or 38.5°C) fever lasts for more than three weeks or is accompanied by pain, swollen joints, a stiff neck, vomiting, diarrhea, or rash.

Flatfootedness

(Pes planus)

The human foot is an engineering marvel, made up of 26 bones, 33 joints, 19 muscles, and more than 100 ligaments. Two arches—a longitudinal one in the midfoot and a short one in the forefoot—act as bony bridges to support the foot and function as shock absorbers.

Flatfootedness occurs when the longitudinal arch is flattened, so that the entire sole of the foot rests on the ground. The condition is common during early childhood, when the arch is filled in with baby fat. As the ligaments in the foot grow stronger, however, the arch normally develops to the point at which a wet imprint on a flat surface will show an empty space between the ball of the foot and the heel. This space is bounded only by an impression of the outer edge of the foot. In flatfooted individuals, the space does not exist.

A flat foot with a flexible arch does not usually cause problems, but rigid, or structural, flatfootedness—in which the arch is nonexistent because the foot bones are improperly aligned—may be disabling. Flat feet resulting from the abnormal development of a bony bridge in the place where a normal joint or space should form can also cause walking difficulties. These unusual conditions generally become apparent between the ages of 8 and 15.

Diagnostic Studies and Procedures

Many primary-care doctors can diagnose flatfootedness on the basis of X-rays and close examination of the bare foot. Podiatrists and orthopedists who specialize in foot problems sometimes use a computerized gait analysis in assessing bone alignment during walking and other foot movement. Other procedures used in diagnosing flatfootedness, especially in children, include checking the flexibility of the arch after taking a footprint and examining the pattern of wear on shoes.

Medical Treatments

Most flatfootedness does not require medical treatment. However, some conditions that develop during childhood may need surgical correction. For example, if misaligned bones are creating flatfootedness, they can be surgically realigned. Similarly, abnormal bony growths can be removed. The earlier an operation is performed, the better the results will be.

Podiatrists often prescribe orthotic devices for flat feet, especially for runners and others whose feet are subjected to considerable stress. Made from metal and rigid plastic, these devices can support weak ligaments, muscles, and foot joints. Some types can also alleviate pain or compensate for legs of uneven length. The devices are custom-made from plaster molds of the feet.

Alternative Therapies

Foot Massage and Reflexology. Treatments that combine massage, hydrotherapy, and reflexology can alleviate foot pain.

Physical Therapy. Exercises designed to strengthen the muscles in the foot may be combined with orthotics.

Self-Treatment

If flatfootedness is causing discomfort, orthotic inserts, foot cushions, pads, supports, and lifts can help to alleviate it. Before investing in custom-made devices, however, try creating your own by cutting and reshaping nonprescription foot products, available in drugstores and shoe-repair shops.

Make sure your shoes fit properly and have built-in arch supports. This is especially important for exercise shoes. Also, select shoes designed specifically

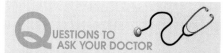
for your physical activity; running shoes are not appropriate for extensive walking and vice versa.

Women with flat feet should avoid high heeled shoes. Ideally, the heel should be one inch high or less. If you feel compelled to wear shoes with higher heels, at least make sure they have an arch support and are large enough to accommodate a half insole to help keep your foot in place.

Whenever possible, walk barefooted. Walking in the sand is especially good for strengthening foot muscles.

Do foot exercises that are designed to strengthen arch muscles. Wiggle your toes and then rotate your ankles 10 times to the left and 10 times to the right. Practice picking up a marble or cotton ball with your toes, doing it 20 times with each foot.

You can also try foot massage methods used by reflexologists and massage therapists. After soaking your feet in warm water or a foot jacuzzi, manipulate the soles and heels with firm circular motions. "Walk" your thumb across the sole horizontally, pressing firmly at the base of each toe.

Other Causes of Flat Feet

Some circumstances contribute to so-called fallen arches. These include obesity, arthritis, fractures, and a job that requires long hours of standing.

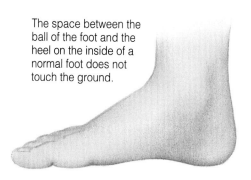

The space between the ball of the foot and the heel on the inside of a normal foot does not touch the ground.

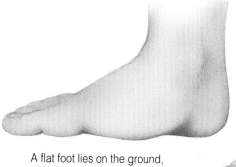

A flat foot lies on the ground, with no arch between the ball of the foot and the heel.

Orthotic devices, which are custom-made, or nonprescription foot cushions can be used to create an arch that supports foot muscles and ligaments.

Flatulence

(Intestinal gas)

Flatulence means having gas, or flatus, in the intestinal tract; the gas passes out of the body through the anus when the rectal muscles relax. Healthy people produce from 6 to 64 ounces of flatus daily. In most cases, flatulence is normal and the gas has no odor.

Most intestinal gas consists of carbon dioxide, hydrogen, nitrogen, and methane, which are created when complex carbohydrates are broken down. Any swallowed air adds oxygen to the mixture. When unabsorbed nutrients undergo fermentation by intestinal bacteria, the resulting by-product can contribute not only to the volume but also to the odor of intestinal gas. In particular, an unpleasant smell is often produced by beans, dried peas, lentils, and other legumes.

It's not just what you eat but also how you eat that can create a problem. People who swallow a lot of air when eating or drinking may pass more than the usual amount of intestinal gas.

There is also a hereditary component; some people simply produce more methane and other gases than others do in the course of normal digestion.

Diagnostic Studies and Procedures

If you have what seems to be excessive flatulence along with any other digestive symptoms—such as abdominal pain or cramps, bloating, diarrhea, and weight loss—consult a physician. Blood tests, stool cultures, intestinal X-rays, and endoscopy may be necessary to rule out a digestive disorder, such as intestinal parasites or diverticulitis.

Medical Treatments

Normally, treatment is necessary only if a gastrointestinal disorder, a rare occurrence, causes the excessive flatulence. However, if a change in lifestyle does not sufficiently reduce a flatulence problem, a doctor may recommend a nonprescription product containing simethicone, an agent that breaks up small gas bubbles that form in the stomach and intestines.

Alternative Therapies

Herbal Medicine. European herbalists often recommend angostura bitters or a tincture of gentian root. A teaspoon of bitters one or more times a day is said to ease flatulence; it can be taken straight or in sparkling water to make a refreshing beverage to drink before

The knee-to-chest yoga position—reclining on your back with one or both knees bent and held to the chest—often helps relieve flatulence (see more explicit directions, below).

or after meals. Other herbal remedies include teas made from crushed and steeped anise seeds, basil leaves, cinnamon, hyssop, and peppermint.

Homeopathy. Practitioners may prescribe nux vomica for gas.

Nutrition Therapy. Large doses of vitamin C can cause flatulence as well as diarrhea. If you are taking supplements of more than 500 milligrams, reduce the amount and increase dietary vitamin C by eating more citrus fruits and other fresh fruits as well as potatoes, sweet peppers, and other vegetables.

Yoga. The knee-to-chest position (see illustration, above) can be helpful in relieving flatulence. While reclining on your back, bend your knees, bringing them up to your chest. Grasp the knees and rock gently, then lower the legs. Repeat the movement, but this time move one leg at a time. Inhale as you begin. When the knee is fully bent, lift your head to touch your nose to that knee, and hold for a count of 10. Exhale as you lower the head and return the leg to the floor. Do this five times with each leg. Then raise both knees again, lift your head until your nose touches your knee, and breathe as instructed for the single leg lift.

Self-Treatment

You can control your gas production to some extent by dietary changes. Through trial and error, identify foods that cause excessive gas in your intestinal tract, then reduce or eliminate them. For example, certain dried beans can result in flatulence because the intestinal bacteria needed for their digestion give off methane. In particular, soybeans and pink beans tend to

produce more methane than Anasazi and black beans. Other foods associated with increased gas include cabbage, spinach, cauliflower, broccoli, Brussels sprouts, eggplant, onions, celery, carrots, raisins, apricots, wheat germ, prune juice, and bran and other high-fiber foods. You may also want to try the following tactics:

▶ Reduce fat intake. The digestion of fats sometimes contributes to the problem.

▶ Eliminate dairy products if you are unable to digest lactose (milk sugar). Alternatively, use products in which lactose has already been partially broken down, as in Lactaid milk. You can also take lactase pills, which contain enzymes needed to digest lactose.

▶ Minimize the swallowing of air by eating more slowly and not talking with food in your mouth. Some doctors also suggest eliminating carbonated beverages because they introduce extra air into the gastrointestinal tract.

▶ Avoid overeating. Eating too much at one time or eating while under stress can also inhibit normal digestion and lead to excessive gas production.

Other Causes of Flatulence

Sometimes flatulence is caused by a digestive disorder, such as lactose intolerance or celiac disease.

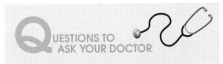

QUESTIONS TO ASK YOUR DOCTOR

▶ Is it possible that my gas problem is caused by lactose intolerance?
▶ Can you suggest a nonprescription remedy to reduce flatulence?

Flu

(Grippe; influenza)

An influenza virus causes the flu, a very common and highly contagious respiratory infection. Some people mistakenly refer to a cold or any upper respiratory disorder as the flu. But in reality, the flu is a more severe illness than the common cold (page 143). Not only can it lead to pneumonia, but some types of the disease are even fatal. For example, the great epidemic of Spanish flu in 1917 killed millions of people throughout the world.

A bout of flu confers immunity against that particular virus strain, but because these viruses quickly change, or mutate, new strains emerge every few years. In general, however, a flu virus falls into one of three categories. Type A, the most common, is responsible for the serious and widespread epidemics; Type B also causes epidemics, but with milder cases than those of Type A; Type C is relatively uncommon, but sometimes causes outbreaks of mild flu.

Diagnostic Studies and Procedures

Your own observation of symptoms is usually enough to tell you that you have the flu, particularly if there has been an epidemic in your area. Flu symptoms are similar to those of a bad cold—fever, sore throat, muscle aches,

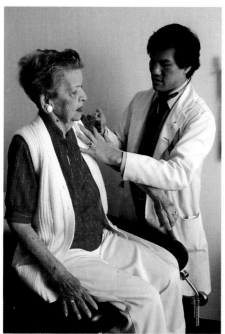

Flu shots are recommended for people over age 65, as well as those with diabetes, heart disease, and other chronic illnesses.

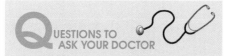
QUESTIONS TO ASK YOUR DOCTOR

▶ Should I have a flu shot? If so, will it protect against all the different strains of flu in my area?

▶ Should I keep my child home from school during a flu epidemic?

running nose, cough, and headache—but they come on more suddenly, are more severe, and last longer. If you consult a doctor, she will do a physical examination and possibly order blood tests and a sputum culture. A chest X-ray may also be necessary if the symptoms suggest the presence of flu-related pneumonia.

Medical Treatments

A physician's care is usually not needed unless you are part of a group with a high risk for developing serious complications (the vulnerable groups are listed in the first paragraph of the box, below). In such cases, if a Type A virus is involved, a doctor may prescribe amantadine (Symmetrel), an anti-Parkinson's disease drug that has an antiviral effect. Or he may prescribe an antibiotic to prevent secondary pneumonia, especially if you suffer from asthma, emphysema, chronic bronchitis, or another lung disorder.

Alternative Therapies

Although they are unlikely to shorten the course of the flu, a number of alternative therapies may alleviate the symptoms of the illness.

Aromatherapy. Therapists recommend placing 5 drops of cinnamon oil in 1 tablespoonful of water and inhaling the scent three times a day; they also advise massages or baths using lemon, pine needle, or rosemary oil.

Herbal Medicine. Boneset has long been advocated to relieve the so-called breakbone fever caused by influenza. Herbalists today still use it to treat fevers resulting from a cold or the flu. It is most often given in an infusion of 1 to 2 teaspoons of dried flowers and leaves in 1 cup of water, to be drunk hot at intervals of 30 minutes until the fever abates. It is also available in capsules and tinctures. A mixture of boneset, elder flowers, licorice, and peppermint can also be taken as a hot tea every two to three hours or consumed in capsule or tincture form.

Homeopathy. Aconite and nux vomica are recommended during the early stages of flu. One dose a week of bacillinum 30 and influenzinum 30, given separately or in combination, may be advised for severe cases. Baptisia is used for headache, aching limbs, and fever, and arsenicum album for chills and diarrhea.

Hydrotherapy. For the achiness of flu, take a hot shower or bath; also try soaking your feet in a basin of hot water for 20 minutes twice a day.

Self-Treatment

Bed rest, while your body fights the virus, is the best medicine. If you have a fever, drink extra fluids, including fruit juice, tea, and broth, to prevent dehydration. Extra fluids also help thin any lung secretions.

For a sore throat, try gargling with warm, double-strength tea, or warm salt water. Acetaminophen, aspirin, nasal sprays, and decongestants may relieve minor discomfort; however, do not give aspirin to anyone under the age of 18 who has a viral infection, because it increases the risk of Reye's syndrome (page 437).

See a doctor if you have fever and are pregnant; or if a fever rises to 103°F (39.5°C) in anyone under age 60, 102°F (39°C) in an adult over 60, or 100°F (38°C) in an infant.

Other Causes of Flu Symptoms

Symptoms similar to those caused by the flu may occur with a bad cold, strep throat, scarlet fever, mild meningitis or encephalitis, or a sinus infection. A high fever accompanied by a cough that produces bloody, brown, or greenish mucus, points to bronchitis or possibly pneumonia.

SHOULD YOU HAVE AN ANNUAL FLU SHOT?

Immunization can prevent the most prevalent kinds of flu, which are caused by the Type A virus. Yearly flu shots are recommended for everyone over the age of 65 and for people of any age if they have heart disease, diabetes, kidney disease, asthma, or a chronic lung disorder, such as emphysema or cystic fibrosis.

Flu shots are also advised for health care workers and people who live in close quarters, such as military barracks.

Annual shots are necessary because the flu virus keeps mutating. The best time for immunization is in October or early November.

Food Poisoning

(Botulism; gastroenteritis; salmonella)
Gastroenteritis, the medical term for food poisoning, covers a number of intestinal disorders contracted from contaminated food. Symptoms usually appear within one to six hours after eating, and include nausea, vomiting, abdominal cramps, and diarrhea. The cause can be a bacterium, protozoan, or toxin. This last may occur naturally in certain plants, mushrooms, fish, or shellfish, or it may be a byproduct of improper canning techniques.

Outbreaks of food poisoning often happen among people who have eaten contaminated food in a restaurant or at a party or picnic. Staphylococcus or salmonella is frequently the culprit.

Food poisoning does not normally pose a threat to healthy people, but it can be serious in an elderly person, a very young child, or anyone debilitated by another medical problem. A new strain of *E. coli* bacterium, found particularly in undercooked ground beef, is especially dangerous to children.

Even healthy people are susceptible to botulism, caused by a toxin created by *Clostridium* bacteria. Though rare, it differs from other forms of gastroenteritis in that symptoms may not appear until several days after infection and do not always include nausea or vomiting. General weakness and blurred vision are typical; difficulty in swallowing and paralysis may follow. Botulism is often fatal.

Diagnostic Studies and Procedures
The broad diagnosis is generally easy, because the diarrhea and other symptoms come on rapidly and are unmistakable. Identifying the responsible organism, however, usually requires a laboratory culture of stool and vomit samples. If a poisonous plant or animal has been ingested, diagnosis rests on identifying the source of the poison.

Medical Treatments
Mild cases usually subside within a few days. If vomiting is severe, it's best to see a doctor, who may seek to control it with injections of an antiemetic drug. He may also prescribe medication for severe abdominal cramps. Antibiotics are not often used, since they may not be effective and can even prolong the problem. Diarrhea may not be treated either, as it helps remove the causative organism from the intestinal tract.

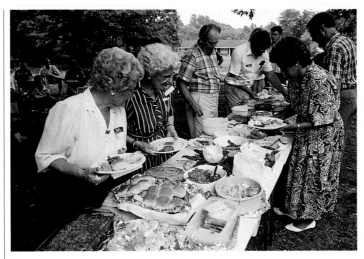

To prevent food poisoning, watch what you eat at picnics and other gatherings where food may have lain unrefrigerated for several hours. Cured foods and dishes high in vinegar or lemon juice are usually the safest, because salt and acid work as preservatives.

E. coli, which can cause a severe type of anemia and kidney failure, and botulism are medical emergencies that require hospitalization and close monitoring of vital signs. Because botulism causes progressive paralysis, which can impair breathing, the patient may have to be put on an artificial respirator and cared for in an intensive care unit.

Alternative Therapies
Various alternative therapies may help alleviate nausea, cramps, and other food poisoning symptoms.
Aromatherapy. Aromatherapists advise inhaling geranium, camphor, or chamomile oils twice a day to relieve nausea and cramps. Inhaling cypress oil is said to aid in reducing diarrhea.
Herbal Medicine. Chamomile tea may help calm the stomach. To stop nausea and vomiting, herbalists suggest steeping cloves in boiling water for five minutes, then drinking the strained tea. A cinnamon stick or 1 teaspoon minced ginger can be used in the same way.

Parsley tea can help settle a stomach, but it is also a diuretic and so is likely to increase urination. Do not employ this remedy if you are dehydrated from vomiting or diarrhea.
Naturopathy. A Native American remedy for an upset stomach is a drink made by pouring 1 cup of boiling

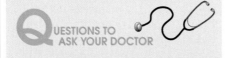

Q UESTIONS TO ASK YOUR DOCTOR

▶ Is it ever safe to eat rare or raw meat?
▶ What foods are most likely to harbor the bacteria that cause botulism?

water over 1 teaspoonful of cornmeal. Let the mixture sit for five minutes, add salt to taste, and then drink.

Self-Treatment
Prevention is the best way to deal with food poisoning. Except for cured products, such as salami, keep fish, poultry, meat, milk and other dairy items, eggs, and gravies refrigerated until cooking and/or serving time. To kill harmful bacteria, cook eggs until no longer runny and meat and poultry until the juices run clear. If you take such foods to a picnic, pack them in containers that keep them cool. Except when they are part of a salad, even rice and beans can cause food poisoning if kept at a warm temperature for more than two hours. Serve them soon after cooking or refrigerate them.

Salmonella from contaminated foods, such as raw chicken, easily spreads to anything with which it comes in contact. Wash your hands and all surfaces and utensils scrupulously.

To prevent botulism, discard any canned foods that have a broken seal, bulging top, or strange color or odor. Infants can develop a type of botulism from honey; thus, a baby under one year should never be given honey.

To combat nausea, drink flat ginger ale or other sweet carbonated beverage. Avoid solid foods until the diarrhea is gone, but drink extra fluids to prevent dehydration. (See Diarrhea, page 161.)

Other Causes of Food Poisoning Symptoms
Some medicines—laxatives, antibiotics, digitalis, and chemotherapy drugs—can produce nausea, diarrhea, and vomiting. Food allergies and excessive alcohol use can have these effects too.

Fractures

Any break or crack in a bone is called a fracture. With a simple, or closed, type, the skin remains intact. By contrast, in an open, or compound, fracture, the skin is broken, either from the injury that caused the fracture or by a piece of the bone itself. Compound fractures are especially dangerous, because they usually involve extensive tissue damage, heavy bleeding, and the possibility of infection.

In a complex, or comminuted, fracture, the bone is broken into several pieces or part of it is shattered. It may be either closed or open. Greenstick fractures are cracks that do not go all the way through the bone. They occur mostly in young children, whose bones are still relatively pliable. Stress fractures are also bone cracks; they usually develop in the legs of runners, dancers, and other athletes who regularly do strenuous weight-bearing exercise.

Diagnostic Studies and Procedures

Although a broken bone is often obvious, X-rays taken from different positions can confirm the exact nature of the fracture. In addition, a doctor may order a CT scan or MRI, especially if the injury involves the head or spine.

Medical Treatment

Treatment begins with setting the bone—a process called fracture reduction, in which the broken pieces are restored to their normal position. If this can be done by simple manipulation, it is referred to as closed reduction.

If an operation is necessary, the procedure is called open reduction. Such surgery requires anesthesia and an incision that allows the doctor access to the fracture. Surgery may also be necessary to mend tissues damaged by a broken bone. For example, a fractured rib that penetrates a lung can cause a collapsed lung, or pneumothorax, which may require surgical repair.

When a dislocation accompanies the fracture, as it often does with a joint bone, the displaced bones must also be returned to their original position; otherwise, the joint cannot function normally. If a fracture extends into a joint, a plate, pin, or screw may be used to keep the parts in place. Such devices are especially common in the repair of a hip fracture. Dislocations involving the wrist, shoulder, and elbow are relatively easy to reposition and can usually be treated in the emergency room or doctor's office using local anesthesia.

Once a fractured bone has been set, immobilization, usually with a cast, is essential to promote healing. If the fracture is only a hairline break, a cast may not be necessary. For a hairline break in the shoulder, for example, a sling will support the arm and keep it raised, thus relieving the shoulder of stress during healing. For a hairline fracture of the hip in an older person, treatment may be limited to extended bed rest until the break has healed.

When a rigid cast is necessary, the physician first covers the area to be immobilized with soft bandaging to protect the skin. He then saturates the wrapping with wet plaster, which hardens within minutes. The cast often extends beyond the area of the fracture. For example, a fractured wrist may need a plaster cast that extends from the knuckles to the elbow. A fractured ankle may require immobilization of the entire leg, so that the person must use crutches to move around.

A cast should never be so tight that it impairs blood flow. This is why toes or fingers are left exposed when a limb is put in a cast; if they turn blue, it's an indication that the cast must be removed and replaced with a looser one.

A physician uses X-rays, taken every few weeks, to monitor the healing of a

FIRST AID FOR FRACTURES

In general:
1. First call the emergency medical service for an ambulance, especially if the victim has sustained multiple injuries, is bleeding, or possibly has a back or neck injury.
2. Prevent the onset of shock by providing a blanket or other covering to conserve heat in the body.
3. If there is any likelihood of a neck or spine injury, DO NOT move the victim at all, unless absolutely necessary. (See Head, Neck, and Back Injuries, page 211.)

For an open fracture:
1. Cut away or remove clothing.
2. Control bleeding by applying pressure directly over the wound with a clean, preferably sterile, dressing. If necessary, a dressing can be improvised—use a towel, sheet, shirt, or other clean material.
3. Cover the protruding bone part with a large, sterile bandage or with some kind of clean material.

For a shoulder fracture:
1. Improvise a sling to support the arm.
2. Bandage the upper arm to the chest.

For an elbow fracture:
1. Handle the arm carefully, since forearm bones may be involved.
2. Place the arm in a sling, and bind the sling to the chest.

For wrist and forearm fractures:
1. Immobilize the limb by applying padded splints on both sides of the arm. (Splints

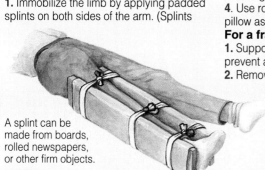

A splint can be made from boards, rolled newspapers, or other firm objects.

After splinting a broken arm, fashion a sling to hold the limb at a slightly raised angle.

can be made of tightly rolled newspaper, layers of cardboard, or other firm material.)
2. Bend the elbow slightly, and place the splinted arm in a slightly raised sling with the thumb pointing upward.

For a leg fracture:
1. Keep the patient lying down with the leg extended and flat.
2. If the break is in the lower part of the leg, also splint the knee and ankle. If the knee or thigh is involved, splint the entire leg.

For ankle and/or foot fractures:
1. Keep the patient lying down with the injured leg slightly elevated.
2. Remove shoes and hose.
3. For an open wound, apply large bulky dressings—sterile, if possible.
4. Use rolled newspapers, a blanket, or a pillow as a splint.

For a fractured jaw:
1. Support the injured person's head to prevent airway obstruction.
2. Remove any broken teeth and foreign matter from the mouth.
3. If there is no indication of a neck or back injury, prop the person up so that he is leaning forward.

FRACTURES (CONTINUED)

fracture. If healing is progressing properly, a plaster cast may at some point be replaced with a lighter, fiberglass type.

Some fractures cannot be immobilized with a cast, so other methods are used to keep the broken bone in place while it heals. For example, a broken rib is usually taped. A broken thigh may be immobilized with the use of traction, which depends on a system of weights and pulleys to keep a limb elevated, while fractured neck bones generally require a rigid steel brace to hold them steady.

A broken bone can be very painful, so codeine or another narcotic painkiller may be prescribed for a few days.

preserve muscle tone without interfering with healing. Exercise is even more important as part of rehabilitation after the cast is removed, especially when a joint is involved. In this case, it is critical to the process of completely restoring a normal range of motion.

After months in a cast, muscles will shrink and weaken; they need a graduated program of resistance and weight-bearing exercises to regain strength and function. A physical therapist can prescribe home exercises to augment sessions at a rehabilitation center. Physical therapy for re-establishing hip function usually involves the transitional use of crutches, a walker, and perhaps a cane.

tation. Music also reduces the perception of pain by stimulating an increase in the production of endorphins—brain chemicals that function as natural painkillers and mood elevators.

Nutrition Therapy. Healing of a broken bone generally demands extra calcium, vitamin D, and protein. A nutritionist may recommend supplements, as well as a diet rich in these nutrients.

Occupational Therapy. For a patient confined to a bed or wheelchair while recovering from a fracture, an occupational therapist can provide ingenious ways of managing daily self-care tasks, such as bathing, dressing, and eating.

Self-Treatment

Be sure to keep weight off the broken bone until it is fully healed. Follow your prescribed exercise regimen, but avoid unnecessary risks; you don't want to break the bone again. Bone tissue regenerates itself, so a healed bone is often stronger than it was before the fracture. Remember, however, that it takes a broken bone about a year to completely heal.

Most people who have worn a cast describe infuriating itching underneath it. Resist the temptation to use a knitting needle or other such implement to scratch under a cast. If you break the skin, you may develop an infection. Instead, try placing an ice pack over the area—cold often eases itchiness.

If you must use crutches, be sure they are adjusted to fit your height and arms. DO NOT rest your weight on the underarm portion—this can compress the nerves to your arm. Instead, use the hand rests to bear your weight.

Other Causes of Fractures

Most broken bones result from falls and accidents; however, osteoporosis (bone thinning that may occur with age) and other bone diseases sometimes cause spontaneous fractures, especially of the hip and back.

| Compound | Simple | Greenstick | Transverse | Oblique | Comminuted |

The different types of fractures illustrated above are most commonly sustained in long, weight-bearing bones; such fractures are casted until healing is complete.

After that, an over-the-counter pain reliever, such as aspirin or acetaminophen, is usually sufficient. Medications to reduce blood clotting and prevent any serious complications, such as a pulmonary embolism, may be prescribed, especially if a broken hip or leg necessitates bed rest. A compound fracture also requires taking antibiotics to prevent infection.

Alternative Therapies

Rehabilitation is an essential aspect of recovery from any fracture, and it often incorporates a combination of conventional and alternative therapies.

Exercise Therapy. Movement is essential to reduce the risk of a blood clot. A physical therapist or doctor will give specific instructions for exercises that

As hip function returns, such movement therapies as t'ai chi and dance therapy may help.

Hydrotherapy. Exercise in water may be easier than other forms of exercise, especially during the early stages of rehabilitation. Whirlpools and underwater massage can alleviate the muscle spasms and soreness that often occur after a long period of disuse.

Massage. As soon as physical therapy for the restoration of muscle function begins, it may be combined with various types of massage to stimulate circulation and overcome muscle spasms.

Music Therapy. Therapists sometimes encourage patients to do their exercise to certain types of music to help improve coordination during rehabili-

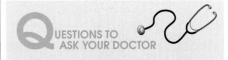

QUESTIONS TO ASK YOUR DOCTOR

▶ What can I do to minimize loss of muscle tone and strength?
▶ What is the best way to bathe without getting my cast wet? What should I do if I accidentally get it wet?
▶ When can I expect bruising or swelling in the area to go away?

Frostbite

(Chilblains)

Frostbite occurs when body tissues freeze, forming ice crystals within them and damaging the smaller blood vessels in the area. As tissue debris accumulates, it increasingly blocks circulation; this causes more injury to surrounding tissues, eventually killing them by depriving them of oxygen.

In less severe conditions, the cold may produce chilblains, in which the exposed parts become red, painful, and swollen. Subsequent exposure to cold causes recurrent symptoms.

The tissues most likely to be affected by both frostbite and chilblains are the skin and muscles of the hands and feet, because the body diverts blood flow from these areas to provide heat to the vital internal organs. The ears, nose, and cheeks are also vulnerable.

Diagnostic Studies and Procedures

Just before frostbite takes hold, the skin may be slightly flushed. As the condition develops, the area becomes cold, white, smooth, shiny, and numb. The person may not be aware of impending danger because she may feel no sensation of pain, but companions may notice the pale, glossy skin, as well as signs of mental confusion.

Medical Treatments

Emergency first aid. Cover the person with blankets and/or loose layers of clothing, and seek shelter. As soon as possible, call for an emergency medical team and ambulance. If the skin is still soft, rewarm the frozen area by immersing it in warm—not hot—water, 105°F to 110°F (40.5°C to 43°C). If the skin is hard or if no water is at hand, warm the frostbitten part with your own body—for example, cover ears with your warm hands.

Stop warming procedures as soon as the area becomes flushed, and help the patient change into warm, dry clothing, if available. (Caution: If the area may become frostbitten again, use skin-to-skin warming, not water. It's dangerous to "thaw" an area that may refreeze.)

There are several things you should not do. DO NOT rub the frozen area; this can cause further tissue damage. DO NOT apply a heating device of any kind. DO NOT permit the victim to place the affected area close to a hot stove or an open fire. DO NOT break any blisters that form. DO NOT allow the person to walk on recently thawed feet, but see that the feet remain elevated. Give warm drinks, but DO NOT permit alcohol consumption.

Emergency hospital treatment. Medical care begins with evaluating the patient's overall condition and taking steps to restore damaged blood vessels and repair damaged tissues.

After the initial warming procedure is completed, the affected area is kept warm, clean, and exposed to air.

Treatment may include administering antibiotics and a tetanus shot to prevent infection, and giving aspirin or ibuprofen to alleviate pain and decrease the danger of blood-clot formation. Intravenous fluids and drugs may be given as well.

In some cases, reserpine may be injected directly into an artery. This drug, used to treat high blood pressure, dilates blood vessels and helps prevent thickening of the blood.

Physical therapy takes place as soon as possible to speed rehabilitation of affected muscles and to restore joint movement. Surgery, if considered, is generally postponed until the extent of irreversible tissue damage is clear. The exception would be a severe case of gangrene; with this condition, prompt amputation is essential.

Alternative Therapies

Long-term management for physical and psychological recovery may employ several alternative therapies.

Hydrotherapy. Warm baths, including underwater-exercise and whirlpool baths, are a major aspect of treatment and rehabilitation.

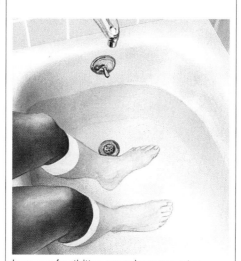

Immerse frostbitten areas in warm water (105°F to 110°F) to thaw them. When an immersed part becomes flushed, remove it.

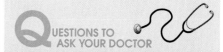

Nutrition Therapy. A high-protein diet may be devised to increase the nutrients necessary for rebuilding tissues damaged by frostbite.

T'ai Chi. The gentle range-of-motion exercises of this ancient discipline can easily be integrated into a program of physical therapy following frostbite.

Self-Treatment

If you must spend time outside during very cold weather, follow these precautions to avoid frostbite.

▶ Listen to weather forecasts and be guided not only by the temperature, but also by wind-chill and humidity factors, which can increase the danger of frostbite significantly.

▶ Wear protective clothing, including thermal underwear, a loose shirt, loose trousers, wind- and moisture-repellent outer garments, wool socks, fleece-lined boots, wool gloves under water-repellent gloves, close-fitting ear coverings, and a face mask. A hat is very important—30 percent of body heat escapes through an uncovered head.

▶ Limit your exposure time.

▶ Maintain general circulation by moving about, but avoid overexertion.

▶ Try to stay out of the wind.

▶ Provide occasional additional warmth for your fingers by crossing your arms and placing your hands in your armpits.

▶ Know the early symptoms of frostbite. If you experience any of them, seek shelter promptly and, if possible, change into dry, warm clothes.

▶ Do not rub any part of your body with snow—this only hastens freezing. Also, do not drink an alcoholic beverage before going out in the cold or while exposed to the cold.

Other Causes of Cold Injuries

Conditions that increase vulnerability to cold injuries include anemia, alcoholism, atherosclerosis, coronary artery disease, heart failure, and such circulatory disorders as Raynaud's disease.

Frozen Shoulder

(Adhesive capsulitis)

The condition called frozen shoulder begins as a slight pain and progresses to severe discomfort, which becomes worse when the shoulder is moved. Eventually, the shoulder stiffens to the point that it cannot be moved at all.

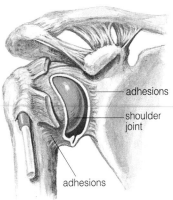

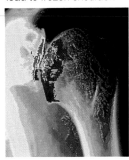

When a painful injury or inflammation prompts a person not to move his shoulder, this inactivity can allow adhesions to form, and these in turn lead to frozen shoulder.

adhesions

shoulder joint

adhesions

The scar tissue from adhesions eventually causes the joint capsule to shrink.

This disorder is not well understood, but it typically starts with a minor injury that leads to inflammation. The normal response is not to move the painful joint, thus allowing adhesions, constricting bands of tissue, to form. Adhesions make it even more difficult and painful to move the shoulder, and a vicious cycle develops. Eventually, the capsule lining the shoulder joint shrinks because of scar tissue resulting from the adhesions.

Diagnostic Studies and Procedures

A diagnosis is often based on symptoms and their progression, as well as a physical examination of the affected shoulder. To confirm the presence of adhesions, a doctor may order an arthrogram, a type of X-ray taken after a dye (to increase the contrast of soft tissues) is injected into the joint. The doctor may also examine the inside of the joint by inserting an arthroscope, a periscope-like instrument with a lighted tip, through a small incision.

Medical Treatments

Doctors usually recommend aspirin, ibuprofen, or prescription-strength nonsteroidal anti-inflammatory medications to alleviate pain. Sometimes cortisone, injected directly into the joint, causes a dramatic reduction in pain and inflammation. Injections have the added advantage of not producing the undesirable side effects associated with oral cortisone and other steroids.

Restoring mobility to the shoulder may require manipulating it to break up the adhesions. This is usually done under general anesthesia, and can be an outpatient procedure or one that requires a brief hospital stay. Once the adhesions have been broken and the pain controlled, a course of physical therapy will be prescribed to rehabilitate the shoulder.

Alternative Therapies

Medical treatment is usually required to overcome a frozen shoulder; the longer such care is delayed, the more difficult a complete cure will be. However, alternative therapies may help.

Chiropractic. Chiropractors treat shoulder pain and stiffness with manipulation techniques similar to those used for back problems. For frozen shoulder, a chiropractor may combine this approach with heat therapy and an exercise program.

Hydrotherapy. Water massage, needle showers, and other types of hydrotherapy may be used in rehabilitation efforts following medical treatment.

Massage. Rolfing or other deep massage techniques may help in treating the early stages of the disorder. Other massage methods can alleviate muscle tension in the upper neck and shoulder area that extends to the base of the shoulder blade. Pressure-point massage techniques, such as shiatsu and reflexology, may also ease shoulder pain.

Osteopathy. Osteopaths, doctors who have special training in manipulation techniques, often use a combination of physical therapy, massage, electrical stimulation, and ultrasound to relax tense muscles and relieve pain. An osteopath is just as qualified as an orthopedist or other medical doctor to break up the adhesions that are responsible for frozen shoulder.

Self-Treatment

If you experience shoulder pain, stop whatever physical activity is triggering it. Rest your shoulder for at least a day, and take aspirin or ibuprofen to ease pain and reduce inflammation.

Apply an ice pack (or ice wrapped in a towel) to the painful area for 20 minutes, remove it for 10 minutes, and reapply it for another 20 minutes. Repeat this as often as possible for the first day or two. The cold helps diminish the swelling and inflammation; after the first 48 hours, however, heat may be more beneficial.

If the pain and stiffness continue or worsen after a few days of self-care, see a doctor, especially if the pain is affecting shoulder mobility. Otherwise, the condition may become permanent.

Following treatment for a frozen shoulder, special weight-lifting exercises can help in regaining strength. But any exercise regimen should be undertaken only with the approval of a physician or physical therapist. A session of weight training should be preceded by range-of-motion exercises to warm up, and followed by muscle stretches to cool down. If your doctor or physical therapist approves, try doing these exercises two or three times a day:

▶ While holding a one- to five-pound weight, let your arm hang loosely at your side. Swing the arm back and forth gently, gradually increasing the range of the swing each day. You can also lean forward and swing the arm in small circles.

▶ Standing with your injured shoulder toward a wall, reach out with your arm until your hand is touching the wall. Keeping your elbow straight, walk your fingers slowly up the wall until you feel tension in the shoulder. Hold for 10 seconds, then walk your fingers back down. Repeat 10 times, trying to walk your fingers up a little more each time.

Other Causes of Shoulder Stiffness

Arthritis and muscle strain or sprain can bring about shoulder pain and stiffness, as can bursitis or tendinitis when caused by the excessive repetition of a motion, such as a golf swing.

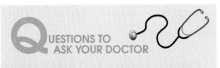

Q UESTIONS TO ASK YOUR DOCTOR

▶ What is the underlying cause of my condition? Is it likely to recur?
▶ What are the chances of a complete cure? About how long will it take?

Fungal Infections

(Mycoses; yeast infections)

Fungal infections are caused by tiny parasitic yeasts and molds. Though the human body hosts a variety of fungi, bacteria, and other organisms on the skin, mucous membranes, and other body tissues, these microscopic beings normally keep each other in check, so that they don't adversely affect your health. When something upsets this natural balance, or your resistance is lowered, some of these microorganisms can multiply unhindered.

Fungal infections range from minor skin problems to life-threatening systemic diseases. The most common minor invasions are ringworm, or tinea, infections, caused most frequently by the *Trichophyton* species and less commonly by *Microsporum* organisms. These fungi can infect the scalp (*tinea capitis*), the beard (*tinea barbae*), the skin (*tinea corporis*), the feet (*tinea pedis*, better known as athlete's foot), the groin area (*tinea cruris*, or jock itch), and the fingernails and toenails (*onychomycosis* and *tinea unguium*).

Among dozens of other fungal infections, the most prevalent are:
Aspergillosis, which can lead to pneumonia in people with lowered immune resistance, for example, anyone with AIDS or cancer chemotherapy patients.
Candidiasis, manifested as vaginitis, oral thrush, bladder infections, or skin infections similar to those of tinea. AIDS patients and others with weakened immune systems may develop disseminated candidiasis, which affects the heart, kidneys, and other vital organs. Recurrent, localized candidiasis, especially in the mouth or vagina, is common in people with diabetes.
Coccidioidomycosis, contracted by inhaling fungi spores in dust. It causes a mild lung infection, called San Joaquin, or Valley, fever because it occurs mostly in the California desert.
Cryptococcosis, which can evolve into a life-threatening form of meningitis, as well as infections of the heart, skin, lung, intestines, and other organs.
Histoplasmosis, which affects mostly the lungs. Fungi in soil contaminated by bat, bird, or chicken droppings bring about this disorder.
Sporotrichosis, caused by a soil mold that often infects the hands of gardeners and others who work with dirt.

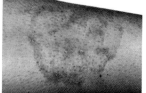

Tinea often produces a round lesion, hence the name ringworm.

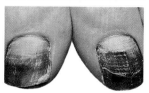

A fungal nail infection causes thickening and discoloration.

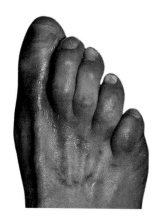

A red, scaling rash is the hallmark of athlete's foot, a highly contagious form of tinea.

Diagnostic Studies and Procedures

Some fungal infections, such as ringworm, can be identified on sight because of the distinctive appearance of the lesions. (Certain other fungal diseases of the scalp and skin have an identifiable appearance under a Wood's lamp, a special kind of ultraviolet light.) But a microscopic study or culture of skin scrapings, pus, or other infected tissues is usually necessary to accurately identify most fungi.

X-rays and other tests, including a biopsy, may be ordered if the lungs or other internal organs are affected.

Medical Treatments

Virtually all fungal infections are treated with antifungal drugs. Mild forms of tinea can be cured with antifungal ointments and creams, such as clotrimazole (Mycelex), nystatin (Mycostatin), and miconazole (Monistat and others). Depending upon the site of the infection, some of these drugs may also be administered as suppositories, eye drops, or pills. Most tinea infections clear up after a few weeks of treatment, but others, especially those involving the nails, may linger or recur.

Widespread infections that involve internal organs require the patient to be hospitalized for several days and given powerful intravenous or oral antifungal drugs, such as amphotericin B (Fungizone), fluconazole (Diflucan), griseoful-

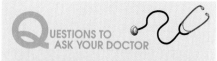

QUESTIONS TO ASK YOUR DOCTOR

► How long does it usually take to clear up a superficial fungal infection like athlete's foot or jock itch?
► At what point should I see a doctor for a prescription drug?

vin (Fulvicin), and ketoconazole (Nizoral). Surgery may be necessary to remove abscesses or pockets of fungi, especially from lungs and sinus cavities.

Alternative Therapies

In general, alternative therapies cannot substitute for antifungal drugs, especially with cases of severe internal fungal infections. In some instances, however, alternative remedies may be used in combination with medical treatment to relieve symptoms.
Aromatherapy. For scalp ringworm, athlete's foot, and other tinea infections of the skin, therapists recommend rubbing essence of geranium in an olive oil base onto the affected areas daily.
Herbal Medicine. Garlic, which is said to have potent antifungal properties, is recommended by herbalists to treat a nail infection. The best approach is to make a paste of crushed garlic in an olive oil base, allow it to age for four days, and then apply the mixture to the affected nails and cover with a bandage. Repeat this daily for 15 to 30 minutes until the infection clears. Practitioners also advocate eating fresh garlic or taking odorless garlic capsules.

Tea tree oil is also said to be effective when rubbed directly on the infection.

Pau d'arco, a South American herb, is yet another antifungal remedy. A cottonball that has been dipped in pau d'arco tea can be applied to the area, or even a tea bag itself.
Homeopathy. Practitioners may prescribe tellurium to relieve symptoms of ringworm of the skin and sepia paste for scalp ringworm.
Naturopathy. Apple cider vinegar is advocated for simple skin infections. For example, naturopaths recommend treating athlete's foot by rubbing apple cider vinegar onto the affected skin each day and letting it dry. Other tinea

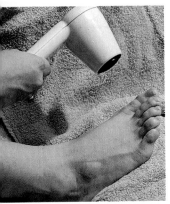

To prevent as well as treat athlete's foot, you should dry your feet thoroughly after bathing. A hair dryer is useful for this purpose.

FUNGAL INFECTIONS (CONTINUED)

skin infections are treated by soaking for 15 to 20 minutes in bathwater to which 3 cups of apple cider vinegar have been added. Rinsing the mouth and gargling with cider vinegar may help control oral thrush.

Naturopaths also recommend eliminating alcohol, sweets, and citrus fruits and other acidic foods from the diet for several weeks or until the fungal infection clears up. Acidophilus, in capsules or in yogurt containing live acidophilus cultures, is also believed to help control vaginal and oral yeast infections.

A word of caution: Although some practitioners advise a restrictive low-carbohydrate diet, there is no evidence that such a diet can prevent or treat systemic candidiasis and other internal fungal infections. Since these disorders usually occur in people with weakened immune systems, conventional medical treatment, along with testing to rule out an underlying disease, is best.

Self-Treatment

If you have a simple infection, such as athlete's foot or jock itch, an over-the-counter antifungal cream or powder may cure it. All products do not work equally well on all people, so if you are unsuccessful with the first one you try, select another.

The key to both prevention and treatment of athlete's foot is to keep your feet as dry as possible. After bathing, dry them thoroughly, especially between the toes and around the nails, and then dust with unscented powder to absorb moisture. It's a good idea also to air your feet as often as possible and wear sandals whenever practical.

When you have an active case of athlete's foot, wash and dry your feet once or twice a day and apply antifungal medication, instead of powder, between the toes and all over the feet. Keep using the product for a while after your symptoms go away. To avoid spreading the fungus to other parts of the body, put on clean, white cotton socks before stepping into your underclothes. Do not share towels (or other personal items), and launder them after each use in hot, soapy water; you may want to add chlorine bleach, which will kill the fungal spores.

You can prevent many fungal infections by following simple precautions. For example, wear rubber gloves when working with soil, and use a dust mask when cleaning up bird droppings to keep from inhaling fungal spores.

If you have a weakened immune system or diabetes, or if you are taking corticosteroids, anticancer drugs, or other agents that lower resistance, you are generally more susceptible to fungal infections. Under these circumstances, you should exercise extra precaution against infections of all kinds, and pay special attention to your foot, mouth, and skin hygiene.

Other Causes of Similar Symptoms

Bacterial and protozoal infections are sometimes mistaken for fungal infections, especially when internal organs are involved. Skin rashes and lesions may come from allergies or other forms of dermatitis. The round rash that occurs in Lyme disease is often confused with ringworm.

A CASE IN POINT

Myra Glenn's problems with a fungal nail began with two trivial toe injuries. First she stubbed her toe on her son's tricycle, and then, a few days later, she dropped a heavy book on the same toe. Within a week, the toenail had darkened and loosened. Glenn wrapped a piece of tape around the toe to keep the loose nail from snagging her stockings. After a couple of weeks, the nail was more firmly fixed, so she dispensed with the taping.

A month later, the toenail was still discolored, and it appeared to have stopped growing. Glenn also noticed between her other toes a recurrence of athlete's foot, a condition she had treated with an over-the-counter medication several months earlier. The athlete's foot cleared up after a few weeks, but the toenail hardly grew and most of it had turned a dull, chalky yellow. It was also thicker than normal, with bits of flaking nail under its edge. Although Glenn's dermatologist immediately suspected a fungal nail infection, he sent some sample scrapings to a laboratory for analysis.

"Repeated toe injuries or shoes that are too short can cause what we call dystrophic nails," the doctor explained. "The nails look like they have a fungal infection, but it's really a problem of a horn-like nail growth rather than a fungus."

Despite this possibility, Glenn's case was indeed a fungal infection. Her toenail disorder may well have been promoted by the injuries and the taping, which provided a moist environment for the fungus. The dermatologist warned Glenn of the difficulty of eradicating such infections. Even when the nail is removed and the underlying tissue treated with antifungal medication, the condition recurs in half or more of all cases. Oral antifungal medications, such as ketoconazole, work better than this procedure but can also cause liver damage.

Instead of either of these treatments, the doctor recommended daily application of a nonprescription cream for athlete's foot and periodic paring of the thickened nail to control the fungus.

From a friend, Glenn learned about an alternative remedy: daily treatment with garlic paste. To make the paste, she put a head of garlic through the food processor and added a few drops of olive oil. Each day, she applied it to her toenail and wrapped the toe with gauze to keep the paste in place for 15 minutes. She then bathed her feet in warm, soapy water, dried them thoroughly, and applied an antifungal cream to the entire foot.

After three months of this routine, the toenail began to return to its normal color and thickness. Not wanting to risk a recurrence, Glenn continued the daily garlic and antifungal treatments another three months, after which time her doctor could find no evidence of infection.

Gallbladder Cancer

(Carcinoma of the gallbladder)
The gallbladder, a small organ under the liver, stores the bile juices manufactured by the liver and released during digestion. If it becomes cancerous, there may be no symptoms early on. Later, however, abdominal pain, jaundice, loss of appetite and weight, and widespread itching may develop. These symptoms are often mistakenly thought to indicate liver disease.

Gallbladder cancer mainly afflicts people in their late sixties and seventies and is somewhat more common among women than men. Between 70 and 80 percent of those who have the cancer also have chronic gallstones and cholecystitis (gallbladder inflammation). The relationship between gallstones and cancer is not clearly understood, but doctors often advise people with the stones to undergo gallbladder removal to prevent a later malignancy.

Diagnostic Studies and Procedures

Because gallbladder cancer can be difficult to diagnose, doctors who suspect it usually order several procedures. An ultrasound examination of the gallbladder may show a thickening or an unusual mass in one area. CT scans and MRI may also reveal abnormalities. To arrive at a definitive diagnosis, a biopsy is necessary; this commonly involves inserting a long, hollow needle into the suspicious area and withdrawing tissue samples for microscopic examination.

When a biopsy confirms cancer, additional diagnostic procedures can determine if it has spread to other organs. These include CT scans and contrast X-ray studies, in which a special dye is used.

Medical Treatments

Treatment depends upon the stage of the disease when it is identified. In stage I, the cancer is confined to the gallbladder, and removal of the organ may be the only treatment needed. (Surgeons often find such a tumor when removing the gallbladder because of stones or chronic inflammation.)

In a stage II malignancy, the cancer has invaded the gallbladder muscle tissue and mucous membranes, but it has not spread to the bile ducts, liver, and nearby lymph nodes. This cancer can also be cured by removing the gall-

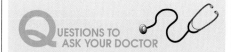

QUESTIONS TO ASK YOUR DOCTOR

▶ Should I have my gallbladder removed to prevent gallbladder cancer?
▶ If surgery is not feasible, can chemotherapy or radiation treatments control my gallbladder cancer?

bladder. As an extra precaution, the adjacent lymph nodes and a portion of the liver may also be excised, along with the lymphatic tissue that surrounds the bile ducts and the major blood vessels serving the liver.

Gallbladder removal is a relatively simple procedure. Loss of the organ poses no lasting problems, as the flow of bile can be redirected during surgery so that it passes directly from the liver into the intestine. Chemotherapy is sometimes used in addition to surgery.

Unfortunately, the majority of gallbladder cancers are not detected until they reach a more advanced stage, by which time large portions of the liver may also be cancerous. When this happens, chemotherapy is likely to be the sole form of treatment.

If the cancer is confined to the bile ducts, radiation may be combined with surgery or used instead of surgery. If a duct is blocked and surgical removal is not possible, a tube may be inserted to bypass the duct and allow bile to flow from the gallbladder to the intestine.

Medications, including painkillers and drugs to reduce itching, may be prescribed to alleviate symptoms.

Alternative Therapies

No known alternative approach can cure this or any other type of cancer. However, certain therapies can help reduce pain and the stress that comes with having a life-threatening disease.

Acupuncture and Acupressure. Acupuncture is often incorporated into pain management for cancer patients and is generally agreed to be effective.

Hypnotherapy. Hypnosis and self-hypnosis are also well-accepted means of managing pain. Patients who are taught self-hypnosis can often lessen the amount of medication they need to control their pain.

Meditation and Visualization. These techniques may be employed to reduce stress and to make the persistent itching that often accompanies gallbladder cancer more tolerable.

Nutrition. Because loss of appetite is common with gallbladder cancer, a nutritionist may help to plan small, highly nutritious meals that can be eaten frequently. She might also recommend that the patient take special enriched supplements to prevent excessive weight loss, since fats could be difficult to digest. Some patients may require a special feeding tube or intravenous feeding of predigested food.

Self-Treatment

Self-care is not effective in treating gallbladder cancer, but you can take measures to prevent gallstones, which are often related to the cancer (see Self-Treatment, page 198).

Other Causes of Gallbladder Symptoms

Hepatitis and other liver disorders can produce symptoms similar to those of gallbladder cancer. Acute abdominal pain is often present in appendicitis, attacks of gastritis, or inflammatory intestinal disorders and other digestive problems. Persistent itching is also associated with allergic reactions, dry skin, liver disease, and leukemia.

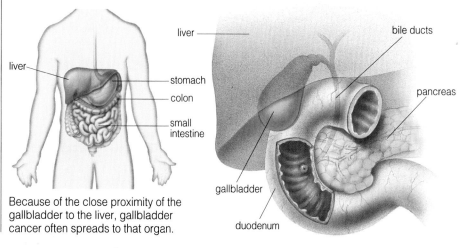

Because of the close proximity of the gallbladder to the liver, gallbladder cancer often spreads to that organ.

Gallstones

(Biliary calculus)

Gallstones are small, hard pellets that form in the gallbladder, the pouchlike organ situated just under the liver, in the upper-right portion of the abdomen. Most gallstones are composed of cholesterol crystals, although some are made of bile salts, which are digestive substances manufactured in the liver and stored in the gallbladder.

The stones can be as tiny as the head of a pin or as large as a walnut. It is not clear why they form, but it may be because of an imbalance in the substances that make up bile; excess cholesterol in the bile juices seems to be an important contributing factor.

If a gallstone blocks one of the ducts that carry bile from the gallbladder to the intestine, the result can be an attack of biliary colic, producing such symptoms as severe abdominal pain, nausea, vomiting, bloating, belching, sweating, and jaundice. The presence of gallstones can also cause gallbladder inflammation and infection, a condition known as acute cholecystitis. More often, however, the gallbladder harbors stones without causing any symptoms; an estimated 16 to 20 million Americans over the age of 40 have gallstones, but only a million experience attacks in the course of a year.

Gallstones most often afflict middle-aged, overweight females. Women taking birth control pills or replacement estrogen also have an increased risk of the condition. For unexplained reasons, about 70 percent of Navajo Indians of both sexes have gallstones.

Diagnostic Studies and Procedures

A doctor usually makes the initial diagnosis of an acute attack on the basis of symptoms. During an attack, abdominal pain occurs suddenly, soon after eating, and continues in waves as the duct contracts to get rid of the stone.

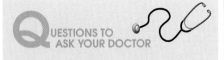

Q UESTIONS TO ASK YOUR DOCTOR

▶ Is estrogen replacement therapy during and after menopause likely to bring on gallstones even though I have not had problems in the past?
▶ If there is a family history of gallstones, should I avoid oral contraceptives?

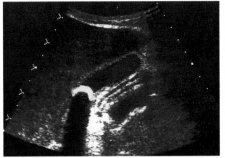

With an ultrasound scan, it is possible to determine if a gallbladder harbors stones, even when there are no symptoms.

An episode may last for several hours, stopping abruptly when the gallstone passes into the intestine.

Diagnostic studies include blood tests and imaging the gallbladder with X-rays, ultrasound, and CT scanning.

Medical Treatments

"Silent," or asymptomatic, gallstones do not require treatment. Those that cause recurrent painful attacks are most often treated by removing the gallbladder, an operation called a cholecystectomy. During this procedure, the bile is redirected so that it flows directly from the liver to the intestines.

A relatively new type of surgery, called laparoscopic cholecystectomy, reduces the length of a patient's hospital stay and speeds convalescence, though it is not recommended for persons who have had prior abdominal surgery. This operation involves making four small punctures in the abdomen and inserting a laparoscope, a catheter with a miniature television camera. The surgical team passes its special operating instruments through the laparoscope, and performs the surgery while viewing the gallbladder and the surrounding organs on a video monitor. The team then removes the gallbladder through the laparoscope.

Instead of taking out the gallbladder, a physician may advise pulverizing the gallstones with shock-wave treatment, known as lithotripsy.

Medications, such as ursodiol (Actigall) or chenodiol (Chenix), can dissolve gallstones, but these drugs take months to work and must then be taken for life to prevent more of the stones from forming.

Alternative Therapies

Alternative therapies are unlikely to cure gallstones, but they may alleviate the colicky pain of an attack.

Acupuncture and Acupressure. Pain may be relieved by stimulating points on the meridians that serve the gallbladder, stomach, and liver.

Herbal Medicine. Herbalists recommend alfalfa tablets or dandelion, either in capsule form or as an extract mixed with water, to enhance gallbladder function. Turmeric capsules are also thought to have a protective effect. European herbalists advocate peppermint oil capsules.

Homeopathy. Homeopaths often prescribe celedonium, podophyllum, and berberis. Taken in highly diluted form, these are said to be similar to the substances that cause gallstones.

Nutrition. In addition to advising a low-fat, high-fiber diet, nutrition therapists may recommend vitamins E and D, lecithin, and bran supplements to reduce blood cholesterol levels.

Shiatsu. Practitioners of this Japanese form of pressure-point massage apply rhythmic pressure in circles around the abdominal area of the gallbladder to alleviate pain.

Self-Treatment

Self-care can often prevent gallstones. If you have an elevated cholesterol level, adopt a cholesterol-lowering diet that is high in starches and fiber, and limit fat intake to 20 percent or less of your total calorie intake.

If you are overweight, try to lose excess pounds gradually through a sensible combination of diet and exercise. Avoid crash diets, however, because rapid weight loss sometimes precipitates a gallstone attack.

Refrain from cigarette smoking, which has been implicated in the formation of gallstones (as well as many other health problems). Women who have had the stones should avoid birth control pills and estrogen replacement, because high levels of this hormone have been associated with gallbladder disease.

When an attack does occur, do not eat, but do take a nonprescription pain medication and rest in bed. Call a doctor if the attack lasts more than three hours. You should also see a doctor if you have recurrent attacks.

Other Causes of Abdominal Pain

Recurring pain in the upper abdomen may also come from ulcers, gastritis, or cancer of the stomach, liver, or pancreas. Pancreatitis, inflammation of the pancreas, also produces pain in this section of the abdomen.

Ganglion

A ganglion is a harmless, although annoying, noncancerous growth that forms directly under the skin. Ganglia usually occur in clusters, on or near tendon sheaths and joint capsules. (These benign growths should not be confused with the cluster of nerve cells that is also referred to as a ganglion.) Formed of the same jellylike substances found in fibrous tissue, ganglia may feel either hard or soft to the touch. A typical ganglion is the size of a pea, but some grow as large as a walnut, especially if they become inflamed.

Most often, ganglia develop along the wrist, especially on the back of the hand; less often, they form on the fingers, palm, or around the ankle. The underlying cause is unknown, but in some cases their occurrence seems to be associated with repetitive stress injuries, as from playing tennis or practicing certain musical instruments.

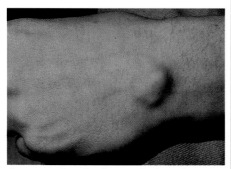

A common location for ganglia is on the wrist, near tendon sheaths or joint capsules.

Ganglia occur most frequently in children, teenagers, and young adults. Unfortunately, they often recur even after removal; for example, about 10 percent of wrist ganglia grow back after surgical excision.

Diagnostic Studies and Procedures

A doctor can usually tell by visual and tactile inspection whether a lump or swelling is a ganglion or a group of ganglia. For further confirmation, an X-ray of the affected area and possibly a sonogram, or ultrasound scan, may be ordered. To ensure that the lump is noncancerous, the physician may decide to submit a sample of the fluid from it for laboratory analysis. To obtain the sample, a doctor or nurse inserts a needle into the lump and withdraws a small amount of the fluid

into the syringe; this procedure is called needle aspiration or needle biopsy.

Medical Treatments

Most small ganglia do not require treatment. If a ganglion becomes inflamed and painful, a doctor may inject it with cortisone. Alternatively, she may withdraw as much of the jellylike substance as possible and then inject the ganglion with cortisone in the hope of preventing its regrowth.

Another treatment, called sclerosing, involves injecting a solution that causes the ganglia to dry up and turn into scar tissue. This procedure must be done carefully, because it can damage the joint lining or nearby nerves, and result in a loss of function.

Surgical Treatment. If you have a ganglion that is unsightly or interferes with normal activities, you may want to consider surgical removal. The procedure, called a ganglionectomy, is considered minor surgery, which usually requires only a local anesthetic and can be done in the doctor's office. For a wrist ganglion, however, a surgeon trained in hand operations should perform the ganglionectomy, since expertise is needed to avoid damaging the nerves that control the fingers. With all such procedures, a magnifying device should be used to ensure that tiny satellite ganglia are removed, reducing the chance that growths will recur.

Following the operation, expect the hand to swell. You will probably wear a wrist splint for a week to allow healing. Stitches will then be removed, but you should use the wrist cautiously for yet another two weeks, taking care to avoid lifting or any sudden twisting movement that can interfere with healing. The operation will leave a small scar, and when the tissues are completely healed, a few sessions with a physical therapist may be required to restore the joint's range of motion.

Alternative Therapies

In some parts of the world, ganglia are known as "Bible bumps." This odd term came about because there were people who once believed that the best way to eliminate a ganglion was to whack it with the family Bible or any heavy book. Traditional though it may

be, this method is dangerous; it can damage surrounding tissues and fracture the small bones of the wrist and hand. Sound alternative treatments are available; those that are effective with joint problems work especially well.

Acupuncture. A few sessions with an acupuncturist may result in rupture of a ganglion. If this happens, the substance inside it will be reabsorbed by the body, although the growth may eventually recur.

Shiatsu or acupressure. These and other forms of massage therapy may have the same effect as acupuncture.

Self-Treatment

In many instances, ganglia rupture spontaneously and disappear. But do not attempt to rupture a ganglion by squeezing or pressing it; you may end up with painful inflammation.

If a ganglion does become inflamed, an over-the-counter anti-inflammatory medication such as aspirin or ibuprofen should provide relief from both the pain and swelling.

Other Causes of Hand Growths

The hand is especially vulnerable to benign growths that resemble ganglia. These include cysts, nerve tumors, warts, fibromas, and bony growths, spurs, and bosses (swellings).

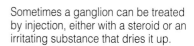

Sometimes a ganglion can be treated by injection, either with a steroid or an irritating substance that dries it up.

Gastritis

(Erosive and nonerosive gastritis)
Gastritis is a stomach inflammation that may produce bleeding, ulceration, and erosion of the lining. Typical symptoms include upper abdominal pain, nausea, vomiting, bloating, heartburn, and sometimes bleeding.

With acute gastritis, the symptoms occur suddenly, caused by an infection, a toxic substance, aspirin and similar drugs, a food allergen, or severe stress from burns, surgery, kidney or liver failure, and other serious conditions.

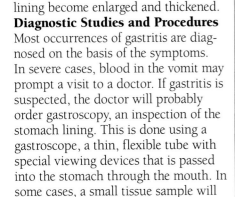

Normally, the stomach lining is a light pink. With gastritis, it turns bright red, and sometimes areas of tissue erode.

esophagus

healthy stomach

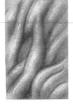

The mucous membrane lining the stomach has numerous folds and small glands.

In hypertrophic gastritis (right), the lining folds are thick and enlarged.

Chronic gastritis often results from alcohol abuse or long-term use of aspirin or another nonsteroidal anti-inflammatory drug used to treat arthritis and other painful conditions. Sometimes it is linked to an underlying disorder, such as Crohn's disease (in which the large and small intestines become inflamed and ulcerated).

In hypertrophic gastritis, a rare disorder, the mucosal folds and the stomach lining become enlarged and thickened.

Diagnostic Studies and Procedures
Most occurrences of gastritis are diagnosed on the basis of the symptoms. In severe cases, blood in the vomit may prompt a visit to a doctor. If gastritis is suspected, the doctor will probably order gastroscopy, an inspection of the stomach lining. This is done using a gastroscope, a thin, flexible tube with special viewing devices that is passed into the stomach through the mouth. In some cases, a small tissue sample will be removed through the gastroscope and sent for laboratory studies.

Other diagnostic measures may include an upper GI series of X-rays, taken after the patient drinks barium, a chalky substance that coats the stomach and other digestive organs to make them visible on film. A sample of stomach fluids may also be taken for laboratory analysis of the acid level, since reduced secretion of gastric juice is often associated with gastritis. Generally, this sample is drawn out with a tube that is passed through the nose and esophagus to the stomach.

Medical Treatments
Treatment will vary according to the symptoms and the underlying cause. Gastritis from a viral infection is self-limiting and does not require any medical intervention.

An over-the-counter antacid may alleviate mild symptoms. If an underlying cause has been found, treating it will usually clear up the stomach problem as well.

Severe erosive gastritis calls for prompt treatment to stop any bleeding. When bleeding is profuse, a stomach tube may be inserted and ice water passed through it to constrict any leaking blood vessels. A blood transfusion may be required, though this is rare. If severe bleeding persists, an emergency operation may be performed to remove the eroded part, or, in some cases, the entire stomach.

Alternative Therapies
Alternative approaches are usually not appropriate for acute gastritis that involves bleeding. They may, however, be useful in treating and preventing chronic, nonerosive gastritis.

Herbal Medicine. To alleviate the inflammation, many herbalists recommend marsh mallow root, which may be taken as a tincture or in capsules. Meadowsweet tea or diluted tincture is said to reduce stomach inflammation; licorice sticks or tea and slippery elm capsules are other remedies. Peppermint tea aids digestion and may help settle an upset stomach. Ginger extract and alfalfa-seed tea may also alleviate a mildly upset stomach.

Some herb books recommend angelica tea for gastritis, but recent studies question its safety. Certain toxic herbs

such as European mandrake, arnica, and tansy can cause severe gastritis (see Poisoning Emergencies, page 339).
Homeopathy. Practitioners often recommend ipecacuanha to ease the pain and other symptoms of gastritis.
Naturopathy. Sometimes reduced production of hydrochloric acid, one of the stomach's digestive juices, promotes gastritis. Naturopaths advise taking a tablespoon of apple cider vinegar during a flare-up. If you find that it helps, sip a little with meals. If, on the other hand, it makes the symptoms worse, discontinue use and avoid digestive aids that contain hydrochloric acid.

Self-Treatment
You can usually treat mild attacks of gastritis yourself with nonprescription antacids, but see a doctor if symptoms last more than a day or two or if they recur frequently. Seek immediate medical attention if you vomit blood.

Since smoking and excessive use of alcohol are often linked to gastritis, abstain from both, as well as from beverages that contain caffeine.

Try to determine whether a particular food triggers the problem. If something does, avoid it in the future. In any event, stay away from spicy dishes and fatty or fried foods. Eating frequent, small meals may also help.

Stop taking aspirin and other nonsteroidal anti-inflammatory drugs. If you need these drugs for a concurrent medical problem, such as arthritis, ask your doctor about taking them in enteric form. These pills have a coating that allows them to pass undissolved into the small intestine, where they are unlikely to cause irritation. In the meantime, take uncoated forms with food or milk, which minimizes their contact with the stomach lining.

Other Causes of Stomach Pain
Heartburn and peptic ulcers produce many of the same symptoms as gastritis. In a few cases, stomach cancer may be responsible for the symptoms.

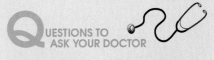

QUESTIONS TO ASK YOUR DOCTOR

▶ Could stress be causing my recurrent bouts of gastritis?
▶ If my arthritis medication is causing my gastritis, can I take an alternative drug that will be easier on my stomach?

Genital Warts

(Condylomata acuminata; venereal warts)
Similar to those that appear on other parts of the body, genital warts may be flat or raised, single or clustered. However, they are much more contagious, spreading easily through sexual contact, and developing within two or three months after sexual relations with an infected person. The causative agents are several papilloma viruses, which come from the same virus family that causes other types.

In women, genital warts occur on the vulva and cervix, in the vagina, and on or near the anus. Sometimes vaginal and cervical warts are so small that they go unnoticed, thus increasing the risk of infecting a partner. In men, the warts most often occur on the penis, but also sometimes in the anal area, on the scrotum, or inside the urethra.

More than 40 million Americans have had genital warts, and about one million new cases are diagnosed each year. These numbers are of concern because genital warts appear to increase the risk of vulvar and cervical cancer.

Diagnostic Studies and Procedures
Sometimes the patient or a sexual partner first notices genital warts. But more often, because they can be miniscule and usually do not cause obvious symptoms, the warts are diagnosed by a physician during a routine physical or gynecologic examination. The doctor may use a magnifying device, such as a colposcope, to examine the warts. She may also order a blood test to differentiate the warts from the skin lesions caused by syphilis. Warts with an

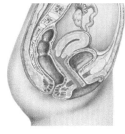

In men, genital warts usually occur on the penis, but may also form inside the anus or urethra or on the scrotum (blue areas).

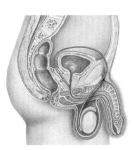

Warts may go unnoticed in a woman because they are often small and internal—located on the vagina and cervix (highlighted in blue).

A CASE IN POINT

When Leroy Hobbs, a 26-year-old computer programmer, learned that he had genital warts, he immediately realized their source—a casual sexual encounter with a woman he had met at an out-of-town business conference. Laser surgery cleared up his warts, but now he faced the problem of breaking the news to his fiancée. He knew he may have passed the infection on to her and that it was important for her to see a doctor.

Hobbs tried to bring up the subject several times, but he simply couldn't admit that besides being unfaithful, he might have given his fiancée a sexually transmitted disease. Finally, he turned to his doctor for guidance.

"Ask your fiancée to come see me, and I'll explain the situation," the doctor told Hobbs. He also suggested that the couple seek counseling to learn how to communicate better.

Hobbs's fiancée did have genital warts, which were also treated with laser surgery. Because of her increased risk of cervical cancer, she was also instructed to have more frequent pap smears.

The next few months were difficult for the couple, but they were determined not to let the incident destroy their relationship. Through premarital counseling offered by their church, they gained new skills in talking to each other. In the end, both of them felt that the unfortunate experience had actually strengthened the bonds between them.

---

unusual appearance and those that persist despite treatment should be biopsied to rule out cancer.

If a woman has warts on the cervix, a pap smear and perhaps a biopsy of cervical tissue should be done to check for precancerous changes in the cells. In addition, any woman who has ever had genital warts should have more frequent pap smears—as often as every three to six months—because of her increased risk of cervical cancer.

Medical Treatments
Single warts or small groups of warts can sometimes be removed with caustic chemicals, such as podophyllin or trichloroacetic acid. This approach often requires several applications and is not

---

always successful. In another technique, cryosurgery, the warts are frozen off with liquid nitrogen. This treatment may cause temporary blistering of the surrounding tissue. Yet another method is cauterization, in which an electric needle is used to burn off the warts after applying a local anesthetic.

Warts in the urethra may be treated with a topical medication several times a day, but this presents a slight chance of urethral obstruction. Removing these warts under general anesthesia may be the most definitive method. In uncircumcised men, performing a circumcision during the same operation may prevent urethral warts from recurring.

Laser surgery, a method of applying a strong light beam to vaporize small amounts of tissue, is being used against genital warts with increasing frequency.

With all treatments, the warts often come back and require more therapy.

Alternative Therapies
Although numerous folk remedies are said to remove ordinary warts, none appear to clear up genital warts.

Self-Treatment
Never attempt to remove genital warts with nonprescription wart preparations; they are ineffective against these types, and can damage genital tissue.

After chemical removal of genital warts, you will be instructed to wash off the caustic medication after a specific time. Until the warts fall off, wear loose-fitting cotton underwear and keep the skin clean and dry. Avoid sexual activity until healing is complete.

If you have warts, your sexual partner should see a doctor. Because of the high recurrence rate, it is important to use a condom during sexual intercourse to avoid reinfection.

Other Causes of Genital Growths
Genital herpes can produce a reddish lesion that may resemble a wart, but, unlike most warts, it is usually quite painful. Vulvar cysts and cancer may begin as wartlike growths.

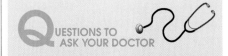

QUESTIONS TO ASK YOUR DOCTOR

▶ How often should I be examined to see if the warts may have returned?
▶ If genital warts are healed and have not recurred, do I still need to tell my partner about having had them?

German Measles

(Rubella; three-day measles)

German measles, or rubella, is a mild, highly contagious childhood disease that lasts about three days as a rule, hence its popular name, three-day measles. It is caused by a virus and is sometimes confused with measles, or rubeola; both conditions produce a fever, a sore throat, and a splotchy red rash, but the symptoms are more severe and long-lasting in measles.

Two to three weeks following exposure to the virus, the person typically develops a slight fever, headache, sore throat, swollen lymph nodes, and loss of appetite. These early symptoms may be so mild, however, that it is difficult to be sure the individual has German measles until the rash appears one to five days later. It usually starts behind the ears or on the face, rapidly spreads to the trunk and sometimes to the arms and legs, and disappears entirely within three or four days (the lymph nodes may remain swollen longer). Adults who contract German measles may have continuing joint pains for a few weeks after the rash has cleared up.

Once a very common children's disease, rubella can now be prevented through routine vaccination, which is usually given around a child's first birthday. (Younger babies cannot be vaccinated successfully, because they still carry antibodies from their mother's immune system and these keep the vaccine from working.) A second dose is given with the measles booster vaccine when the child is 11 or 12.

Teenagers and adults who lack immunity against the disease can also contract it. The greatest danger of German measles, however, is to a developing fetus. If a pregnant woman becomes infected with the virus, it can cause congenital rubella in the child she is carrying. This can be particularly devastating if the infection occurs during the first trimester of pregnancy. Possible consequences include stillbirth or serious birth defects, especially impaired hearing or deafness, eye defects or blindness, heart defects, mental retardation, and behavioral problems.

Diagnostic Studies and Procedures

A doctor can usually diagnose German measles by physical examination.

If an expectant mother believes she has contracted rubella, she may have a

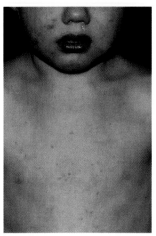

The rash of German measles generally starts on the head, quickly spreads to the trunk and limbs, and is gone in about three days.

prenatal ultrasound examination, which can detect some birth defects, such as a malformed heart, but not neurological complications. A physician may suspect congenital rubella in a newborn, if there is a possibility that the mother was exposed to the disease during pregnancy and if the baby exhibits certain birth defects. Laboratory tests of the baby's throat secretions, urine, or blood can confirm the diagnosis.

Medical Treatments

Home care is all that is necessary, because rubella is normally mild and self-limited. A doctor may recommend acetaminophen to reduce fever, but aspirin should not be given to anyone under the age of 18 who has a viral infection because of the risk of Reye's syndrome, a serious illness characterized by severe vomiting, lethargy, personality changes, and damage to the liver and brain (see box, page 437).

The situation is much different for babies born with rubella. They usually require intensive treatment, especially if they contracted the virus during the first three months of gestation, when the various organ systems are developing. These babies often have severe heart defects that may require surgical

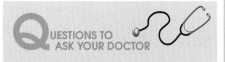

QUESTIONS TO ASK YOUR DOCTOR

▶ How long should I wait after rubella immunization before attempting to become pregnant?
▶ If I develop rubella during pregnancy, what are the odds that my baby will have serious birth defects?

repair early in life. In addition, many rubella children need lifelong specialized treatment, depending upon the type and extent of their birth defects. Those with hearing impairment, for example, may have to be provided with special devices and instruction to learn how to talk. A child with mental retardation will probably require special-education services as well.

Prevention is the best approach to congenital rubella. Studies show that 10 to 20 percent of women lack antibodies against the disease. Some experts urge that every woman be tested for rubella antibodies before becoming pregnant, even if she was once immunized or had the disease. A simple blood test can determine whether a woman has this immunity. If not, she should be vaccinated before becoming pregnant. Immunization cannot be administered during pregnancy because the fetus can contract congenital rubella from the live-virus vaccine.

A woman who is already pregnant should also have a rubella antibody test. If she lacks immunity, she must avoid exposure to German measles, particularly during the first trimester.

Alternative Therapies

Homeopathy. A number of substances are used to treat the symptoms of German measles; they include aconite, belladonna, camphor, and sulphur. The specific medication chosen will depend upon the constellation of symptoms and their severity.

Reflexology. When lymph nodes are tender and swollen, pressing specific points on the hands and feet may be recommended to promote the flow of lymph. This should be done twice a day, for three minutes each time, for a duration of three weeks.

Self-Treatment

Bed rest is not necessary unless there is a high fever. Sponging or bathing the child with tepid water can lower a fever. The patient should drink plenty of fluids and eat light meals.

Other Causes of Skin Rashes

An allergic reaction to any number of substances can cause a rash that looks like that of German measles, as can a hypersensitive reaction to a medication. Prickly heat can also produce a reddish rash, but usually without any other symptoms. A rash accompanied by fever can stem from another viral infection such as chickenpox.

Gestational Diabetes

(Pregnancy-related diabetes mellitus)
Gestational diabetes develops during pregnancy and disappears almost immediately after the baby is delivered. As in other forms of diabetes (page 158), blood sugar levels are too high, because the woman does not properly metabolize carbohydrates, due either to inadequate insulin or an inability to fully utilize the hormone. The symptoms are often so mild that they may not even be noticed unless her blood sugar is checked periodically.

When the mother's blood sugar levels are too high, the fetus produces extra insulin, which acts like a growth hormone during fetal development. The result is an oversized and sickly baby. Excessive fetal insulin also interferes with potassium metabolism, which can lead to potentially fatal arrhythmias, or irregular heartbeats.

Gestational diabetes is the most common cause of stillbirths and late fetal death. The disorder also increases the possibility of birth defects.

Factors contributing to the risk of gestational diabetes include pregnancy after the age of 35, obesity, and having had an earlier baby larger than nine pounds. Women who themselves weighed more than nine pounds at birth also have an increased incidence of gestational diabetes, which in turn carries a risk of eventually developing either Type I or Type II diabetes.

Diagnostic Studies and Procedures

A doctor can detect gestational diabetes by screening for elevated levels of blood sugar between the 24th and 28th weeks of pregnancy. Medical personnel give the expectant mother a sugar drink and measure her blood sugar level an hour later. If the level is elevated (over 150 mg/dl), the doctor will order a three-hour glucose tolerance test; the woman consumes 100 grams of oral glucose, after which her blood sugar levels are monitored hourly three times.

Most obstetricians recommend that all pregnant women be screened for gestational diabetes. They also advise that those who fall into a high-risk group be tested more often. Such women might, for example, undergo screening in the 12th, 18th, and 32nd weeks of pregnancy.

Medical Treatments

After a woman has been diagnosed, treatment should begin immediately to normalize blood sugar levels. Proper diet and exercise can often accomplish this, but some women may need to be hospitalized initially to bring the diabetes under control.

Once the level of blood glucose has been normalized, it is critical to keep it under control to reduce risks to the fetus. This usually involves careful self-monitoring of the glucose levels several times a day, as well as keeping up the diet and exercise regimen.

If adjusting the diet and exercise are not enough, the doctor may prescribe one or more daily injections of insulin. The woman will also need to see her obstetrician more often, usually weekly during the last two or three months of pregnancy, to make sure the fetus is continuing to grow normally.

Alternative Therapies

No alternative methods can be used to treat gestational diabetes effectively, but appropriate nutrition and a regular exercise program to maintain ideal weight before becoming pregnant can help to prevent the condition. Also, aspects of these therapies can be adopted into the medical regimen with the obstetrician's knowledge and approval.

Herbal Medicine. Ginseng tea is believed to reduce blood glucose levels. Other herbs recommended to treat diabetes include dandelion root and uva-ursi. However, check with your doctor before taking these, or any other herbal remedies.

Naturopathy. Practitioners recommend consuming a diet high in starches and fiber and shunning sugars. Spirulina, a type of warm-water algae especially high in protein, is said to help lower the blood sugar.

Self-Treatment

Self-care is the key to preventing or controlling gestational diabetes and increasing the chances of having a healthy baby. If you are overweight, try to achieve your ideal weight before you conceive. Do not attempt to lose weight during pregnancy; doing so could deprive the fetus of necessary nutrients.

If you do develop gestational diabetes, maintaining normal blood glucose levels is critical. This usually requires distributing your food intake over four to six small meals a day and reducing your total number of calories.

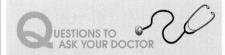
QUESTIONS TO ASK YOUR DOCTOR

▶ If I've had gestational diabetes during one pregnancy, what is my risk of developing it in a subsequent pregnancy?
▶ If the fetus seems to be too big, should an early labor be induced?

You may have to monitor your blood glucose levels six to eight times a day. Fortunately, you can do this with a simple, electronic blood glucose monitor now available for home use. If you must use insulin, learn to administer these injections yourself, and ask your doctor to help you develop a system for rotating injection sites.

As your delivery date nears, your obstetrician may ask you to pay special attention to fetal activity and to report promptly any decrease in the baby's kicks and other movements.

Other Causes of Abnormal Blood Glucose Tests

Ordinary blood glucose tests fail to detect gestational diabetes when pregnant women fast before seeing their doctors for fear that they are gaining too much weight. This practice temporarily lowers blood glucose levels and masks gestational diabetes.

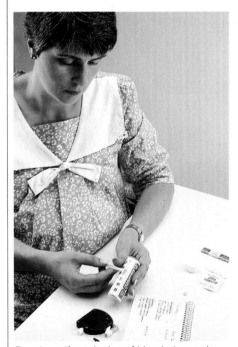

Regular self-monitoring of blood glucose is an important part of managing gestational diabetes. Electronic blood glucose monitors make the job easier.

Gingivitis

Gingivitis is an inflammation or infection of the gums, particularly the tissue around the teeth, that is characterized by swelling and bleeding when teeth are being brushed or flossed. The condition can affect anyone at any age but usually appears first during puberty and then persists throughout adult life.

Most often, the cause is irritation from plaque, a sticky substance produced by bacteria that live in the mouth. Plaque can form on any tooth surface, but the accumulation is heaviest between the teeth and along the gum line, areas that are not self-cleaning. In time, plaque hardens into calculus, or tartar, and layers of new plaque form over it, causing further irritation.

If gingivitis is allowed to progress, pockets form between the swollen gums and teeth, and plaque penetrates deeper into the tissue. As food and bacteria become trapped in these pockets, infection may develop, leading to periodontitis, a more serious infection that is a leading cause of adult tooth loss in the United States. At this stage, the gums are red, swollen, painful, and fragile. As pockets deepen, abscesses may form. The infection will gradually destroy the underlying bone, causing the teeth to loosen and fall out.

Diagnostic Studies and Procedures

Either a doctor or a dentist can diagnose gingivitis by inspecting the gums. If gums are badly infected, a sample of the plaque may be removed and cultured to identify the bacteria. X-rays can determine whether any loss of the jawbone has occurred.

Gingivitis and periodontitis may be associated with an underlying disease, such as diabetes or leukemia. If this is suspected, the patient will be referred to a physician for diagnosis.

Medical Treatments

A thorough cleaning and removal of plaque and tartar is the essential first step. In a mild case of gingivitis, this may be done in one visit to a dentist

or dental hygienist. In more advanced cases, treatment will probably require more than one visit and may include replacing fillings, excising gingival tissue, operating on the gums, or even removing loose teeth. Antibiotics, as well as a special mouthwash, may be prescribed to fight the infection.

Alternative Therapies

Herbal Medicine. Western herbalists recommend using a diluted tincture of myrrh or self-heal (*Prunella vulgaris*) as a mouthwash for bleeding gums. Some also suggest massaging the gums with

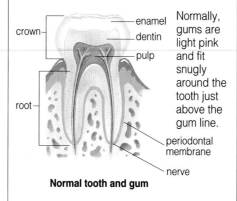

Normally, gums are light pink and fit snugly around the tooth just above the gum line.

Normal tooth and gum

crown — enamel, dentin, pulp
root — periodontal membrane, nerve

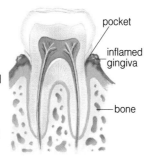

Gingivitis is marked by red, swollen gums that bleed easily and pull away from the tooth, allowing bacteria to form pockets under the gum line.

pocket
inflamed gingiva
bone

eucalyptus oil at bedtime. Chinese herbalists advocate taking a combination of pinellia, ginseng, and ginger twice a day, either as a tea or in tablet form.

Homeopathy. Staphysagria (stavesacre) is often prescribed for gingivitis, to be used in tincture three times daily. Borax (borate of sodium) may be used to treat bleeding ulcers on the gums.

Naturopathy and Nutrition Therapy. A diet high in vitamins B and C—or supplements of these vitamins plus zinc, calcium, and vitamin A—may be advised. A nutritionist may suggest also increasing your intake of raw fruits and vegetables to exercise the gums more. Massaging the gums with vitamin E oil may also promote healing.

Self-Treatment

Self-care plays an essential role in both the prevention and treatment of gingivitis. Brush thoroughly with a soft toothbrush at least twice a day, and floss your teeth daily. Replace your toothbrush promptly when it becomes worn. Use a wooden pick or irrigation device to stimulate the gums and remove bits of food from between the teeth after each meal. The gums may bleed at first, but with continued care, the bleeding will stop in a few weeks when the gums heal.

Before brushing, rinse the mouth with a product that helps loosen plaque. Some dentists recommend brushing with a paste made of baking soda and 3 percent hydrogen peroxide, but others feel that it's thorough brushing and flossing, not the paste, that's important. After brushing and flossing, rinse the mouth with salt water, a solution of water and baking soda, or an antibacterial mouthwash. A rinse made of one part hydrogen peroxide and four parts water also helps fight gum infection. Use more water if this solution burns or irritates the gum tissue.

Smoking or using tobacco in any other way promotes gingivitis. If you continue smoking, the gum disease may continue to worsen even with improved dental hygiene.

In addition to self-care, you should see a dentist regularly, at least twice a year, or more often if you experience new symptoms of gingivitis or other dental problems.

Other Causes of Bleeding Gums

Some women's gums bleed during pregnancy, but the problem usually disappears soon after the baby is born. Bleeding gums can also be a symptom of thyroid problems and blood-clotting disorders. Grinding the teeth, known as bruxism, and malocclusion (teeth that do not fit together properly) also promote gingivitis.

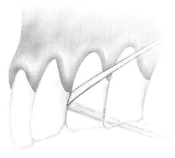

To remove plaque, move dental floss up and down between the teeth and along the line where the gums and teeth meet.

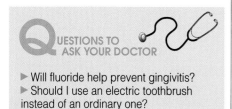

QUESTIONS TO ASK YOUR DOCTOR

▶ Will fluoride help prevent gingivitis?
▶ Should I use an electric toothbrush instead of an ordinary one?

Glaucoma

(Open-angle, closed-angle, or congenital glaucoma)

Glaucoma entails a buildup of fluid pressure in the eye's anterior chamber, which lies between the cornea and iris. The eye disease affects about one in 25 Americans, usually after the age of 40.

About 85 percent of all cases are chronic open-angle glaucoma, in which the outflow of the clear fluid, called aqueous humor, gradually declines. As the pressure within the anterior chamber increases, the tiny blood vessels that nourish the optic nerve become pinched, causing the nerve to slowly wither and die; the eventual result is blindness. This type of glaucoma may start in one eye and then affect the other eye, with no early warning signs.

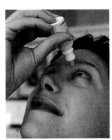

Eye drops that are applied daily can control most glaucoma.

Closed-angle, or congestive, glaucoma, which accounts for less than 10 percent of occurrences, comes on rapidly when the iris is so expanded that it blocks the outflow of fluid. Within days, the eye becomes very red, hard, and painful, causing nausea, and severely disturbed vision, including blurring and halos. Such an attack must be treated as a medical emergency, because the high pressure quickly damages the retina and optic nerve, causing permanent blindness.

Congenital, or infantile, glaucoma, a rare birth defect, can also result in blindness if it is not treated early.

In some unusual cases, glaucoma is secondary to an infection, tumor, injury, or other circumstance that blocks the outflow of aqueous humor.

Diagnostic Studies and Procedures

Because open-angle glaucoma generally has no obvious symptoms until it has already damaged the eye, about half of those with the disease do not know they have it. Early diagnosis, essential to prevent vision loss, is possible with a simple procedure called tonometry, in which a probe touches the eyeball to measure pressure in the anterior chamber. Tonometry should be part of a routine eye examination at least every

other year after the age of 35. Although a puff of air may be used to measure eye pressure, this test is not as accurate as the probe. When pressure is abnormally high, further tests are necessary, including an evaluation of peripheral vision.

An ophthalmologist diagnoses acute congestive glaucoma on the basis of the sudden onset of symptoms, an eye examination, and tonometry. A doctor may suspect congenital glaucoma when a baby is born with or soon develops an enlarged, protruding eyeball.

Medical Treatments

Eye drops that keep the pressure at a safe level can usually control chronic open-angle glaucoma. The drops most often prescribed are timolol maleate (Timoptic), which reduces fluid production and increases its outflow, and pilocarpine (Pilagan and others), which increases outflow by reducing the size of the pupil. Alternatively, acetazolamide (Diamox), an oral medication, may be prescribed. Marijuana also reduces fluid pressure, but the medicinal use of this illegal substance is reserved for acute cases that cannot be treated by conventional means.

If medication alone fails or creates a problem with side effects, surgery may be performed, either traditionally or with a laser beam, to create an enlarged exit route for the aqueous humor. Or surgery may be used to implant a drainage valve. Sometimes a freezing probe is applied briefly to the portion of the eye that produces the fluid to decrease its output.

With acute glaucoma, the immediate objective is to reduce pressure. This is done with eye drops to constrict the pupil, thereby moving the iris away

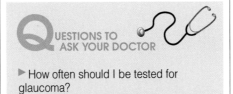

QUESTIONS TO ASK YOUR DOCTOR

▶ How often should I be tested for glaucoma?
▶ Could my high blood pressure cause the eye disease?

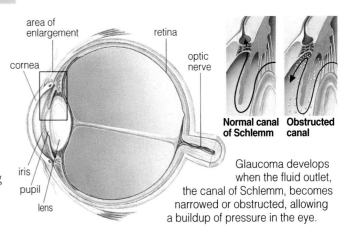

Normal canal of Schlemm **Obstructed canal**

Glaucoma develops when the fluid outlet, the canal of Schlemm, becomes narrowed or obstructed, allowing a buildup of pressure in the eye.

from the outflow ducts. Massage of the eye may also stimulate fluid outflow. These simple measures tend to provide only temporary relief; usually another attack will occur unless surgery is performed. The most common operation is an iridectomy, in which a small hole is made in the iris to allow fluid to exit. A doctor may also advise this surgery for the unaffected eye, since anyone who has had an acute attack in one eye is likely to have one in the other.

Congenital glaucoma is also treated with surgery to correct the defect and preserve vision.

Alternative Therapies

Alternative therapies cannot cure glaucoma. People with chronic glaucoma should use alternate methods only to complement medical treatment.

Nutrition Therapy. Some studies indicate that vitamin C supplements and bioflavonoids, especially the anthocyanidin compounds found in red and blue berries, may be useful adjunctive therapies for glaucoma.

Self-Treatment

The most important aspect of self-care with chronic glaucoma is to take all medications, including eye drops, precisely as prescribed.

Avoid taking medications that raise intraocular pressure. These include tranquilizers and nonprescription cold and allergy pills and other drugs containing antihistamines or cortisone.

Other Causes of Vision Disturbances

Many disorders can cause halos, tunnel vision, blurred vision, and other symptoms similar to those of glaucoma; they include a detached retina, macular degeneration, a stroke or mini-stroke, and a tumor of the eye or brain. An eye injury or infection or the presence of a foreign object can also disturb vision.

Gonorrhea

Gonorrhea is a sexually transmitted disease, caused by the gonococcus bacterium *Neisseria gonorrhoeae*. This organism, which thrives in delicate, moist tissue, affects the reproductive tract. But if untreated, it may enter the circulatory system, spreading throughout the body and causing gonococcal arthritis. It can infect the heart, liver, kidneys, and other vital organs as well.

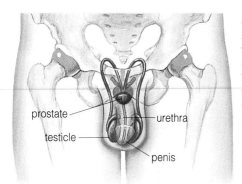

prostate
testicle
urethra
penis

Gonorrhea in men affects the urethra, which carries urine and semen through the penis, and may cause discharge of a pus-like fluid and burning on urination.

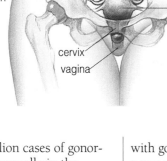

In women, gonorrhea typically attacks the cervix, and may spread to the fallopian tubes and uterus. Symptoms are dull pain in the lower abdomen, burning in the vagina, and a cloudy discharge.

fallopian tube
ovary
uterus
cervix
vagina

More than 2 million cases of gonorrhea are reported annually in the United States. These numbers include children, who may be infected as a result of sexual abuse, and newborn babies, who can contract the disease during birth if the mother is infected. In newborns, the infection often settles in the eyes and can cause blindness.

Oral or anal sexual activity can transmit infection to either of these areas, producing gonococcal pharyngitis (infection of the throat) or gonococcal proctitis (infection of the rectum).

A man who becomes infected with gonorrhea usually experiences burning pain when urinating and a discharge of pus from the penis. A woman often has no early symptoms except perhaps an abnormal discharge. This lack of symptoms sometimes allows the disorder to progress undetected to an advanced stage, at which point it may result in pelvic inflammatory disease (PID), a serious infection of reproductive organs that can cause infertility. Some women also become asymptomatic carriers.

Diagnostic Studies and Procedures

A diagnosis in men is based on symptoms and a microscopic examination of any discharge. A more definite diagnosis requires a culture of the discharge. Making the initial diagnosis in women is more difficult, because the symptoms are often mild or non-existent. In addition, discharge that may be present can be misleading, since bacteria that normally live in the vagina might be mistaken for the gonococcus. Thus, diagnosis usually must await the results of a culture.

No reliable blood tests exist for gonorrhea, but a blood sample will probably be tested for other sexually transmitted diseases, including syphilis and chlamydia, which are commonly found along with gonorrhea. A woman may undergo a pap smear to test for a cervical infection from the human papillomavirus (HPV), the organism that causes genital warts. Tests for HIV, the virus that causes AIDS, may also be advisable, because people with one sexually transmitted disease are often infected with others contracted in that manner.

Medical Treatments

Antibiotics can quickly eradicate gonorrhea, but there is a growing problem of drug resistance among certain gonococcal strains. For example, some are totally resistant to penicillin, which heretofore was the standard treatment. The Centers for Disease Control and Prevention now recommend as the first-choice an injection of ceftriaxone (Rocephin), along with an oral antibiotic, such as doxycycline. Treatment of gonorrhea that has spread to other organs is more complicated and may require a regimen of intravenous antibiotics for 3 to 10 days. In all cases, follow-up culture studies should be performed to make sure that the gonococcus has been fully eradicated.

Alternative Therapies

Home remedies and folk medicine treatments for gonorrhea are not effective. Antibiotics provide the only cure.

Self-Treatment

Over-the-counter drugs, such as aspirin and acetaminophen, can relieve discomfort; they may be taken in addition to antibiotics.

It is vital to refrain from sexual relations until the infection is fully cured. All sex partners who may have been exposed to gonorrhea must also be checked for the disease.

Gonorrhea can be prevented by adopting safer sexual practices. This means using a rubber condom during intercourse, even if you also use other means of birth control; refraining from oral and anal sex unless you are confident of your partner's sexual health; and not sharing such personal items as douche equipment.

Although sexual contact is by far the most common means of transmitting gonorrhea, it can be spread in other ways. Studies show that the gonococcal bacterium can survive for up to four hours on inorganic surfaces, such as toilet seats, bedding, and clothing.

Other Causes of Gonorrhea Symptoms

Reiter's syndrome and nonspecific urethritis, which are also sexually transmitted diseases in men, can produce symptoms similar to those of gonorrhea, as can chlamydia infections in both men and women. Bladder infections and interstitial cystitis cause painful urination. The joint pain and swelling that often occur in gonococcal arthritis may be mistaken for other forms of arthritis.

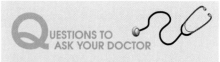

QUESTIONS TO ASK YOUR DOCTOR

▶ Is there a government agency that can help notify previous sexual partners? And is the information kept confidential?
▶ If you have gonorrhea once, are you more susceptible to getting it again?

Gout

(Crystal arthritis)

With gout, a type of arthritis, tiny mineral, or urate, crystals collect in certain joints, causing an intense inflammatory reaction. The crystals are composed of uric acid, a metabolic waste product normally excreted in the urine.

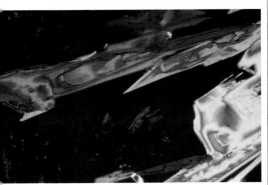

Crystals of uric acid have knifelike projections that cause intense joint pain.

In people with a hereditary metabolic defect, uric acid builds up in the blood and other body fluids. Most people with this condition, called hyperuricemia, do not develop gout, but those who do experience recurring attacks in the affected joints and may also suffer kidney stones.

Gout is primarily a male disease, and the big toe is its most common site, although it may affect other foot joints as well as the fingers, ankles, elbows, wrists, and knees. During an attack, the joint becomes painful, red, swollen, and hot to the touch. Attacks come on suddenly but pass quickly. The intervals between vary from a few days to years.

When gout goes untreated, attacks become increasingly frequent and eventually damage the affected joints and sometimes the kidneys and other internal organs. In addition, deposits of urate crystals, called tophi, may occur under the skin near affected joints, over the elbow, or on the outside edge of the ear. These may eventually break through the skin and become infected.

Diagnostic Studies and Procedures

A doctor can usually diagnose gout on the basis of the symptoms and the appearance of the afflicted joint. A definitive diagnosis can be established by examining a sample of the joint fluid under a microscope with polarizing lenses. During an acute attack of gout, the uric-acid crystals can be seen in the fluid, surrounded by white cells summoned by the immune system.

Medical Treatments

A combination of medical treatment and self-care can completely control gout.

Doctors most often recommend colchicine to counter an attack. At the first sign, the drug is injected into a vein, or it may be taken orally every few hours for a day or two. It is highly toxic, however, and should be stopped as soon as diarrhea and other intestinal symptoms develop; by that time, the attack is usually over. Certain nonsteroidal anti-inflammatory drugs, especially phenylbutazone (Butazolidin) and indomethacin (Indocin), are sometimes prescribed as an alternative. These medications can also cause some adverse effects, including bone marrow suppression and bleeding.

With most patients, acute attacks can be prevented with daily doses of a uricosuric agent, such as sulfinpyrazone (Anturane), to improve the body's elimination of uric acid, or allopurinol (Lopurin or Zyloprim), which reduces uric-acid production. If these drugs do not work, a doctor may prescribe a low daily dosage of colchicine and closely monitor the person for side effects.

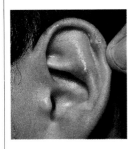

The ears are a common site of tophi deposits, which are made up of urate crystals.

Alternative Therapies

For those who cannot take antigout medication, other therapies may help.

Acupuncture. Acupuncture and acupressure may ease the pain of an attack.

Herbal Medicine. For joint pain, some herbalists recommend applying fireweed oil or Balm of Gilead ointment. A mixture of burdock root, celery seed, yarrow, and thuya is advocated for gout and may be taken as an infusion, in capsule form, or as a tincture. A word of caution: Although the antigout drug colchicine is derived from the autumn crocus, which is used by some herbalists, this plant is highly toxic. Use only the FDA-approved drug.

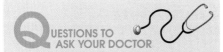

QUESTIONS TO ASK YOUR DOCTOR

▶ Will gout medication interact with any of the other drugs I am taking?
▶ Since gout is hereditary, what are the chances my sons will develop it? Are there any preventive measures?

Homeopathy. Practitioners may prescribe guaiacum, benzinum acidum, belladonna, or, for gout that moves from joint to joint, pulsatilla nigricans. A hot compress with tincture of colchicine may also be applied to the affected joints.

Meditation. Stress can sometimes precipitate an attack of gout. Meditation, yoga, and other relaxation techniques can help prevent a flare-up.

Nutrition Therapy. Many specialists advise avoiding foods high in purine, a substance that raises the uric-acid level in the blood. These foods include organ meats (liver, kidneys, sweetbreads, and brains), sardines, anchovies, meat extracts, and dried peas, lentils, and other legumes. Red wine, beer, and some other alcoholic beverages may also trigger an attack.

Self-Treatment

Anyone with gout should drink at least two quarts of nonalcoholic beverages daily to dilute urine and prevent a buildup of uric acid. An overweight patient should shed excess pounds, since obesity aggravates gout. Do not go on a crash diet, however; an abrupt loss in weight can also precipitate an attack. Regular exercise helps keep joints mobile and flexible, but avoid stressing inflamed joints, which can lead to permanent damage.

Drugs, especially the diuretics used to treat high blood pressure, sometimes cause gout. If you are taking medication for other disorders and suffer an attack of gout, talk to your doctor about an alternative regimen.

Other Causes of Joint Pain

Pseudogout is quite similar to gout, except the attacks are usually less severe and the crystals are composed of calcium pyrophosphate dihydrate. Joint pain may come from another form of arthritis, such as osteoarthritis, rheumatoid arthritis, or lupus. Bunions and other foot disorders produce pain and toe deformity.

Hammertoes

A hammertoe is a deformity in which a toe is raised and bent, giving it the appearance of a claw. The condition most commonly develops in the second toe, but it may affect the others as well, causing the smaller toes to turn under and lie close to each other. A hard corn usually develops at the top of the raised joint. This bump of hardened tissue protects the bones from the constant irritation of a shoe, but it also causes intense pain if it presses upon an underlying nerve.

The deformity may begin in childhood because of an inherited abnormality in the alignment of the foot's metatarsal bones. When it develops in adulthood, the cause is usually poorly fitted footwear, especially high-heeled shoes that force an uneven distribution of weight on the toes. Hammertoes may also be a consequence of the muscle and nerve deterioration that accompanies diabetes, stroke, and such neurologic disorders as Friedreich's ataxia. Structural defects are ocasionally responsible; these include a tight heel cord and weakness of the anterior tibial muscle, the calf muscle whose tendon extends across the top of the foot to the toes. In addition, hammertoe is sometimes associated with arthritis, corns and calluses, and obesity.

Diagnostic Studies and Procedures

A hammertoe is readily apparent by visual examination, but the underlying cause may be more elusive. When visiting a podiatrist or a physician who specializes in foot disorders, take along an old pair of shoes so that the patterns of wear can be examined. These patterns provide clues to many foot problems, including a walking style that contributes to hammertoe.

An important new diagnostic aid is the computerized gait analysis. A patient's feet are connected with a computer. As the patient walks about the room, the computer provides a print-out showing the weight-bearing distribution on the foot during contact with the ground. The doctor then has a clearer picture of how the toes have been distorted by undue stress.

Medical Treatments

Drug Therapy. Lidocaine, a local anesthetic, sometimes provides long-term relief when given by injection two or three times a week. If not, it may be combined with a cortisone injection.

Orthotics. If gait is a factor, a doctor may advise custom-fitted orthotics. These are plastic and metal shoe inserts designed to relieve pressure on the

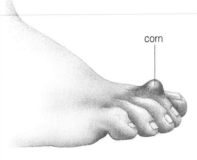

Painful corns often form on a hammertoe, prompting a person to seek treatment.

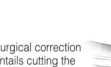

corn

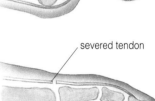

A tight, short tendon can bend the toe to form a hammertoe.

severed tendon

Surgical correction entails cutting the tendon, allowing the toe to straighten itself out.

toes. They can be designed from the computerized gait analysis or fashioned from plaster molds of the feet.

Surgical Treatment. If an operation is needed, it can usually be done in an outpatient setting under local anesthesia. Surgery consists of cutting the toe tendons, which releases the soft tissue and lets the curled toe relax. As tendons heal, the severed ends reattach and lengthen, so that the toe straightens out. In severe cases, a small part of the metatarsal bone may be removed.

Full recovery from surgery takes about a week, during which time a cane should be used. Soft shoes should be worn until the foot is fully healed. Individually fitted orthotics are essential for maintaining the correction.

Alternative Therapies

Alternative therapies may alleviate the symptoms and sometimes remedy an underlying cause, but they cannot correct the actual deformity.

Alexander Technique. This postural treatment can help when an abnormal gait and improper weight distribution are contributing to the problem.

Hydrotherapy. Soaking one's feet in warm water for at least 20 minutes is the first step in softening a troublesome corn. The layers of dead skin can then be rubbed away with a pumice stone or fine emory board.

Massage. Foot massage using reflexology techniques may temporarily alleviate the pain of a hammertoe.

Self-Treatment

To ease discomfort, cover the toe with mole skin or an unmedicated corn pad. Make sure your shoes have a toe box deep enough to comfortably accommodate your toes. Alternatively, wear open-toed sandals. Some people have had success with improvising their own orthotics by taking several shoe pads and cutting, shaping, and fitting them into their shoes.

To prevent the development of hammertoes, follow these guidelines:

▶ Get rid of shoes that don't fit properly. Remember that feet get a bit larger with age, so you may not be able to wear shoes from several years ago.

▶ Buy new shoes late in the day, when your feet are likely to be somewhat larger than in the morning.

▶ Reserve high heels for occasions when you won't be doing much walking. Avoid pointed toes; you should be able to wiggle your toes comfortably.

▶ Don't buy shoes that feel too tight with the expectation that they will grow more comfortable with wear.

▶ Use every opportunity to walk barefooted. Second best is wearing thong sandals whenever possible.

Other Causes of Deformed Toes

Foot injuries and congenital bone diseases may cause toe deformity, although in the latter case, other bones will be affected as well.

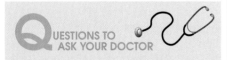

Q UESTIONS TO ASK YOUR DOCTOR

▶ If I have diabetes, is it safe for me to have foot surgery?
▶ Could there be undesirable side effects if I have frequent cortisone shots to ease the pain in my toe?

Hardening of the Arteries

(Arteriosclerosis; atherosclerosis)
Hardening of the arteries is the common term for arteriosclerosis, which refers to any condition in which the walls of arteries thicken and lose their elasticity. To some degree, this disorder is a natural consequence of aging. Often, however, it stems from atherosclerosis, the accumulation of fatty material in the inner surfaces of arteries. These deposits, or plaque, are composed mostly of cholesterol, a waxy substance that circulates in the blood and is an essential component of cell membranes and several hormones.

Although it can occur in an artery anywhere in the body, atherosclerosis is especially common in the coronary arteries and the carotid artery, which supplies blood to the brain. Fatty deposits in these critical blood vessels can result in a heart attack or stroke.

What triggers atherosclerosis is unknown, but many scientists think it begins when the innermost layer of the artery, the endothelium, is damaged, perhaps by a virus or immune response that causes inflammation. Although the consequences generally manifest themselves later in life, studies show that the process may begin in early adulthood or even childhood. As deposits of cholesterol, calcium, and other substances accumulate along the walls of an artery, the vessel becomes progressively narrowed, reducing blood flow. Depending upon what vessels are affected, symptoms may include angina, high blood pressure, reduced mental function, leg pains, and kidney failure.

Diagnostic Studies and Procedures
Nearly everyone who is middle-aged or older has some degree of hardening and narrowing of the arteries. In many cases, obvious symptoms don't occur until the condition is well advanced. During a routine physical examination, the doctor may detect signs of arteriosclerosis by listening to the carotid pulse in the neck for whooshing sounds (bruits), or by feeling for a weakened pulse and noting coldness in the feet.

Blood studies to measure cholesterol levels also yield important diagnostic information. In addition to measuring the total amount of cholesterol, these tests should determine the ratio of the

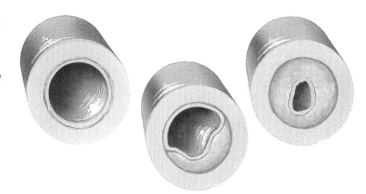

Normally, an artery's inner lining is smooth and elastic, allowing the vessel to dilate and constrict. Fatty deposits progressively narrow and stiffen the artery, resulting in arteriosclerosis.

protective HDL cholesterol to the detrimental LDL component. HDLs (high-density lipoproteins) carry cholesterol away from the artery walls, whereas LDLs (low-density lipoproteins) deposit cholesterol there.

The patient's medical history also provides important diagnostic clues. For example, diabetes increases the risk of premature hardening of the arteries. The doctor will ask whether muscle cramps have been felt in the legs, a sign that the femoral arteries may be affected. Of course, the presence of angina suggests involvement of the coronary arteries. The doctor will also ask about lifestyle, as smoking, excessive use of alcohol, and lack of regular exercise contribute to arteriosclerosis. The medical history of close relatives is important as well, because the more severe forms of this condition, which are associated with early death from heart attacks, tend to run in families.

If serious arteriosclerosis involving atherosclerosis is suspected, a doctor may order various X-ray studies to identify the sites of dangerous narrowing. These might include:
Angiography, in which a contrast dye is injected into the bloodstream to make the arteries visible on film.
Positron emission tomography, or PET scanning, which produces three-

dimensional pictures of the blood flow to and from the heart.
Cardiac catheterization, in which a narrow tube is inserted into the heart and coronary arteries and a dye or radioactive material is injected.
Doppler ultrasonography, in which echoes from high-frequency sound waves allow a study of the blood flow through specific arteries.

Medical Treatments
Most experts consider arteriosclerosis incurable, but the progress of the disease and its symptoms can be controlled by a combination of medications or other medical approaches, alternative therapies, and self-care.
Drug Therapy. For people who have a high level of blood cholesterol, a doctor may prescribe medication, when diet and other lifestyle measures have not helped to lower it (see Cholesterol Disorders, page 130). Recent studies suggest that a major decrease in cholesterol can slow down and may even reverse the process of atherosclerosis.

If a patient has high blood pressure, a physician will prescribe medications to lower it. The control of diabetes and other contributing diseases is important as well.

Various drugs may alleviate symptoms from narrowed blood vessels. These include nitroglycerin, beta blockers, or calcium channel blockers to control chest pain; low-dose aspirin (one tablet a day or every other day) to reduce the risk of blood clots; and other medications to increase blood flow to the brain and legs.

If drugs do not work, surgery is often the next recourse. Procedures include:
Balloon angioplasty, in which a catheter, with a deflated balloon at its tip, is inserted into a narrowed artery and then inflated. This widens the artery by flattening plaque against its walls.

Q**UESTIONS TO ASK YOUR DOCTOR**

▶ If atherosclerosis runs in my family, should I follow a diet more stringent than the one recommended by the American Heart Association? Should my children also have a special diet?
▶ Must I undergo an exercise stress test before starting a fitness program?

HARDENING OF THE ARTERIES (CONTINUED)

The progress of the catheter through the artery is monitored by fluoroscopy, a moving X-ray technique, and the balloon is inflated at the site of narrowing.

Angioplasty is most commonly performed on narrowed coronary arteries, the renal artery in the kidney, and vessels in the lower leg. In some cases, it is combined with laser surgery to destroy the plaque. Alternatively, a special device with tiny rotating blades may be inserted through the catheter to shave away the plaque, in a manner similar to the corkscrew action of implements used to unclog plumbing drains.

Bypass surgery, in which a graft, made from a section of a vein or artery removed from somewhere else in the patient, is used to carry blood around portions of narrowed vessels. Coronary bypass surgery is the most common procedure of this type, but bypass operations may also be done on the carotid artery and vessels in the legs.

Endarterectomy, in which the clogged vessel is opened up and fatty deposits are surgically removed. This operation is common on the carotid artery in the neck and arteries in the legs. A patch of Dacron or other synthetic material may be inserted to strengthen the vessel.

Gene therapy, in which genes that direct the growth of new blood vessels are surgically inserted into the blocked artery to encourage formation of a natural bypass around the blockage. This technique is highly experimental, but might someday replace bypass surgery.

Alternative Therapies

Most alternative therapies are directed to modifying the risk factors that underlie atherosclerosis.

Acupuncture. This may be employed to help smokers who cannot break their habit by more conventional means.

Exercise Conditioning. Physicians and alternative therapists alike recommend a program of aerobic exercise to improve circulation, reduce cholesterol, and control obesity, diabetes, and other factors that contribute to atherosclerosis. Walking, cycling, stair climbing, and other activities that use the leg muscles are especially beneficial in alleviating leg pain from reduced circulation. A word of caution, however: Before embarking on any exercise program, have a doctor determine your safe level of physical activity.

Herbal Medicine. Herbalists advocate a number of herbs to reduce cholesterol

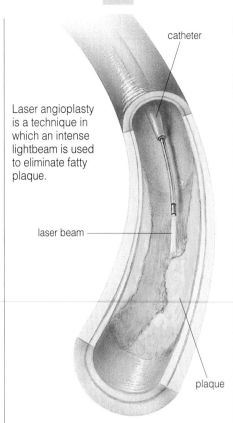

Laser angioplasty is a technique in which an intense lightbeam is used to eliminate fatty plaque.

catheter

laser beam

plaque

and improve blood flow. These include American ginseng, taken as capsules, powder, or tea; garlic, in either natural or capsule form; and oil of evening primrose in capsules. Ginger, boiled or consumed as an extract, may be helpful in alleviating leg pain from reduced circulation, and ginkgo tincture or tablets are said to improve general circulation.

Chinese herbalists also recommend the bupleurum and dragon bone combination (bupleurum, pinellia rhizome, skullcap root, ginger, jujube, ginseng, cinnamon, oyster shell, China root, rhubarb, rhizome, and dragon bone, which is pulverized fossil bones) or the major bupleurum combination (bupleurum, skullcap root, pinellia rhizome, peony root, citrus peel, rhubarb rhizome, jujube, and ginger).

Naturopathy and Nutrition Therapy. Practitioners espouse many of the dietary and exercise recommendations made by the medical establishment, but some naturopaths may take diet a step further. They advocate eliminating virtually all dietary fats and oils, meat, and all dairy products other than nonfat milk and yogurt, and at the same time increasing consumption of grains, fruits, vegetables, legumes, and fiber. A few practitioners recommend daily helpings of alfalfa sprouts, wheat germ,

and various supplements, especially vitamins E and C, beta carotene, lecithin, niacin, calcium, and magnesium. Some also advocate fish oil, or omega-3 fatty acid capsules; however, scientific studies of these substances have produced mixed results, with some showing a lowering of cholesterol levels and others finding no benefit or an increased risk of bleeding problems.

Some naturopaths also recommend chelation to remove minerals from the blood, but there is no evidence that this procedure improves atherosclerosis.

Yoga and Meditation. These and other relaxation therapies can reduce stress, which may raise blood pressure and cholesterol and have other detrimental effects on circulation.

Self-Treatment

Lifestyle plays a major role in preventing the premature development of arteriosclerosis and atherosclerosis. Losing excess weight, quitting smoking, exercising regularly, and following a prudent diet, such as that recommended by the American Heart Association (AHA), are the essence of prevention and self-care for hardening of the arteries. The AHA diet is similar to the government's Dietary Guidelines for Healthy Americans, as well as diets advocated by the American Cancer Society (see box below).

As far as exercise is concerned, walking or engaging in another aerobic activity for 15 to 30 minutes three or four times a week is needed to maintain fitness and promote good circulation.

Other Causes of Arteriosclerosis

Familial hypercholesterolemia is a genetic disease characterized by extremely high cholesterol levels. People with this condition often have heart attacks early in life, sometimes even during childhood.

AMERICAN HEART ASSOCIATION DIETARY RECOMMENDATIONS

Percentage of Daily Calories	Source
55-60%	Carbohydrates
12-15%	Protein
Less than 30%	Total fat
No more than 10%	Saturated fat
Dietary cholesterol limit:	300 milligrams per day
Dietary sodium limit:	3 grams per day (about 1½ teaspoons of salt)

Head, Neck, and Back Injuries

Accidents that involve the head, neck, and back are invariably serious because of the dangers they pose to the central nervous system; namely, the brain and spinal cord. Because these injuries often occur together, the presence of a serious head injury should be assumed to involve also the neck or back (and vice versa) until proven otherwise.

The severity of a head, neck, or back injury is often difficult to judge. Superficial scalp wounds tend to bleed profusely and may look more serious than they are. In contrast, a seemingly minor blow to the head or a fall can cause serious brain damage or a broken back.

Diagnostic Studies and Procedures

Upon arrival at the hospital, the victim's vital signs (blood pressure, pulse, respiration), state of consciousness, and neurological responses are evaluated, and X-rays are taken to look for fractures. A doctor may order CT scans or MRI, especially if a brain or spinal-cord injury is suspected.

The Glasgow Coma Scale measures the patient's eye responses, verbal ability, and nerve reflexes. The scale is used during the emergency room evaluation, and then regularly in the days that follow. The results are especially useful in predicting the extent of a patient's recovery from a serious brain injury.

Medical Treatments

Painkillers, excluding morphine and other drugs that depress the central nervous system, are given as necessary. For severe head injuries, anticonvulsants may be administered to protect against seizures, and diuretics may be given to reduce brain swelling.

For a serious head injury, care during the first week is critical. There is often bleeding inside the skull or a swelling of brain tissue. In either instance, the

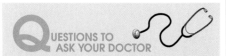

QUESTIONS TO ASK YOUR DOCTOR

▶ How long should a child be observed for warning signs after a minor fall or bump on the head?
▶ What are the chances of regaining nerve function after suffering a broken neck or back?

ADMINISTERING FIRST AID

For Head Injuries:

A person who has suffered a head injury should be transported by trained paramedics to the closest hospital, preferably one with a trauma center. As a first step, call your local emergency number (usually 911) and ask for an ambulance and emergency medical service. Tell the operator that the person has a possible brain or spinal-cord injury. While waiting for help, administer the following first aid:

1. If the person is unconscious, check for breathing and pulse. If necessary, perform artificial respiration or CPR, but be careful not to rotate or turn the head. Instead of the usual backward head tilt, gently elevate the chin only enough to open the airway.

2. If the person is conscious, keep him lying quietly until the ambulance arrives.

3. Cover and keep the victim comfortably warm to help prevent shock.

4. Do not give the injured person anything to eat or drink.

5. Do not attempt to raise the victim's head, but if necessary, gently turn the entire body to the side so that secretions

brain will become compressed, which could possibly result in coma. During this period, the intracranial pressure requires constant monitoring, and if it should rise, emergency measures must be taken to prevent any permanent damage. One approach entails draining away small amounts of cerebrospinal fluid to reduce the pressure inside the skull.

Breathing must also be monitored to prevent hyperventilation, or overbreathing. Rapid, shallow breathing may help reduce the intracranial pressure by lowering blood flow, but it can be dangerous if the brain becomes deprived of vital oxygen.

A spinal-cord injury also requires immediate action and constant monitoring. A severed spinal cord results in permanent paralysis of the body served by spinal nerves below the point of injury. Artificial respiration is necessary if the breathing muscles are paralyzed. When the spinal cord is compressed but not severed, varying degrees of nerve function may return as swelling subsides and healing takes place.

In some cases, emergency surgery can minimize the long-term effects. Advances in microsurgery techniques make it possible to repair many nerve injuries once considered hopeless.

can drain from the mouth. Be sure to support the head and neck so that the neck does not twist.

6. Report unusual behavior, a state of unconsciousness, convulsions, or other symptoms to the ambulance crew.

For Neck and Back Injuries:

If there is any possibility of a neck or back injury, DO NOT move the victim unless there is an immediate danger of death from an explosion, a fire, or similar hazard. (Even then, follow the steps outlined in Moving an Accident Victim, page 212.) If a vertebra is dislocated or broken, any movement of the head, neck, or back can sever the spinal cord and result in permanent paralysis or death. Call for an ambulance, and while waiting, carry out these first-aid procedures:

1. If the person is unconscious, follow Step 1 as described for head injuries.

2. Immobilize the head, neck, and trunk until emergency help arrives. You can do this by placing rolled-up clothing, blankets, or other firm objects close to both sides of the body.

3. Cover the victim with blankets or coats to keep him warm and prevent shock.

Rehabilitation, which includes intensive physical and occupational therapy, ideally begins as soon as the patient's condition is stable. The person must do

IMPORTANT WARNING SIGNS

The presence of any of these signs and symptoms demands extra caution:

Head injury:

▶ A depression in the skull, or a cut or bruise in the scalp
▶ Bleeding or clear discharge from the nose or ears
▶ Bleeding from the mouth
▶ Pupils of different sizes
▶ Speech or vision disturbance
▶ Altered mental state, such as drowsiness, confusion, or unconsciousness
▶ Muscle twitching
▶ Convulsions
▶ Altered pulse rate (more than 80 beats or less than 60 beats per minute)
▶ Vomiting
▶ Unusual pallor or reddish skin tone
▶ Headache

Neck and back injury:

▶ Head resting in an abnormal position
▶ Stiff neck
▶ Tingling sensations in the hands and feet
▶ Loss of feeling
▶ Paralysis of the arms, legs, or other parts of the body
▶ Loss of bladder control

MOVING AN ACCIDENT VICTIM

If it is absolutely essential to move an accident victim with a suspected head or spinal injury, make every effort to keep the head, neck, and back in a straight line.

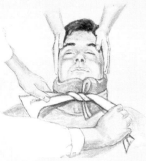

1. If time allows, stabilize the neck with an improvised collar, using a towel, clothing, or other material that can be worked under the neck without moving the head.

2. If a board or other firm object is available, slide it under the victim, taking care to keep the head, neck, and back in alignment. This is best done with the aid of three or four helpers, who can carefully roll the person onto the board without any twisting of the head, neck, or back. If possible, tie the victim securely to the board, and then move him to safety by dragging or carrying the board.

3. If a board is not available, substitute a blanket. To move the victim onto the blanket, fold it in wide pleats, and place it against the person's body. Work a few inches of the pleated part under the victim, then place one hand under the shoulders and the other under the buttocks. Roll the person a quarter turn toward you on the side opposite the blanket, making sure that the back remains straight. Push the blanket under the raised portion, then roll the victim a quarter-turn away from you and pull the blanket through. Roll the blanket firmly around the person, and move to safety by pulling the blanket from the top.

4. If others are available to help but you have no object to place under the victim, have the rescuers kneel on either side of the person. Instruct these carriers to place their hands under the victim's head, neck, back, and hips. If possible, have each carrier grasp the hands of the person directly opposite to form interlocking grips to bear the weight. Work as a team, with a leader calling out instructions: "All ready...lift...step forward one, two..."

5. If you alone must drag the person from danger without the aid of a board or blanket, use your body to support the head, neck, and trunk. Kneel at the victim's head, and while keeping his body in a straight line, work your arms under the armpits and use your thighs and chest as support while you move to safety.

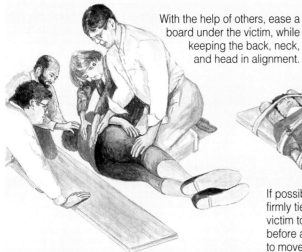

With the help of others, ease a board under the victim, while keeping the back, neck, and head in alignment.

If possible, firmly tie the victim to the board before attempting to move him.

If it's absolutely necessary to drag the person from danger, use your body as a support.

HEAD, NECK, AND BACK INJURIES (CONTINUED)

assisted range-of-motion exercises several times a day to preserve muscle tone and prevent contractures. Learning new ways to do simple tasks may take months or even years, but electronic devices enable some patients to walk and carry out tasks despite paralysis.

Alternative Therapies

Many rehabilitation programs include a variety of alternative approaches.

Acupuncture. This ancient Chinese therapy helps with pain management.

Biofeedback Training. Using electronic monitors, patients are taught to control involuntary functions, such as breathing, that are disrupted by their injuries.

Hydrotherapy. Whirlpools and underwater exercise help patients to regain muscle tone and strength.

Music Therapy. Music encourages movement, and exercising to music can improve coordination and gait. Music also prompts the brain to increase production of endorphins, the body's natural painkillers and mood enhancers.

Pet Therapy. Animals can help paralyzed people achieve greater self-sufficiency. For example, monkeys trained to perform simple tasks are sometimes sent home with patients. Other rehabilitation programs use horses; a horse's gait is similar to that of a human, so a patient who can master riding a horse can often relearn how to walk.

Self-Treatment

Recovery from a head or spinal-cord injury can be arduous and frustrating, and success often depends upon the patient's persistence and determination. Numerous accounts of miraculous recoveries can be explained only by the person's tremendous willpower and effort. Experts agree that starting with an optimistic attitude is a big plus.

Other Causes of Head, Neck, and Back Injuries

Most of these injuries are accidental, but child abuse is also a major cause.

POSTCONCUSSION SYNDROME

A mild head injury that causes a person to feel stunned, disoriented, and dizzy usually indicates a mild concussion. Though tests may fail to detect any anatomical brain damage, the brain tissue may be "shaken up," which can result in postconcussion syndrome. Common symptoms include attacks of nerve pain, headaches, memory loss, difficulty in concentrating and learning, and possible personality changes. In time, these symptoms usually disappear, but if a child is afflicted, some difficulties, such as hyperactivity and learning problems, may linger or become permanent.

Headaches

A headache is any pain in the head, the discomfort of which can vary greatly. It may be dull or sharp, throbbing or constant, localized to a small area or engulfing the entire head. Some people suffer headaches only occasionally, while for others the problem is chronic.

Although a headache is often the symptom of an underlying problem such as the flu, and may be temporarily debilitating, it is rarely associated with a serious condition. Nevertheless, for some 20 million Americans each year, the pain of headache is severe enough to warrant a visit to a doctor. And according to government estimates, some 64 million workdays are lost annually due to various types of headaches.

Simple tension is the leading cause of headaches, and the basis for the tension very often is stress. Other possible causes include fatigue, blocked sinuses, allergies, and irritated or inflamed blood vessels in the scalp. Overuse of alcohol and tobacco can bring on a headache, and so can adverse reactions to medications. Some women experience this symptom just before or during menstruation. Changes in the weather and other environmental factors can also trigger the affliction.

Diagnostic Studies and Procedures
Often, a doctor can tell what kind of headache you are suffering simply by asking you to describe when and how it develops. He will inquire about any triggering factors, the patterns of frequency, and the nature and duration of pain. Questions might include: Can it be controlled with nonprescription painkillers, such as aspirin or acetaminophen? Does it change when you move your head? Is there a family history of similar headaches?

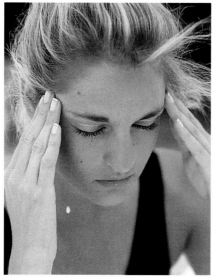

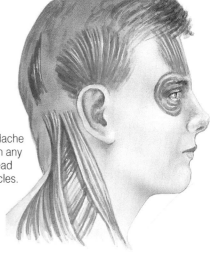

Massaging the temples may alleviate a simple tension headache.

A tension headache can originate in any of the major head and neck muscles.

The next step is a physical examination, paying special attention to the eyes and ears. The doctor will feel the head itself for bumps, tensed muscles, or an unusual throbbing of blood vessels in the temple and neck.

Blood and urine tests, as well as X-rays of the skull and sinuses, may be ordered. Imaging studies of the brain, using CT scanning techniques or MRI, could be necessary to rule out a tumor or other structural abnormality. Some cases require vision and other eye tests. If meningitis or brain infection is suspected, a sample of cerebrospinal fluid will be obtained for analysis.

Medical Treatments
A doctor may recommend a decongestant to reduce swelling if blocked sinuses are responsible for a headache, or antibiotics if there is an infection. Other possible medications depend upon the type of headache involved; they include muscle relaxants for tension headaches, antihistamines for allergies, and tranquilizers or antidepressants for headaches related to psychiatric disorders.

For the vascular headaches, cluster (page 136) and migraine (page 298), a variety of treatments is available.

In unusual cases in which headaches stem from tumors or brain abnormalities, surgery may be indicated. If fluid builds up in the brain, a drainage tube may be implanted to shunt the excess fluid to another area of the body.

Alternative Therapies
In recent years, headache clinics have incorporated a number of alternative therapies into their medical regimens,

especially in dealing with chronic headaches that have no obvious organic cause. These therapies may include:
Acupuncture and Acupressure. A series of acupuncture treatments to stimulate points on the head, neck, hands, and feet may be recommended. Alternatively, practitioners advise applying pressure to the web between the thumb and forefinger.
Alexander Technique. Chronic headaches are often traced to poor postural habits that create muscle tension. An Alexander technique instructor observes your normal posture and movements and then teaches you ways to change any bad habits.

HOW TO SPOT A SERIOUS HEADACHE
In general, you should see a doctor about any unexplained change in the nature and frequency of your headaches. Although most types are not serious, seek immediate medical attention for any headache that is:
▶ Especially severe and comes on suddenly, without warning.
▶ Accompanied by confusion, blurred vision, partial paralysis, loss of consciousness or sensation, and other neurological changes.
▶ Accompanied by a fever and stiff neck or difficulty turning the head.
▶ Recurring frequently in the same place, such as above or in an eye.
▶ Recurring with increasing frequency or intensity, or its pattern of recurrence changes without apparent cause.
▶ Is the cause of your awakening in the middle of the night.

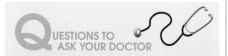

Q **UESTIONS TO ASK YOUR DOCTOR**

▶ What should I do to alleviate a child's headache safely?
▶ Certain changes in the weather seem to give me a headache. Are there any preventive measures I can take?

HEADACHES (CONTINUED)

Aromatherapy. A facial massage using clary sage or rose oils can relax tensed muscles and thereby alleviate a headache related to tension.

Biofeedback. Patients are taught to divert some blood flow from vessels in the scalp to the hands or elsewhere. Biofeedback training can also be used to counter muscle tension.

Chiropractic. Practitioners use neck adjustments to treat simple headaches. Treatments may also include massage and electrical stimulation techniques.

Herbal Medicine. Herbalists recommend numerous preparations to treat headaches, including feverfew capsules, mint tea, white willow bark tablets or capsules, and rosemary tea.

Homeopathy. Practitioners may prescribe nux vomica, sepia, or belladonna preparations, depending upon the nature of the headache.

Hypnosis. Self-hypnosis is taught as a way to treat various pain syndromes, including headaches. While the patient is hypnotized, a hypnotherapist implants instructions of specific actions to take in order to stop a headache. When the patient awakens, the therapist repeats these instructions and then instructs the person what to do when a headache develops.

Massage. This is an age-old technique to alleviate head pain. Massaging the back of the neck, temples, scalp, and face can relax tensed muscles, thereby relieving a simple tension headache.

Music Therapy. Listening to soothing music not only is relaxing but it also increases the brain's production of endorphins, which are natural painkillers.

Nutrition Therapy. Caffeine and alcohol trigger many headaches. Try eliminating these substances from your diet. MSG, artificial sweeteners, and other food additives also cause headaches in some people. Nutritionists recommend keeping a careful food diary, looking for links between headaches and foods, and then performing trial eliminations of suspect foods from your diet.

Osteopathy. In addition to medications recommended by other doctors, osteopaths may also use massage and manipulative methods to treat headaches.

Yoga and Meditation. These relaxation techniques are especially beneficial in treating tension headaches.

Self-Treatment

Simple self-care measures can alleviate most headaches. If the headache is related to tension or fatigue, resting in a darkened, quiet room with a cool compress on your forehead may cure it. Otherwise, nonprescription painkillers, such as aspirin, acetaminophen, and ibuprofen, work for most people.

Other Causes of Headaches

Many diseases, ranging from the common cold and flu to stroke and brain tumors, can produce headaches. However, the presence of additional symptoms usually distinguishes headaches that are secondary to other ailments from primary headaches.

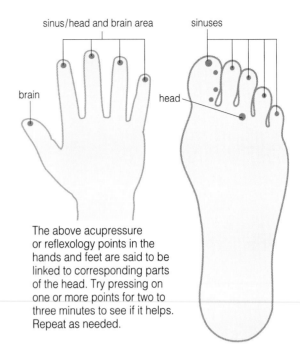

The above acupressure or reflexology points in the hands and feet are said to be linked to corresponding parts of the head. Try pressing on one or more points for two to three minutes to see if it helps. Repeat as needed.

A CASE IN POINT

Alex Stone, a 44-year-old architect, was suffering from frequent headaches that lasted for days or even weeks at a time. Typically, the pain would develop slowly, starting at the base of the skull. Within hours, Stone's entire head would feel as if it were being squeezed in a vice, with a dull ache extending from the upper neck, up the back of his head, and across his scalp. Sleep failed to solve the problem; even after 10 or 11 hours of sleeping, his head would still ache.

Nonprescription painkillers provided little relief, and a stronger nonsteroidal anti-inflammatory drug usually upset his stomach. Codeine did not have much effect either, and Stone was reluctant to take it on a regular basis anyway.

During one particularly relentless episode, Stone decided to turn to a headache clinic for help. "For the first time," he said later, "I underwent a thorough neurological workup that included a CT scan."

No organic abnormalities were found, but the specialist who questioned Stone uncovered some important clues as to what was causing the headaches.

A pattern of excessive sleepiness, steady weight gain, a persistent feeling of sadness, and difficulty in concentrating and making decisions pointed to undiagnosed depression, a common component of tension headaches.

"This doctor came up with an entirely different approach," Stone said. "First, he advised me to stop taking painkillers. Instead, he prescribed an antidepressant drug (Prozac) and recommended that I join the clinic's group therapy sessions."

The doctor also recommended that Stone cut back on his sleep to no more than eight hours a night, explaining that both too much and too little sleep can trigger tension headaches.

After a fellow patient in group therapy described how the Alexander technique had helped her headaches, Stone also tried this alternative approach.

In the end, he was unable to say what aspect of his treatment had helped the most. The antidepressant and the group therapy certainly helped brighten his outlook, resulting in renewed self-esteem and decisiveness. Now he woke up feeling more refreshed, even though he was sleeping fewer hours each night. After altering his posture and changing his work space as suggested by the teacher of Alexander technique, Stone felt less tired at the end of the day. Perhaps all of these elements contributed to making his prolonged headaches disappear.

Hearing Loss

(Otosclerosis; presbycusis)

Aging is the most common cause of hearing loss, but the degree of deficiency varies greatly from person to person and affects men more than women. Presbycusis, a type of sensory-neural hearing loss that is particularly prevalent in the elderly, is due to deterioration of the tiny hair cells that line the cochlea in the inner ear. These cells send electrical sound impulses to the part of the brain where sounds are received and processed. Accidents and exposure to excessive noise can also damage these cells.

Hearing deficits present at birth may stem from a congenital or hereditary disorder, or to a birth defect caused by drug use or illness, such as rubella, during pregnancy. A doctor will suspect hearing impairment in an infant who fails to respond to sound or does not begin talking by age two.

Childhood diseases, especially chronic middle ear infections, and less commonly, complications from chickenpox, mumps, or measles, can cause hearing loss. Untreated childhood hearing disorders may lead to later speech, reading, behavioral, and learning problems.

Gradual hearing loss that begins between the ages of 20 and 40 may be caused by otosclerosis, a degeneration of the stapes bone in the ear.

While the above conditions are mostly irreversible, hearing loss from an excessive buildup of earwax (page 169) or the side effects of some medications, such as aspirin, antibiotics, quinine, and certain diuretics, is usually temporary.

Diagnostic Studies and Procedures

Hearing is tested in a soundproof booth, with the patient wearing special earphones. A variety of tones are broadcast at different pitches through the earphones, and the person signals if he hears them. Hearing comprehension is tested by broadcasting different words through the earphones. After a doctor

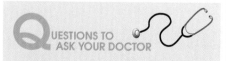

▶ Will a hearing aid help me?
▶ What is the best type of hearing aid for my particular needs?
▶ Will surgery restore my normal hearing?

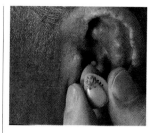

New types of hearing aids are not as unwieldy as older models and they produce fewer sound distortions.

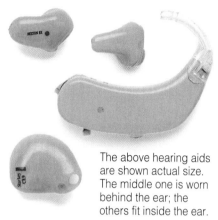

The above hearing aids are shown actual size. The middle one is worn behind the ear; the others fit inside the ear.

has assessed the hearing loss, further tests may be performed to determine its cause. These may include X-rays and a CT scan of the head to detect bone loss or deformities.

Medical Treatments

Depending on the extent of the loss, a hearing aid can often partially or completely restore hearing, but about 70 percent of people with hearing impairments do not seek help.

If a hearing aid is necessary, a health professional, rather than a salesperson, should select and fit it because the cause of the hearing impairment determines the type of aid. For example, hearing loss that is equally distributed throughout sound frequencies is best treated with a device that magnifies any sound. Presbycusis, which often entails hearing loss in the higher frequencies only, responds better to a hearing aid designed to amplify only the lost sounds. Audiologic rehabilitation, including auditory training and lip-reading, is sometimes needed in addition to a hearing aid.

Surgery may remedy some cases of otosclerosis. In one procedure, called a stapedectomy, the diseased stapes bone is removed and replaced with a prosthesis that conducts sound vibrations to the inner ear.

When there is severe or total hearing loss, special implants can permit the perception of some sound, although they cannot restore the ability to distinguish ordinary speech sounds.

Alternative Therapies

Nutrition Therapy. Some practitioners believe that certain types of hearing loss from inner ear disease may be caused by atherosclerosis. They advocate the same type of low-fat, low-cholesterol diet—with plenty of fresh fruits and vegetables and whole grains—recommended for people with heart disease. If you have a high cholesterol level, and especially if you are overweight and have diabetes, this healthful lifestyle adjustment may not only protect your hearing, but also prevent a heart attack or stroke.

Music Therapy. Through music, children with impaired hearing or speech difficulties have been helped to discover new ways of communicating.

Self-Treatment

If a buildup of earwax is responsible for diminished hearing, you may be able to remove it using a home kit available in most pharmacies. A warm solution, usually glycerol and an antiseptic, is inserted into the ear to soften the wax, which can then be removed with a syringe or flushed out with warm water. If this doesn't work, see a doctor. Never attempt to remove wax with a hairpin or other sharp object. Such tactics are likely to drive the wax in deeper, and can also damage the ear.

If ringing in the ears or any hearing loss develops while you are taking a medication, call your doctor to discuss discontinuation or a lower dosage.

Excessive noise is a leading cause of hearing loss. Wear earplugs when you are using noisy equipment. Even a hair dryer, according to some doctors, makes enough noise over time to impair hearing. If you are unavoidably exposed to a loud noise, such as a siren or subway train, press your fingers against the flap of tissue that covers each ear opening until the sound abates. If you work in a noisy environment, such as an airport or a printing shop, ask about occupational protective ear muffs. Remember, any noise that provokes pain can cause hearing loss.

Other Causes of Hearing Loss

Headsets, a popular means of listening to music while drowning out other sounds such as traffic, can themselves be detrimental to your hearing, especially if you turn the volume up high. Ménière's disease, brain tumors, strokes, head injuries, and viral infections may also result in hearing loss.

Heart Attack

(Coronary thrombosis; myocardial infarction)

A heart attack, or myocardial infarction, involves the death of heart muscle (myocardium). Most heart attacks result from blockage in one of the coronary arteries, blood vessels that encircle the heart and supply oxygen and other nutrients to the myocardium.

Often, a heart attack is the first obvious symptom of heart disease, but it usually culminates a lengthy process in which the coronary arteries have become clogged with fatty plaque, which is mostly cholesterol. As these arteries progressively narrow, blood flow to the heart muscle is reduced. If a vessel closes completely, the heart muscle it nourishes dies. The restricted blood flow encourages formation of a blood clot, or coronary thrombosis, which may cause the final blockage. Less often, the plaque itself closes the artery.

Some heart attacks are painless and not discovered until an electrocardiogram is taken at a later date. More often, however, a heart attack produces distinct symptoms. These may include:
▶ A feeling of discomfort, pressure, fullness, or squeezing in the center of the chest, lasting for two minutes or more.
▶ Pain that spreads throughout the chest and radiates to the shoulders, neck, jaw, arms, or back.
▶ Dizziness, fainting, sweating, clamminess, nausea, vomiting, and/or shortness of breath.

Not every symptom is always present; in some cases, symptoms subside only to return later. All too often, they are ignored or attributed to indigestion. Studies show that half of heart attack victims wait more than two hours before getting help—a delay that frequently proves fatal. Each year, about 500,000 Americans die from heart attacks, 60 percent within the first hour. Most of the early deaths are from ventricular fibrillation, an uncoordinated, spasmodic twitching of heart muscle that makes pumping blood impossible.

Diagnostic Studies and Procedures
Emergency care for a patient who may be having a heart attack is a fight for time, with diagnosis and treatment taking place virtually simultaneously. Even before reaching the hospital, an emergency medical team may perform cardiopulmonary resuscitation (CPR).

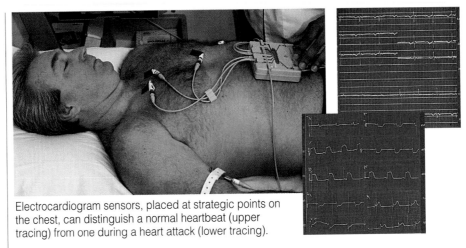

Electrocardiogram sensors, placed at strategic points on the chest, can distinguish a normal heartbeat (upper tracing) from one during a heart attack (lower tracing).

Many hospital emergency rooms have a coronary-care area for people with suspected heart attacks. There, a special team first makes sure that the person is breathing and has an adequate pulse rate and blood pressure. Then they perform any necessary life-saving maneuvers; these may include defibrillation, the administering of an electric shock to the heart to stop ventricular fibrillation. They then connect the patient to a heart rhythm monitor, so that an electrocardiogram (ECG) can show the pattern of the heartbeat. The team also administers oxygen, drugs to restore normal heart rhythm, and perhaps a pain medication.

Further diagnostic measures are likely to include an angiogram, a special X-ray study of the arteries, to determine whether one or more coronary arteries is blocked. Blood tests include measurement of enzymes released by damaged muscle. A rise in these enzymes helps confirm a heart

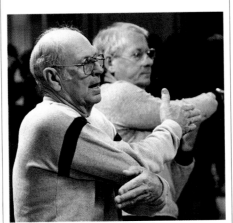

Exercise is an important part of rehabilitation after a heart attack. Initially, it may be carried out in a group setting, under the supervision of a doctor or an exercise physiologist.

attack in cases for which symptoms and the ECG are not so clear-cut.

Medical Treatments
In recent years, the use of thrombolytic drugs to dissolve clots has greatly improved the long-term outlook for heart attack victims. These drugs include streptokinase (Streptase and Kabikinase), urokinase (Abbokinase), tissue plasminogen activator (t-PA), and anistreplase (Eminase). When given intravenously during the first hour or two of a heart attack, thrombolytic agents can literally stop the attack and prevent heart muscle death; this technique is called reperfusion therapy. Consequently, many patients can now leave the hospital having suffered little or no damage to the heart.

To prevent formation of new clots, heparin may be given intravenously. Or, aspirin may be used, often with equally good results and a lower risk of serious side effects. Other drugs that may be given early in the course of a heart attack include beta blockers, to limit the attack and prevent recurrence, and antiarrhythmia drugs, to correct or prevent abnormal heart rhythms that may accompany the attack.

If drugs are not sufficient to restore blood flow and a normal heartbeat, surgery may be necessary. Emergency coronary bypass surgery involves implanting grafts to restore blood flow to areas of heart muscle. Another procedure is balloon angioplasty, which increases blood flow through narrowed arteries (see Angina, page 80).

After emergency treatment, the patient is transferred to the hospital's cardiac care unit (CCU), where doctors, nurses, and technicians with special training monitor heart function.

As soon as heart function is stable, the patient may be moved to a standard hospital room. There, ongoing therapy includes continued monitoring to measure recovery rate and to guard against another heart attack. Medication may include aspirin, beta blockers, and drugs to prevent angina and heart enlargement, common complications of a heart attack. A rehabilitation program will be designed to help the patient gradually increase activity and resume a normal lifestyle. Surgery may be considered if angina continues or if an artery becomes reblocked.

The average hospital stay is five to seven days but can vary, depending on the patient's overall health, the extent of damage done by the heart attack, and the development of complications. Before being discharged, the patient may undergo a modified stress test to determine a safe level of physical activity.

After the patient leaves the hospital, frequent checkups are necessary for the first few months to watch for signs of late complications, including heart failure. Continuing treatment often includes medication to lower blood pressure, reduce high cholesterol levels, and strengthen the heartbeat.

Alternative Therapies

Alternative therapies can be invaluable in recovering from a heart attack. In particular, exercise conditioning is an integral part. Many hospitals offer such programs, as do heart and cardiofitness clinics. A physical therapist can also provide guidance and supervise a therapeutic exercise regimen. The goal is to develop a life-long exercise routine that can be done safely at home or in a health club without medical supervision. Other helpful approaches include:

Meditation. Stress reduction is an important aspect of cardiac recovery. Some hospitals and many rehabilitation programs offer instruction in meditation, yoga, biofeedback training, and other relaxation techniques.

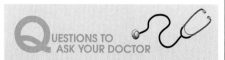

QUESTIONS TO
ASK YOUR DOCTOR

▶ After leaving the hospital, how soon will I be able to resume driving? Return to work? Have sexual relations?
▶ What can I do to avoid having a second heart attack?

THE BASICS OF CARDIOPULMONARY RESUSCITATION (CPR)

CPR is an emergency measure to supply oxygen and circulate the blood until medical help arrives. It can be used in any situation in which a person's respiration and heartbeat have stopped. The techniques are best learned in a course approved by the Red Cross, American Heart Association, or similar group, but it is still useful to familiarize yourself with the basics.

▶ Try to rouse the person and check for breathing and a carotid pulse (1); if there are none, call your local emergency medical system (EMS). Be sure to give your location, phone number, a description of what has happened, and what is being done.
▶ Remember the ABC's of CPR: Airway, Breathing, and Circulation, and proceed in that order.
▶ Airway: Position the victim on his back on a hard, flat surface, with arms alongside his body. If you are alone, situate yourself at the victim's side so you can do both the mouth-to-mouth breathing and chest compressions. Open the airway by lifting the chin and applying pressure to the forehead, moving the head back slightly (2). This maneuver moves the tongue out of the airway, and may be enough to restart breathing. Check for this and also feel again for a carotid pulse.
▶ Breathing: If the victim still is not breathing, begin mouth-to-mouth respiration. Pinch the victim's nostrils shut, take a deep breath, seal your mouth over the victim's, and deliver two slow breaths of 1½ to 2 seconds each (3). Watch the victim's chest to make sure it rises and falls, indicating that air is reaching the lungs.
▶ Circulation: If there is no pulse, position your hands as illustrated and begin chest compressions (4). Apply enough pressure to compress the sternum 1 to 1½ inches (in an adult). After each compression, allow the sternum to return to its normal position. Establish a rhythm by counting: One (push down) and (let up) two (push down) and (let up)—until you have done 15 compressions.
▶ Check for a pulse and breathing; if they are still absent, do two full lung inflations, followed by 15 chest compressions. Keep up this rhythm until breathing and a pulse return, help arrives, or you are unable to continue.
▶ If a helper is available, one of you should do the chest compressions, the other the rescue breathing. Establish a rhythm of five chest compressions after each mouth-to-mouth ventilation.

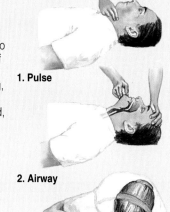

1. Pulse

2. Airway

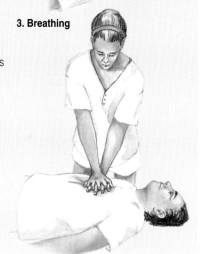

3. Breathing

4. Circulation

Nutrition Therapy. Even before leaving the hospital, a heart-attack patient will be given specific dietary instructions. Depending upon individual factors, these may include a reduced-calorie diet to lose excess weight; reductions in fat and cholesterol to help prevent atherosclerosis; sodium restriction to help control blood pressure; and vitamin E supplements, believed to reduce the risk of a future heart attack.

Self-Treatment

Changes in lifestyle are usually central to successful recovery and prevention of subsequent heart attacks. These include giving up smoking, limiting consumption of alcohol, engaging in regular exercise, and eating healthfully. Altering basic habits is often difficult. Joining a support group, such as the American Heart Association's Mended Hearts Club, can provide the motivation for permanent change.

Other Causes of Acute Chest Pain

An anxiety or panic attack can closely mimic a heart attack. Chest pain with shortness of breath, fever, and a cough can be a sign of pneumonia or pleurisy. A pulmonary embolism or a collapsed lung can also cause chest pain. Pain that is worse when bending over or lying down may come from heartburn.

Heart Enlargement

(Dilated congestive cardiomyopathy; hypertrophic cardiomyopathy)
An enlarged heart is the most common manifestation of heart muscle disease, or cardiomyopathy. Even so, there are only about 50,000 new cases in the United States annually.

Any abnormality of the heart muscle can cause cardiac enlargement, because the heart increases in size to compensate for the muscle weakness. If the expanded muscle is also abnormal, it further reduces the heart's ability to pump blood. Although the entire heart can be affected, the left ventricle, the main pumping chamber, usually becomes the most enlarged part.

If allowed to progress, the enlargement will eventually cause heart failure, in which the weakened muscle pumps ineffectively. Because blood then flows more slowly through the heart, clots tend to form; they can lead to pulmonary embolism, a stroke, a heart attack, or another circulatory blockage.

The underlying cause of an enlarged heart often cannot be identified, but possibilities include a heart attack, high blood pressure, heart valve disease, a sustained fast heartbeat, alcoholism, radiation therapy, anticancer drugs, inflammation of the heart muscle, infection, malnutrition, complications of pregnancy, and genetic, metabolic, or neurological disorders.

Diagnostic Studies and Procedures
A chest X-ray will usually detect an enlarged heart and the accompanying fluid-filled lungs. Echocardiography, an examination using ultrasound, provides a more detailed image of the heart's chambers and how well they are functioning. Various scanning techniques can measure stroke volume and cardiac output, the amount of blood that is pumped with each heartbeat and during one minute. An MRI study may be ordered to obtain a three-dimensional picture of the heart.

If the diagnosis is still in doubt, an imaging study called cardiac catheterization may be necessary. During this examination, which involves threading a long, thin, flexible tube through a blood vessel and into the heart, a small sample of heart muscle may be collected for laboratory analysis.

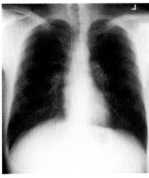

The above chest X-ray shows a heart that is normal size.

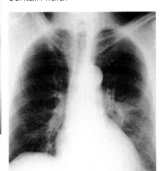

In the X-ray below, the heart is enlarged and the lungs contain fluid.

Medical Treatments
Treatment depends on the stage and nature of the enlargement. Sometimes correcting the underlying cause, such as lowering high blood pressure, can halt further heart expansion. In many cases, however, treatment focuses on relieving the symptoms of heart failure. A doctor may prescribe digitalis and other medications to strengthen the heartbeat and increase the efficiency of the heart's pumping action. Diuretics can reduce fluid retention and lessen lung congestion. (See opposite page.) Steroids may be necessary if the heart muscle is inflamed.

If drug therapy does not succeed in controlling heart failure and the enlargement progresses, a heart transplant may be considered.

Alternative Therapies
Although the role of alternative therapies in treating an enlarged heart is limited, some can be useful adjuncts to medical treatment.

Herbal Medicine. Hawthorn berries are thought to strengthen the heart, lower blood pressure, and dilate blood vessels, thereby increasing blood flow.

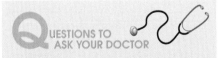

QUESTIONS TO ASK YOUR DOCTOR

▶ Should I take a daily aspirin or other blood-thinning medication to reduce the risk of blood clots?
▶ If I take digitalis, what other medications should I avoid?
▶ If I have chemotherapy or radiation treatments for cancer, what are the chances of my heart enlarging?
▶ How often do I need tests to monitor the condition?

Available in capsule form, hawthorn is also a mild diuretic. Anyone with heart disease should check with a doctor before taking hawthorn, however, because it may interact with other medications. Herbalists also contend that garlic, consumed raw, cooked, or in capsule form, strengthens the heart muscle.

Nutrition Therapy.
A low-salt diet is recommended to help prevent retention of fluid. Thiamine supplements may also be advocated if alcoholism is responsible for the enlargement.

Self-Treatment
Self-care alone cannot manage an enlarged heart, but lifestyle can play an important role in alleviating symptoms and perhaps halting progression of the disorder. Total elimination of alcohol is imperative. Alcohol is toxic to heart muscle cells, so even small amounts can worsen the condition. If you smoke, now is the time to quit. And avoid secondhand smoke, which is also detrimental to the heart.

Consult a nutritionist or doctor before making any major dietary changes. Losing excess weight and keeping it off reduces the heart's workload and can help relieve symptoms. However, crash diets can be dangerous for anyone with heart disease, because the body metabolizes its own muscle tissue, including the heart, when calories are overly restricted.

Learn to pace yourself. Regular exercise can help improve endurance, but it must be adapted to the limitations of an impaired heart. A doctor, in consultation with an exercise physiologist, can work out an appropriate regimen.

Avoid becoming overly tired; if necessary, take frequent rest breaks while working or doing exercises.

Simple measures, such as propping the head and back with extra pillows, may help reduce lung congestion.

Other Causes of an Enlarged Heart
Athletes sometimes develop an enlarged heart because of the extra demands that intense exercise workouts place on their heart muscle. However, this type of enlargement usually does not cause problems.

Heart Failure

(Congestive heart failure)

Contrary to popular belief, heart failure does not denote cardiac arrest; rather, it refers to the heart's inability to pump enough blood to meet the body's need for oxygen and other nutrients. The reduced circulation also allows metabolic waste products to collect in the body's tissues. As the disease progresses, blood that the heart would normally pump into circulation instead builds up in the lungs, a condition referred to as congestive heart failure with pulmonary edema.

In the early stages, patients often complain of awakening during the night with a choking sensation, which they relieve by sitting at the edge of the bed with their feet dangling down. Reclining makes the lungs waterlogged. During the day, the extra fluid pools in the legs, causing swollen ankles and feet. Other symptoms include shortness of breath, a bluish cast to the lips and nails, coughing up sputum tinged with blood, and persistent fatigue.

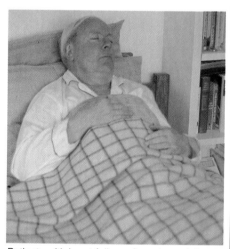

Patients with heart failure often sleep sitting up to keep lungs clear of fluid.

The American Heart Association estimates that between 2.3 and 3 million Americans suffer from heart failure, which can be caused by a narrowing of the coronary arteries, diseased heart muscle, faulty heart valves, or high blood pressure. It can also result from a heart attack or congenital heart disease.

Diagnostic Studies and Procedures

The diagnostic process starts with a physical examination, during which a doctor uses a stethoscope to listen for

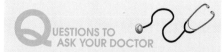

crackling noises, called rales, in the lungs; these indicate excess fluid. She will also listen for sounds of abnormal functioning of the heart's chambers and valves. A chest X-ray will show whether the heart is enlarged, and an electrocardiogram will provide data on the heart's electrical impulses.

If heart failure is suspected, additional tests may include an echocardiogram, an ultrasound examination of the heart; a radionuclide angiogram, in which a radioactive isotope is injected into the bloodstream and tracked as it moves through the heart; and cardiac catheterization, in which a thin tube is inserted through a vein or artery into the heart to determine whether blood vessels are blocked and to measure the pressure in the heart's chambers.

Medical Treatments

The goal of treatment is to improve the heart's ability to pump blood, thereby reducing lung congestion and fluid retention. Digitalis, the oldest heart medication, is often given to strengthen the heart's pumping action. A diuretic may be prescribed to help the kidneys eliminate excess fluid. Or angiotensin converting enzyme (ACE) inhibitors, which work by widening the small peripheral arteries, may be the drug of choice. Two examples are captopril (Capoten) and enalapril (Vasotec).

When possible, the underlying cause of heart failure will be treated; for example, lowering high blood pressure will improve the chances of success.

Surgery is used to treat heart failure from a congenital heart defect or diseased heart valve. In a few severe cases, heart transplantation is a last resort.

Alternative Therapies

Alternative remedies should be considered an adjunct rather than primary therapy for heart failure.

Exercise Conditioning. A medically supervised cardiovascular exercise program can improve circulation and increase endurance and the body's effi-

cient use of oxygen. A typical exercise prescription calls for 15 to 30 minutes of moderate exercise, such as walking or using a stationary cycle, three or four times a week.

Herbal Medicine. Garlic and onions are said to strengthen the heart. Garlic may be taken in capsule form, used in cooking, or eaten raw in salads. Raw onions are more beneficial than cooked, but cooking may be necessary to prevent indigestion. Other herbal remedies include alfalfa pills and rose petals, eaten raw or brewed as a tea. A word of caution: Although digitalis is derived from the foxglove plant, use only a commercial preparation. Herbal or homemade digitalis can be lethal.

Naturopathy and Nutrition Therapy. A low-salt diet is advised to reduce fluid accumulation. Some nutritionists also recommend supplements of vitamin E to reduce coronary artery disease, one of the underlying causes of congestive heart failure. Foods high in potassium—whole grains, legumes, bananas, tomatoes, and other fresh fruits and vegetables—are suggested for patients who are taking diuretic drugs, as some of these medications increase potassium excretion.

Yoga and Meditation. Because stress can aggravate heart failure, yoga, meditation, and other relaxation therapies can be helpful. Deep-breathing yoga exercises in particular may calm the panic that comes from breathlessness.

Self-Treatment

Self-care is directed toward reducing any unnecessary strain on the heart. If you are overweight, make every effort to shed the excess pounds. Abstain from smoking and alcohol; both contribute to heart failure.

Regular exercise is important, but you should follow a regimen prescribed by a doctor or physical therapist. You may need to rest in bed during periods when symptoms worsen. Avoid lifting, straining, and doing isometric exercises, which can strain the heart and reduce its pumping action.

Other Causes of Heart Failure Symptoms

Lung disorders such as bronchitis, lung cancer, pneumonia, and emphysema can cause breathing difficulties. Kidney failure can cause swelling of the ankles and legs. Anemia and other blood disorders can also produce symptoms similar to those of heart failure.

Heart Valve Disorders

(Mitral, aortic, tricuspid, and pulmonary stenosis and regurgitation)

The heart has four valves that control the flow of blood passing in and out of its chambers. A defect or disease in any

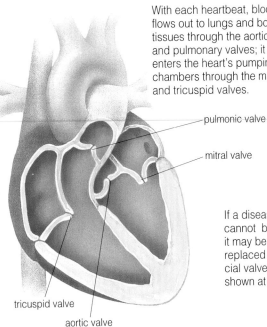

With each heartbeat, blood flows out to lungs and body tissues through the aortic and pulmonary valves; it enters the heart's pumping chambers through the mitral and tricuspid valves.

pulmonic valve

mitral valve

tricuspid valve

aortic valve

one of them will disrupt normal flow. There are two categories of disorder: stenosis, in which a valve fails to open fully, and insufficiency, or regurgitation, in which it does not close properly.

Congenital heart defects often produce valve problems; valves can also be damaged by coronary artery disease, heart attacks, and infections, especially rheumatic fever (page 361) and endocarditis (page 178). In elderly people, calcium deposits may narrow the aortic valve. And many women have mitral valve prolapse (page 300), in which one or more of the mitral valve's leaflets fail to close completely.

Valvular disease can exist for years without causing symptoms or requiring treatment. When symptoms do develop, they may include breathlessness, fatigue, angina, and dizzy spells.

Consequences of a diseased heart valve vary. Mitral valve stenosis and regurgitation can cause congestive heart failure. A diseased aortic valve can lead to enlargement and weakening of the left ventricle.

Diagnostic Studies and Procedures

An initial diagnosis is made when a doctor hears a heart murmur through a stethoscope. An electrocardiogram and a chest X-ray will provide important information about heart size and function, but to make a precise assessment, a physician will order echocardiography, an ultrasound examination that provides images of the valves and other heart structures. Doppler echocardiography, in which the blood flow is measured, can be particularly useful when assessing valve disorders.

If these noninvasive procedures are not sufficient, or if valve replacement surgery is being considered, cardiac catheterization will

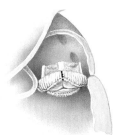

If a diseased valve cannot be repaired, it may be surgically replaced with an artificial valve, like the one shown at the right.

Artificial mitral valve

be employed. This procedure, which involves inserting a catheter into an artery and then into the heart, will help pinpoint the valve problem and other abnormalities.

Medical Treatments

Symptoms can often be alleviated with medications, though they cannot cure the disease. The most frequently prescribed drug is digitalis, which helps the heart beat more forcefully. Diuretics may be given to reduce the body's fluid volume and ease the heart's workload. Vasodilators might be prescribed to widen small arteries. These include nitroglycerin; prazosin (Minipress); calcium-channel blockers, such as nifedipine (Procardia); and ACE inhibitors, such as captopril (Capoten). Anticoagulant drugs may also be needed to prevent blood clots, and antiarrhythmia drugs to control irregular heartbeats.

Balloon valvuloplasty is sometimes used to open a narrowed, or stenosed, valve. A balloon-tipped catheter is inserted through an artery into the heart and narrowed valve. The balloon

is then inflated to widen the valve's opening. Although valvuloplasty is not as effective as surgical repair, it is safer and less expensive, and may be advised for elderly patients who are unlikely to tolerate heart surgery. It is most effective in treating a narrowed mitral valve and, to a lesser degree, the aortic valve.

Surgery is reserved for severe, progressive cases. Sometimes the damaged valve can be repaired, but more often it must be replaced with one made from synthetic materials or from animal or human tissue. If a synthetic valve is implanted, the patient must take anticoagulant drugs to prevent blood clots.

All forms of valvular disease increase the risk of endocarditis, a serious infection of the heart's lining. Prophylactic antibiotic therapy is often recommended, especially before dental or surgical procedures that involve bleeding.

Alternative Therapies

Alternative approaches should be used only as additions to medical therapy.

Nutrition Therapy. A low-salt diet can reduce fluid accumulation. When taking diuretics, a patient should consume high-potassium foods to replace the excreted potassium. Good choices include bananas, tomatoes, potatoes, legumes, and whole-grain products. A low-fat diet that is high in fiber and carbohydrates is recommended for all heart patients. Supplements of vitamins E and C may also be advised.

Self-Treatment

Moderate exercise can usually be tolerated, but not strenuous physical activity. It is important to refrain from smoking, to abstain from alcohol or use it in moderation, to maintain ideal weight, and to control other cardiovascular disorders, such as high blood pressure and elevated cholesterol.

Other Causes of Breathlessness

Numerous lung diseases, including emphysema and tuberculosis, can cause shortness of breath, as can anemia and congestive heart failure.

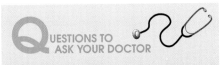

QUESTIONS TO ASK YOUR DOCTOR

▶ If I have a heart murmur but no symptoms, should I cut down on exercise or alter my lifestyle in any other way?
▶ Is pregnancy risky for a woman with a heart murmur?

Heartburn

(Esophageal reflux)

This ailment is so common that 25 to 50 million Americans regularly endure its discomforts. It has nothing to do with the heart, but involves a burning pain in the chest that radiates upward into the neck and throat and sometimes the face. Heartburn usually occurs after a meal, especially if the person lies down, and is often accompanied by belching and regurgitation into the mouth of bitter gastric juices, which prompt a flow of extra saliva. Some people also have difficulty swallowing, experience mild abdominal pain, and in a few cases, vomit.

The most frequent cause is a weakening of the opening, or sphincter, located at the lower end of the esophagus. This sphincter, which connects the esophagus and stomach, opens when food moves down the esophageal tube, permitting it to enter the stomach. It then closes to prevent stomach acid (needed for digestion) from splashing up, or refluxing, into the esophagus.

If muscle tone in the sphincter is lost and it remains open when it should be closed, the result is acid reflux and the painful sensations of heartburn. This action occurs after a meal because that is when the stomach secretes acidic gastric juices. Also, pressure inside the stomach builds when it is full, making it more likely that stomach contents will be pushed back through the sphincter.

Diagnostic Studies and Procedures

A doctor normally makes a diagnosis on the basis of the patient's description of symptoms. If the heartburn has continued for some time, the lower esophagus may have become inflamed. This can be detected by examination with an esophagoscope, a long, slender tube with magnifying and lighting devices. A doctor may also order an upper GI series—X-rays taken after the patient has swallowed barium, a chalky substance that coats the esophagus and stomach to make them show up on film. Because heartburn can mimic the pain of angina, an electrocardiogram and other heart studies may also be ordered to rule out heart disease.

Medical Treatments

If heartburn is severe and chronic, prescription medication may help to alleviate it. Among the commonly used agents are a class of drugs known as

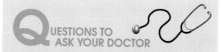

H₂ blockers, antihistamines that decrease production of stomach acid. They include cimetidine (Tagamet), ranitidine (Zantac), and famotidine (Pepcid). To create a barrier between the esophagus and the stomach, a drug called sucralfate (Carafate) may be prescribed. To improve sphincter tone and hasten the emptying of the stomach into the small intestine, metoclopramide (Reglan) may be administered.

In a few cases, severe heartburn may require surgery to correct such complications as narrowing of the esophagus due to chronic inflammation.

Alternative Therapies

Homeopathy. Homeopathic practitioners often recommend nux vomica to treat heartburn.

Naturopathy. Numerous natural remedies are said to help heartburn. One calls for drinking ½ cup of raw potato juice diluted with ½ cup of water after each meal. To make the juice, simply put a washed potato through a juicer. Another remedy is made by mixing 1 tablespoon each of honey and apple cider vinegar in 1 cup of warm water and drinking it at the first hint of discomfort. Papaya tablets might also alleviate an attack of heartburn.

Self-Treatment

There is much you can do to prevent heartburn, starting with modifying your eating habits. Consume small frequent meals, eat slowly, and chew each bite thoroughly. Avoid alcohol, caffeine, and fatty or highly spiced foods, and keep a food diary to identify foods that trigger an attack. Drink liquids between meals, rather than while you are eating; water with meals

dilutes and increases the volume of the stomach's contents, making it easier for acid reflux to occur.

Avoid stooping, bending over, or lying down for at least an hour after meals. If heartburn is bothersome at night, do not eat for a few hours before bedtime, and try sleeping with your upper body in an elevated position, using a wedged pillow or placing books or bricks under the head of your bed to raise it a few inches.

For temporary relief of symptoms, use an over-the-counter antacid. Ask your doctor or pharmacist to recommend a product, because some ingredients should be avoided if you have certain disorders. For example, sodium bicarbonate antacids are high in sodium and should not be used by people with high blood pressure. Other products contain calcium and should not be taken by anyone with kidney stones.

Other Causes of Heartburn

Stomach ulcers, gallbladder disease, and other gastrointestinal disorders may bring about discomfort similar to heartburn. A hiatal hernia can result in an esophageal reflux. Esophageal spasm or stricture can cause difficult or painful swallowing and a burning sensation in the upper chest.

A heart attack can easily be confused with heartburn. Any chest pain that radiates to the jaw or an arm should be investigated by a doctor, especially when accompanied by other symptoms, such as sweating, nausea, dizziness, shortness of breath, and fainting. Do not take a chance, as prompt action may save your life. Go immediately to the nearest hospital emergency room, or call your local emergency number (usually 911) for assistance.

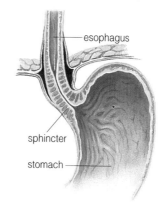

esophagus

A weakened sphincter allows stomach acid to back up into the esophagus (below).

sphincter

stomach

Normally, the sphincter at the lower end of the esophagus (above) closes after food enters the stomach, preventing a reflux of acid.

Heat Exhaustion/ Heatstroke

(Heat prostration; sunstroke)
Heat exhaustion and heatstroke are medical emergencies brought on by exposure to more heat and humidity than the body can adapt to. Although the two terms are sometimes used interchangeably, they are distinctly different conditions.

Heat exhaustion is caused by dehydration, usually the result of sweating heavily and not consuming adequate replacement fluids. Warning signs include increasing fatigue, weakness, and feelings of anxiety, along with a drenching sweat. As the condition worsens, blood pressure drops, the pulse slows, and the skin becomes pale and clammy. The person could be confused and might faint.

Heatstroke develops when the body's ability to cool itself by sweating fails during very hot, humid weather. It is potentially more serious than heat exhaustion because it can quickly lead to a fever of 104°F (40°C) or higher. Unlike heat exhaustion, heatstroke comes on suddenly, but is sometimes preceded by a headache, dizziness, and

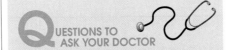

QUESTIONS TO ASK YOUR DOCTOR
▶ Should I stop using antiperspirants during hot weather?
▶ Are some people more prone to heat exhaustion than others?
▶ If it occurs once, is it likely to recur?

fatigue. The person's skin will be hot, flushed, and dry. The pulse may rise as high as 160 to 180 beats per minute, and breathing may be rapid and shallow. Confusion and disorientation may occur, followed soon by unconsciousness or convulsions and a collapse of the circulatory system.

The most common victims of heatstroke are the elderly, the obese, and people who consume too much alcohol or who are weakened by chronic illness. Certain drugs, such as the phenothiazines used to treat mental illness or the diuretics used to reduce body fluids, also increase the risk.

Diagnostic Studies and Procedures
Heat exhaustion and heatstroke are both diagnosed by the symptoms. Once the immediate emergency has been brought under control, a doctor will order blood and urine tests and take a complete medical history to determine whether drug toxicity could have contributed to the episode.

Medical Treatments
Most cases of heat exhaustion do not need treatment beyond first aid measures. But if the episode is severe or the person does not respond to first aid, a doctor should be seen immediately, preferably in the nearest hospital emergency room. It may be necessary to administer intravenous fluids or give medication to stimulate the heart.

Heatstroke requires immediate hospitalization so that the patient's temperature can be continuously monitored and controlled. If convulsions continue, an intravenous sedative, usually diazepam (Valium) or a barbiturate, will be given. Bed rest is necessary for several days after an episode of heatstroke, and temperature may be erratic for weeks.

Alternative Therapies
Hydrotherapy. If it is necessary to perform physical labor in hot weather, use cool water to keep your temperature from rising to dangerous levels. A cool shower or a swim in a pool, pond, lake, or other body of readily accessible water will do. Alternatively, soak a towel in a bucket of cool water and apply it as a compress.

Self-Treatment
Common sense prevention is the best approach. Keeping the body well hydrated helps avoid heat exhaustion. Drink water, fruit juice, broth, or other nonalcoholic beverages every hour or so, even if you do not feel thirsty. Beverages that contain contain caffeine are not recommended because of their diuretic and stimulatory effects.

Avoid strenuous outdoor activities in hot and humid weather, particularly between 10:00 A.M. and 4:00 P.M. If your job demands that you work under these conditions, wear lightweight, light-colored clothing, try to stay out of the sun, drink plenty of liquids, and eat light meals. Rest frequently in a cool, shady place. If you have a chronic cardiovascular, neurological, or skin disease, seek your doctor's advice about working outdoors in the heat.

Other Causes of Symptoms
An insulin overdose, poisoning, hemorrhage, or traumatic shock can produce symptoms similar to those of heat exhaustion. Food, chemical, or drug poisoning may mimic heatstroke.

FIRST AID

For heat exhaustion
▶ Take the person to a cool, shady place or an air-conditioned room, and have him lie down with feet propped up.
▶ Remove or loosen tight clothing.
▶ Give small amounts of cold fluid, preferably plain water or fruit juice, every few minutes. If possible, add about ½ teaspoon of salt per quart of beverage. Do not offer iced drinks.

For heatstroke
▶ Immediately call your emergency number (usually 911) to request an ambulance or an emergency medical team.
▶ Cool the person as rapidly as possible by any available means, preferably by immersing in cold water, or placing ice packs under the arms, in the groin, and around the neck, knees, and ankles, to cool large blood vessels. If neither of these measures is possible, wrap the person in cold, wet sheets or towels. Fan vigorously to help bring down temperature, but be careful not to induce shivering, which generates heat.
▶ Take the patient's temperature about every 10 minutes, and stop the cooling measures when it comes down to 100°F (38°C). Continue to keep the person quiet until the ambulance arrives.

A person suffering from heatstroke can be cooled off by covering him with a wet sheet, and creating a breeze with an electric fan, newspaper, or whatever is available.

Heat Rash

(Miliaria; prickly heat)

Heat rash, or prickly heat, consists of clusters of tiny blisters filled with perspiration. It forms when pores become blocked and prevent the sweat glands from releasing perspiration, or when heat and humidity exceed the ability of the sweat glands to cool the body. The rash itches but does not become inflamed. It usually develops in the armpits and groin, and sometimes also on the chest, waist, and back.

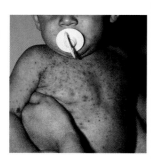

Infants and young children are especially prone to heat rash, but people of all ages may be affected.

Babies are especially vulnerable because their ability to sweat is not fully developed, and because they often wear or lie on waterproof materials, which intensify the effects of heat.

A similar rash, caused by sensitivity to ultraviolet light, may accompany prickly heat or occur independently. Referred to as a polymorphic light eruption, it produces itchy red spots within 24 to 48 hours of exposure to the sun. The rash appears mostly on the body, rarely on the face. Although children sometimes develop the rash, it is more common in young adults, especially Caucasians.

Diagnostic Studies and Procedures

In most cases, a doctor can diagnose heat rash by looking at the affected areas. If the rash looks infected, she may send a skin scraping to be cultured to determine whether a fungus or bacterium is causing the eruption.

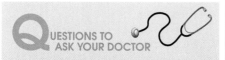

QUESTIONS TO ASK YOUR DOCTOR

▶ How can I keep a young child from scratching prickly heat and making it worse or causing infection?
▶ How long should I treat a rash myself before seeking medical attention?

Medical Treatments

A doctor may advise applying an over-the-counter cortisone lotion or cream two to three times daily (always check with your physician before using these products on a baby). He may prescribe antihistamines for severe itching or an antifungal medication containing cortisone, such as clotrimazole and betamethasone dipropionate (Lotrisone), if a secondary fungal infection has developed. A severe polymorphic light rash may require treatment with an oral steroid drug, such as prednisone.

Alternative Therapies

Remedies that alleviate itching and cool the skin usually work well.

Herbal Medicine. Herbalists often recommend adding thyme tea to bathwater. Thyme contains thymol, an antiseptic substance that eases itching.

Hydrotherapy. Soaking in a tepid or cool bath is a soothing remedy. Do not apply soap to the rash. Instead, add 1 cup of oatmeal, 1 cup of baking soda, 2 cups of apple cider vinegar, or 2 cups of laundry starch to the bathwater. (A word of caution: Bathe a baby only in plain water.) Soaking in a whirlpool bath of cool water is also helpful. Alternatively, take one or two cool showers a day.

After bathing, gently pat the skin dry rather than rubbing it, then dust the affected areas lightly with cornstarch or baby powder. Do not apply moisturizing creams and lotions or use bath oil. These products may further clog pores.

Self-Treatment

You can usually prevent heat rash by staying out of the sun and heat as much as possible, using air conditioning whenever available, and wearing lightweight, loose-fitting, cotton garments. If a rash does develop, calamine lotion may ease the itching. Do not scratch. Expose the affected areas to the air when you can. Avoid strenuous exercise or any activity that causes sweating.

When a baby has heat rash, change diapers as soon as they are wet; then pat the skin dry and apply a dusting of cornstarch. Avoid laying an infant on a plastic-covered mattress or pad; instead, use a cotton sheet or towel.

Other Causes of Itchy, Red Rashes

Intertrigo, an inflammatory skin condition that is also aggravated by heat, produces a rash in areas where the skin rubs against itself, such as the groin and under the breasts and arms.

People with lupus often develop a splotchy red rash after exposure to the sun. Certain drugs also increase sun sensitivity and can cause a rash similar to that of a polymorphic light reaction. Other causes of red, itchy rashes include skin allergies, contact dermatitis, and eczema. In babies, a diaper rash can resemble prickly heat.

Hemophilia

(Factor VIII or IX deficiency; hereditary coagulation disorders)

Hemophilia is an inherited disorder in which the blood fails to clot normally. It is characterized by heavy bleeding after a minor injury, spontaneous bruising, and frequent nosebleeds. Joints, particularly the knee and elbow, are often swollen and painful due to bleeding into the joint space.

A person with hemophilia lacks a clotting factor, a protein that goes into action when the wall of a blood vessel is damaged. In hemophilia A, about 80 percent of all cases, the deficiency is in clotting factor VIII. In hemophilia B, clotting factor IX is lacking. Both produce the same symptoms, but treatment differs in that the specific missing clotting factor must be replaced.

The disease is an X-linked type; that is, the mother carries the defective gene but does not have the disorder. A son who inherits the gene will develop the disease; a daughter who inherits it will become a carrier who is not likely to be affected. As with other X-linked disorders, the hemophilia gene cannot be passed from father to son (see box, below). There are rare cases in which a defective gene seems to develop spontaneously without a hereditary history.

Diagnostic Studies and Procedures

A review of symptoms can provide a tentative diagnosis of hemophilia, but blood tests are necessary to confirm it.

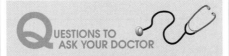

Clotting time will be determined, and other blood studies will be done to measure for the factors VIII and IX.

Medical Treatments

At the first signs of bleeding, the missing clotting factor is administered. (The concentrated clotting factor is obtained from many units of blood that are frozen until needed, then thawed and reconstituted with plasma.) The frequency of transfusions depends on the severity of the disease and the particular circumstances. For example, extra transfusions may be given before surgery or dental work.

Because the clotting factor for even one transfusion is derived from dozens of donors, hemophiliacs face a high risk of hepatitis and other blood-borne diseases. Before a screening test for HIV, the virus that causes AIDS, was developed in 1986, a tragically high number of hemophiliacs contracted this deadly disease. Clotting factor transfusions are now heat-treated to kill HIV, but hepatitis remains a risk; hepatitis immunization is advocated for all hemophiliacs.

Any bleeding episode is potentially an emergency for a hemophiliac. Controlling bleeding requires the care of a hematologist who is trained in the management of the disease.

Alternative Therapies

Alternative therapies should be used only to supplement conventional medical treatment.

Hydrotherapy. Pain and swelling in joints may be alleviated by applying ice packs, which can also slow bleeding. Once bleeding has stopped, soaking in a tub of warm water may be soothing. (Avoid hot packs or warm water

during a bleeding episode because heat increases the flow of blood.) The gentle swirling of a whirlpool or Jacuzzi may also help to reduce pain.

Exercises performed in water not only relieve joint pain, but are also among the safest forms of physical activity for a hemophiliac. Many communities now offer therapeutic swimming sessions with a physical therapist or sports medicine specialist.

Nutrition Therapy. Supplements of calcium, niacin, and vitamins C and K, essential to clotting, may be advocated.

Physical Therapy. Physical therapists can design specific exercise programs to help maintain full range of motion and prevent disability.

Self-Treatment

The most important aspect of self-care is prevention of bleeding episodes. Learn the early warning signs of dangerously low levels of clotting factor, such as joint and muscle pain, swelling, and bruising. Avoid contact sports and other activities that carry a high risk of injury. And always wear a protective helmet and knee and elbow pads when engaging in any activity that carries the risk of a fall or blow.

Learn emergency techniques for controlling bleeding and take immediate first aid action if it occurs. If the site of bleeding is accessible, apply direct pressure to it with your hand. As quickly as possible, apply an elastic bandage and an ice pack. If ice is not available, press the flat side of a knife or spoon to the bruised area for 5 to 10 minutes. If bleeding persists, or there is evidence of internal bleeding, seek emergency treatment.

A person with hemophilia should never take aspirin or other medication that interferes with blood clotting. Acetaminophen for pain relief is usually safe, but a doctor should always be consulted before taking any nonprescription remedy or vitamin supplements. Preventive dental care is also very important to avoid the potential problems of dental surgery.

Hemophiliacs should at all times wear a medical identification bracelet or pendant detailing their condition.

Other Causes of Easy Bleeding

Aspirin and steroids cause bleeding and easy bruising. Platelet disorders, such as thrombocytopenia, can cause bleeding, as can infections, anemia, leukemia, and vitamin deficiencies.

HEMOPHILIA INHERITANCE PATTERN

Hemophilia is an X-linked genetic disorder, in which the disease is passed from mother to son. A daughter may inherit the gene and become a carrier. Any son has a 50-50 chance of inheriting the gene for hemophilia on the mother's X chromosome and developing the disease.

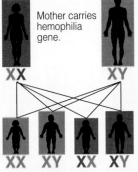

Mother carries hemophilia gene.

One daughter inherits gene and is a carrier.
One son inherits gene and has the disease.

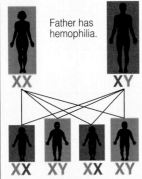

Father has hemophilia.

Sons are normal.
Daughters inherit gene and become carriers.

Hemorrhoids

(Anal varicosities)

Hemorrhoids are varicose veins in the anal area that cause pain, itching, and bleeding. (The three veins that serve the anal area normally expand, or dilate, during bowel movements and shrink afterward. Repeated straining to pass hard stools can result in permanent swelling. The enlarged veins then press on surrounding nerves, thus producing the itchiness and discomfort.) They may be located inside or outside the anal opening; external ones tend to be more painful and the internal type bleed more easily.

Usually, hemorrhoids are uncomfortable and annoying but not serious. For some people, however, they can cause extreme pain, particularly when defecating. The swollen veins may also rupture and bleed.

Hemorrhoids are very common, afflicting about one-third of Americans, or some 75 million people. They tend to run in families, but millions with no family history develop them. Contributing factors include excessive sitting, constipation, obesity, and pregnancy.

Diagnostic Studies and Procedures

External hemorrhoids can easily be seen; internal ones are readily detected by a rectal examination, in which a doctor inserts a gloved finger into the rectum. To confirm the diagnosis, anoscopy or sigmoidoscopy may be ordered. For both procedures, a thin, flexible tube with a lighted tip and magnifying devices is inserted through the anus and used to examine its interior (anoscopy) or the lower part of the colon (sigmoidoscopy).

Medical Treatments

If constipation is part of the problem, a doctor may recommend use of a stool softener, as well as anesthetic sprays or creams to alleviate pain and itching.

If these approaches are ineffective, removal of the hemorrhoids may be advisable. The simplest procedure is to strangle the hemorrhoid by using a small rubber band to cut off its blood supply. As the varicosed portion of the vein dies, the tissue sloughs away.

When rubber band ligature is not possible, a relatively painless alternative is laser surgery, in which intense light beams are used to vaporize the tissue. Conventional surgery may be done in severe cases. The operation,

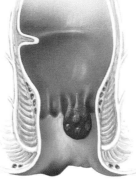
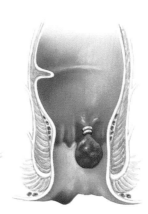

The simplest way to eliminate a hemorrhoid (above) is by cutting off its blood supply with a rubber band (right).

which involves removing dilated veins from around or inside the anus, usually is performed on an outpatient basis.

Alternative Therapies

Acupuncture and Acupressure. Points for the treatment of hemorrhoids are located on the top of the head and at the base of the spine. Applying needles or finger pressure to these points may help relieve pain.

Aromatherapy. A bath with aromatic oils can help relieve pain and itching, particularly when combined with other remedies. Equal amounts of cypress, frankincense, and juniper oils are recommended. The patient should remain in the bath for 10 to 15 minutes.

Herbal Medicine. Western herbalists recommend astringent herbs, such as pilewort, which is taken as a tea or applied as an external ointment. Witch hazel may be combined with pilewort and used as a tincture or an ointment.

Sitting for 15 minutes twice a day in a basin of warm water to which ¼ cup of witch hazel has been added has been reported to alleviate hemorrhoids.

Chinese herbalists recommend a tea called Itsuton, consisting of rhizoma rhei, radix angelicae sinensis, radix scutellariae, radix glycyrrhizae, radix bupleurui, and rhizoma cimicifugae.

QUESTIONS TO ASK YOUR DOCTOR

► Are hemorrhoids that develop during pregnancy likely to cause continued problems after childbirth?
► What nonprescription products do you recommend? What adverse effects should I watch for?

Homeopathy. Practitioners recommend sulphur if hemorrhoids are itchy but not bleeding and if constipation is a problem. Aloe gel is prescribed for use three times daily when hemorrhoids protrude and there is itching, bleeding, and diarrhea. Nux vomica is advocated when there is constipation.

Naturopathy and Nutrition Therapy. A high-fiber diet helps prevent constipation. Some naturopaths recommend taking two tablespoons daily of bran, mixed with yogurt or a fresh fruit salad. They also advocate a diet that includes at least four to six servings of whole-grain cereals, breads, and other complex carbohydrates, and four to six servings of fruits and vegetables a day.

Self-Treatment

To alleviate pain and shrink swollen tissue, use an ice pack made by putting several ice cubes in a plastic bag and wrapping a cloth around it. Apply this for 20 minutes, remove it for 10 minutes, then reapply it for another 20 minutes. Do not apply ice directly to the skin, as you may damage delicate tissue. You can also try nonprescription hemorrhoid products that contain astringents and ingredients to shrink hemorrhoids. Sitting in a tub of tepid water may also bring some relief.

Refrain from inserting any object into the rectum. After a bowel movement, wipe with moistened tissue or an anal cleansing pad sold in drugstores. Avoid scratching or rubbing.

If constipation is a problem, use a stool softener but avoid long-term laxative use. Don't stay on the toilet any longer than necessary, since this position places a strain on anal veins. If possible, adopt a squatting position, or place the feet on a low stool to relieve pressure on the veins around the anus.

If your job involves sitting for long periods, walk around at least once an hour, and stand whenever possible.

Other Causes of Anal Itching and Bleeding

Colitis, diverticulitis, colon polyps, and colon or rectal cancer can produce blood in the stool. Anal bleeding, pain, and itching may be due to an anal fissure, infection, or injury.

Hepatitis

(Viral hepatitis)

Viral hepatitis is an inflammation of the liver caused by one of four hepatitis viruses—A, B, C, or D. In its earlier stages, the disease may be mistaken for flu, with fever, fatigue, nausea, diarrhea, loss of appetite, and muscles and joint aches the major symptoms. These are followed by the characteristic jaundice, or yellowing of the eyes and skin due to a buildup in the blood of bile, a digestive substance that the liver normally controls. Excessive bile can also cause severe itchiness and a darkening of urine; the stool becomes light colored.

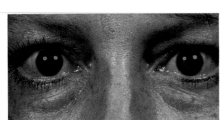

Jaundice, or yellowing of the skin and whites of the eyes, is a hallmark of hepatitis.

Hepatitis A is the most common strain, infecting tens of thousands of Americans each year. The virus is shed in the stool, and is usually contracted by consuming food or fluids that have been contaminated by human feces.

The virus that causes hepatitis B, once known as serum hepatitis, is found in blood, semen, saliva, and other body fluids. It is spread by blood transfusion, sharing of contaminated hypodermic needles, sexual contact, and other exposure to bodily fluids. Worldwide, there are some 200 million carriers of hepatitis B, who can pass the disease to others without experiencing any symptoms themselves.

Hepatitis C, formerly referred to as non-A, non-B hepatitis, is spread mostly through blood transfusion. Hepatitis D is spread by close personal contact in endemic areas such as the Mediterranean countries. In the United States and other nonendemic areas, most cases of hepatitis D are contracted through frequent blood transfusions, such as those required by people with hemophilia, or by drug users who share needles.

Most people with hepatitis A recover completely in one to two months. The other forms of viral hepatitis may lead to chronic liver disease and increased risk of liver cancer.

Diagnostic Studies and Procedures

When hepatitis is suspected, a doctor will palpate the liver during a physical examination for signs of enlargement. The liver will be tender to the touch and the spleen may also be enlarged. Laboratory analyses of blood and urine samples confirm the diagnosis. A liver biopsy is rarely needed unless other liver disorders are suspected.

Medical Treatments

The majority of people with hepatitis do not require extensive medical treatment, although hospitalization may be necessary for elderly patients or those with concomitant diseases. Fulminant hepatitis, a serious complication of hepatitis B in which large portions of the liver are destroyed (hepatic necrosis), generally requires hospitalization. With intensive supportive care, there is a possibility that the damaged liver will regenerate itself.

To alleviate severe itching, cholestyramine (Questran), a drug normally taken to lower blood cholesterol, may be prescribed. This drug binds with bile salts, which are the cause of the itchiness, and helps the body rid itself of them.

Persons who have been exposed to hepatitis may be given immune globulin containing hepatitis antibodies. Hepatitis A, B, and D can now be prevented with vaccines. The American Academy of Pediatrics recommends hepatitis B immunization for all babies. Immunization is also advocated for health-care workers, family members or sexual partners of people with the disease, and others who are at high risk of contracting hepatitis.

Alternative Therapies

Some alternative therapies may help speed recovery from mild hepatitis, but a physician should oversee treatment of severe or chronic cases.

Herbal Medicine. Herbalists recommend turmeric capsules to reduce liver inflammation and jaundice. Milk thistle capsules are a popular tonic among European herbalists. Artichokes steamed with garlic, as well as dandelion capsules or extract, are also promoted as liver tonics.

Nutrition Therapy. Proper nutrition plays a critical role in recovery from viral hepatitis. Usually, extra calories

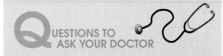

are needed, but meals should be small, frequent, and low in fat. Intravenous feeding may be necessary if persistent nausea and vomiting interfere with eating. Naturopaths recommend lecithin supplements to promote normal liver function, but its value is unproved.

Self-Treatment

Most cases of hepatitis can be treated at home, provided that proper precautions are taken to prevent the spread of the disease. The person who is ill should have a separate set of eating and drinking utensils and these should be boiled before being used again. The alternative is to use disposable ones. Also, she should not handle food or beverages intended for others.

The patient (and anyone who has contact with him) must be scrupulous about washing the hands thoroughly and frequently, particularly after a bowel movement.

In mild cases, it is not necessary to stay in bed, but frequent naps or rest periods are important to speed recovery. The disease usually resolves itself in four to eight weeks, but people vary widely as to when they can return to work and other activities.

Alcohol and medications that are potentially toxic to the liver must be avoided. These include acetaminophen, birth control pills, methyldopa (a blood pressure medication), phenytoin (an anticonvulsant), and certain antibiotics. Check with your doctor before taking any medications, including nonprescription drugs.

Other Causes of Liver Inflammation

Alcoholism can cause a chronic form of hepatitis, as can exposure to a number of chemicals and toxic fumes. Wilson's disease, a genetic disorder in which copper builds up in the liver, is also a cause of hepatitis. Jaundice may develop as a complication of mononucleosis, pancreatitis, gallbladder disease, cancers of the liver and pancreas, bacterial or parasitic infections, and yellow fever.

Hernia

A hernia develops when an organ or tissue pushes through a weakness in supporting muscles, encroaching on other organs or body structures. There are dozens of different hernias, but those involving the small intestine are the most common. These include:

Abdominal, in which a portion of small intestine pushes through the abdominal muscle wall.

Femoral and inguinal, in which the small intestine protrudes into the musculature of the groin, the scrotum in men, or the vagina or other parts of the genitalia in women.

Rectal, in which the small intestine protrudes into the wall of the rectum.

Other common hernia types include:

Diaphragmatic, in which the stomach or some other abdominal organ pushes through the diaphragm into the chest (see Hiatal Hernia, page 229).

Incisional, which develops at the site of an old surgical wound.

Umbilical, a swelling near or within the navel, usually in a baby.

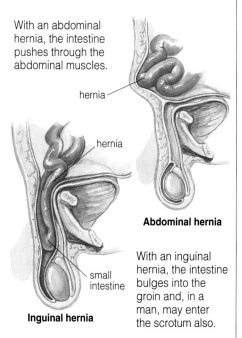

With an abdominal hernia, the intestine pushes through the abdominal muscles.

hernia

hernia

Abdominal hernia

hernia

small intestine

Inguinal hernia

With an inguinal hernia, the intestine bulges into the groin and, in a man, may enter the scrotum also.

Not all hernias are obvious, but those protruding through the abdominal wall usually produce a visible swelling. Mild pain at the site of swelling is common. Men with inguinal hernias may also have swelling in the scrotum.

Most hernias are not serious. But one can be life threatening if a protruding portion of intestine becomes trapped or

ABDOMINAL STRENGTHENING EXERCISES

After hernia surgery, any exercise program should be approved by a doctor or physical therapist. The exercises below are among those often recommended. All should be done on the floor, using an exercise mat if you like.

▶ **Back Arch.** Kneel on all fours with arms and thighs straight and hands flat on the floor. Slowly tighten your abdominal muscles and, at the same time, bend your head downward. Using your abdominal muscles, hunch your back upward. Hold for a count of four, and slowly relax. Repeat six to eight times. If your abdominals are especially weak, this exercise is a good starter because it builds their strength gradually without straining other muscles.

▶ **Modified Leg Lifts.** Lie on your back with your arms at your side, knees bent, and feet flat on the floor. To a count of four, slowly bring one knee up toward your chest and, while exhaling, lift your head and try to touch your forehead to your raised knee. You should feel a pulling of the abdominal muscles. Hold for a count of five, then slowly return your head and foot to the floor. Repeat with the opposite leg. Gradually work up to 15 lifts per session.

▶ **Curl Downs.** Sit with knees bent and feet flat on the floor about 12 inches from your buttocks. Tuck your chin in and bend your head forward, then lean back until you feel your abdominal muscles begin to pull. Cross your arms in front of your chest and slowly uncurl as far as you can without falling backward, then move back up to the starting position.

▶ **Bent-Knee Sit-Ups.** As you gain strength in your abdominal muscles, try this more advanced exercise. Lie on your back with knees bent and feet flat on the floor. By flexing your abdominal muscles, slowly pull yourself up. In the beginning, extend your arms straight in front of you. As strength increases, clasp your hands behind your head.

strangulated and the blood supply is cut off, thus leading to tissue death.

Hernias are more prevalent in premature infants, the elderly, the obese, and people with chronic coughs. A person with bulimia (page 170) may develop a hernia from repeated vomiting.

Diagnostic Studies and Procedures

A hernia can usually be detected by physical examination. A doctor will press it to determine whether it can be manipulated back to its normal position. X-rays and an ultrasound examination may be ordered to rule out other causes of swelling.

Medical Treatments

Even if a hernia is not producing significant symptoms, doctors generally recommend surgical repair to avoid its enlargement and serious complications. The exception is an umbilical hernia, which almost always disappears on its own by the age of four.

Hernia surgery involves removing the hernia's sac and repairing and strengthening the weakened muscle wall. In certain cases, the muscle will be knit together with permanent nonabsorbable stitches. Some hernia surgery can be performed on an outpatient basis; sometimes, however, a short hospital stay is necessary.

Alternative Therapies

Alternative therapies are of little value in treating hernias involving the small intestine. If obesity is a factor, a weight-loss diet combined with an exercise program may have a preventive effect.

Physical Therapy. Once recovery from surgery is complete, a physical therapist or sports medicine specialist can design an exercise routine to strengthen abdominal muscles, which will help prevent recurrence. (See box, above.) These practitioners also teach posture and lifting techniques to avoid straining the abdominal and back muscles.

Self-Treatment

Do not wear a hernia truss unless instructed to do so by a doctor. If your hernia protrudes while you await surgery, gently push it back into place. This is best done when lying down. Avoid heavy lifting, straining, and sudden movements. Try to suppress sneezing and coughing; if that is impossible, tightly hug a firm pillow or a rolled-up piece of clothing to your abdomen until the coughing or sneezing spell passes.

Other Causes of Hernia Symptoms

Severe abdominal pain and swelling may be due to an intestinal obstruction. Abdominal pain and swelling in a woman could be caused by an ovarian cyst. Both conditions are potential medical emergencies.

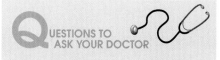

QUESTIONS TO ASK YOUR DOCTOR

▶ Is it safe to apply pressure to a baby's umbilical hernia?
▶ What will happen if I decide not to have hernia surgery?

Herpes

(Genital herpes; herpes simplex type 2)
The herpes simplex virus infects skin and mucous membranes, causing painful, recurrent outbreaks of sores. There are two major strains: Type 1 generally causes cold sores and fever blisters (page 137); type 2 commonly affects the genital and anorectal area. Genital herpes is usually spread through sexual contact, and some 500,000 Americans contract it each year.

Symptoms of genital herpes usually appear two to seven days after contact with an infected sexual partner. Typically, the first sign of infection is itching and irritation in the genital area, followed by especially painful blisters, which rupture in a few days. These then turn into painful, shallow skin ulcers that last from one to three weeks. In women, sores may be present in the vagina, cervix, and urethra. Blisters may also develop on the hands or mouth if these were used during sexual activity. Other possible symptoms are painful urination, enlarged lymph nodes, fever, and general malaise.

Although the sores and other symptoms disappear in a few weeks, the virus lingers in the body and may flare up from time to time. The frequency with which it recurs varies widely, but stress and lowered immunity can lead to more flare-ups.

Diagnostic Studies and Procedures

A doctor can usually diagnose genital herpes by reviewing the symptoms and inspecting the blisters. Examining cells from one or more of the lesions under a microscope usually confirms the presence of type 2 herpes. A laboratory culture of a tissue sample from one of the blisters is sometimes needed.

Medical Treatments

At present, there is no cure, but the symptoms can be alleviated. The first attack is likely to be the most severe, and a doctor may prescribe acyclovir (Zovirax), an antiviral drug that is taken orally or used as a topical cream. Acyclovir reduces the intensity and duration of the symptoms but does not prevent recurrent herpes outbreaks.

A woman who is pregnant and has had herpes or contracts it during pregnancy should inform her obstetrician at once. Although it is not life threatening to adults, an active infection in the mother at the time of birth can be transmitted to the baby. Herpes in a

---

A CASE IN POINT

Ruth Gregory, a 29-year-old lawyer, contracted genital herpes while in college. After several painful flare-ups, the disease became quiescent, although it occasionally reemerged during periods of unusual stress.

Gregory's doctor instructed her to protect any sexual partner by avoiding direct genital contact during a flare-up and always using a condom, regardless of whether or not she had a herpes sore. She followed this advice, even when she married. After two years of marriage, however, Gregory and her husband wanted to have a baby, so she asked her gynecologist how best to achieve this while still avoiding giving herpes to her husband.

After a thorough pelvic examination showed no evidence of an active herpes lesion, the doctor outlined a simple strategy: "Use a home ovulation test to determine when you are most likely to conceive and if you have no signs of a flare-up, have unprotected sex at that time."

Gregory became pregnant in the third month of trying this approach, but worried that her baby might contract herpes if she developed an active herpes sore around the time of delivery. She was so concerned, her doctor agreed to do a cesarean delivery, thus removing any possibility that the baby might pick up herpes during vaginal delivery. The pregnancy proceeded normally, ending with the birth of a healthy 7½-pound boy.

---

newborn can cause blindness; systemic herpes can cause retardation, neurological damage, and even death. These complications can be prevented by a cesarean delivery or other precautions.

Alternative Therapies

Although alternative therapies cannot cure genital herpes, some may alleviate pain and other symptoms.

Aromatherapy. A daily bath in water containing six drops of geranium oil of 2 percent strength is recommended. The treatment should be continued until the skin ulcers disappear.

Herbal Medicine. Herbalists recommend aloe vera gel to soothe and dry the sores. An alternative is a poultice made with powdered slippery elm or comfrey root. Make a paste of one of these, put it between layers of gauze, and apply it to the sores.

Visualization. This technique is said to help prevent recurrences. The patient learns to visualize the immune system successfully fighting off the virus.

Yoga and Meditation. Because stress can precipitate an attack, practicing these and other relaxation techniques may help prevent recurrent flare-ups.

Self-Treatment

For generalized pain, take aspirin or acetaminophen. To soothe localized pain and itching, use compresses soaked in cool milk or water. Vitamin E oil or A and D ointment applied to the sores may also alleviate pain, though some experts believe these remedies slow healing by keeping sores moist; they suggest cornstarch instead. You can also try taking several sitz baths a day; use tepid water and add ½ cup of baking soda per gallon. Pat the sores dry or use a hair dryer set on low.

Women can reduce pain during urination by relieving themselves in the shower or urinating through a tube to keep the urine stream from contacting the lesions. A small plastic cup with the bottom removed can serve the purpose.

Keeping the sores dry and exposed to air speeds healing. Wear cotton underclothes and avoid nylon pantyhose and tight-fitting jeans. Also, do not douche without consulting a doctor.

To avoid passing on the virus, abstain from sexual contact for at least one month after recovery. To prevent further attacks, do not engage in oral, genital, or anal sex if one partner has sores in the genital area or on the mouth. When either partner has had genital herpes, a rubber condom should always be used.

Other Causes of Genital Sores

Type 1 herpes can cause lesions similar to those of genital herpes if the virus infects this area. Blistering and ulceration can be due to gonorrhea, syphilis, and genital warts.

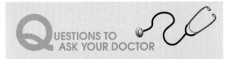

QUESTIONS TO ASK YOUR DOCTOR

► How can I tell if my sexual partner has herpes if there are no blisters or sores?
► What precautions should a woman with herpes take when giving birth?

Hiatal Hernia

(Diaphragmatic hiatus hernia)

All hernias involve the protrusion of a body organ through its surrounding wall of muscle. A hiatal hernia occurs when the stomach pushes up through the hiatus, which is an opening in the diaphragm, the muscle that separates the abdomen from the chest cavity. Normally, the diaphragm holds the stomach in place. But a weakening in the hiatus allows the upper portion of the stomach to bulge into the space ordinarily occupied by the esophagus.

Although hiatal hernias are quite common, occurring in about 40 percent of the population, most do not cause symptoms. Some people, however, may experience heartburn, as well as belching and regurgitation of stomach acid into the throat. This happens when the hernia prevents a full closure of the lower esophageal sphincter, thus allowing stomach contents to flow back up into the esophagus.

Some hiatal hernias result from a congenital defect that causes an inborn weakness of the diaphragm. Obesity, aging, and alcoholism can be contributing factors. So too can an abdominal injury that creates enough pressure to tear a hole in some part of the diaphragm. In most cases, however, a cause cannot be identified.

Diagnostic Studies and Procedures

If a hiatal hernia produces no symptoms, it may never be identified. But when a patient complains of heartburn, acid reflux that causes a burning sensation, and excessive belching or burping, a doctor may suspect hiatal hernia and order X-rays with a contrast medium such as barium, which will readily reveal the condition in most cases.

Endoscopy may also be employed to view the esophagus and the stomach, especially if surgery is being considered. In this procedure, usually performed with local anesthesia, a thin, flexible tube with a lighted tip is passed down the throat and into the esophagus and stomach. Endoscopy is usually done to rule out other disorders, such as ulcers, gastritis, or an esophageal abnormality.

Medical Treatments

In rare cases, a hiatal hernia may strangulate the lower esophagus and block the blood supply. This is a medical emergency that requires immediate

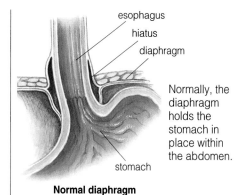

Normal diaphragm

Normally, the diaphragm holds the stomach in place within the abdomen.

esophagus
hiatus
diaphragm
stomach

Hiatal hernia

A hiatal hernia occurs when a portion of the stomach pushes up through the hiatus, an opening in the diaphragm.

esophagus
stomach

surgery. Call your doctor right away if you have the sensation that food is not going down but is stopping around the area of the breastbone, and pain is accompanied by shortness of breath, sweating, or nausea. These are symptoms of a possible strangulated hernia.

Otherwise, most hiatal hernias do not need medical treatment, although persistent or severe heartburn may require medication. A drug that hastens the emptying of the stomach into the small intestine might be prescribed. In most cases, however, a doctor will suggest using an over-the-counter antacid, to be taken an hour before each meal and at bedtime. A stool softener may also be recommended, because straining can worsen the hernia.

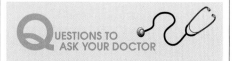

QUESTIONS TO ASK YOUR DOCTOR

▶ Does a hiatal hernia worsen intestinal problems, such as gallbladder disease?
▶ What types of exercise should I avoid? What about contact sports?

Alternative Therapies

Alternative therapies cannot cure a hiatal hernia itself, but the following can help alleviate symptoms.

Aromatherapy. To minimize belching, therapists suggest sniffing essential oils of basil and sandalwood, either singly or in combination.

Herbal Medicine. Belching is treated by drinking a tea made by boiling a teaspoonful of dill seeds in 1 cup of water for 15 minutes and straining it. To relieve the discomfort of heartburn and acid reflux, try fennel tincture or tea, chamomile tea, or papaya tablets.

Homeopathy. Practitioners use nux vomica to treat heartburn.

Naturopathy and Nutrition Therapy. A light, bland diet is recommended to avoid heartburn. Stay away from fatty foods, which remain in the stomach longer than other types, and increase your fiber intake, which speeds the digestive process. Abstain from alcohol and beverages and foods that contain caffeine, such as chocolate, coffee, tea, and cola drinks. Alcohol and caffeine can impair closure of the sphincter between the esophagus and stomach.

Self-Treatment

Avoid large meals; instead, consume four to six small meals a day. Also, do not bend over or lie down for at least two hours after eating.

To prevent the stomach from moving upward at night, raise the head of your bed four to six inches.

If you are overweight, consult a nutritionist to work out a sensible weight-loss diet. Do not wear tight clothes or belts that bind the abdomen.

Regular exercise is important, but avoid weight lifting and other activities that require straining. For lifting heavy objects, learn techniques that do not put extra strain on the diaphragm.

Other Causes of Abdominal Discomfort

Indigestion, ulcers, and gastritis can cause discomfort similar to that of a hiatal hernia, as can inflammation, narrowing, and other disorders of the esophagus. Remember, too, that a heart attack is often mistaken for a digestive problem. Chest pain that persists for more than a few minutes, radiates to the arms, neck, jaw, or back, and is accompanied by shortness of breath, sweating, nausea, and vomiting demands prompt medical attention to rule out a heart attack.

High Blood Pressure

(Hypertension)

High blood pressure, or hypertension, occurs when excessive force is exerted against artery walls as the heart pumps blood. This silent disease has no symptoms until it has reached an advanced and dangerous stage, at which point it may produce headache, lightheadedness, ringing in the ears, and rapid heartbeat. If uncontrolled, hypertension can lead to a heart attack, stroke, or kidney failure. It can also damage the eyes and other organs.

In most people, the cause is unknown and the hypertension is classified as primary, or essential. In about 5 percent of cases, it may result from kidney disease, a hormonal imbalance, or some other identifiable factor. This is known as secondary hypertension.

Predisposing risk factors have been identified; these include obesity and a family history of hypertension or stroke at an early age. A high-salt diet contributes to the condition in genetically susceptible people. African-Americans have a higher incidence of hypertension than whites. Women are less prone than men to high blood pressure, but pregnancy and use of oral contraceptives increase their risk. The disease affects an estimated 50 million Americans.

Diagnostic Studies and Procedures

Because there usually are no symptoms, hypertension is most often diagnosed during a routine medical examination or a special screening program.

Blood pressure is normally measured with a sphygmomanometer (pronounced sfig/moe/ma/NOM/a/ter). This device consists of an inflatable cuff, an air pump, and a column of mercury. The cuff is wrapped around the upper arm and inflated. The objective is to measure the amount of pressure needed to stop the flow of blood through an artery. As the air pressure in the cuff increases, it drives up the column of mercury. By listening through a stethoscope placed over the artery at a point below the cuff, a doctor or nurse can quickly determine when the flow of blood has stopped. The cuff is then decompressed, and the height of the mercury at the first thumping sound is noted. This is the systolic pressure, which is the peak

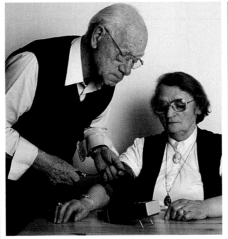

Regular blood pressure checks, which can be done at home, indicate how well medication and/or lifestyle changes are working to keep blood pressure at desirable levels.

force exerted against the artery wall when the heart contracts to push blood out. More pressure is released from the cuff, and a different sound is heard. This is the diastolic pressure, which occurs when the heart muscle relaxes to allow blood from the veins to flow in. Thus, in a blood pressure reading of 120/80, the 120 represents systolic pressure and 80 is diastolic pressure.

During the course of a day, blood pressure varies considerably. It is generally lowest during sleep and highest in the early morning. Anger or stress sends blood pressure up; caffeine, nicotine, and alcohol can do so also.

A resting blood pressure of 120/80 is considered normal for adults; a consistent reading of 140/90 or higher is classified as hypertension. To make a diagnosis, however, blood pressure should be measured a number of times over several weeks, unless the initial reading is dangerously high—160/110, for example. Wearing a 24-hour blood pressure monitor may be recommended in some cases. This device continually measures and records blood pressure. If a complication related to hypertension, such as an enlarged heart, is suspected, additional tests, including a chest X-ray and electrocardiogram, may be done.

Medical Treatments

The choice of treatment is determined by the severity of the disease and the presence of complications. Mild to moderate hypertension, generally defined as readings of 140-149/90-104, is initially treated by lifestyle changes (see Self-Treatment, facing page).

Antihypertensive drugs are prescribed when lifestyle changes fail to achieve the desired lowering or when blood pressure is diagnosed in the moderate to severe range of more than 160/105. Although high blood pressure almost always can be controlled, there is no single antihypertensive drug that works for everyone.

Treatment may involve taking one or several medications. The classes of antihypertensive drugs are as follows: ***Diuretics,*** also called water pills, work by increasing excretion of sodium and water through the kidneys, thereby reducing the total volume of blood. Thiazide diuretics such as hydrochlorothiazide are most commonly used, but in some cases, loop diuretics, such as furosemide (Lasix), are prescribed. These drugs work in a part of the kidney called the loop of Henle and they are generally more potent than thiazide diuretics. Both types of drugs can cause such side effects as lethargy, dizziness, and urinary frequency. ***Beta blockers*** lower blood pressure by slowing the heartbeat and reducing the amount of blood pumped during each beat. Propranolol (Inderal), the oldest beta blocker, is still widely used. In addition, there are at least a half-dozen newer ones, including atenolol (Tenormin), metoprolol (Lopressor), nadolol (Corgard), and timolol (Blocadren). ***ACE (for angiotensin converting enzyme) inhibitors*** lower blood pressure by blocking the production of angiotensin II, a body chemical that constricts, or narrows, blood vessels. ACE inhibitors include captopril (Capoten) and enalapril (Vasotec). ***Calcium-channel blockers*** work by preventing the entry of calcium into the muscle cells that control the arterial walls. This dilates, or opens, the blood

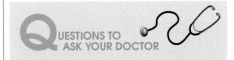

QUESTIONS TO ASK YOUR DOCTOR

▶ How long does it usually take to decide if lifestyle changes are effective enough to control high blood pressure?
▶ How often should my blood pressure be monitored?
▶ What are the most common side effects with my particular drug regimen?
▶ Will I have to take antihypertensive medication for the rest of my life? (The answer is usually yes.)

vessels, making it easier for blood to flow through them. Drugs in this category include verapamil (Calan) and diltiazem (Cardizem).

Vasodilators widen, or dilate, arteries. Hydralazine (Apresoline), the oldest antihypertensive drug, is a fast-acting vasodilator; another member of this class is minoxidil (Loniten). These drugs are usually prescribed along with other antihypertensives.

Alpha-blocking agents work through the autonomic nervous system. They block the alpha receptors on the blood vessel walls, which, when stimulated, cause a narrowing of the vessels. Thus, they lower blood pressure by allowing the arteries to open more widely. Two examples are prazosin (Minipress) and terazosin (Hytrin).

Peripheral adrenergic antagonists block the release of norepinephrine, a hormone that raises blood pressure. Reserpine, which is made from rauwolfia, an Indian herb, is the major drug in this category. It is usually prescribed in small doses and used in conjunction with a diuretic.

Centrally acting drugs lower blood pressure by reducing nerve impulses from the brain. These agents include methyldopa (Aldomet), clonidine (Catapres), and guanabenz (Wytensin). They, too, are combined with other drugs, usually diuretics.

Side effects are often a problem with blood pressure medications. However, they can almost always be minimized by changing either the dosage or the medication itself. Among the common side effects are unusual tiredness, dizziness or feeling faint upon standing up, nightmares, impotence, and depression. These and any other lingering problems should be reported to a doctor as soon as possible so that the dosage can be changed or an alternative drug can be prescribed.

When arteries are constricted, blood pressure rises. — artery

blood

Vasodilator drugs, which widen arteries, are one approach to lowering blood pressure. artery —

vasodilator effect

blood

Alternative Therapies
Poorly controlled high blood pressure can have serious consequences; it is vital to see a doctor regularly and take any prescribed medications. Alternative therapies cannot cure the condition, but some can reduce or even eliminate the need for drugs. When using an alternative therapy, be sure to let your physician know, so medical treatment can be adjusted appropriately.

Acupuncture. Therapists may stimulate meridians for the liver and bladder, as well as certain ear points. Blood pressure should be monitored during every session, and these techniques should not be used for any patient whose blood pressure is higher than 160/100.

Biofeedback. Patients are taught to lower their heart rate and control other normally involuntary responses. This method is especially useful for reducing stress, which raises blood pressure.

Exercise Conditioning. A program of aerobic exercise designed to improve cardiovascular fitness can help to lower blood pressure. Before embarking on such a program, it may be advisable to have an exercise stress test.

Herbal Medicine. Dandelion tea or capsules may be recommended as a natural diuretic. Garlic, either natural or in capsule form, is also said to lower high blood pressure. Because licorice raises blood pressure, capsules, teas, candy, and other products that contain the natural form should be avoided. The artificial flavoring that is used in most licorice candy in the United States is a safe substitute.

Homeopathy. Thyroidinum, prepared from the thyroid gland, is sometimes recommended; nux vomica is also prescribed for intermittent hypertension.

Nutrition Therapy. Mild to moderate hypertension can often be controlled through diet alone. Add minimal or no salt to your food, especially if you are salt sensitive. Use herbs for flavorings or ask your doctor about using potassium chloride as a salt substitute. Also, avoid processed foods that contain any form of sodium. Increase your consumption of vegetables, fruits, and whole-grain products, while reducing intake of red meat and other fatty foods.

Yoga and Meditation. These and other relaxation techniques can lower blood pressure. The effects tend to be temporary, so the chosen method should be practiced at least daily.

Self-Treatment
In addition to dietary adjustments, other lifestyle changes that should be incorporated into a prevention or treatment program include:
▶ If you smoke, stop now. Also, avoid exposure to second-hand smoke.
▶ Lose excess weight. Staying within 15 percent of your ideal weight is the single most effective thing you can do to control blood pressure.
▶ Avoid alcoholic beverages.

Other Causes of High Blood Pressure
An adrenal tumor called a pheochromocytoma produces adrenaline-like hormones that can cause very high blood pressure. A narrowing of the renal artery to the kidney can also raise blood pressure, as can pre-eclampsia, or toxemia of pregnancy, a serious complication that sometimes develops during the final trimester.

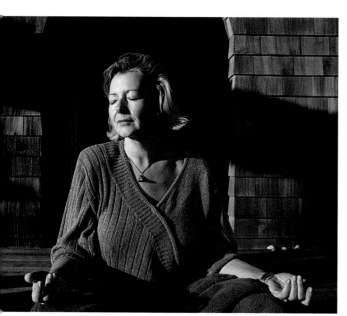

Yoga and meditation are useful adjuncts to medication in the control of hypertension.

Hirsutism

(Constitutional or male-pattern hirsutism)
Hirsutism is the medical term for excessive hair, or hairiness, particularly in women. When a woman grows hair on her face, trunk, and limbs that is similar to a man's, the condition is called male-pattern hirsutism.

Humans appear to be fairly hairless, but in reality we have as many hair follicles as apes. However, most human follicles produce vellus hair, which is colorless and fine. Some vellus hair, though, is converted into the coarser, more visible terminal hair during puberty, when testosterone—a male sex hormone—stimulates its growth. Males produce more testosterone than females; thus, men normally have more visible facial and body hair.

Excessive hair growth does not always signal a medical problem. It may be seen instead as constitutional hirsutism, or hair growth that is normal for a person's age or racial and ethnic heritage. Women of Mediterranean and Near Eastern ancestry, for example, have more visible hair than their North European counterparts. Caucasians have more hair than Africans; and both Asians and Native Americans have less than other peoples.

Following menopause, women normally grow more facial hair. But the sudden development of male-pattern hirsutism in a younger woman often indicates an imbalance of sex hormones, especially if there are other signs of virilization, such as a deepening of the voice and increased muscle growth. Porphyria, a genetic disease marked by extreme sun sensitivity, can cause hirsutism, as can tumors of the ovaries or adrenal glands. If a cause cannot be identified the condition is called idiopathic hirsutism.

In both sexes, hirsutism may develop from certain medications: these include prednisone and other corticosteroids;

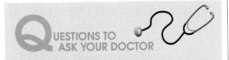

QUESTIONS TO ASK YOUR DOCTOR

▶ Will estrogen replacement therapy prevent development of unwanted facial hair following menopause?
▶ What are the chances of hirsutism being linked to cancer?

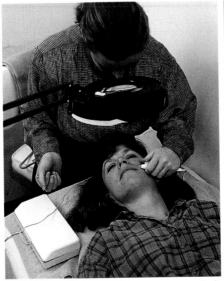

The only permanent way to remove unwanted hair is to destroy the root with electrolysis. This job should be done by a professional.

phenytoin (Dilantin), an anticonvulsant medication; and minoxidil (Loniten), an antihypertensive agent.

Diagnostic Studies and Procedures

A general physical examination will reveal the extent and pattern of hairiness, as well as any signs of masculinization. Specific tests will be done to rule out an underlying medical cause.

A gynecological examination, including a pap smear, should be done. The ovaries may be examined at that time for abnormalities, and vaginal and cervical cells may also be analyzed to determine whether normal amounts of female hormones are being produced. In addition, a urine analysis may be ordered, and blood tests to study hormone levels, especially testosterone.

If a hormone-producing tumor is suspected, ultrasonography and a CT scan may be recommended. When an ovarian tumor is a possibility, laparoscopy—an examination using a viewing instrument inserted through a small incision near the navel—may be ordered.

Medical Treatments

When constitutional hirsutism is the problem, no medical treatment is required. Treatment of male-pattern hirsutism depends upon the underlying cause. If there is excessive production of testosterone, spironolactone (Aldactone) may be prescribed to block it.

Surgery may be necessary if a hormone-producing tumor is present. When surgery is not possible, it may be destroyed by radiation therapy.

Removing the underlying cause of hirsutism will halt the conversion of vellus to terminal hairs, but it will not eliminate existing unwanted hair. Physical removal is necessary.

Alternative Therapies

Electrolysis. This is the only permanent method of hair removal. It is a time-consuming procedure that requires a skilled operator, known as an electrologist. Each hair is removed by the insertion of a fine probe into the hair follicle. An electrical current of low voltage passes through the probe and destroys the hair root.

Nutrition Therapy. If obesity is contributing to a hormone imbalance that is causing excessive hair growth, a qualified nutritionist can devise a long-term weight-loss program.

Self-Treatment

There are numerous ways to remove unwanted hair temporarily or to make it less noticeable.

Bleaching. This makes hair less visible. Use a commercial product or make your own by mixing one ounce of 6-percent hydrogen peroxide, 10 drops of household ammonia, and enough baking soda to form a paste. Before using the mixture, do a small patch test on the inside of your wrist.

Depilatories. These chemicals dissolve hair into a gelatinous mass that can be removed with a washcloth. Do a patch test and follow instructions carefully.

Plucking. This is a quick way to remove small amounts of body hair temporarily. Use care, however, as plucking can injure follicles and trigger infection, especially on the face.

Shaving. This is the quickest and most widely used method for removing hair from the underarms and legs. Although men regularly shave their faces, women hesitate to do so, as they mistakenly think that shaving will stimulate the growth of their hair. It only appears to, because all of the shaved hair grows back at the same time.

Waxing. Warm melted wax is applied to the skin, allowed to cool, and then peeled off, taking with it any embedded hairs. Wax treatments are available in salons and there are also wax products for home use.

Other Causes of Hairiness

Thyroid disease, ovarian cysts, and pituitary tumors are among the endocrine disorders that can cause excessive hairiness.

Histoplasmosis

Histoplasmosis is a disease caused by the fungus *Histoplasma capsulatum*. The plant-like fungus gives off microscopic spores—its counterpart of seeds—that are light enough to float in the air. Once inhaled, these spores take root in the lungs, growing and multiplying rapidly and causing symptoms that range from mild to life threatening, depending on the number of spores inhaled and the person's general health. In rare cases, months or even years after the original infection, the disease infects the eyes, producing ocular histoplasmosis syndrome.

Histoplasmosis spores are most frequently found in the droppings from bats, chickens, and pigeons and other birds. They flourish in the warm, moist, dark places where these droppings accumulate: barns, pigeon roosts, chicken houses, belfries, caves, and the undergrowth of city parks where starlings are abundant.

Four types of histoplasmosis exist:

Mild histoplasmosis has symptoms similar to those of a benign case of the flu—fatigue, a slight fever, and occasional coughing. Many infected people don't even notice them. This is the least serious of the four forms of histoplasmosis, and it commonly disappears after a few days without the need for any treatment.

Acute pulmonary histoplasmosis produces labored breathing, recurring fever and chills, and persistent coughing. It is confined to the lungs and is usually self-limiting. Even without

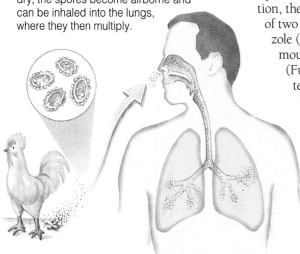

Histoplasmosis spores are found in bird and bat droppings. When the droppings dry, the spores become airborne and can be inhaled into the lungs, where they then multiply.

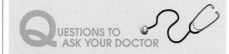

treatment, this variation of the disease is likely to clear up, although it may take a month or more.

Chronic pulmonary histoplasmosis is characterized by weight loss, recurring fever, malaise, and coughing that may produce blood. About one-third of these patients improve spontaneously, whereas the remaining two-thirds tend to worsen gradually.

Disseminated histoplasmosis occurs when a large number of spores have spread beyond the lungs, settling in various organs, including the liver, spleen, gastrointestinal tract, bone marrow, lymph nodes, eyes, and in rare cases, the brain. This form usually affects only people with immune systems weakened by immunosuppressive drugs, or by AIDS, cancer, or some other disease. Without treatment, 10 to 30 percent of patients with disseminated histoplasmosis die within 4 to 10 months of contracting the disease.

Diagnostic Studies and Procedures
The goal of diagnostic procedures is to differentiate histoplasmosis from other diseases. In addition to chest X-rays, studies may include skin and blood tests. Laboratory examinations of sputum, urine, bone marrow, and a liver biopsy may also be ordered.

Medical Treatments
Depending on the extent of the infection, the medication of choice is either of two antifungal agents: ketoconazole (Nizoral), which is given by mouth, or amphotericin B (Fungizone), which is administered intravenously. If the infection has reached the central nervous system, as might happen in people who have AIDS, amphotericin B is injected into the spinal column.

While the adverse side effects of ketoconazole—nausea, diarrhea, abdominal pain, and itching—are minor when compared with those of amphotericin B—weight loss, anemia, fever, and kidney disorders—both of these drugs must be monitored closely because of their potential to produce liver toxicity.

Antifungal medications are not effective for treating the histoplasmosis syndrome that affects the eyes. In these instances, treatment consists of a combination of corticosteroids, laser surgery, and radiation therapy, all directed to the retina.

In cases of extensive lung damage, the affected portions of the lung may be surgically removed.

Alternative Therapies
The chief role of alternative therapies in treating these diseases is the strengthening of the immune system to help fight the infection.

Herbal Medicine. Herbalists recommend echinacea (purple coneflower) tea, black walnut extract, or pau d'arco, available as capsules, extract, and tea.

Nutrition Therapy. A nutritionist may recommend a diet rich in vitamin A and beta carotene to boost immunity; vitamin C, which is said to increase levels of interferon, a group of proteins that fight infections; vitamin B_6 (pyridoxine), to maintain a proper level of antibody production; and zinc supplements, which are also thought to strengthen the immune system.

Self-Treatment
Milder forms of histoplasmosis are treated with bed rest, extra fluids, abstaining from smoking, and avoidance of secondhand smoke.

To reduce the possibility of infection, city dwellers should avoid pigeon and starling roosts. Rural residents have a more difficult problem because they are likely to be surrounded by the airborne spores. The American Lung Association recommends taking the following preventive measures:
▶ Keep farm buildings, especially chicken houses, as clean and dry as possible. Before sweeping them out, wet down the floor to reduce dust.
▶ Wear a facial mask to keep from inhaling spores in areas where there are bat or bird droppings.
▶ Keep storm cellars clean and dry.

Other Causes of Lung Symptoms
Mild forms of the disease are often attributed to a cold or flu. Various other fungal infections can also be confused with histoplasmosis.

Hives

(Angioedema; urticaria; wheals)
Hives, an allergic skin disorder, are raised round pink or red lesions with flat tops. Itchy and warm to the touch, they range in size from ¼ to 1½ inches or sometimes larger. More severe hives, called angioedema, tend to be larger and linked to one another; they also penetrate more deeply into the skin. In rare cases, hives can develop in the mouth and throat, obstructing breathing or heralding a life-threatening anaphylactic reaction.

Most often, hives are caused by food allergies, with the most frequent culprits being chocolate, shellfish, nuts, eggs, strawberries and other fruits, as

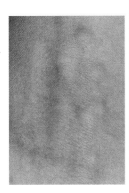

Typically, hives are round bumps that are pink or red. They normally range in size from ¼ to 1½ inches.

well as food preservatives, dyes, and other food additives. Some people develop hives after eating even a minute amount of the offending food, while others break out only when they overindulge in it.

Certain drugs, especially penicillin, can also cause hives, as can aspirin and numerous other medications.

There are people who develop hives in response to contact with cats or other animals, insect bites, extreme temperatures, or exposure to detergents or dry cleaning chemicals on clothes. In others, hives appear as part of a photosensitive reaction to sun exposure, especially if certain medications are being taken. The role of stress in hives has been much debated; some allergists say it can be a factor, but other experts dispute this claim.

Diagnostic Studies and Procedures

Hives are easily self-diagnosed on the basis of their appearance and feel. If you have recurrent hives but do not know what triggers them, skin tests performed by an allergist can help identify the offending substances. If allergies are not responsible for persistent hives, more extensive testing will be necessary to identify their cause.

Medical Treatments

Hives usually disappear on their own within one to seven days of their development. In the meantime, if the cause is not obvious and you are taking any medication, call your doctor to ask if you should discontinue it.

To alleviate itching and discomfort, a physician may prescribe an antihistamine in prescription-strength, such as diphenhydramine (Benadryl), cyproheptadine (Periactin), or hydroxyzine (Atarax). In mild cases, a nonprescription antihistimine may be sufficient. (Caution is needed when taking these drugs because they produce drowsiness.) If hives are widespread and severe, a doctor may prescribe a corticosteroid drug such as prednisone.

If symptoms of an anaphylactic reaction develop (page 71), or if there is a "lump" in your throat or a choking sensation, get immediate help by calling an ambulance or having someone take you to the nearest emergency room. In such a situation, an injection of epinephrine (adrenaline) is life saving.

Alternative Therapies

Herbal Therapy. Herbalists recommend a tea made from *Urtica dioica*, the stinging nettle plant, as a natural alternative to antihistamine drugs. This herb is also available as capsules made from a freeze-dried extract.

Hydrotherapy. Bath additives can often help ease the itching and discomfort of hives. Try cornstarch, baking soda, or colloidal oatmeal. If you have hives that are induced by exposure to cold temperatures, you may be able to build up your tolerance by taking a cool shower once or twice a day.

Nutrition Therapy. Try to identify the foods that you believe trigger your hives and then eliminate them from your diet. Follow up by returning the suspected offenders, one at a time. If hives reappear, then you know you have correctly identified an offending food that you should avoid in the future.

Self-Treatment

A topical treatment such as calamine lotion can ease the itching of hives, and an over-the-counter antihistamine can speed healing.

If you suffer with chronic hives, your doctor may also recommend the following preventive measures:
▶ Avoid aspirin and other nonsteroidal anti-inflammatory drugs, such as ibuprofen. These medications sometimes provoke hives and other allergic reactions involving the skin.
▶ Avoid these food additives: tartrazine, a common food and drug coloring; the food dye FD&C Yellow No. 5; benzoate food preservatives; and the preservatives BHA, BHT, and nitrates.

Other Causes of Hives

In unusual cases, hives may be the first sign of a viral infection, such as hepatitis, rubella, or mononucleosis, as well as serious illnesses, such as lymphoma, lupus, hyperthyroidism, or cutaneous vasculitis. In rare instances, chronic angioedema is caused by a hereditary enzyme deficiency.

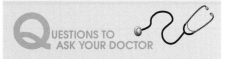

QUESTIONS TO ASK YOUR DOCTOR

▶ Should I carry an anaphylaxis prevention kit in case my hives develop into a more serious hypersensitivity reaction?
▶ Should I undergo allergy skin tests?

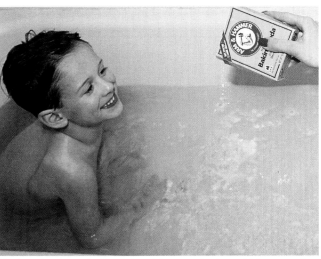

Soaking for several minutes in a lukewarm bath to which a cup of baking soda has been added can help relieve the itching of hives.

Hydrocele and Varicocele

Hydroceles and varicoceles are two relatively common disorders affecting the male reproductive tract. Specifically, a hydrocele is a pear-shaped cyst in the groin. It develops when there is a buildup of the fluid that is normally found between the two layers of membrane that enclose the testicles. A varicocele is a tangle of varicose veins surrounding a testicle. It can usually be felt as a lump or swelling, most commonly on the left side of the testicle.

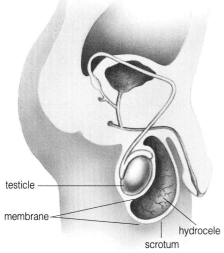

A hydrocele develops as a fluid-filled cyst between the two layers of membrane that enclose the testicle.

Hydroceles are often present at birth or develop shortly thereafter, occurring in about 10 percent of all boys. They may be located on one or both sides of the groin and are caused during birth by pressure on the abdomen; it pushes amniotic fluid down to the testicles through the channel surrounding the spermatic cord and blood vessels. These cysts are generally harmless and painless. If pain does develop, it is usually a sign that the hydrocele is infected.

A hydrocele in an adult male may be secondary to epididymitis, an inflammation of the tubes that carry sperm from the testes. Other possible causes include a testicular tumor, injury, or infection. A sexually transmitted disease, especially gonorrhea, can also cause a hydrocele to develop.

Varicoceles are exceedingly common, affecting 10 to 15 percent of all adult men, and 20 to 40 percent of those with fertility problems. Although they do not affect general health, they impair a man's fertility because the accumulation of blood in the swollen vein raises the temperature of the affected testicle, thereby hampering sperm production.

Diagnostic Studies and Procedures

A doctor can detect a hydrocele or varicocele during a physical examination of the groin and testicles, but additional tests are needed to rule out tumors and other causes of swelling. A hydrocele can usually be diagnosed by transillumination, a procedure in which a strong light is passed through the swelling to show that it is filled with fluid. Ultrasound is also used to differentiate a hydrocele from a solid mass, and also to diagnose a varicocele. If there is suspicion of a tumor, a biopsy is necessary to rule out testicular cancer, a relatively common malignancy in young men (page 403).

Medical Treatment

In most cases, a hydrocele in a newborn will resolve itself by the time a baby is 12 to 15 months old, as fluid is reabsorbed into the body. In the meantime, the lump should be checked regularly to make sure that the swelling is not expanding. If it becomes enlarged or tender, a doctor should be seen to rule out a hernia.

Aspiration of the fluid is not recommended because it increases the risk of infection. In some cases, however, surgery may be necessary. In infants and young children, the operation is performed through an incision in the groin, and may require general anesthesia and an overnight hospital stay. If the baby has a hernia, as is often the case, it can be repaired at the same time.

In adults, surgery is done through an incision in the scrotum. Part of the double membrane that holds the excess fluid is cut away, and the fluid is drained. The operation may be performed with local anesthesia on an outpatient basis.

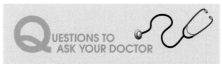

QUESTIONS TO ASK YOUR DOCTOR

► Can surgery to remove a hydrocele or varicocele affect sexual function?
► What is the likelihood that removal of a varicocele will increase fertility?

A varicocele usually does not require treatment unless it is causing fertility problems, such as a low sperm count or a large number of defective sperm. In such a case, a simple procedure to remove it may be recommended.

Alternative Therapies

Hydroceles and varicoceles do not lend themselves to alternative therapies.

Self-Treatment

There is no self-treatment for these conditions, but beginning with the late teens, all males should examine their testicles monthly for the presence of lumps, swelling, or other abnormalities. This is done by slowly rolling each testicle between a thumb and forefinger. If a lump or other change is noted, a doctor should be consulted.

Other Causes of Testicular Swelling

In babies, an inguinal hernia can cause swelling similar to that of a hydrocele. In older males, cancer, an injury, or infection can produce testicular lumps.

Hydrocephalus

(Congenital, normal pressure, and obstructive hydrocephalus)

Hydrocephalus is the buildup of fluid in the spaces, or ventricles, within the brain and skull. Normally, the body produces about a pint of cerebrospinal fluid each day; after circulating through these spaces, the fluid is reabsorbed into the bloodstream and replaced by a fresh supply.

Most often, hydrocephalus develops when a ventricle becomes blocked. The blockage may be the result of an overgrowth of tissue, a cerebral hemorrhage, inflammation, or a head injury. In rare cases, hydrocephalus results from an overproduction of cerebrospinal fluid caused by a brain tumor.

Congenital hydrocephalus is quite common in newborn babies, especially premature ones. Worldwide, approximately one infant in a thousand is born with it. Premature babies are particularly vulnerable, because they often develop bleeding into the brain's ventricles, resulting in inflammation and scar tissue that blocks the fluid outflow. Other causes include viral infections transmitted by the mother to her fetus during pregnancy, birth defects, or an injury during birth.

A baby who is born with congenital hydrocephalus often has an abnormally large and deformed head. The infant may also cry constantly, vomit frequently, and exhibit spastic movements. If the condition occurs early in fetal development, major brain damage is always a consequence.

Hydrocephalus that develops after age five, when the skull bones have knit together and closed permanently, results in increased pressure within the skull on the brain itself. This type of hydrocephalus may be caused by diseases affecting the brain, including meningitis (page 289), encephalitis (page 177), or a brain abscess or

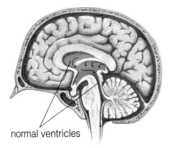 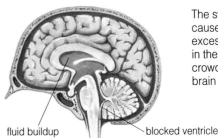

normal ventricles

fluid buildup · blocked ventricle

The swelling caused by excessive fluid in the ventricles crowds normal brain tissue.

tumor. The symptoms might include a severe headache, mental changes, blurred vision, vomiting, dizziness, and impaired coordination.

A condition known as normal pressure hydrocephalus sometimes occurs in elderly persons. It produces mental changes and a shambling gait that is often mistaken for Alzheimer's disease or other degenerative brain disorders. The cause of the disorder is unknown, although some patients have a history of head injuries or meningitis.

Diagnostic Studies and Procedures

A doctor will suspect congenital hydrocephalus if a baby has been born with an oversized head and some of the other symptoms. Blood tests will be ordered to rule out an infection, and electroencephalography will be done to determine if seizures are due to epilepsy. Other procedures include examination of the head with ultrasound; transillumination, in which the brain is examined by using a bright light; tapping the head to see if it produces a characteristic "cracked pot" sound; and listening for abnormal sounds typically produced by deformed blood vessels.

After the age of one, a diagnosis of hydrocephalus can be confirmed by CT brain scans or MRI. These imaging studies can also detect possible causes, such as a brain cyst, abscess, or tumor. The scans are especially important in elderly patients to rule out Alzheimer's disease and other forms of dementia.

Medical Treatments

Prompt treatment is critical in all types of hydrocephalus to prevent permanent brain damage and even death. Among babies born with the condition, about half die without treatment. Among those who do receive prompt surgery and survive, about 40 percent will have normal intelligence; the remaining 60 percent are likely to suffer from varying degrees of mental or neurological impairment.

In some instances, giving a combination of acetazolamide (Diamox) and glycerol will reduce the production of

cerebrospinal fluid. The majority of cases, however, are treated surgically.

Treatment may begin with punctures in the lumbar region of the spine to remove some of the fluid. But the standard operation consists of implanting a shunt into the ventricle to reroute the fluid from the head, under the skin, and into the peritoneal cavity of the abdomen, where it is reabsorbed into the bloodstream. The shunt is made of silastic rubber, which does not deteriorate nor interact with body tissues. In a baby, the neurosurgeon will insert extra tubing to accommodate growth. A shunt may malfunction or become blocked and thus require removal or replacement. Otherwise, these devices are usually left in place for years.

Surgical shunting for normal pressure hydrocephalus in the elderly is most successful when it is done within one year of the appearance of symptoms. In such cases, surgery often succeeds in reversing the mental deterioration.

Alternative Therapies

Although alternative therapies cannot be used to treat hydrocephalus itself, some can help patients improve their impaired coordination.

Dance and Music Therapy. When used as a movement therapy, these modalities can improve coordination and gait.
T'ai Chi. The range-of-motion exercises that are incorporated into this movement therapy can help older patients overcome the shuffling gait seen in normal pressure hydrocephalus.

Self-Treatment

Hydrocephalus does not lend itself to self-treatment.

Other Causes of Brain Symptoms

Reye's syndrome, a rare childhood disease that causes brain swelling, can cause symptoms similar to those of hydrocephalus. In older people, Parkinson's disease causes a shuffling gait. In addition to disorders mentioned earlier, chronic alcoholism and severe malnutrition can lead to mental deterioration and gait disturbances.

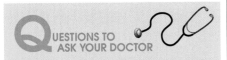

QUESTIONS TO ASK YOUR DOCTOR

▶ Can hydrocephalus that is detected in a fetus by ultrasound during pregnancy be treated before birth?
▶ How often should a brain shunt be checked? How is this done?

Hyperactivity

(Attention-deficit/hyperactivity disorder; hyperkinesis)

After many years of research and debate, hyperactivity is now classified as an aspect of disruptive behavior disorders; the preferred medical term is attention-deficit/hyperactivity disorder, or ADHD. It has previously been called minimal brain dysfunction, hyperkinesis, and hyperactive child syndrome.

The name may have changed, but the characteristics have remained the same—hyperactive children have an abnormally short attention span, are impulsive, and in constant motion. They often have explosive tempers, but no mood lasts for long; they can

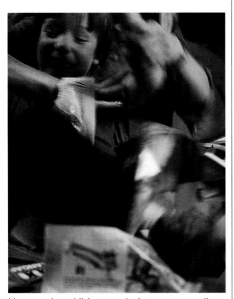

Hyperactive children are boisterous, usually accident prone, and difficult to control.

go from laughter to tears in an instant. These children are also excessively accident prone. As they grow older, about three-fourths of hyperactive youngsters become unusually defiant and aggressive. Part of their antisocial behavior may reflect low self-esteem.

Now considered the most common developmental disorder among American children, it affects 3 to 5 percent of those in elementary school; boys outnumber girls about five to one.

Symptoms typically appear before the age of four and always by age seven. Many parents report, however, that their hyperactive children were somehow different from infancy. They may have slept poorly, cried a good deal,

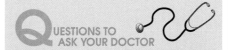

▶ What are the chances that my child will outgrow symptoms of hyperactivity after reaching puberty?
▶ What are the long-term effects of Ritalin and other stimulant drugs?

moved about more than average, and been hypersensitive to noise, light, and other environmental changes.

In rare cases, hyperactive children exhibit early behavior that fits an opposite extreme: They are unusually placid, sleep a good deal, and develop at a slower than average pace.

No one knows for certain what is the cause of this disorder, but it is presumed to result from an immaturity in brain development. Some researchers believe that an imbalance of brain chemicals is responsible. There may also be a genetic predisposition, since it seems to be more common in children whose parents were themselves hyperactive and who also have various neurological or psychological problems.

Having one child who is hyperactive increases the risk that siblings will also be affected. There is some evidence that exposure during pregnancy to alcohol, cigarette smoking, and certain drugs increases the incidence of hyperactivity. Babies born addicted to crack cocaine suffer from a unique form of hyperactivity, in which they develop a high pitched, mewing cry and cannot tolerate being touched or cuddled.

Diagnostic Studies and Procedures

In many instances, a parent or teacher labels a child as hyperactive, when, in fact, the youngster is simply talkative and rambunctious. Before assuming a child is hyperactive, parents should seek a professional evaluation.

As a first step, the child should be examined for a possible organic disorder. For example, certain brain studies, including CT scans and an electroencephalogram, may be ordered to look for structural brain damage. Ideally, the child should be evaluated by a team of specialists that includes a child psychiatrist, developmental pediatrician, and, if possible, a neuropsychologist. The evaluation will be based on descriptions of the child's behavior at home and in school, an examination to rule

out vision and hearing disorders, and tests to measure intelligence, memory, and other mental capabilities. After organic disorders and other problems have been eliminated, a diagnosis of hyperactivity requires the presence of specific characteristics (see box, below).

Medical Treatments

When treatment with medication is recommended, it should be undertaken as part of a complete program that includes behavior modification, counseling, and special education. The administering of medication is usually postponed until the child starts school. Ironically, the drugs that are the most effective are stimulants, such as methylphenidate (Ritalin), pemoline (Cylert), and dextroamphetamine (Dexedrine). About 80 percent of all hyperactive children benefit from these medicines, showing an increased ability to focus their attention on learning and a reduction in compulsive movement.

DIAGNOSING HYPERACTIVITY

According to the diagnostic guidelines of the American Psychiatric Association, a diagnosis of ADHD requires that six of the following symptoms of inattention (or six from the hyperactivity/impulsivity list) have developed before age seven, have persisted for at least six months, and are severe enough to interfere with normal social or school activities.

Inattention
▶ Pays little attention to details and makes careless mistakes.
▶ Has difficulty paying attention.
▶ Does not listen when spoken to.
▶ Fails to follow through or finish tasks.
▶ Has difficulty getting organized.
▶ Avoids tasks requiring sustained mental effort or concentration.
▶ Often loses things needed for school or other daily activities.
▶ Is easily distracted.
▶ Is often forgetful in daily activities.

Hyperactivity/Impulsivity
▶ Often fidgets or squirms.
▶ Often leaves seat when staying put is expected.
▶ Runs about or climbs on things in inappropriate settings.
▶ Has difficulty engaging in quiet play or other activities.
▶ Is constantly on the go or appears to be driven by a motor.
▶ Talks excessively.
▶ Blurts out answers prematurely.
▶ Has difficulty awaiting turn.
▶ Often interrupts or intrudes on others.

Ritalin, given in small daily doses, is the most frequently prescribed drug because it has fewer side effects than Dexedrine and Cylert. Although its side effects differ among children, a major drawback is possible suppression of growth. It can also cause headaches, stomach pain, sleep disturbances, loss of appetite, and depression. Many doctors recommend that Ritalin be taken only on school days, with weekends, school holidays, and summer vacations considered drug holidays. Unfortunately, when the effects of Ritalin wear off, hyperactive symptoms return.

If stimulants do not work, an antidepressant, imipramine (Tofranil), may be prescribed. It works by blocking the action of catecholamines, body chemicals related to adrenaline. However, this drug is usually not given before age six, and because it can damage the heart, it requires careful physician monitoring.

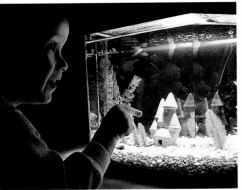

Watching the movements of fish can be both fascinating and calming.

Alternative Therapies
Although controversial, several alternative therapies appear to help some children who are hyperactive, and have the added benefit of avoiding the adverse effects of drugs.
Music Therapy. Regular exposure to music is likely to be part of the special education program for a hyperactive child because of its calming effects. Parents can ask a qualified music therapist to suggest kinds of music to be played at home. Also, having a child make music on his own may help him to expand his attention span.
Naturopathy and Nutrition Therapy. Although they concede that other factors may be involved, numerous naturopaths and nutritionists believe that food sensitivities, sugar, and chemical

food additives play a role in many cases of hyperactivity, a theory first put forth in 1973 by Dr. Benjamin Feingold, an allergist. But carefully controlled studies have shown no connection between diet and hyperactivity. Some nutritionists believe that eliminating sugar helps. Others think that hyperactivity comes from specific food allergies. Parents who wish to test this approach should consult a qualified nutritionist for a plan that eliminates suspected foods while providing essential nutrients.

Some naturopaths treat hyperactivity with high doses of vitamins. Not only are the benefits unproven, but the supplements can also cause nutritional imbalances.
Pet Therapy. Supervised contact with and caring for an animal can have a calming effect and also foster improved self-esteem and a sense of responsibility. A hyperactive child is likely to benefit more from being around a docile animal, such as an older cat, than a frisky dog or kitten. A bowl of goldfish may be an even better choice.

Self-Treatment
Parents need all the help they can get in meeting the challenge of a hyperactive child. Since parental understanding and an orderly home environment play a critical role in helping a child overcome hyperactivity, it is doubly important that parents keep calm. Here are some guidelines to follow:
► Accept the fact that hyperactivity is a chronic condition that needs special attention. Don't blame yourself for your child's problems, but do seek help.
► Join a support group to obtain practical advice and information.

ADULT HYPERACTIVITY
There is mounting evidence that childhood hyperactivity can persist into adulthood. Called residual hyperactivity, its symptoms are similar to those of the childhood form. Such adults often have trouble holding a job because they have difficulty in concentrating and are impulsive, restless, and easily distracted. Low doses of Ritalin or amphetamines may help, but require careful monitoring. Behavior modification and psychotherapy are also recommended.

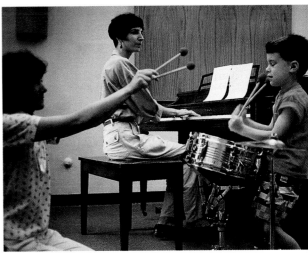

Music therapy can help a hyperactive child to relax and concentrate and also build self-esteem.

► Accustom the child to a consistent daily routine with specific times for meals, naps, play, snacks, and going to bed.
► Be alert to fatigue. Hyperactivity increases when a child is tired. Suggest a rest and a quiet story or warm bath.
► Make simple rules and enforce them without physical punishment. Discipline should be prompt and matter-of-fact, relying heavily on sending the child to a quiet place for "time out."
► For a preschool child, provide simple, safe, unbreakable toys to be played with one at a time.
► Keep the TV off except for carefully chosen nonviolent programs.
► Allocate an open space for active play to get rid of excess energy. Do not allow roughhousing, especially indoors, with siblings or friends.
► Always be quick to praise the child for obeying or playing quietly.
► Do what you can to increase the child's attention span before he enters school. Choose age-appropriate games, picture books, and puzzles. As soon as the child begins to fidget, switch to a physical activity.
► Investigate preschool programs that cater to children with special needs. Find out what provisions your public school has for children with learning disabilities. Ask that your child be tested by the special education team, and as soon as he is enrolled in school, request regular conferences with teachers and the school psychologist.
Other Causes of Hyperactivity
Hyperactive behavior is a component of some types of mental retardation and genetic neurological syndromes.

Hypochondria

(Hypochondriasis)

Hypochondria is a preoccupation with symptoms of an illness when there is no physical evidence of disease. In some people, it is a chronic state but with others, it is sporadic, occurring mostly during periods of depression, anxiety, or stress. Hypochondria is thought to be slightly more common in men than women. The condition affects all age groups, with the peak of incidence in men during their thirties, and in women during their forties.

Unlike most people, individuals with this disorder are not reassured when a doctor tells them there is no cause for worry. Instead, they go from doctor to doctor in the hope that an illness will be diagnosed. They rarely consult a mental health professional.

The causes of hypochondria are unknown, but predisposing factors have been identified. In some cases, a real medical disorder paves the way for later hypochondria. An asthmatic child, for example, is more likely to develop an

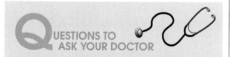

imagined problem, with symptoms unrelated to asthma, than a healthy youngster. In other instances, retreating into sickness allows a person to avoid certain obligations and postpone or escape making decisions. Some studies indicate that people with hypochondria are overly sensitive to physical sensations; what one person may perceive as a minor pinprick, a hypochondriac may feel as a sharp, stabbing pain.

Diagnostic Studies and Procedures

Even when doctors suspect hypochondria, they will order a thorough physical examination and tests because there is always the possibility that the complaints are indeed due to some organic illness. Routine tests usually include blood and urine studies, a chest X-ray,

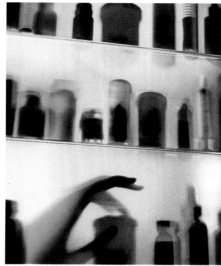

People with hypochondria often resort to self-treatment with myriad medications, thus risking dangerous drug interactions.

electrocardiogram, and, depending on the symptoms claimed, various imaging scans and other procedures.

A patient may be asked to fill out a prepared questionnaire containing a long list of symptoms. Checking off an unusually large number of symptoms that have no medical foundation alerts the doctor to the possibility that the person is prone to hypochondria.

Under diagnostic criteria established by the American Psychiatric Association, the following must be present—in addition to preoccupation with symptoms and a fear of serious disease that persist for at least six months:

▶ Appropriate physical examination and tests fail to find any organic explanation for the symptoms.
▶ The symptoms are not due to panic attacks or other mental disorders.
▶ The fear of having the disease persists despite a doctor's reassurances.
▶ The preoccupation causes significant distress and impairs normal social and occupational functioning.

Medical Treatments

If a doctor believes that the symptoms mask underlying anxiety or depression, he may prescribe antianxiety or antidepressant medications. Otherwise, hypochondria is generally not responsive to medical treatment.

Alternative Therapies

Although people with hypochondria typically resist seeking psychological counseling, treatments involving some form of psychotherapy are most likely to work against the disorder.

Dance Therapy and T'ai Chi. These movement therapies may be especially beneficial when depression is contributing to the problem.

Yoga and Meditation. The deep-breathing exercises of relaxation techniques are helpful in reducing anxiety that may underlie hypochondria.

Self-Treatment

Persons suffering from hypochondria are likely to try any number of treatments, both self- and medically prescribed, and are unlikely to accept the futility of such attempts. Family members and friends can help by responding in an appropriate manner. Many specialists believe that hypochondria should be thought of as a handicap that can be controlled, even if it can't be cured. Here are some helpful tactics:

▶ *Listen.* Show a sincere, sympathetic interest in the person's complaints, so that the need for gaining special attention is diminished.
▶ *Don't argue.* Take the symptoms seriously, but explain that stress can make them seem worse.
▶ *Talk about your own feelings.* By discussing your anger and frustration and revealing your own emotional upsets, you may be able to lessen the other person's focus on symptoms.
▶ *Do not recommend any new tests or medicines.* Instead, suggest that over-medication or drug interactions may be responsible for the symptoms.
▶ *Suggest group therapy.* People with a profound need for attention and understanding sometimes benefit from airing their complaints to each other.

Other Causes of Hypochondriacal Symptoms

In addition to depression and anxiety, schizophrenia and other psychological disorders should also be ruled out before diagnosing hypochondria.

REVERSE HYPOCHONDRIA

Some doctors refer to denial of illness as reverse hypochondria. In this situation, patients attribute their symptoms to psychological factors in order to avoid coming to terms with illness. Such patients believe that a neurotic illness is easier to cure than a physical one. Reverse hypochondria, which is thought to stem from a fear of helplessness, is potentially much more dangerous than hypochondria because it keeps patients from seeking necessary treatment.

Hypoglycemia
(Reactive hypoglycemia)

Hypoglycemia is a general term used to describe an abnormally low level of glucose, or blood sugar. This is defined as a glucose level of less than 60 milligrams per deciliter of blood (mg/dl). The normal range of blood sugar levels, taken while fasting, is between 80 and 120 mg/dl.

Symptoms include hunger, weakness, nervousness, difficulty concentrating, and mood swings. A more severe reaction is characterized by excessive sweating, a pounding heartbeat, and cold and clammy skin, along with growing weakness, difficulty in walking, and increasing confusion. If uncorrected, a severe hypoglycemic reaction can progress to convulsions, loss of consciousness, coma, and even death.

Hypoglycemia most often occurs in people who have diabetes, and results from taking too much insulin or too high a dose of a hypoglycemic drug, a medication prescribed for type II, or adult-onset, diabetes, in which the body still produces some insulin. Despite a popular belief that hypoglycemia is a common and frequently unrecognized condition responsible for a whole host of vague symptoms, it is rare in people who do not have diabetes. However, the condition sometimes occurs during a prolonged fast, and some people develop it in response to alcohol or as a side effect of certain medications.

Diagnostic Studies and Procedures
Hypoglycemia is readily identified by a check of blood sugar levels. This can be done with a self-monitoring kit that analyzes a drop of blood obtained with a simple finger prick. Anyone with diabetes should know how to perform this self-test, and do it regularly at home, usually several times a day.

In a patient who does not have diabetes, laboratory studies of blood sugar levels will be performed. The most frequently used test is an oral glucose tolerance test, or OGTT, in which blood sugar levels are measured after the patient has fasted and then remeasured hourly for the next several hours, after the person consumes a sugar drink.

Medical Treatments
Hypoglycemia usually does not require special medical treatment, other than adjusting the medication regimen in people who use insulin or oral agents

for diabetes. The proper balance of medication, diet, and exercise is the key to its control. A person who is experiencing a mild hypoglycemic reaction is helped by eating a simple sugar, such as honey, orange juice, or hard candy. A severe hypoglycemic reaction is a medical emergency that must be treated with intravenous glucose and other measures to raise blood glucose levels.

Alternative Therapies
Anyone with diabetes should be under the care of a medical specialist and use alternative therapies only with the approval of a physician.

Exercise Conditioning. Regular aerobic exercise is an important aspect of stabilizing blood glucose levels. Exercise also contributes to general feelings of well-being, and thus may control some of the vague symptoms, such as fatigue and depression, that are often attributed to hypoglycemia.

Naturopathy and Nutrition Therapy. A diet of five or six small meals a day is recommended, with emphasis on low-fat sources of protein, including fish, skinless white meat of chicken or turkey, and skim milk and other low-fat dairy products. Candy and other sugary foods should be avoided. Alcohol and caffeine should be minimized.

Yoga and Meditation. These and other relaxation techniques can be useful in reducing stress, which may contribute to nervousness and other symptoms attributed to hypoglycemia.

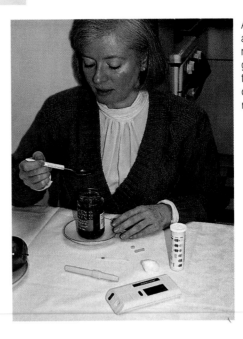

A home monitoring kit allows a person to measure her blood glucose levels and, if they are too low, take a concentrated sugar to reverse hypoglycemia.

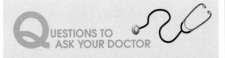

▶ Is recurring hypoglycemia a sign that my dosage of diabetes medication needs to be changed?
▶ How is true hypoglycemia differentiated from psychological disorders?

Self-Treatment
Self-treatment is the key to controlling hypoglycemia. Symptoms can be relieved within 10 to 15 minutes if the proper action is taken.

At the first signs of a hypoglycemic reaction, eat six or seven hard candies, or two teaspoons of honey, syrup, or sugar. Alternatively, drink ½ cup of orange juice or any sugary soft drink. Wait for 10 to 15 minutes, measure your blood sugar, and repeat the process if necessary.

When symptoms are more severe, eat or drink something sugary and then eat a high-carbohydrate food, such as an apple or banana, a slice of bread, a few crackers, or a bowl of cereal. These foods supply both simple and complex carbohydrates, and help to stabilize blood glucose levels.

Avoid alcohol if it is clearly the cause of hypoglycemia. If your medication brings on a hypoglycemic reaction, discuss alternatives with your doctor.

Other Causes of Hypoglycemia Symptoms
Faintness, weakness, and dizziness can also be signs of a heart condition. Excessive sweating may be due to anxiety, menopause, hyperthyroidism, or even a heart attack. Increasing confusion could indicate the onset of a stroke, a transient ischemic attack (TIA), excessive drinking, or an adverse reaction to a drug. Emotional problems, including depression and anxiety, can also lead to symptoms similar to those of hypoglycemia.

Hypothermia

Hypothermia is a life-threatening drop in the body's internal temperature to below 95°F (35°C); this occurs when the body loses heat faster than it can generate it. Although hypothermia is associated usually with prolonged exposure to very cold weather outdoors, most cases actually occur indoors with room temperatures ranging from 50° to 60°F (10° to 15.6°C).

It is estimated that as many as 50,000 elderly Americans are hospitalized every winter for what is presumed to be a stroke or other illness, when they are actually suffering accidental hypothermia. Older people are at special risk because of poor circulation, illnesses, and medication use. In addition, sensitivity to cold decreases with age, as does the ability to shiver, the body's way of quickly generating heat.

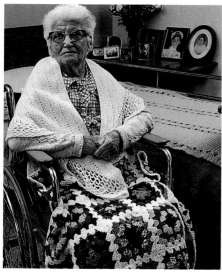

Simple measures like dressing warmly can prevent hypothermia in the elderly.

Someone afflicted with hypothermia appears to be semiconscious and has uncoordinated movements, slurred speech, confused responses, slow breathing, and a weak pulse. Without treatment, the death rate from this condition is about 50 percent.

Diagnostic Studies and Procedures

Hypothermia can be quickly verified by taking a person's temperature. In the absence of a thermometer, place the back of one hand on the individual's bare abdomen. If the skin feels unusually cold, presume that the person does have hypothermia and either call for an ambulance or take her to the nearest emergency room. While waiting for help, begin first aid (see box, below).

When the patient is eventually seen by a doctor, blood pressure, pulse, and other vital signs will be quickly evaluated. She will be examined for possible tissue damage, and an electrocardiogram taken. After the patient is stabilized, blood tests may be ordered to check for anemia and other disorders that can contribute to hypothermia.

Medical Treatments

The first priority is to bring body temperature back to normal, then treat frostbite (page 193) and other underlying or precipitating conditions. Medications, alcohol use, and nutrition are reviewed to make sure they are not contributing factors.

Alternative Therapies

Any alternative approach should be directed to preventing hypothermia. Even people with limited mobility can benefit from therapies that improve circulation and mental outlook.

T'ai Chi. These gentle exercises are usually within the capability of anyone who can walk. They improve coordination, help overcome joint stiffness, and foster an enhanced sense of well-being.

Meditation. The deep breathing used in meditation can help counteract both anxiety and depression, emotional problems that can lead to self-neglect.

Nutrition Therapy. Many older people who live alone have little incentive to prepare balanced meals; they may subsist on such foods as canned soup, tea, and toast. Programs such as Meals on Wheels, which deliver nutritious meals to the homebound or infirm, can help. The elderly of limited means should use the information and referral services of their local agency for the aged.

Self-Treatment

Older people can limit the risk of hypothermia by taking these precautions:
▶ If you live alone, arrange to have a neighbor or relative phone or drop by in the morning and evening.
▶ If you have a live-in health aide, make sure that this person is informed about the potential danger of hypothermia and how to deal with it.
▶ Don't put your life at risk by economizing on fuel. Set the thermostat at 68°F (20°C) during the day, and no lower than 60°F (15.6°C) at night. If you rent, keep a reliable thermometer in the bedroom and another in a different regularly used room. If the temperature drops below 68°F (20°C), contact the proper authority to complain. If possible, stay with a relative or friend until the situation at home improves.
▶ Dress in layers, even indoors. If the inside temperature goes down to 50°F (10°C) at night, wear long underwear, socks, and a nightcap and woolen gloves if necessary; place one wool blanket under your body and as many as you need over it.
▶ When out-of-doors in cold weather, wear waterproof, windproof garments over layered sweaters, fleece-lined rubber boots, wool gloves, and a hat that protects the ears. Stay in the sun as much as possible, and head for warm, dry shelter at the first sign of snow.
▶ When taking an auto trip in cold weather, keep several blankets in the trunk. Buy a cellular phone for the car in case you become stranded in snow.

Other Causes of Hypothermia

Contributing factors include impaired circulation, prolonged immobility, excessive alcohol consumption, malnutrition, and overuse of tranquilizers, sedatives, and antidepressant drugs.

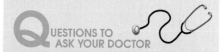

QUESTIONS TO ASK YOUR DOCTOR

▶ Am I taking any medications that could increase my risk of hypothermia?
▶ Can young children develop accidental hypothermia?

FIRST AID FOR HYPOTHERMIA

To administer help while waiting for professional assistance, the following first-aid procedures are recommended:

▶ Check for a pulse and breathing. Begin cardiopulmonary resuscitation (CPR) if they are absent (page 217).
▶ If possible, move the person to a warm room and cover him with a blanket to prevent further heat loss. Rewarming should proceed very slowly, no faster than one degree per hour.
▶ Do not attempt to rewarm any part of the body by rubbing or by using a heating pad. Rapid warming of the skin is dangerous because it carries blood away from vital organs.
▶ Give nothing by mouth unless the person is conscious and able to swallow. If so, offer warm clear soup or tea, but DO NOT give any alcoholic drinks.

Hysteria

(Hysterical conversion disorder)

In everyday parlance, hysteria refers to any emotional extreme; for example, an episode of hysterical weeping or laughter. When used medically, the word refers to a disorder, formerly called hysterical neurosis, in which unconscious psychological conflict is transformed into physical, or somatic, symptoms.

The most common conversion symptoms suggest a neurological disorder, such as paralysis, seizures, blindness or tunnel vision, deafness, or an inability to smell, feel, or speak. Less commonly,

ORIGINS OF HYSTERIA

Historically, hysteria has been a female disorder. In fact, the widespread female invalidism of the 19th century, in which thousands of seemingly healthy women took to their beds, was later seen as an unconscious attempt to call attention to their emotional and intellectual needs.

Physicians assumed that hysteria was caused by "disturbances in the womb." In fact, hysteria is the Greek word for uterus, and until this century, hysterectomy was a common treatment for it.

The breakthrough that removed hysteria from the realm of gynecology was the 1895 publication of Sigmund Freud's *Studies on Hysteria*, in which this father of modern psychiatry described the celebrated case of Anna, and her cure of hysteria with a new form of treatment. This "talking cure" soon became known as psychoanalysis.

symptoms may appear to originate in the endocrine system; for example, a false or hysterical pregnancy. In one form, called globus hystericus, the person has difficulty swallowing because of a nonexistent lump in the throat. Vomiting and fainting can also be expressions of a conversion disorder.

In some cases, symptoms are brought on by extreme psychological stress. In hysterical amnesia, for example, loss of memory is a way of suppressing events that are too painful to recall.

Psychiatrists cite two subconscious mechanisms that seem to be involved in hysterical conversion reactions. One is avoidance of psychological conflict. For example, a sudden inability to hear or speak may follow an intense argument and reflect the person's inability to otherwise confront his anger. The

other is avoidance of a dreaded activity. Examples include the child who vomits when it is time to set off for school or the soldier who suddenly goes blind, exempting him from battle.

Diagnostic Studies and Procedures

Before making a diagnosis of hysteria, a thorough medical workup that includes a complete physical examination, blood and urine studies, and a neurological evaluation is needed. Additional tests depend on symptoms, but may include CT scans or MRI and other imaging studies to rule out an organic cause, such as a stroke or tumor. If hysteria is suspected, then psychological testing is in order (see Diagnostic Criteria, below). Once a doctor determines that the problem is psychological, hypnosis may be used to search for the underlying emotional cause.

Medical Treatments

An attack, or fit, of hysterics, in which the individual alternates between uncontrolled crying and laughter, is usually treated with a sedative or tranquilizer. This loss of control is generally triggered by an emotional trauma and is unlikely to become chronic.

Some psychiatrists prescribe tranquilizers during treatment of chronic conversion disorder, but psychotherapy is the main approach. Although this is lengthy, it usually produces results because it helps patients come to terms with the underlying emotional cause for physical symptoms. Dream analysis may play a role in treatment. In some cases, short-term goal-oriented therapy may suffice, especially if there is a clear link between the symptoms and their psychological cause.

Alternative Therapies

Alternative therapies can help patients confront experiences and memories that they have buried.

Art Therapy. An art therapist can guide a patient in recreating scenes from childhood or in making sketches that express hidden feelings. Combined with psychotherapy, this approach can be highly beneficial.

Hypnosis. During hypnosis, some patients have been able to recall and eventually come to terms with the circumstances that led to their physical symptoms. This technique has been especially useful in helping adults overcome psychological problems stemming from childhood sexual abuse and other traumatic or frightening events.

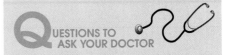

Self-Treatment

A conversion disorder is unlikely to be resolved by self-treatment without the help of a mental-health professional. Individuals suffering from hysteria are too willing to take all kinds of medicines, and even to undergo surgery, for nonexistent illnesses. Family members and friends should discourage this behavior. Although they might try to be sympathetic and listen to complaints, they should encourage the person to seek professional help.

Other Causes of Hysteria Symptoms

Many specialists find it difficult to establish clear boundaries between hysteria and other psychological problems, including hypochondria, anxiety, panic attacks, phobias, and depression. Some are convinced that chronic fatigue syndrome and severe multiple allergies—two prevalent disorders that lack any identifiable physical cause—are manifestations of a conversion disorder.

In addition, a number of organic diseases produce symptoms that may be attributed to a conversion disorder. These include multiple sclerosis, systemic lupus erythematosus, and various neurological diseases.

DIAGNOSTIC CRITERIA

To diagnose a conversion disorder, the American Psychiatric Association has established the following guidelines:
► The person has one or more symptoms or deficits affecting voluntary motor or sensory function that suggests a neurological or other medical disorder, but there is no evidence of an underlying organic disorder.
► Psychological factors are associated with the symptoms. For example, stress may initiate or worsen symptoms.
► The symptoms are not intentionally feigned, as in malingering.
► The symptoms cause significant psychological distress or impair the ability to function normally.

Impetigo

(Bullous and nonbullous; ecthyma)

Impetigo is a common, contagious skin infection that causes a painless red rash with many small, itchy blisters, some of which contain pus. When the blisters break, characteristic yellow crusts form. Some people also have a slight fever with impetigo. Occasionally, bullous skin ulcers develop, creating a condition called ecthyma, which is likely to cause scarring.

The infection, which is most common in infants and children, is caused by either streptococcal or staphylococcal bacteria. In some instances, the bacteria come from an infection elsewhere in the body, usually the nose or ears. In other cases, the bacteria invade the skin through a minor cut or an insect bite that has become infected by scratching. Less commonly, it can be contracted by direct contact with an infected person or a shared personal item, such as a razor or washcloth. Other precipitating factors that increase a person's risk of infection with impetigo include:

▶ Skin sensitivity to friction, chemicals, sun, and other irritants.
▶ Resistance weakened by fatigue, poor nutrition, or illness, especially diabetes or leukemia.
▶ Use of steroids or anticancer drugs.
▶ Poor hygiene and crowded, unsanitary living conditions, especially in a moist and warm climate.

Most impetigo infections are mild and easily cured. In some cases, however, streptococcal impetigo can result in kidney inflammation, a serious condition called acute glomerulonephritis, which can be life threatening if it is not treated immediately.

Staphlococcal bullous impetigo can lead to scalded skin syndrome, in which large areas of skin separate and are shed, leaving raw, oozing patches. This complication occurs most often in babies, especially newborns.

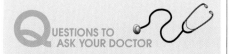

▶ What can I do to prevent scarring and other skin complications?
▶ Are there precautions that will prevent kidney involvement?

Diagnostic Studies and Procedures

A doctor can make an initial diagnosis of impetigo by inspecting the lesions, but confirmation requires scraping a sample of cells from the sores for laboratory examination.

Medical Treatments

If the infection is in an early stage at the time of diagnosis and affects only a small area, removal of the scabs with a coarse gauze sponge followed by application of a topical antibiotic ointment may be sufficient. The ointment must be applied as instructed, which is usually at least three applications a day. Mupirocin (Bactroban), an antibiotic ointment, is particularly effective with certain staphlocccal and streptococcal strains.

In some cases, however, a topical antibiotic is not enough, and an oral medication, such as a cephalosporin or a penicillin, is prescribed. As an alternative, some doctors treat the infection with a single injection of long-acting penicillin. In addition, a doctor may also recommend use of a nonprescription antibiotic ointment containing bacitracin or neomycin.

Antibiotic therapy should completely cure the infection within about 10 days. (During that period, the patient usually cannot spread it to others by direct contact.) If it persists longer, or if the sores continue to spread or don't start to heal within three days of the beginning of treatment, the causative organism may be antibiotic resistant. Trying a different antibiotic usually works.

Alternative Therapies

Herbal Medicine. Garlic, eaten raw or swallowed in capsule form, has natural antibacterial effects. Applications of aloe vera gel soothe skin sores and promote healing.

Nutrition Therapy. Some nutritionists advocate high doses of vitamin C to strengthen the immune system and fight infection. They often recommend high doses of vitamin B complex when antibiotics are being taken, and also yogurt that contains natural cultures or acidophilus capsules or liquid to prevent digestive problems and an overgrowth of yeast. Vitamin E oil applied to the sores may hasten healing.

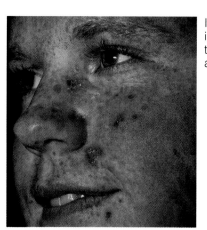

In its early stages, impetigo can be treated with topical antibiotics alone.

Self-Treatment

Self-care is unlikely to cure the infection, but it can speed healing when antibiotics are used, and prevent spreading of the infection to others.

▶ Wash the rashy areas with antiseptic soap. Use disposable gauze or paper towels instead of a washcloth or towel. The causative bacteria can spread to others on shared towels.
▶ When blisters break open, remove crusting areas to expose and cleanse the lesions. Then cover the sores with gauze to keep from touching or scratching them.
▶ Women with blisters under their arms or on their legs and men with facial blisters should refrain from shaving or do so carefully. While the infection persists, use a new blade every day, rather than an electric razor, and use an aerosol shaving cream, instead of a shaving brush. These measures help avoid possible reinfection. Even if you discontinue using an electric razor and shaving brush until the infection clears up, be sure to wash them thoroughly in an antibacterial solution, such as Betadine or Hibiclens, before resuming their use after the infection has been cured.
▶ Never use an over-the-counter cortisone cream on any skin rash that might be impetigo. Cortisone can worsen it.
▶ To protect other household members from infection, wash the infected person's bed linens and clothing separately, using the hottest water available; if possible, presoak the articles in boiling water. All other household members should bathe daily with an antibacterial soap or solution.

Other Causes of Skin Infections

A herpes infection can cause skin lesions similar to those of impetigo.

Incontinence

(Urinary incontinence)

Incontinence, the inability to control the flow of urine, affects about 10 million Americans. Between 10 and 30 percent of people over the age of 65 who are living independently are incontinent, as are more than 50 percent of those who live in nursing homes and other long-term care institutions. The problem, which is more common in women, may be transient or chronic, depending upon its cause.

Urge incontinence is characterized by a sudden, overwhelming desire to urinate and an inability to hold the urine long enough to get to a toilet. This may be due to a disorder or obstruction of the bladder or a neurologic problem, such as stroke, multiple sclerosis, or

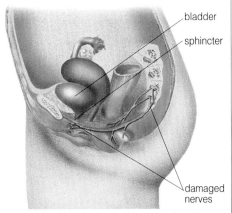

Normally, bladder control is maintained by involuntary muscles. Nerve deterioration in these muscles (inset), caused by a disease such as multiple sclerosis, may lead to their malfunction and thus, incontinence.

Parkinson's disease. In many cases, however, a cause cannot be identified. Then the condition is referred to as idiopathic incontinence.

Stress incontinence is an involuntary loss of a small amount of urine as a result of coughing, sneezing, laughing, lifting, straining, or any other motion that increases pressure in the abdominal cavity. Especially common in older women, it is due to a weakening of the muscles that support the bladder and control the urine flow. These muscles can lose tone as a result of repeated pregnancies, obesity, or hormonal changes during menopause. In men, stress incontinence is most common after prostate surgery.

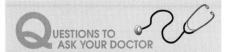

QUESTIONS TO ASK YOUR DOCTOR

▶ Would switching from a diuretic to some other type of medication help my urinary problem?
▶ Am I a candidate for surgical correction of a displaced bladder?

Diagnostic Studies and Procedures

The type of incontinence is usually apparent from the patient's description of the symptoms. In addition, a urine analysis will be ordered to rule out a urinary tract infection, which can cause transient incontinence.

Other tests depend on the possible cause. If a stroke or other neurological problem is suspected, an electroencephalogram and a brain scan may be ordered. Sometimes the bladder is filled artificially and a catheter placed in it so that pressures can be observed and function monitored by a computer.

Medical Treatments

Treatment can cure or significantly improve about two-thirds of all cases. Antibiotics will be prescribed when a urinary infection has been identified.

For stress incontinence, a pessary—a donut-shaped device—may be inserted into the vagina to support the uterus and bladder. Urge incontinence may be treated with medications that prevent the bladder from contracting.

In cases where no underlying problem can be identified, alpha-adrenergic drugs may be given to help close the neck of the bladder. (Many older patients cannot take these medications, however, because they tend to elevate blood pressure.) Or surgery may be performed to restore the neck of the bladder to its normal position.

Estrogen cream is often prescribed to help restore muscle tone in menopausal and postmenopausal women, even if they are taking oral estrogen.

Alternative Therapies

Biofeedback Training. Behavior modification using biofeedback to train the bladder to wait a certain length of time before emptying is sometimes helpful. The goal is to gradually lengthen the intervals between urinating until a normal pattern is established.

Herbal Medicine. Herbalists may recommend extracts of horsetail or sweet sumac, or huang chi, a Chinese herb available in capsule and tincture forms. Chinese herbalists also suggest the Rehmannia Eight formula and cervus with powdered deer antler added as treatments for incontinence.

If a urinary tract infection is responsible, drinking diluted marsh mallow root extract may help. Saw palmetto tea or capsules are also recommended.

Homeopathy. For nocturnal incontinence, practitioners recommend belladonna, to be taken every four to six hours. Causticum is advocated for stress incontinence, and gelsemium is used when the prostate is enlarged or a bladder stone is obstructing the flow of urine. For constant dribbling of urine, verbascum thapsus may be prescribed.

Naturopathy. Eliminating coffee, tea, and other sources of caffeine from the diet is helpful in controlling urge incontinence. Drinking cranberry juice is said to deodorize the urine, minimizing the odor problems.

Self-Treatment

Women often find Kegel exercises helpful for strengthening the muscles of the pelvic floor to allow greater control over urination. The exercises involve the pubococcygeus muscle, which controls the bladder sphincter. To practice, imagine that you are stopping the flow of urine in midstream. Start by tightening this muscle, then squeeze your vagina, and finally, tighten the anus as if you are holding back a bowel movement. Hold each contraction for a slow count of three. Repeat the exercise 10 to 20 times, three or more times a day. You can do it while standing, sitting, or lying down.

Rather than waiting for the urge to urinate, go to the bathroom every two or three hours. Use sanitary napkins or disposable adult diapers to catch small amounts of leaking urine. Various types of adult diapers are available, including nonbulky ones that fit under clothing.

When caring for a person who is incontinent, provide a portable urinal or commode. Either can be purchased or rented from a medical supply company or through a pharmacy. Make sure that the patient's clothing is easy to remove and keep the skin clean and dry to prevent sores and rashes.

Other Causes of Incontinence

Diuretic medications increase urine output and can cause incontinence. Emotional stress can also cause incontinence, especially in children.

bladder
sphincter
damaged nerves

Indigestion

(Dyspepsia)

Indigestion is the general term for an upset stomach that stems from no identifiable cause or physical abnormality. Symptoms typically develop during or soon after eating or drinking, with the most common complaints being stomach pain, a sensation of fullness or bloating in the upper abdomen, gas, and possibly belching. Some people also experience mild nausea and heartburn, a burning sensation accompanied by an acid taste in the mouth.

Indigestion can be triggered by foods, especially high-fat or gas-producing types, such as beans. It may also be due to a food allergy or overindulging in alcohol or caffeine. Sometimes it's related to smoking, constipation, or swallowing air while eating. Stress can also bring on or worsen the condition.

Normally, indigestion is no cause for alarm; simple measures can alleviate it (see Self-Treatment). But if it persists for more than a week or two, you should seek a doctor's care, especially if the pattern of symptoms changes, or you experience vomiting, unexplainable weight loss, appetite loss, fever, vomiting of blood, severe diarrhea, or black, tarry stool—all indications of a potentially serious intestinal disorder.

Diagnostic Studies and Procedures

The physical examination and medical history are of primary importance, particularly the patient's description of stressful situations, habits, or foods that seem to bring on the symptoms. Although a doctor can usually diagnose simple indigestion with this information, additional tests may be ordered to rule out digestive disorders.

Studies may include an upper GI series, which consists of X-rays of the esophagus, stomach, and intestines taken after the patient swallows barium, a chalky substance that coats these organs to make them visible on film.

The interior of the stomach or the intestines may also be examined using endoscopy. This involves passing a long, slender, flexible tube with a lighted tip through the esophagus and into the stomach and duodenum, the uppermost segment of the small intestine.

Medical Treatments

If there is no underlying disease, medical treatment is usually unnecessary. For severe cases, an antispasmodic

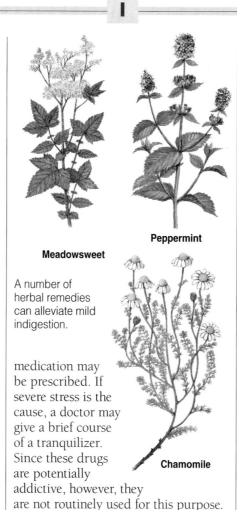

Meadowsweet

Peppermint

Chamomile

A number of herbal remedies can alleviate mild indigestion.

medication may be prescribed. If severe stress is the cause, a doctor may give a brief course of a tranquilizer. Since these drugs are potentially addictive, however, they are not routinely used for this purpose.

Alternative Therapies

Indigestion can usually be eliminated by a combination of alternative therapies and self-care.

Aromatherapy. Therapists advise putting two drops of oil of basil on the back of the wrist and inhaling it three times a day. The basil oil can also be combined with black pepper, chamomile, and lavender oils.

Bach Flower Remedies. If indigestion is related to stress or anxiety, try three to five drops of tincture of agrimony.

Herbal Medicine. Western herbalists advocate meadowsweet to reduce stomach acid. Before a meal, drink a tea made with one teaspoonful of the herb, steeped for 10 minutes in a cup of boiling water and strained. Add honey if desired. Take this mixture no more

than twice a day. Peppermint or fennel extracts can be added to alleviate gas. Lavender and chamomile teas are also said to relieve stress-related indigestion. Garlic may help stimulate the secretion of digestive juices. If the garlic itself produces indigestion, take it in pill form. Chinese herbalists recommend hoelen in tablet form or as a tea.

Homeopathy. Amonium crudum is often prescribed for indigestion with nausea, or natrum phosphoricum for indigestion with belching.

Naturopathy. To sooth the digestive system, naturopathists advocate drinking distilled water and eating light, bland foods. To prevent indigestion, some practitioners suggest the following: add 1 cup miller's bran and 1 cup oatmeal to 1 gallon of water; allow it to stand for 24 hours, then strain. Drink a cup of the liquid 15 minutes before eating. Also, eating some form of papaya, either fresh, as juice, or in pill form, is said to combat indigestion through the action of an enzyme called papain.

Yoga and Meditation. Yoga breathing methods can help overcome stress that contributes to some cases of indigestion. Also, positions such as the knee-to-chest (page 188) and the spine twist are said to tone the digestive system.

Self-Treatment

Indigestion usually can be prevented by paying attention to what and how you eat. Avoid large, high-fat meals. Eat slowly and chew each bite thoroughly. To reduce the swallowing of air, avoid carbonated beverages and chew with your mouth closed.

Strive to make mealtimes a relaxed, pleasant part of the day, avoiding arguments or discussion of upsetting news. Also, avoid excitement or strenuous exercise just after eating, especially after a heavy meal. If indigestion does develop, a nonprescription antacid liquid or tablet usually brings relief.

Other Causes of Indigestion

Lactose intolerance and malabsorption syndromes can cause indigestion. Upper abdominal pain that is worsened by eating could be due to gallbladder disease, whereas pain that lessens after eating may indicate gastritis or an ulcer. Other causes of abdominal pain include gastroenteritis, irritable bowel syndrome, colitis, infection, and emotional stress. Symptoms of indigestion may also be due to a parasitic disorder, such as giardiasis or amebiasis.

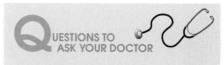

QUESTIONS TO ASK YOUR DOCTOR

▶ Is it harmful to take nonprescription antacids on a long-term basis? Will they interact adversely with other medications I am taking?

Infertility

A couple is considered infertile if they have been unable to conceive after one year of regular sex without contraceptives. It is estimated that 20 percent of American couples have some sort of fertility problem, almost double the percentage of a few decades ago.

Some experts believe that at least part of this increase reflects a growing number of people who are seeking help for infertility, rather than an actual doubling of the incidence. Another contributing factor is that so many couples are delaying parenthood until their peak fertility is past. Sexually transmitted diseases also take a toll.

New techniques now make it possible to find and correct the cause of many couples' infertility. Experts stress the importance of evaluating both partners —in about 40 percent of cases, the problem lies with the male; in another 40 percent, it is traced to the female; and in the remaining 20 percent, both partners may have abnormalities or no cause can be found. (See box on facing page for specific causes of infertility.)

Diagnostic Studies and Procedures

A workup for infertility can be lengthy, emotionally trying, and expensive. A gynecologist, urologist, or primary-care doctor might quickly determine the cause, but in complicated cases, it may be necessary to seek help from a fertility specialist or reputable fertility clinic.

A diagnostic study should start with a detailed medical history and a thorough physical examination of both partners that includes basic blood and urine studies. Screening for sexually transmitted diseases and other infections is important, because these can affect fertility of both sexes.

Male Studies. Early in the detection process, the male's semen is analyzed for the number of sperm, which are also studied for their ability to move (motility). The woman's cervical mucus is usually sampled and studied several hours after the couple has had intercourse, to detect whether the sperm are moving. If they are not, the mucus may be too thick or damaging to the sperm.

A vasogram, X-rays of male reproductive organs after injection of a dye, may be done to determine if a blockage is preventing the passage of sperm. A testicular biopsy may also be performed.

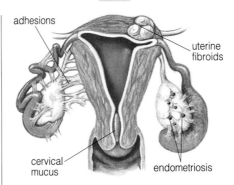

Female infertility can result from uterine tumors or conditions that alter the positions of the ovaries and fallopian tubes.

Female Studies. These usually start with ovulation tests to see whether the woman is producing eggs normally. Her blood will be tested for hormone levels at specific times during her menstrual cycle. Other hormone studies depend on results of the physical examination and medical history.

An ultrasound examination of the woman's reproductive organs may show pelvic abnormalities, such as uterine fibroids or polyps.

A hysterosalpingogram, an X-ray of the uterus and fallopian tubes taken after injecting a dye, may be made. A doctor may also use a hysteroscope to view the uterus directly. This long, slender tube with viewing devices is inserted into the uterine cavity through the cervix. During this examination, tissue can be collected for a biopsy of the uterine lining (endometrium) to detect abnormalities that prevent implantation of a fertilized egg.

Laparoscopy is another diagnostic tool. A laparoscope, a tube similar to the hysteroscope, is inserted through a small incision in the abdomen to view the uterus, fallopian tubes, and ovaries. During this examination, a doctor will look for endometriosis (page 179), a disorder in which endometrial tissue

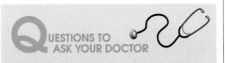

UESTIONS TO ASK YOUR DOCTOR

► What are the potential side effects of hormone treatment? Will it affect my potency or sex drive?
► Based on your experiences, what are our chances for achieving pregnancy?
► If surgery is recommended, what are its potential complications?

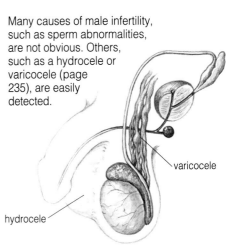

Many causes of male infertility, such as sperm abnormalities, are not obvious. Others, such as a hydrocele or varicocele (page 235), are easily detected.

grows outside the uterus, often causing adhesions and distortion of the reproductive organs and leading to infertility.

Both Partners. Chromosomal studies may be ordered if an inborn condition that affects fertility is suspected.

Medical Treatments

If either partner has an infection that affects the genital tract, both will be treated with antibiotics to clear it up. Once the condition is corrected, other treatments may begin.

Male Treatments. The most common correctable cause of male infertility is a varicocele (page 235), a swelling in the scrotum caused by varicose veins that have dilated and filled with blood. The increased blood flow brings extra heat to the area, slowing sperm production and resulting in a low sperm count. Varicoceles are corrected by minor surgery to remove the abnormal veins.

If infertility is a result of a low sperm count, hormonal therapy can sometimes be used to increase it.

Microsurgery may be done to remove or bypass obstructions in the tubes that convey sperm from the testicles to the penis. If the blockage cannot be corrected, other methods will be employed to remove sperm from the male and fertilize the woman's egg in the laboratory.

Female Treatments. Hormonal abnormalities can be treated, but the specific regimen depends upon identifying the underlying endocrine problem. For example, if the woman is not ovulating despite having normal estrogen levels, clomiphene (Serophene) may be prescribed. This drug stimulates the ovaries to ripen an egg, thereby allowing ovulation to occur. Several cycles of the drug may be needed, but about 30 percent of women with ovarian failure can be helped with this regimen.

If clomiphene fails to stimulate the ovaries, injections of menotropins (Pergonal) may be tried. This drug must be administered by an expert in its use, however, because even a minute overdose can stimulate the ovaries to produce far too many eggs, which can lead to a multiple pregnancy.

Microsurgery may be done to correct obstructions in the fallopian tubes, or to reverse sterilization in women who have had a tubal ligation. Adhesions in the uterus may also have to be removed. A deficiency of progesterone, a hormone needed to establish pregnancy, can be treated with hormonal suppositories. Endometriosis may be treated with drugs, surgery, or both.

When none of these approaches works, a couple may turn to artificial insemination or high-tech procedures such as in vitro fertilization—in which drugs are given to stimulate the ovaries, several ripened eggs are harvested and mixed with sperm, and the fertilized eggs are returned to the uterus.

A newer technique called GIFT, for gamete intrafallopian transfer, has a higher success rate than in vitro fertilization. With GIFT, the fertilized eggs are returned to the fallopian tubes and proceed naturally to the uterus. An even newer approach is microinjection of a single sperm into the egg.

Alternative Therapies
Stress may be a factor in infertility; if so, massage and aromatherapy may help. Other alternative approaches are:
Herbal Medicine. Chinese herbalists prescribe the cinnamon and hoelen formula for infertility due to infection or a malpositioned uterus. Both Western and Eastern herbalists recommend ginseng to treat impotence.

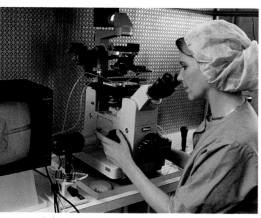
A fresh semen sample is examined to observe the number and motility of sperm.

Nutrition Therapy. Some therapists recommend vitamin E and zinc supplements to stimulate production of sex hormones. (Women should avoid high doses of vitamin A—if pregnancy does occur, high reserves of the vitamin can cause serious birth defects.) Women may be advised to forego caffeine and both males and females should abstain from alcohol when trying to conceive. If either partner is seriously over- or underweight, a nutritionist can plan an appropriate diet.

Self-Treatment
A young woman's choice of birth control can affect future fertility. In some women, for example, it can take months or years for normal ovarian function to resume after stopping birth control pills. An IUD may reduce fertility by damaging the uterus wall. These devices also increase the risk of pelvic inflammatory disease, a common cause of infertility.

Both partners should stop smoking, which has a marked effect on fertility. In women, it diminishes the production of estrogen and sometimes leads to early menopause. In men, smoking reduces the sperm count.

Men should not wear tight-fitting underwear; it can raise the temperature of the scrotum and adversely affect sperm production. A few months before a couple begins trying to conceive, the man should cease taking hot baths, saunas, and lengthy hot showers.

A woman trying to conceive should exercise in moderation. Strenuous workouts can result in excessive loss of body fat, menstrual irregularity, and cessation of ovulation.

If a woman's cervical mucus is too thick, some doctors advise taking Robitussin, a cough medication that thins all body secretions.

In some cases, a woman develops antibodies against her partner's sperm. This can sometimes be overcome by using condoms for several months, thus reducing the woman's exposure to the sperm and allowing the antibodies to weaken. The couple can then try to conceive by having unprotected intercourse only at the time of ovulation.

Timing of intercourse is especially important because sperm are viable for a limited time—usually only 24 to 48 hours. To increase chances that sperm and an egg can meet, some experts advise having it every other day during

COMMON CAUSES OF INFERTILITY
In about 10 percent of all cases, there is no identifiable cause for infertility, and in a small number, the problem is related to infrequent or poorly timed intercourse. Otherwise, the most common causes of infertility include the following:

Both Sexes
▶ Hormonal disorders (ovarian or testicular abnormalities, pituitary failure, adrenal or thyroid disease)
▶ Gonorrhea, chlamydia, and other sexually transmitted diseases
▶ Obesity and excessive thinness
▶ Alcoholism and other drug abuse, and excessive smoking
▶ Genetic disorders
▶ Immunological factors

Female
▶ Failure to ovulate (including menopause)
▶ Pelvic inflammatory disease and tubal scarring
▶ Endometriosis
▶ Uterine fibroids
▶ Uterine and cervical malformations
▶ Hostile cervical mucus
▶ Prenatal exposure to DES, a synthetic estrogen prescribed to prevent miscarriage until the late 1960s
▶ Turner's syndrome, a genetic disorder in which a woman has three rather than two X chromosomes

Male
▶ Low sperm count or other sperm abnormalities
▶ Hydrocele or varicocele
▶ Undescended or underdeveloped testicles
▶ Impotence or ejaculatory disorders
▶ Prostatitis
▶ Testicular injury or inflammation
▶ Klinefelter's syndrome, a genetic disorder in which a man has more than one X chromosome

the week when ovulation is likely. For more precision, use a home ovulation testing kit, or chart the woman's basal temperature—the body's temperature when awakening in the morning and before getting out of bed—to detect changes (a slight decline followed by an abrupt increase) that occur with ovulation. Intercourse at this time is most likely to result in conception.

Other Causes of Infertility
A woman with irregular or no menstrual periods due to being over- or underweight may experience a temporary fertility problem, but a normal menstrual cycle usually reappears when weight returns to normal.

Inflammatory Bowel Disorders

(Crohn's disease; ulcerative colitis)
The term inflammatory bowel disease describes a chronic condition of intestinal inflammation and ulceration that has no identifiable cause. The two most common examples are Crohn's disease and ulcerative colitis.

Crohn's disease, also called ileitis or regional enteritis, can affect any part of the gastrointestinal system, from the mouth to the anus, but most often attacks the lowermost portion of the small intestine, or ileum, and the colon. The disease usually appears early in life, commonly between the ages of 14 and 24. Men and women are equally affected and, for unknown reasons, there has been a worldwide increase in the disease since it was first described by Dr. Burrill B. Crohn, a New York gastroenterologist, in the 1930s.

Ulcerative colitis also causes inflammation and often severe ulcerations as well, but it is confined mostly to the lining of the colon and rectum.

More than 2 million Americans suffer from one of these disorders. The main symptoms of both conditions are persistent diarrhea, rectal bleeding, fever, abdominal cramps, and weight loss. A number of nonintestinal symptoms are also associated with inflammatory bowel disorders, including eye inflammation, arthritis, skin and mouth ulcers, and liver disease.

Although no cause for inflammatory bowel diseases has been identified, certain predisposing factors are known. For instance, researchers believe that susceptibility is inherited, because there is a tendency for the disorders to run in families, with people of Jewish descent the most vulnerable. They also suspect that the disorders might be triggered by an infectious organism or immune system reaction, but this theory remains unproved. Psychological factors also may play a role, as the conditions often develop during periods of high stress and emotional turmoil. But exactly how stress triggers the inflammatory response is unknown.

Diagnostic Studies and Procedures

The characteristic symptoms will prompt a doctor to suspect inflammatory bowel disease, but the diagnostic process requires a thorough physical

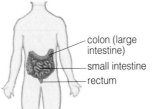

colon (large intestine)
small intestine
rectum

Following removal of the colon and part of the rectum, an ileo-anal anastomosis may be created. In this procedure, muscles of the rectum are attached to the ilium (lowermost portion of the small intestine), thus permitting fecal waste to exit through the anus. (A less desirable alternative is a stoma, an opening in the abdominal wall for eliminating waste.)

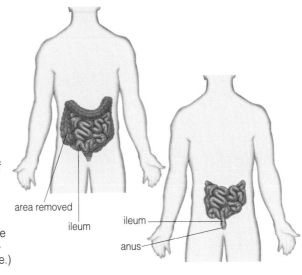

area removed
ileum
ileum
anus

examination and tests to rule out other intestinal problems. Blood tests are conducted to look for signs of infection as well as anemia, a common consequence of intestinal bleeding. X-rays of the colon taken after a barium enema will also be ordered.

An examination of the colon using a colonoscope, a viewing instrument with special lights and magnifying devices, is the next diagnostic step. During this procedure, tissue samples are removed for biopsy studies.

In ulcerative colitis, the mucous membrane lining the entire colon will be seen as uniformly inflamed and ulcerated. A portion of the small intestine that adjoins the colon may also be inflamed, but this is not a major characteristic. In addition, the lining might show evidence of dysplasia, precancerous changes that eventually develop into invasive colon cancer.

In its early stages, Crohn's disease can be difficult to differentiate from ulcerative colitis, but the colonoscopy and biopsies usually reveal some significant differences. In Crohn's disease, the inflammation involves all layers of the intestine, not just the lining, but is often confined to specific areas interspersed between normal sections. Laparoscopy, in which a viewing device is inserted into the abdominal cavity through a small incision, may show that the tissue surrounding the intestines, the mesentery, as well as nearby lymph nodes, are also swollen and inflamed. As the disease progresses, the intestine becomes thickened and leathery, and the channel through which food and waste must flow becomes

progressively narrowed and stiff. Extensive ulcerations often lead to the formation of fissures, or tears, and fistulas, abnormal channels between segments of the intestine.

Medical Treatments

Inflammatory bowel disorders cannot be cured by medications, although in some cases, they will disappear for long periods or even for life. The goal of treatment is to alleviate symptoms and, if possible, achieve a remission. Mild cases can be treated on an outpatient basis, but severe flare-ups require hospitalization for intravenous fluids, drugs, and in cases where there is significant bleeding, blood transfusions.

Sulfasalazine (Azulfidine), a combination of a sulfa drug and a compound similar to aspirin, and corticosteroids are the principal drugs used to control inflammatory bowel diseases. Steroids may be given by mouth or by injection during a flare-up and then tapered off slowly. They also may be administered as an infusion into the lower colon and rectum. This enema form has fewer side effects than systemic steroids.

In some cases, medications that suppress the immune system may be prescribed. Broad-spectrum antibiotics may also be administered, especially in severe cases in which perforation of the intestine is a possibility.

Surgery is often required to treat severe Crohn's disease, especially if there is an intestinal obstruction or other complication. Usually, the operation involves removing the diseased section of intestine and joining together the two healthy ends, a procedure called resection and anastomosis. This often improves the patient's condition dramatically, with the symptoms disappearing for many years. It is not a cure, however, as the disease frequently recurs at or near the site where the two healthy sections were joined.

In cases of ulcerative colitis, surgery to remove the entire colon and rectum affords a permanent cure. However, the treatment is one of last resort because it usually means that the patient must eliminate solid wastes through a stoma (page 141), an artificial opening in the abdominal wall. To avoid this, a new procedure called ileoanal anastomosis is used. It involves retaining the rectum but stripping off its innermost layer and inserting, just above the anus, a pouch made from the ileum portion of the small intestine. Because the rectal muscles are preserved, the patient can have normal bowel movements.

Alternative Therapies

Inflammatory bowel diseases require expert medical care. In general, any alternative therapies should be directed to reducing stress or devising a diet that minimizes symptoms.

Aromatherapy. Massages or relaxing baths incorporating basil, bergamot, and jasmine oils are recommended by aromatherapists to reduce stress.

Nutrition Therapy. Proper nutrition is probably the single most important nonmedical treatment for inflammatory bowel disease; patients should consult a clinical dietitian trained in their management. Although foods play no role in causing these disorders, the typical symptoms of reduced appetite, poor

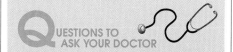

QUESTIONS TO ASK YOUR DOCTOR

▶ Is pregnancy dangerous for a woman who has inflammatory bowel disease? Can it affect her fetus?
▶ If colon removal is necessary, can normal bowel function be preserved?
▶ How often should I be screened for colon cancer?

absorption of nutrients, and diarrhea rob the body of essential fluids, nutrients, vitamins, and minerals.

Nutrition therapy is aimed at restoring a proper nutritional balance and, in severe cases, resting the bowel to give it a chance to heal. Thus, bland, low-fiber foods are recommended during a flare-up. Foods that are difficult to digest, such as raw vegetables, raw or dried fruits, nuts and seeds, bran, and whole grains should also be avoided.

Patients with Crohn's disease are often put on a high-protein diet, and many require nutritional supplements and concentrated liquid feedings, or an elemental diet, which does not produce any solid wastes. Intravenous feedings may be necessary, especially for children who cannot otherwise eat enough for proper growth and development.

Psychotherapy. Inflammatory bowel diseases are not psychosomatic, but emotional problems are a precipitating factor in both their instigation and flare-ups. Also, coping with a serious chronic illness is stressful in itself.

Some form of counseling or therapy is often helpful, particularly if the therapist has a special interest in dealing with patients who have these disorders. *Yoga and Meditation.* The breathing, meditation, and gentle exercises of yoga are helpful in controlling stress and perhaps preventing recurrences.

Self-Treatment

Most people with these diseases can lead productive lives, even though symptoms may flare up periodically and possibly require hospitalization. Doctors stress that patients should continue with school, work, and other activities as much as possible, but in moderation, to minimize undue stress and to conserve weight and strength.

During a flare-up, self-care can reduce complications. To combat dehydration, a potentially serious side effect of diarrhea, increase your fluid intake. Drink water, clear broth, or a rehydration fluid such as Gatorade, which also helps replace the electrolytes that are lost during bouts of diarrhea. Try the BRAT diet—bananas, rice, applesauce, and toast—to reduce diarrhea. Also keep a list of foods that seem to be associated with worsening the symptoms, and avoid them.

Other Causes of the Symptoms of Intestinal Inflammation

Diarrhea and cramping can be due to irritable bowel syndrome, a viral or bacterial infection, intestinal parasites, lactose intolerance, and malabsorption syndromes. Blood in the stool may be caused by hemorrhoids, colon polyps, or intestinal cancer.

A CASE IN POINT

Jessica Myers was diagnosed as having colitis midway through her freshman year in college. At first, she attributed her diarrhea, cramps, and fever to a bad bout of stomach flu. But when bright red blood appeared in her stool, she was promptly hospitalized.

Colonoscopy revealed inflammation and ulcerations along her colon wall and Myers was started on intravenous fluids, a sulfa drug, and prednisone, a steroid, to stop the inflammation and promote healing. After two weeks in the hospital, she was sent home to begin recuperating. By the fall, Myers was off the steroids and again enrolled for classes; then she

suffered a relapse during finals week. This time she recognized the warning symptoms, and her doctor immediately resumed her steroid medication—a treatment that Myers dreaded. "Prednisone gave me terrible acne and made me gain weight," she explained. "It also sent me into an emotional tailspin."

Over the next year, she suffered two more flare-ups. Each time, she was put back on prednisone. After the second occurrence, her parents sought help from a support group for colitis patients and their families. At one of the meetings, she met a young attorney who had experienced similar bouts of colitis and had

been helped by a holistic nutritionist. Myers consulted the same nutritionist, who provided much more than dietary advice. "She taught me meditation, relaxation, and visualization," Myers said. "For the first time, I felt that I had some control over this frustrating disease."

By the time Myers returned to college, she had made peace with the fact that she had a chronic condition that could be exacerbated by stress. "I no longer worried that it was going to take me six years to graduate," she explained. "I had learned to set realistic goals. Daily meditation, a healthy diet, and a new outlook gave me a new lease on life."

Ingrown Toenail

(Onychocryptosis)

An ingrown toenail occurs when one side at the top of a nail turns under and cuts into the skin that surrounds it, causing the area to become very sensitive to pressure from a shoe. The nail of the big toe is the one affected most often. If untreated, the tissue around the ingrown nail becomes swollen and inflamed. Continued pressure may also cause small, painful corns to develop in the groove of the nail.

An ingrown toenail is usually the result of cutting the nail on a curve instead of straight across, or cutting it too short. Shoes that are too short or narrow can also contribute to the problem. Other precipitating factors include a foot injury or faulty foot structure that leads to an uneven distribution of body weight.

Diagnostic Studies and Procedures

Ordinarily, an ingrown nail is immediately obvious and does not require any other diagnostic procedure. If there are complications, such as an abnormal gait, X-rays of the foot may be ordered.

Medical Treatments

When circulation is poor due to diabetes or some other chronic condition, it is important that an ingrown toenail be treated by a podiatrist or a medical doctor who specializes in foot disorders, especially if there are signs of infection. If the area is badly infected, an antibiotic should be administered.

In severe cases, a portion of toenail may require surgical removal. This can be done as an outpatient procedure by a podiatrist or a general surgeon. The doctor first numbs the area with a local anesthetic, then removes the part of the nail that has grown inward. If some surrounding soft tissue has to be cut away, a few stitches may be necessary.

If infection is severe, it is sometimes advisable to remove the nail itself and the matrix (or nail bed) from which it

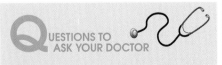

QUESTIONS TO
ASK YOUR DOCTOR

► Should I try cutting a notch in the middle of the affected nail?
► What protective measures should I take if the nail is permanently removed from my big toe?

REMOVING A MILDLY INGROWN TOENAIL

1. Soak the affected foot for 10 minutes in two quarts of warm water to which 2 tablespoons of mild detergent have been added.
2. After drying the foot, place an ice cube against the toe for about three minutes to numb the surface (A).
3. Using a toenail clipper that has been sterilized by rinsing with alcohol or wiping with Betadine solution, insert the clipper under the border of the nail at a slight angle and clip out the ingrown part (B). Hold the clippers as close to the nail as possible to avoid cutting into surrounding flesh.
4. With sterilized tweezers, carefully remove the loose portion of the nail (C).
5. If the area is bleeding slightly, keep the foot raised and apply an ice pack, taking care not to put too much pressure on the toe.
6. Dry the foot, apply Betadine solution to the toe with a cotton swab, and cover it with a wide adhesive bandage.
7. During healing, soak the toe in the morning and again at bedtime in warm water, and after drying, apply Betadine solution.
8. If necessary during healing, wear a shoe that has been cut open at the toe. Or weather permitting, wear sandals.

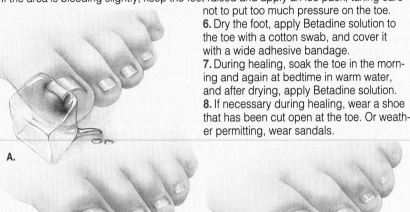

A.

B.

C.

grows. This is accomplished by making a small incision at the base of each side of the toenail. The flap of skin is pulled back so that the matrix is exposed. The entire nail is removed and the matrix is destroyed by cauterizing (burning) it, or by applying an acid solution that disintegrates it. (If the matrix is not completely destroyed, the nail may grow back in the same distorted way. Once a matrix has been fully removed, the nail will never grow back.) After destroying the matrix, the doctor then reattaches the skin flap to the surrounding tissue with small stitches.

Following this operation, the toe is wrapped in a soft dressing, and the patient wears a surgical shoe or uses crutches until the foot can bear full weight. Oral antibiotics are usually given, and medicated toe soaks may be advised. Two days after the operation, the toe is examined to check on healing. Stitches are removed in a week. Healing progresses more quickly if the patient keeps the foot elevated whenever possible. The toe should be healed completely in six weeks.

Sometimes laser surgery is an acceptable alternative, but its merits are open to debate. Proponents claim that laser

surgery is faster and less painful than conventional methods. Its detractors believe that conventional surgery is more likely to produce a cure because laser surgery may leave behind a few matrix cells, thus allowing the regrowth of the ingrown nail.

Alternative Therapies

Alternative therapies are of little value in treating an ingrown toenail.

Self-Treatment

If the problem is due to improper toenail cutting and involves only a small portion of the nail, cutting a notch in the middle of the nail may be sufficient. This redirects nail growth from the edge to the center. You can also cut out the ingrown portion (see box, above). However, this approach is advisable only in the earliest stage of the condition and should not be attempted if the surrounding area is inflamed, markedly swollen, or infected.

To prevent ingrown toenails, cut nails straight across. Also, wear shoes that are comfortably wide and round-toed rather than narrow and pointed. Avoid wearing extremely tight socks.

Other Causes of Ingrown Nails

A fungal infection can cause misshapen and ingrown nails.

Intermittent Claudication

(Arteriosclerosis obliterans)

Intermittent claudication refers to impaired blood circulation in a muscle during exercise. It develops commonly in the legs, causing symptoms that can range from a tired feeling to a crampy ache, a burning sensation, or severe pain. The discomfort occurs most often in the calf but also may arise in the foot, thigh, hip, or buttocks.

Symptoms usually develop after walking for a time. People with this condition can avoid them by resting before pain would normally occur. When discomfort does develop, it often disappears after a few minutes of rest.

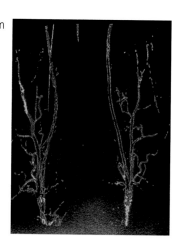

The arteriogram on the right shows extensive blockage of an artery in the lower leg.

As the disease worsens, however, the distance one can walk before pain occurs decreases, and eventually, pain may be felt even during rest. At this stage, the foot might be painful, cold, or numb, and the skin dry and scaly. The poor circulation may result in skin ulcers on the lower leg or foot and, in the worst cases, gangrene.

Intermittent claudication is caused by atherosclerosis, the buildup of fatty deposits, or plaque, on the inner lining of artery walls. Other contributing factors include smoking, hypertension, diabetes, and inactivity.

Diagnostic Studies and Procedures

A doctor immediately suspects intermittent claudication when a patient describes the typical characteristics. Also, the pulse over the arteries in the leg or ankle may be weak. The areas of blockage can be identified by Doppler ultrasonography, the use of sound

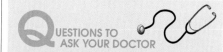

QUESTIONS TO ASK YOUR DOCTOR

▶ What can I do to avoid leg pain at night, especially if it interrupts my sleep?
▶ Do support hose hurt or help?

waves to study blood flow, and an arteriogram, an X-ray of the blood vessels, taken after injection of a dye.

Medical Treatments

Many doctors recommend daily low-dose aspirin (one-half to one regular 325 milligram tablet) to help reduce the risk of blood clots, which develop commonly in arteries narrowed by atherosclerosis. A doctor may prescribe pentoxifylline (Trental), a drug that thins the blood so that it flows more easily through smaller blood vessels. However, this medication helps only about one-third of patients, and many are unable to tolerate its side effects.

In severe cases where pain occurs during rest, invasive procedures are recommended. If there is only a single blockage or a small number of isolated ones, angioplasty is the treatment of first choice. Or surgery might be suggested. One common operation is an endarterectomy, in which the artery is opened, fatty plaque removed, and the vessel reclosed. Alternatively, the affected arteries may be bypassed, which is done by inserting a vein taken from elsewhere in the body or a graft made from synthetic material.

Alternative Therapies

Exercise Conditioning. Mainstream physicians and alternative practitioners alike recommend daily exercise as an integral component of treating intermittent claudication. Most regimens call for walking at least 35 minutes daily, working up to an hour a day. Stop as often as necessary and wait for discomfort to abate. Practiced daily, this program will increase the distance you can walk before pain begins. Using a stationary exercise cycle is an acceptable alternative to walking.

Herbal Medicine. A salve of horse chestnut extract is said to benefit poor circulation. It can be applied directly to the legs to ease leg cramps. Other possible herbal remedies include butcher's broom capsules or tea, gingko

extract, and hawthorn berry capsules—all said to improve circulation.

Nutrition Therapy. Vitamin E supplements are recommended to improve circulation in cases of extensive atherosclerosis. Some nutritionists theorize that the vitamin enables muscles to do more work before pain occurs. Lecithin capsules or powder may reduce buildup of fatty plaque; chlorophyll (liquid or pills) is said to enhance circulation.

Self-Treatment

In addition to daily exercises, self-care includes the following:

▶ Do not smoke, and avoid second-hand smoke. Smoking contributes to atherosclerosis and also reduces the amount of oxygen available to muscles.
▶ Follow a low-fat, high-fiber diet that emphasizes whole grains, fruits, and vegetables, which can reduce cholesterol levels. Maintain your ideal weight; obesity puts an extra burden on legs.
▶ Do not wear garters or socks with tight elastic bands, which can further impair blood flow. Choose cotton or wool socks in cold weather to keep feet warm. Make sure that your shoes fit properly and are made of leather or a fabric that allows air to circulate.
▶ Wash feet gently every day with lukewarm water and mild soap and apply a moisturizer. Have corns, calluses, and other foot problems treated by a podiatrist or doctor to avoid infections.

Other Causes of Leg Pain

Phlebitis, varicose veins, certain types of arthritis, and sports-related injuries can also cause leg pain.

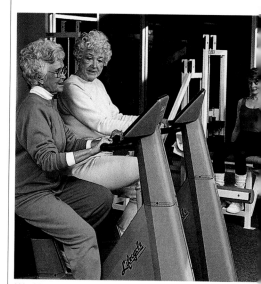

Working out on a stationary exercise cycle improves circulation in the legs and increases endurance as well.

Interstitial Cystitis

(Painful bladder syndrome)
This painful, chronic inflammation of the bladder varies considerably in its severity and symptoms, depending upon the form of the disease. Nonulcerative interstitial cystitis—by far the most common type—develops mostly in young to middle-aged women, and is marked by intermittent episodes of abdominal and bladder pain, urinary urgency, and painful sexual intercourse. Bladder capacity remains constant or perhaps slightly increased, in marked contrast to the more severe ulcerative form, which occurs mostly in older women and accounts for only 5 to 10 percent of cases. In this latter type, the bladder holds less urine than normal, and cracks, scars, and star-shaped sores called Hunner's ulcers, which sometimes bleed when the bladder is full, develop in the muscular wall. In time, the bladder wall becomes thickened and stiff.

The incidence of interstitial cystitis is unknown, but it's been estimated that it afflicts 500,000 Americans, 90 percent of them women. Unlike ordinary cystitis (page 152), which is usually caused by a bacterial infection, interstitial cystitis has no known cause. Possible predisposing factors are under study, including frequent childhood urinary tract infections, bladder damage from surgery, and toxic substances in the urine. Stress appears to trigger flare-ups.

Diagnostic Studies and Procedures
There is no single test to diagnose interstitial cystitis, but a doctor suspects it when a patient describes symptoms of cystitis but a urine culture fails to grow bacteria and antibiotics do not alleviate discomfort. Before concluding that a patient has interstitial cystitis, however, a doctor must rule out other conditions, including urinary tract or genital infections, cancer, kidney or bladder stones, and neurological disorders.

The doctor may inspect the bladder by cystoscopy, in which a lighted viewing device is inserted into the urethra and bladder. In nonulcerative cystitis, the bladder may appear normal. (In the ulcerative form, cystoscopy usually reveals the characteristic scarring and ulcers.) Even if the bladder appears normal, tiny areas of pin-point bleeding

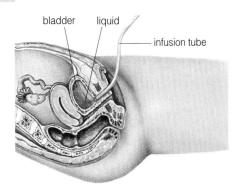
bladder   liquid
infusion tube

To diagnose non-ulcerative interstitial cystitis, the bladder is filled artificially and the distended walls are then inspected for tiny bleeding sores.

called glomerulations are often revealed after the organ is distended by filling it with water or gas. Both cystoscopy and bladder distention are painful procedures that are performed after administering local anesthesia.

Medical Treatments
A doctor may start with aspirin or ibuprofen and move to stronger nonsteroidal anti-inflammatory agents such as naproxen (Naprosyn) or piroxicam (Feldene). Sodium pentosanpolysulfate (Elmiron), an experimental drug used for bladder washes, may restore the bladder lining. Another experimental drug called nalmefene (Incystene) may block off pain receptors, thus alleviating this symptom. Amitriptyline (Elavil), an antidepressant drug, may also alleviate pain and night voiding.

In some cases, bladder distention may be tried, as some patients have noticed an improvement in symptoms following the procedure.

Another approach involves periodically instilling RIMSO-50, a compound made from the industrial solvent DMSO, into the bladder. (This is the only FDA-approved medical use of DSMO.) The substance passes into the bladder wall, reducing inflammation and perhaps halting painful muscle contractions. Its major drawback is that it produces a strong, garlic-like breath and skin odor for up to 72 hours.

In severe cases, surgery may be considered. However, the results vary and symptoms sometimes recur. Laser

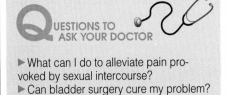
QUESTIONS TO ASK YOUR DOCTOR
▶ What can I do to alleviate pain provoked by sexual intercourse?
▶ Can bladder surgery cure my problem?

surgery may be used to seal off ulcerated areas; alternatively, resection consists of removing ulcers by cutting around them. In intractable cases, approaches may include: denervation, in which some nerves to the bladder are cut to alleviate pain; augmentation, which enlarges the bladder, usually by adding a section of the patient's small intestine; and cystectomy, in which all or part of the bladder is removed. After a cystectomy, a stoma is needed to reroute urine. Or the bladder may be replaced with a pouch made from a piece of the large intestine.

Alternative Therapies
Although alternative therapies cannot cure the syndrome, some can alleviate its most troublesome symptoms.
Acupuncture and Acupressure. These techniques may be helpful in alleviating chronic pain.
TENS. In this approach, which stands for transcutaneous electrical nerve stimulation, mild electrical impulses are sent into the skin, creating a sensation that distracts from the pain impulses.
Yoga and Meditation. These and other relaxation techniques can help reduce stress, which aggravates symptoms.

Self-Treatment
Bladder retraining sometimes helps. For a week or two, keep a careful diary of how often you urinate daily. Then try to extend the typical time between voidings by 10 or 15 minutes.

Experts recommend experimenting with the diet to identify foods that provoke symptoms. Acidic and highly spiced foods often cause problems. Keep a food diary, then eliminate likely offenders, returning them one at a time.

Abstain completely from smoking, alcohol, and artificial sweeteners; reduce or eliminate caffeine. Also, use caution when taking supplements, especially vitamin C, which irritates the bladder.

Other Causes of Bladder Inflammation
A bacterial urinary tract infection is the most common cause of bladder inflammation. Symptoms may also be produced by bladder stones, urethritis, or an enlarged prostate.

252

Intestinal Cancer

(Adenocarcinoma; carcinoid; intestinal lymphoma; leiomyosarcoma)

Intestinal cancer usually refers to a malignancy of the small intestine. It is relatively rare in the United States, with only about 3,600 new cases a year. (In contrast, cancer of the colon, or large intestine, is second only to lung cancer in prevalence.) When intestinal cancer does occur, it is often in conjunction with other disorders. For example, persons with inflammatory bowel disease (page 248) have an increased risk of adenocarcinoma, a cancer in which the malignant cells function like glands and produce hormones, mucus, or other glandular substances.

The risk of intestinal lymphoma, a cancer of the lymph structures, increases with the presence of celiac sprue, a type of malabsorption disorder (page 283). In many cases, neither adenocarcinoma nor intestinal lymphoma have any symptoms until they begin to spread. Then, there may be pain, bleeding, and an intestinal obstruction.

A rare type of cancer, leiomyosarcoma, develops in the smooth muscle cells of the intestine, and sometimes produces large tumors that can be felt by pressing on the abdomen.

Still another type of intestinal cancer is a carcinoid tumor, a slow-growing malignancy that secretes a number of hormones and other body chemicals, resulting in a constellation of symptoms known as the carcinoid syndrome. These include diarrhea, cramps, hot

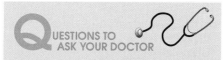
flashes, and skin flushing. Some patients may also develop asthma and heart valve disease. These cancers commonly arise in the appendix and often spread to the liver.

Diagnostic Studies and Procedures

X-rays taken after swallowing barium can be helpful as an initial study. However, if intestinal cancer is suspected, the primary diagnostic technique is enteroscopy. In this procedure, a thin, flexible tube with lighting and magnifying devices is inserted through the mouth, esophagus, and stomach, into the small intestine, allowing the doctor to view its inner lining. The enteroscope also has attachments that make it easier to suction off secretions or take tissue samples for biopsy studies.

Imaging studies, such as CT scans, MRI, or ultrasonography, may be called for when a carcinoid tumor is suspected. The blood and urine will also be analyzed for the presence of specific chemicals produced by the tumor.

Medical Treatments

Adenocarcinomas and leiomyosarcomas are removed surgically, often followed by radiation therapy. As intestinal cancers tend to recur, repeated operations may be necessary. Chemotherapy also may be administered if the cancer has spread beyond its original site. With intestinal lymphoma, the tumor is removed and follow-up treatment includes abdominal radiation therapy and chemotherapy.

Carcinoid tumors are also taken out, followed by chemotherapy. If the cancer has spread to the liver, the diseased portion of that organ is also removed, if

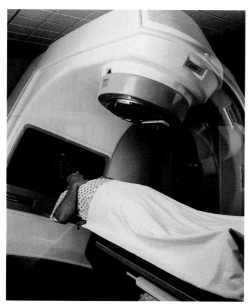

Radiation therapy is often part of treatment for intestinal cancer. Because high-technology X-ray machines can administer precise doses of radiation to very small areas, damage to the healthy tissue surrounding a tumor is usually minimal.

possible. To treat carcinoid syndrome symptoms, various drugs are prescribed, including cimetidine (Tagamet) or ranitidine (Zantac) for flushing, as well as drugs to control diarrhea.

Alternative Therapies

These should be used only as adjuncts to medical treatments for controlling pain and other symptoms.

Hypnotherapy. This technique has proved useful in pain management, particularly for advanced cancer.

Meditation. Meditation can reduce stress, help control pain, and improve the quality of life for cancer patients.

Nutrition Therapy. Normal eating may be difficult following intestinal surgery, especially if a large portion of the small intestine has been removed. A clinical dietitian or nutrition therapist who is trained in working with cancer patients should be consulted.

Visualization. This therapy employs guided imaging techniques to visualize the body's white cells fighting the invading cancer cells. It is taught in many cancer centers as a way to help patients cope with the disease.

Self-Treatment

There are measures you can take to help insure that you maintain good nutrition while undergoing treatment.

▶ Eat small, frequent meals, timed to coincide with periods free of nausea and vomiting. For example, if you normally feel best in the morning, have your main meal then.

▶ Emphasize bland, easily digested foods that provide maximum nutrition and calories. Good choices include puddings made with whole milk that is enriched with powdered milk, cream soups, puréed or creamed vegetables, ice cream, and milk shakes.

▶ Food odors often provoke nausea. Stay out of the kitchen as much as possible, and serve foods either cold or at room temperature.

▶ If diarrhea is a problem, eat a low-residue diet of BRAT (bananas, rice, applesauce, and toast). Or try an oral nutritional supplement that is formulated not to produce solid wastes.

Other Causes of Intestinal Symptoms

Bleeding, with or without pain, may be due to some other type of cancer, inflammatory bowel disease, or a peptic ulcer. Diarrhea and cramping may also be the result of inflammatory bowel disease, irritable bowel syndrome, or a gastrointestinal infection.

Iritis

(Anterior uveitis)

Iritis is an inflammation of the iris, the two-layered, pigmented tissue of the eye that defines its color. Lying under the cornea, the translucent tissue that covers the eyeball, the iris separates the front of the eye from the back. It's often likened to the diaphragm of a camera,

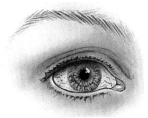

Normally, the iris appears to have straight lines radiating through it.

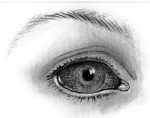

With iritis, the iris is swollen and red, and its lines are obscured.

because it functions as a shutter, responding to varying light conditions by opening or contracting the pupil.

When the iris is inflamed, the eye is red, painful, teary, and sensitive, especially to bright light. The condition can can cause severe headaches that intensify when the eyes are used continuously for several hours. If the inflammation is acute, vision will be blurred. Myopia, or nearsightedness, may also develop, although this tends to be temporary.

Iritis may follow an eye injury, in which case the entire eye is likely to be affected because of a process called sympathetic ophthalmia. But more often, it is secondary to other disorders, including nose infections, corneal ulcers, tuberculosis, and syphilis.

As part of the body's network of connective tissues, the iris is also vulnerable to inflammatory changes caused

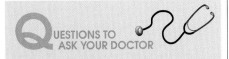

QUESTIONS TO ASK YOUR DOCTOR

▶ Are there steps I can take to reduce the chances of a recurrence?
▶ Do I have to stop wearing my contact lenses permanently? Do they increase the risk of iritis?

by autoimmune diseases in which the immune system attacks the body's healthy tissues. Thus, it is one of the manifestations of juvenile rheumatoid arthritis (page 259) and systemic lupus erythematosus (page 278), and it often occurs in conjunction with spinal arthritis (page 387). In more than half of all cases, however, an underlying cause cannot be found.

Like all eye disorders, iritis produces symptoms that require prompt medical care. If neglected, the inflammation may lead to secondary glaucoma and cataract formation.

Diagnostic Studies and Procedures

An ophthalmologist, by inspecting the eye with various magnifying instruments, can readily diagnose the condition. The iris will be swollen and the lines that normally radiate through it may be obscured. An internist or other primary-care physician should also be seen for a careful physical examination and tests to determine whether the iritis is related to some other disorder.

Medical Treatments

When iritis is secondary to a systemic disease, the underlying condition will be treated. At the same time, corticosteroid eye ointment or drops will be given to reduce the inflammation. Oral steroids may also be prescribed.

To relieve pain, eye drops containing atropine may be used. This drug keeps the pupil dilated, thereby immobilizing the inflamed iris. The dilation also reduces the risk that the back of the iris may adhere to the lens and cause irreversible eye damage.

Occasionally, iritis is traced to a parasitic infection, such as toxoplasmosis. In such cases, drugs to eradicate the organism will also be prescribed.

Alternative Therapies

Alternative therapies are not recommended to treat iritis itself. However, some naturopaths and other alternative practitioners advocate iriscopy, or iridology, a diagnostic tool using a lighted magnifying device to evaluate the condition and appearance of an iris. This approach is based on the fact that an estimated half-million nerve filaments of the iris are connected to the cervical ganglia of the sympathetic nervous system. The neuro-optic reflex is said to produce changes in the color of the iris that indicate systemic disorders before they can be detected by conventional diagnostic techniques. Iridology is used

A CASE IN POINT

When 23-year-old Hope Jackson developed a red, sore eye, she at first thought it was from chlorine in her health club's swimming pool. But eye drops and a break from daily swimming failed to help; in fact, over the next week, the eye pain worsened and evolved into a dull headache. Light hurt her eye so much that she wore dark glasses even indoors.

Jackson's boss finally insisted that she see an ophthalmologist, who quickly diagnosed iritis and prescribed steroid and atropine eye drops. He also suggested that she have a checkup, explaining that iritis may signal an undiagnosed disease.

A few days later, Jackson's doctor performed a complete physical, paying special attention to her joints because iritis is sometimes linked to arthritis or lupus. He also ordered a chest X-ray and blood and urine studies, but all were normal.

In the meantime, her ophthalmologist stopped the atropine, and over the next three months, slowly tapered her off the steroid drops as well. After the drops were halted, she had a monthly checkup for the next three months. She was also cautioned to watch for any recurrent reddening, pain, or light sensitivity, but no further problems arose. In the end, she concluded: "I guess I'm one of the lucky ones whose iritis has no apparent cause, and does not recur."

more widely in Europe than the United States, though some alternative practitioners have learned its basic methods.

Self-Treatment

Avoid exposure to bright light by wearing sunglasses outdoors and dimming the lights when indoors.

Take aspirin or acetaminophen to alleviate pain. When reading or using your eyes for other tasks, take breaks often to rest your eyes.

Do not wear contact lenses until an ophthalmologist says it's safe to do so. Have frequent eye checkups, especially if using steroid eye drops.

Other Causes of Eye Redness

Disorders with pain and redness similar to those of iritis include ocular herpes, conjunctivitis, and acute glaucoma.

Iron Overload

(Hemochromatosis)

Iron overload, medically known as hemochromatosis, is an inherited metabolic disease in which the body absorbs too much iron from food. Normally, the body recycles iron from old red blood cells and absorbs new iron when its reserves are low. In hemochromotosis, this natural control goes awry, and the body both recycles its own iron and extracts more from food. Eventually, deposits of iron in many of the body's organs and tissues become dangerously high, resulting in possible diabetes and damage to the heart, liver, pancreas, joints, and testicles. Congestive heart failure is a leading cause of death among people with hemochromatosis.

Symptoms rarely appear before age 20 and are observed most commonly between ages 40 and 60. Manifestations include chronic fatigue, aching joints, gastrointestinal pains, jaundice, an enlarged liver, and cardiac arrhythmias. Many people also develop abnormally ruddy skin, especially on the face.

About one person in 10 carries the responsible gene, but to develop the disease, a person must inherit it from both parents, who may themselves be asymptomatic carriers. Hereditary, or primary, hemochromatosis is far more common than previously thought, affecting more than 1 million Americans. Men outnumber women five- to tenfold; this is attributed to the fact that women lose iron periodically through menstruation or pregnancy.

Diagnostic Studies and Procedures

Too much iron in the blood can be verified through blood tests and a liver biopsy, which will reveal the excessive iron deposits. A liver specimen is obtained by means of a thin, hollow aspiration needle.

Unfortunately, the disease often goes undiagnosed until it causes widespread damage, because early symptoms are easily mistaken for those of rheumatoid arthritis, hepatitis, or heart disease, and doctors often order extensive tests for these other diseases. With increasing awareness of hemochromatosis, however, a number of diagnostic laboratories have added a screening test for high iron levels to their list of routine blood studies. Patients who are experiencing symptoms of mysterious origin, or are visiting a doctor for a routine checkup, should request this blood test.

Medical Treatments

The only effective treatment is bloodletting, or phlebotomy. In times past, this procedure was widely practiced to treat a variety of ailments, often with disastrous results. With the advent of more effective treatments, bloodletting was deemed a form of quackery, so today, many patients with iron overload are skeptical when their doctors prescribe it. But removing a pint of blood once or twice a week for several weeks usually brings iron levels down to normal. More severe cases may require removal of larger amounts over two or three years. (The blood can be donated to a blood bank if the patient has no blood-borne diseases.) Bloodletting is then repeated from time to time whenever it's necessary.

In most cases, bloodletting therapy can reverse some heart damage, reduce the size of the liver and spleen, and return liver function to normal. Drugs may be prescribed, depending upon manifestations of the iron overload.

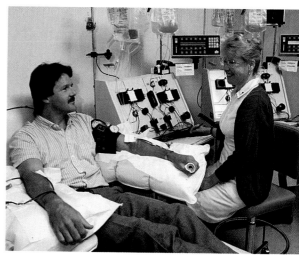

Periodic blood donation is one way to control hemochromatosis and, at the same time, possibly help others in need of blood.

For example, deferoxamine (Desferal) is prescribed to remove excessive iron in patients with severe heart disease.

Alternative Therapies

Nutrition therapy is an important adjunct to medical care. People who are genetically predisposed to conserve iron should consult with a clinical dietitian or qualified nutritionist, who will design a diet that incorporates substitutes for high-iron foods, especially red meat, liver, egg yolks, and cereals fortified with iron. Persons with iron overload should also avoid vitamin C supplements, which increase the body's iron metabolism.

Self-Treatment

Read all food labels carefully, and avoid products, especially cereals and breads, that are fortified with iron. If you are taking a daily multiple vitamin, make sure it does not contain iron. Check with your doctor to ascertain that other supplements are safe.

Other Causes of Iron Overload

Frequent blood transfusions, liver disease, or prolonged and excessive intake of iron supplements can result in iron overload without the inherited gene.

IRON IS NOT A TONIC

Contrary to popular belief, iron is not a tonic, nor is it a cure for "tired blood" or fatigue. Iron supplements should never be taken without a doctor's diagnosis of anemia. If they have been prescribed, store them in a container with a child-proof cap where children cannot reach them. Iron pills are a leading cause of accidental poisoning in children.

The possible role of iron in heart disease is under intensive study. A 1992 report by Finnish researchers suggested that high levels of iron promote heart attacks and low levels are protective. These findings support the theory that iron contributes to the formation of plaque in the artery walls, thereby interfering with the flow of blood to the heart. It is also believed that excess iron is involved in the injury and destruction of heart muscle cells during a heart attack.

Our Western diet, which is high in iron-rich red meat, may be a factor. And some researchers theorize that dietary iron, more than fat and cholesterol, may explain the diet-heart disease link.

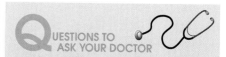

QUESTIONS TO ASK YOUR DOCTOR

▶ Should my blood be tested to see if I have high iron level?
▶ Is it possible to screen a child for the presence of the iron overload gene?
▶ Can early dietary reduction of iron prevent symptoms?

Irritable Bowel Syndrome

(Spastic colon; mucous colitis)

Irritable bowel syndrome, or IBS, produces myriad symptoms that affect mostly the large intestine. Abdominal pain and cramping, bouts of diarrhea alternating with constipation, gas, bloating, and nausea are among the complaints that make IBS the third most common intestinal disorder seen by doctors; it is exceeded only by heartburn and indigestion. An estimated 40 million Americans have the syndrome, with women outnumbering men two to one. Often associated with stress, IBS usually appears first in late adolescence or early adulthood.

The disorder affects peristalsis, the intestinal contractions that move digested food and waste through the digestive system. Normally, these contractions are gentle and well coordinated. In a person who has irritable bowel syndrome, however, peristalsis is irregular and poorly coordinated, with contractions alternating between overly forceful and too weak. This irregularity produces the characteristic symptoms.

No anatomical abnormality causes the condition, but emotional factors, diet, drugs, and hormones can precipitate or aggravate it. Some doctors believe that food allergies or sensitivities may also be involved.

Diagnostic Studies and Procedures

One key to an accurate diagnosis is a thorough medical history, including an account of the patient's medications and

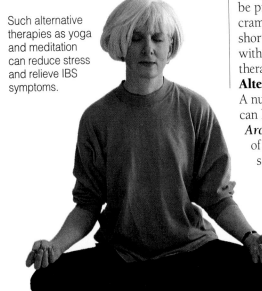

Such alternative therapies as yoga and meditation can reduce stress and relieve IBS symptoms.

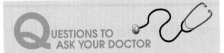
diet. The doctor will also ask about any personal problems, emotional concerns, and such habits as smoking, drinking, and recreational drug use.

Diagnostic studies are aimed at ruling out any other conditions that could cause similar symptoms. A physical will include a rectal examination, as well as a pelvic examination in women. Using a slender tube with lighting and magnifying devices, a doctor will inspect the inner lining of the rectum and the lower segment of the large intestine in a procedure called proctosigmoidoscopy. Endoscopy, a similar examination of the esophagus, stomach, and duodenum portion of the small intestine, may also be performed. And stool samples will be studied for the presence of blood and parasites.

Other tests may include an ultrasound examination of the abdominal area and barium studies of the upper and lower gastrointestinal tract. The latter tests involve taking X-rays after barium, an opaque substance, is swallowed and also infused into the colon.

Medical Treatments

Once organic disease has been ruled out, the goal of treatment is to alleviate symptoms. Antispasmodic drugs may be prescribed to relieve abdominal cramps. Some patients may be given a short course of tranquilizers to cope with a period of severe stress. Psychotherapy may also be recommended.

Alternative Therapies

A number of alternative approaches can help to control IBS.

Aromatherapy. To promote a sense of well-being, therapists recommend soaking three or four times a week in a bath with rose oil added to the water. To treat diarrhea, they advocate inhaling two drops of rosemary oil and then two drops of black pepper oil. Their remedy for constipation is to inhale two or three drops of marjoram oil.

Herbal Medicine. Cascara sagrada, or buckthorn, may promote normal digestive function, especially during a bout of constipation. It is available in capsules and tablets. Care is needed to avoid an overdose, which can cause diarrhea. Other herbs that are said to promote normal digestion are chamomile and pau d'arco, which can be taken as pills, extracts, or teas.

Hypnotherapy. Some people find this approach beneficial in dealing with the symptoms of irritable bowel syndrome, as well as for stress reduction.

Nutrition Therapy. Diet is crucial in controlling IBS. Nutritionists suggest keeping a diary to identify foods that may trigger symptoms. During a flare-up, a bland diet that eliminates fatty or spicy foods may help. Some naturopathic nutritionists recommend charcoal tablets to alleviate gas.

After symptoms subside, a low-fat, high-fiber diet is prescribed. Drinking three glasses of unsweetened black currant juice a day is said to help regulate bowel function. To minimize gas and bloating, such foods as beans, cabbage, and onions should be avoided.

Reflexology. Practitioners use foot massage to treat diarrhea and constipation, as well as cramping and bloating.

Yoga and Meditation. These and other relaxation techniques can help counter the stress that often precipitates IBS.

Self-Treatment

Self-care emphasizes a lifestyle of moderation. Abstain from alcohol and caffeine, or use these substances only occasionally and in small amounts. Exercise regularly, and make sure you get enough sleep. Strive to manage stress; if you find this difficult, try the alternative therapies described above. Or experiment with progressive relaxation exercises, in which you alternately contract and relax muscle groups, starting with the toes and working upward; whenever stress mounts, take 10 to 15 minutes to go through this routine. During a flare-up, alleviate pain and cramping with a heating pad, hot water bottle, or warm bath.

Other Causes of Irritable Bowel Symptoms

Inflammatory bowel disorders and diverticulosis can produce similar symptoms. Intestinal parasites, particularly giardia, may also be responsible, as may lactose intolerance or various malabsorption syndromes.

Itching

(Pruritus)

From time to time, everyone develops an itching sensation, which prompts an instinctive desire to scratch. Most itches are caused by localized skin conditions, that range from insect bites or dry skin, to allergic reactions or rashes resulting from chickenpox, athlete's foot, and other infectious diseases. A maddening and persistent itch characterizes some skin disorders, especially eczema, and stress can either produce or aggravate it.

Diagnostic Studies and Procedures

The presence of an itch is readily apparent, but tracking down the cause often requires some medical detective work, such as a review of recent activities. If there is no evidence of dry skin, a rash, or another type of skin lesion, a doctor may order blood and urine studies to identify an underlying cause (see Other Causes of Itching, below.)

Medical Treatments

Simply eliminating an underlying disorder usually solves the problem. In the meantime, a cortisone cream or topical antihistamine/antipruretic (anti-itching) product may be advised, depending

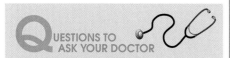

QUESTIONS TO ASK YOUR DOCTOR

▶ Do you think my itching is due to an underlying disease? If so, what tests might pinpoint the cause?
▶ How can I prevent a young child from scratching an area that itches?

upon the reason for the itching. For example, cortisone eases itching from insect bites and allergies but should not be used for fungal infections.

If itching is interfering with sleep, an oral antihistamine, such as astemizole (Hismanal), may be prescribed. For severe, chronic itching, a tranquilizer, such as hydroxyzine (Atarax), may provide relief.

Alternative Therapies

Numerous alternative remedies can alleviate itching; they include:

Biofeedback Training. This approach may be advised for chronic itching that does not appear to be caused by an underlying disease.

Herbal Medicine. Creams or lotions containing aloe vera can stop itching brought on by dry skin. For itching eczema, try chickweed applied as an ointment or cream or in oil form added to bathwater. Herbalists also recommend urtica dioica (stinging nettle) capsules for localized itching. Chinese herbalists advocate pueraria (arrow root vine) for generalized itching.

Hydrotherapy. Topical poultices or bath additives can often ease itching. Try adding cornstarch, baking soda, or colloidal oatmeal to bathwater. Alternating cold and hot water sprays may also bring relief. Be aware, however, that too much bathing can aggravate dry skin, especially in winter.

Meditation and Visualization. These and other relaxation techniques, including self-hypnosis, may help prevent itching related to stress.

Nutrition Therapy. Food allergies and sensitivities provoke hives and itching in many people. If itching appears to be related to your diet, keep a food diary to help identify likely culprits. Then eliminate these foods for two or three weeks to see if the itching abates. Return the foods, one at a time; should itching recur, avoid that food.

Self-Treatment

Scratching results in an "itch-scratch-itch" cycle that intensifies the itching and can lead to an infection. Try a counterirritant ointment instead.

When bathing, wash with warm, rather than hot, water. Choose a soap formulated for dry skin, avoiding deodorant soaps and others that may contain harsh chemicals. After bathing, pat your skin dry; don't rub it. Before you are totally dry, apply a moisturizing lotion containing lactic acid or 10 percent urea to your whole body.

Should you develop itchy skin when you are wearing a new garment or one that has just been washed, you may be reacting to the fabric or to chemicals in the detergent. Try washing the garment in a mild soap. If it still provokes itching, suspect the material itself.

Other Causes of Itching

Generalized itching can stem from an obstruction of the bile ducts, jaundice, thyroid disease, uremia, lymphoma, leukemia, or polycythemia, a blood disorder in which the body produces too many red blood cells. Pregnancy is occasionally associated with itching. Some drugs also cause itching.

Each winter, Barbara Caldwell suffered from dry, itchy skin, and each year, the problem got worse. Finally, Caldwell mentioned the itchiness to her family doctor, but he dismissed it as simply dry skin and aging.

"As we grow older, our skin gets thinner and dryer," he said. "Keep using lotion and hope for an early spring." As a lifelong resident of Maine, the 64-year-old Caldwell knew that spring seldom came early. One blustery January day, therefore, she decided it would be worth making the 50-mile drive to see the nearest dermatologist.

The dermatologist diagnosed her problem as xeroderma, the medical term for winter itch and chapping. In many cases, winter itch is related to eczema; the skin is always vulnerable to scaling and itchiness, but the condition worsens when the air is cold and dry. In other instances, the problem develops only during the winter. Caldwell fell into this latter category.

The next step was to find out what was aggravating the itching, so the dermatologist asked Caldwell about her habits and how her house was heated. The answers provided several avenues of attack.

The doctor advised Caldwell to take a tepid shower every other day instead of her long, hot, nightly baths. "Hot water draws oil and water from the skin," she explained, "and it also increases surface blood circulation, which can add to itchiness." The dermatologist also recommended using a nondrying soap substitute and, afterward, applying an emollient containing lactic acid, as well as a nonprescription hydrocortisone cream for especially itchy places.

The Caldwells relied on central heating, which makes winter air even dryer than normal, promoting further evaporation of moisture from the skin. The doctor suggested putting pans of water on each radiator to add moisture to the air and taking up indoor winter gardening, since house plants give off moisture.

A few weeks of this routine brought marked improvement in Caldwell's skin condition. And she discovered a new hobby—growing fresh herbs and salad greens in her indoor window boxes.

Jaundice

(Hyperbilirubinemia)

Jaundice is a yellowing of the skin, whites of the eyes, and mucous membranes. The discoloration results from a buildup in the blood of bilirubin, a pigment produced when the hemoglobin in worn-out red blood cells is broken down so that its iron can be recycled to make new blood cells.

Normally, the liver metabolizes and converts bilirubin into substances that are transported with bile into the intestinal tract to be eliminated. These by-products give feces its brown color.

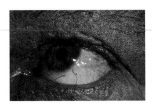

An individual with jaundice may have yellow tinges in the whites of the eyes.

Thus, jaundice is typically accompanied by light stools and dark urine, resulting from the kidneys' attempt to eliminate excess bilirubin from the body.

Various conditions can cause the buildup of bilirubin and different types of jaundice, including the following:

Hemolytic jaundice develops when an unusually large number of red blood cells are destroyed at the same time and the liver is unable to metabolize all of the resulting bilirubin.

Obstructive jaundice, or cholestasis, occurs when the bile ducts to the intestine are blocked, causing the bilirubin to be reabsorbed into the bloodstream.

Hepatic jaundice is caused by hepatitis and other disorders that not only reduce the liver's ability to process bilirubin, but also produce inflammation, which blocks bile channels and prevents the exit of bile that is processed.

Neonatal jaundice often develops in the first few days of life because of the liver's immaturity. About half of all newborns develop this type of jaundice. It usually clears up by the time a baby is 7 to 10 days old but may linger in premature infants. Mild jaundice is not serious, but very high bilirubin levels may require treatment.

Diagnostic Studies and Procedures

This condition should always receive prompt attention by a doctor, who will begin by noting skin color and asking questions about lifestyle, chronic ill-

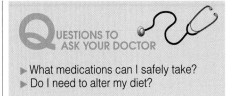

QUESTIONS TO ASK YOUR DOCTOR

▶ What medications can I safely take?
▶ Do I need to alter my diet?

ness, medications, alcohol consumption, and possible exposure to harmful chemicals. The doctor will also inquire about itchiness, the color of urine and stools, and digestive problems—all of which are common aspects of jaundice.

Urine, stool, and blood samples may be sent to a laboratory for special tests, which can be used to diagnose many liver disorders, including hepatitis and damage from drugs, chemicals, and other toxic substances. However, a liver biopsy may be needed to diagnose liver cancer and other conditions.

If obstructive jaundice is suspected, further diagnostic procedures may include abdominal X-rays, sonography, and CT scans or MRI. In some cases, laparoscopy, an examination in which a viewing tube is inserted into the abdominal cavity through a small incision, is necessary to make a diagnosis.

Medical Treatments

Medical treatments for jaundice are determined by the underlying cause. Obstructive jaundice usually requires some sort of intervention—surgery, endoscopy, or the insertion of drainage tubes—to unblock the bile ducts.

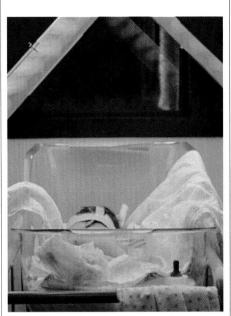

Newborns with jaundice are treated with exposure to ultraviolet light.

Rest and avoidance of alcohol and other toxic substances are the main treatments for many types of liver disease. The liver has remarkable regenerative capabilities and often heals itself, at which time the jaundice disappears.

Mild neonatal jaundice can usually be minimized by frequent feedings to increase excretion of bilirubin in the stools. In more severe cases, exchange transfusions of blood may be necessary.

Alternative Therapies

After a medical diagnosis has been established, various alternative therapies may be useful.

Herbal Medicine. Herbalists recommend milk thistle extract, dandelion extract or tea, and black radish extract to strengthen and rebuild the liver. Tea made from dried wild Oregon grape is also said to help overcome jaundice.

Light Therapy. Exposing a jaundiced newborn to ultraviolet light speeds clearance of bilirubin from the blood.

Nutrition Therapy. Consult a clinical nutritionist if jaundice is the result of liver disease, which often causes loss of appetite. Try frequent small meals, with emphasis on complex carbohydrates and a moderate amount of fat (30 percent or less of calories) and protein (about 10 percent of calories). A proper balance of the amino acids that make up protein is especially important. Generally, protein from plants and milk is better tolerated than that from meat. Severe cases may require tube feeding or enriched liquid supplements.

Self-Treatment

Self-treatment usually involves easing the liver's workload by reducing the amount of chemicals it must process. Abstain from alcohol and take only those nutritional supplements and medications specified by your doctor. Avoid exposure to potentially harmful chemicals and gases, especially carbon tetrachloride, benzene, paint strippers, and cleaning fluids. Women should not use birth control pills.

Other Causes of Jaundice

Gallbladder disease, yellow fever, and pancreatic or liver cancer may cause yellow skin. Some women develop jaundice during pregnancy. Some 3 to 5 percent of the population may develop mild, asymptomatic jaundice. If liver-function and other laboratory tests turn out to be normal, the jaundice is probably due to slower than usual processing of bilirubin.

Juvenile Rheumatoid Arthritis

(Pauciarticular, polyarticular, or systemic JRA)

Juvenile rheumatoid arthritis, or JRA, is the most common type of arthritis in children. (See page 85 for other forms of arthritis.) It develops before the age of 16 and can take one of three forms: *Pauciarticular JRA*, the mildest type, affects only a few joints, especially large ones such as the knees, ankles, and elbows. Different joints on either side of the body are usually involved. *Polyarticular JRA,* a more severe type, generally attacks five or more joints, often those of the fingers and hands, as well as weight-bearing joints, such as the hips, knees, and ankles. This form of JRA affects the same joints on both sides of the body. *Systemic JRA, or Still's disease,* the most severe form, attacks many joints, usually the large ones, as well as some organs, often the heart and eyes.

The first typical symptoms are joint stiffness and discomfort upon arising in the morning. Systemic JRA, however, may begin with symptoms like those of an infection: high fever, especially at night; a rash on the chest and thighs; and swollen lymph nodes.

As in the adult form of rheumatoid arthritis, symptoms may come and go over many months or years. In severe cases, the swollen, inflamed joints become distorted. Though the disorder may disappear by early adulthood, in some people it recurs throughout life.

The cause is unknown, but many medical researchers believe it is an autoimmune disease, in which the immune system attacks normal body tissue as if it were a foreign invader.

Diagnostic Studies and Procedures

There is no single test that can diagnose juvenile rheumatoid arthritis. When doctors suspect the disease, they usually refer the child to a rheumatologist for additional blood tests, X-rays, and an analysis of synovial fluid taken from the affected joints.

Medical Treatments

Treatment depends on the type and severity of the disease. If only a few large joints are mildly affected, a doctor may inject cortisone or another steroid drug directly into them. This can reduce inflammation and alleviate pain without the growth problems, weight gain, bleeding problems, and other side effects of taking oral steroids.

In most cases, aspirin is the drug of choice. However, it must be taken on a regular schedule and in high doses, which can cause ringing in the ears and possible hearing loss. Because a young child may not be able to report such problems, parents should be alert for signs, such as tugging of the ears and poor response to normal sounds.

If aspirin proves insufficient, a doctor may recommend stronger nonsteroidal anti-inflammatory drugs, such as ibuprofen or naproxen, available in both prescription and over-the-counter strength. For severe cases, the more potent drugs used to treat adult rheumatoid arthritis, such as injections of gold salts and systemic steroids, may be tried. Because steroids interfere with normal growth and development, their use must be carefully monitored.

The child should be checked every few months for any complications of the disease. These include pericarditis, inflammation of the outer lining of the heart; pleuritis, inflammation of the membrane covering the lungs; and blood abnormalities, such as anemia. Because the eyes are often affected, an ophthalmologist should be seen regularly. A pediatric orthopedist may be called in to evaluate joint deformity and if necessary, do corrective surgery.

Alternative Therapies

Although medical treatment is essential to control the disease, supplemental techniques can be helpful.

Herbal Medicine. Herbalists often recommend capsules of evening primrose oil to control joint inflammation; feverfew tea to alleviate fever and other symptoms; and garlic, fresh or in capsules, to reduce joint damage.

Hydrotherapy. Hot baths or cold compresses help many patients. For others, contrast baths work best; these involve sitting in a hot tub for about

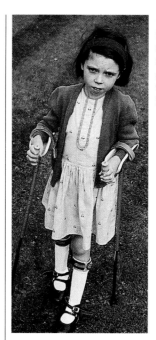

In all of its forms, juvenile rheumatoid arthritis usually affects the weight-bearing joints.

10 minutes, then standing in a cool shower for 2 or 3 minutes.

Pet Therapy. A child with JRA often lacks self-esteem and becomes lonely and withdrawn. Providing a gentle, companionable pet can foster a sense of responsibility and help compensate for not being able to engage in overly strenuous activities.

Physical and Occupational Therapy. Physical therapists teach patients special exercises that can strengthen muscles and help maintain mobility without causing joint damage. They also provide splints and other devices to protect inflamed joints.

Occupational therapists teach new approaches to daily tasks, such as getting dressed, that minimize aggravation of painful, inflamed joints.

Self-Treatment

Children with JRA should be encouraged to take part in physical activities, but these may have to be modified. Finding the right balance of rest and exercise is important. See that the child sleeps at least eight hours each night and takes a nap during the day.

Make sure that the child maintains normal weight, because excess weight increases the burden on joints. To help prevent stomach irritation, always give aspirin or nonsteroidal anti-inflammatory drugs with milk or food.

Other Causes of Joint Pain

Rheumatic fever, Lyme disease, and bone or joint infections can produce joint pain and inflammation.

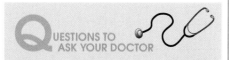

QUESTIONS TO ASK YOUR DOCTOR

▶ What side effects can occur with drugs used to treat JRA?
▶ What steps can we take to avoid permanent joint damage?

Kaposi's Sarcoma

(K.S.)

Kaposi's sarcoma (K.S.) is a cancer in which malignant cells appear as red or purple patches under the skin or the mucous membranes. These lesions most commonly originate on the legs and, depending upon their type, may spread to the lymph nodes, lungs, liver, or intestinal tract.

The disease is named for Dr. Moritz Kaposi, a Hungarian-born dermatologist who first described it in 1872 as a rare disease afflicting older Italian and Middle Eastern Jewish men. By the early 20th century, a somewhat different form was identified in Africa; it was found mostly among young men and children and was generally more lethal than the European type.

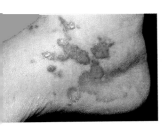

The distinctive purple and red lesions of Kaposi's sarcoma frequently appear first on the legs and feet.

In the past, Kaposi's sarcoma was a rare disease in the United States, affecting mostly recipients of kidney transplants or others with reduced immunity. This situation changed drastically with the beginning of the AIDS epidemic in 1981. Within a few years, nearly half of homosexual men who were infected with the AIDS virus also had this form of cancer. Given the pattern of the disease in Africa and its prevalence among homosexual men with AIDS, some experts believe that this aggressive form of K.S. is a sexually transmitted disease that spreads more readily among persons with lowered immunity. This theory is bolstered by research indicating a type of herpes virus may cause Kaposi's sarcoma.

In its European form, K.S. develops slowly, with an average survival rate for patients of 10 to 15 years. Otherwise, this cancer progresses rapidly and the outlook is poor, especially if it occurs along with AIDS or another condition that lowers immunity. The skin lesions themselves are painless, but they are often accompanied by widespread swelling, or edema, caused by blocked

lymph channels. Other symptoms of Kaposi's sarcoma include low-grade fever, and difficulty swallowing or breathing if there are internal lesions.

Diagnostic Studies and Procedures

The appearance of painless purple or red skin patches or nodules raises the suspicion of Kaposi's sarcoma, especially among high-risk groups, such as male homosexuals. A biopsy of the skin lesions will confirm the diagnosis. The task then is to classify the disease into one of the following categories:

Classic, or European, which progresses slowly and is confined to the legs for a number of years.

African, typically an aggressive disease affecting children and adult males.

Immunosuppressive-related, which occurs mostly among transplant patients who must take drugs that weaken the immune system to prevent rejection of the donor organ.

AIDS-related, or epidemic, which affects mostly HIV-positive males and progresses rapidly.

Medical Treatments

Treatment varies according to the type of disease. The classic and African forms are usually treated with anticancer drugs, especially vinblastine (Velban), which is given alone or in combination with vincristine (Oncovin and others). Doxorubicin (Adriamycin) and other chemotherapy agents have also produced good results. Care is needed when using a combination of anticancer drugs, however, as some of them suppress immunity.

An HIV-positive patient with only a few lesions may be treated mostly with interferon or the antiviral drug AZT, both of which are used to slow the progression of AIDS. Radiation therapy might also be used; it reduces edema and improves general appearance as well.

Experimental treatments are available to many Kaposi's sarcoma patients, especially those who have not been

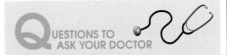

Q UESTIONS TO ASK YOUR DOCTOR

► Can radiation treatments improve the appearance of K.S. lesions?
► Am I a good candidate for any experimental treatments?
► Does K.S. increase my vulnerability to serious infection?

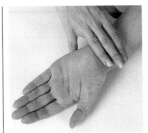

To find the acupressure point for relieving nausea caused by anticancer treatments, measure three finger widths up from the inner wrist.

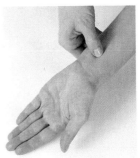

Apply steady pressure to this point until the nausea is eased. An alternative is to wear an antinausea acupressure bracelet like the one shown on page 310.

helped by standard therapies. (See Health Resources, page 465.)

Alternative Therapies

A growing number of studies show that using alternative therapies to bolster the immune system increases survival among Kaposi's sarcoma patients. The greatest benefits are noted with visualization, imagery, meditation, and other relaxation techniques that increase the production of endorphins. These are natural body chemicals that are thought to boost immunity in addition to elevating mood and dulling pain perception.

Acupressure. Persons undergoing cancer chemotherapy or radiation treatments may be able to reduce nausea by pressing on a point or the inner wrist (see photographs, above).

Self-Treatment

Regular exercise may help reduce the swelling from blocked lymph channels. If Kaposi's sarcoma is a component of AIDS, a support group of other patients with similar problems can provide valuable insight and suggestions on coping with the disease.

A consultation with a cosmetician experienced in working with people who have disfiguring skin lesions can be helpful. Numerous skin products are formulated to cover K.S. lesions, especially on the face.

Other Causes of Skin Lesions

Other types of skin cancer can bring about disfiguring lesions. Certain blood-clotting disorders can produce bruises that resemble Kaposi's sarcoma patches and nodules.

Kidney Cancer

(Renal cell carcinoma; renal pelvic carcinoma; Wilms' tumor)

Kidney cancer is relatively uncommon in the United States, accounting for about 29,000 new cases and 12,000 deaths a year. In patients of all ages, males outnumber females about two to one. There are several types of kidney cancer; the most common are:

Renal cell carcinoma, which most often originates in the nephrons, the filtering units of the kidney, and accounts for 85 percent of cases. This cancer can strike at any age, but it most common between ages 40 and 60.

Cancer of the renal pelvis, which starts in the central part of the kidney, and frequently spreads to the ureter, the tube that carries urine from the kidney, and to the bladder.

Wilms' tumor, a rare childhood malignancy, which usually occurs before the age of five years and often spreads to other abdominal organs. Wilms' tumor is quite different from adult kidney cancer. It produces a large abdominal swelling that grows rapidly. There may also be a low-grade fever, weight loss, fatigue, and other symptoms.

In adults, kidney cancer in its early stages usually does not produce symptoms, but may be detected during an examination for another problem. When symptoms do occur, they are often vague and misleading. As the cancer progresses, it may produce persistent flank pain, bloody urine, weight loss, fatigue, and malaise.

The cause of most kidney cancer is unknown, although heredity is thought to play a role. Cigarette smoking increases the risk of renal cell carcinoma, as does exposure to asbestos. Persons on long-term kidney dialysis also have an increased incidence of kidney cancer.

Diagnostic Studies and Procedures

Unexplained blood in the urine should prompt a doctor to investigate the possibility of kidney cancer, especially in an older adult. CT scanning is now the most accurate method of detecting the disease. In the past, an intravenous pyelogram—X-rays taken after an iodine solution had been injected into the bloodstream—was the major diagnostic study, and may still be ordered along with angiography, dye-enhanced X-rays of the renal blood vessels.

An ultrasonogram helps to differentiate between a fluid-filled cyst and a solid tumor. If a tumor is discovered, a biopsy will be necessary to find out if it is malignant; this is usually done by using a hollow needle to withdraw cells for laboratory analysis.

If kidney cancer is detected, additional CT scans will be done to determine whether or not it has spread to other parts of the body. At the time of diagnosis, about one-third of all renal cell carcinomas have already metastasized.

Procedures for diagnosing Wilms' tumor are essentially the same as those for adult kidney cancer. Because this cancer often spreads to the lungs, liver, and adrenal glands, the child may have to be hospitalized for special scans and liver studies.

Medical Treatments

Surgical removal is the usual treatment, most often a radical nephrectomy, in which the diseased kidney, surrounding fat and tissue, and nearby lymph nodes are excised. In 3 to 5 percent of cases, both kidneys are cancerous and must be taken out, necessitating at least two years of dialysis treatment. If there is no sign of cancer after that time, a kidney transplant may be considered.

Chemotherapy is sometimes used, especially if the cancer is inoperable or has metastasized, but only about

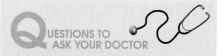

QUESTIONS TO ASK YOUR DOCTOR

▶ If I need dialysis, should I be tested for kidney cancer?
▶ What are the chances that my child's Wilms' tumor will recur?

10 percent of patients improve with it. Radiation treatments are also of little use in treating adults. More benefit has been achieved with immunotherapy, in which vaccines and other substances are given to stimulate the immune system to fight the cancer. For unexplained reasons, metastatic tumors sometimes disappear after the diseased kidney has been removed.

Unlike adult kidney cancers, Wilms' tumor is highly treatable with a combination of surgery and chemotherapy. Recent studies show that 80 to 90 percent of children survive at least two years with this combined regimen, and many of these survivors are eventually cured. The younger the child at the time of diagnosis, the better the chance of a complete cure.

Alternative Therapies

Imagery and Visualization. Because renal cell carcinoma often responds to anything that bolsters the immune system, these techniques may be especially beneficial. For added stress reduction, they are often combined with meditational yoga.

Nutrition Therapy. Although diet has no impact on kidney cancer itself, dietary changes may reduce the risk of contracting it among people who have chronic kidney stones (page 264).

Self-Treatment

Self-care is directed mostly to prevention. Do not smoke; this is especially critical. Wear a protective mask if you work with naphthalene, aniline dyes, and other potentially harmful gases or chemicals. Everyone with congenital kidney or urinary-tract abnormalities should undergo frequent screening examinations to detect possible kidney cancer in an early, more treatable stage.

Other Causes of Kidney Symptoms

Nephritis and other kidney infections can cause flank pain, bloody urine, and other symptoms similar to those of kidney cancer. Bladder and urinary tract infections also cause such symptoms and sometimes mask kidney cancer.

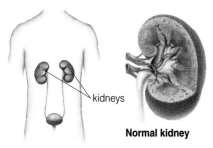

Normal kidney

Most kidney cancers start at the top of the organ in the nephrons, the organ's filtering units. Less often, they begin in the central renal pelvis and may spread to the ureter.

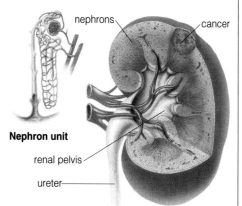

nephrons

cancer

Nephron unit

renal pelvis

ureter

Kidney Failure

(Acute or chronic renal failure)
Kidney failure occurs when these organs cease to remove toxic wastes from the blood and excrete it in the urine. There are many causes of kidney failure but it follows one of two courses:
Acute kidney failure comes on suddenly. There is an abrupt decrease in urination and widespread swelling, or edema. Warning signs include unexplained weight gain of two or more pounds a day, facial puffiness, nausea, and marked weakness. As the failure progresses, the breath may have a urine odor. This is a life-threatening medical emergency, yet most patients eventually recover kidney function.

About 60 percent of cases are associated with surgery or an injury that causes shock. Other precipitating conditions include severe kidney infection or injury, dehydration or heatstroke, poisoning, extensive burns, and failure of other organ systems. Acute kidney failure can also be a complication of pregnancy, especially if the woman has pre-eclampsia, or toxemia.
Chronic kidney failure develops slowly and is usually irreversible. The early stages may produce no noticeable symptoms. As the condition worsens, fatigue, lethargy, and headaches occur, possibly with muscle twitches, cramps, numbness, or pain in the arms or legs. In contrast to the weight gain of acute failure, the patient experiences loss of appetite and weight, nausea, vomiting, and a bad taste in the mouth.

Glomerulonephritis, in which the kidney's filtering units (nephrons) are gradually destroyed by chronic inflammation, is the most common cause of chronic kidney failure. Other causes include diabetes, high blood pressure, and such kidney disorders as hereditary polycystic kidney disease.

Diagnostic Studies and Procedures
Diagnosis requires a complete physical examination, as well as urine and blood tests, X-rays, kidney scans, and in some cases, a kidney biopsy.

Medical Treatments
Whatever the type and cause of kidney failure, renal dialysis must be performed to remove the buildup of waste products in the blood, a process called uremia. In acute failure, treatment of the underlying cause usually allows the kidneys to recuperate and return to

normal function, thus ending the need for dialysis. In the case of chronic progressive failure, however, dialysis must continue for the rest of a patient's life, unless a kidney transplant is undertaken. There are two major types of dialysis: hemodialysis and peritoneal dialysis.

In hemodialysis, the blood is filtered through a membrane in an artificial kidney machine. First, an artery and vein in either an arm or a leg are joined under the skin to form a fistula. Then a small tube, or shunt, is inserted into the fistula so that the machine can be attached to the body. During the procedure, blood is drawn from the artery, through the shunt, and into tubes that take it to an artificial kidney, where it is cleansed by a fluid called dialysate and then returned to the body through the vein.

Depending on the level of kidney failure and the machines being used, a hemodialysis session can take from three to eight hours and generally must be performed several times a week. It can take place in a hospital, an outpatient kidney dialysis center, or the patient's residence with a home dialysis machine. The last usually requires the assistance of someone who is trained in the use of the machine. Even so, most people find home dialysis less expensive than going to a dialysis center and also more convenient, as it can be done at night while they sleep. An added convenience is that a portable home machine can be used when traveling. Otherwise, advance arrangements must be made to have dialysis performed at

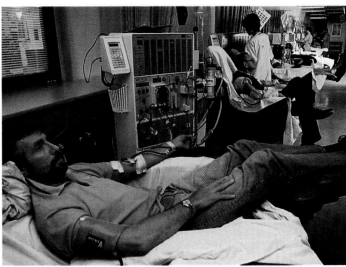
Hemodialysis, which is often done in a clinic or outpatient unit, must be performed three or four times a week as a rule.

an out-of-town site when a patient travels for more than two or three days.

Peritoneal dialysis involves using the peritoneum, the membrane that lines the abdomen, for filtering wastes. To provide access to it, a small incision is made in the wall of the abdomen and a permanent opening is established with a soft plastic tube. During dialysis, the peritoneal sac is filled with a special fluid that helps draw off waste material. This fluid is washed in and out of the abdomen in cycles.

Three techniques are used for this type of dialysis. Intermittent peritoneal dialysis (IPD) lasts 10 to 14 hours and is done in a hospital or clinic three times a week. Another method, continuous ambulatory peritoneal dialysis (CAPD), can be performed at home. This is an ongoing process in which the person always has about two quarts of dialysis fluid in the abdomen. The fluid is changed manually three or four times a day, with each fluid exchange taking 20 to 40 minutes. In automated peritoneal dialysis (APD), a more recent innovation, a cycler machine performs the dialysis while the patient sleeps. This system usually eliminates the need for fluid exchanges during the day.

A doctor must monitor blood levels of phosphate, potassium, and other electrolytes at regular intervals, because these substances, essential to maintaining normal body chemistry, often become imbalanced during kidney failure. The physician will recommend supplements as needed. Because kidney failure also increases the risk of anemia,

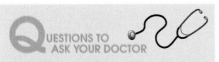
QUESTIONS TO ASK YOUR DOCTOR
▶ Do you think that my kidney failure is likely to be reversible?
▶ What out-of-hospital dialysis options are available in this community?
▶ Am I a good candidate for a kidney transplant operation?

blood tests must be done frequently, and erythropoietin may be prescribed. This hormone, which is normally produced by the kidneys, helps prevent anemia by stimulating the bone marrow to make red blood cells.

A kidney transplant is an alternative to long-term dialysis. This is the treatment of choice for chronic kidney failure, but donor kidneys can be difficult to find. The best chance for achieving a successful transplant rests with receiving a kidney from a living donor, preferably a relative whose body tissues are genetically compatible so that the chances of rejection are reduced.

Healthy people require only one kidney to function, but only 20 percent of those needing a kidney transplant have a relative who is an acceptable donor. Most transplant candidates go on a waiting list to receive a healthy cadaver kidney taken from someone within minutes of dying, usually as the result of an accident. A shortage of cadaver kidneys forces many transplant candidates to wait years for one.

The transplanting of a kidney is major surgery, requiring general anesthesia and lasting two to three hours. After removal from a donor, a kidney must be transplanted within 18 hours. In most cases, the failed kidneys are left in place, with the transplanted kidney positioned much lower in the abdomen than normal. The donor kidney also must be attached to blood vessels—the internal iliac artery, which supplies blood to the pelvic organs, and the external iliac artery and vein, which serve the legs.

The majority of kidney transplants are successful, allowing the recipient to lead a relatively normal life. But about one-third of transplanted kidneys temporarily cease to function for a time ranging from a few days to two weeks. In a few cases, the kidneys will never resume functioning, necessitating continued dialysis or a second transplant.

Most transplant recipients leave the hospital in two to three weeks to continue recuperation at home. In the first few weeks after surgery, patients have blood tests several times a week to monitor for signs of organ rejection. They must also take powerful immunosuppressive drugs for the rest of their lives to prevent rejection. Because these drugs increase the risk of infection and cancer, regular checkups are necessary.

Alternative Therapies
Kidney failure always requires careful medical treatment directed by a nephrologist, a specialist in kidney disease. Thus, any alternative practitioners should be a part of the treatment team.
Herbal Medicine. Uva-ursi, or bearberry, is an old remedy for irritation and inflammation of the urinary tract. Practitioners recommend one or two capsules of uva-ursi extract three or four times a day to treat nephritis, which can cause kidney failure.
Nutrition Therapy. A nutritionist or clinical dietitian trained in treating kidney failure should be enlisted to plan a diet. In particular, protein intake must be carefully regulated because too much places a heavy burden on the kidneys. Fluids may be restricted. Also, the diet should be low in salt and phosphorus, and potassium levels must be carefully monitored. Vitamin and mineral supplements may be advised.

Some dietary restrictions might be adjusted for patients who undergo a kidney transplant. For example, protein intake should actually be increased after surgery to prevent a breakdown of muscle tissue caused by steroid medications, which are often given to help prevent rejection.
T'ai Chi. This or some other gentle exercise program can help counter the loss of muscle mass and weakness that often accompanies kidney failure. Exercise is also important to prevent bone loss caused by steroids and other drugs given to kidney transplant patients.

Self-Treatment
In addition to adhering consistently to any dietary restrictions, self-care centers on maintaining overall good health and controlling any underlying condition that contributes to kidney failure.
▶ If you have high blood pressure or diabetes, two common causes of chronic kidney failure, be especially diligent about keeping them in check.
▶ If you require long-term dialysis, learn how to do home dialysis.
▶ If you have flaky skin, a common problem for people with chronic kidney failure, apply a moisturizer after bathing and bathe in lukewarm, rather than hot, water.
▶ If you are a woman suffering from chronic kidney failure, practice scrupulous birth control because pregnancy presents an increased risk of complications for both you and the fetus.

Other Causes of Kidney Failure
A number of conditions can cause urinary symptoms, including an enlarged prostate, bladder or kidney stones, urinary tract infection or tumors, and an obstruction of the ureters, the tubes that carry urine from the kidneys to the bladder. If untreated, these disorders can damage the kidneys.

Kidney Stones

(Renal calculi)

Kidney stones are accumulations of minerals and crystallized salts that form in the upper part of the urinary system. Most remain in the kidney, but some dislodge and move down the ureter into the bladder.

Small stones may pass unnoticed through the urinary tract, but larger ones make their presence known with severe colicky pain. The onset of an attack may be mild, but the pain intensifies rapidly, disappearing only when the stone is passed. If a stone becomes lodged along the way, the resulting pain is extreme and immobilizing.

Each year, approximately 1 in 1,000 Americans is hospitalized with kidney stones; men outnumber women about three to one. At least half of those who suffer one attack will have a recurrence.

Although about 80 percent of kidney stones contain calcium, the role of this mineral in their formation is unclear. Doctors believe that the problem could

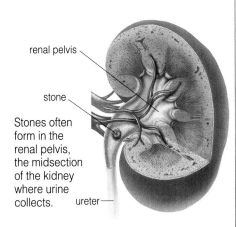

renal pelvis

stone

Stones often form in the renal pelvis, the midsection of the kidney where urine collects.

ureter

be connected to the faulty metabolism of calcium. Perhaps more calcium than the body needs is absorbed from food, and some of the excess remains in the kidneys rather than being excreted in the urine. Or a metabolic problem may prompt the bones to release excessive calcium into the bloodstream.

Stones that contain uric acid are frequently due to a metabolic disorder (gout, for example) that results in overproduction of uric acid.

In about 10 percent of cases, a bacterial infection prompts stone formation.

Diagnostic Studies and Procedures

Diagnostic tests include blood and urine studies and X-rays of the kidney, ureters, and bladder. An ultrasound examination of the kidneys and urinary tract may also be ordered; for this test, high-frequency waves are used to create an image of internal structures. When the stone or stones are passed or removed, they should be collected for analysis to find the underlying cause.

Medical Treatments

Most stones eventually pass on their own; painkillers and perhaps antibiotics are prescribed while waiting for this to happen. If a stone is blocking the ureter, a device called a ureteral stent may be used to widen the tube and allow urine to pass through it. Stones that cannot be passed naturally must be removed. In the past, this often required major surgery. Today, less invasive treatments are available.

Laser surgery offers one of the safest and least invasive ways to remove stones lodged in the ureter. The procedure entails inserting a hair-thin optical fiber into the ureter. When the fiber reaches a stone, it releases a burst of energy in the form of a very intense light beam, which breaks up the stone without harming surrounding tissue. The stone fragments are then passed in the urine or extracted through a urinary catheter. Laser surgery takes about a half hour, but a few days of hospitalization may be needed.

Percutaneous surgery is a minor operation in which an endoscope is inserted into the kidney through a small incision. If the stone is small enough, it can be snared and removed. A larger stone will be broken up by shock waves, allowing its natural passage.

Lithotripsy uses shock waves to break up the stone. The patient sits in a tub of water positioned under a lithotripter, which delivers shock waves to the kidneys and pulverizes any stone into tiny fragments. Some specialists discourage this procedure because the shock waves may damage the kidneys, and any stone fragments remaining in the kidneys can lead to new stones.

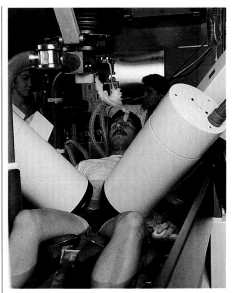

In lithotripsy, a relatively new treatment for kidney stones, the patient sits in a tub of water while shock waves are delivered to the kidneys to break up the stones, which can then be passed in the urine.

After an acute attack, treatment involves preventing new stones. Thiazide diuretics, such as hydrochlorothiazide (Esidrix, HydroDIURIL), may be prescribed to lower the amount of calcium excreted in the urine. Allopurinol (Zyloprim) and/or potassium citrate may be used to prevent uric acid stones.

Alternative Therapies

Herbal Medicine. Juniper berry extract or tea may be advocated for its diuretic properties to flush out the kidneys.

Nutrition Therapy. Dietary changes depend upon the type of stone. If excessive calcium absorption is a factor, moderate restriction of calcium intake (to about 600 milligrams a day) may help. Because high doses of vitamin C can precipitate stone formation, supplements should be avoided.

Self-Treatment

Drink at least eight 8-ounce glasses of water every day; some urologists recommend even more. Plain water is best. Avoid sugary soft drinks, as well as carbonated beverages high in phosphates. Foods high in oxalates, salts that promote stone formation by binding with calcium ions, may have to be limited. These include green leafy vegetables, chocolate, tea, and many nuts.

Other Causes of Renal Colic

Nephritis can cause severe flank pain. Bladder stones, which are similar to kidney stones in composition, may obstruct urine flow.

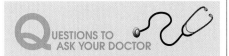

QUESTIONS TO ASK YOUR DOCTOR

► What type of kidney stones do I have?
► Should I reduce my calcium intake?
► Should I drink more than the recommended amount of water on hot days or when I perspire a lot?

Lactose Intolerance

(Lactase deficiency)

People who are lactose intolerant are unable to digest milk and milk products because they have insufficient amounts of lactase, the enzyme needed for digesting lactose, or milk sugar. Instead of being broken down and converted into glucose, or blood sugar, the lactose remains intact in the intestines, absorbing large amounts of water. This accumulation of fluid stimulates peristalsis, the rhythmic intestinal contractions that move material through the intestines, and results in gas, cramps, and diarrhea. In addition, certain bacteria that inhabit the colon ferment the lactose, leading to an even greater buildup of gas, and the passage of watery, acidic stools.

Typically, the discomfort and diarrhea hit within an hour after consuming milk products and disappear within a day after eliminating them from the diet.

The degree of lactose intolerance varies among individuals. Some have problems only when they consume large quantities of milk, while even small amounts trigger symptoms in others. Many people are unaware that they are lactase deficient until they abruptly increase their milk consumption. This often happens when older women start drinking more milk to obtain more calcium.

About two-thirds of the world's population suffer some degree of lactose intolerance. Lactase production gradually declines after infancy, when the diet no longer depends solely on milk. This natural occurrence is especially common among Native Americans and people of African, Mediterranean, Asian, and Middle Eastern descent. These persons can usually tolerate small amounts of lactose as children, but they have increasing difficulty in doing so as they grow older.

A small number of infants are born with congenital lactase deficiency. Some adults have other types of intestinal disease that hinder lactase production, making them lactose intolerant.

Diagnostic Studies and Procedures

Many people are never diagnosed with lactose intolerance because they normally avoid milk products. For anyone who is suffering symptoms, a doctor can usually pinpoint the condition by instructing the patient to abstain from milk products for a few days to see if symptoms disappear.

If this procedure is inconclusive, he may order a lactose intolerance test. This involves having the patient ingest an oral dose of 50 grams of lactose and then taking blood samples to measure glucose levels at specific intervals for the next two hours. The development of abdominal bloating and discomfort within a half hour and a below-normal rise in blood glucose indicate lactase deficiency. Another diagnostic test measures the amount of hydrogen exhaled before and after ingesting lactose.

Congenital lactase deficiency in an infant may require a biopsy of the small intestine to pinpoint the cause.

Medical Treatments

Medical care is usually not needed except for babies, who must be given a lactose-free formula. A doctor will also prescribe calcium supplements for a lactose-intolerant child, to ensure proper growth and development.

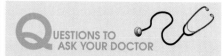

Alternative Therapies

Nutrition therapy is the mainstay of treatment. A nutritionist can help plan a diet that provides adequate amounts of calcium while avoiding milk. Foods other than milk contain small amounts of calcium; good sources are dark green vegetables, sardines with bones, tofu (soybean curd), and legumes. But supplements will probably be needed if all milk and milk products are eliminated.

Self-Treatment

Most people who are lactose intolerant can consume small amounts of milk and milk products without developing symptoms. To find your level of tolerance, first eliminate all milk products from your diet. (Check labels carefully for whey and other hidden sources of milk or milk sugar.) Then try ¼ to ½ cup of milk with a meal to see if it produces symptoms. Some people handle chocolate milk better than plain milk.

Those with lesser degrees of lactose intolerance can consume products whose lactose levels have been reduced by bacterial cultures that partly predigest it. Aged cheeses, buttermilk, sour cream, yogurt made with live cultures, and acidophilus milk have reduced lactose levels and are usually tolerated better than untreated milk.

People who are highly sensitive to lactose but still want to drink milk, can try taking it with lactase, available in tablets or liquid form. If this does not work (the enzyme may become neutralized in the stomach), a more satisfactory alternative might be lactose-free soy milk or milk with reduced lactose and added lactase. These products are usually available in large supermarkets and health food stores.

Other Causes of Intestinal Symptoms

Other food intolerances or malabsorption problems can produce bloating, gas, and diarrhea similar to those of lactose intolerance. Irritable bowel syndrome is also a possibility.

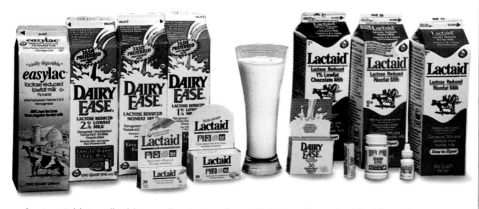

Lactase tablets or liquid, as well as lactose-free milk, buttermilk, and acidophilus milk are among the alternatives to regular milk that are available to those individuals who are lactose intolerant.

Laryngitis

Laryngitis is an inflammation of the larynx, or voice box, that interferes with speech. Early symptoms include a tickling dry cough, hoarseness, and a sore throat. In more serious cases, a person may have no voice at all, and both swallowing and breathing may also be difficult.

The cause is usually a viral infection that begins as a cold or sore throat and travels down to the voice box. As the vocal cords and surrounding tissues become irritated by the infection, they swell and can no longer vibrate freely to produce the sounds of speech. In young children, a similar infection may produce croup (page 150) and its characteristic barking cough.

Laryngitis can also result from strep throat or another bacterial infection, or from irritation caused by alcohol, very hot beverages, toxic vapors, dust, and tobacco smoke, including secondhand smoke. Screaming and yelling produce inflammation of the larynx, and such misuse of the voice can cause hoarseness and the development of vocal cord nodules. Without treatment, these nodules can permanently distort the voice.

Diagnostic Studies and Procedures

A doctor should be consulted if the laryngitis is accompanied by a fever, becomes acutely painful, or lasts more than two weeks. He can usually gauge the cause and seriousness simply by inspecting the throat with a bright light and tongue depressor. When a physician suspects a bacterial infection, he

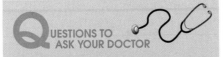

QUESTIONS TO ASK YOUR DOCTOR

▶ Is viral laryngitis contagious?
▶ Will I get my voice back faster if I stay on a liquid diet?

will collect a throat-sputum specimen for a laboratory culture to identify the causative organism.

When closer inspection is needed, indirect laryngoscopy may be done. In this examination, a tube with fiberoptic viewing devices is inserted into the throat and a tiny camera inside takes video pictures that are projected onto a monitor. Using this apparatus, a doctor can determine whether a tumor, polyps, or nodules are causing the hoarseness. If the lower part of the larynx is to be inspected, the tongue and throat are first sprayed with a local anesthetic to prevent gagging. Biopsy samples of any growths or nodules can be collected during this examination.

Medical Treatments

Viral laryngitis does not require drug therapy, but if a bacterial infection has been diagnosed, ampicillin, tetracycline, or another broad-spectrum antibiotic will be prescribed, typically for 10 days. Laryngitis due to vocal abuse or irritants is best treated with rest and inhalation of moistened air.

A singer, actor, or public figure who must use his voice during a bout of mild laryngitis may be helped by spraying a few drops of epinephrine directly onto the vocal cords. This is especially effective in countering allergic laryngitis, the condition that plagued President Clinton during his 1992 campaign. It can, however, also produce numerous side effects, especially headaches, irregular heartbeat, and nervousness. Therefore, it is not always the most suitable approach to treatment.

Hoarseness due to polyps, nodules or other benign growths on the vocal cords may be treated by surgical removal of

the growths. (See Larynx Cancer, opposite page, for information on voice problems related to cancer.)

Alternative Therapies

Herbal Medicine. To reduce inflammation in the larynx, herbalists advise gargling several times a day with sage tea mixed with a teaspoon of cider vinegar. Sucking on honey and eucalyptus lozenges may also help.

Speech Therapy. Professional voice training may help to prevent chronic laryngitis from overuse or misuse of the voice. This may involve learning to speak or sing at a lower pitch and learning proper breathing and voice-projection techniques.

Self-Treatment

Self-care based on common sense is all that is needed for most cases of laryngitis. The most effective measure is to rest the vocal cords by not talking at all. You should also avoid whispering, which is even harder on vocal cords than ordinary speech, because it puts stress on the cords by forcing them together. If you must communicate by speaking instead of writing, try to use your voice as normally as possible, despite the hoarseness.

Drink plenty of warm fluids. Try chewing sugarless gum to stimulate saliva flow and moisten the vocal cords. Use a cool-mist humidifier to keep the air moist. Do not take cold pills that contain antihistimines. These medications have a drying effect and therefore increase hoarseness.

Other Causes of Hoarseness and Laryngitis

Smoking and heavy use of alcohol irritate the vocal cords, sometimes resulting in hoarseness. Hay fever and other allergies may also bring about hoarseness and other vocal changes.

THE DANGER OF EPIGLOTITIS

Sometimes infection and inflammation of the vocal cords spread to the epiglottis, the leaf-shaped bit of cartilige that functions as a trap door to prevent food and fluids from entering the larynx and windpipe, or trachea. A swollen epiglottis can block the flow of air into the airways, resulting in suffocation. Any difficulty breathing during a bout of laryngitis is a medical emergency that demands immediate treatment. If necessary, a breathing tube may be inserted into the trachea until the swelling subsides.

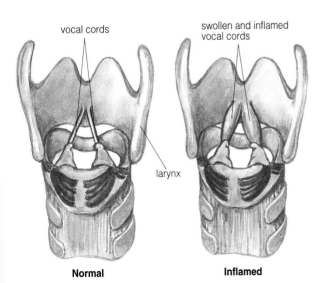

vocal cords

swollen and inflamed vocal cords

larynx

Normal   **Inflamed**

In laryngitis, the vocal cords and surrounding tissues swell, so that they can no longer vibrate.

Larynx Cancer

With cancer of the larynx, or voice box, malignant cells develop in or near the vocal cords. The disease usually occurs after age 55; males with this cancer outnumber females four to one. The condition is most common among smokers, and those who also consume large amounts of alcohol suffer the highest incidence. Some studies have suggested that long-term asbestos exposure may also increase the risk.

An early symptom is a voice change, especially increasing hoarseness. As the cancer progresses, it may also cause a sore throat, difficulty in swallowing, a chronic cough, bloody sputum, ear pain, and a lump in the neck.

Diagnostic Studies and Procedures

A doctor begins by feeling the patient's throat for lumps and examining the larynx through a lighted tube inserted into the throat. At this time, a small biopsy sample can be taken from any suspicious-looking tissue. If malignant cells are detected, additional tests will be ordered to determine the extent or stage of the cancer. These tests usually include X-rays, blood studies, and MRI or other imaging studies.

Medical Treatments

Treatment depends on what part of the larynx is affected and whether the cancer is strictly localized or has spread. The patient's age and general health are also important considerations. Often treatment is carried out by a team of specialists that includes a surgeon, a cancer specialist (oncologist), an ear-nose-throat specialist (otolaryngologist), a radiation oncologist, speech pathologist, nurse, dietitian, and dentist.

Treatment options should be discussed with the patient so that he can make informed choices, especially because these choices may affect the way he will look and speak. A speech pathologist is usually present at these

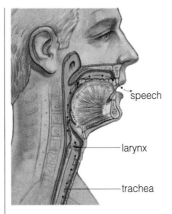
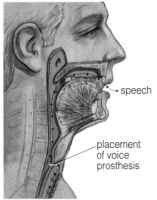

speech

larynx

trachea

speech

placement
of voice
prosthesis

Normally, speech is produced as air passes through the larynx into the trachea (far left). After a laryngectomy, a voice prosthesis may be inserted into the trachea (left), and speech produced by closing the opening with the thumb or a valve (insets, below).

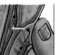

preliminary discussions to answer questions and help plan later rehabilitation and speech therapy techniques. The following treatments may be used separately or in combination:

Radiation therapy is used to kill the cancer cells and shrink tumors. This approach is tried first whenever possible, especially for early, localized cancer, because it preserves normal speech.

Surgery is often combined with radiation. The type of surgery is determined by the extent of the cancer. A small tumor on the vocal cord can often be removed by laser surgery, leaving all or most of the cord intact.

More extensive cancer may require complete surgical removal of the larynx, a procedure called a laryngectomy. In such cases, a tracheostomy, an opening in the front of the neck, will be made to allow air to pass through the windpipe, or the trachea, on its way to and from the lungs, and a prosthetic speech devise may be inserted. In addition to learning how to breathe through the opening, the patient must also learn a new way to speak with the prosthesis (see illustrations, above).

If only part of the larynx is removed to facilitate breathing, a temporary tracheostomy will be created. Eventually, the tracheostomy tube will be removed, allowing the patient to breathe normally. Most patients also regain their ability to speak normally, although the voice may be weak and hoarse.

Chemotherapy is used if the cancer has spread to other parts of the body. It may also be employed to shrink a large tumor before further treatment with surgery or radiation.

Alternative Therapies

There are no effective alternative therapies for larynx cancer itself, but they can play a critical role in rehabilitation

and adjustment during and after treatment. In particular, speech therapists can help patients regain the ability to speak, even after a total laryngectomy.

Nutrition Therapy. During treatment, it may be difficult to eat. In such cases, intravenous feeding may be necessary until it's possible to swallow normally again. After first resuming eating, the patient may need a liquid diet to reduce the risk of choking. A dietitian or pharmacist can recommend an enriched product to maintain good nutrition.

Speech Therapy. A technique called esophageal speech allows people who have had a total laryngectomy to speak again. A speech therapist teaches the patient how to trap air in the upper esophagus and use it to form sounds. If this cannot be learned, mechanical devices or an artificial larynx may help the person regain speech.

Self-Treatment

If you have been treated for larynx cancer, avoid strong chemical fumes and secondhand smoke, which will irritate the vocal cords. Above all, abstain from using alcohol and tobacco. After a partial laryngectomy, avoid shouting and other activities that tax your voice.

A consultation with a speech therapist can provide guidance in protecting your remaining voice. Joining a self-help support group, such as the Lost Chords or New Voice clubs sponsored by the American Cancer Society, can help in adjusting to life if you have had a total laryngectomy.

Other Causes of Voice Loss

Larynx polyps, nodules, and chronic laryngitis can produce hoarseness and other symptoms similar to those of larynx cancer. The accidental swallowing of lye or another caustic substance can also damage the larynx, and result in loss of voice.

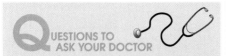

QUESTIONS TO ASK YOUR DOCTOR

▶ Can my cancer be treated without removing my larynx?
▶ If radiation therapy is recommended, how will it affect my voice?
▶ What are the hazards of living with a tracheostomy?

Lead Poisoning

(Plumbism)

Lead interferes with several vital enzyme activities if it is chronically inhaled or ingested in sufficient quantity to accumulate in the blood. Developing fetuses, infants, and young children are most vulnerable to damage from lead; even small amounts can cause harm. Some 2 million preschool children are afflicted by varying degrees of lead poisoning in the United States each year.

Severe childhood lead poisoning can cause neurological and kidney damage, anemia, and even death. Moderate poisoning can produce stomach upsets, vomiting, convulsions, an abnormal walk, headaches, irritability, hyperactivity, learning and behavioral disorders, delayed mental development, and perhaps retardation.

In adults, toxic levels of the metal can do extensive damage, especially to the nervous system and kidneys. Its symptoms include high blood pressure, headache, loss of appetite, intestinal upset, memory loss, an impaired gait, and a metallic taste in the mouth. During pregnancy, lead poisoning can cause miscarriage, severe congenital defects, or death of the fetus.

Although laws now ban lead in gasoline and other products, large amounts still remain in the environment.
Paint. Before 1971, lead was used in most paints. Toddlers may eat chips of old paint from peeling walls or inhale lead dust when walls are scraped or sanded. Youngsters may also chew on lead-painted toys and furniture.
Drinking water. Lead can leach from plumbing and brass fittings, especially if water is hot or naturally corrosive.
Leaded glassware, ceramics, and china dishes. Foreign imports or U.S. products made before 1971 may contain problematic amounts of the metal.

Soil. Lead from water and other sources can accumulate in soil, posing a hazard to children who play in it.
Manufacturing processes and miscellaneous products. Emissions from can-manufacturing plants, foundries, and smelters may contain lead. Less potent sources include food from cans sealed with lead, lead foil at the tops of wine bottles, and antique pewter.

Diagnostic Studies and Procedures

A simple blood test detects the presence of lead. Many states now require pediatricians and health clinics to screen young children for lead levels. Testing is recommended when a child develops any of the symptoms listed earlier. Some obstetricians advise women planning to become pregnant to have a blood test for lead exposure.

Medical Treatments

Moderate lead poisoning can be treated with an oral chelating drug, such as succimer (Chemet), that binds to the lead, which is then excreted in the urine. The pills must be taken for 19 days and may cause a rash, loss of appetite, nausea, vomiting, diarrhea, and a metallic taste in the mouth.

Severe lead poisoning requires taking one or more intravenous drugs, usually dimercaprol (BAL) and calcium disodium-EDTA. Regimens vary, but the medication is usually given several times a day for five to seven days, and the therapy is repeated every two to three weeks until blood tests are normal.

Alternative Therapies

Chelation is the only effective therapy. However, because it may also remove other metals from the body, zinc and iron supplements may be needed to restore these minerals.

Self-Treatment

There are several measures you can take to prevent lead exposure.
▶ If your house was built before 1971, you almost certainly have lead-based

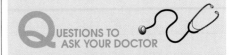
paint. You can seal off painted surfaces with plasterboard, paneling, or wallpaper. If you are doing renovations, anyone in the house during sanding or stripping must wear a filtering facial mask. Pregnant women and children should stay elsewhere until several days after all renovation is completed.
▶ If children play in the soil around your home, have it tested for lead. Cover soil that contains high lead levels with a hard-top surface or at least eight inches of low-lead top soil.
▶ Test water, ceramics, china, and glassware for lead contamination. Some state and local health departments offer water testing, or you can go to a private lab. Home kits are available to test dishware.
▶ If testing reveals a high level of lead in your tap water, have pipes replaced or purchase a home water-purifying system. Until you do this, do not use water from the hot-water faucet for drinking or cooking. Instead, let the cold-water tap run for a few minutes or until water reaches its maximum coldness before using it.
▶ Look for lead-free labeling when buying ceramic, china, or glass tableware, especially if it is manufactured abroad.
▶ Save leaded crystal glassware for special occasions. Don't store wine or any other beverages in leaded crystal, or acidic foods in glazed ceramic ware.

Other Causes of Metal Poisoning

Numerous minerals and heavy metals, including iron pills, arsenic, and mercury, can cause metal poisoning.

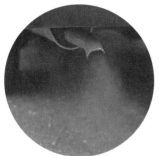
Auto exhaust

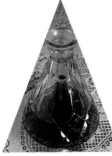
Crystal

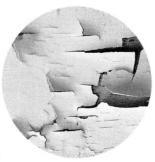
Paint

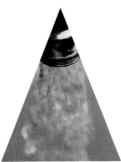
Tap water

Potentially dangerous levels of lead can be found in many common objects, most notably auto exhaust, crystal made with lead, old paint, and tap water that flows through plumbing that contains the metal.

Learning Disabilities

(Developmental disorders; dyslexia)
Learning disabilities are generally defined as developmental problems that interfere with a child's ability to process information. In the broadest sense, this definition covers mental retardation (page 296) and such neurological disorders as hyperactivity (page 237), but this discussion focuses on difficulties that disappear in time or are highly treatable. Although there may be some overlap, most learning disabilities fall into three categories:
Disorders affecting academic skills, most commonly reading or math.
Included are such perceptual problems as dyslexia, which causes difficulty in learning to read; excluded are blindness and other sensory impairments.
Disorders affecting language and speech. The milder forms, which include lisping and stuttering, are probably the most common of all learning disabilities, as well as the most benign. More serious, but less common, examples include an inability to form sentences or difficulty in understanding certain sounds or words.
Disorders affecting coordination or other motor skills in the absence of neurological, muscular, or other physical problems. These include difficulty learning to write, tie shoelaces, work puzzles, and perform other tasks that require fine coordination.

Some learning disabilities, such as poor coordination and language problems, are obvious at an early age. The child may be slow in starting to walk or have unusual trouble in learning to talk. Those disabilities affecting academic skills usually do not show up until the child starts school.

At one time, these learning disabilities were attributed to low intelligence. Experts now know that many children with these problems are highly intelligent but may have a subtle brain or nerve abnormality that interferes with information processing. Heredity is believed to be a major factor, especially in dyslexia. One study found that 60 percent of dyslexic children had parents or siblings with the same problem.

Other factors that are sometimes associated with learning disorders include low birth weight, nutritional deficiencies, and drug or alcohol abuse during pregnancy. Parental neglect or sensory deprivation during infancy can also contribute to later learning problems.

Some researchers theorize that certain difficulties stem from over- or underdevelopment of one side, or hemisphere, of the brain. For example, a higher-than-average incidence of left-handedness occurs among learning-disabled children; this could indicate overdevelopment of the brain's right hemisphere.

Diagnostic Studies and Procedures
Evaluation of a child with a suspected learning disability begins with ruling out physical and neurological disorders, including mental retardation. This is best done by a child psychologist, developmental pediatrician, or other qualified health professional. In addition to a physical and neurological examination, studies are likely to include vision and hearing tests and perhaps a CT brain scan and electroencephalogram, a study of the brain's electrical patterns.

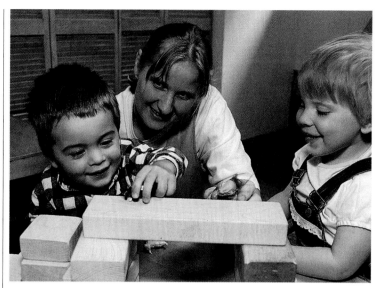
Working with blocks and other playthings can help children with poor motor skills improve eye-hand coordination.

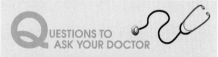
QUESTIONS TO ASK YOUR DOCTOR

▶ What is the best way to help a learning-disabled child without giving the problem undue attention?
▶ If I have dyslexia, what are the chances that my children will have it too?
▶ How reliable are IQ tests for learning-disabled children? Is it possible that such tests can be used to misdiagnose a child as mentally retarded?

To find out whether the child is performing below potential, an IQ test will be administered. A standard IQ test evaluates a child's memory, language skills, and ability to organize information. Specific learning disabilities may also be diagnosed by a speech pathologist and an occupational therapist.
Medical Treatments
In general, children with learning disabilities do not require any special medical treatment unless an underlying disorder, such as anemia or nutritional deficiency, is a factor.
Alternative Therapies
A number of alternative therapies can often reach children with learning disabilities and provide ways of overcoming them. Multisensory approaches are especially helpful; for example, a child of normal or higher-than-average intelligence who has trouble reading or writing is encouraged to learn by seeing, hearing, and moving. Techniques that may be employed include:
Art Therapy. How a child uses art materials is often a clue to specific learning and perception difficulties. Art may also be the medium in which a youngster reveals special talents that may hold a key to overcoming some learning disabilities.
Dance Therapy. Especially clumsy youngsters can improve their coordination by dancing and engaging in other types of movement therapy. Older children may benefit from t'ai chi, judo, or another martial art.
Music Therapy. Group singing, playing a musical instrument, listening to tapes, and identifying musical compositions

LEARNING DISABILITIES (CONTINUED)

to foster musical memory are more than socially enriching activities; they also provide an alternative means of expression and learning. Children who stutter or lisp can often learn to form words normally by singing. By memorizing a song, a child may grasp how to form a sentence. Music can also be used to teach math and other skills.

Pet Therapy. Animals have become an integral part of many programs for the learning disabled. Mimicking their sounds may help children with speech problems. Learning to ride a horse is a valuable means of improving coordination. Pets can also foster a sense of responsibility and improved self-esteem—both important advantages for the learning disabled.

Special Education. It is increasingly clear that many, if not most, learning disabilities can be overcome through special teaching techniques. Dyslexics, for example, can usually be taught to read by teachers using special methods. Federal legislation requires that all public school systems evaluate children at risk for learning disabilities and provide special education programs for those who need them.

Speech Therapy. There are several new methods for overcoming speech problems. Ask your pediatrician or teacher for a referral to a qualified therapist.

Self-Treatment
Patience, understanding, and realistic expectations should form the basis of parental help for a child with learning disabilities. Specialists agree on the following guidelines for parents:

▶ Encourage academic accomplishment, but don't push. Meet regularly with the child's teachers and supervisors, and participate in developing an individualized plan that builds on the child's strengths and devotes more time to reducing weaknesses.

▶ Be helpful with homework, but resist doing it for the child. Instead, allow the child time to produce the right answers by asking a series of leading questions.

▶ Provide a good role model by letting the child know how much pleasure you get from reading. Read to a young child at bedtime, and encourage older children to read books that are of special interest to them. To help the child get accustomed to using the local library, go there together on a regular basis.

▶ Be sensitive to the child's feelings. If a youngster gets frustrated and angry, let him know that adults share the same feelings and have appropriate means of dealing with them.

▶ Set time aside for sharing a hobby, special outings, or other enjoyable pursuits that foster the child's self-esteem.

▶ Above all, accentuate the positive and praise strong points. Help your son or daughter take pride in any accomplishments, even if ordinary.

Other Causes of Learning Problems
Numerous neurological and physical conditions can cause or contribute to learning disabilities. These include autism, brain tumors, cerebral palsy, depression, fetal alcohol syndrome, head injuries, hearing loss, lead exposure, hydrocephalus, hyperactivity, mental retardation, schizophrenia, and severe uncontrolled epilepsy.

A CASE IN POINT

Nine-year-old Ed hated school, and with good reason; he was failing most of his subjects and was almost certain to have to repeat the fourth grade.

Ed's parents and teachers were puzzled by the boy's learning problems. Repeated testing showed above-normal intelligence. The child was well-behaved, attentive, and tried hard. His hearing and eyesight were normal, and there was no evidence of a neurological problem.

Ed's performance in reading, history, art, and sports were average, but he was failing science, spelling, and arithmetic. The last subject was Ed's special nemesis, a difficulty reflected in all of his achievement tests. His most recent tests put Ed's reading ability slightly above grade level, spelling slightly below, and his arithmetic scores in the second-grade range.

At the urging of school officials, Ed's parents took him for an evaluation by a psychologist who specialized in learning disorders. The psychologist's report described Ed as "a quiet but personable boy who expresses concern about his schoolwork and says he 'just really hates to go to school.'" Further probing again identified arithmetic as the problem.

Ed explained that the numbers get "all jumbled up." When the psychologist gave Ed the simple problem of adding three and four, the boy laboriously counted out the answer on his fingers, gave the correct oral answer, but then wrote down two instead of seven. Mathematical concepts such as multiplication and division were beyond Ed's grasp, even though his teacher had spent extra time trying to teach them.

After a careful evaluation of Ed's other academic skills, the psychologist concluded that the boy had what is classified as a developmental arithmetic disorder (formerly called acalculia). Criteria for such a diagnosis include arithmetic skills that are consistently below intellectual ability and that interfere with overall academic performance.

Some children with developmental arithmetic disorder also have reading, behavior, and coordination problems. Because Ed's difficulties did not extend to these areas, the psychologist thought that intensive remedial instruction might help. He urged Ed's parents to look into Project MATH, a multimedia program that their son could use on their home computer. He also suggested enlisting a child a year or two older than Ed as a math tutor. "Some children who have problems learning from an adult do much better with a peer as a teacher," the psychologist explained. "This is why it's vital to integrate children with learning disorders into regular classes."

The psychologist cautioned Ed's parents not to expect overnight miracles, stressing that no one fully understands why some children have so much trouble learning arithmetic. "Some seem to outgrow the problem," he said, "but others always have difficulty with numbers."

In Ed's case, his determination and the support of his parents and teachers helped considerably. The Project MATH program turned out to be not only educational, but also fun. Ed's teacher arranged for a fifth-grader to tutor him three times a week.

Although progress was generally slow, his teachers felt that it was significant enough for Ed to advance to the next grade. In return, he agreed to spend part of the summer continuing his remedial work so that he could keep up with his fifth-grade classmates.

Legionnaire's Disease

(Legionella pneumophilia *broncho-pneumonia; legionellosis*)

Legionnaire's disease is a pneumonia caused by the bacterium *Legionella pneumophila*. The organism, which normally dwells in pond water, was given its popular name after being identified as the cause of an outbreak of a mysterious, highly virulent pulmonary infection among 200 people attending a 1976 American Legion convention in Philadelphia. Since that time, nearly 20 species of the disease-causing bacterium have been identified.

These organisms are transmitted through the air. In the 1976 epidemic, the bacteria were present in a hotel air-conditioning system. Since then,

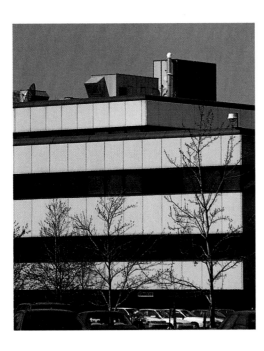

The water tank of an air conditioner provides an ideal breeding environment for *Legionella* bacteria, which can then spread throughout the building by way of the ducts.

numerous smaller outbreaks have been traced to central air-conditioning systems, where the bacteria thrive in pools of stagnant water and are circulated through air ducts.

Symptoms of Legionnaire's disease come on suddenly after an incubation period ranging from 2 to 10 days. Characteristic indications include general malaise, chills, nausea, vomiting, diarrhea, headache, muscle aches, disorientation, a fever that may rise as high as 105°F (40.5°C), and a cough. The cough usually starts out dry but gradually progresses to produce gray

or blood-streaked sputum. About 15 percent of all untreated cases are fatal.

Diagnostic Studies and Procedures

If Legionnaire's disease is suspected, a chest X-ray will be taken; it may reveal fluid in one or both lungs and perhaps lung abscesses. Laboratory cultures of sputum must be done to identify the organisms that are causing the disorder. To collect the tissue samples and secretions for these studies, bronchoscopy may be used. This procedure involves passing a long, flexible viewing tube through the mouth and windpipe and into the bronchial tubes, thus enabling the doctor to study the interior of the airways as well as to collect tissue and fluid samples. Blood tests may detect antibodies to the bacterium.

Medical Treatments

Antibiotic therapy is the cornerstone of treatment, erythromycin being the drug of first choice. In addition to erythromycin, seriously ill patients might receive rifampin, an antibiotic most commonly used to treat tuberculosis. The drugs may be given intravenously at first, then by mouth, once a patient's condition has improved. Treatment usually continues for three weeks or more, and all prescribed medication should be taken, even when symptoms abate.

Severely ill patients may be hospitalized in an intensive care unit, where oxygen can be administered and vital signs monitored continuously. These precautions help prevent such complications as shock, delirium, heart failure, kidney failure, and development of an irregular heartbeat.

Alternative Therapies

Only antibiotic treatment can cure Legionnaire's disease, but alternative therapies may help relieve symptoms.

Herbal Medicine. To treat pneumonia of all types, Western herbalists recommend tea made of giant Solomon's seal, an herb that may also be used to make a poultice for application to the chest

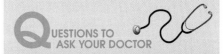
two or three times a day. Other herbal remedies include hyssop tea and garlic, boneset, or mullein capsules.

Homeopathy. Among the substances practitioners use in treating pneumonia are aconitum, arsenicum album, and the ABC formula. Bacillinum may be given once a week but should not be repeated if the first dose brings no improvement. Hepar is said to be effective when phlegm is thick, greenish, or foul-smelling.

Self-Treatment

Complete bed rest until acute symptoms abate is the most important aspect of self-care, even for mild cases. Until the illness is over, which can take two to four weeks, do not try to exercise other than to practice deep breathing and gentle range-of-motion exercises of the limbs, neck, and shoulders.

A cool-mist humidifier increases the moisture in the air, which helps thin lung secretions so they can be coughed up more easily. Drinking extra fluids also helps thin mucus. A heating pad can relieve chest pain, but be sure to turn it off before going to sleep. Keep warm. Avoid singing and talking loudly, both of which can trigger coughing.

If your cough is painful but produces no sputum, ask your doctor about a nonprescription cough suppressant. If it does produce sputum, an expectorant makes the secretions easier to cough up. To reduce a mild fever, take aspirin or acetaminophen.

Call your doctor immediately if any of these symptoms appear:
▶ A fever of 102°F (38.9°C) or higher.
▶ Severe chest pain.
▶ Increased shortness of breath.
▶ Bloody sputum.
▶ Bluish color of the nails, lips, or skin.

Other Causes of Pulmonary Symptoms

Similar symptoms occur in other lung infections, especially other types of bacterial pneumonia.

Leukemia

(Acute and chronic lymphocytic and myelogenous leukemias)

Leukemia, a term used to describe several types of blood cancer, comes from the Greek words for "white blood." The name refers to the whitish or pale-pink blood leukemia patients have because of high numbers of abnormal white cells. Although leukemia affects all types of blood cells, as well as bone

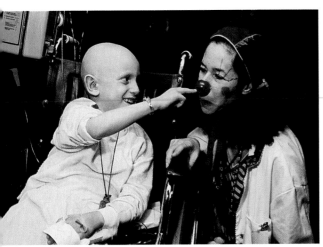

Recognizing the healing value of laughter, some hospitals employ clowns to work with young cancer patients.

marrow and other blood-producing structures, the white cells, or lymphocytes, are involved the most.

The types of leukemia are broadly classified as follows:

Acute lymphocytic or lymphoblastic causes a rapid increase in abnormal lymph cells, or lymphocytes. It occurs most commonly in children.

Chronic lymphocytic entails a slow increase in abnormal lymphocytes and generally affects older people.

Acute myelogenous progresses rapidly and involves increased numbers of abnormal myelocytes, or granulocytes, the white cells that fight bacteria. It is rare in children and becomes increasingly common with advancing age.

Chronic myelogenous progresses slowly at first and most frequently strikes middle-aged people.

Leukemia is further classified according to cell size, rate of proliferation, and such characteristics as the appearance and immunologic features of the proliferating cells. Acute leukemias are the most serious; they appear abruptly and worsen rapidly.

Common symptoms of leukemia include easy bruising and bleeding, fatigue, pallor, weakness, fever, shortness of breath, joint pain, and abdominal swelling and tenderness.

Chronic leukemia may be present for years without producing noticeable symptoms. As the disease worsens, however, it may cause a low-grade fever, night sweats, loss of appetite and weight, and fatigue that comes on quite easily. Unless diagnosed and treated, the disease eventually enters an acute stage, producing more pronounced symptoms and a rapid decline.

Leukemia is the most prevalent childhood cancer, with about 2,500 new cases and 600 deaths a year. The incidence is even higher among adults, however, with some 26,000 new cases and 20,000 deaths a year. Radiation exposure greatly increases the risk of leukemia, as does contact with benzene and the use of anticancer and some other drugs. Several genetic disorders, including Down's syndrome, also seem to increase its risk.

Diagnostic Studies and Procedures

Abnormal cells, found in a microscopic examination of blood, raises the suspicion of leukemia, which is confirmed by a bone marrow biopsy. (This study entails removing a sample of bone marrow with a hollow needle inserted into the breastbone or hip.) The specific type of leukemia can also be established this way. Additional blood studies and bone marrow biopsies will be performed during treatment to monitor its effectiveness and adverse side effects.

Medical Treatments

Acute leukemias are usually treated with intensive chemotherapy, using various combinations of anticancer drugs. Radiation treatment is often used also. It is sometimes directed at the brain to eliminate any leukemia cells that may elude anticancer drugs, which ordinarily do not cross the protective blood-brain barrier. Even after a remission has been achieved, chemotherapy, using lower doses of anticancer drugs, is continued to help prevent a recurrence.

Transfusions of red cells, platelets, and sometimes white blood cells may be part of the treatment. Because leukemia makes infections difficult to control, patients may be placed in a special germ-free room, especially during certain phases of treatment. Visitors must wear gowns and masks.

Relapses are common in all types of acute leukemia, so frequent follow-up is necessary. If a relapse occurs, the patient will begin a new course of chemotherapy, perhaps using a different combination of drugs.

For a growing number of patients, doctors are recommending bone marrow transplants, preferably after the first or second remission. This procedure involves destroying the patient's diseased marrow with drugs or intensive radiation and then replacing it with healthy marrow from a donor. Usually the donor must be a close relative to achieve a good genetic match and reduce the risk of rejection.

An alternative approach calls for removing bone marrow from the patient during a remission, treating it with drugs to kill any cancer cells, and then freezing it for possible future use if a relapse occurs. This is referred to as an autologous marrow transplant.

The treatment for chronic leukemia is different from that of acute forms of the disease. Often, treatment is not even advised during the early, asymptomatic stages. Instead, the patient is closely monitored with periodic blood tests and marrow biopsies. If these tests indicate that the disease may be getting worse, chemotherapy is started. A bone marrow transplant may also be tried, especially in patients under 40 who have chronic myelogenous leukemia.

Alternative Therapies

Any alternative therapy should be employed as an adjunct to, rather than a substitute for, medical treatment. Imagery, visualization, hypnosis, and meditation and other relaxation techniques are examples of safe alternative therapies that enhance feelings of well-being and may promote healing by strengthening the immune system. Other alternative therapies include:

Acupressure. Practitioners recommend pressing a point on the underside of the wrist to counter nausea (page 260). Alternatively, you can wear an acupressure bracelet, such as that promoted for preventing motion sickness (page 310).

Herbal Medicine. Madagascar periwinkle is the source of vinblastine and vincristine, potent anticancer drugs that are often used to treat leukemia. Western herbalists may advocate taking periwinkle extract, but doctors discourage this practice, as the herb can interact with the chemicals of chemotherapy, increasing the risk of side effects. However, other herbs, such as ginger, ginseng, sarsaparilla, and wild Oregon grape, can reduce nausea. Garlic pills may be recommended to bolster the body's immune system.

Nutrition Therapy. Sound nutrition is especially important during chemotherapy, which often causes nausea and loss of appetite. Patients are encouraged to eat their largest meals when they feel best, which is usually in the morning. The emphasis should be on bland, high-calorie foods that are easy to swallow and digest. Scrambled eggs, cream soups, and enriched milk shakes will be better tolerated than spicy or fried foods. Any supplements need the approval of an oncologist; high doses of some vitamins can cause digestive problems that could be serious in a leukemia patient.

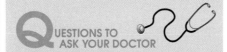

QUESTIONS TO ASK YOUR DOCTOR

▶ Am I a candidate for a bone marrow transplant? If so, is it possible to use my own marrow?
▶ How often will I need follow-up examinations? What signs and symptoms indicate a possible relapse?
▶ How can I minimize the side effects of my treatment?
▶ Will I be susceptible to possible long-term complications of chemotherapy? Of radiation?

A word of caution: In the past, laetrile, a toxic substance that is obtained from apricot pits and other seeds, was promoted as a cure for leukemia and other cancers. Numerous studies have failed to prove that it is of any benefit; in fact, it may do considerable harm. One reason is that laetrile contains cyanide and can cause cyanide poisoning when taken in high doses, especially if it is combined with vitamin C. Other strategies that should be avoided are fasting and strict macrobiotic diets, which can exacerbate weight loss.

Self-Treatment
Because even a cold can be a serious threat to anyone undergoing intensive chemotherapy, leukemia patients should try to avoid contact with anyone who has an infectious disease. It's best to stay away from crowds as much as possible, especially during the flu and cold season, wash hands often to decrease the chances of contracting an infection, and try not to become chilled.

Leukemia and its treatment accelerate dental and oral problems. Consult a dentist before beginning treatment, and schedule dental checkups at least every three months. For mouth ulcers, rinse often with a solution of 1 tablespoon of salt in 8 ounces of warm water. Use a soft toothbrush; if this still provokes bleeding gums, clean your teeth with a soft cloth dipped in 3-percent hydrogren peroxide. Do not take aspirin because it increases bleeding.

Other Causes of Leukemia Symptoms
Anemia, mononucleosis, bleeding disorders, and chronic infections such as tuberculosis can produce a constellation of symptoms that can be confused with those of leukemia.

A CASE IN POINT

Janis Hines discovered that she had leukemia when she underwent routine blood tests as part of a preemployment checkup. Although she felt fine and was in apparent good health, the tests showed an abnormally high count of white blood cells, with a large number of precursor cells that indicate chronic myelogenous leukemia—a diagnosis confirmed by additional blood studies.

The doctor explained that this type of leukemia can smolder for several years without causing serious problems, but that eventually a crisis develops and the disease enters an acute stage. When that happens, chemotherapy may produce a brief remission, but the long-term outlook is generally poor.

"The news is not all grim," the doctor added. "More than half of patients who undergo a bone marrow transplant while the leukemia is in a chronic stage are cured," meaning apparently free of cancer five years after treatment.

The doctor referred Hines to an oncologist who specialized in treating leukemia. This specialist quickly determined that Hines was an ideal candidate for a marrow transplant. At age 28, she was much younger than the average patient, and the disease was still in an early, asymptomatic stage. She also had both parents living and six healthy brothers and sisters. "There's a good chance that one will be a suitable genetic match," the doctor said. "If not, your name will be added to our computerized register for bone marrow transplants."

The oncologist told Hines to stay as healthy as possible in the meantime by getting adequate rest and consuming a nutritious diet. He also put her on alpha interferon, an experimental drug that seems to delay onset of acute leukemia.

The next task was to test family members to see if any were suitable marrow donors. None were, so Hines's name was added to the transplant register.

Over the next year, she participated in several public events aimed at encouraging more people to be tested and donate bone marrow. "Even if I didn't succeed in finding a donor, at least I was doing something to help other people in my situation," she explained.

Her oncologist also referred her to a counselor who taught guided imagery, a technique that gave Hines a positive focus to help ease her worries. Fortunately, her health held up, and a bone marrow donor was found eventually.

"The next few months were hard," she recalls, "but by then, things were out of my hands." Her own bone marrow was destroyed and the donor marrow injected into her body. Until it started to function, she was especially vulnerable to infection, so she stayed in a special germ-free hospital room until blood tests showed that her own immune defenses were returning. Even then, she had to be very careful to avoid infection.

A year after the transplant, tests showed no sign of the leukemia, and Hines was again leading a normal life. In fact, she was so preoccupied with planning her wedding that at times she even forgot about this dark period.

Lice

(Pediculosis; crabs)

Lice are tiny parasitic insects that live on blood. In humans, they infest primarily the scalp, hair, and genital area, but also other parts of the body. The most common types are:

Head lice (Pediculus humanus capitis), usually less than ⅛ inch long and almost as wide. They are most often spread through direct contact, but can also be picked up by sharing brushes, combs, and other head gear. Schools are a common source of outbreaks because lice spread easily on hats, scarves, and jackets in coat closets.

Pubic lice (Phthirus pubis), shorter and fatter than head lice. Their resemblance to tiny crabs, complete with claws, has given rise to their popular name, "crabs." They are usually transmitted by sexual contact.

Body lice (Pediculus humanus corporis), longer and thinner than pubic lice. Infestation is common among people who live in crowded, unsanitary conditions.

Although unpleasant, head and pubic lice don't carry disease, whereas body lice may transmit typhus, relapsing fever, and other disorders.

In all lice infestations, the primary symptom is intense itching, a reaction to the insect's saliva. Head lice tend to cause itching behind the ears and along the hair line at the back of the neck. Pubic lice, which sometimes also infect beards and eyebrows, typically produce itching in the genital area. Itching from body lice occurs mostly on the shoulders, trunk, buttocks, and abdomen.

Diagnostic Studies and Procedures

Detection is based on spotting the parasites. Although lice can be observed with the eye, a magnifying glass may

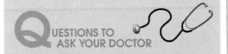

be needed to tell one type from another. Head lice also leave telltale eggs, or nits, which appear as tiny, silvery clumps attached to the hair shaft near its root. They are easy to differentiate from dandruff because the nits do not flake off, but are virtually cemented to the hair shaft and must be removed by combing (see Self-Treatment and the photograph, below). Pubic lice also leave eggs attached to the base of pubic hairs. Body lice and their eggs tend to live in the seams of underclothing rather than on the skin.

Medical Treatments

Until recently, the preferred treatment for all types of lice infestations was lindane (Kwell), a DDT- derivative available as a prescription shampoo, cream, or lotion. Although lindane is highly effective, its use has become controversial because of the risk of central nervous system damage and other side effects. Most experts now recommend reserving Kwell for severe infestations that cannot cleared up by safer nonprescription products. If you are using Kwell, be sure to follow your doctor's instructions to the letter.

In some cases, itching is so severe that an antipruritic medication is necessary. For this problem, a doctor may prescribe a topical steroid or an oral medication such as clemastine (Tavist).

Alternative Therapies

Herbal Medicine. Although herbal therapy cannot destroy lice, such preparations as capsules of stinging nettle extract can ease severe itching.

Self-Treatment

In recent years, researchers discovered that chrysanthemums produce pyrethrin, a natural pesticide, that is deadly to all types of lice yet safe for humans. Today, nonprescription pyrethrin shampoos, available at pharmacies, are as effective as lindane while being much safer, especially for children.

Start by killing adult lice with a pyrethrin shampoo, following package directions carefully. Then use a fine-toothed metal comb to remove eggs bonded to the hair shaft. Part wet hair into sections and carefully comb, from base to tip, one-inch wide tufts. Wipe nits from the comb frequently. A week to 10 days later, repeat the entire process. If lice have settled on the eyelashes, applying petroleum jelly three or four times a day should banish them within a week. (If this technique fails, consult your doctor; do not apply pyrethrin or any other lice-killing product around the eyes.)

Body lice are eliminated by bathing and discarding or fumigating infested clothing. To prevent reinfestation of all types of lice, you must rid your home of the pests. While adult head and body lice die after 48 hours without a blood meal, nits may not hatch until a month later, restarting the infestation. To avoid this, wash all personal clothing, bed linens, and other potentially infested items in hot water (at least 130°F or 49°C) and put them in a hot clothes dryer for at least 20 minutes. Dry cleaning also kills lice and nits. Disinfect combs and brushes. Vacuum upholstered furniture and rugs.

Although self-treatment clears up most lice infestations, see your physician if scratching has caused open, infected sores. To alleviate itching, try soaking in a bath containing cornstarch or colloidal oatmeal. Also, consult a doctor if a child under the age of two years is infested or if over-the-counter treatment has been ineffective.

Other Causes of Itching

There are many causes of itching skin. Conditions to rule out include scabies, which is also produced by a skin parasite; ringworm and other fungal infections; and skin allergies.

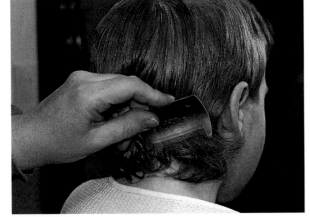

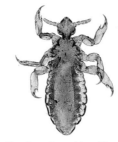

Greatly enlarged head louse

Although the eggs (nits) from head lice can be hard to detect with the naked eye, they must be carefully removed with a comb.

Liver Cancer

(Hepatic carcinoma)

Cancer that originates in the liver is relatively rare in the United States; worldwide, however, it is one of the most common malignancies. The precise cause of the cancer is unknown, but chronic hepatitis is a major precipitating factor, as is cirrhosis, a disease in which scar tissue replaces normal liver

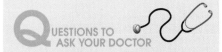

Liver cancer may originate in the organ itself, but more frequently, it spreads to it from other sites in the body.

cells. Other contributing factors include occupational exposure to vinyl chloride and similarly toxic chemicals, the use of synthetic testosterone and other anabolic steroids to build muscle mass, and alcoholism. Because liver cancer is more prevalent in sub-Saharan Africa and the Far East, some experts theorize that environmental and cultural factors play a strong role in its development.

In its early stages, liver cancer usually has no noticeable symptoms. When symptoms develop, they initially include fatigue, loss of appetite and weight, and vague discomfort in the upper-right abdomen, possibly with a spread of pain to the shoulder and back. As the cancer progresses, jaundice—a yellowing of the skin, whites of eyes, and mucous membranes—develops. In its advanced stages, liver cancer produces ascites, noticeable swelling caused by fluid retention in the abdomen.

Diagnostic Studies and Procedures

Palpating, or pressing, on the upper abdomen may reveal that the liver is enlarged and hard, forming a lump below the rib cage on the right side. A doctor may employ various methods to visualize the liver, including X-rays, CT scans, MRI, and ultrasound studies. But a biopsy is necessary for a firm

diagnosis. This can be done by inserting a needle into the liver to remove a small sample of tissue.

A doctor may order ultrasound or laparoscopy to locate suspicious areas that should be biopsied. For the second procedure, a viewing tube is inserted through a small incision in the abdomen, allowing examination of the liver and other abdominal organs. A biopsy sample can be taken at the same time. Angiography, special X-ray studies of blood vessels after injection of a dye, can provide important information about the type and size of the tumor.

Medical Treatments

Surgical removal of a localized tumor, such as hepatocellular carcinoma, the most common type of liver cancer, sometimes produces a cure. Because the liver has a remarkable ability to regenerate itself, a fairly large portion can be removed without threatening life. Chemotherapy may follow the operation. For advanced or inoperable cancer, radiation therapy may alleviate pain and prolong survival.

A liver transplant is another option, especially if the cancer has not spread. The major difficulty lies in finding a healthy, genetically compatible liver from a recently deceased donor.

If fluid retention is a problem, a drainage tube may be inserted into the abdomen to reduce its accumulation. Diuretics may also be prescribed.

Alternative Therapies

Although alternative therapies cannot cure liver cancer, they may help to lessen pain and other symptoms.

Acupuncture and Acupressure. These techniques can be useful for controlling pain. Pain management specialists often employ one or both as an adjunct to surgery, radiation, and chemotherapy. Acupressure using a point on the inner wrist (see page 260) is also helpful for controlling nausea from chemotherapy.

Hypnotherapy. Self-hypnosis is another way to relieve pain and nausea. It may be taught with other methods, such as meditation, visualization, and guided imagery, to promote a sense of well-being, even if a cure is not possible.

Naturopathy and Nutrition Therapy. A low-salt diet can help to reduce fluid accumulation. Many nutritionists advocate supplements of beta carotene,

a precursor of vitamin A that is said to suppress cancer cells, but studies indicate that food sources are more effective than pills. These include deep green or orange vegetables, such as broccoli, spinach, sweet potatoes, and carrots. Some experts also recommend tomatoes, watermelon, and red peppers, as they contain lycopene, which seems to have some anticancer potential.

Yoga. This is useful in pain control and relaxation and can be of value to persons coping with the stress of living with cancer. Although there is no scientific proof, some people believe that yoga meditation, combined with other techniques such as visualization, can improve the body's ability to heal itself, possibly by boosting the immune system.

Self-Treatment

As much as possible, reduce demands on the liver. First and foremost, abstain from alcohol, which is highly toxic to this organ. This step is important, even if you do not have liver cancer but fall into a high-risk group for developing it or some other form of liver disease. In addition, ask your doctor if you need immunization against hepatitis. This vaccine is recommended for the sexual partners of all people who have chronic hepatitis B, as well as healthcare workers, male homosexuals, and others at risk of contracting the disease. Hepatitis immunization is also recommended for all infants.

Other Causes of Liver Cancer Symptoms

Metastatic cancer that starts elsewhere in the body and spreads to the liver is more common than cancer that arises in that organ. Symptoms of liver cancer should initiate a search for cancer elsewhere. Jaundice, a common symptom of liver cancer, can result from hepatitis, cirrhosis, and other liver diseases.

Lung Cancer

(Pulmonary carcinoma)

Lung cancer is any malignancy that originates in the lungs, in contrast to cancers that arise elsewhere and then spread to the lungs, as many do. It is the most common fatal malignancy in the United States, with about 170,000 new cases annually, and accounting for 153,000 deaths every year.

Smoking is the main cause of lung cancer. However, one in eight occurrences are in people who have never smoked. In these cases, the direct cause is unknown, but long-term exposure to such environmental elements as air pollution, asbestos, secondhand tobacco smoke, or radon (a colorless, odorless gas that can accumulate to unhealthful levels in a home) seem to increase the risk. Continuous occupational exposure to certain chemicals, radiation, and chromium compounds is also

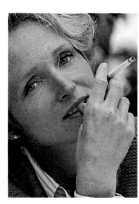

Smoking is by far the leading cause of lung cancer. Studies have shown that secondhand smoke also increases the risk of this and other respiratory disorders.

believed to play a role in inducing some lung cancers. And evidence suggests that a diet high in saturated fats may be a factor, especially in women.

Four major types are described below: The first two are the most common; the last two are relatively rare. *Squamous cell carcinoma,* also known as epidermoid carcinoma, usually begins in the larger bronchial tubes. *Adenocarcinoma* usually starts in the smaller, more distant bronchial tubes. These cancers frequently spread to the lymph nodes and then to the brain and other organs. *Small-cell carcinoma,* also known as oat cell carcinoma, is the most aggressive type of lung cancer; it is often fatal within a year of diagnosis. *Large-cell carcinoma* tends to spread or metastasize through the bloodstream

to other parts of the body, in particular the adrenal glands, brain, and bones.

Lung cancer often mimics other pulmonary disorders, especially in the early stages. Symptoms include a persistent cough, an aching chest pain, shortness of breath, and the spitting up of bloody sputum. They may develop slowly and are often mistakenly attributed to chronic bronchitis or another condition. As the cancer advances, it causes extreme weakness and fatigue, loss of appetite and weight, and swollen, tender lymph nodes, usually in the neck or under the arm.

Diagnostic Studies and Procedures

Unfortunately, lung cancer is rarely discovered early, because there are no effective screening tests and symptoms do not usually occur until the disease is well advanced. Sometimes a laboratory examination of sputum can detect abnormal cells when the disease is in its earliest stages, but at that point it may be extraordinarily difficult to pinpoint the site. Often, by the time lung cancer can be seen on a chest X-ray, it has spread, or metastasized, to other parts of the body.

If symptoms indicate the possibility of lung cancer, diagnostic studies begin with a complete physical examination that includes blood tests, laboratory analysis of a sputum sample, chest X-rays, a CT scan, and bronchoscopy. For this last test a flexible tube, or bronchoscope, is inserted down the throat to enable direct examination of the lung itself. Using the tube, doctors can also extract a sample of tissue for a biopsy, though they may instead use a large-bore needle if the site is difficult to reach.

When lung cancer is diagnosed, additional tests and scans may be done to see if it has spread to other areas.

Medical Treatments

Treatment depends on the size of the cancer and whether it has spread. Surgery is often the first step; removal of all or part of the lung in which the

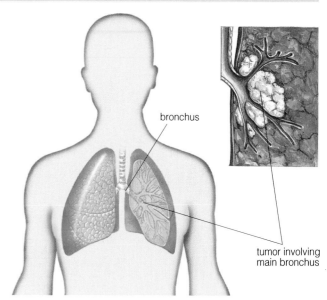

bronchus

tumor involving main bronchus

In stage I lung cancer, illustrated above, the tumors are small and localized, with no evidence of spread to lymph nodes.

tumor is located can sometimes cure a small, localized cancer. For example, squamous cell cancer grows slowly in its initial stages, so surgery alone may produce a cure if it is detected early.

Unfortunately, most lung cancer has spread by the time it is diagnosed. If the disease is in both lungs or has spread to nearby lymph nodes, radiation therapy may be used to shrink tumors or slow their growth. When the cancer has spread beyond these areas, chemotherapy may be best, using such drugs as cyclophosphamide, cisplatin, vinblastine, and/or methotrexate.

In many cases, a combination of approaches may be used. For example, for those with oat cell cancer, chemotherapy combined with radiation may produce an extended remission. Or if the cancer has spread to the brain (a common occurrence), radiation treatment of the head may be tried.

While aggressive therapy can often produce a remission, lung cancer usually recurs. Only about 13 percent of patients survive five or more years after treatment. In the 16 percent of patients whose disease is diagnosed when it is still localized, the five-year survival rate is considerably higher, at 46 percent. In those with localized small-cell lung cancer, the two-year survival rate has risen from 40 percent to 75 percent because of treatment with the relatively new combination of chemotherapy and radiation. However, when the cancer has already spread to the lymph nodes or into the mediastinum (the part of the chest containing the heart and other organs), the cure rate is only 5 percent.

Antibiotics may be prescribed to counter the increased risk of infection from the bone-marrow suppression caused by chemotherapy and radiation. Drugs like ondansetron (Zofran) or metoclopramide (Reglan) may be used to reduce the attendant nausea.

Alternative Therapies

Lung cancer requires intensive medical and surgical treatment to prevent or delay death. Nonetheless, alternative therapies may play an additional role both in its care and prevention.

Meditation, Self-Hypnosis, and Visualization. Cancer patients who participate in group support sessions that include these techniques may experience longer-than-average survival. A number of researchers believe that these therapies help mobilize the immune system to fight cancer.

Nutrition Therapy. Some nutritionists recommend daily supplements of beta carotene (a precursor to vitamin A) and vitamins C and E to help prevent cancer, but studies indicate that food sources of these antioxidants are more protective than vitamin pills. Foods rich in these nutrients include yellow and orange fruits and orange and dark-green vegetables, especially cruciferous vegetables, such as broccoli, Brussels sprouts, cabbage, and cauliflower. Studies at Johns Hopkins University showed that sulforaphane, a chemical in broccoli, lowered the incidence of lung cancer among smokers. The role of other dietary components remains controversial, although some studies suggest that a low-fat diet can reduce the risk of lung cancer.

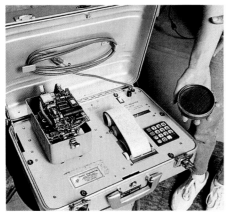

Radon, which is implicated as a risk factor in lung cancer, can be measured using a do-it-yourself kit or by calling in a professional.

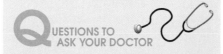

Self-Treatment

Prevention is the best approach to lung cancer. If you smoke, quitting is the most important measure. Studies show that within weeks of stopping cigarette use, suspicious precancerous lesions begin to heal, and in 5 to 10 years, the risk of lung cancer in ex-smokers is only slightly higher than that of people who have never smoked. Even if you already have lung cancer, quitting smoking and keeping your environment as free of smoke and other pollutants as possible may help slow its growth and improve chances of a cure.

Another preventive approach is to check your home for the presence of radon. If tests show radon levels above government standards, hire a qualified firm to improve ventilation, thereby preventing a buildup of the gas.

If you are undergoing treatment for lung cancer, a balance of rest and exercise is important to maintain strength and foster a sense of well-being. A daily walk or other exercise appropriate to your physical condition may help boost the immune system by releasing endorphins, chemicals produced by the brain that affect mood and diminish pain.

In many cases, patients die of starvation rather than cancer itself, because both the disease and its treatment can cause severe loss of appetite and weight. You can best deal with nausea from the side effects of chemotherapy and radiation by avoiding situations that worsen it. For example, stay out of the kitchen and away from cooking odors that may trigger nausea. If you must cook, avoid aromatic foods, such as cabbage and onions, and fatty, spicy, or other strongly flavored dishes. Foods served cold or at room temperature have less smell than those served hot, and they are usually better tolerated. Eat slowly in a relaxed, pleasant atmosphere, avoiding a room that is stuffy or too warm.

Eat dry, bland foods, such as crackers and toast, before meals. Plan to have your largest meal in the morning, when you are less likely to experience nausea, or eat small meals throughout the day, stopping if nausea hits. When it does develop, breathe deeply and sip small quantities of flat ginger ale or chew ice chips until it passes.

Rest for a half hour after eating; if possible, sit in an upright position, because reclining may trigger reflux of stomach contents into the esophagus, as well as nausea and vomiting.

If you know when nausea and vomiting are likely to occur, such as after a treatment, eat a bland, easy-to-digest meal several hours beforehand. Avoid milk and milk products, which may be difficult to digest. Many cancer patients find that red meat takes on an unpleasant taste. Chicken or turkey may be more palatable. If poultry cannot be tolerated, try eating combinations of grains and legumes, which provide equally high-quality protein and meet other nutritional requirements.

After an episode of vomiting, sip a clear liquid, such as tea or broth, every 10 minutes. Gradually increase the amount until you can hold down two tablespoonfuls every 30 minutes. Other liquids can then be added until you feel well enough to resume a regular diet.

Enriched nutritional supplements may be recommended for patients who suffer from lack of appetite. Maintaining an adequate food intake is essential, especially if surgery is part of the treatment.

In some cases, cachexia, a severe form of malnutrition and weight loss, appears to result from the body's response to the cancer itself. Some oncologists caution against trying to force-feed cachectic patients with supplemental nutrition, because their condition may reflect the body's attempt to "starve" the tumor. Although family members may find it difficult to watch a patient eat minimally and progressively lose weight, it may be wise to allow this person to limit food intake while aggressive cancer therapy is undertaken to destroy the tumor.

Other Causes of Pulmonary Symptoms

Persistent coughing, wheezing, and chest pain may be signs of asthma, congestive heart failure, tuberculosis, chronic bronchitis, or a lung abscess.

Lupus

(Systemic lupus erythematosus)

Lupus, frequently referred to as SLE for systemic lupus erythematosus, is a chronic rheumatic disease in which connective tissue throughout the body becomes inflamed. It is an autoimmune disorder in which inflammation is caused by antibodies that attack normal body tissue as if it were an outside invader. The precise cause is unknown, but researchers believe that certain people inherit a genetic predisposition to the disorder, which is then triggered by a virus or some other unidentified environmental factor.

The disease strikes women about 10 times as often as men. It can develop at any age, but is most common in young adults. Symptoms range from so mild that SLE goes undetected for long periods to disabling, even life threatening.

Lupus is often described as the great pretender among diseases because it causes such a wide range of symptoms, the most common of which are fatigue and joint pain. But other manifestations may include a chronic low-grade fever, hair loss, weakness, weight loss, dry eyes and mouth, muscle aches, swollen lymph nodes, loss of appetite, nausea, and mouth ulcers.

About half of all patients develop a butterfly-shaped rash over the nose and cheeks. Depending upon the organs affected, SLE may also cause severe headaches, anemia, inflammation in the lining of the heart or lungs, kidney failure, and mental disorders.

A variation—discoid lupus erythematosus—affects mainly the skin. A rash may appear not only on the face but also on the neck, scalp, and other areas. It ranges from a mild scaliness to a widespread blistery eruption.

As in many other rheumatic disorders, symptoms come and go unpredictably. Sun exposure or stress often produces a flare-up. During pregnancy, symptoms can worsen and cause miscarriage.

Diagnostic Studies and Procedures

Any unexplained joint pain and stiffness accompanied by other vague signs warrant seeing a rheumatologist for lupus testing. The workup should include blood tests to determine if the body is producing substances called antinuclear antibodies (ANA) and, more specifically, antibodies against your own DNA. If lupus seems likely,

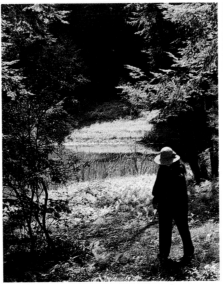

Because sun exposure can worsen lupus symptoms, it's critical to cover up and protect yourself from the sun when outdoors.

further tests will be done to evaluate the kidneys, lungs, and other organs that are frequent targets of the disease.

Medical Treatments

You and your doctor may have to experiment with various drug regimens over a period of months to find the right one for you. Possibilities include:

Aspirin and other nonsteroidal anti-inflammatory drugs (NSAIDs), such as ibuprofen (Motrin and others), naproxen (Naprosyn and Anaprox), indomethacin (Indocin), sulindac (Clinoril), tolmetin (Tolectin), and piroxicam (Feldene). They are the first line of treatment and may be all that is necessary to control relatively mild forms. NSAIDs ease pain by interfering with the body's production of prostaglandins, chemicals involved in the inflammatory process. However, they can cause stomach irritation and ulcers, and should always be taken with food and perhaps antacids.

Even if you do not take any of these drugs for pain, your doctor may recommend taking one baby aspirin daily to reduce your risk of blood clots because lupus can also increase the risk of heart attack and stroke.

Antimalarials, such as hydroxychloroquine (Plaquenil). These help control lupus by suppressing the immune system. They are particularly useful in preventing rashes and joint pain. However, it may take two to six months before benefits are noted, especially disappearance of a nightly low-grade fever. Because these drugs cause eye

damage in a small percentage of patients, anyone using them on a long-term basis must have an eye examination every three to six months.

Oral corticosteriods, such as prednisone and methylprednisolone, synthetic versions of cortisone (one of the body's own steroid hormones). They reduce inflammation by suppressing the immune system. Steroids are often a mainstay of treatment for people with lupus-related kidney, blood, and neurologic disorders, but they cause unwanted side effects, including weight gain and lowered resistance to infections. Therefore, they should be taken only for limited periods, at the lowest possible dosage and, preferably, on alternate days. Because steroids taken long term increase the risk of osteoporosis, daily calcium supplements are recommended. When steroids are to be discontinued, the dosage should be reduced slowly over a period of several weeks to months, because sudden cessation can cause a lupus flare-up or life-threatening adrenal gland failure.

Topical steroids, such as hydrocortisone creams and ointments, carry fewer side effects than oral steroids and may be useful in the treatment of lupus rashes. Continuous use should be limited to no more than two weeks.

Cytotoxic drugs, such as azathioprine (Imuran) and cyclophosphamide (Cytoxan or NEOSAR), were developed to suppress the immune system in patients undergoing organ transplants. Subsequently, doctors discovered that they are also useful for treating severe lupus. They may be prescribed instead of, or in addition to, steroids. However, because of their potentially severe side effects, including possible liver damage and a slightly increased risk of cancer, frequent blood and urine tests are necessary to detect such problems early.

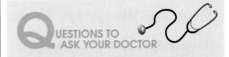

QUESTIONS TO ASK YOUR DOCTOR

► What symptoms of a flare-up should prompt me to call you?
► What side effects may be caused by the drugs I am taking?
► How often should I visit you for regular checkups to monitor my condition?
► Should I forego having children, or are there measures I can take to reduce the risk of a flare-up during pregnancy?

Alternative Therapies

Herbal Medicine. Feverfew, which is available in capsule form and as a tea, has been shown to have an anti-inflammatory effect and some studies have reported benefits in the treatment of autoimmune joint pain.

Hydrotherapy. Contrast baths can alleviate severe generalized pain. Sit in a bath that is as hot as you can stand for 5 to 10 minutes, then take a cold shower for 2 to 5 minutes. If pain is in only one or two joints, an ice pack may be sufficient; or use a plastic bag filled with frozen peas or corn that can be molded around the joint. Wrap the pack in cloth before placing it on the skin.

Meditation and Self-hypnosis. These and other relaxation techniques are helpful in controlling stress, which can aggravate lupus.

Nutrition Therapy. Nutritionists recommend a diet low in protein, and high in starches (complex carbohydrates), fresh fruits, and vegetables. Alfalfa sprouts and seeds, which may trigger a flare-up, should be avoided. Some people find that milk, beef, and certain vegetables can also intensify symptoms. It may be wise to keep a food diary and eliminate from your diet any food that causes problems.

Antioxidant vitamins, especially beta carotene (a precursor to vitamin A) and vitamins C and E, have been reported to help alleviate lupus. Vitamin E applied directly to the skin may help mitigate a lupus rash.

Studies suggest that gamma linoleic acid (GLA) and other omega-3 fatty acids may decrease the inflammatory response. Good sources of and recommended dosages include capsules of evening primrose oil (1000 milligrams twice a day) or black currant oil (500 milligrams twice a day). Other good sources of omega-3 fatty acids are flaxseed oil and cold-water fish such as salmon and sardines. In general, lupus patients should avoid such polyunsaturated oils as corn, safflower, sunflower, and soybean, which are high in arachidonic acid, a fatty acid that may contribute to inflammation. Better are canola, olive, and other monounsaturated oils.

Self-Treatment

As a starting point, try to identify any factors that worsen the condition. Keep a daily diary of symptoms and your evening temperature (when elevated, it can be an early sign of an impending flare-up. At the first indication of an increase in symptoms, see your doctor; aggressive treatment with more potent medications may head them off.

To lessen fatigue, get at least nine hours of sleep at night, and during the day, take half-hour rest breaks between periods of activity. Reorganize your home and work space to decrease unnecessary energy expenditure. When energy levels permit, exercise regularly, but avoid jarring movements that stress joints. Walking, swimming, and stretching movements seem to be best.

When the disease is active, arrange a less demanding schedule and try not to make plans that cannot be easily canceled, because you never know how you will feel from one day to the next. If you are planning a vacation, purchase trip cancellation insurance. If your symptoms are worsened by the sun, try to avoid exposure between 10 A.M. and 4 P.M. and always use a sunscreen and wear protective clothing.

Because estrogen may be implicated in the development of lupus, women with the disease are often advised not to use birth control pills. After menopause, estrogen replacement therapy may not be advisable for such women.

Certain drugs, including antibiotics and sulfa drugs, can provoke a lupus flare-up. In general, do not take any medication without checking first with your rheumatologist.

If your medication regimen includes NSAIDs and/or steroids, after meals take two antacids that contain calcium to lessen stomach irritation and the risk of osteoporosis.

If you have dry mouth, sip water or sugarless soda throughout the day. Try sugarless gum to stimulate production of saliva. Or use a nonprescription saliva substitute. Remember, too, that dry mouth increases the risk of cavities and gum disease. Brush and floss regularly, see a dentist at least every six months, and ask about fluoride treatments and antibacterial dental products.

Find out about lupus support groups in your area. Meeting with others who have the disease can alleviate a sense of isolation and provide you with information for enhancing your life.

Other Causes of Lupus-like Symptoms

Chronic fatigue syndrome and Lyme disease and other rheumatic disorders can cause symptoms like those of lupus.

A CASE IN POINT

In retrospect, Diane Bradley realizes she had been suffering with lupus for 10 years before her diagnosis. At one point, she had described her symptoms—joint and muscle pain, constant fatigue, hair loss, increasing dental problems—to her internist, who said: "These things happen to women in their forties."

A sudden escalation of her joint pain accompanied by a low-grade fever prompted Bradley to see a rheumatologist, who diagnosed the lupus and prescribed naproxen, an NSAID; prednisone, a corticosteroid; and Plaquenil, an antimalaria drug. This regimen alleviated the pain, but did not bring remission of the disease.

"I suffered from toxic fatigue," Bradley recalls, "that would come on suddenly; I could do nothing but go to bed, sometimes for two or three days." Hair loss, dry mouth, and dental problems persisted, as did bouts of diarrhea and muscle and joint achiness.

The inactivity and long-term prednisone resulted in a 60-pound weight gain in less than two years. But each time her rheumatologist tried to lower the dosage, the symptoms worsened. Bradley decided to try alternative therapies. Her doctor expressed doubts, but told Bradley to go ahead, and keep her informed.

"I changed only one thing at a time," Bradley says, "continued it for a month, and kept a careful diary of results—good or bad. I then stopped the therapy for a month to see if that made any difference." After months of trial and error, here's what seemed to work: a low-calorie, low-protein diet with little or no meat and other animal products; four 1,000 milligram capsules of evening primrose oil a day, and 30 minutes of meditation and visualization each evening.

As Bradley's symptoms disappeared, her rheumatologist slowly reduced her prednisone dosage, and Bradley increased physical activities. In the year it took to be weaned off prednisone, Bradley lost more than 60 pounds. She continued to take Plaquenil and an NSAID, but reduced the dosage of the latter. Minoxidil (Rogaine) stimulated hair growth.

Now she tells her friends, "I can truly say 'life begins at 50!'"

Lyme Disease

Lyme disease is a tick-borne infection that can cause serious illness. Named after the Connecticut town where a cluster of cases were diagnosed in the mid 1970s, the disorder has now been reported throughout much of the United States, with the highest levels of infection on the East Coast, from Maine to Maryland, in the Upper Midwest, and in California.

The cause is a type of screw-shaped bacteria, known as a spirochete, that is transmitted by several species of tiny ticks. Although these ticks are most often found on deer, rodents, and other wild animals, they also bite humans.

The first sign of Lyme disease usually is a painless, donut-shaped red rash that develops at the site of the tick bite within a few weeks, although in some cases it shows up sooner. It is often

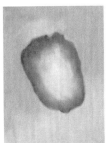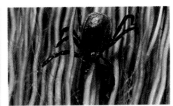

Lyme disease, carried by the deer tick (magnified above), initially may cause a red, circular rash (left).

accompanied by headache, low fever, achiness, and other flu-like symptoms.

Many people do not know that they have been infected with Lyme disease because they are unaware of having been bitten by a tick. (Up to half of those who are bitten fail to develop the warning rash.) Without treatment, weeks or even months after the bite, arthritic, cardiac, and/or neurological complications may occur. The most common manifestations are joint swelling, pain, and stiffness. Less common complications include cardiac arrhythmias, meningitis, neurological disorders including paralysis, and depression and other psychological problems. Infection in pregnant women may lead to fetal death and miscarriage.

Diagnostic Studies and Procedures

There are blood tests for Lyme disease, but they have limitations. For example, it may take months for an infection to produce a positive result using antibody tests. This situation is expected

to change if experimental tests fulfill their initial promise. In the meantime, a diagnosis can often be made on the basis of symptoms and the likelihood of exposure to a tick bite.

Medical Treatments

Lyme disease usually can be cured with antibiotics, especially if treated in its earliest stages, before complications occur. In the past, penicillin or tetracycline were the drugs of choice, but current therapy favors doxycycline, a more readily absorbed tetracycline, or amoxicillin, a penicillin derivative that has increased potency. Doxycycline is most commonly used because it has to be taken only twice a day and causes fewer gastrointestinal side effects than amoxicillin, which must be taken three times a day. More serious infections, especially those involving the central nervous system, may be treated with ceftriaxone (Rocephin); this is a new antibiotic that is given by injection or intravenously.

Approaches for later and more severe manifestations of Lyme disease remain controversial. Generally, treatment at this stage is longer and more intensive. It may be necessary to undergo two to four weeks of intravenous therapy with ceftriaxone or penicillin G, especially for central nervous system complications such as meningitis. Intravenous therapy may be given in the hospital, an outpatient clinic, or at home by a visiting nurse or IV therapist.

If symptoms persist despite a course of IV antibiotics, some doctors recommend long-term intravenous therapy. Others feel this approach is futile.

Other medical treatments depend upon symptoms. For example, Lyme arthritis generally responds to aspirin, ibuprofen, and other nonsteroidal anti-inflammatory drugs.

People with certain types of cardiac arrhythmias may be treated with antiarrhythmia drugs; others may benefit from implantation of a pacemaker. Eye inflammation can be treated with antibiotic eye drops. Medication may also be prescribed to treat depression.

Vaccines against Lyme disease are being tested in areas of Connecticut where the disease is widespread. If these prove effective, Lyme disease will become a preventable disorder.

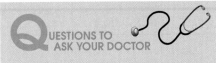

Alternative Therapies

Physical Therapy. A physical therapist can suggest exercises that will help inflamed joints retain function and maintain mobility, but at the same time will not damage them. An occupational therapist can teach new ways to perform daily tasks with minimal pain.

T'ai Chi. The gentle movements of this ancient exercise routine can help maintain flexibility and may also promote healing and a sense of well-being.

Self-Treatment

The ideal self-treatment is to prevent Lyme disease by avoiding tick bites. When walking in tick-infested areas, wear light-colored clothes on which ticks will be more visible, and spray them with permethrin. Apply an insect repellant that contains DEET—preferably in a concentration of less than 35 percent—to exposed skin. (Check with your doctor before using DEET on a young child; it may cause seizures.) Also, try to avoid brush and leaf litter.

Shower as soon as possible after any outing into an area known to be populated by ticks, and then examine yourself carefully. If you find a tick attached to your body, remove it promptly by grasping it with a pair of tweezers as close to the skin as possible and tugging gently. The sooner it is removed, the lower the risk that it will transmit infection. Place the tick in a closed container so that it can be examined if you develop any symptoms.

Make sure that all cats and dogs wear tick collars, and comb pets regularly to remove any ticks.

Other Causes of Lyme Symptoms

Arthritis symptoms similar to those of Lyme disease may be caused by rheumatoid arthritis, lupus, and Reiter's syndrome, a type of infectious arthritis. Neurological symptoms may be due to encephalitis and other central nervous system infections. Depression and chronic fatigue syndrome may also be mistaken for Lyme disease.

Lymphoma

(Hodgkin's disease; non-Hodgkin's lymphoma; Burkitt's lymphoma)
Lymphomas are malignant tumors of the lymph system, the network of nodes and glands that produce infection-fighting substances. In the United States, there are about 58,000 new cases each year.

The most common general symptom is a painless enlargement of one or more lymph nodes in the neck, groin, or armpit. Additional indications of Hodgkin's disease include a chronic low-grade fever and night sweats. Some people with non-Hodgkin's lymphoma also develop skin rashes, enlarged tonsils, and abdominal swelling.

Although the cause of most lymphomas is unknown, some are strongly linked to viruses. In Africa, Burkitt's lymphoma is associated with the Epstein-Barr virus and chromosomal abnormalities. In recent years, the AIDS (HIV) virus has been linked to a type of non-Hodgkin's lymphoma.

Diagnostic Studies and Procedures

A doctor who suspects lymphoma will carefully palpate, or feel, all lymph nodes that lie close to the surface of the body. Any suspicious areas will be biopsied, which may entail removal of several lymph nodes.

If Hodgkin's disease seems probable, diagnostic procedures may include laparotomy, in which a viewing tube is inserted through a small incision near the navel, allowing a doctor to collect tissue samples from abdominal organs that lymphoma often attacks.

Lymphangiography may also be done. In this procedure, a radiopaque dye is injected into the lymph system where it reveals abnormalities under X-ray examination.

If non-Hodgkin's lymphoma is diagnosed, bone marrow studies and CT scans can detect any spread.

Medical Treatments

Until recently, most lymphomas were invariably fatal. Today, many can be cured, especially when treated early. Hodgkin's disease, for example, often responds to radiation therapy alone. Or the patient may undergo a combination of radiation and chemotherapy and possibly surgery. Hodgkin's disease is now one of the most treatable forms of cancer; 77 percent of patients are still living five years after the diagnosis.

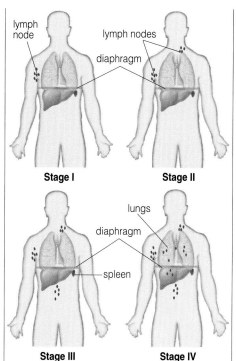

The various stages of Hodgkin's disease are determined by the location of the cancer. Stage I is confined to a single lymph node either above or below the diaphragm; stage II involves two or more nodes on the same side of the diaphragm; stage III affects lymph nodes both above and below the diaphragm, and perhaps the spleen as well; and in stage IV, the disease has spread from the lymph nodes to nearby organs.

For non-Hodgkin's lymphoma, radiation therapy is often employed. Chemotherapy may also be used, particularly if the disease has spread. When remission has been achieved, a bone marrow transplant may be tried. This involves destroying the patient's bone marrow with drugs or radiation and replacing it with healthy marrow from a donor. Marrow may also be collected from the patient during a remission, treated to destroy any lingering cancer cells, and then frozen for use later should there be a relapse. Marrow transplants may cure lymphoma, but there is an increased

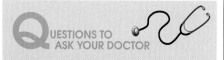

QUESTIONS TO ASK YOUR DOCTOR

▶ Am I a candidate for a bone marrow transplant? If so, at what stage of treatment should it be attempted?
▶ What are the long-term complications of my therapy? Are there any preventative measures I can take?

risk of infection due to the use of immunosuppressive drugs that prevent rejection of the donor marrow.

New approaches are also being developed to treat lymphoma patients after a relapse. These include the use of highly specific monoclonal antibodies that are directed against lymphoma cells, and improved methods for preserving and transplanting bone marrow.

Alternative Therapies

Acupuncture and Acupressure. These techniques are generally accepted by physicians as an adjunct to medical therapy to ease pain and stress.
Herbal Medicine. Teas or extracts of Siberian ginseng, sarsaparilla, and wild Oregon grape may help minimize the negative side effects of chemotherapy. Chinese herbalists may use ginseng, bupleurum, and the Longan herbal combination to treat manifestations of lymphoma, including anemia, fatigue, and an enlarged spleen. An herbal preparation called Golden Yellow powder is used to counteract skin inflammation caused by radiation therapy.
Hypnotherapy. Hypnosis and self-hypnosis are employed to control pain and to impart a positive attitude, which many experts believe facilitates medical treatment. These methods, along with meditation, can also reduce stress.
Nutrition Therapy. Nutritionists recommend foods that may have an anticancer effect. High on the list are those that contain beta carotene, a precursor to the antioxidant vitamin A, which studies suggest may help the body fight off cancer. Foods high in beta carotene include yellow and dark green vegetables, such as carrots and broccoli. Although some nutritionists also advocate supplements of antioxidants, food sources are more effective.
Visualization. This fosters relaxation, which is thought to have a positive effect on the immune system. It may be combined with guided imagery, which involves imagining the body's immune system destroying the cancer cells.

Self-Treatment

Self-care is directed toward coping with the side effects of treatment. Fatigue is common, so it is important to schedule frequent rest periods.

Other Causes of Lymphoma Symptoms

Enlarged lymph nodes, fever, and other lymphoma symptoms also occur in leukemia, mononucleosis, and AIDS.

Macular Degeneration

(Atrophic or exudative macular degeneration)

Macular degeneration entails gradual destruction of the macula, the tissue that makes up the central portion of the retina (see illustration, below). It generally strikes the elderly, and among older Americans, it is one of the most common causes of legal blindness.

Researchers believe that a hereditary predisposition is involved, but the precise cause of the condition is unknown. Typically, both eyes will be affected—either at the same time or sequentially. Because the disorder tends to develop

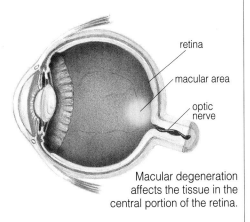

Macular degeneration affects the tissue in the central portion of the retina.

very slowly and is painless, a person may not realize that there is a problem until considerable vision has been lost.

There are two types of the disease. In the most common form, known as exudative (wet) macular degeneration, small blood vessels grow abnormally in the macular region beneath the retina. As these blood vessels become narrowed and hardened, the blood supply to the macula is impaired. If these vessels leak blood, the retinal cells in the macula can be damaged, resulting in blurred and distorted central vision.

The second type, atrophic (dry) macular degeneration, is caused by a disturbance of pigment cells in the macular region, without the hemorrhaging that occurs in the wet type.

Both types lead to increasingly impaired central vision. Initially, a person may notice difficulty in reading or in seeing distant objects such as street signs. If both eyes are affected, any activities that require sharp central vision eventually become impossible.

Diagnostic Studies and Procedures

Macular degeneration can be detected easily by an ophthalmologist (eye specialist) as part of a regular examination with an ophthalmoscope. This instrument has a bright light and a magnifying device that allows a doctor to view the inside of the eyes. By focusing on the macula, the doctor can detect any abnormalities in the pigment, as well as pinpoint small areas of bleeding and scarring. With another procedure called fluorescein angiography—a special X-ray study of the blood vessels in the retina—a doctor can also detect an overgrowth of blood vessels.

Medical Treatments

Until recently, little could be done to treat macular degeneration. Now, laser surgery has brought dramatic advances in treating the exudative type, but to prevent vision loss, therapy must begin early in the course of the disease, preferably even before symptoms occur.

To seal off newly formed abnormal blood vessels, doctors use a technique called laser photocoagulation. They focus the laser, a very narrow beam of extremely intense light, on the retina, where it makes a tiny circular burn that blocks the blood vessels crossing that area. Depending on the number of abnormal blood vessels, a doctor may make dozens or even hundreds of such minute burns on the retina. Drops are inserted into the eye to prevent movement during the procedure, but it is entirely painless. The patient remains conscious, and will see a bright flash of light with each burn.

Alternative Therapies

There are no alternative therapies that can restore vision lost to macular degeneration, but research indicates that zinc may help prevent the disease or slow its progress. Some nutritionists also recommend extra vitamin C for the same purpose.

Self-Treatment

If you have been diagnosed with the exudative, or wet, form of macular degeneration, you should check your vision daily for any further deterioration. To do this, your ophthalmologist will give you a card that is imprinted with the Amsler grid (see illustration, right). Even if you have normal vision, the periodic use of an Amsler grid can detect some early signs of vision loss.

During the early stages of macular degeneration, magnifying glasses may

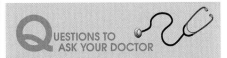

▶ Do I have the form of macular degeneration that can be treated by lasers?
▶ At what stage should I consider embarking on vision retraining?

be prescribed to help you read. Even if vision deteriorates markedly, special eyeglasses and other devices can significantly improve the quality of life.

Contact your local association for the blind for information on counseling and training to adapt to impaired vision. People who lose their central vision completely can be helped by retraining their eyes to more fully use their side vision. This should be taught by an occupational therapist who works with the visually impaired.

Other Causes of Vision Loss

Poorly controlled diabetes can cause a loss of vision due to an overgrowth of blood vessels in the retina, a condition called diabetic retinopathy. Vision loss similar to that of macular degeneration can result from a detached retina, although the onset will be sudden.

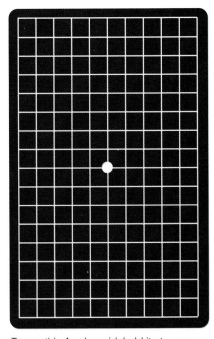

To use this Amsler grid, hold it at a comfortable reading distance from your face. (Wear your glasses if you normally need them for reading.) Look at it, one eye at a time, in both verticle and horizontal positions. See your ophthalmologist if there is any blurring or distortion of lines.

Malabsorption Syndromes

(Celiac disease; sprue; Whipple's disease)
All malabsorption disorders involve an inability to absorb one or more nutrients from the small intestine into the bloodstream. Many conditions can cause this problem (see box, far right), and the specific nutrients that cannot be utilized vary according to the cause.

In a common form, celiac disease, a hereditary defect prevents a person from absorbing gluten, a protein found in wheat, rye, and to a lesser extent, other cereal grains. This disorder usually shows up at an early age, often when a baby starts eating solid foods, but it may not appear until adulthood.

People with the less common tropical sprue, seen mostly in the Caribbean, India, and Southeast Asia, usually cannot digest and absorb many foods. As a result, they suffer numerous vitamin and mineral deficiencies.

Whipple's disease, a rare intestinal disorder affecting mostly middle-aged men, also involves a variety of nutrients. For these people, intestinal abnormalities prevent proper absorption, but the underlying cause is unknown.

Typical symptoms include weight loss, flatulence, abdominal bloating, and sometimes diarrhea. Nutritional deficiencies caused by malabsorption can result in anemia, childhood growth problems, neurological symptoms, and other signs of deficiency diseases.

Diagnostic Studies and Procedures
When a malabsorption disorder is suspected, blood studies will be ordered to look for nutritional deficiencies. A stool sample will also be examined for a high fat content, a common finding.

If symptoms suggest celiac disease, tropical sprue, or Whipple's disease, a biopsy of the small intestine will be

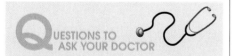

QUESTIONS TO ASK YOUR DOCTOR
▶ If I have one child with celiac disease, what are the chances that my other children will also develop it?
▶ Will I have to eat a special diet for the rest of my life?
▶ Are there measures I can take to prevent sprue when visiting tropical areas?

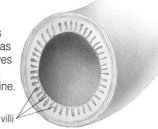

Digestion is completed as a meal moves through the small intestine.

villi

Small intestine

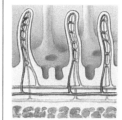

Nutrients are absorbed through the hair-like villi that line the small intestine.

Normal villi

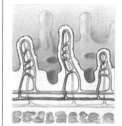

With a malabsorption syndrome, the villi may be either wide or flat, preventing normal absorption of nutrients.

Abnormal villi

done to look for characteristic abnormalities in the intestinal villi, the tiny finger-like structures through which nutrients are absorbed. Other possible tests include X-rays and endoscopy, in which the intestinal tract is inspected through a fiberoptic viewing tube.

Medical Treatments
For malabsorption caused by another disease, the underlying problem will be tackled. Primary malabsorption syndromes are treated as follows:
Celiac disease requires scrupulous avoidance of foods that contain gluten (see Nutrition Therapy, below). Vitamin and mineral supplements are usually prescribed to counter nutritional deficiencies. Severely ill adults may need intravenous feeding. If dietary measures fail to improve absorption, prednisone or another steroid may be given to induce a remission.
Tropical sprue can be cured by several months of antibiotic therapy, even when there is no apparent bacterial infection. Folic acid and possibly other nutritional supplements may also be prescribed. Another round of antibiotics will be ordered if a relapse occurs.
Whipple's disease is also cured with antibiotics. A typical regimen calls for 10 to 14 days of a high-dose antibiotic

such as penicillin, followed by 10 to 12 months of a lower dose. Improvement is usually seen within two weeks, although full recovery may take two years. Recurrences are treated with renewed antibiotics.

Alternative Therapies
Nutrition Therapy. A clinical nutritionist or dietitian should be consulted. Sometimes diet is the sole treatment, especially for celiac disease, in which consuming even a small amount of gluten can produce symptoms. Gluten is widely used in processed foods, so labels must be checked carefully.

Self-Treatment
Self-care should be directed to preventing a flare-up by following your recommended diet. If diarrhea is a problem, increase fluids to prevent dehydration. Tea, apple juice, broth, and water are good choices for mild diarrhea. Eliminate solid foods until bowel function normalizes, then gradually resume a normal diet, starting with bland foods like rice, bananas, or mashed potatoes.

Other Causes of Malabsorption Symptoms
Irritable bowel syndrome, diverticulosis, food poisoning, stress, or simple indigestion can cause diarrhea and other symptoms of malabsorption.

CAUSES OF MALABSORPTION
Disorders that damage the intestinal lining:
Amyloidosis
Celiac disease
Crohn's disease
Tropical sprue
Whipple's disease
Conditions that impair digestion:
AIDS
Bacterial overgrowth
Biliary obstruction
Congestive heart failure
Cystic fibrosis
Intestinal infection
Lactose intolerance
Liver failure
Lymphoma (intestinal)
Nutritional deficiencies
Pancreatitis
Scleroderma
Zollinger-Ellison syndrome
Structural problems:
Diverticulosis
Shortened intestine
Volvulus
Miscellaneous:
Alcoholism
Neomycin and certain other drugs

Malaria

Malaria is an infectious disease caused by any of four strains—*P. falciparum*, *P. malariae*, *P. vivax*, and *P. ovale*—of the *Plasmodium* protozoan, a single-cell parasite. Once the parasites enter the body, they travel via the bloodstream to the liver, where they multiply rapidly. After an incubation of one to two weeks, thousands of parasites reenter the blood, where they destroy red cells. The parasites then invade and destroy red blood cells in regular cycles.

Each wave of destruction produces a flare-up of symptoms, which vary according to the specific *Plasmodium* strain. Attacks typically include intermittent fever, chills, sweating, achiness, throbbing headache, and a generally ill feeling. Within a week, the typical pattern of the disease is established, which usually entails a short period of malaise or a headache followed by chills and a fever lasting up to several hours. Once the fever subsides, the patient will feel well until the onset of the next attack, which may come within 48 to 72 hours.

If the infective organism is *P. falciparum*, the typical pattern of attacks may be absent. Instead, there may be

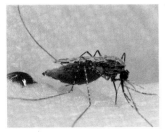

The female *Anopheles* mosquito is the vector, or carrier, of malaria.

a sensation of chilliness followed by a gradually rising fever that can last from 20 to 36 hours, with an accompanying headache. After this, for a period of 36 to 72 hours the patient feels ill and has a low-grade fever. A life-threatening complication of infection with *P. falciparum* is cerebral malaria. This is characterized by a fever, which may reach as high as 104°F (40°C), accompanied by severe headache, drowsiness, delirium, and confusion.

When the agent is *P. malariae*, the illness begins suddenly as a rule, with a paroxysm that recurs every 72 hours.

Malaria is usually transmitted by a bite from an infected *Anopheles* mosquito, but it can also be contracted from a

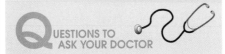

QUESTIONS TO ASK YOUR DOCTOR

▶ If I live in an area where malaria is common, do I have to take antimalaria drugs for the rest of my life? If so, what are their side effects?
▶ Is it possible to get malaria more than once? Are subsequent attacks likely to be more or less severe?

contaminated blood transfusion or by needle-sharing among intravenous drug abusers. Malaria is rare in the industrialized countries, but is common in undeveloped tropical areas.

Diagnostic Studies and Procedures

Periodic attacks of chills and fever with no apparent cause alert a doctor to the possibility of malaria, especially if the person has traveled recently to an area where malaria is endemic. The physical examination will include palpating the spleen to determine if it is enlarged, one sign of the disease.

To confirm the diagnosis, a blood sample will be examined for the parasite. More than one sample may be required, however, because the number of parasites present in the bloodstream varies according to the organisms' life cycle. The strain of *Plasmodium* must also be identified to select the most effective treatment.

Medical Treatments

Malaria treatment is complicated by increasing *Plasmodium* resistance to the most common antimalaria drugs. This is especially true of *P. falciparum*, the most dangerous form of malaria, which has developed resistance to chloroquine (Aralen) in much of the world. In these particular areas, a few days of quinine sulfate therapy followed by an oral antibiotic such as tetracycline or pyrimethamine/sulfadoxine (Fansidar) may be sufficient to treat a mild, uncomplicated case of *P. falciparum* malaria. In more severe cases, hospitalization to give intravenous quinidine is necessary. Left untreated, *P. falciparum* malaria has a 20 percent mortality rate.

An uncomplicated case of *P. vivax*, *P. malariae*, or *P. ovale* may be treated with several days of chloroquine.

Because all antimalarial drugs can cause serious side effects, their use must be carefully monitored by a doctor. Call your physician immediately if

you develop nausea and vomiting, blurred vision, or hearing loss, all signs of potentially serious drug side effects. Taking the drugs with milk or food reduces intestinal upset.

Alternative Therapies

Herbal Medicine. Years ago, herbalists discovered that tea brewed from Peruvian bark, or cinchona trees, could cure malaria. Scientists later extracted quinine from cinchona bark. Today, this mainstay in the medical treatment of malaria is synthesized artificially, but resistance to these drugs is a growing problem. A Chinese herb called ginghaosu appears to be a promising alternative, and pharmaceutical researchers are studying its potential as a new antimalaria drug.

Self-Treatment

Prevention is the best self-care for malaria. Before visiting an area where the disease is common, ask your doctor about taking an antimalaria drug as a preventive measure. Chloroquine is often prescribed prophylactically where resistance is not a problem. Mefloquine (Lariam), another antimalaria drug, may be prescribed as an alternative. Be sure to take the full course of pills, even after returning home.

When in a mosquito-infested area, protect yourself by using fine-mesh window screens and mosquito netting over your bed. Apply insect repellent before going out. Some doctors also recommend carrying a few pills of pyrimethamine/sulfadoxine to take, should a fever and other symptoms of malaria develop in a remote area where medical care is not readily available.

If you contract malaria, drink large amounts of nonalcoholic liquids to replace fluids that are lost through sweating. During a prolonged period of very high fever, take a cool bath to lower the body's temperature.

Alternating hot and cold compresses on the forehead and the base of the skull can help ease headaches. Do not take aspirin or other nonprescription drugs, however, because they may interact with malaria medication.

Other Causes of Fever and Chills

Many infections, including Lyme disease and AIDS, can cause recurrent chills and fever. Recurrent fever is also a sign of some cancers, especially those that affect the blood and lymph systems, such as Hodgkin's disease, leukemia, and multiple myeloma.

Mastitis

Mastitis is an inflammation of the breast that occurs primarily in nursing mothers, although it can develop as a result of a breast injury. The condition is usually caused by *Staphylococcus aureus* bacteria, which are ubiquitous in our environment. In healthy people, they generally cause no problems, so long as they remain on the skin. But these organisms can start an infection when they enter the breasts through tiny skin cracks or fissures. Nursing mothers are susceptible because cracked nipples are common during the first month of breast-feeding. Improper nursing techniques or the use of a breast pump increases the risk.

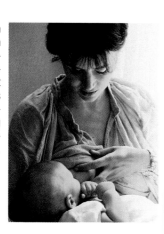

Although mastitis can make nursing uncomfortable, it usually does not necessitate giving up breast-feeding.

In acute mastitis, one or both breasts become sore and swollen. The nipple may give off a yellow pus-like secretion, and the skin may be red and warm. There may also be a low-grade fever. The infection usually remains confined within an abscess.

Diagnostic Studies and Procedures

In nursing mothers, doctors usually diagnose mastitis on the basis of the symptoms. In some cases, however, it may be necessary to culture a sample of the breast discharge to identify the causative bacteria. In women who are not pregnant or breast-feeding, diagnosis may be more complicated. Blood tests and analysis of any breast discharge are usually required, and mammography and a breast biopsy may be indicated if something other than an infection is suspected.

Medical Treatments

Mild mastitis usually responds to self-care within a few days (see Self-Treatment). If the breast becomes painful or develops a discharge, or body temperature rises above 102°F (39°C), an antibiotic may be prescribed. However, many strains of staphylococcus are now resistant to penicillin, the former drug of choice. Thus, severe or chronic mastitis may require an alternative antibiotic. An abscess should be lanced and drained.

Alternative Therapies

Hydrotherapy. Take a hot shower and, while under the water flow, massage the breasts gently from their base toward the nipple. This can help open the milk ducts, expel infectious material, and restore the flow of milk. Warm compresses may also alleviate pain.

Self-Treatment

Self-care can resolve most mild cases.
► To ease pain and keep milk flowing, apply moist heat packs for 10 minutes every few hours and before nursing.
► Take acetaminophen for pain.
► Drink extra fluid to avoid dehydration, especially if you have a fever.

Nursing can usually continue because bacteria or other infectious material is destroyed by the infant's digestive juices. If the mother is taking an antibiotic, some can pass into her breast milk, but is not likely to harm the baby. However, he may develop diarrhea or other intestinal problems from it.

If an abscess develops, it might be necessary to discontinue nursing at that breast until it heals. To maintain the flow of milk and prevent engorgement, be sure to express milk from it.

Other Causes of Breast Soreness

It is important to differentiate the swelling and soreness of mastitis from engorgement, an uncomfortable fullness in the breasts that develops two or three days after birth, signaling that the breasts are producing milk. This is normal and usually disappears as mother and infant develop their nursing skills.

Some women have more severe engorgement, leading to breasts that are

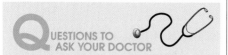

QUESTIONS TO ASK YOUR DOCTOR

► Should I stop nursing if antibiotics give my baby an upset stomach? If so, will I be able to resume nursing after the infection has cleared up?
► If expressing milk is necessary, what is the best type of breast pump to use in order to minimize breast problems?

A CASE IN POINT

At age 27, Sandra Small had her first baby, a healthy girl named Heather. Like so many of her friends, Small was determined to breast-feed. The nurse-midwife who had overseen her pregnancy and delivery also instructed the new mother in breast-feeding.

All went well until Heather was five weeks old; at that time, Small developed flu-like symptoms and a tender, feverish breast. She immediately called her nurse-midwife, and was told she undoubtedly had mastitis.

"Does this mean I have to stop nursing?" Small asked. She was pleasantly surprised when the midwife instructed her to continue nursing, explaining that the germs causing the infection normally live on the skin and mucous membranes of the mouth and nasal passages. "In fact, they may have come from Heather."

The nurse outlined a simple home treatment: "Stay in bed as much as possible. Apply warm compresses or a heating pad to your breast for 10 to 15 minutes every hour or two. When you nurse, offer the sore breast first to empty it more completely."

When Small asked about antibiotics, the midwife said that they were not advisable for mild mastitis, because most strains of the causative bacteria are now resistant to antibiotics. Even so, she instructed Small to call her if there was no improvement within a few days.

As it turned out, Small's mastitis cleared up in less than a week of self-care. "At first, the baby didn't seem to like the milk from the sore breast," Small said. The nurse explained that mastitis may give milk a salty flavor that babies don't relish. But it does not alter the milk's nutritious quality. Unless an abscess develops, nursing can continue without problems.

tense, tight, painful to touch, and lumpy in some areas. The absence of redness and fever helps rule out mastitis.

Mild to moderate breast swelling every month as part of premenstrual syndrome is not unusual. Unexplained or persistent breast swelling and soreness may be a sign of breast cancer or other disease and warrants prompt consultation with a physician.

Measles

(Rubeola)

Measles is a highly contagious disease caused by a paramyxovirus. Medically known as rubeola, in the past it was referred to as nine-day measles to distinguish it from the milder, three-day German measles, or rubella. Measles was once exceedingly common during childhood, occurring often in local epidemics. Today, it is rare in most industrialized countries, thanks to widespread immunization during infancy.

From 10 to 14 days after exposure to the virus, flu-like symptoms develop, including fever, runny nose, red watery eyes, and a dry cough. Some children also have diarrhea. The disease is at its most contagious during this phase.

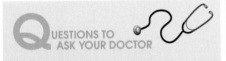

Q UESTIONS TO
ASK YOUR DOCTOR

▶ What should I do if my baby is exposed to measles before being immunized?
▶ How can I tell if my earlier measles immunization is still effective?

Within one to two days, tiny white dots (called Koplik's spots) appear on the lining of the mouth. A day or two later, the characteristic skin rash of measles appears. It starts behind and below the ears and, within another day or two, spreads to cover the entire head and body. The rash begins as tiny, slightly raised red spots that gradually increase in size and often join together to form large splotches. Any itching is

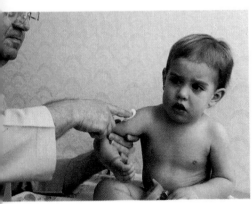

The first measles shot should be given between 12 and 15 months, with a second between ages 4 and 6 or 12 and 14 years.

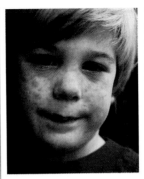

The measles rash consists of widespread red spots that may converge to form large splotches.

usually mild. From three to five days after the appearance of the rash, all of the symptoms start to disappear.

Although measles itself is generally mild, it carries a high risk of complications, such as pneumonia, ear infections, and encephalitis.

Diagnostic Studies and Procedures

A doctor can usually diagnose measles simply by observing the characteristic rash and other symptoms. If there is any doubt, laboratory evaluation of the nasal discharge can sometimes identify the virus. Or blood tests can be done to look for antibodies to the virus.

Medical Treatments

When an unimmunized child or immunocompromised person has been exposed to the measles virus, an injection of measles immune globulin or immune serum globulin might be administered. These shots will bolster immunity, and thus may prevent the disease or reduce its severity.

Antibiotics, although ineffective against the virus, may be prescribed to prevent or treat a secondary infection. Otherwise treatment is aimed at making the child more comfortable (see Self-Treatment).

You should watch for signs of complications and call a doctor immediately if any arise. These would include complaints of eye pain from bright light, unusual sleepiness or stupor, severe headache, and convulsions. At particular risk for complications are infants, persons who are taking steroids or immunosuppressive drugs, and children who have diabetes, asthma, or other chronic diseases.

Alternative Therapies

Herbal Medicine. Herbalists frequently recommend drinking saffron tea to promote perspiration and help lower the fever that accompanies measles.

Nutrition Therapy. One study showed that vitamin A supplements reduced complications and the death rate

among malnourished third-world children with measles. However, high doses of vitamin A are not generally recommended for children because of the danger of toxicity from them.

Self-Treatment

No one should ever have to suffer from measles, because a vaccination is available to prevent it. A child should be immunized shortly after his first birthday and again during the school years. The age for the second shot varies because some areas require the immunization before the child starts school (see box, below).

Children who do contract the disease should be kept at home to prevent spreading the infection and to allow for adequate rest to aid in recuperation. Although total bed rest is not necessary, only quiet activities should be allowed. Contrary to past advice, it is not necessary to keep a child in a dark room to protect his eyes.

You may give a child acetaminophen to ease the fever, headache, and other discomforts, but not aspirin, which is associated with an increased risk of Reye's syndrome, a severe brain and liver disorder (page 437). Be sure to offer the patient plenty of liquids, but do not force him to eat, especially when fever or diarrhea is present.

If itching is a problem, applications of calamine lotion to rashy areas may ease it. Taking a bath in lukewarm water to which cornstarch or colloidal oatmeal has been added also alleviates itching.

Other Causes of Rashes and Fever

Symptoms similar to those of measles may be caused by other viral infections that produce a splotchy rash, such as chickenpox, rubella, and scarlet fever.

IMMUNIZATION CHECKLIST

In recent years, there have been several serious measles epidemics on college campuses and among inner city schoolchildren. In addition to routine immunization of all children between 12 and 15 months of age and again between ages 4 and 6 or 12 and 14, the American Academy of Pediatrics recommends measles immunization for the following:
▶ Anyone born since 1957 who has not had measles or proven immunization.
▶ Persons of any age who were immunized before their first birthday.
▶ Anyone immunized between 1963 and 1967, at which time an ineffective vaccine may have been given.

Melanoma

Melanoma, the most lethal form of skin cancer, develops when pigment-producing cells (melanocytes) undergo malignant changes. Unlike other types of skin cancer, melanoma frequently metastasizes, spreading to the lungs, brain, liver, or other internal organs.

The incidence of melanoma has increased about 4 percent every year since 1973. In 1995, there were more than 34,500 new cases and over 7,000 deaths. Excessive sun exposure is by far the leading cause, especially among light-skinned people who sunburn easily. Heredity is also thought to play a part, and so is occupational exposure to coal tar, pitch, creosote, arsenic compounds, and radium.

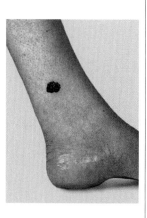

A change in the appearance of a mole is often an early sign of melanoma.

A mole (nevus) or other darkly pigmented spot that changes in size or color is a common warning sign. Large moles are especially associated with an increased risk of melanoma; they should be examined periodically. Other warning signs include scaling, oozing, bleeding, or a change in the appearance of a bump or nodule, and pigmentation that spreads from the border of a mole or bump into the surrounding skin.

Although most melanoma originates on the skin, in rare cases it arises in the pigment cells of the eyes. Melanoma of the choroid—the layer of tissue that lies between the retina and the eye's outer covering—often metastasizes.

Diagnostic Studies and Procedures

New techniques have been developed to screen for early melanoma. One is epiluminescence microscopy, in which the outer layer of a lesion is coated with mineral oil to make it translucent. Then a magnifying instrument, called a dermatoscope, is used to examine skin for abnormalities. Computerized image analysis, in which a computer is used to study details that the human eye cannot see, is another experimental technique of screening for melanoma.

Any suspicious mole or skin lesion should be biopsied.

Medical Treatments

Surgery is almost always the most effective treatment. In addition to the tumor, a surgeon will remove a margin of tissue around and underneath it to excise any additional cancer cells. Skin grafts will be used to cover large incisions. Melanoma that has spread to internal organs may require additional surgery.

Chemotherapy may be used in addition to surgery. When melanoma is confined to an arm or a leg, a technique called isolation perfusion is sometimes tried. This treatment entails briefly isolating the blood supply of the limb from the rest of the circulation, and allowing a higher concentration of anticancer drugs in that area.

High-dose radiation therapy can control the spread of melanoma and also alleviate pain from metastases.

Experimental immunotherapy shows promise against some types of metastic melanoma. The goal is to stimulate the body's white blood cells, or lymphocytes, to fight the cancer cells.

Alternative Therapies

Alternative therapies should be limited to controlling pain, coping with the stress of cancer therapy, or strengthening the body's immune system.

Imagery and Visualization. These techniques are taught in many cancer centers to help patients cope with both cancer and its treatment. Some people

STAGING OF MELANOMA

Of the several methods for determing the stage of a melanoma, the Clark's system, which measures the tumor's depth of penetration, is the one most commonly used.

Clark's Level	Depth	Percent Curable
I	Epidermis	100%
II	Papillary dermis	92%
III	Junction of papillary and reticular dermis	65%
IV	Reticular dermis	54%
V	Below subcutaneous fat	45%

believe that such methods can also boost the immune system to fight the cancer. *Nutrition Therapy.* A diet high in antioxidant nutrients—beta carotene, vitamins A, C, and E—is believed to protect against cancer, including melanoma. Fish oil and other substances high in gamma linoleic acid may also be recommended.

Yoga and Meditation. These and other relaxation techniques such as deep-breathing exercises can help control pain and reduce stress.

Self-Treatment

The most effective preventive measure is to limit sun exposure. Using a sunscreen with an SPF of at least 15 may help reduce the risk of some skin cancers, but experts warn that it does not prevent melanoma. If possible, stay out of the sun between 10 A.M. and 3 P.M., or at least wear protective clothing.

Perform a monthly self-examination of your skin. Use mirrors to examine parts of your body that are difficult to see; for example, the back of your neck, scalp, and buttocks. Take careful note of the size and location of freckles, moles, bumps and other such features.

When inspecting moles, remember the ABCD description of the typical melanoma lesions: They are **a**ssymetrical; they have irregular **b**orders and multiple **c**olors (usually combinations of brown, red, gray, or black); and their **d**iameters are larger than 5 to 10 millimeters (1/5 to 2/5 inch). During subsequent examinations, look for any changes in the number, size, shape, and color of moles or other blemishes. If you see any, consult your doctor at once.

Other Causes of Melanoma Symptoms

The warning signs of basal cell and squamous cell carcinomas, less aggressive forms of skin cancer, are sometimes similar to those of melanoma.

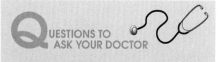

QUESTIONS TO ASK YOUR DOCTOR

▶ Do medications that increase the skin's sensitivity to the sun also raise the risk of acquiring melanoma?
▶ Do I have any moles that bear special watching? If so, should they be removed? If not, how often should I have them checked?

Ménière's Disease

Ménière's disease is a disorder of the inner ear. An attack most often starts with ringing in the ears (tinnitus) and a sensation of fullness or pressure in one or both ears. Then severe vertigo, nausea, vomiting, and possibly a migraine headache usually occur. There may also be some hearing loss, especially if the episodes are prolonged and frequent. Occurrences can be incapacitating, lasting from several hours to several days and recurring with varying frequency.

An attack is precipitated by a rise in fluid in the labyrinth area of the inner ear, causing increased pressure and a disrupted sense of balance. Although the underlying cause of the disease is unknown, some experts think that degeneration of hair-like structures in the inner ear, which transmit sound waves, may be responsible. Ménière's usually begins in mid-life and occurs about equally in men and women.

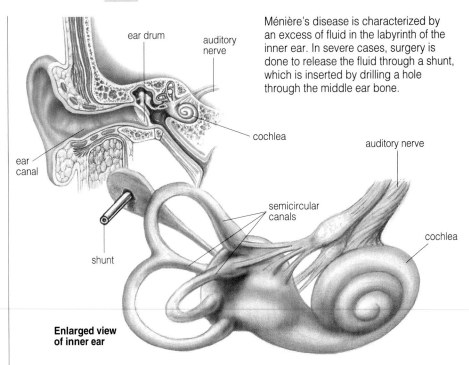

Ménière's disease is characterized by an excess of fluid in the labyrinth of the inner ear. In severe cases, surgery is done to release the fluid through a shunt, which is inserted by drilling a hole through the middle ear bone.

Enlarged view of inner ear

Diagnostic Studies and Procedures

Diagnosis starts with a complete physical, which includes a careful examination of the ears and hearing tests. You may be instructed to restrict fluid or to take a diuretic to lower the body's fluid volume before taking the hearing test.

In another procedure, the ears are irrigated with water at different temperatures, which causes a whirling sensation and makes the eyes flicker. These eye movements can indicate whether or not the labyrinth is diseased.

In some cases, a doctor may order electrocochleography, a test performed under general anesthesia, in which a probe is inserted through the eardrum to measure electrical activity.

Medical Treatments

Medication cannot cure Ménière's disease, but taking a diuretic to rid the body of excess fluid may help prevent attacks. To alleviate an episode, a doctor may prescribe:

Antihistamine drugs, such as diphenhydramine (Benadryl), meclizine (Antivert), or cyclizine (Marezine), which can help to ease the vertigo. Tranquilizers such as diazepam (Valium) may have a similar effect.

Antinausea drugs, such as dimenhydrinate (Dramamine) or scopolamine (Transderm Scōp), to ease nausea and vomiting.

Steroids, such as prednisone, if an autoimmune cause is suspected. Since taking anything by mouth can be

impossible during an attack, drugs may be given in the form of a skin patch, a suppository, or an injection.

Surgery is sometimes recommended if attacks are disabling. The simplest procedure involves drilling a hole through the bone of the middle ear into the labyrinth to release the excess fluid. Removal of a nerve in the ear's vestibular system may alleviate the vertigo and usually does not damage hearing. However, if total hearing loss has already occurred, complete removal of the labyrinth may be recommended to eliminate the vertigo.

Alternative Therapies

Acupuncture. Symptoms are sometimes alleviated in a single session, and a series of treatments may reduce the frequency of attacks.

Herbal Medicine. Ginger tea is said to alleviate nausea and dizziness. Butcher's broom and betony, taken in extract or capsule form, may also help.

Nutrition Therapy. A low-salt diet can reduce excess body fluid, which may in turn reduce the frequency and severity of Ménière's attacks. Caffeine, alcohol,

and chocolate can worsen symptoms and should be avoided. Some people have been helped by reducing fat intake to less than 10 percent of calories and increasing their consumption of fresh vegetables and fruits and whole grains. Improvement may be seen within two to three weeks.

Self-Treatment

During an attack, you should stay in bed in a darkened room, lying as still as possible. Sip flat ginger ale to help alleviate nausea and dry mouth.

It is extremely important to protect the ears from any further damage to the hair-like structures that are instrumental in hearing. Wear earplugs when you are in a noisy environment or when using noisy equipment or appliances, including a vacuum cleaner and hair dryer. If your job involves using a jackhammer or other noisy machine, wear protective occupational earmuffs. Do not subject your ears to any device that delivers sound directly into the ears through earphones or plugs.

Other Causes of Vertigo and Hearing Loss

Vertigo may also be the result of an inner ear infection, motion sickness, allergic rhinitis, high doses of aspirin and other drugs that damage the inner ear, a blow to the head, a vascular disorder in the brain or, less commonly, multiple sclerosis. Hearing loss also may be caused by a brain tumor, a stroke, trauma, a viral infection, or nerve damage.

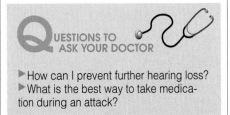

QUESTIONS TO ASK YOUR DOCTOR

▶ How can I prevent further hearing loss?
▶ What is the best way to take medication during an attack?

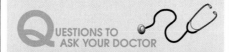

Meningitis

(Acute bacterial; aseptic viral; and subacute meningitis)

Meningitis is an inflammation of the meninges, the membranes that surround and protect the brain and spinal cord. The most common and acute types are caused by bacteria, typically meningococcus, *Haemophilus influenzae* type B (HIB), or pneumococcus.

When meningitis is caused by something other than bacteria it is called aseptic meningitis. Viruses, including Coxsackie and herpes, are the most frequent causes of aseptic meningitis. In some cases, the brain also becomes inflamed, a condition referred to as encephalitis (page 177). Subacute meningitis is usually secondary to other disorders, including tuberculosis, Lyme disease, syphilis, leukemia, lymphoma, AIDS, and brain cancer.

All forms of acute meningitis produce similar symptoms—fever, headache, a stiff neck, and vomiting. The onset can be rapid, quickly evolving into confusion, drowsiness, stupor, and coma.

Diagnostic Studies and Procedures

Prompt and accurate diagnosis and treatment are essential, because acute bacterial meningitis can become life-threatening within hours. As part of the physical examination, a complete neurological workup will be performed. The head, throat, ears, and skin will be inspected for sources of infection.

The most important test, however, is a lumbar puncture, or spinal tap, in which a hollow needle is inserted between two vertebrae in the lower spine to aspirate a small amount of spinal fluid. Cloudy fluid that contains white blood cells strongly suggests bacterial meningitis, but laboratory analyses and culture will confirm the diagnosis and identify the causative organism. Other tests may include a CT scan or MRI to look for a possible brain abscess or other cause of inflammation.

Medical Treatments

Drug Therapy. If bacterial meningitis is suspected, the person will be hospitalized immediately and started on intensive intravenous antibiotics, even before the diagnosis is confirmed. Initially, a broad-spectrum antibiotic, such as cephalosporin or penicillin, may be given, although identification of the organism may require a later switch of drugs. Recently, the pneumococcus

---

QUESTIONS TO ASK YOUR DOCTOR

► If I have been exposed to meningitis, should I be immunized or take prophylactic antibiotics?
► If my baby receives the HIB vaccine to prevent meningitis, does it carry any risks or side effects?

---

organism that causes some cases of meningitis has developed resistance to a number of antibiotics, greatly limiting choices of treatment.

Deciding upon treatment is even more difficult if viral meningitis is a possibility. In such cases, antibiotics have no effect, and the risk of their side effects, especially anaphylaxis, must be considered. Depending on the patient's condition, a doctor may delay starting antibiotics for 8 to 12 hours to await results of culture studies. If a herpes virus is responsible, intravenous acyclovir (Zovirax) will be administered. Similarly, intravenous antifungal drugs will be given if a fungus is the cause.

Subacute meningitis may be treated with steroids, antibiotics, or other drugs. In all forms of the disease, drugs may be prescribed to reduce fever and alleviate nausea and head pain. Intravenous fluids are usually given, but care is needed to avoid giving too much, which can lead to brain swelling.

Surgical Treatment. In unusual cases, parasites form a brain abscess that can cause meningitis. Such an abscess may require surgical removal and drainage.

Alternative Therapies

Alternative therapies cannot cure meningitis and should never be substituted for prompt medical treatment.

Aromatherapy. During convalescence, a lavender bath or massage with lavender, rosemary, marjoram, or peppermint oil is soothing.

Herbal Medicine. Western herbalists may recommend black horehound for headaches with nausea and vomiting. It can also be combined with meadowsweet and chamomile tea.

Physical and Occupational Therapy. Sometimes severe meningitis causes tremor, palsy, and other neurologic problems, requiring rehabilitation under the guidance of physical and occupational therapists.

Self-Treatment

While undergoing medical therapy, the patient should stay in bed. Because light sensitivity is likely, a darkened room is advisable. During recovery, adequate rest is important, as is a nutritious diet and at least eight glasses of fluids per day. Do not take any medication, even aspirin or acetaminophen, without first checking with your doctor. Intensive antibiotic therapy carries a risk of possible drug fever, which is worsened by additional medications.

Epidemics of meningococcal meningitis sometimes occur in military barracks and similar settings. During such an outbreak, immunization can help stop the spread. Anyone exposed to the disease may also need preventive antibiotic treatment with rifampin.

Meningitis caused by *Haemophilus influenzae* type B can be prevented by HIB vaccine, now recommended for all infants, beginning at age two months.

Other Causes of Meningitis Symptoms

Lead poisoning can cause inflammation of the meninges; Rocky Mountain spotted fever produces symptoms similar to those of meningitis.

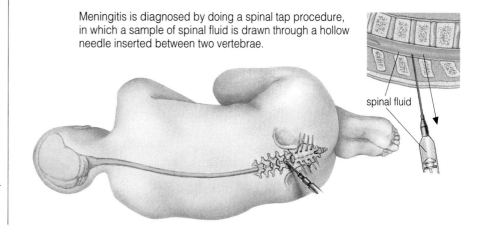

Meningitis is diagnosed by doing a spinal tap procedure, in which a sample of spinal fluid is drawn through a hollow needle inserted between two vertebrae.

spinal fluid

Menopause

(Female climacteric)

Menopause marks the end of a woman's natural ability to conceive and bear a child. Technically, menopause occurs when she ceases to menstruate, but the biological mechanisms and symptoms leading up to it begin several years earlier, during the pre- or perimenopausal period. (The exception involves women who have had their ovaries removed surgically; for them, menopause occurs immediately.) Similarly, menopausal symptoms may continue for several years after menstruation ends.

The age at which menopause occurs varies, with some women entering it as early as 40 and others not until their mid-fifties. On average, however, menopause occurs by age 52, and virtually all women have completed the process by the age of 58.

Menopause is triggered by a decline in estrogen, the ovarian hormone that controls female reproduction and gives a woman her female characteristics. Estrogen production peaks during a woman's twenties, starts a gradual decline after age 30, and then drops sharply at menopause.

A change in the menstrual cycle is the primary indicator of approaching menopause, with specifics differing from one woman to another. Menstrual cycles and periods become shorter or longer, and bleeding heavier or lighter. Sometimes several months elapse between periods, followed by several cycles of two or three weeks. These changes may shift from month to month, until menstruation ceases altogether. After a full year without menstruation, menopause is complete and a woman enters her postmenopausal stage, which today is about one-third of her total life expectancy.

In addition to the cessation of menstruation, menopause brings numerous physical and psychological changes. The two most common are:

Hot flashes, marked by a sudden sensation of heat, usually in the upper body, and perhaps accompanied by a reddish blush and sweating that are followed by chills. Most episodes last only a few minutes, but they vary considerably in intensity and frequency. Some women experience frequent and intense hot flashes, especially at night, often waking up drenched in perspira-

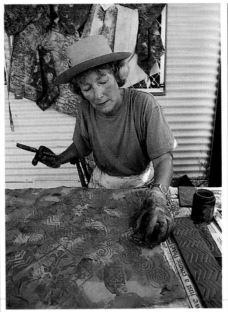

Many older women find that developing new pursuits brings new zest to life.

tion. As the body adjusts to its new hormone levels, the flashes subside, and most end by age 60.

Vaginal dryness and atrophy, caused by thinning of the outer layer of the mucous membrane that lines the vagina. These changes can lead to painful intercourse and persistent vaginitis. Similar tissue thinning in the lower urinary tract increases the incidence of bladder infections, and leads to other problems such as incontinence.

Other symptoms associated with menopause include heart palpitations, skin dryness and itchiness, headaches, insomnia, weight gain, thinning scalp and pubic hair, and increased growth of facial hair. There might also be marked mood swings, perhaps due to lack of sleep or changing hormone levels. Many women develop memory problems, especially in the area of verbal fluency. A number also experience changes in sexual drive, with some reporting increased sexual interest and others a lessening of desire.

Diagnostic Studies and Procedures

Menopause is a normal part of every woman's life, not an illness, and usually does not require diagnostic tests other than a pelvic examination and pap smear. In some instances, however, a doctor may order an FSH test to confirm that symptoms are in fact due to menopause. This blood study measures the body's level of follicle stimulating hormone, a substance produced by the

pituitary gland to stimulate ovulation. As estrogen levels decline, the pituitary secretes more FSH; thus, a high level may herald the onset of menopause.

Blood and urine tests also can determine whether a woman is continuing to ovulate, an important issue for women seeking to avoid pregnancy.

Medical Treatments

Most gynecologists now advocate estrogen replacement therapy (ERT) to halt or ease menopausal symptoms, as well as to help prevent osteoporosis and heart disease later in life. Studies show a 50 to 80 percent reduction in hip, wrist, and vertebrae fractures—some of the common consequences of osteoporosis—among women who start taking replacement estrogen within three to five years of menopause.

Similarly, estrogen replacement cuts the risk of a heart attack in half, a benefit attributed to estrogen's role in raising levels of protective HDL cholesterol. Studies also indicate that estrogen may also protect against Alzheimer's disease, a devastating form of mental decline that is much more common in women than in men.

The estrogen may be taken systemically, either by a pill, such as Premarin or Estrace, or by wearing an Estraderm skin patch. If vaginal dryness is the primary concern, localized therapy with an estrogen vaginal cream is usually sufficient. Another localized application, a cervical ring that is impregnated with a time-release estrogen, is expected to become available soon.

Doctors remain divided as to how long estrogen replacement should continue. Some feel that it should stop after two or three years when the body adjusts to its altered hormone levels. In contrast, a growing number of doctors advocate long-term or life-long ERT, especially for women with a high risk of osteoporosis or heart disease. However, even the most ardent advocates of

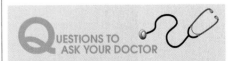

QUESTIONS TO ASK YOUR DOCTOR

▶ Am I a candidate for estrogen replacement? If so, what form do you recommend? For how long?
▶ If I do take estrogen, how often should I have a pelvic examination and pap smear? (Most doctors recommend every six months.)

At the age of 37, Heather Johnson had both her ovaries removed as part of a radical hysterectomy after developing endometrial cancer—a malignancy of the uterine lining. The surgeon had recommended this approach because Johnson had already completed her family and her mother had died of ovarian cancer, increasing her risk of this lethal disease.

"I vaguely knew that removal of the ovaries would throw me into menopause," Johnson commented later, "but I had no concept of what this really meant. All at once, I started having a dozen or more hot flashes every day. I'd also wake up drenched with sweat two or three times each night."

Normally, estrogen replacement is prescribed to ease the symptoms of an abrupt surgical menopause. Unfortunately, Johnson's history of high blood pressure and phlebitis precluded this approach. "My doctor assured me that the symptoms would eventually lessen," Johnson recalls, "but the opposite seemed to be happening."

Her hot flashes continued and, over the next few months, she suffered several bouts of vaginitis. Up until that time, Johnson and her husband had enjoyed a pleasurable sex life, but for Heather, this ceased because of vaginal dryness. She tried various vaginal lubricants, but none of them were adequate.

"I was feeling increasingly depressed," she says, "but I didn't know if this was hormonal or a consequence of my other symptoms. In retrospect, it was probably a combination of factors." In desperation, Johnson sought help from a gynecologist who was a specialist in menopause.

This doctor agreed that Johnson probably should not take replacement estrogen, but felt that localized applications of an estrogen vaginal cream could solve the vaginitis and dryness problems without undue risk. "Some estrogen is absorbed into the bloodstream," she cautioned, "but the dosage is small compared to what is administered through pills or a medicated patch." Even so, Johnson was instructed to take 200 milligrams of vitamin E a day to protect against possible clotting problems. Fortunately, she seemed to tolerate the cream well, and the vaginal problems quickly improved.

The frequent hot flashes and night sweats were more difficult to alleviate. The gynecologist suggested various lifestyle measures—for example, cool showers, fanning, layered clothing, and cutting back on alcohol and caffeine—which produced little improvement.

At that point, Johnson decided to join a menopause self-help group. "I stood out on two counts," Johnson remembers. "I was the youngest woman in the group and my symptoms were the most severe." An older woman credited herbal medicine with reducing her hot flashes to a tolerable level, and Johnson decided to give this approach a try.

"I met with her herbalist, who seemed to be very knowledgeable about the medicinal properties of different plants. When I told her I couldn't take estrogen replacement, she said that this eliminated two popular herbs for menopause—dong quai, or female ginseng, and black cohosh—because both contained substances similar to estrogen." In addition, Johnson's history of high blood pressure was a contraindication for licorice, another herb that is often used to treat menopausal symptoms.

As an alternative, the herbalist recommended a daily cup of tea brewed from a combination of herbs—squaw weed, red raspberry leaf, motherwort, and cramp bark. Johnson was instructed to try this for six weeks to see if there was any improvement. She kept a careful diary of hot flashes and night sweats; at the end of six weeks, there was a slight reduction in their frequency, but not enough to make much difference.

Johnson returned to the herbalist, who added two more herbs to the brew—goldenseal and gotu kola, an Indian herb commonly used by practitioners of ayurveda. She also recommended a teaspoon of evening primrose oil to be taken three times a day, and suggested that Johnson take up yoga and meditation. Several of the other women in Johnson's menopause support group were practicing yoga, so she added this alternative therapy to her regimen.

Again, Johnson kept a diary of her symptoms. After six weeks, she managed to sleep through an entire night without experiencing any sweating. Over the next few months, the night sweats all but disappeared and the number of hot flashes diminished to one or two a day. "While still bothersome, these I can live with," Johnson says.

ERT recognize that there are adverse side effects and risks. The possible side effects include weight gain, fluid retention, increased vaginal secretions, breast tenderness and enlargement, altered libido, nausea, vomiting, bloating, cramps, headaches, dizziness, high blood pressure, uterine bleeding, and depression. Use of the estrogen patch may lessen some of these problems but it can also cause skin irritation or rash at the application site.

Even more worrisome is the fact that estrogen replacement increases the risk of uterine cancer. This became apparent in the late 1960s, when estrogen was being prescribed routinely. Almost immediately, ERT dropped dramatically, but returned to favor in the late 1980s when new research showed that uterine cancer could be prevented by lowering the estrogen dosage and adding another hormone, progesterone, to the regimen. Used as part of ERT, progesterone causes a periodic, menstrual-like shedding of the uterine lining. It is theorized that preventing an overgrowth of the endometrium is what reduces the risk of uterine cancer.

There is still an unresolved question of whether or not ERT increases the risk of breast cancer. Studies to date have produced conflicting results, but one long-term study of 140,000 nurses found a significant increase in breast cancer among women taking estrogen.

Estrogen replacement causes blood clots in some women, and should not be used by anyone who has had thrombophlebitis, stroke, or other clotting disorders. It can also cause gallstones and damage the liver, but this last problem probably can be avoided by using an estrogen patch, which allows the hormone to bypass the liver and go directly into the bloodstream.

Other women who may have problems with estrogen replacement include those who have diabetes, migraines, asthma, uterine fibroid tumors, endometriosis, hypertension, and lupus or other disorders that are treated with corticosteroid drugs. Although ERT reduces the risk of heart attack, it may

MENOPAUSE (CONTINUED)

actually be hazardous for a woman whose heart muscle has already been damaged, because starting estrogen may provoke congestive heart failure.

Other drugs that are sometimes prescribed to treat menopausal symptoms for women who cannot take estrogen include the following:

▶ Low doses of a beta blocker such as propranolol (Inderal) to alleviate any heart palpitations.

▶ Diuretics to reduce fluid retention.

▶ Antidepressants such as fluoxetine (Prozac) to ease severe depression.

▶ Low doses of oral contraceptives for premenopausal women who experience heavy bleeding.

▶ Tamoxifen, an antiestrogen drug that appears to protect against osteoporosis and breast cancer.

▶ Dehydroepiandrosterone, or DHEA, an adrenal hormone that the body converts to androgens, male sex hormones, and estrogen. This experimental hormone therapy is under study as an alternative to ERT.

In certain cases, dilation and curettage (D&C), a scraping of the uterine lining, may be recommended, especially when a woman is experiencing irregular and/or very heavy periods and anemia. Or a hysterectomy may be advised in some instances of severe and unrelenting anemia.

Alternative Therapies
Numerous alternative therapies can alleviate menopausal symptoms and reduce or eliminate the need for ERT.

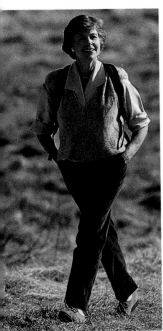

Regular physical activity can help control weight and retain a more youthful figure and outlook.

POSTMENOPAUSAL PREGNANCY
Medical technology makes it possible now for a woman to have a baby long after menopause. Although her own ovaries no longer have viable eggs, a postmenopausal woman can undergo intensive hormone therapy to prepare her body for pregnancy, and then have a fertilized donor egg inserted into her uterus.

The first reported postmenopausal pregnancies involved American women acting as surrogates to carry their own grandchildren. In at least two such cases, the younger women could not bear children themselves because they did not have a uterus, although they did have functioning ovaries. This use of postmenopausal pregnancy did not raise a public outcry, but the story was different when the technology was used by women in their late fifties and sixties who wanted babies of their own. Reports of these births sparked widespread debate over the ethics of using costly medical services to produce pregnancies for women beyond the natural age for reproduction. The question remains unresolved, but worldwide, an increasing number of postmenopausal women are embarking on motherhood.

Herbal Medicine. Herbal teas said to alleviate hot flashes and other symptoms include red raspberry leaf, dong quai, damiana, sarsaparilla, licorice, and valerian. Ginseng and black cohosh capsules or extracts are sometimes recommended because they contain estrogen-like substances. Capsules of evening primrose or black current oil may prevent bloating, and marigold ointment stops vaginal itching.

Nutrition Therapy. Many doctors and nutritionists recommend that postmenopausal women get 1,000 to 1,500 milligrams of calcium and 400 to 800 IU of vitamin D a day to protect their bones, and 200 to 400 milligrams of vitamin E to help prevent heart disease. A diet that includes three or four servings of low-fat milk or milk products can provide adequate calcium, but it is virtually impossible to get 200 milligrams of vitamin E without taking supplements. Extra vitamin C and beta carotene may also be advocated for their antioxidant effects. Studies indicate, however, that eating fruits and vegetables high in these nutrients is more protective than taking high-dose supplements, which may actually

increase damage from by-products of oxygen metabolism. A low-fat diet that emphasizes fruits, legumes, grains, and vegetables, provides balanced nutrition with minimal calories, thereby helping also to prevent weight gain.

Yoga and Meditation. These and other relaxation therapies can help counter depression and mood swings, as well as prevent hot flashes by lowering stress.

Self-Treatment
To minimize the discomfort of hot flashes, wear layers of lightweight clothing that can be shed quickly as the need arises. Work and sleep in a cool environment, since a warm room itself can bring them on. To help prevent night sweats, take a cool shower before going to bed and cover yourself with only a sheet or light blanket.

Abstain from nicotine, alcohol, and caffeine, which can aggravate hot flashes. If you smoke, now is the time to stop. Women who smoke enter menopause an average of two to four years earlier than nonsmokers; they also have an increased risk of osteoporosis, heart disease, and many cancers.

Regular exercise, such as a brisk 15- to 20-minute walk four or five times a week, can elevate mood, ease fluid retention, prevent weight gain, build stronger bones, and reduce the risk of heart disease.

Regular sexual activity helps to prevent vaginal dryness and thinning. A vaginal lubricant specially formulated for use after menopause can also prevent painful intercourse. Some women find that vitamin E oil or unscented vitamin E cream applied to the vaginal area provides similar benefits.

Finally, consider joining a menopause support group, especially if you are troubled by entering this stage of life. The rapidly expanding population of older women has brought a new openness about menopause, and many women can benefit from sharing their worries and experiences.

Other Causes of Menstrual Irregularities
Pregnancy, the most common cause of cessation of menstruation, should always be ruled out in a sexually active woman. Irregular periods may also be caused by uterine or cervical tumors, ovarian cysts, thyroid or other hormone disorders, diabetes, anemia, depression, excessive weight gain or loss, and alcoholism.

Menorrhagia

(Anovulatory vaginal bleeding; menometrorrhagia)

Menorrhagia is excessive menstrual bleeding due to a prolonged period, very heavy flow, or a combination of the two. Doctors generally define menstrual bleeding as excessive if the woman must change her tampon or pad at least every hour.

On average, a woman discharges four to six tablespoons of blood during menstruation, but this volume may be doubled by mucus, cells, and bits of membrane from the endometrium that resemble clots. (Menstrual blood normally does not clot because the uterus produces an enzyme that destroys clotting mechanisms.) This other material may lead a woman to believe that she is bleeding more profusely than she is.

Menstruation in the absence of ovulation, or anovulatory bleeding, is a common cause of menorrhagia, especially during adolescence and in the period approaching menopause—times when ovulation may be sporadic. In an anovulatory cycle, estrogen stimulates growth of the endometrium, the tissue lining the uterus, which is normal during the first, or proliferative, phase of a woman's cycle. When ovulation does not take place, there is no surge of progesterone, the hormone that prompts the endometrium to enter its second (luteal) phase, in which the lining thickens and fills with fat and other nutrients to nourish a fertilized egg.

Without progesterone, the proliferative phase continues, with the endometrium continuing to grow and increase its supply of blood vessels. After a week or two, estrogen levels fall, causing the endometrium to break down and shed as menstruation. These cycles tend to be shorter than normal, with much heavier bleeding because the endometrium has undergone a prolonged proliferative phase.

Other causes of menorrhagia include the use of an IUD for birth control, the presence of fibroid uterine tumors, uterine cancer, and hormonal disorders that are marked by excessive estrogen production. Women who smoke have a five-fold increase of menorrhagia over nonsmokers; the reason for this is not known, although some researchers believe it may be because smoking can suppress ovulation.

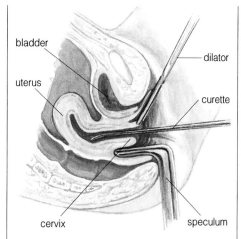

During a D&C, a dilator is used to open, or dilate, the cervix, and a curette is employed to scrape the uterine lining.

Diagnostic Studies and Procedures

Persistent, heavy menstrual bleeding warrants a complete checkup that includes a pelvic examination, pap smear, and blood and urine tests. Hormone studies can determine whether or not ovulation is taking place and detect hormonal imbalances.

Other tests may include a pelvic sonogram; hysteroscopy, in which the uterus is examined with a fiberoptic viewing tube; and a D&C (dilation and curettage), in which the cervix is widened, or dilated, and a curette, a spoon-shaped instrument, is used to scrape away part of the uterine lining.

Medical Treatments

Treatment is determined by the underlying cause. If an IUD is responsible, periods usually return to normal after it is removed. Women using oral contraceptives usually have light periods, so this method of birth control may be recommended if the woman is not trying to conceive and there is no medical cause for the menorrhagia.

Sometimes, a D&C cures the problem, especially in a woman who is nearing menopause, or who has had an incomplete miscarriage or abortion. Fibroid tumors can sometimes be

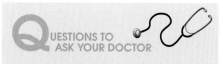

QUESTIONS TO ASK YOUR DOCTOR

▶ Can my type of heavy bleeding be treated with a D&C?
▶ What level of menstrual bleeding warrants seeing a doctor?

removed surgically. A hysterectomy is considered only if bleeding is due to cancer or is causing severe anemia.

Alternative Therapies

An organic cause of heavy menstruation, such as a tumor, must be ruled out before trying alternative therapies.

Herbal Medicine. Uva-ursi, or bearberry, is said to reduce heavy menstruation by constricting blood vessels that line the uterus. It is available in tincture and capsule form.

Nutrition Therapy. Vitamin C taken with foods high in bioflavonoids, substances found in buckwheat, fruits, nuts, and seeds, is said to reduce heavy menstruation by strengthening the capillary walls. Women who bleed heavily after stopping birth control pills are sometimes helped by vitamin A supplements, but vitamin A can build to toxic levels if high doses are consumed. An excess also causes severe birth defects, so supplements should be stopped at least three months before attempting to conceive.

Heavy menstruation can lead to iron deficiency anemia; if this is diagnosed, iron supplements may be needed. Iron-rich foods include liver and other organ meats, red meat, legumes, shellfish, fish, dried apricots, and fortified breads and cereals. Acidic foods such as tomatoes and applesauce, when cooked in a cast iron pot, will leach iron from it.

Self-Treatment

The first step is to make sure that you really are bleeding excessively. If you have recently changed from using pads to tampons or vice versa, or chosen a less absorbent type, your flow may seem heavier than normal. Switch back to your former product to see if bleeding still seems excessive.

Also, consider lifestyle factors that may impact on your menstrual cycle. Stress, heavy alcohol use, crash dieting, and overexercise can lead to menstrual irregularity, cessation of ovulation, and periods that are heavier or lighter than normal. Excessive use of aspirin or other blood-thinning medications may also induce abnormally heavy periods.

Other Causes of Heavy Bleeding

A miscarriage can cause heavy bleeding, and if it occurs early in pregnancy, the woman may mistake it for heavy menstruation. Heavy bleeding also may be associated with a tubal pregnancy, endometriosis, hypertension, diabetes, or blood disorders.

Menstrual Cramps

(Dysmenorrhea)

Many women experience discomfort, usually abdominal cramps and a sensation of heaviness in the pelvic area, just before or during menstruation. Typically, symptoms subside after a day or two of menstrual flow. When cramps are severe and prolonged, however, the condition is called dysmenorrhea.

Not so long ago, dysmenorrhea was dismissed as psychological or simply a natural aspect of womanhood. We now know that it is caused mostly by prostaglandins, hormone-like chemicals that produce the muscle contractions needed to rid the uterus of menstrual fluid. (Prostaglandins produce similar contractions during labor and childbirth.) Some women find that their cramps lessen after they've had a baby. For others, the problem worsens.

Diagnostic Studies and Procedures

Persistent, severe cramps warrant seeing a gynecologist who will, at the very least, perform a pelvic examination and take a pap smear. Additional tests may include blood and urine studies, an ultrasound evaluation, hysteroscopy to examine the inside of the uterus, and laparoscopy, a procedure that involves inserting a viewing instrument into the abdominal cavity to look for such abnormalities as tumors and adhesions.

Medical Treatments

Primary dysmenorrhea can usually be alleviated or prevented by taking a nonsteroidal anti-inflammatory drug (NSAID), which will block excessive prostaglandin production. Aspirin and ibuprofen are the most widely used. If these do not work, a doctor may prescribe one of a dozen stronger NSAIDs. Often, several must be tried because their effectiveness varies from person to person. To prevent cramps, start taking the medication a day or two before a period is expected, and continue it until a day or two after menstruation begins. This regimen will also help to prevent headaches, back pain, and other discomfort.

Five to 10 percent of women with severe dysmenorrhea fail to get adequate relief from NSAIDs. In such cases, a doctor may prescribe codeine or a similar pain reliever. Birth control pills are

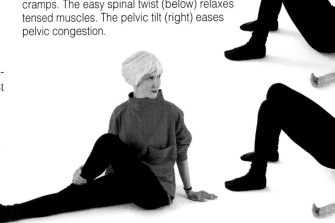

The two yoga exercises shown here are among those said to alleviate menstrual cramps. The easy spinal twist (below) relaxes tensed muscles. The pelvic tilt (right) eases pelvic congestion.

another approach; many women who use them find that menstrual cramps abate. Although dysmenorrhea is not considered an adequate reason to take an oral contraceptive, it may play a role in selecting a method of birth control.

Alternative Therapies

Herbal Medicine. Raspberry leaf tea is often recommended for relieving cramps. Other remedies are chamomile or valerian tea, extract, or capsules. Ginger tea, extract, or candy may help alleviate the nausea and vomiting that sometimes accompany dysmenorrhea. White willow bark tea or capsules contain a salicylate, the major ingredient in aspirin, but are less likely to cause stomach upset. Some women report that taking two or three capsules of evening primrose oil or black currant oil each day prevents menstrual cramps as well as symptoms of premenstrual syndrome.

Hydrotherapy. Soaking in a tub of warm water that contains a few drops of juniper oil may ease cramps.

Self-hypnosis and Visualization. These techniques help overcome pain by focusing the mind on it in a way that makes it manageable. One begins by closing the eyes and then concentrating on the color, shape, and size of the pain. By visualizing it, the color or shape may change, and as it does, the discomfort may disappear.

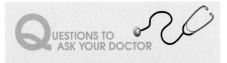

Q UESTIONS TO ASK YOUR DOCTOR

▶ Should I be concerned that my cramps indicate some kind of disorder?
▶ How often can I take an NSAID?

Massage. This age-old remedy may be combined with acupressure or aromatherapy. Exerting gentle pressure on acupoints just below the breast bone, the bottom of the tailbone, the back of the neck, and the pelvic area is said to alleviate cramps. Aromatic oils reputed to ease menstrual cramps and headaches include chamomile, tarragon, marjoram, and juniper.

Yoga. Positions that can help ease menstrual cramps include the corpse pose (lying flat on the back with legs slightly apart and arms at the sides, palms facing up), cat stretch (page 91), pelvic tilt, and easy spinal twist (see photos above).

Self-Treatment

Distraction often helps; try listening to music, watching a movie, or losing yourself in a good book. Other measures that help many women include:

▶ A heating pad or hot water bottle applied to the crampy area.
▶ Moderate exercise, such as a brisk walk or aerobic dance.
▶ Sexual activity that produces orgasm.

Other Causes of Pelvic Cramps

Five to 10 percent of menstrual pain is secondary to such disorders as endometriosis, in which tissue that normally lines the uterus grows elsewhere. Secondary dysmenorrhea, which tends to begin after age 30 and progressively worsen, may also be caused by fibroid tumors. Sudden, severe pelvic pain could indicate a tubal pregnancy or ruptured ovarian cyst, which are both medical emergencies. Pain and tenderness in the lower abdomen, especially if accompanied by a fever, vaginal discharge, irregular bleeding, or backache, may be a sign of pelvic inflammatory disease, a serious infectious condition.

Menstrual Irregularity

(Oligomenorrhea)

In theory, the typical menstrual cycle lasts for 28 days. In real life, however, menstrual cycles range from 25 to 30 days, although anything between 20 and 40 days (even longer) is normal so long as the pattern is reasonably consistent. A marked variation that produces a missed period or an abnormally short or long cycle is classified as oligomenorrhea, the medical term for menstrual irregularity. Circumstances that contribute to oligomenorrhea include:

Stress, perhaps the most common cause of menstrual irregularity in a healthy woman.

Hormonal factors, with adolescents and women approaching menopause especially vulnerable to shifting levels of estrogen and other hormones. Diabetes and thyroid disorders may also cause irregular menstrual periods.

Rapid weight change, which also affects hormone levels.

Excessive exercise, which alters the ratio of body fat to lean tissue. Menstrual irregularities are common among women who take up endurance sports such as marathon running.

Tumors of the reproductive tract or hormone-producing organs. These include both benign and cancerous growths of the uterus, ovaries, cervix, and thyroid and pituitary glands.

Use of alcohol and drugs, including illegal substances, anticancer medications, and oral contraceptives.

Miscellaneous disorders, including anemia and depression.

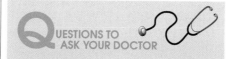

QUESTIONS TO ASK YOUR DOCTOR

▶ Could stress or other emotional problems account for my irregular periods?
▶ After stopping contraceptive pills, how long does it usually take for a normal menstrual cycle to return?

Diagnostic Studies and Procedures

Persistent menstrual irregularities at any age warrant a complete physical examination, preferably by a gynecologist. Take with you a chart of your menstrual history, showing how periods vary from one month to another. The evaluation will include a pelvic examination, a pap smear, and routine blood and urine tests. Depending upon the symptoms and preliminary findings, other tests may include X-rays, ultrasonography, and hormone studies. In certain cases, laparoscopy—an examination in which a viewing instrument is inserted into the abdominal cavity through a small incision near the navel—may be ordered.

Medical Treatments

Treatment depends upon the underlying cause. In some cases, time resolves the problem, especially if the irregularity is due to the erratic ovulation of adolescence. If a tumor is found, surgical removal may be warranted in some cases. Hormonal therapy may be necessary to correct imbalances to establish more regular periods. Irregularity caused by drugs may respond to a change in medication. Depression may warrant drug therapy, psychotherapy, or both.

Alternative Therapies

These should be tried only after serious organic causes, for example, a tumor or thyroid disorder, have been ruled out.

Herbal Medicine. Dong quai capsules, an ancient Chinese herbal remedy, are used for irregular menstruation. Both Chinese and Western herbalists also recommend elecampane tea.

Light Therapy. Some researchers have experimented with using light to shorten or regulate long or irregular cycles, but its effectiveness is unproven.

Nutrition Therapy. If anemia is causing irregular periods, treatment may include iron supplements as well as a diet that contains liver, lean red meat, seafood, fish, and legumes—all good sources of iron. Oligomenorrhea linked to weight problems calls for a sensible diet that allows a woman to achieve and then maintain her ideal weight.

Yoga and Meditation. These and other relaxation methods may clear up menstrual irregularities caused by excessive stress.

Self-Treatment

First, make sure that your menstrual cycles are actually abnormal. For several months, mark a calendar with your cycles, noting any unusual circumstances that might account for irregularity.

Most menstrual irregularities are just temporary responses to unusual stress, weight change, exercise, and other factors. Thus, self-treatment calls for examining your lifestyle and taking some corrective action. Have you recently gone on a diet? Dramatically increased your exercise? Started taking birth control pills or other medication that may affect menstruation? Overindulged in alcohol? If so, try to alter these circumstances and see if your periods return to normal.

Other Causes of Menstrual Irregularities

Abnormal cycles or bleeding between periods that is accompanied by pain, fever, or a vaginal discharge may be caused by infection or pelvic inflammatory disease (PID); both of these warrant prompt antibiotic therapy. Failure to menstruate for more than two months calls for a medical evaluation.

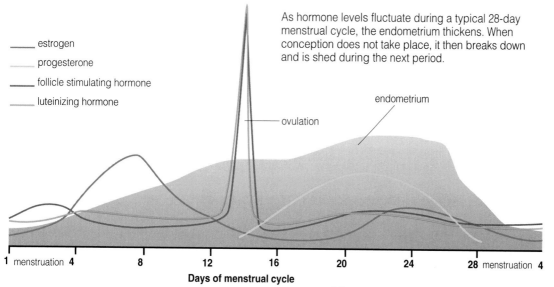

As hormone levels fluctuate during a typical 28-day menstrual cycle, the endometrium thickens. When conception does not take place, it then breaks down and is shed during the next period.

estrogen
progesterone
follicle stimulating hormone
luteinizing hormone

ovulation

endometrium

1 menstruation 4   8   12   16   20   24   28 menstruation 4

Days of menstrual cycle

Mental Retardation

(Down's syndrome and other chromosomal abnormalities; mental deficiency)

In general, mental retardation is characterized by subnormal intelligence, defined as an IQ of 70 or lower, that prevents a person from functioning normally in society. The impairment often becomes evident during infancy or early childhood; sometimes the signs first manifest themselves after the child enters school and is unable to keep up with other children.

About 1 percent of the population is classified as retarded, with the degree of impairment ranging from mild to profound (see box at right). Males are affected one and a half times more often than females. In about 75 percent of all cases, no identifiable biological cause can be found for the retardation. In the remaining 25 percent, the most common causes are:

Chromosomal abnormalities, with Down's syndrome, formerly called mongolism, being the most familiar. Children with this syndrome have Mongoloid features, including slanted eyes, a flat nose, and epicanthal eyelids, the folds that are normal among Asians. It has been determined that the abnormalities are caused by an extra chromosome 21.

About one in 700 babies born in the United States has Down's syndrome; however, the incidence rises to one in 100 when the mother is over the age of 32. The frequency continues to increase with advancing age.

Genetic metabolic disorders, such as phenylketonuria (PKU), in which the baby inherits a gene that precludes normal metabolism. Often, such a child lacks one essential enzyme; PKU babies, for example, are missing a liver enzyme necessary to metabolize phenylalamine, an essential amino acid.

Alcohol use during pregnancy, when it results in fetal alcohol syndrome (FAS). In addition to mental retardation, FAS children may have severe heart defects, deficient growth, slow motor development, and a variety of facial and skeletal malformations.

Malnutrition that results in a premature or low birth-weight baby. This problem is most common among teenagers from economically deprived families.

DEGREES OF MENTAL RETARDATION

DEGREE OF RETARDATION	IQ* (% OF RETARDED)	CHARACTERISTICS
Mild	50-70 (85%)	Most can develop social and communication skills and achieve sixth grade level by late teens. They may achieve minimal self-support, but will probably need guidance and assistance when under social or economic stress.
Moderate	35-49 (10%)	Most can communicate, but have poor social awareness and are unlikely to go beyond second grade level. Most achieve self-maintenance in a sheltered unskilled or semi-skilled work environment.
Severe	20-34 (3-4%)	Most can learn to talk or communicate and can be trained in basic self-care, but they do not benefit from vocational training. Some can develop minimal skills in a controlled environment and may become partially self-sufficient.
Profound	Below 20 (1-2%)	Many may achieve some motor skills and speech, but only very limited self-care, and they require lifelong nursing or custodial care.

*IQ ranges are plus or minus five at lower end.

Thyroid deficiency, which can cause cretinism, profound retardation, and growth problems if it is not detected and corrected shortly after birth.

Infections, such as rubella, AIDS, toxoplasmosis, syphilis, systemic herpes, meningitis, encephalitis, and other diseases, that have been contracted before birth or during early childhood.

Lead poisoning and exposure to other toxic substances, either before birth or during childhood.

Head trauma, most often from falls and other accidents, as well as child abuse. Brain damage also may occur from lack of oxygen during birth, near drowning, or other mishaps.

Diagnostic Studies and Procedures

Down's syndrome, severe brain deformity, and certain other defects can be detected before birth by amniocentesis, ultrasound, and other prenatal examinations. Doctors generally recommend these tests for women over age 35 or those of any age with a family history of certain genetic disorders.

Some forms of retardation are apparent immediately after birth, but others may not show up until the child's development begins to lag.

During an examination, a doctor will look first for such characteristic physical features as a head that is too large or too small. In addition, she will order routine blood and urine tests, and perhaps chromosome analyses, enzyme analyses, and hormone studies. X-rays or a CT scan may also be needed to see if there are abnormalities such as excessive fluid in the brain. A complete neurologic examination will be done, which may include an electroencephalogram, the measuring of electric impulses in the brain cells.

Hearing should definitely be tested; some children assumed to be mentally retarded turn out to have a hearing problem and normal intelligence. As the child grows, intelligence will be assessed, although the results of early IQ tests do not necessarily predict the achievable level of later functioning.

Medical Treatments

Some forms of retardation can be prevented by early medical intervention. For example, if the abnormalities of PKU and low thyroid hormone levels are detected at birth, they can be corrected by early dietary treatment and hormone replacement. In some cases, excessive brain fluid (Hydrocephalus, page 236) can also be corrected, minimizing the extent of brain damage.

The physical defects that often accompany mental retardation can be similarly treated. For example, cleft palate, heart abnormalities, and the deformities common in fetal alcohol syndrome may be repaired surgically.

Later, drug therapy may be prescribed to treat hyperactivity, anxiety, depression, and other problems related to mental deficiency. Otherwise, treatment generally centers on helping the child achieve his fullest potential. In the past, retarded children were often warehoused in institutions because it was generally assumed that they could never achieve self-sufficiency. We now know that up to 85 percent of the mentally retarded are capable of developing social and vocational skills that will allow them to become at least partially self-supporting. And the more supportive and enriched their environment, the better their outlook will be.

Many learn to read up to a sixth grade level. Behavior is often a problem, but with proper guidance and understanding, they can also achieve necessary social skills.

People who work with the mentally handicapped generally agree that, even though these children require special education and will never catch up with their normal peers, they do best if they are taught in a regular school setting where they can imitate and learn from other children. Of course, the child is not the only one who needs help; parents and other family members also benefit from support and psychological counseling (see Self-Treatment).

Alternative Therapies

Increasingly, psychologists, teachers, and parents are employing alternative therapies to help retarded children overcome physical and social handicaps. Some of the more useful include:

Art, Dance, and Music Therapy. These modalities, when instituted at an early age, give the child additional means of expression and also help to improve motor skills and behavior. These and other forms of creative or play therapy

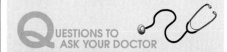

are not only enjoyable, but can also help the child to express feelings of frustration and anger.

Nutrition Therapy. Some metabolic disorders require a special diet, which should be devised by a clinical dietitian experienced in treating such problems. Parents should resist the temptation to give high-dose vitamins and other nutrition remedies without checking with a doctor or a registered dietitian. Excessive amounts of some nutrients can exacerbate a metabolic condition.

Some types of mental retardation result in compulsive eating habits. In such cases, food intake must be controlled to prevent severe obesity. Some parents are forced to keep refrigerators and food cabinets locked.

Physical Therapy and Exercise Conditioning. Mental retardation is often accompanied by poor muscle tone, lack of coordination, and slow development of motor skills. The

parents of such an infant are often instructed to exercise the child's limbs passively and to encourage as much movement as possible. A physical therapist can teach parents the best way to exercise a child at different ages to improve muscle tone, strength, and coordination. In some cases, braces or other devices may be needed to help the child learn to walk.

Pet Therapy. Numerous special education programs employ animals to help improve motor development and social skills, and build self-esteem by introducing the child to a loving and accepting living creature. Animals used in pet therapy with the retarded range from dolphins and horses to cats and goldfish. A pet for a retarded child should be gentle and yet tolerant of rough handling—a large dog that likes children is a better choice than a small, nervous lap dog or a cranky cat.

Self-Treatment

Parents of a retarded child often harbor feelings of anger and guilt; others are simply overwhelmed by the extra responsibilities, especially if they have other children. Counseling, family therapy, and support groups can help all family members deal with their own feelings and also gain insight into how to help the handicapped child.

Teaching good behavior can be one of the most trying aspects of bringing up a retarded child. Of course, even highly intelligent children can develop behavior problems, but learning social skills is especially difficult for the mentally retarded, because usually they cannot tolerate frustration and are unable to control their impulses. Experts agree that positive reinforcement works best. Reward good behavior, while ignoring or gently correcting the bad.

If a child is engaging in dangerous or destructive activities, you can resort to the same time-out technique that works for normal children. Remember, however, that it takes longer for a retarded child to learn (or unlearn) behavior, so don't expect that one or two time-outs will do the trick.

Other Causes of Mental Deficiency

Mental retardation is sometimes a component of autism. Parental neglect, failure to thrive, extreme malnutrition, a prolonged high fever or other serious illness, and/or sensory deprivation can lead to diminished intelligence in children who were normal at birth.

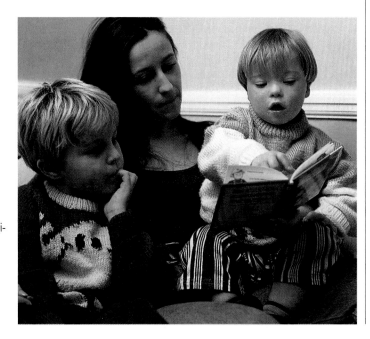

In a supportive environment, retarded children are more likely to fulfill their learning potential. Eventually, many learn to read up to a sixth grade level.

Migraine Headaches

(Vascular headaches)

A migraine is a severe, throbbing headache that lasts anywhere from a few hours to several days. There are two general types: classic and common. A classic migraine is heralded by a warning aura, or prodrome, of dizziness, mood changes, loss of appetite, and visual distortions such as flashing lights and blind spots. This prodrome stage is lacking in a common migraine, which develops suddenly when the blood vessels open up, or dilate, thus resulting in expanded flow of blood and producing the throbbing pain that is typical of this headache.

In both types, the pain generally begins in the temple area, and may quickly engulf one side of the head. In some cases, the pain will spread to the other side, or alternate from one side to the other. It is often accompanied by loss of appetite, nausea and vomiting, and increased sensitivity to light.

Migraines occur at any age, but are most common between ages 25 and 55. Women migraine sufferers outnumber men by about three to one, and there is a family history of the headaches in up to 60 percent of cases. Fluctuating levels of serotonin, a hormone-like body chemical that acts on blood vessels, sets a migraine in motion, but exactly how is unknown. Migraine triggers, which vary from person to person, include hormonal changes related to a woman's menstrual cycle, the weather, bright lights, stress, odors, alcohol, and chocolate and certain other foods.

Diagnostic Studies and Procedures

A doctor can usually diagnose migraines by questioning the patient about the nature of the headaches and what brings them on. However, he may order blood and urine studies and a CT scan or MRI to rule out a brain tumor and other possible causes.

Medical Treatments

There are three approaches to the medical treatment of migraines:

Prophylactic drugs are taken daily to prevent the headaches. These include low doses of beta blockers, usually propranolol (Inderal); calcium-channel blockers such as verapamil (Calan) or diltiazem (Cardizem); tricyclic antidepressants such as amitriptyline (Elavil)

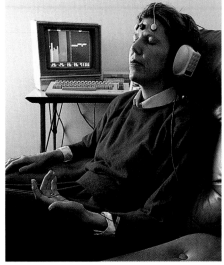

Using biofeedback monitors, a patient learns to increase blood flow to the hands and thus alleviate the excessive flow in the head.

or doxepin (Sinequan); anticonvulsants such as valproic acid (Depakene); and methysergide (Sansert).

Abortive medications are taken at the first warning signs to ward off a full-blown headache. These include sumatriptan (Imitrex), a newer injectable drug that works specifically on the receptors in the brain. Older abortive drugs include ergot alkaloids, such as Cafergot and Wigraine, which also contain caffeine, and Ergomar and Ergostat, which can be taken by placing a pill under the tongue. For some people, naproxen (Naprosyn), a nonsteroidal anti-inflammatory drug, also works. Fiorinal, a combination of butalbital, aspirin, and caffeine, is another alternative, but many doctors do not prescribe it because of its habit-forming barbiturate component.

Drugs that relieve symptoms are used for severe, prolonged headaches. Commonly given by injection, they include Imitrex, dihydroergotamine (D.H.E. 45), prochlorperazine

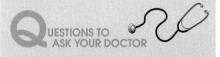

Q UESTIONS TO ASK YOUR DOCTOR

▶ What are the side effects of the drugs I'm taking for migraine?
▶ Am I a candidate for Imitrex? If so, is it difficult to inject myself? (The answer to the second part is usually no because the drug is prepackaged in a disposable syringe.)

(Compazine), and a narcotic painkiller such as meperidine (Demerol). Many people try a combination of treatments before finding a regimen that works.

Alternative Therapies

Biofeedback. Patients are taught to redirect some blood flow from the head by learning to raise the temperature of their hands. Biofeedback also promotes relaxation, thereby reducing the stress that is related to headaches.

Herbal Medicine. Feverfew capsules, taken daily, have been shown to reduce the frequency of migraines in some people. Peppermint tea may help to relieve the nausea that often accompanies a migraine headache.

Nutrition Therapy. Keeping a food diary may help to identify foods that trigger migraines. Although caffeine is highly effective in aborting a migraine, it is also a common trigger and should be eliminated from the diet. Headache specialists also advise avoiding wine, anchovies, strong cheeses, processed meats and other foods that contain nitrites, fermented foods such as soy sauce, and anything prepared with MSG. A few studies have found that high-dose vitamins, especially vitamin A, can trigger a migraine. In contrast, taking 100 milligrams of niacin (nicotinic acid) during the prodrome stage may abort one by causing a brief dilation of constricted blood vessels.

Yoga and Meditation. Some people have learned to abort a migraine by practicing these relaxation techniques during the prodrome period.

Self-Treatment

The best approach is to identify and then avoid as much as possible factors that trigger migraines. Often, adopting a lifestyle that provides adequate rest, regular exercise, and a meal schedule that prevents getting overly hungry goes a long way toward averting them. A strategy that can abort a migraine during the prodrome period is to take aspirin or ibuprofen with caffeine—a cola or cup of strong coffee—then lie down in a quiet, darkened room.

Other Causes of Headaches

Cluster headaches are similar to migraines, but tend to be more severe and shorter in duration and occur one after another. Other types of headaches are caused by tension and sinusitis. A number of diseases, ranging from the common cold to brain tumors, also produce headaches.

Miscarriage

(Spontaneous abortion)

Doctors generally define a miscarriage as the natural termination of a pregnancy during the first 20 weeks of gestation. (Delivery between the 21st and 38th weeks is considered a premature birth, even if the fetus does not survive.) At least 20 percent of all pregnancies end in a miscarriage between the sixth and tenth weeks. Recent studies indicate, however, that the figure may be as high as 50 percent, but that many go unnoticed because women don't always realize they are pregnant.

Typically, a miscarriage begins with vaginal bleeding or a brownish discharge, which may be accompanied by cramps and lower back pain. If the woman is unaware of being pregnant, she may simply assume that she is having a heavy menstrual period.

The majority of miscarriages are caused by a problem in fetal development, most often chromosomal abnormalities or structural malformations. For example, fertilization toward the end of the 24-hour period after ovulation can cause these abnormalities. Some researchers believe late fertilization is the major cause of miscarriage.

Other possible causes include maternal hormone imbalances, such as those caused by thyroid disease or diabetes; a structural defect in the uterus or cervix; poor attachment of the placenta to the uterine wall; rubella or other infectious illnesses, including sexually

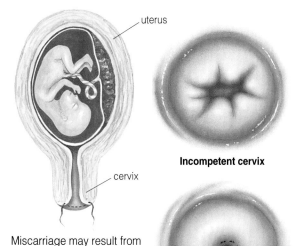

Miscarriage may result from an incompetent cervix, which dilates prematurely. It can be stitched closed temporarily, and the stitches removed as birth approaches to permit a normal delivery.

Incompetent cervix

Cervix closed with suture

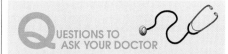

QUESTIONS TO ASK YOUR DOCTOR

▶ Do I have an increased risk of another miscarriage?
▶ How long should I wait before attempting another pregnancy? (The answer is usually at least two months, and preferably longer.)

transmitted diseases; complications from kidney disease; the presence of an IUD in the uterus; or severe emotional shock. Lifestyle factors that increase the risk of miscarriage include smoking, use of alcohol, poor nutrition, and exposure to radiation, hazardous chemicals, or lead. For many miscarriages, however, a cause cannot be found.

Diagnostic Studies and Procedures

Vaginal bleeding may prompt a woman to think she has had a miscarriage when, in fact, the fetus is still in the uterus. This type of threatened miscarriage can sometimes be stopped.

If a miscarriage has taken place, a woman should undergo a careful physical examination, which may include viewing of the uterus by ultrasound. The uterus may also be examined by hysteroscopy using a lighted magnifying instrument inserted through the cervix. If possible, the fetus and other material expelled from the uterus should also be examined for abnormalities that might explain what went wrong.

Repeated miscarriages call for other tests to seek a possible cause; these might include:
▶ Genetic and chromosomal studies.
▶ Hormonal evaluations to check for thyroid disease and diabetes, or, more importantly, the presence of hormones needed for normal ovulation.
▶ Blood tests to identify possible immunologic abnormalities, such as production of antibodies that can cause a miscarriage.
▶ Hysterography or hysteroscopy to assess the anatomy of the uterus.

Medical Treatments

If minor bleeding signals that a miscarriage is imminent, a doctor is likely to recommend bed rest to save the pregnancy. If bleeding stops and the fetus appears to be normal, the pregnancy may still continue to term.

When a miscarriage has truly begun, however, it usually cannot be prevented. If it is incomplete, then the remaining fetal and placental material must be removed from the uterus. In first-trimester miscarriages, this can be accomplished by suctioning the uterus or performing a D&C, in which the cervix is widened (dilated) and the uterus is scraped with a curette.

An incomplete miscarriage during the second trimester may be treated by giving the woman an intravenous infusion of oxytocin, a hormone that causes uterine contractions to expel all the remaining tissue in a process similar to that of normal labor. In some cases, antibiotics are prescribed to treat or prevent infection.

If there is a risk of future miscarriages, these preventive steps may be taken, depending upon the cause:
▶ When certain antibodies have been found in the blood, anticoagulant drugs are given, generally either low-dose aspirin or heparin.
▶ When uterine abnormalities, such as polyps or fibroids, have been found, corrective surgery may be undertaken before attempting another pregnancy.
▶ When the cervix has opened prematurely, the incompetent cervix may be stitched closed during the next pregnancy (see illustration, at left).

Alternative Therapies

Although no alternative therapies can prevent a miscarriage, psychotherapy may be beneficial as part of aftercare. It is normal to feel sad after a miscarriage, and psychological counseling or participation in a support group can help ease unwarranted feelings of guilt as well as anxiety about future pregnancies.

Self-Treatment

Many women have some vaginal bleeding during the early months of pregnancy. This does not necessarily signal a miscarriage, but it should always be reported to a doctor. Complete bed rest for a week or longer may stop a threatened miscarriage from progressing. Also, sexual intercourse and strenuous physical activity should be avoided until the crisis is past.

Other Causes of Pregnancy Loss

A pregnancy may be terminated intentionally in an induced abortion.

Mitral Valve Prolapse

(Click murmur; floppy valve; or balloon mitral syndrome)

Mitral valve prolapse is a minor heart defect that prevents the valve linking the two left chambers—the atrium and ventricle—from closing properly. After blood receives fresh oxygen in the lungs, it passes into the left atrium, through the mitral valve (shaped like a bishop's miter), into the left ventricle, which pumps it out of the heart into the aorta. In mitral valve prolapse, one or both

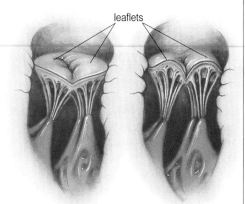

leaflets

Normal mitral valve   Prolapsed mitral valve

The heart's mitral valve has two leaflets that open and close to regulate blood flow from the left atrium to the left ventricle. A prolapsed mitral valve has bulging leaflets that allow blood to leak back into the atrium.

leaflets—the flaps that open and close to form the valve—bulge into the atrium during each heartbeat, and a little blood heading for the ventricle may leak (regurgitate) back into the atrium.

In most people, this is a harmless, symptomless condition. When symptoms do occur, they usually take the form of palpitations, fatigue, shortness of breath, chest pains, dizziness, and a tendency to faint. Stress appears to bring on or exacerbate these problems.

Serious complications are rare, but mitral valve prolapse can increase clot formation, leading to a stroke. People with this condition are also at greater risk of endocarditis, an infection of the membrane that lines the heart and its valves. And the condition can set the stage for serious disturbances in the heart's normal rhythm, especially ventricular tachycardia, which may lead to sudden death. In rare cases, the valve may rupture, which is also fatal.

In the past, mitral valve prolapse was considered primarily a congenital disorder of women. However, research shows that men and women are about equally affected.

Diagnostic Studies and Procedures

A characteristic clicking sound heard through a stethoscope placed over the left side of the heart and the back tips off a doctor to the possibility of mitral valve prolapse. Tests include an electrocardiogram and chest X-ray; an echocardiogram revealing abnormal mitral leaflets gives a definitive diagnosis.

Medical Treatments

Mitral valve prolapse seldom requires treatment, but periodic heart checkups are advisable because the degree of prolapse can progress with age.

Drug Therapy. Frequent palpitations and chest pain can be treated with low doses of a beta-blocking drug such as propranolol (Inderal) to slow the heart rate. If the heart is unable to pump sufficient blood, other drugs can be prescribed to make it beat more forcefully.

Because any valve abnormality carries an increased risk of endocarditis, prophylactic antibiotics should be taken before any dental procedure or surgery that involves bleeding and a risk that bacteria may invade the bloodstream and be carried to the heart.

Surgery. In unusual cases, the mitral valve becomes so diseased that it allows blood to back up into the lungs. When this happens, the defective valve can be replaced with an artificial one.

Alternative Therapies

Exercise Conditioning. A program of gradual exercise conditioning can improve stamina and alleviate fatigue.

Yoga and Meditation. Because stress can provoke symptoms, these and other relaxation techniques are often recommended to counteract it.

Self-Treatment

Many people with mitral valve prolapse experience orthostatic hypotension— brief periods of dizziness and faintness

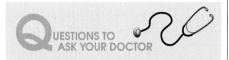

QUESTIONS TO ASK YOUR DOCTOR

▶ Are there any sports in which I can safely participate? Which ones should I avoid?
▶ How often should I see a cardiologist for evaluation?

when getting out of bed or rising from a chair. This can be prevented by avoiding sudden changes in position. For example, when you arise in the morning, slowly sit up and let your feet dangle over the side of the bed for a minute before standing. When getting out of a chair, sit forward with your feet on the floor for a few seconds, then stand up slowly.

You may be advised to avoid any strenuous activities that place particular strain on the heart, especially if you have severe symptoms.

Other Causes of Cardiac Symptoms

Other types of heart valve disease, angina, and congestive heart failure can cause symptoms similar to those of mitral valve prolapse, as can panic attacks.

Mononucleosis

(Epstein-Barr infection)

Mononucleosis is a highly contagious disease that strikes mostly adolescents and young adults. It is sometimes called the kissing disease, because it is transmitted by direct contact with saliva or nasal secretions infected with the causative organism—the Epstein-Barr virus (EBV). However, kissing an infected person is not necessary; mononucleosis is easily transmitted by sharing personal items such as a drinking glass, eating utensils, or a toothbrush.

In most cases, exposure to Epstein-Barr virus does not cause symptoms. By the age of five, about half of all children have already contracted the virus and developed immunity to it, even though most do not get sick. Studies among Peace Corps volunteers and military recruits have similarly shown that 90 percent of those who are infected do not develop symptoms.

When symptoms do occur, they begin 30 to 60 days after exposure with fatigue, headache, and chills, followed a day or two later by fever, sore throat, and swollen glands, especially in the neck. Some people also complain of weakness, loss of appetite, and muscle and joint pain. In severe cases, the spleen becomes swollen, and jaundice may develop if the liver is involved. Symptoms typically persist for one to four weeks, but full recovery may take two or three months.

Mononucleosis itself is generally not serious, but sometimes life-threatening complications develop, especially among people with AIDS or other conditions that lower immunity. Complications include hepatitis; obstructed breathing from throat swelling; meningitis, seizures, and psychosis, if the brain and nervous system are infected; blood disorders such as hemolytic anemia; and a ruptured spleen.

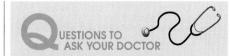

QUESTIONS TO ASK YOUR DOCTOR

► What signs of possible complications should prompt me to see a doctor?
► When can I resume regular activities, including participation in sports?

Diagnostic Studies and Procedures

A complete blood count usually shows abnormal white blood cells. Antibodies to Epstein-Barr antigens may also be present. An initial negative blood test does not necessarily rule out mononucleosis; when tests are repeated later, they are often positive.

Medical Treatments

In most cases, mononucleosis is self-limiting. Because it is a viral illness, antibiotics are not effective. In some cases, however, a corticosteroid drug is prescribed if there is a severe sore throat and swelling that threatens breathing. AIDS patients and others with lowered immunity may be given oral or intravenous acyclovir (Zovirax). Otherwise, acetaminophen is recommended, if needed, for headaches, fever, or achiness.

In rare cases, hospitalization is necessary. For example, a ruptured spleen is a medical emergency that demands immediate blood transfusions and surgery to prevent death.

Alternative Therapies

Aromatherapy. Inhaling vapors of lavender, eucalyptus, peppermint, or bergamot are said to alleviate fatigue and other symptoms.

Herbal Medicine. Tea or capsules made from echinacea and marigold are often recommended to fight the Epstein-Barr infection. Some herbalists also suggest taking teas or capsules of pau d'arco, dandelion, or goldenseal.

Homeopathy. Homeopaths advocate carcinosin as the remedy of first choice for the infection itself, and phytolacca for swollen glands.

Nutrition Therapy. Some nutritionists recommend taking extra vitamin C plus bioflavonoids—substances believed to enhance the effectiveness of the vitamin—to help speed recovery. Mononucleosis can lower resistance to other infections. A high-protein diet that includes lean meat, poultry, fish, or a combination of grains and legumes is said to help boost immunity. Some therapists prescribe oral spleen extracts, but their value is doubtful.

Self-Treatment

Staying in bed is usually advised as long as there is fever; after that, normal activities can be resumed, but frequent rest periods are needed to counter fatigue. Because the spleen remains vulnerable even after symptoms subside, contact sports should be avoided for at least two months following recovery.

Care should be taken to avoid the spreading of the disease to others. A person is considered contagious until all symptoms have disappeared. Even after that, the virus remains in the body and can be detected in saliva and nasal secretions of about one-fourth of otherwise healthy adults.

Even after recovery, a patient should be alert for symptoms of late complications, especially hepatitis. Jaundice—a yellowing of the skin and white portion of the eyes—warrants calling a doctor.

Other Causes of Mononucleosis Symptoms

Flu produces many of the same symptoms as mononucleosis. Cytomegalovirus, related to the herpes virus that commonly infects newborns, and toxoplasmosis, a parasite, also cause symptoms similar to those of mononucleosis. Mononucleosis can also resemble lymphoma, cancer of the lymph system.

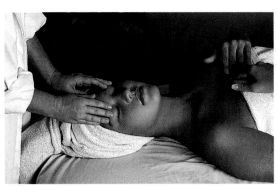
A facial massage using aromatherapy can help fight fatigue and other symptoms of mononucleosis.

CHRONIC EPSTEIN-BARR INFECTION

In recent years, there has been speculation that mononucleosis sets the stage for chronic fatigue syndrome (page 133), an illness characterized by extreme tiredness, inability to concentrate, persistent fever, and swollen lymph nodes.

Researchers have discounted any association between the Epstein-Barr virus and chronic fatigue syndrome. In rare cases, however, chronic Epstein-Barr infection develops. This disorder is marked by fever, eye inflammation, blood abnormalities, and an unusual type of pneumonia called interstitial pneumonitis. A lingering fever or any other symptom following a bout of mononucleosis warrants a doctor's investigation.

Mountain Sickness

(High-altitude sickness; cerebral and pulmonary edema)

Mountain sickness develops when the body is unable to adapt to an abrupt increase in altitude. Atmospheric pressure declines with increasing altitude; though the percentage of oxygen in the air remains constant, less oxygen enters the bloodstream through the lungs. To compensate, the heart and lungs work harder and the body gives off more carbon dioxide, which can upset its biochemical balance and cause fluid to accumulate between cells. Symptoms include headache, fatigue, nausea, rapid heartbeat, and breathlessness.

This illness is most common among people who travel to high altitudes without allowing time for their bodies to adjust. Typically, a person will fly to a high destination and set out to ski, sightsee, or engage in other strenuous activities, attributing tiredness, headache, insomnia, and other symptoms to jet lag. Exertion worsens the problem and can lead to buildup of fluid (edema) in the brain or lungs. The latter is signaled by breathlessness that persists even during rest, a cough that may produce frothy, blood-tinged sputum, and blueness of the lips. Indications of cerebral edema include an unsteady or drunken gait, eye hemorrhages, headache, drowsiness, and coma.

Some 20 to 25 percent of people who travel from a low altitude to 9,000 feet or higher in less than a day develop

HIGH-ALTITUDE DESTINATIONS

The following are popular vacation destinations and their altitudes:

City	Altitude in feet
Albuquerque, N.M.	4,945
Aspen, Col.	7,773-11,212
Cheyenne, Wyo.	6,100
Darjeeling, India	7,431
Denver, Col.	5,280
Flagstaff, Ariz.	6,900
LaPaz, Bolivia	12,001
Lhasa, Tibet	12,002
Machu Picchu, Peru	8,003
Mexico City	7,347
Mount Everest	18,000-29,028
St. Moritz	6,089-10,837
West Yellowstone, Mont.	6,644

mild mountain sickness. Other persons develop symptoms at only 6,500 feet; children, women who are premenstrual, and people over age 40 seem to be the most vulnerable.

Diagnostic Studies and Procedures

Mountain sickness and its complications can usually be diagnosed on the basis of symptoms. When pulmonary or cerebral edema are suspected, blood and spinal fluid analyses may be ordered to rule out pneumonia and other disorders.

Medical Treatments

Simple mountain sickness does not require medical treatment, although it might be a good idea to return to a lower altitude. Bed rest and extra fluids are also advisable. Acetazolamide (Diamox), a medication with a diuretic effect, may be prescribed to speed recovery and help prevent pulmonary edema. Aspirin also helps alleviate headache and may reduce the risk of lung clots (pulmonary emboli) as well.

Pulmonary and cerebral edema are emergencies that call for immediate descent. If this is not possible, the best procedure is to take the person to a high-altitude first aid center where there is equipment to raise air pressure to simulate that of a lower altitude. Diuretics may be administered, but care must be taken to avoid dehydration. Sometimes, administering intravenous steroids helps to lessen cerebral edema.

Alternative Therapies

Nutrition Therapy. When traveling to a high altitude, increase your intake of water to replace the fluid lost during rapid breathing of dry air. Reduce salt intake, and abstain from caffeine, which can worsen sleep disturbances, and alcohol, which exacerbates the sickness. Eat frequent, small meals that are low in fat and high in easily digested carbohydrates, such as fruits and starches.

Self-Treatment

To prevent mountain sickness, ascend gradually—no more than 2,000 feet a day at elevations of 5,000 to 10,000 feet, and 1,000 feet a day at greater heights. Plan to spend each night at an elevation of 8,000 feet or lower until your body is fully acclimatized. Rest frequently, and limit vigorous activity such as skiing, hiking, or climbing to a half day for the first two or three days.

Should you develop mild symptoms, balancing frequent rests with moderate activity will help your body adjust more quickly than taking to your bed.

If you want to speed acclimatization, talk to your doctor about a prescription for Diamox. Studies show that starting this drug two days before arriving at a high altitude may prevent mountain sickness. Carefully follow directions for its use; abruptly stopping the drug can lead to pulmonary or cerebral edema.

Some Himalayan climbers take the steroid dexamethasone (Decadron) to prevent cerebral edema, but its long-term use is discouraged because of its many possible side effects—bleeding problems, lowered immunity, muscle weakness, and ulcers, among others.

Other Causes of Altitude Problems

Persons with pulmonary hypertension or congestive heart failure are especially susceptible to mountain sickness. Some who live at high altitudes develop chronic mountain sickness, or Monge's disease, marked by shortness of breath, fatigue, and clotting problems. Bloodletting may help, but recovery usually requires descending to sea level.

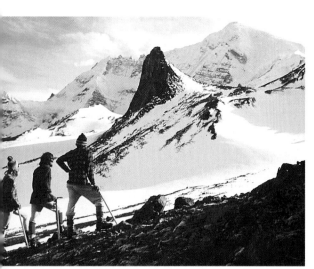

A gradual ascent to give the body time to adjust to high altitudes is the key to preventing mountain sickness.

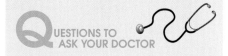

QUESTIONS TO ASK YOUR DOCTOR

▶ Should I take Diamox as a preventive measure?
▶ Do I have any conditions that make travel to a high altitude inadvisable?

Multiple Sclerosis

(MS; disseminated sclerosis)

Multiple sclerosis, a chronic, slowly progressive disease of the central nervous system, is characterized by patchy destruction and scarring (sclerosis) of myelin, the fatty sheath surrounding nerves in the spinal cord and brain. In time, the sclerosis interferes with transmission of nerve signals, producing a wide range of symptoms that vary from person to person. These commonly include numbness, weakness, tremor, poor coordination, an abnormal gait, loss of bladder and bowel control, and impotence in men. Vision and hearing may be impaired and there might be memory loss, confusion, and speech problems. Symptoms lessen or disappear during periods of remission, but relapses occur in which old problems worsen and new ones develop.

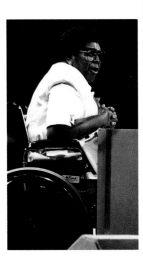

The former congressional representative Barbara Jordan, a MS patient, addressed the 1992 Democratic Convention from her wheelchair.

About 250,000 Americans have MS, with women outnumbering men about two to one. The cause is unknown, but some researchers theorize that a slow-acting virus may be responsible; others believe that MS is an autoimmune condition in which the immune system attacks healthy tissue. Still others think that a combination of factors, including genetic susceptibility, may be involved.

Diagnostic Studies and Procedures

There is no specific test to detect multiple sclerosis, so diagnosis entails investigating and eliminating other possible causes of symptoms. In addition to a physical examination and blood and urine analyses, studies may include a neurological workup that tests reflexes, equilibrium, sensory function, and

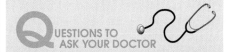

QUESTIONS TO ASK YOUR DOCTOR

▶ Can you put me in touch with a support group for MS patients and their families?
▶ Can my type of multiple sclerosis be helped by Betaseron? If so, what are my chances of obtaining it?

emotional stability. A sample of cerebrospinal fluid may also be obtained. As the disease progresses, MRI is used to locate lesions along nerve paths.

Medical Treatments

Betaseron, a genetically engineered form of human beta interferon, is the only medication to date that reduces the frequency and severity of MS attacks. When the drug was approved for general use in 1993, demand for it far exceeded production. A lottery system was set up to select patients to receive the drug until supply catches up with the demand.

Otherwise, treatment is directed to alleviating symptoms. During a flare-up, ACTH, a synthetic hormone normally produced by the pituitary gland, sometimes induces a remission. It is given intravenously in high doses at first, then in smaller intramuscular injections. After a few weeks, the hormone is tapered off and stopped. Relatively few patients respond to this treatment, however, and side effects such as intestinal bleeding and edema generally limit its use.

Corticosteroid drugs may also be used, but they do not always help; even when they do, they are not recommended for long-term treatment. Antibiotics may be prescribed to treat or prevent bladder infections, a common problem in multiple sclerosis. Depending upon the specific problem, devices such as a hearing aid, special eyeglasses, and leg braces or a wheelchair may be needed.

Alternative Therapies

Individuals with multiple sclerosis can be helped by a variety of alternative therapists, who can also teach appropriate approaches to self-treatment.

Nutrition Therapy. There is some evidence that the progression of MS can be slowed by limiting intake of saturated fats to less than 5 percent of total calories, or about 10 grams a day, while increasing corn, safflower, canola, and

other polyunsaturated oils to 40 to 50 grams a day, or 20 to 25 percent of calories. Having several servings a week of mackerel, salmon, and other fatty cold-water fish, which are high in omega-3 oils, is said to help maintain nerve function. Increasing fiber and fluid intake can alleviate constipation, a common problem with MS. Full-strength cranberry juice protects against cystitis, which is another frequent complication. Patients who have difficulty chewing or swallowing may need liquid nutritional supplements.

Physical Therapy. Stretching exercises, moderate physical activity, massage, and manipulation help sufferers retain muscle strength. Canes, braces, orthotics, and other devices can stabilize gait, although the occasional use of a wheelchair may be advisable to conserve energy. Recent studies show that horseback riding, or equine therapy, carried out under the supervision of a specially trained physical therapist can improve both gait and strength.

Occupational Therapy. Practical ways for simplifying self-care to conserve energy are taught by these specialists. Speech and bowel therapists may be enlisted to deal with special problems.

Yoga and Meditation. Deep breathing exercises, visualization, and relaxation therapies not only alleviate the stress of living with this chronic, debilitating disease, but they may also strengthen the immune system and prevent some complications of MS.

Self-Treatment

Specialists agree that active involvement in self-care is the best way to maintain a positive attitude. Start by adopting a realistic view of your capabilities so that you can set achievable goals. Whenever possible, seek out enjoyable new experiences that expand your horizons without increasing physical demands; for example, consider learning a foreign language or a new craft. A support group can provide an invaluable outlet for your feelings of frustration as well as practical pointers in self-sufficiency.

Other Causes of Progressive Paralysis

Amyotrophic lateral sclerosis, or Lou Gehrig's disease, may be mistaken for multiple sclerosis. Hereditary diseases such as muscular dystrophy produce progressive muscle weakness, as can infections like chronic Lyme disease.

Mumps

(Epidemic parotitis)

Mumps is a viral disorder that causes painful swelling of the salivary glands in the neck and jaw. The causative paramyxovirus is highly contagious and easily spread in droplets expelled into the air by sneezing, coughing, even breathing, or by sharing a drinking glass, food utensils, or other items that have come in contact with the saliva of an infected person.

Typically, a low-grade fever, chills, loss of appetite, sore throat, and general malaise begin about 18 days after exposure to the paramyxovirus. Within a day or so, the parotid salivary gland, located between the ear and jaw, begins

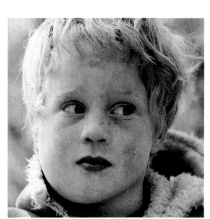

The classic symptom of mumps is painfully swollen salivary glands in the neck and jaw.

to swell, first on one side, and then usually on the other as well. The fever subsides in about a week, but the parotid swelling may persist for a few more days. As long as the glands are swollen, chewing and swallowing will be painful, especially when eating acidic foods such as citrus fruits.

About one-third of affected males who have completed puberty also develop inflamed and swollen testicles, a complication that sometimes results in sterility. Rare complications that may occur at any age in both sexes include deafness (if the auditory nerve becomes damaged), meningitis, encephalitis, arthritis, pancreatitis, heart inflammation, and blood disorders.

Until the 1970s, mumps was an extremely common childhood disease. This began to change with the introduction of an effective mumps vaccine in 1967. By 1977, use of the vaccine had become widespread throughout the United States and the disease had

entered the category of rare. Sporadic cases still occur, however, among children and adults who have not been immunized or those exposed to the virus before they are old enough to be vaccinated. In addition, the vaccine fails to confer immunity in about 5 percent of those who receive it.

Diagnostic Studies and Procedures

Mumps usually can be diagnosed by reviewing the symptoms and noting the swollen salivary glands. In some cases, a blood test may be ordered to detect antibodies to the virus.

Medical Treatments

There are no drugs that can shorten the course of mumps, so treatment is aimed at alleviating symptoms. The disease usually can be treated at home, although the patient should be isolated from anyone who may lack immunity until all neck swelling and other signs of the illness have totally disappeared.

Acetaminophen can be given to ease discomfort, but aspirin should be avoided if the patient is under the age of 18 because of an increased risk of Reye's syndrome, a rare but serious disease that affects the liver and brain (see box, page 437). In some cases, a stronger prescription painkiller such as codeine may be needed, and corticosteroids might be prescribed to reduce severe swelling.

Parents should be alert to symptoms of serious complications, and seek immediate medical attention if any develop. A fever higher than 103°F (39.5°C), severe or persistent vomiting, inflamed or swollen testicles, unusual lethargy, ringing in the ears, and a severe headache accompanied by neck stiffness and pain are among the signs of possible complications requiring prompt medical treatment.

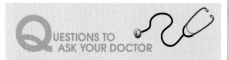

QUESTIONS TO ASK YOUR DOCTOR

▶ What symptoms should prompt me to seek medical attention?
▶ If I cannot recall having had mumps, should I be immunized?

MUMPS IMMUNIZATION

A single shot of mumps vaccine is administered at the age of 15 months, as part of the MMR shot that protects against mumps, measles, and rubella. A booster MMR shot is now recommended at age 10 or 11. Immunization is also advisable for adults who lack immunity and plan travel to areas where exposure to mumps is a possibility.

Adverse reactions to the vaccine are rare, but it should not be given to anyone who is allergic to eggs or whose immunity is lowered. The vaccine is also contraindicated during pregnancy.

Alternative Therapies

Herbal Medicine. Echinacea tea is said to reduce swelling of the salivary glands.
Hydrotherapy. Warm or cold compresses on the swollen neck may make a youngster feel more comfortable. Try both to see which works best.

A cool sponge bath can lower a fever. Sponge with plain water instead of rubbing alcohol, which gives off potentially irritating fumes.
Nutrition Therapy. Sucking on zinc lozenges, which are sold at health food stores, may aid healing.

Self-Treatment

Whether or not the child should stay in bed depends upon the severity of symptoms. Anyone who has a mild case does not necessarily need bed rest, but should be encouraged to rest often, and engage in quiet activities such as reading, listening to music, and playing word or board games.

Encourage the child to drink extra fluids and offer broth, soups, and soft, bland foods that are easy to swallow. Mashed banana, scrambled eggs, puddings, frozen yogurt, and fruit-flavored gelatin are good choices.

Avoid orange juice or other sour or acidic foods, which stimulate the flow of saliva and worsen pain.

Males who develop swollen and painful testes require complete bed rest. Ice packs should be applied to the scrotum.

Other Causes of Neck Swelling

Many infectious diseases can trigger swelling of the lymph glands in the neck, but the swelling is rarely as marked as that seen in mumps. Other conditions in which the parotid gland may be swollen include severe malnutrition, liver or kidney disease, and cystic fibrosis.

Muscle Cramps

(Muscle spasms)

A muscle cramp is a sudden, sharp pain caused by involuntary muscle spasms. These spasms happen most often in the limbs, but they also occur in certain internal organs. Among the more common causes are:

Inadequate flow of blood to muscles, often resulting from hardening of the arteries (arteriosclerosis).

Exhaustion and cold, which cause the type of cramps suffered by swimmers.

Minor muscle injuries that cause spasmodic contractions. Athletes are especially vulnerable.

Poor posture that strains specific muscles. People who work at poorly designed computer work stations frequently experience muscle cramps in their hands, arms, neck, and shoulders.

Chronic overuse of certain muscles, such as those of the hand that produce a writer's or tailor's cramp.

Excessive loss of sodium and perhaps potassium and magnesium. Heat cramps caused by profuse sweating during vigorous exercise in hot, humid weather are the most common.

Unaccustomed pressure on back and leg muscles during pregnancy.

Pains may also be caused by spasms of the tiny muscles in internal organs. Examples include menstrual cramps, angina due to coronary artery spasms, and cramps related to a spastic colon.

Diagnostic Studies and Procedures

Muscle cramps are usually self-diagnosed, but if the cause is not apparent and the condition persists, a doctor should be consulted. A doctor's prompt evaluation is especially important if:

▶ Uterine cramps occur at any time during pregnancy.

▶ Muscle cramps in the lower back or legs impede movement.

▶ Abdominal cramps are accompanied by vomiting and diarrhea.

Medical Treatments

Drug Therapy. Most muscle cramps respond to self-treatment, but those that persist or are immobilizing may call for medication. The simplest, most common approach is the use of drugs that block prostaglandins, hormone-like chemicals that cause inflammation and muscle contractions. These include aspirin, ibuprofen, and other nonsteroidal anti-inflammatory drugs. Diphenhydramine, an ingredient in

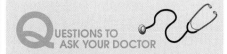
combination sleeping aids and painkillers for use at night, may alleviate muscle cramps that occur during sleep.

An injection of cortisone or a local anesthetic may help bring relief from more severe cramps, such as those causing back or neck pain. Diazepam (Valium) or similar tranquilizers, which also relax muscles, can alleviate severe cramping in the back and neck. Anticholinergic drugs, such as Librax or Donnatal, can relieve abdominal pain from colon spasms.

Calcium-channel blockers such as verapamil (Calan) ease chest pains due to coronary spasms. Imbalances in body chemistry are treated with intravenous potassium, sodium, or other substances, depending upon the cause.

Surgical Treatment. Surgery to increase blood flow through arteries clogged by fatty plaque may be recommended for chronic leg cramps. Procedures include balloon angioplasty to flatten fatty deposits, bypass surgery to redirect blood flow around blockages, and laser surgery to destroy plaque.

Alternative Therapies

Alexander Technique. People who work at computers often benefit from sessions with an instructor of the Alexander technique, who can teach proper posture and suggest how to set up a work environment that minimizes this type of muscle tension.

Hydrotherapy. A whirlpool bath or underwater massage eases muscle cramps that occur from either overuse or tension.

Massage. Deep massage or rolfing can help to alleviate muscle cramps in the legs and back. Other therapeutic techniques include acupressure and shiatsu.

Nutrition Therapy. Leg cramps are said to be relieved by 300 to 400 IU of vitamin E each day. A 500-milligram calcium pill at night also may help.

Self-Treatment

Most cramps can be eased by gently massaging or compressing, and then extending and stretching the contracted muscle. If the cramp recurs, try an ice pack or heating pad. A contrast bath may help: Soak in hot water for 10 to 15 minutes, then stand under a cold shower for two or three minutes.

To prevent cramps while exercising, always warm up and cool down by stretching before and after workouts.

If nighttime leg cramps are a problem, do this calf stretching exercise before retiring: Stand two to three feet from a wall. Lean forward, extending your arms straight from the shoulders and placing your palms on the wall. Keeping your back and legs straight and your heels on the floor, slide one leg backwards until you feel a pulling sensation along calf muscles. Maintain this stretch for a slow count of 10. Relax and repeat with the other leg. Do three sets and follow by massaging.

Other Causes of Muscle Cramps

Muscle cramps are associated with tetanus, muscular dystrophy, multiple sclerosis and other neuromuscular disorders, and food poisoning and other poisoning emergencies.

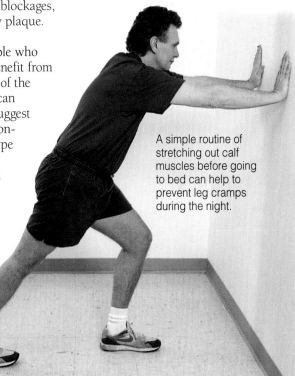

A simple routine of stretching out calf muscles before going to bed can help to prevent leg cramps during the night.

Muscle Strain

(Pulled or torn muscle)

A strain is an injury to muscles and perhaps tendons—fibrous bands that connect muscles to bones. It should not be confused with a sprain, which involves stretching or tearing of ligaments—the fibrous bands that connect bones and strengthen and stabilize joints.

There are two general categories of muscle strain: acute injury from sudden and excessive pressure in which muscle fibers tear, resulting in bleeding, swelling, pain, and loss of strength and function; and overuse injury, in which muscles become stretched from chronic stress. In the latter, muscles are sore, but they are not ruptured and there is no loss of strength.

Tears are likely to occur as muscles are subjected to sudden and extreme stress when cold, fatigued, or weak from disuse. The hamstrings (at the back of the thigh) are susceptible to such injury. For example, a torn hamstring might result when a normally sedentary person plays an intense game of tennis.

In contrast, overuse injuries result from muscles being repeatedly stressed over a longer period, such as when gardening. Back and groin muscles are commonly affected, although the legs and shoulders are also vulnerable.

Diagnostic Studies and Procedures

A doctor usually can diagnose a muscle strain by examining the area, but may order an X-ray to rule out a fracture or

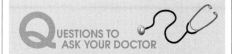

other bone injury. In unusual cases, an MRI will be ordered to rule out a torn ligament. Another diagnostic tool is electromyography (EMG), in which needle electrodes are inserted into muscles to measure responses electrically.

A chronic muscle problem may also be assessed by a specialist in sports medicine or a physiatrist, a doctor who specializes in physical rehabilitation.

Medical Treatments

Self-treatment is sufficient for most simple strains (see below). However, a doctor should be seen if there is no improvement after three or four days, or as soon as possible if there is marked swelling and loss of muscle function. In such cases, a nonsteroidal anti-inflammatory drug such as indomethacin (Indocin) may be prescribed to reduce inflammation and swelling and alleviate pain. Research suggests that these drugs should not be taken immediately after an injury; waiting at least one day allows the inflammation to help rid the injured area of damaged cells.

A muscle relaxant may provide added relief if spasms are a contributing factor. An injection of cortisone into the injured area can also reduce both the swelling and inflammation.

Surgical repair might be necessary if a tendon has been ruptured or torn.

Alternative Therapies

Acupuncture. This therapy may reduce soreness of a pulled muscle, but it is unlikely to be helpful for a ruptured muscle or tendon.

Alexander Technique. This approach is of greatest benefit as a preventive measure. A therapist will study the individual's body

movements and provide instruction in correcting any habits that could contribute to an injury.

Chiropractic. These practitioners treat strained muscles in the neck, back, and shoulders by manipulating and realigning the spinal column. They may also use diathermy to relax tensed muscles.

Massage Therapy. Swedish massage and similar therapeutic techniques are favored by many athletes, professional dancers, and others whose muscles are often strained by overuse. The massage is sometimes combined with heat treatments or hydrotherapy in the form of hot and cold soaks, whirlpool baths, underwater massage, and needle showers.

Rolfing. This method of deep, often painful manipulation is intended to break down excessive connective tissue that interferes with the proper alignment of the body.

Yoga and Meditation. These and other relaxation techniques can help alleviate muscle soreness due to stress.

Self-Treatment

RICE, an acronym for **r**est, **i**ce, **c**ompression, and **e**levation, is the preferred self-treatment for a pulled muscle. The injury should be rested immediately, and ice packs applied for 10 minutes every half hour during the first day. (To create a soft ice pack, fill a plastic bag with crushed ice or frozen peas or corn.) Compression is accomplished by wrapping the injured part in an elastic bandage. Depending upon the site of the injury, it can be elevated by using a sling, pillow, or other support.

After 24 to 36 hours, you may switch to a heating pad or hot packs. (These should not be used sooner, because heat increases blood flow to the area and may contribute to bleeding and swelling.) At this time, it is all right to take an anti-inflammatory medication that contains aspirin or ibuprofen. Acetaminophen will reduce pain but not the inflammation.

Ointments, liquids, and other rubbing agents such as Sloan's Liniment or Ben-Gay may ease pain by producing a sensation of warmth and numbness. However, these preparations are not as effective as anti-inflammatory agents in healing a strained muscle.

Other Causes of Muscle Pain

Sprains, tendonitis, shin splints, dislocations, stress fractures, and other sports or work injuries also produce pain and swelling.

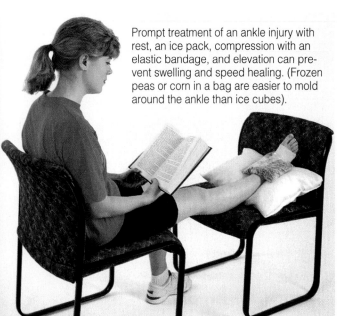

Prompt treatment of an ankle injury with rest, an ice pack, compression with an elastic bandage, and elevation can prevent swelling and speed healing. (Frozen peas or corn in a bag are easier to mold around the ankle than ice cubes).

Muscular Dystrophy

(Duchenne, fascioscapulohumeral, and myotonic dystrophies)

Muscular dystrophy is the general term for hereditary muscle diseases characterized by progressive weakness and disability. There are numerous forms, but the most common are:

Duchenne dystrophy, the most severe type. It strikes boys who inherit the gene from their mothers. The progressive muscle weakness, usually apparent by age three, is caused by a lack of the protein dystrophin in muscle cells. The disability affects mainly the torso and limb muscles, and by age 12, most patients are confined to a wheelchair. Progressive weakening of the chest muscles usually results in respiratory failure or fatal pneumonia by age 20.

Fascioscapulohumeral (FSH) dystrophy, which occurs in both sexes, with onset during adolescence. Typically, there is difficulty in raising the arms overhead, changing facial expression, and perhaps closing the eyes due to muscle weakness. The back and shoulders become progressively curved. Although the person appears deformed, he or she can still walk, and life expectancy is close to normal.

Myotonic dystrophy, which affects various organs as well as muscles. The symptoms vary from person to person. In most patients, muscles fail to relax after use—a condition called myotonia. In some cases, there is obvious wasting of facial and neck muscles, which may impair swallowing and blinking. Complications can range from increased miscarriages in women and sterility in men to cataracts and personality changes. However, many people with myotonic dystrophy live normal lives, often unaware of the disease.

GENETIC COUNSELING

Couples with a family history of muscular dystrophy may benefit from genetic counseling. For example, a woman who carries the gene for Duchenne dystrophy has a 50-50 chance of passing the disease to a male offspring. Counseling can also alert a couple to the patterns of inheritance. The discovery, for instance, that the gene for myotonic dystrophy becomes more dominant each time it is inherited means the disease itself will become more severe in new generations.

Diagnostic Studies and Procedures

A family history of muscular dystrophy plus a gradual weakening and shrinking, or atrophy, of muscles points to the possibility of dystrophy. A diagnostic workup will include blood, urine, and spinal fluid studies, and electromyography to assess muscle responses.

Muscle biopsy helps to identify the type of dystrophy. In Duchenne dystrophy, a biopsy will show the presence of excessive fat and connective tissue, which weaken muscle fibers. In FSH dystrophy, it will reveal abnormal muscle fibers and cell structure.

Because myotonic dystrophy can affect organs as well as muscles, it is often misdiagnosed. However, electromyography will show abnormal muscle function, and an electrocardiogram may reveal abnormal heart function.

Medical Treatments

As yet, there is no cure, so treatment is concentrated on easing symptoms and preventing complications. If the chest muscles are weakened, antibiotics may be prescribed to prevent pneumonia and other respiratory infections.

Digitalis and other heart medications are used to strengthen the heartbeat and to steady cardiac arrhythmias.

Quinine, used to treat malaria, is sometimes given to prevent the muscle contractions of myotonic dystrophy. Androgens, male sex hormones that promote muscle-building, may be used to relieve some of its symptoms, but do not seem to help other types of dystrophy.

Surgery may be recommended to forestall certain disabilities or alleviate symptoms. For example, a procedure to lengthen leg tendons and cut the fascia, fibrous tissue that encases the muscles, sometimes prolongs mobility.

An experimental treatment for Duchenne dystrophy entails injecting millions of healthy muscle cells into the patient's diseased muscles. Some patients appear to improve, but long-term benefits are doubtful. Researchers hold the most hope for advances in genetic engineering that will enable doctors to replace the defective gene.

Alternative Therapies

A controversial alternative therapy, developed by the parents of a boy who suffered from muscle disease, is said to delay the progression of some types of

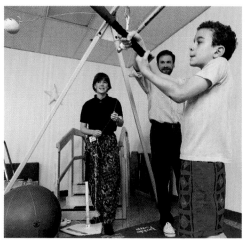

Physical therapy that is designed to preserve muscle strength and tone is helpful in some forms of muscular dystrophy.

dystrophy. However, its benefits have not been proven. A commercial version (known as Lorenzo's oil), made from purified olive and rape seed oils, is under development.

Nutrition Therapy. A high-protein, low-fat diet is advocated, and vitamin E supplements may be recommended. It's important to maintain normal weight; extra pounds can strain weak muscles further and exacerbate spinal deformity.

Physical Therapy. All patients can benefit from intensive physical therapy. Special leg braces and crutches help to retain mobility, and passive and active stretching exercises help to prevent muscle shortening and contractures. These exercises may be combined with therapeutic massage and music therapy.

Self-Treatment

The goal is to stay active and keep a positive attitude. Prolonged bed rest should be avoided, as it hastens muscle wasting. Regular exercise, though difficult, is essential to forestall disability.

Other Causes of Muscle Weakness

Multiple sclerosis, myasthenia gravis, amyotrophic lateral sclerosis (Lou Gehrig's disease), and polio are among the disorders causing muscle weakness.

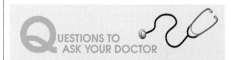

QUESTIONS TO ASK YOUR DOCTOR

▶ If I have one child with muscular dystrophy, what are the chances that future children will be similarly affected?
▶ Are there tests to determine if I carry the gene for myotonic dystrophy, even though I do not have symptoms?

Myasthenia Gravis

Myasthenia gravis is a relatively rare neuromuscular disease characterized by increasing weakness of voluntary muscles, especially those controlling the eyelids and the parts of the mouth and throat used in speaking and swallowing. Typically, the first symptoms are droopy eyelids and double vision. As the disease progresses, facial expressions become difficult to control; for

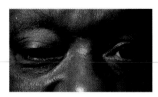

Drooping eyelids appear early in the course of myasthenia gravis.

example, a person trying to smile may appear to be snarling. Chewing, swallowing, and speaking are also impaired.

Problems eventually develop in the arms and legs, which can lead to difficulty in walking and lifting objects. In about 10 percent of sufferers, breathing muscles are affected, in which case an artificial respirator may be needed. The rate of progression varies greatly; about 25 percent of patients go into spontaneous, often permanent remission, while others decline rapidly and experience widespread muscle weakness.

Women are stricken more often and at a younger age than men. Babies born to women with the disease frequently develop symptoms at an early age.

What triggers myasthenia gravis is unknown, but it is classified as an autoimmune disease, in which the immune system destroys cells located at the junction of muscles and nerves. People with other autoimmune diseases appear more susceptible to myasthenia gravis, as are those with a history of a thymus tumor or lung cancer.

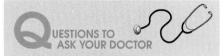

QUESTIONS TO ASK YOUR DOCTOR

▶ How long do remissions of myasthenia gravis usually last?
▶ Should I refrain from having children? If I do have a baby, what are the chances that he will develop the disease?

Diagnostic Studies and Procedures

If symptoms raise a suspicion of the disease, blood tests may be done to look for antibodies to acetylcholine, a body chemical that transmits nerve messages. Diagnosis can be confirmed by the person's response to an intravenous anticholinesterase drug, such as edrophonium, which produces an immediate, albeit temporary, improvement in muscle strength in people with myasthenia gravis. Additional tests may include electromyography to measure electrical activity in muscle cells, and a CT scan to look for a thymus tumor.

Medical Treatments

Anticholinesterase medications such as pyridostigmine (Mestinon) or neostigmine (Prostigmin) are the first line of treatment. Dosages and timing vary according to needs. For example, a person with swallowing problems may benefit by taking the medication before meals. Most patients improve with these drugs, but few recover completely.

A blood cleansing technique called plasmapheresis is often used during a crisis or to strengthen a patient for surgery. The person is hooked up to a machine that separates plasma from other blood components. Once separated, the cleansed plasma is returned to the patient's bloodstream. Plasmapheresis usually produces marked short-term improvement.

In some cases, the thymus is taken out, even if the gland is free of a tumor, because the operation prompts a remission in some patients. Those who benefit most are under age 55 and have only recently developed symptoms.

Steroids and other drugs that suppress the immune system can slow progression of the disease, but their many side effects—lowered immunity, easy bleeding, mood swings, weight gain, and thinning of bones, skin, and other tissues—preclude their long-term use.

A myasthenic crisis, during which difficulty in breathing or swallowing becomes life threatening, requires hospitalization for artificial respiration and intravenous feeding, if necessary.

Alternative Therapies

Alternative therapies should be adjuncts to conventional treatments and used only with the approval of a specialist in neuromuscular disorders. Therapies most likely to help are those that reduce stress and strengthen the immune system, such as meditation

and visualization. The gentle exercises of yoga and t'ai chi are particularly suitable, because they build strength and endurance without undue exertion.

Self-Treatment

Adequate rest is essential, as weakness is less pronounced after resting or sleeping. Set aside several rest periods each day, but strive for balance; too much rest accelerates muscle weakness.

Because a myasthenic crisis can come on suddenly, you should carry an anticholinesterase drug with you at all times. Also, wear a medical bracelet to alert emergency personnel to your condition.

Other Causes of Muscle Weakness

Symptoms suggesting myasthenia gravis may be caused by drugs such as penicillamine and some types of antibiotics. Thyroid disease should also be ruled out.

Nail Disorders

Fingernails and toenails can speak volumes about the state of your health. Inspecting them, a doctor can find important clues to many diseases (see Other Causes). Nails themselves also are vulnerable to a host of common, albeit minor, problems—splitting, hangnails, discoloration, ingrown toenails, and infections, among others.

Healthy nails are smooth, shiny, and a somewhat translucent pink. (The visible nail plate is composed of keratin, a hard protein formed in the matrix, which is protected from infection and damage by the cuticle.) The pink color comes from blood vessels in the underlying nail bed; a bluish color indicates inadequate oxygen in the blood.

A healthy fingernail grows about ⅛ inch a month; toenails grow more slowly, taking two months to grow the same amount. In older people, the rate of growth slows and the nails become thinner and develop vertical ridges.

Many nail problems are due to overuse of, or sensitivity to, nail polish and remover, adhesives, and nail extenders. Overexposure to water and/or harsh chemicals can also damage nails, causing them to chip, split, or break. Tight, pointed shoes can lead to ingrown toenails (page 250), as can improper cutting and injuries. Nail biting and overly aggressive removal of cuticles promote bacterial infections (paronychia). In rare cases, the infection spreads from the rim of the nail plate into the tissue below.

Diagnostic Studies and Procedures

Simple nail problems usually can be diagnosed by inspection. If a fungal infection is suspected, a scraping from the nail will be sent for a laboratory culture to identify the organism. The appearance of such abnormalities as red streaks, discoloration, pitting, or an unusual shape calls for additional tests to detect a possible underlying disease.

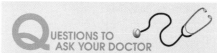

Q UESTIONS TO ASK YOUR DOCTOR

► Do my nails indicate a possible disease elsewhere in my body?
► What can I do to improve the condition of my nails?

Medical Treatments

Nail infections can be difficult to treat, and may require both topical and oral medication. A bacterial infection that has begun to spread from the nail bed is often treated with broad-spectrum oral antibiotics. Pockets of pus should be lanced and drained.

Fungal nail infections are very difficult to cure, though topical ointments and, in some cases, the oral antifungal medication griseofulvin (Fulvicin P/G) may be prescribed (see page 195).

Warts can form around the base and sides of a nail; most eventually disappear on their own. Those that persist can be removed by freezing with liquid nitrogen. Alternatively, daily applications of a topical combination of salicylic acid and lactic acid softens a wart, making it possible to peel it away.

Alternative Therapies

People who bite or pick their nails because of nervousness or stress may benefit from deep breathing, meditation, and other relaxation techniques.
Nutrition Therapy. Extra vitamin A and B complex are recommended to counter dry, brittle nails. Gelatin capsules have been promoted to strengthen nails, but there is no scientific evidence that they do. Calcium is said to make nails grow faster, but again, research has failed to substantiate the claim.

Self-Treatment

Simple nail problems can be remedied by home care.
► Wear gloves when doing household cleaning to keep nails dry and protect them from unnecessary wear and tear. After handwashing or bathing, gently rub a lotion or moisturizer that contains 10 percent urea into the nail plate and surrounding tissue.
► Try to minimize the use of polishes and removers. Dermatologists stress that they cause dry, brittle nails. (Repair chips rather than stripping and repolishing.) Check their ingredients and avoid those that contain formaldehyde, which is especially damaging. Remember, too, that chemicals in nail products can provoke allergic reactions in many people. Whenever possible, use hypoallergenic products, and even then, keep your fingers away from the face, neck, and eyelids until the substances are completely dry.
► Limit use of artificial nails. All have hazards and drawbacks. Press-on nails cause fewer problems than other types, but many women find them inconvenient as they can be worn for only a few hours at a time. Of the longer lasting nails, silk ones carry the lowest risk of infection and allergic reactions.
► Resist the temptation to use your nails as a convenient tool.
► Removing the cuticles with chemical solutions or with clippers deprives the nails of a tough and effective barrier against infection. Instead, dermatologists recommend pushing the cuticles back with an orange stick after soaking the fingers in warm water.

Other Causes of Nail Problems

The following nail abnormalities, may reflect serious underlying diseases:
Unusual color. Yellow, thick nails may be the result of chronic lung disease, a thyroid disorder, or a fungal infection. A bluish color indicates possible anemia or circulatory problems.
Pitting. Psoriasis, eczema, and fungal infections are possible causes.
Horizontal ridges, or beau's lines, may result from a serious infection, malnutrition, or certain hormonal disorders.
Streaks. Vertical red streaks might be caused by psoriasis, rheumatoid arthritis, or high blood pressure. Horizontal white streaks may be caused by sickle cell disease, heart disease, Hodgkin's disease, or kidney failure.
Spoon-shaped nails. Anemia or thyroid disease can produce depressed, spoon-shaped nails.
Clubbing. Nails that rise upward and curl around the finger tip can signal lung, liver, colon, or heart disorders.

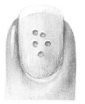

Pitting is associated with psoriasis, eczema, and fungal infections.

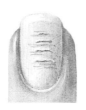

Horizontal ridges signal a serious medical condition.

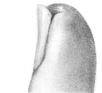

Spoon-shaped nails may be due to iron deficiency anemia or thyroid disease.

Thickened nails may be caused by an allergy to polishes or a fungal infection.

Nausea and Vomiting

Nausea and vomiting—a feeling of queasiness followed by the forcible ejection of the contents of the stomach—are not themselves disorders, but rather are common symptoms that may signal anything from pregnancy or overindulgence in food or alcohol to poisoning or a life-threatening disease. The two usually, but not always, occur together.

Nausea can originate in the labyrinth part of the ear, the brain, or gastrointestinal tract. Vomiting is a reflex (controlled by the vomiting center in the brain stem), in which the muscles controlling the esophageal sphincter relax, the diaphragm and abdominal muscles contract, the opening to the larynx, or windpipe, closes, and the lower portion of the stomach contracts and forces the contents upward and out of the mouth.

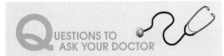

QUESTIONS TO ASK YOUR DOCTOR

▶ Is it safe to give a young child medication to prevent carsickness?
▶ What steps might lessen nausea and vomiting during cancer chemotherapy?

Diagnostic Studies and Procedures
In most instances, nausea and vomiting are responses to an obvious, self-limiting circumstance, such as motion sickness, overeating, or exposure to an unpleasant odor, that does not require diagnosis or treatment. But if they develop along with other symptoms, such as fever, pain, swellings, or dizziness, a careful workup should be done to find the cause. Blood and urine tests are sometimes sufficient, but if an intestinal disorder such as gallbladder disease, pancreatitis, hepatitis, an ulcer, or a tumor is suspected, X-rays, ultrasound, a CT scan, MRI, and other imaging studies will likely be ordered.

Medical Treatments
A doctor may prescribe preventive medications to be taken before travel, surgery, or other events that are likely to provoke nausea and vomiting. If the drugs cannot be taken orally, they will be administered by injection, suppository, or a medicated patch.

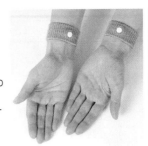

Acupressure bracelets help prevent or allay nausea by applying constant pressure to the inner wrists on the point corresponding to nausea control.

Drug Therapy. The following antinausea drugs, or antiemetics, suppress the vomiting center:
▶*Antihistamines,* such as dimenhydrinate (Dramamine and others), meclizine (Antivert and Bonine), and promethazine (Phenergan), reduce the sensitivity of the vomiting center of the brain. They also cause drowsiness.
▶ *Metoclopramide (Reglan)* controls peristalsis, the wave-like action that propels food through the intestinal tract. It is prescribed to prevent nausea and vomiting that commonly occurs during cancer chemotherapy, radiation treatment, or general anesthesia.
▶ *Phenothiazines,* such as fluphenazine (Permitil), perphenazine (Trilafon), and prochlorperazine (Compazine and others), are primarily antipsychotic agents that also block impulses to and from the brain's chemoreceptor center, which stimulates the vomiting center. These drugs are especially useful in preventing or stopping nausea and vomiting associated with chemotherapy, severe migraine headaches, and general anesthesia.
▶ *Scopolamine (Transderm Scōp),* which is administered as a medicated patch placed behind the ear, is prescribed to prevent motion sickness or treat vertigo.

Alternative Therapies
Acupressure. Pressing on a point located on the inner wrist can help prevent or ease nausea (see page 260). There are also special bracelets that apply constant pressure to this point (see photograph, above).
Aromatherapy. Facial massages or inhaling essences of basil, fennel, lavender, lemon, peppermint, rose, and sandalwood are said to alleviate nausea.
Biofeedback Training. Many people undergoing chemotherapy or radiation therapy suffer from nausea and vomiting prompted by anticipation rather than the effect of the treatment itself. Biofeedback training, hypnosis, and visualization help prevent this reaction.

Herbal Medicine. Gingerroot is the most popular herbal remedy for nausea and vomiting. It is available as capsules, tea, or ginger sticks that are chewed. Drinking tea made from peppermint or crushed anise seeds or chewing caraway seeds also may reduce nausea. For morning sickness, basil tea or raspberry leaf tea are recommended.

Self-Treatment
Common sense and prudence can go a long way toward preventing nausea and vomiting, especially when the cause is overindulgence.

During a bout of vomiting, avoid solid foods, milk, and citrus juice; instead, sip flat ginger ale, water, sweet fruit juice, bouillon, or a softened popsicle. If these provoke more vomiting, try sucking crushed ice.

After symptoms subside, gradually add bland, fat-free foods such as applesauce, bananas, dry toast, clear soup, rice, pretzels, or soda crackers. As you recover, try skinless chicken, lean beef, puddings, and similar foods.

To prevent pregnancy-related morning sickness, eat small, frequent meals throughout the day, and have a banana or something starchy such as rice pudding before going to bed. Keep some crackers at your bedside to eat before getting up in the morning.

Other Causes of Nausea and Vomiting
Reye's syndrome causes a persistent type of forceful vomiting. Babies born with pyloric stenosis, a defect in which food cannot pass from the stomach into the small intestine, also vomit forcefully after eating.

THE SPECIAL CASE OF MOTION SICKNESS
Nausea and vomiting triggered by motion are caused by a disturbance of the vestibular apparatus, or balance center, in the inner ear, which is closely linked by nerves to the brain's vomiting center. The symptoms, which stop when motion ceases, are exacerbated by anticipation, anxiety, fumes, poor ventilation, and looking at a horizon that appears out of sync with one's sense of balance.

Although motion sickness occurs at any age, children are especially susceptible. Most outgrow the problem by age five or six. Simple strategies like sitting in the front seat of a car and focusing on a stable object on the horizon will often prevent motion sickness.

Neck Pain

(Cervical syndromes)

Neck pain, ranging from a steady, dull ache to incapacitating spasms, is a very common complaint, with many causes and manifestations. The pain may originate in any of the neck structures—muscles, ligaments, tendons, and the disks that cushion the seven cervical vertebrae, as well as bony overgrowths and spurs. Or it can originate elsewhere; for example, the shoulders or the temporomandibular joint (TMJ) of the jaw—and radiate to the neck along nerve pathways that serve both areas.

Increasingly, chronic neck pain is due to occupational demands on the upper musculoskeletal system, such as long hours spent driving or working at a computer display terminal. Psychological stress is still another common cause. Or a whiplash injury that seems inconsequential initially may produce chronic pain weeks later.

Diagnostic Studies and Procedures

After asking questions about the onset and nature of the pain and doing an examination, a doctor will order X-rays. If he suspects a disk problem, he may also recommend a CT scan or MRI. When the sufferer is an athlete or a gymnast, dancer, or instrumentalist, a video of the patient at work may reveal biomechanical problems.

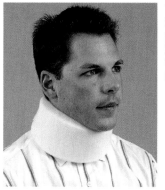

Treatments for neck pain might include wearing a brace.

Medical Treatments

When neck pain is treated with drugs, the first choice is one that combines analgesia and anti-inflammatory properties, such as aspirin or ibuprofen. Where pain is immobilizing, an injection of cortisone may help. Neck pain caused by muscle spasms may be treated with baclofen (Lioresal), chlorzoxazone (Paraflex), or diazepam (Valium).

However, long-term use of any of these drugs is discouraged as a rule, because they can become habit forming.

In some cases, wearing an orthopedic neck brace helps. An acute strain of the muscles and tendons is treated with rest. Surgery may be recommended for a herniated disk or bony overgrowths.

Alternative Therapies

Appropriate alternative therapies are often combined with or substituted for conventional treatments.

Acupuncture. A series of treatments may be all that is needed to provide lasting relief, especially for neck pain caused by muscle spasms and stress.

Alexander Technique. Learning new postures and ways of moving are helpful for people whose neck pain is job related. Many professional musicians, for example, benefit from this technique.

Aromatherapy. Combined with massage, this is a good way to relax muscles.

Biofeedback. Training in biofeedback skills can help overcome muscle spasms. Biofeedback may also be useful in stopping tooth grinding and other habits that cause TMJ problems.

Chiropractic. Treatments are concentrated on the neck and upper back to alleviate pressure on nerves in the neck.

Meditation and Yoga. Breathing exercises, relaxation methods, and focused meditation can ease stress-related pain.

Self-Treatment

A heating pad can be helpful, but even more effective is the wet heat provided by special pads such as Thermaphore. Otherwise, self-care centers on exercises to relieve tension at the back of the neck. The following routine can be done several times a day, at home or at work. To increase their effect, do the first two exercises as slowly as possible, and when you drop your head, drop your lower jaw too and close your eyes.

▶ Roll your head slowly three times clockwise, then three times counterclockwise, dropping its full weight at the end of each cycle.

▶ Drop your head forward, without moving your shoulders, then from one side to the other; next, tilt it backward as far as you can. Do this 10 times.

▶ Without tilting your head, swivel it slowly from side to side 10 times, and then repeat the exercise more quickly.

▶ To relax neck and shoulders, sit in a chair with good back support. With your feet about 18 inches apart and flat on the floor, stretch your arms and

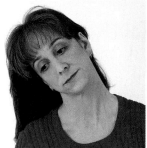

Begin this exercise by dropping your head forward, then in a smooth gentle movement, roll your head to the right.

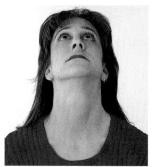

Slowly move your head back and to the right without moving your shoulders.

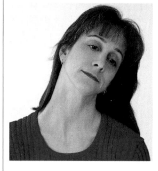

Finally, move your head to the left, then bring it back to the center and drop it forward.

trunk upward. With buttocks firmly placed on the seat, drop your body forward, letting head and arms dangle.

▶ Standing straight, with feet parallel and about 12 inches apart, stretch arms high above your head, then drop your upper body forward from the hips so that your arms, head, and shoulders are hanging loose. Keep this position for about 30 seconds, then shake arms, shoulders, and head, and raise your body slowly. Repeat several times.

Other Causes of Neck Pain

Arthritis, structural defects, and wry neck are a few causes of neckaches. Pain also may be referred to the neck during earache, headache, or toothache.

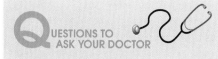

QUESTIONS TO ASK YOUR DOCTOR

▶ How long can I take strong painkillers?
▶ Should I consider wearing a neck brace? How long will I need it?

Nephritis

(Bright's disease; glomerulonephritis; pyelonephritis)

Nephritis is the general term for acute or chronic inflammation or impairment of the kidneys caused by infection, a degenerative process, or vascular damage. The disorder is always serious because it can set the stage for kidney failure. Two of the most common forms of nephritis are:

Pyelonephritis, caused by an acute or chronic bacterial infection. High fever, chills, severe flank pain, and an increased need to urinate, accompanied by burning pain, are typical symptoms.

Glomerulonephritis, which can be caused by a variety of disorders that damage the glomeruli, kidney structures that filter waste from the blood. Children, for example, sometimes develop acute glomerulonephritis after

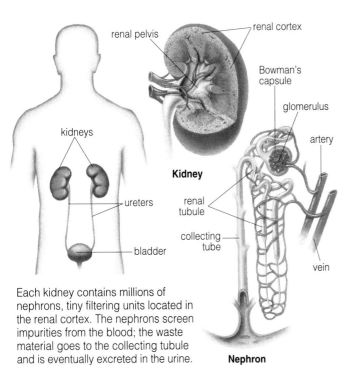

Kidney

Nephron

Each kidney contains millions of nephrons, tiny filtering units located in the renal cortex. The nephrons screen impurities from the blood; the waste material goes to the collecting tubule and is eventually excreted in the urine.

a strep throat infection. Symptoms include headaches, blurred vision, generalized aches and pains, and fluid retention marked by facial puffiness in the morning, swollen ankles in the evening, and decreased urination. The urine may be amber or rusty in color, because it contains blood and protein.

Chronic glomerulonephritis develops slowly and without obvious symptoms until it reaches an advanced stage. It is sometimes secondary to diabetes or a

disease such as lupus (page 278), which can damage the kidneys.

Diagnostic Studies and Procedures

The presence of blood and protein in the urine typically points to a kidney disorder. Other tests will be needed to look for the underlying cause, and may include blood studies and cultures, a 24-hour urine collection and analysis, X-rays, and such imaging procedures as a CT scan, ultrasound, and an intravenous pyelogram, in which a dye is injected into the kidneys before X-rays are taken. A kidney biopsy also may be ordered in some cases.

Medical Treatments

Bacterial pyelonephritis is treated with a combination of antibiotics, usually for several weeks, to prevent recurrence. Antibiotics are also prescribed for acute glomerulonephritis due to an infection. If necessary, kidney dialysis may be ordered temporarily until the kidneys have had a chance to recover. With chronic glomerulonephritis, diuretics may be necessary to remove any excess fluid from the body. Blood pressure should be regularly monitored; if it is too high, antihypertensive drugs will be prescribed.

Some studies have shown that the gradual development of glomerulonephritis caused by diabetes, one of the most common causes of chronic kidney failure in the United States, can be prevented by taking captopril (Capoten), which inhibits the angiotensin converting enzyme, a body chemical that helps to regulate blood pressure.

When nephritis results in chronic kidney failure, long-term dialysis is necessary. Erythropoietin, a hormone that increases production of red blood cells, is given to counteract the anemia that commonly accompanies kidney failure. A kidney transplant is an alternative to dialysis for treating chronic kidney failure (see page 262).

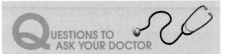

Alternative Therapies

Nephritis is a serious disorder that mandates careful medical treatment and monitoring. Before initiating any dietary change or other alternative therapy, be sure to check the procedure with your doctor.

Herbal Medicine. A few of the herbs that have a diuretic effect and thereby reduce the kidneys' workload are red clover, goldenrod, juniper berries, nettles, marsh mallow root, and uva-ursi. These are taken as teas.

Nutrition Therapy. A clinical dietitian experienced in working with kidney patients can work out an appropriate diet. The goal is to limit the buildup of waste products and fluids in the blood.

Generally, restriction of protein, phosphorus, sodium, potassium, and sometimes fluids is recommended. Calcium supplements may be needed, along with supplements of vitamins B_6, folic acid, and C, if the diet does not supply the recommended dietary allowances (RDAs) of these essential nutrients. However, high doses of vitamin C can damage the kidneys further and should be avoided by anyone with reduced renal function.

Self-Treatment

Avoid nonprescription painkillers, especially acetaminophen and combinations of aspirin and acetaminophen; these can worsen nephritis.

Individuals with chronic kidney disease can benefit from participation in a self-help group where members can discuss stress management and their emotional problems.

Other Causes of Kidney Inflammation

In addition to infections, nephritis may be caused by drugs and numerous toxic substances, especially solvents, pesticides, and arsenic, lead, and other heavy metals. Glue sniffing or inhaling benzene and other toxic fumes also causes nephritis.

Neuropathy

(Peripheral neuropathy; peripheral neuritis)
Inflammation involving nerves that serve parts of the body outside the brain and spinal cord are referred to as peripheral neuropathy or neuritis. Because the inflammation interferes with the transmission of messages along these nerves, symptoms, in addition to pain, may include numbness, weakness, and tingling sensations.

Mild peripheral neuropathy may arise from poor posture, repetitive motions, or activities that require maintaining a cramped position for long periods, such as squatting while gardening. Nerve damage from an accident or surgery, an infection, alcoholism, and lead poisoning and exposure to other toxic agents can cause persistent or severe neuropathy. Another cause, especially in the lower legs, feet, and hands, is diabetes.

Other disorders commonly associated with neuropathy include hardening of the arteries (arteriosclerosis), AIDS, multiple myeloma and certain other types of cancer, and disorders such as rheumatoid arthritis, scleroderma, Lyme disease, and lupus. Shingles can cause neuropathy that lasts for a year or more after the rash clears up.

Certain medications can cause neuropathy, especially isoniazid (Nydrazid), used to treat tuberculosis; phenytoin (Dilantin), an anticonvulsant; and some anticancer agents. Other causes include nutritional deficiencies, such as those that develop in alcoholics; or chronic overdoses of B vitamins, especially vitamin B_6.

Diagnostic Studies and Procedures

The diagnostic challenge is to track down the underlying cause. This starts with a complete physical examination that includes blood and urine tests, and possibly X-rays to detect bone changes impinging on nerves. A neurologic workup may be done to check reflexes and look for any muscle weakness or atrophy and impaired sensory function. Nerve tests may include electromyography and nerve conduction studies, which can pinpoint the nerves causing the symptoms.

Medical Treatments

Neuropathy resulting from an accident or nerve damage during surgery will improve or disappear as healing takes place. Similarly, nerve pain caused by an infection or toxic agent usually goes away after recovery.

Studies have shown that diabetic neuropathy can be prevented or even reversed by maintaining normal levels of blood glucose. Circulation to areas affected by arteriosclerosis or other obstructions also may improve with treatment of the underlying cause.

Taking corticosteroids or other drugs that suppress inflammation and the immune system sometimes prompts healing of nerve damage due to rheumatic disorders such as rheumatoid arthritis, lupus, and scleroderma.

High doses of intravenous antibiotics may help to ease symptoms of chronic Lyme disease, but will not always halt neuropathy. Even so, nerve pain that is linked to the disease usually lessens with time.

Halting high doses of vitamin B_6 can prevent further nerve deterioration caused by the excess, but it may not reverse existing damage.

Alternative Therapies

Prompt diagnosis and medical treatment of underlying causes of persistent neuropathy are essential. Meanwhile, the following alternative therapies may help to alleviate symptoms.

Acupuncture. This technique is one of the most effective alternative therapies for alleviating nerve pain, especially the kind that often follows shingles.

Alexander Technique. Neuropathy stemming from poor posture and work habits may be reversed by correcting the faulty body mechanics (see photo, above right).

Aromatherapy. Massaging the painful area with oil of peppermint is said to alleviate nerve pain.

Herbal Medicine. A poultice, made with fresh chopped or grated horseradish mixed with water to form a paste, creates a sensation of heat that may counter neuropathy temporarily. Some herbalists also suggest black cohosh, or squaw root, especially if pain is caused by rheumatoid arthritis or other inflammatory conditions. It is available as a tea, tincture, or powder capsules.

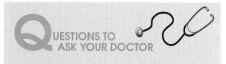

QUESTIONS TO
ASK YOUR DOCTOR

▶ Is my neuropathy likely to disappear, stay the same, or worsen?
▶ What can I do to prevent neuropathy caused by muscle contractures?

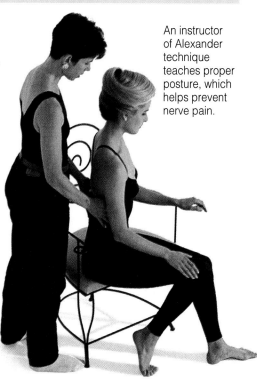

An instructor of Alexander technique teaches proper posture, which helps prevent nerve pain.

Massage. Neuropathy that is caused by muscle contractions or impinged nerves may be alleviated by massage and other manipulative techniques.

Physical and Occupational Therapy. These adjuncts to conventional medicine are especially beneficial in dealing with progressive or permanent nerve damage, because the therapists can teach ways to compensate for lost mobility. They may also recommend splints, braces, and other devices to ease the pain of compressed nerves.

Self-Treatment

If you develop mild symptoms of peripheral neuropathy, such as "pins and needles" tingling or numbness, try to analyze your body mechanics for a possible cause. Take frequent breaks from tasks that place extra or repetitive stress on one part of the body.

Lifestyle changes can also prevent or alleviate conditions that contribute to neuropathy. Avoid self-treatment with megadose vitamins, use alcohol only in moderation, and if you smoke, make every effort to stop.

Other Causes of Nerve Pain

An unusual type of neuropathy called phantom limb pain sometimes occurs following amputation; the person experiences pain, tingling, or other sensations at the site of the missing limb. Multiple sclerosis and other neuromuscular disorders that produce muscle contractures can cause neuropathy, as can a stroke or other brain damage.

Night Voiding

(Bed-wetting; enuresis)

Night voiding, or enuresis, refers to urinary incontinence while asleep. When this occurs in children under age six, it is called bed-wetting and usually is not considered abnormal. Some youngsters continue to wet the bed, perhaps infrequently, until the teen years; the problem usually disappears by adulthood.

Theories abound as to why some children continue to bed-wet long after achieving daytime bladder control, but the reason remains unknown. Boys outnumber girls, and there may be a hereditary link because, in many cases, their fathers were also bed-wetters. Some experts think that bladder size and maturation play a role. Foods that cause bladder irritation may promote night voiding. Occasionally, an emotional upset can prompt a previously toilet-trained child to revert to bed-wetting, but only temporarily as a rule.

In adults, night voiding is generally due to an underlying medical disorder such as diabetes, chronic urinary tract infections, or a structural or nerve problem. In older men, an enlarged prostate (page 351) is a common cause. Older women often develop urge incontinence, or spastic bladder, a condition that is characterized by a sudden and overwhelming need to urinate. The problem is caused by instability of the bladder's detrusor muscle, which contracts unpredictably, releasing urine.

Diagnostic Studies and Procedures

The process will begin with a complete physical that includes a pelvic examination in women and a rectal exam of the prostate gland in men. Blood and urine tests, X-rays, and an inspection of the bladder with a cystoscope, a magnifying instrument that is inserted into the urethra, can sometimes identify the underlying problem.

Other studies may include a cystogram, a dye-enhanced X-ray of the bladder as it is emptied; nerve and sphincter studies; and perhaps tests to measure the bladder's capacity and its ability to empty completely.

Medical Treatments

A toilet-trained child who reverts to bed-wetting may be treated with counseling if no physical cause for the problem can be identified. If a urinary tract infection is responsible, antibiotics may be prescribed.

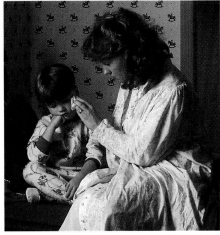

An emotional upset may cause a toilet-trained child to revert temporarily to bed-wetting.

Anticholinergic medications, which block certain nerve impulses, may be prescribed to treat night incontinence; these include flavoxate (Urispas), or imipramine (Tofranil), an antidepressant drug that has an anticholinergic effect. Prostate problems are also treated with drugs, and perhaps surgery. If an undersized bladder is responsible for night voiding, balloon dilation to expand the bladder and increase its capacity helps overcome the problem. When weak pelvic muscles are at fault, some urologists use electrical stimulation to strengthen them and prevent the involuntary release of urine.

Alternative Therapies

Biofeedback. This technique can be used to help train the bladder if urge incontinence is the problem. The training involves filling the bladder with sterile water by means of a catheter. An electrical monitoring device measures bladder pressure and tells the patient when the bladder is preparing to contract. The person then learns how to control the bladder contractions to allow time to get to the bathroom before voiding. Typically, training takes weeks or even months, but once mastered, it produces lasting results.

Herbal Medicine. Chewing on a piece of cinnamon bark several times a day is said to reduce the need for night voiding. Another time-honored remedy calls for taking cornsilk extract just before bedtime. Some herbalists also advocate uva-ursi tea or elcampane decoction.

Homeopathy. Gelsemium or belladonna may be prescribed, particularly for children. Ferrum phosphorica is used to treat a weak sphincter muscle.

Hypnosis. This technique sometimes works well, particularly with children, who are taught to hypnotize themselves at bedtime to avoid bed-wetting.

Self-Treatment

If a child continually wets the bed, refrain from scolding, punishing, or embarrassing him. Instead, give a reward for staying dry.

If you have a night voiding problem, drink fluids during the day and cut back a few hours before going to bed. If you invariably have to go the bathroom in the middle of the night but wake up too late, set an alarm clock. The same tactic may help a child.

Some people find that avoiding certain foods reduces urinary urgency. Acidic juices are a common bladder irritant. Coffee, tea, and other sources of caffeine not only may irritate the bladder, but they also act as diuretics, increasing output of urine. Nicotine is another bladder irritant, as is alcohol, which also has a diuretic effect. If you are taking a diuretic for high blood pressure, ask your doctor about an alternative drug or about taking your medication in the morning.

Self-help groups often benefit people who have incontinence problems. Adult diapers, waterproof bed pads, and similar products can help in coping with night voiding. For men, a shield or sheath that covers the penis can be worn to bed, but must be held in place by underwear.

Pay extra attention to skin care if you sleep with a device that brings the skin in contact with urine. Shower in the morning, dry the area thoroughly, and apply cornstarch or talcum powder. You can also ask your pharmacist about special skin care products for incontinence problems.

Other Causes of Night Voiding

Loss of urinary control is common in Alzheimer's disease and other dementias. Multiple sclerosis, stroke, and spinal cord injuries can also lead to loss of bladder control.

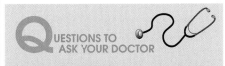

QUESTIONS TO ASK YOUR DOCTOR

► At what point should I worry about my child's bed-wetting?

► Am I a candidate for bladder training? If so, what method do you recommend?

Obesity

(Overweight)

Being overweight is the most prevalent nutrition-related health problem in the United States, affecting about half of all adults. Of these, 30 percent are obese, defined as being 20 percent or more above desirable weight (see box).

In addition to creating psychological and self-image problems, obesity increases the risk of some of our most lethal disorders, including diabetes and heart disease, and has been linked to an increased risk of cancers of the breast, uterus, ovaries, colon, prostate gland, and gallbladder. Excess weight also contributes to arthritis, back and foot pain, and respiratory disorders. In women, obesity can lead to menstrual irregularity and fertility problems.

The more you weigh, the greater the danger. One long-term study of several thousand men found that every pound over their ideal weight increased their mortality rate by 1 percent between ages 30 and 49, and 2 percent per pound among those 50 to 62.

Until recently, being overweight was thought to be a simple matter of consuming more calories than the body burned during daily activities. We now know that weight problems are more complex, involving heredity, hormones, psychological makeup, and ethnic and cultural background, among other factors. Heredity is especially important; for example, a study of identical twins who were raised by different families revealed that they tended to develop about the same weight by adulthood, regardless of their eating habits and other environmental factors.

Recognizing that the problem of obesity goes beyond willpower, it is not surprising that about 90 percent of dieters regain within five years all or most of any weight lost. However, this does not mean that attempts at weight loss are hopeless. Long-term weight-control programs that take a slow but steady approach are most likely to bring lasting success. Even if people do not achieve their ideal weight, modest reductions may still lower their risks of some disorders, such as diabetes.

Diagnostic Studies and Procedures

A certain body weight alone does not necessarily indicate a problem; what's important is whether or not you have too much body fat. An objective look

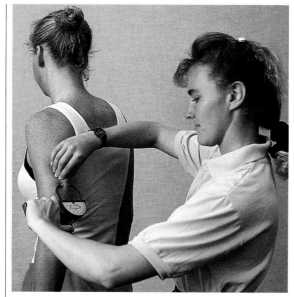

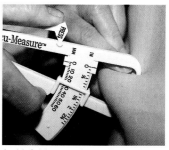

A skinfold test using calipers is done to assess body fat levels. A skinfold of more than an inch in certain areas of the body indicates excess fat.

in the mirror can be more telling than a scale—if you look fat and flabby, you probably are overweight. In contrast, if you are big boned and muscular, your weight may exceed what is considered ideal, but you will still look trim and fit, because muscle and bone weigh more than fat.

To determine if you have too much body fat, a doctor may use calipers, instruments that measure the thickness of a skinfold—the amount of skin and underlying fatty tissue that you can pinch together. About 50 percent of body fat lies just below the skin; thus skinfolds more than an inch thick on your underarm or the area just above your hip bone indicate excess body fat.

An even more accurate measurement of body fat is obtained by underwater weighing. You are weighed on land, and again while submerged in water. A formula based on these two weights gives the percentage of body fat.

Additional tests that may pinpoint the cause of excess weight include blood, urine, and hormone studies. A doctor will also want to review your eating habits and activity levels, which are important not only in finding the cause of weight gain, but also for devising a regimen to lose the excess pounds and then keep them off.

Medical Treatments

Many weight specialists now consider obesity a chronic disease that calls for lifelong treatment with a combination of lifestyle changes, alternative therapies, and perhaps drugs. Indeed, some doctors say that treating obesity without drugs will some day be viewed as archaic, like telling a person to control hypertension simply by cutting down on salt and staying in bed.

Mild obesity—when weight is 20 to 40 percent above what is considered ideal—usually can be self-treated, perhaps with the assistance of nutrition and exercise professionals (see Self-Treatment, page 317).

Moderate obesity, defined as weight 40 to 100 percent above normal, is likely to require treatment with a medication to suppress appetite, a diet planned by a dietitian or nutritionist, and possibly behavior modification, assisted by a psychiatrist or psychologist (see Alternative Therapies).

Severe obesity of more than 100 percent above normal may require surgical

---

WHAT'S YOUR IDEAL WEIGHT?

You can use this formula to determine your ideal weight:

Females

Allow 100 pounds for the first 5 feet of height, and 5 pounds per inch over 5 feet. Thus, if you are 5 feet, 6 inches:

100 + (6 x 5) = 130 pounds

Add 5 to 10 pounds if you are large-boned and/or very muscular.

Males

Allow 106 pounds for the first five feet of height, and 6 pounds per inch over 5 feet. Thus, if you are 5 feet, 10 inches:

106 + (10 x 6) = 166 pounds

Add 10 to 15 pounds if you are large-boned and/or very muscular.

treatment in addition to drugs, diet, and behavior modification.

Drug Therapy. Historically, most doctors viewed diet pills, or anorectics, as unnecessary and potentially addictive crutches. This attitude changed with the introduction of safer drugs that can be used long-term. But even proponents of these drugs stress that relying on pills alone does not break bad eating habits or teach new ones. Thus, most physicians prescribe diet pills as a temporary aid to promote weight loss while the person adopts new eating and exercise habits.

The major function of diet pills is to suppress appetite and, in some cases, to reduce cravings for certain high-calorie foods. For example, some people turn to sweets when they feel depressed or

HOW MANY CALORIES DO YOU NEED?

If you are a healthy adult, use this formula to calculate how many calories you need per day:

Basic needs—10 calories per pound of body weight
Normal activities—3 calories per pound of body weight plus extra calories used for exercise
Adjustment for age—Subtract 2 percent of total calories for each decade after age 30.

Example: If you are a 55-year-old man who weighs 160 pounds and walks 3 miles a day:

Basic needs:	10 x 160	=	1600
Normal activities:	3 x 150	=	450
3-mile walk:	3 x 100	=	300
			2350
Age adjustment	.06 x 2250	=	−135
Total calories per day		=	2215

tense. Simple carbohydrates raise levels of tryptophan (a natural amino acid) in the bloodstream; the tryptophan, in turn, increases the production of serotonin, a brain chemical that improves mood. Thus, people who habitually turn to carbohydrates to improve their moods may have trouble shedding pounds without the aid of diet pills.

Most diet pills have similar side effects, which may include nervousness, high blood pressure, palpitations, headaches, dizziness, insomnia, mood

swings, tremor, dry mouth, diarrhea, constipation, itching, and rashes.

It is necessary to abstain from alcohol while taking any type of diet pill, and restrict caffeine, which can add to the nervousness. Also, these drugs cannot be prescribed for more than 12 consecutive weeks because they are classified as potentially addictive. Diet pills include the following:

▶ *Stimulants, such as dextroamphetamines (Dexedrine and Adderall),* which are the oldest types of diet pills and the most addictive; their use is now discouraged. Amphetamines, commonly called uppers, work by suppressing the appetite. They may also speed up metabolism, but this is unclear. After a few weeks, however, a tolerance for the drugs develops, thus decreasing their benefit and raising the risk of addiction should the dosage be increased.

▶ *Fenfluramine (Pondimin),* a drug that is chemically similar to amphetamines but with fewer stimulant and dependency problems. It suppresses appetite by raising the level of serotonin in the brain. It also increases the body's utilization of glucose.

▶ *Phentermine (Fastin and Adipex-P),* also chemically similar to amphetamines. It carries somewhat less risk of dependency, however.

▶ *Fluoxetine (Prozac),* one of the newest diet drugs; it is better known as an antidepressant. Prozac effectively increases levels of serotonin in the brain, where it helps curb appetite and elevate mood.

▶ *Phenylpropanolamine (Dexatrim and Control),* an over-the-counter drug that shares many of the stimulatory effects of amphetamines. It is also used in medications designed to relieve allergies and bronchial asthma.

Surgical Treatment. Several operations have been developed for treating life-threatening severe obesity. Some involve reducing the size of the stomach so that a person feels full after eating only small amounts of food. Others entail removing parts of the small intestine, thus reducing the absorption of nutrients. People who have such operations usually show a rapid weight loss, which then tapers off after a few years.

These major surgical techniques are recommended only for people with severe weight problems who have failed to lose weight by all other means. Afterwards, patients must undergo frequent checkups because of an increased risk

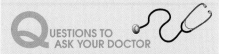

QUESTIONS TO ASK YOUR DOCTOR

▶ If I use diet pills, how long can I take them without the risk of developing an addiction problem?
▶ Is it safe for me to begin an exercise program? If so, what kind of activities do you recommend?

of metabolic disorders and other serious health problems that can result from the operation.

Alternative Therapies

Many of the alternative therapies promoted for weight loss either do not work or are potentially dangerous. Liquid protein diets, for example, have been linked to fatal cardiac arrythmias that develop when the body metabolizes lean tissue, including heart muscle. Ephedra, or ma-huang, a popular herbal remedy, raises blood pressure and can cause stroke and nerve damage.

Exercise Therapy. All successful weight-loss programs include exercise to help regulate appetite and stabilize the metabolic rate. Walking one mile at any pace burns up about 100 calories. It's best to start by walking a half-mile in 15 minutes every day, and with time, build up the pace and increase the distance to 3 miles in 45 minutes. Taking a brisk walk before a meal has the added benefit of curbing appetite.

A markedly overweight person should consult a doctor before undertaking an exercise program. If there is no heart disease or other problem that precludes vigorous exercise, a trained exercise physiologist can help plan a progressive conditioning regimen to burn calories and build muscle and strength. Initially, exercising in water may be recommended because it is easier on weight-bearing joints than other activities. As weight is lost, walking and other low-impact aerobic exercises can be added to the plan.

Nutrition Therapy. This remains the mainstay of all weight-loss programs. A nutritionist or registered dietitian can help plan a healthy diet that allows a gradual weight loss while adopting new eating habits. Any weight-loss diet should include a variety of foods and provide at least 1,000 calories a day. Even then, a multiple vitamin may be needed to ensure adequate nutrition.

Crash diets should be avoided. Any eating plan that restricts calories will result in weight loss, but a rapid shedding of pounds is self-defeating. When calories are overly restricted, your body lowers its metabolic rate to conserve energy. Even after you have achieved your weight goal, your body will continue to run at a slower pace, meaning that it needs fewer calories than normal. So just to avoid regaining weight, you must continue to restrict calories.

Self-hypnosis and Visualization. These techniques can help prevent overeating. For example, if a person frequently turns to chocolate or some other high-calorie sweet, a hypnotist can implant a suggestion that makes such foods undesirable and foster a craving for a low-calorie substitute.

Self-Treatment

Before undertaking any significant changes in your eating or exercise habits, consult your doctor if you:

▶ Have any chronic health problem, such as diabetes, gallstones, glaucoma, depression, or heart, kidney, liver or thyroid disease.

▶ Are taking any sort of medication on a regular basis.

▶ Want to lose more than 15 pounds.

▶ Are under age 21 or over age 35.

▶ Are pregnant.

Your goal should be to lose two or three pounds a week, and then to maintain the loss. This means bringing about a permanent change in your eating and exercise habits.

Start by keeping a careful food diary for at least two weeks (see sample, above). Be sure to write down everything you eat and drink immediately; it's difficult to reconstruct a day's total intake if you wait until evening. Note what prompts you to eat; this helps identify habits that might need adjusting. If, for instance, you tend to nibble on whatever is handy while studying or watching TV, you should keep on hand low-calorie foods such as fat-free crackers, raw vegetables, or unbuttered popcorn, instead of potato chips and nuts.

Successful weight loss invariably requires some change in eating behavior. You may need to eat more slowly, or you might have to adopt new attitudes toward food. Joining a self-help group such as Weight Watchers or Overeaters Anonymous may provide the motivation you need. The following principles of good nutrition can also help.

SAMPLE FOOD DIARY

DATE

FOOD	SERVING SIZE	CALORIES	CIRCUMSTANCES
Cereal	½ cup	140	Breakfast
Milk (1%)	¼ cup	25	"
Banana	1 small	80	"
Coffee: 1 tablespoon milk	1 cup	13	"
Bran muffin	medium	105	Snack
Cream cheese	2 teaspoons.	28	"
Sandwich: roast beef (3 ounces.), whole-wheat bread, lettuce, tomato, 2 teaspoons mayonnaise		687	Lunch
Apple juice	1 cup	120	"
Raspberry Yogurt (nonfat)	1 cup	125	Snack
Pasta with tomato sauce	(about 2½ cups)	503	Dinner
Salad of mixed vegetables	1 cup	180	"
Italian bread	1 slice	65	"
Chocolate chip cookies	2 medium size	103	"
Total calories for the day		2174	

▶ Make breakfast and lunch your main meals, and end the day with a light dinner. This type of eating schedule provides the most calories when you are active, and prevents you from becoming overly hungry, which can lead to overeating and weight gain.

▶ Reduce your intake of high-fat foods, such as cheese, cream, mayonnaise, luncheon meats, butter, ice cream, nuts, pies, and anything that is fried.

▶ Use low-fat or nonfat dairy products, lean cuts of meat, such as beef round, and reduced fat salad dressings.

▶ Grill, steam, roast, or broil foods, or sauté them in a nonstick pan instead of frying. Remove the skin from poultry.

▶ Increase your intake of complex carbohydrates, especially those that are high in fiber, such as vegetables and whole-grain breads and cereals.

▶ Avoid artificial sweeteners, which have been shown to stimulate appetite.

▶ Take a fiber pill or guar, available in pill or powder form, with a glass of water about 30 minutes before eating to curb your appetite.

▶ At meals, serve yourself moderate portions and don't take seconds, except of vegetables. If you feel deprived, serve your food on a smaller plate, which will make portions look bigger.

▶ For snacking between meals, keep on hand low-fat choices, such as hard pretzels, carrot sticks, rice or soda crackers, fruit, or nonfat yogurt.

▶ When eating out, order a low-fat main course that is broiled, steamed, or roasted, and ask that any sauce or butter be served on the side. Similarly, request that salad be served with the dressing in a separate container. Many ethnic foods, especially those that emphasize grains and vegetables, generally are good choices, but ask how they are prepared. Sautéed Chinese dishes—commonly thought of as being low in calories—have often been cooked with a large amount of oil. Similarly, even plain popcorn served in movie theaters usually contains oil.

Other Causes of Overweight

Unexplained weight gain may be caused by an underactive thyroid gland (hypothyroidism), depression, and conditions such as congestive heart failure, kidney failure, and cirrhosis of the liver that promote excess fluid retention. Long-term use of steroid drugs also causes weight gain.

Occupational Lung Disorders

(Asbestosis; berylliosis; pneumonoconiosis; silicosis)

Numerous occupations expose workers to chemicals, gases, dust, and toxins that can damage the lungs. Asbestos is one of the most familiar of occupational lung hazards, but there are others that are even more lethal. Types of occupational lung disorders include:

Pneumonoconioses, caused by industrial dusts or fibers. Asbestosis, a result of inhaling asbestos particles, falls into this category. Other examples are silicosis, a deadly disease in which nodules of scar tissue containing silica, or quartz dust, form in the lungs; berylliosis, in which the lungs become filled with masses of inflamed tissue called granulomas after exposure to beryllium dust; and black lung disease, which afflicts coal miners.

Workers in many fields are vulnerable to these dust diseases. Construction workers can be exposed to asbestos, but it is also a risk for automobile mechanics who repair old brake linings that were made with asbestos.

Silicosis is a hazard faced by miners of gold, lead, copper, and zinc ores embedded in rock that contains quartz. Other jobs that can lead to silicosis include pottery and china making, sandblasting, stone cutting, and working in foundries.

Berylliosis is caused by exposure to the dust or fumes of beryllium or its alloys, which are toxic metals used in the electronics, aerospace, and nuclear industries. Because beryllium is present in fumes released into the atmosphere during the manufacturing process, persons living near refineries and plants are also at risk.

About 30 percent of coal miners eventually develop black lung disease. The risk is greater among those who work with anthracite, or hard coal, than miners of bituminous, or soft coal.

Organic dust pneumonoconiosis, or farmer's lung, an allergic disorder triggered by inhaling mold or dusts from hay and straw or, less commonly, bark, coffee beans, tobacco, and cork. Textile workers exposed to cotton fibers and dust are also vulnerable to this disease. Although organic dusts are not as deadly as those of metals and inorganic compounds, they still can lead to lung scarring and a loss of elasticity similar to the conditions of emphysema.

Toxic gases and fumes, which can cause serious lung damage when inhaled. People who work in chemical plants, oil refineries, and dry cleaning plants are vulnerable, as are farmers and others who use pesticides and herbicides.

Symptoms of occupational lung diseases vary, depending upon the cause, and may take years to appear. Breathlessness, frequent coughing that usually produces phlegm, loss of appetite and weight, chronic bronchitis, emphysema, fatigue, chills and fever, and sometimes chest pain are common to all of these diseases.

Diagnostic Studies and Procedures

The patient's symptoms and job background provide important clues in diagnosing an occupational lung disease. The doctor will want detailed descriptions of the workplace, the types of substances used, and safety precautions followed. Because occupational lung diseases often take 10 or more years to develop, it is necessary to find out about jobs even in the distant past. Nonoccupational pursuits such as hobbies that involve exposure to toxic substances should also be investigated. Family members may also have been exposed to toxic materials brought home on workclothes, skin, and hair.

Chest X-rays, lung function tests, and biopsies are the mainstays of diagnosis. The X-ray will reveal characteristic opaque areas in the lungs. A biopsy often confirms the type of disease and may also detect the presence of cancer, a common complication of many occupational lung disorders. Phlegm and sputum samples might be studied for the presence of infection.

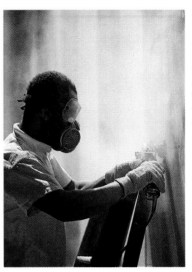

Protective measures such as wearing a mask are essential in preventing exposure to toxic substances that can cause occupational lung disorders.

If berylliosis is suspected, bronchoalveolar lavage will be performed. In this procedure, a bronchoscope, a viewing tube with magnifying devices, is inserted through the mouth and into the lungs. A fluid is then injected through the tube to wash up cells from the bronchial lining. Berylliosis is diagnosed if the cells are found to contain elevated levels of beryllium.

Medical Treatments

For the most part, these diseases are incurable and treatment usually is directed to alleviating symptoms. As lung failure advances, supplementary oxygen may be needed. Preventive antibiotics may be prescribed at the first sign of a cold or flu to head off a secondary lung infection.

Berylliosis is sometimes treated with steroid drugs. Hospitalization may be necessary during an acute episode in which lungs are inflamed. Patients with severely swollen or bleeding lungs may need assistance with a ventilator.

To treat black lung, bronchodilators may be prescribed. These drugs open the airways, making it easier to breathe. Steroids may also be used to prevent bronchospasm, in which the muscles that line the bronchial tubes contract and tighten. Diuretic drugs help control the buildup of fluid in the lungs.

Silicosis is difficult to treat, and there is no cure. Medications for shortness of breath and coughing are prescribed, as are bronchodilators and antibiotics.

Farmer's lung is usually treated with steroids to reduce inflammation, hospitalization may be necessary in severe cases, but the outlook is more optimistic than that of other occupational

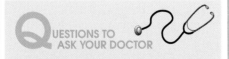

QUESTIONS TO ASK YOUR DOCTOR

▶ What is the likely course of my disease? Can I continue working and caring for myself?
▶ Am I eligible for disability payments? How do I find out more about my legal rights as an employee?

A CASE IN POINT

Frank Oster comes from a long line of Montana ranchers, a life he has always loved. As a boy, when asked what he wanted to be when he grew up, young Frank had only one answer: "A cattle rancher." After graduating from high school, he entered into a full-time partnership with his father, with an eye to eventually taking over the family ranching operation.

"Ranching is in my blood," he often said. Sadly, he was also developing an insidious disease—organic dust pneumonoconiosis, or farmer's lung—that was to threaten his ranching career at the age of 32. By then, Oster was married and had taken over the ranch completely.

He mistook his first symptoms—fever, fatigue, nausea, and a cough that produced large amounts of phlegm—for a lingering case of flu. But his illness worsened over the next few weeks. He now had difficulty breathing, he coughed all the time, and he had lost more than 10 pounds. At his wife's insistence, Oster finally saw a doctor in a nearby town. "This was an old-time family doctor," Oster recalls, "and his advice was: 'You need a vacation. Why don't you take a couple of weeks to visit your folks in Arizona?'" Although ranching is a year-round job, Oster felt he could go away and leave a hired hand in charge.

At first, it seemed that the vacation had done the trick. By the time Oster returned to Montana, his cough had disappeared, his appetite had returned, and he was gaining back his lost weight. But improvement was short-lived; within two weeks, his symptoms had returned.

This time, Oster made a trip to the Mayo Clinic, where he underwent a battery of tests that included a chest X-ray, pulmonary function tests, bronchoscopy, and a lung biopsy. The tests confirmed that Oster was suffering from farmer's lung, an allergic response to mold dusts from hay, silage, grain, and other organic products. If exposure to these dusts continues, the lungs become chronically inflamed and may eventually lose their elasticity, resulting in emphysema.

"The diagnosis was a blow," Oster recalls. "The Mayo doctors said I should quit ranching, but that was the only life I had ever known or wanted."

Fortunately, there were alternatives. A short course of steroid medication cleared the lung inflammation, but it was imperative that Oster avoid further exposure to mold dust. "I turned over most of the barn work to my hired hand, and I wore a special mask whenever I worked with hay or silage," Oster recounts. He also consulted the local farm agent about new silage and hay storage techniques that would reduce mold growth and had new silos and hay bins built.

"This was a major investment," Oster says, "but it paid off; we now have a lot less spoilage." More important, the changes enabled Oster to continue ranching.

lung disorders. In fact, the symptoms often disappear if contact with the offending molds or dust can be avoided.

Alternative Therapies

No alternative therapy can cure serious lung diseases, but some alleviate symptoms and make breathing easier.

Aromatherapy. Inhaling steam to which eucalyptus oil has been added helps to loosen lung secretions and improve breathing.

Herbal Medicine. Drinking a hot tea made from elecampane root thins phlegm and mucus. Horehound, taken as a decoction, syrup, or a tincture, may also help to clear sputum.

Hydrotherapy. A hot, steamy bath or shower helps to open up the airways. Conversely, a cold pack placed on the chest sometimes relieves lung congestion and makes breathing easier.

Physical Therapy. A respiratory therapist teaches special breathing methods and exercises, as well as a postural drainage technique to help clear secretions from the lungs. An occupational therapist may be consulted for ways to conserve energy when performing tasks.

Self-Treatment

Prevention is the best approach to occupational lung disorders. Make sure that your workplace meets mandated safety standards (see box, below), with adequate ventilation and protective gear. Employers should be providing laundered workclothes plus washing facilities and showers so that workers can change into their street clothes at the end of their shift. Also, vacuuming, washdown procedures, and wet sweeping can help reduce the dust.

Do not eat or drink while working. When you take a break, wash your hands thoroughly before touching any food or beverage. Store your belongings away from work areas, in a closed

YOUR RIGHT TO PROTECTION

There are laws to protect workers from occupational hazards. If your job exposes you to toxic substances, make sure that the rules are being followed.

If you feel that safety is lacking or you have not been given proper safety equipment, contact your union representative, supervisor, or local Occupational Safety and Health Administration (OSHA), the federal agency that oversees worker safety standards. Also do your part. Wear protective masks and follow all safety precautions and work practices, even if they seem cumbersome.

space where they are not exposed to dust and other toxic substances. Follow similar safety precautions at home or in your workshop if you are a do-it-yourselfer or hobbyist who regularly works with chemicals and other hazardous substances.

Smoking greatly compounds the risk of occupational lung disorders; if you are a smoker, the single most important thing you can do is to stop. Even a person who has smoked for years can decrease the risk by stopping.

If you should develop an occupational lung disorder, make every effort to avoid any further contact with the offending substance. This is especially important if berylliosis is diagnosed. If possible, change jobs or determine whether you are eligible for disability benefits. Also minimize contact with other substances harmful to the lungs; for example, stay indoors during periods of high air pollution and avoid secondhand tobacco smoke.

Other Causes of Lung Symptoms

Diseases that cause progressive loss of pulmonary function and produce symptoms similar to those of occupational lung disorders include bronchiectasis, sarcoidosis, emphysema, lung cancer, and tuberculosis.

Osteoporosis

Osteoporosis is a disease in which bones lose calcium and other minerals. There are two forms: type 1, the most common, occurs in postmenopausal women or younger ones whose ovaries have been removed; type 2, or senile osteoporosis, develops in both men and women, usually after age 75.

The decline of estrogen, the major female sex hormone, plays a major role in type 1. Up to half of all American women over the age of 45 have some degree of type 1 osteoporosis. Such bone loss is especially pronounced in the first decade following menopause. Other risk factors linked to osteoporosis include cigarette smoking, heredity, and being thin, fine boned, and of Asian or northern European extraction.

Symptoms generally begin with mild back pain, which worsens as the vertebrae become compressed, caused by tiny crush fractures that afflict about one-third of women over age 50. Compression of the spinal column also leads to height loss and a deformity commonly called dowager's hump. Wrist and hip fractures are common.

Diagnostic Studies and Procedures

Standard X-rays can detect decreased bone density of the vertebrae, but only after 25 to 40 percent of calcium has been lost. Bone density studies, such as single-photon absorptiometry, dual-energy absorptiometry, and quantitative computed tomography, provide earlier and more accurate assessments of bone density, but are costly. A scanning technique called X-ray densitometry is less expensive and is gaining wider use.

Medical Treatments

Treatment can usually slow bone loss, and sometimes even reverse it. The earlier that treatment begins, the more likely it is to increase bone density. One or more of the following drug treatments may be combined with the alternative therapies discussed below.

Postmenopausal estrogen replacement therapy lowers the incidence of vertebrae and hip fractures. It is most effective when started within four to six years after menopause (page 290).

Calcitonin, a thyroid hormone that regulates calcium metabolism and inhibits the loss of calcium from bones, shows promise as a drug to halt osteoporosis; it may also increase bone density. Although the hormone must usually

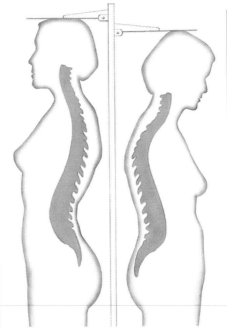

Bone loss in osteoporosis leads to diminished height and often spinal compression fractures.

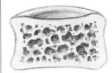 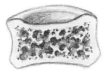

Normal vertebrae   **Osteoporosis**

be administered by injection, a newer form, calcitonin nasal spray appears to be equally effective.

Etidronate (Didronel), a drug first used to treat Paget's disease, another bone disorder, is under study as a treatment for osteoporosis. Research suggests that it can increase vertebral density and reduce the risk of fractures.

Tamoxifen (Nolvadex), an estrogen-blocking drug used for treating breast cancer, also appears to prevent osteoporosis; how it works is unknown. In addition, several promising new drugs are being used experimentally; these include alendronate (Fosamax), a drug that decreases bone demineralization.

Alternative Therapies

Exercise and Physical Therapy. Bones are constantly being rebuilt, a process that requires a certain amount of stress. Thus, walking and other weight-bearing activities are key components of any treatment program. If you already have osteoporosis, a physical therapist can develop an exercise regimen and teach you how to use your body more efficiently to reduce the risk of fractures. Also helpful are an orthopedic support, heat, and gentle massage.

Nutrition Therapy. Calcium and vitamin D are essential to building and maintaining bones. The best dietary sources of calcium are low-fat milk and milk products; canned sardines and salmon with bones; and certain green leafy vegetables such as broccoli and kale. However, beet greens, spinach, and other vegetables high in oxalates bind to calcium and prevent its absorption. Too much bran or other high-fiber food also hinders absorption of calcium, while citric acid enhances it.

Experts recommend that post-menopausal women get at least 1,500 milligrams of calcium a day, especially if they are not taking estrogen or are over age 65. For most women, this means adding supplements. Calcium citrate and calcium carbonate are the most absorbable forms; many brands are combined with vitamin D, which the body needs in order to absorb calcium. Dolomite and bone meal are not recommended because they sometimes contain lead and other contaminants.

Self-Treatment

Preventive self-care measures include:
▶ Do not smoke. Tobacco use appears to lower estrogen production.
▶ Limit caffeine intake to the equivalent of three cups of coffee daily.
▶ Abstain from alcohol, or use it in moderation, defined as no more than two alcoholic drinks a day.
▶ Try to spend 30 minutes in the sun two or three times a week; this enables your body to produce vitamin D. Otherwise, make sure that your calcium supplement or milk is fortified with this vitamin.
▶ If you take antacids, avoid brands containing aluminum salts, which impede calcium absorption, in favor of those containing calcium carbonate.

Other Causes of Bone Loss

Secondary osteoporosis may be caused by endocrine disorders such as diabetes; drug side effects, such as long term use of corticosteroids; rheumatoid arthritis; and prolonged bed rest.

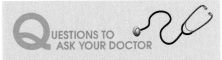

Q UESTIONS TO ASK YOUR DOCTOR

▶ When should I undergo studies for bone density?
▶ Should I take a calcium supplement? If so, what dosage?

Ovarian Cancer

(Ovarian carcinoma)

Ovarian cancer is the most lethal malignancy of the female reproductive organs. According to the American Cancer Society, about 27,000 new cases are diagnosed each year, with a death toll of almost 15,000. The high mortality rate is attributed to the fact that by the time ovarian cancer is detected, it usually has spread.

The cause remains unknown, though it is believed that hereditary factors play a role because ovarian cancer tends to run in families. It can occur at any age, but is more prevalent after menopause. Women who have never had children show a somewhat higher incidence; women who have used oral contraceptives seem to be at lower risk.

In general, early ovarian cancer is asymptomatic, but as the tumor grows, there may be vague abdominal discomfort and gas. As the cancer advances, abdominal swelling, pain, and weight loss often occur. In unusual cases, there may be vaginal bleeding.

Diagnostic Studies and Procedures

Women over age 40 should have a thorough pelvic examination every year or two that includes palpation of the ovaries because any enlargement of an ovary raises a suspicion of cancer.

When ovarian cancer is suspected, ultrasound can be used to detect the presence of a mass. Blood tests using monoclonal antibodies to search for specific substances called tumor markers show promise in screening for ovarian cancer, but are still experimental.

A definitive diagnosis usually requires laparoscopy, a procedure in which a viewing tube is inserted into

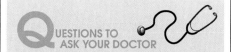

QUESTIONS TO ASK YOUR DOCTOR

▶ What are my treatment options?
▶ If both ovaries are removed, can I take replacement estrogen?
▶ Because ovarian cancer seems to run in families, what preventive measures should my sisters or daughters follow?

the pelvic cavity through a small incision near the navel, to allow examination of the ovaries and collection of biopsy samples. If the biopsy confirms cancer, additional tests will be done to determine whether or not it has spread to other parts of the body. These may include bone and CT scans, a chest X-ray, and laboratory examination of fluid obtained during laparascopy.

Medical Treatments

Surgery to remove one or both ovaries is the first line of treatment. In young women with localized cancer in only one ovary, the operation, an oophorectomy, may be confined to that ovary. More commonly, however, both ovaries are removed, along with the uterus, the fallopian tubes, and adjacent lymph nodes, a procedure known as salpingo-oophorectomy and hysterectomy.

Chemotherapy and/or radiation therapy usually follow surgery. With a new technique, anticancer drugs are infused into the abdominal cavity, a procedure called intraperitoneal administration. This approach not only increases the effectiveness of the drugs, but it also reduces their side effects.

A premenopausal woman who has had both of her ovaries removed will enter menopause immediately and frequently will experience hot flashes and other menopausal symptoms more intensely than a woman in whom it has occured normally. In such a case, estrogen replacement therapy will usually be added to her drug regimen as long as there are no contraindications for its use.

Alternative Therapies

Ovarian cancer always requires intensive medical and surgical treatment, although alternative therapies may play an adjunctive role. In addition to meditation, visualization, self-hypnosis, and other techniques to control pain, alternative therapies may include:

Nutrition Therapy. With ovarian cancer, as with many types of cancer, nutrition may play a role in prevention. In particular, vitamins A, C, and E, the antioxidant vitamins, and beta carotene (a precursor of vitamin A) are believed to help avert genetic changes in cells that contribute to the cancer development. Foods that contain high levels of vitamins A and C and beta carotene include citrus fruits, orange and dark green vegetables, and cruciferous vegetables such as broccoli, cabbage, brussels sprouts, and cauliflower. Those high in vitamin E are wheat germ, vegetable oils, nuts and seeds, green vegetables, and egg yolks. Although the role of other dietary components remains controversial, some studies suggest that a low-fat diet may reduce cancer risk.

Self-Treatment

As noted, removal of both ovaries results in an abrupt menopause. If you are unable to take estrogen, devise other strategies to minimize symptoms. To help mitigate night sweats, lower the thermostat in your bedroom, use light covers, and take a tepid shower before going to bed. During the day, wear light, layered clothing that can be removed easily if hot flashes occur. (For more ideas, see Menopause, page 290.)

While undergoing cancer chemotherapy and radiation treatments, practice visualization, self-hypnosis, or meditation to control side effects such as nausea and vomiting. Distractions such as listening to music or becoming absorbed in a good book or movie can also help. Get adequate rest, but try to exercise for at least a few minutes each day. Simply going for a short daily walk can help.

Consider joining a support group of other cancer patients; it's comforting to know you are not alone, and helpful to share coping tips with others.

Other Causes of Pelvic Symptoms

Abdominal pain and discomfort is most often caused by a gastrointestinal disorder, ranging from simple indigestion to cancer. Ovarian swelling is more often due to a benign cyst than cancer.

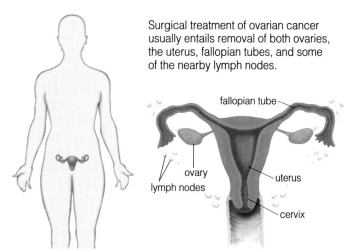

Surgical treatment of ovarian cancer usually entails removal of both ovaries, the uterus, fallopian tubes, and some of the nearby lymph nodes.

fallopian tube
ovary
lymph nodes
uterus
cervix

Ovarian Cysts

(Polycystic ovaries; Stein-Leventhal syndrome)

Ovarian cysts are benign growths that form on the ovaries, the two small, almond-shaped organs located on either side of the uterus. There are many different types, but the most common are functional cysts, which develop in the following way:

During the first half of a woman's menstrual cycle, the ovaries increase estrogen secretion, which in turn signals the pituitary gland to release FSH and LH, hormones that stimulate the ovaries to ripen one or more eggs. The eggs mature in tiny sacs called follicles, which grow to a size of ½ to ¾ inch in diameter. During ovulation, the mature egg bursts from its follicle, which is then replaced by the corpus luteum, a structure that secretes the hormone progesterone. Sometimes the egg is not released from the follicle, which then thickens to form a cyst that continues to pump out estrogen.

A cyst may grow as large as an orange, possibly rupture, and cause severe hemorrhaging and pain. More often, the woman experiences abdominal pain and irregular or abnormally heavy menstruation for a few cycles, but the cyst disappears in time, and normal periods resume.

In the case of polycystic ovaries, multiple cysts have developed, causing the ovaries to enlarge. This condition is associated with failure to ovulate and high levels of male sex hormones, which may lead to masculinization. Women who have polycystic ovaries typically experience menstrual abnormalities and infertility.

Women with endometriosis may develop ovarian chocolate cysts, or endometriomas, which form when tissue similar to the lining of the uterus attaches to the ovaries (see case, right).

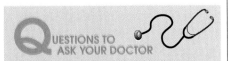

QUESTIONS TO ASK YOUR DOCTOR

▶ Do ovarian cysts increase the likelihood of cancer?
▶ What are my chances of conceiving if I undergo surgery for polycystic ovaries?
▶ If I have a cyst removed, is it likely that another one will develop?

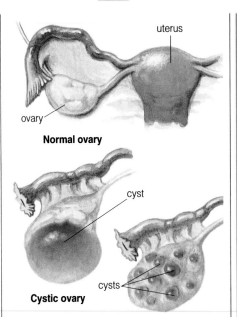

Normal ovary

Cystic ovary

Polycystic ovary

A single ovarian cyst (middle illustration) may grow and rupture. A polycystic ovary (lower right) is enlarged with multiple cysts.

Diagnostic Studies and Procedures

Most ovarian cysts are found when a doctor palpates the ovaries during a pelvic examination. Blood tests may be ordered to measure hormone levels. Ultrasound can determine whether the growth is solid or filled with fluid. For some cases, laparoscopy may be ordered, especially if the cyst appears to be solid. In this procedure, a viewing tube is inserted into the pelvic cavity through a small incision near the navel. The examination is usually done under general anesthesia in a hospital setting.

Medical Treatments

Treatment depends on symptoms, the size and type of cyst, and the woman's age and overall health. A young women with a small functional cyst and no symptoms will probably be told to wait for two or three menstrual cycles to see whether the cyst disappears on its own.

Hormones may be prescribed to stimulate ovulation, especially if the woman wants to conceive. If these do not work, surgery may be performed to remove the cystic portion of the ovary. Surgery may also be advised if the cyst is large or has ruptured, if there is severe pain or bleeding, or if the cyst becomes twisted, cutting off circulation.

It is possible sometimes to remove the cyst while leaving the ovary intact, but in other cases, one or both ovaries may have to be removed completely.

Alternative Therapies

Alternative therapies are not effective in treating ovarian cysts, although acupuncture may alleviate pain.

Self-Treatment

Self-care cannot eliminate an ovarian cyst. If you develop menstrual irregularity or are having trouble conceiving, a home ovulation test can determine if you are ovulating normally. Should symptoms persist for more than three menstrual cycles, see your doctor.

Other Causes of Pelvic Pain

Endometriosis, menstrual cramps, tubal pregnancy, and pelvic inflammatory disease can cause symptoms similar to those of ovarian cysts. Ovarian cancer should be ruled out, especially if the cyst is solid. An adrenal tumor or hormonal disorder should also be investigated as a possible cause of menstrual abnormalities or other symptoms linked to ovarian cysts, particularly if masculinization develops.

Paget's Disease

(Osteitis deformans)

Paget's disease is a chronic disorder in which bone metabolism goes awry. Instead of an orderly, constant process of repair and replacement, there is rapid loss, or resorption, of calcium and other bone minerals. The marrow is then replaced by fibrous tissue and a proliferation of blood vessels, their growth often rapid and chaotic. The new bone has an abnormal structure; it is less compact and contains more blood vessels than normal bone. As a result, the affected bones may, in time, become enlarged and so weak that they break spontaneously.

The disease can exist for years without producing obvious symptoms, so its incidence is difficult to gauge. Experts estimate, however, that about 3 percent of people over the age of 40 have some degree of Paget's disease. The incidence is proportionally higher among older people.

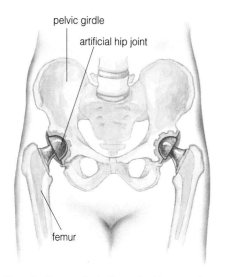

Paget's disease that affects the hips may be treated surgically with removal of the diseased joints and implantation of artificial ones.

The cause of Paget's disease remains unknown, but a genetic predisposition as well as a viral trigger have been implicated. Among candidates for the viral trigger are respiratory syncytial virus, an organism that can cause bronchitis and pneumonia, and the measles virus. Also, an association between dog ownership and Paget's disease in one area of England has led some researchers to speculate that a canine virus may be involved.

Symptoms vary according to the site of the disease, but bone pain is common. The bones most often affected are the tibia (shin bone), femur (thigh bone), pelvis (hip bone), vertebrae, and skull. In some severe cases, thigh bones become so soft that they bend outward and the shins bend forward. In others, the head becomes visibly larger. If the leg and hip bones are deformed, lower back pain often radiates to the buttocks and legs, and walking may be difficult, Bone changes affecting the inner ear may lead to deafness; facial pain and headaches are also common.

The proliferation of blood vessels in pagetic bone increases blood flow to the extremities, which may feel unusually warm to the touch. If the disease affects more than one-third of the skeleton, the heart must pump harder to meet the needs of the extra blood vessels, which can lead eventually to heart failure. In some cases, there are severe deformities of the spinal column, which compress the spinal cord and cause neurological symptoms, such as numbness or paralysis of a limb.

Diagnostic Studies and Procedures

Paget's disease is often discovered when X-rays taken for some other purpose show the characteristic mosaic pattern of bone tissue. In other instances, investigation of hearing loss, facial nerve pain, or other symptoms seemingly unrelated to the bones may uncover the abnormality.

Blood and urine tests also provide clues of abnormal bone metabolism. Bone scans with a radioactive substance confirm a diagnosis. Additional tests or scans may be ordered to look for sarcomas, a type of bone cancer that is a possible complication of Paget's disease. An electrocardiogram and other heart studies may reveal a higher-than-normal cardiac output.

Medical Treatments

Drug Therapy. When Paget's disease is asymptomatic, treatment is unnecessary. If pain is the major problem, large doses of aspirin provide relief and appear to suppress the disease itself. Similar results are achieved with other nonsteroidal anti-inflammatory drugs (NSAIDs), especially indomethacin (Indocin).

Steroids such as prednisone also suppress the disease, but because they must be given in high doses that can produce serious side effects, including lowered immunity, they are not recom-

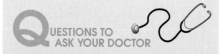

mended except as short-term treatment. A drug used specifically for Paget's disease, etidronate (Didronel), is sometimes prescribed to slow the rate at which bone is broken down and rebuilt.

Injections of calcitonin, a thyroid hormone, decrease resorption of bone that has been broken down by the body. If etidronate and calcitonin are ineffective, plicamycin (Mithracin), an intravenous anticancer drug, may be tried. This drug inhibits bone resorption, but its use in Paget's disease is considered experimental. Long-term calcitonin therapy can reduce bone pain and stabilize cardiac output.

Surgical Treatment. An osteotomy, or bone resection, may be recommended to correct a disabling deformity of the leg bones. Total hip replacement may be considered if the disease has caused serious impairment of those joints.

Alternative Therapies

Meditation and Self-hypnosis. These and other relaxation techniques may be helpful in alleviating pain.

Physical Therapy. A suitable level of physical activity is important in fostering proper bone metabolism and retaining mobility. A physical therapist can provide guidance in developing a realistic exercise program, and also may recommend braces and other protective devices to help prevent fractures.

Tai Chi. These gentle movements are especially appropriate for patients with weakened bones. Some types of dance therapy may have similar benefits.

Self-Treatment

Avoid prolonged bed rest, which will accelerate bone loss and resorption. If your doctor prescribes high-dose aspirin or stronger NSAIDs, make sure that you take the pills with food to minimize stomach upset.

Other Causes of Bone Symptoms

Osteoporosis produces bone changes and pain similar to some aspects of Paget's disease.

Pain Syndromes

(Chronic pain syndrome; somatoform pain disorder)

Chronic pain syndrome is usually defined as pain that lasts longer than six months and does not respond to standard therapies such as surgery, medication, and bed rest. It has been estimated that more than 55 million Americans suffer from chronic pain, and it is the most common reason for lost workdays in the United States as well as a major cause for litigation and disability payments.

Although cancer and numerous other diseases can produce unrelenting pain, chronic pain syndrome has no identifiable physical cause. The average patient is said to have suffered pain symptoms for as long as seven years, undergoing exploratory tests over and over again in a futile search for the source. Pain may have originated with a minor injury or surgical procedure, but it continues long after the condition has healed.

Chronic back pain is one of the most common examples of a pain syndrome. It was a rare diagnosis before World War II, but now the United States leads the world in people who are disabled by lower back pain.

There is increasing evidence that chronic pain is linked to the psychological mechanism called somatization in which bodily complaints are used to express emotional states. Dr. Kathleen Foley, director of the pain service at New York's Memorial Sloan-Kettering Cancer Center, says that chronic pain

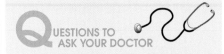

"may be a metaphor for anxiety or depression or spiritual discomfort," rather than actual physical pain.

Regardless of whether or not an organic cause can be found, chronic pain can affect every aspect of an individual's life, impairing ability to work, socialize, and sleep. Feelings of hopelessness and helplessness stemming from the condition lead to depression and isolation. Family members eventually bear a special burden and may unwittingly contribute to the problem by submitting to constant demands for sympathy and special consideration at the expense of the well-being of others.

Diagnostic Studies and Procedures

A complaint of chronic pain was once likely to result in a battery of costly, high-tech tests, and perhaps even exploratory surgery. Now, if a physical examination, blood and urine tests, and perhaps X-rays fail to turn up an organic disorder, additional testing may be considered futile. Instead, the patient will be referred to a clinic or center that specializes in chronic pain.

There, the person will undergo a comprehensive evaluation by a team made up of a physiatrist (a specialist in rehabilitation medicine), psychiatrist, neurologist, and orthopedist.

Medical Treatments

Treatment often begins with weaning patients off such addictive narcotic painkillers as codeine, oxycodone (Percodan, Percocet, and others) or hydromorphone (Dilaudid). This is usually done on an inpatient basis in a hospital or clinic, because close monitoring is necessary during withdrawal. Throughout this period, which lasts two to three weeks, nonaddictive painkillers and an antidepressant may be given. The major focus, however, is instruction in pain management techniques tailored to specific needs.

Even in the absence of painkiller addiction, hospitalization may be considered essential for physical and psychological evaluation and behavior modification. Family counseling is often an important part of the process to help those close to the patient refrain from rewarding chronic pain behavior rather than helping to change it.

Treatment may continue on an outpatient basis, during which a person typically spends two to six hours a week at the pain clinic. Some people master the coping skills within three weeks; others may take up to six months. In both hospital and outpatient programs, the emphasis is on a multidisciplinary approach that includes standard and alternative therapies to enable patients to regain control of their lives.

Many pain clinics employ TENS, or transcutaneous electrical nerve stimulation, illustrated here to treat shoulder and knee pain. The devices work by using low pulses of electrical current to interrupt pain signals before they reach the spinal cord and brain.

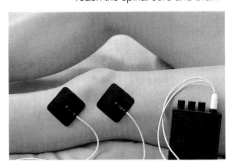

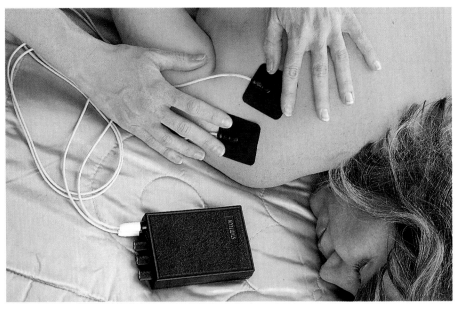

Alternative Therapies

Most of the therapies described below have been incorporated into the comprehensive programs of pain treatment centers, and they are considered alternative only in the sense that they represent a substitute for medication. The most effective approaches provide the individual with self-regulating methods for reducing pain.

Acupuncture and Acupressure. Some people have experienced pain abatement following five or six sessions with a trained acupuncturist. Back and neck pain, headaches, and nerve pain appear especially amenable to such treatment. The patient may then be taught acupressure, in which specific points are pressed to alleviate pain.

Biofeedback and Relaxation Training. Biofeedback training teaches individuals how to manipulate involuntary body processes, such as heart rate and brain-wave patterns. It is possible for a person to learn how to control almost any measurable physiological function when she is fed certain information while hooked up to biofeedback equipment. With a few training sessions, most people produce alpha waves—the brain electrical patterns generally associated with a relaxed and alert frame of mind—at will. This is accomplished by connecting electrodes to the patient and then to an electroencephalograph, which transmits the brain-wave patterns into an oscilloscope so that they can be seen on a screen. A musical tone sounds whenever alpha waves appear on the screen; the patient maintains this tone by concentrating on the images that produce these waves.

Having mastered this skill, a patient is hooked up to various measuring instruments when pain sensations occur. At the same time, measurements of skin temperature, muscle tension, and heartbeat are made visible. The therapist then instructs the patient in deep breathing exercises and encourages her to think calm and pleasant thoughts. Feedback information is accompanied by sounds of changing intensity, indicating changes in heartbeat, muscle tension, and skin temperature, with an accompanying decrease in the sensation of pain.

Chiropractic. Spinal manipulation often alleviates chronic back and neck pain. Treatments may also include the use of electrical stimulation and heat.

Electrical Stimulation. Pulses of low-voltage current may be used to short-circuit pain messages (see illustration on facing page).

Guided Imagery or Visualization. With the guidance of a psychologist or other mental health professional, patients learn how to relax completely and imagine themselves totally free of pain. By concentrating on agreeable images of serenity and natural beauty, a form of self-hypnosis takes place, which can eventually be induced at will as a way of controlling pain.

Hypnosis. During hypnosis, a patient is instructed to focus total concentration on specific suggestions put forth by the hypnotist. Because the sensation of pain is processed in the brain, the hypnotist tries to induce a hypnotic state that will enable the patient to transform that sensation into one of numbness or a slight tingling.

Massage. Pain produces tension in muscles, which in turn intensifies pain. This cycle can be broken by different types of massage and manipulation techniques. An accredited physical therapist is usually trained in these hands-on skills.

Music Therapy. Studies have shown that listening to certains types of music increases the production of endorphins, the body's natural painkillers. Researchers at New York's Rusk Institute of Rehabilitation Medicine have found that patients with arthritis and other painful conditions can reduce their medication dosage with music.

Yoga and T'ai Chi. These classic therapies combine movement and meditation, which results in a renewed sense of calm and well-being.

Self-Treatment

Once mastered, meditation, imagery, biofeedback, and other alternative therapies can be used at home or at work as the need arises. Distraction can also have an analgesic effect. People who suffer chronic pain often find that it seems to disappear when they watch an engrossing movie, lose themselves in a good book, or become immersed in their work or a hobby.

Other Causes of Chronic Pain

Chronic pain may be an aspect of anxiety, depression, hypochondria, or hysteria, or it may originate in a number of physical injuries and disorders, especially arthritis, bursitis, tendinitis, and other inflammatory conditions.

A CASE IN POINT

At the age of 72, Edward Weiss felt his life was becoming increasingly dominated by chronic back pain due to spinal stenosis. Three back operations had failed to solve the problem, but he was determined to remain as active as possible, enjoying his grandchildren, gardening, traveling with his wife of 50 years, and playing an occasional round of golf. Weiss's orthopedist referred him to a pain clinic that offered a range of treatments—everything from acupuncture to physical therapy.

After a careful evaluation, the clinic staff outlined a back rehabilitation program for Weiss. "We can't cure your stenosis," one of the therapists said, "but we can teach you how to live more comfortably with it."

Weiss was scheduled for a series of six weekly acupuncture treatments to see if they might alleviate his back pain. He was evaluated by an Alexander technique instructor who proposed a number of changes: sleeping on his side with a pillow tucked between his knees and another snuggled to his chest, and assuming more relaxed sitting and standing postures to ease back strain. She visited his home to check out his favorite chair and desk, then suggested he invest in ergonomic replacements designed for his height and back problem. After watching him work in his garden, she recommended a kneeling stool to make it easier for him to get up and down. Finally, she urged him to trade in his present car for one with seats that could be adjusted for his back.

The physical therapist designed an exercise routine that emphasized stretching and motions to promote back flexibility. He also advised Weiss to switch from a stationary exercise cycle to a cross-country ski machine.

There were no overnight miracles, but after several months of following new routines, Weiss began to notice improvement. "I know my back will never be pain-free," he says, "but now I feel that I can live with it."

Nerve disorders, such as carpal tunnel syndrome, diabetic neuropathy, postpolio syndrome, post-shingles neuropathy, and Bell's palsy, can also produce chronic pain.

Painful Intercourse

(Dyspareunia)

Painful intercourse, known medically as dyspareunia, is discomfort or pain that accompanies sexual intercourse. Depending on the cause, the pain may be mild or acute; in some cases, it makes sexual intercourse impossible.

For most women, the first experience with sex is uncomfortable, usually due to the tearing of the hymen, perhaps coupled with insufficient vaginal lubrication. After a period of adjustment, according to Dr. Helen Singer Kaplan, director of the Human Sexuality Program at New York Hospital-Cornell University Medical Center, it is abnormal for intercourse to hurt. Dr. Kaplan has found that in about half of her patients who experience painful intercourse, the cause is physical; for the rest, emotional factors or both physical and psychological problems are responsible.

Physical causes of persistent pain during intercourse include genital herpes, vaginitis, pelvic inflammatory disease, endometriosis, a displaced or tipped uterus, thinning of the vaginal tissues following menopause or during breast-feeding, and an allergic response to contraceptives. The problem can also be the result of a poorly sewn episiotomy or scarring from a childbirth injury.

Among the causative emotional factors are anger, fear of pregnancy, and guilt. Childhood sexual abuse or a punitive upbringing in regard to sexual matters may be involved. Also, women who have been raped sometimes develop dyspareunia. When troubled feelings have been deeply repressed, they may lead to vaginismus; these are involuntary contractions or spasms of the vaginal muscles that make penetration impossible.

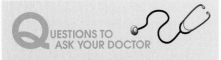

QUESTIONS TO ASK YOUR DOCTOR

▶ Can you recommend any home exercises that I can do to overcome my fear (or distaste) of sexual intimacy?
▶ If I undergo sex therapy, should my partner also participate?
▶ How do estrogen vaginal creams compare with estrogen replacement therapy?

Diagnostic Studies and Procedures

Any continuing discomfort or pain during or after intercourse warrants investigation by a gynecologist, who will ask numerous questions about sexual practices, contraception, pregnancies, and other factors that may contribute to the problem. The questioning will be followed by a pelvic examination, pap smear, and blood and urine studies.

Medical Treatments

Should diagnosis reveal pelvic inflammatory disease or some other bacterial infection, antibiotics will be prescribed. Genital warts will be treated chemically or removed with laser surgery, freezing, or an electric needle. An antiviral drug may be given to help ease the pain from genital herpes. Yeast infections will be treated with antifungal creams or suppositories.

Postmenopausal women may benefit from hormone replacement therapy in the form of an estrogen vaginal cream, pills, or medicated patch to combat vaginal thinning and dryness.

Surgical Treatments. Conditions such as endometriosis, a prolapsed uterus, or postpartum scarring may require surgical correction if more conservative measures fail to help.

Alternative Therapies

Sex Therapy. Since the late 1960s, sex therapy clinics have been helping women and their partners overcome a broad range of sexual problems, including painful intercourse. Most major medical centers and teaching hospitals now have such clinics, usually as part of psychiatric and mental health services. Sex therapy is also offered by some physicians, marriage counselors, and psychologists. A word of caution, however: Anyone can set up practice as a sex therapist, because there are no state licensing or accreditation requirements for doing so. Before embarking on sex therapy, ask about the therapist's training and qualifications and steer clear of anyone who advocates using surrogate sexual partners.

Self-Treatment

Vaginal dryness can be countered by using a lubricating cream or jelly, and by extending the time devoted to foreplay to help increase vaginal secretions.

In some cases, painful intercourse may be due to inexperience or poor positioning, especially if the male is much larger than the female. It might help to experiment with some different

Evelyn Marks felt that her menopause had been easy except for one troubling aspect: Persistent vaginal dryness made intercourse—something she had always enjoyed—painful.

"I tried various lubricants," she confided. "They helped some, but didn't solve the problem. More and more, I found myself avoiding sex. My husband was understanding, but neither of us was ready to close the books on that part of our lives."

Marks found it difficult to discuss such intimate details with her doctor, and was relieved when her gynecologist broached the subject during her annual checkup. Marks described the pain caused by intercourse and added that none of the remedies she tried had been very effective. "I know that estrogen replacement works, but I'm afraid of getting cancer," she added.

The doctor explained that an estrogen vaginal cream might solve her problem. "But you should also know that we have new ways of giving postmenopausal hormone replacement that reduce the risk of cancer." He went on to describe the added benefits—reduced risk of osteoporosis and heart attacks and perhaps protection against Alzheimer's disease. "Of course, there are some women who should not take hormones, but you don't fall into any of the high-risk categories."

He gave her literature describing the pros and cons of hormone therapy, and said to call him after she had assessed the facts for herself. In the end, Marks decided that the benefits outweighed the risks. Just two months after starting the hormone therapy, she was once again enjoying pleasurable, pain-free lovemaking.

positions that will allow the woman to control the depth of penile thrusts.

Vaginismus may be treated by using vaginal dilators, which are inserted into the vagina over a period of weeks, starting with a pencil-thin tube and gradually progressing to larger ones.

Other Causes of Painful Intercourse

Disorders affecting organs near the female genitals sometimes result in painful intercourse. Examples include cystitis, hemorrhoids, and genitourinary fistulas.

Pancreatic Cancer

(Exocrine cancer)

The pancreas is an oblong, pear-shaped organ, about six inches long, that lies within a loop of the small intestine behind the stomach. The exocrine portion of the pancreas, the tissue in which digestive juices and enzymes are produced, is the site of 95 percent of all pancreatic cancers. These cancers typically originate in the ductal cells in the head of the pancreas.

After decades of steadily increasing, the incidence of pancreatic cancer is dropping somewhat, with about 24,000 new cases a year. The higher death toll of 27,000 a year reflects the incidence of the recent past. Men, especially African-Americans, are the most common victims of the disease, although there has been a recent slight rise in cases among African-American women.

The cause is unknown, but smoking has been strongly implicated as a factor because the occurrence among smokers is more than double that of nonsmokers. A high-meat, high-fat diet also has been linked to increased risk of pancreatic cancer, and so has working with dry cleaning agents, benzene, and certain other chemicals.

At one time, chronic pancreatitis, diabetes, and cirrhosis of the liver were considered risk factors, but recent data has rendered these relationships invalid. However, the sudden onset of diabetes in an individual who is not overweight and has no family history of the disease suggests the possibility of pancreatic cancer.

The disease has been called a silent cancer because it develops very slowly and does not produce symptoms in its early stages. As the tumor grows, it often blocks the bile duct, resulting in

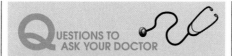
itchiness and jaundice, a yellowing of the skin and the whites of the eyes. Nausea, pain in the middle of the abdomen, lack of appetite, unexplained weight loss, indigestion, and fatty stools (steatorrhea) are other symptoms of pancreatic cancer.

Diagnostic Studies and Procedures

Unfortunately, because there are no effective screening tests, very few pancreatic tumors are being diagnosed in an early, treatable stage. This may change if the current search for a chemical marker for the cancer yields a screening blood test.

Ultrasound or CT scans may be ordered, but normal findings do not necessarily rule out a pancreatic tumor, which may not show up on imaging studies. If a doctor suspects pancreatic cancer, an ERCP, or endoscopic retrograde cholangiopancreatogram, may be performed. For this test, a flexible tube is inserted into the throat and passed through the stomach and small intestine. Dye is then injected into the drainage duct of the pancreas to make its structure show up on X-ray film. During this procedure, samples of pancreatic juice can be obtained and studied for the presence of cancer cells. In some cases, however, a definitive diagnosis of cancer will require laparoscopy. This

surgical procedure involves the use of a viewing instrument that is inserted through an incision near the navel, allowing a doctor to examine the pancreas and take multiple biopsy samples.

Medical Treatments

If the cancer is confined to the head of the pancreas, surgical removal of this portion can sometimes cure the disease. But, according to statistics of the American Cancer Society, only 3 percent of patients survive five or more years after such treatment.

In addition to surgery, chemotherapy and radiation treatments may be employed. New ways of delivering radiation are under study. In one experimental approach, pellets of iridium are implanted temporarily in the pancreas to deliver large doses of radiation directly into the tumor. Administering high-dose radiation at the time of surgery is another experimental technique currently in use.

Palliative surgery—a procedure performed to alleviate symptoms even if a cure is unlikely—may be recommended to relieve obstruction and other complications of advanced cancer.

Alternative Therapies

The use of alternative therapies is generally limited to managing pain and other symptoms. Self-hypnosis, biofeedback, meditation, and visualization may be helpful. Hydrotherapy in the form of contrast baths may be beneficial as well. It consists of 5 to 10 minutes in a hot bath followed by a cold shower for two to five minutes, which may relieve the itchiness that often accompanies chronic jaundice.

Self-Treatment

Because pancreatic cancer often causes severe digestive problems, especially of fats, it's wise to keep a food diary to identify those foods that seem to provoke special problems.

Many patients with advanced cancer and their family members find comfort from joining a support group. Information about such groups can be obtained from a hospital social service office or from the local chapter of the American Cancer Society.

Other Causes of Pancreatic Symptoms

Chronic pancreatitis can cause pain and symptoms similar to those of pancreatic cancer, as can gallbladder disease, an obstructed bile duct, or a liver disorder.

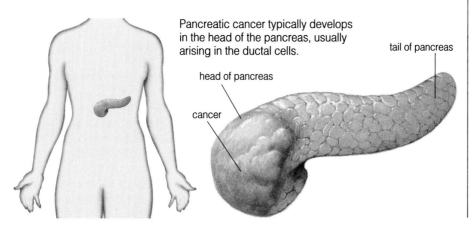

Pancreatic cancer typically develops in the head of the pancreas, usually arising in the ductal cells.

tail of pancreas

head of pancreas

cancer

Pancreatitis

When the pancreas, a digestive organ situated behind the stomach, becomes inflamed, the condition is referred to as pancreatitis. The inflammation may be acute or chronic, and is thought to result from an abnormal activation of certain digestive enzymes produced by the pancreas. Instead of waiting until they reach the small intestine to begin their digestive functions, the enzymes start working in the pancreas itself, leading to swelling, bleeding, inflammation, and sometimes tissue death.

Researchers have identified a number of factors that may trigger the process: alcoholism, gallstones, elevated blood lipids, excessive production of parathyroid hormones, hepatitis and various other viral infections, an adverse drug reaction, and injury to the pancreas, such as from surgery and invasive diagnostic procedures.

An acute attack produces an upper abdominal pain that bores from front to back and often radiates to the chest, flanks, and lower abdomen. The pain intensifies with coughing, deep breathing, and lying supine, and may be alleviated by sitting with the knees drawn up. Other symptoms include nausea, vomiting, abdominal swelling, a rapid heartbeat, low blood pressure, and perhaps shock. Acute hemorrhagic pancreatitis may result in vomiting of blood.

Recurrent attacks of pancreatitis can evolve into a chronic condition marked by abdominal pain, digestive problems, possible nutritional deficiencies, weight loss, diarrhea, and passage of bulky, foul-smelling, fatty stools. Diabetes develops if the islet cells within the pancreas cease to produce insulin.

Diagnostic Studies and Procedures

Various blood tests will be ordered. Elevated blood levels of the digestive enzyme amylase or lipase confirm acute pancreatitis. In chronic pancreatitis, the level of these enzymes might be normal, but there may be other abnormalities, such as elevated blood glucose levels.

X-rays or a CT scan may show areas of calcification, a sign of chronic pancreatitis, or enlargement typical of an acute attack. Endoscopy, an examination using a lighted viewing device inserted through the throat into the stomach and small intestine, may be ordered to determine if gallstones might have triggered the condition.

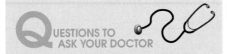

QUESTIONS TO ASK YOUR DOCTOR

► Could any of my medications be responsible for an attack of pancreatitis?
► If alcohol was not a factor in my case, is it still necessary to abstain from even an occasional drink?

Medical Treatments

Acute pancreatitis is a life-threatening emergency that demands immediate hospitalization for intensive care. The goal is to rest the pancreas and allow it to heal itself. The patient is put on a strict fasting regimen in which neither food nor fluids are taken by mouth. Fluids are given intravenously until the inflammation subsides, which usually takes three to seven days, then a clear liquid diet is started; a normal diet can be resumed usually two or three days later. Painkillers are administered as needed and antibiotics are added to the regimen if there is a bacterial infection.

In some cases, a suction tube is inserted through the nose and into the stomach to remove stomach acids, a procedure called nasogastric suction. Severe, unremitting pancreatitis may be treated with washing, or lavage, of the peritoneal cavity to remove damaging secretions from the pancreas. If an obstructive gallstone is responsible for the attack, it can be removed by endoscopy (see Ulcers, page 426).

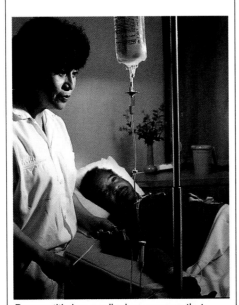

Pancreatitis is a medical emergency that calls for immediate hospitalization and administration of intravenous fluids.

In many cases, chronic pancreatitis can be controlled by diet, as described below, plus painkillers, and large replacement doses of pancreatic enzymes, which are taken with meals. If pancreatic ducts become obstructed, or if a cyst or abscess is present, surgery may be performed to remove the obstruction, cyst, or abscess.

Alternative Therapies

Because alcohol abuse is frequently a contributing factor in both acute and chronic pancreatitis, medical and alternative therapies are directed to helping patients overcome any drinking problem. Acupuncture, self-hypnosis, and meditation may be helpful, not only in abstaining from alcohol but also in alleviating the pain of the disease.

Nutrition Therapy. A clinical dietitian should be consulted to devise a low-fat, nutritionally balanced diet. Small, frequent meals may be advisable to prevent overworking the pancreas. Vitamin and mineral supplements may be needed also to correct any nutritional deficiencies in the diet.

Some naturopathic nutritionists recommend taking pancreatin, a preparation of enzymes made from pig pancreases and other natural enzymes, such as bromelain from pineapples and papain from papayas. You should consult a doctor before taking any enzyme preparations, to make sure that they do not interact with the body's own pancreatic enzymes.

Self-Treatment

As noted earlier, abstaining from alcohol is critical. Joining Alcoholics Anonymous or a similar self-help program can prove life saving. Otherwise, self-care is directed to preventing an acute attack or controlling a chronic condition. Taking sodium bicarbonate and prescribed pancreatic enzymes with meals may alleviate digestive problems. However, antacids that contain calcium carbonate or magnesium hydroxide should be avoided because they may worsen diarrhea.

Other Causes of Pancreatic Symptoms

Disorders that can produce symptoms similar to those of pancreatitis include a perforated ulcer, peritonitis, gallbladder disease, intestinal obstruction, and a dissecting aortic aneurysm. Some inflammatory diseases, such as lupus or inflammation of the aorta, can also mimic pancreatitis.

Paranoia/ Delusional Disorders

(Paranoid personality disorder)
Paranoia is characterized by a pervasive distrust of others. In the past, it has been classified as a manifestation of a relatively rare class of mental illnesses, known as delusional disorders (see box, right), but many psychiatrists

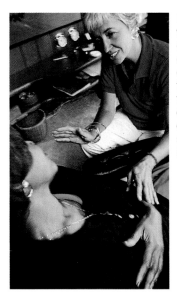

If a person with a delusional disorder can learn to trust a therapist, one-on-one counseling may be helpful.

now regard it as a distinctly separate condition. Regardless of classification, a paranoid personality is beset with delusions that make it impossible to form normal relationships with others.

The cause of paranoia and other delusions is unknown. Their manifestations generally appear in adulthood, but psychiatrists believe they originate in childhood. Mental health professionals theorize that symptoms develop when patients start to attribute their own failings and suppressed negative feelings to outside forces. Thus, a person who is unable to hold a job may become convinced that a neighbor, government agency, or even a space alien is plotting against him rather than face his own shortcomings. This type of thinking also serves as a way to protect an individual from recognizing and dealing with unacceptable impulses.

Diagnostic Studies and Procedures
To determine that delusional or paranoid thinking is not the result of a medical illness, a complete physical

examination will be conducted, and standard mental function tests may be given as well. The American Psychiatric Association lists the following diagnostic criteria for delusional disorders:
► The delusion persists for more than one month and involves a situation that might occur in real life, such as being poisoned, stalked, or secretly loved.
► Aside from the delusion and its ramifications, the person's behavior is not obviously strange.
► There is no identifiable organic basis for the delusions.
To be diagnosed as paranoid, a person:
► Harbors irrational and unwarranted suspicions that others are trying to harm or deceive him.
► Is reluctant to confide in others.
► Bears persistent grudges.
► Mistakenly reads hidden threats into benign remarks.
► Is convinced that a sexual partner is being unfaithful.

Medical Treatments
Once a diagnosis has been established, a doctor then tries to determine if the patient has violent intentions. In making this evaluation, she must decide if hospitalization is advisable and, should the patient refuse to go voluntarily, whether or not legal commitment should be sought.

An antipsychotic drug, usually haloperidol (Haldol), may be prescribed in gradually increasing doses for six weeks. If there is no obvious improvement, another antipsychotic drug may be tried. Patients who respond to such medications usually can maintain their improvement with a long-term, low-dose therapy.

Psychotherapy is successful only when the patient sees the doctor as a helper rather than a foe, a trust that is especially difficult to establish with a paranoid person. Individual, or one-to-one therapy, appears to be more successful at achieving this relationship than group sessions.

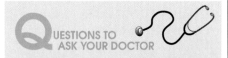

QUESTIONS TO ASK YOUR DOCTOR

► Is hospital treatment advisable? If so, how long will I be hospitalized?
► Could my feelings be caused by a medication or other chemical substance? Will they disappear if I stop taking it?

TYPES OF DELUSIONAL DISORDERS

Type	Characteristics
Erotic	Delusion of being loved, usually by a person of higher status.
Grandiose	Greatly inflated view of ability and self-worth.
Jealousy	Delusion that one's sexual partner is unfaithful.
Persecution	Paranoid delusion of malevolent treatment by others.
Somatic	Conviction that one has a dreaded disease despite lack of medical evidence.
Unspecific	Combination of delusions without a dominant theme.

Other family members may become involved in therapy, but not until the patient knows that the only objective is to help. When psychotherapy works, the patient learns to seek situations that strengthen self-esteem and to avoid those that may reinforce his delusions.

Alternative Therapies
Drama or Dance Therapy. These techniques may be employed to provide the therapist with a deeper insight into the personality problem.
Meditation. Delusions originating from a stressful situation may be alleviated by meditation, visualization, or other relaxation therapies.
Pet Therapy. A paranoid person may be able to establish a trusting relationship with a dog, cat, or other animal, paving the way for human interaction.

Self-Treatment
People who harbor delusions or are paranoid almost always need professional help. Once healing has begun, self-help strategies should be directed to finding enjoyable avenues of expression. For example, a person with past delusions of grandeur may benefit from joining an amateur theater group that provides an outlet for grandiose ideas.

Other Causes of Delusions
Delusions and paranoia may be associated with alcoholism and other addictions, adrenal or thyroid disorders, Alzheimer's disease, brain tumors, stroke, Parkinson's disease, and schizophrenia, depression, and other psychiatric disorders. Some medications and severe nutritional deficiencies can cause delusions.

Parkinson's Disease

(Parkinsonism; paralysis agitans)

Parkinson's disease, also called parkinsonism and paralysis agitans, is a brain disorder that causes progressive muscle stiffening, a rhythmic tremor, and an unstable gait. The disorder has no obvious cause and no known cure. About 1 million Americans have varying degrees of it, with onset typically occurring between ages 50 and 65.

The brain changes that lead to parkinsonism are not fully understood, but it appears that they involve the nerve cells containing melanin, the pigment that gives skin its color. These cells, called substantia nigra, are concentrated in a part of the brain called the basal ganglia. As the cells deteriorate, production of dopamine—a chemical that carries messages within the brain—falls, and the result is the characteristic symptoms.

Initially, a patient may notice a slight tremor of one hand or leg and a slowing or stiffening of muscle movement. Even before tremor becomes apparent, the person may develop a frozen facial expression and slow speech. As the disease progresses, tremor becomes more pronounced and movement more rigid and feeble, and the person walks with a stooped, shuffling gait of short, rapid steps. About one-third of patients eventually suffer mental decline.

Diagnostic Studies and Procedures

A doctor performs a careful neurological examination, looking for the disease's characteristic tremor, shuffling gait, and precarious balance. Reflexes and muscle strength are tested, as is mental function. Blood tests and a CT scan or MRI will be ordered.

Medical Treatments

Patients with mild parkinsonism may not require medication, but as tremors become more pronounced, anticholinergic drugs, thought to reestablish a normal balance of brain chemicals, may be prescribed. These are given in very low doses to minimize side effects such

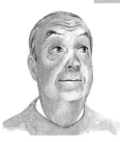

These exercises are designed to help retain facial mobility. Start by raising your eyebrows and wrinkling your forehead.

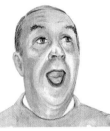

Open your mouth as widely as you can. At the same time, try to raise your eyebrows.

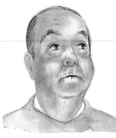

Close your mouth tightly and puff out your cheeks as much as possible. Release the air, and then wiggle your nose.

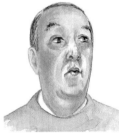

Pucker your lips and try to whistle. Repeat each exercise 10 times at least once a day.

as dry mouth and constipation. Or beta blockers such as propranolol (Inderal) may be prescribed to reduce tremor.

As the disease progresses, other drugs are needed to increase levels of dopamine. Dopamine itself cannot be given, but amantadine (Symmetrel) prompts the release of stored dopamine. And levodopa (Dopar and Larodopa) is converted to dopamine by the body.

Unfortunately, the effectiveness of levodopa eventually wanes, and high doses may produce intolerable side effects, including nausea and cardiac arrhythmia. Giving levodopa along with carbidopa (Sinemet) or selegiline (Eldepryl) allows a lower dosage. Sustained-release carbidopa (Sinemet CR) also reduces side effects of levodopa. Benztropine (Cogentin), bromocriptine (Parlodel), and pergolide (Permax) may be used to supplement levodopa.

There has been renewed interest in the operation called pallidotomy, which entails destruction of small areas of the

brain. First developed in the 1940s, it fell out of favor with the introduction of levodopa. Refined neurosurgical techniques and accounts of remarkable improvement in some patients have led to its resurgence. Unfortunately, some patients quickly regress and others are left worse off because of brain hemorrhages or excessive tissue destruction.

A promising experimental treatment involves implanting fetal brain cells into the adult brain. Because this procedure requires fetal tissue obtained from elective abortions, it remains controversial in the United States.

Alternative Therapies

Alternative therapies play a role in increasing effectiveness of medication and delaying more disabling symptoms.

Meditation. Stress exacerbates parkinsonism; meditation and other relaxation therapies can help reduce it. Combining meditation with yoga or t'ai chi may also improve muscle tone and control. Meditation can be helpful too in inducing sleep, if insomnia is a problem. The focused concentration of self-hypnosis temporarily enables persons with parkinsonism to perform tasks that require fine coordination.

Nutrition Therapy. There have been some reports that a reduced intake of protein may be beneficial. Certainly, a high-fiber diet can help prevent constipation, a common side effect of anticholinergic drugs.

Physical and Occupational Therapy. Therapists trained in these disciplines can instruct patients in ways to help retain self-sufficiency. Patients also should be given an individually designed exercise program which they can follow at home on their own.

Self-Treatment

Although parkinsonism is a progressive disease, it is important to realize that most patients live for many years with little or minimal disability. An optimistic mental attitude appears to play an important role, and many patients and their family members find joining a self-help group especially helpful.

Other Causes of Parkinsonism

Parkinsonism may be caused by certain antipsychotic drugs. The chemical MPTP, a contaminant of street heroin, can cause severe parkinsonism when injected intravenously. Boxers sometimes suffer a type of parkinsonism—the punch drunk syndrome—caused by repeated blows to the head.

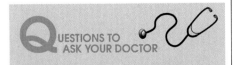

QUESTIONS TO ASK YOUR DOCTOR

▶ How can I best time my medication to reduce nausea and other side effects?
▶ Can you refer me to a physical therapist who will teach me an exercise routine?

Pelvic Inflammatory Disease

(PID; endometritis; myometritis; oophoritis; salpingitis)

Pelvic inflammatory disease, or PID, is an infection of a woman's internal reproductive organs, although doctors generally use more precise terms for specific areas. For example, salpingitis refers to inflammation of the fallopian tubes, oophoritis to the ovaries, endometritis to the endometrium (lining of the uterus), and myometritis to the uterine muscle. Most PID is sexually transmitted, with gonorrhea (page 206) and chlamydia (page 129) as the two most common underlying causes. In the past, intrauterine devices (IUDs) also increased the risk of PID, especially among women with multiple sex partners. However, newer IUDs appear to be much safer in this regard.

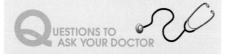

QUESTIONS TO ASK YOUR DOCTOR

► Does one bout of PID make me more vulnerable to subsequent infections? Should I have more frequent gynecologic checkups?
► When can I safely resume sexual relations after treatment for PID?
► When can I attempt a pregnancy?

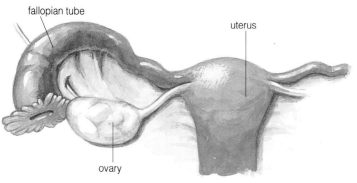

Although PID can attack any of a woman's internal reproductive organs, the fallopian tubes and ovaries are especially vulnerable to permanent damage.

PID has reached epidemic proportions in recent years and public health officials estimate that one in seven American women of reproductive age now has or has had PID. At the current rate of increase, there will be 1 million new cases annually by the year 2,000. Even more worrisome is the fact that only about half of all women with the condition are diagnosed and treated, largely because it is often asymptomatic. Doctors believe that this silent epidemic accounts for a dramatic rise in ectopic, or tubal, pregnancies and infertility. By one estimate, a single episode of PID quadruples a woman's chance of ectopic pregnancy.

Typically, a woman contracts the infecting bacteria during sexual intercourse. When the infection is left untreated, it spreads through her reproductive tract, often causing adhesions and scarring. If the scar tissue blocks a tube, it can prevent conception or keep a fertilized egg from entering the uterus; this last occurrence would result in a tubal pregnancy (page 346).

When symptoms occur, they may be mild or acute depending on the site of the infection and the type of bacteria. A chlamydial infection in the early stages, for example, may cause extensive damage, but produce only a little abnormal discharge and mild backache or pelvic discomfort. In other cases, the woman may have a high fever and severe abdominal pain and tenderness, symptoms that resemble those of appendicitis.

Diagnostic Studies and Procedures

If a doctor suspects PID, she will do a careful pelvic examination to seek the site of infection and order blood and urine tests. Vaginal mucus and secretions will be cultured to identify the specific bacterium.

A pelvic sonogram may also be done to determine whether or not an abscess has formed. In some cases, laparoscopy might be necessary. This procedure, which may be performed in a hospital or a diagnostic clinic, involves inserting a lighted viewing tube into the pelvic cavity through a small incision near the navel.

Medical Treatments

Many specialists believe that any woman who has PID should be hospitalized, while others feel that this is necessary only when there is a high fever, severe abdominal pain, and other acute symptoms. In any event, intensive antibiotic treatment is necessary. If there is no significant improvement within 48 hours, hospitalization for administration of intravenous antibiotics is recommended. Abscess drainage also requires hospitalization.

A woman who undergoes outpatient treatment needs rest. After two weeks, she will be reevaluated to decide when normal activities can be resumed. In the meantime, the woman's sexual partner should be examined and treated if he is found to harbor chlamydia, gonorrhea, or another disease that can be transmitted sexually.

In severe cases that do not respond to drug treatment, surgery may be necessary. This approach may include a hysterectomy, which will end the woman's ability to have a baby.

Alternative Therapies

There is no effective alternative to antibiotics for treating PID, although meditation, visualization, and breathing exercises may help control pain during the process of recovery.

Self-Treatment

A woman with PID should abstain from sexual intercourse during convalescence and until she is sure that her sexual partner is free of disease. Use of a condom is advisable, even if other methods of birth control are being employed. A woman who has had PID should check with her doctor to make sure she has no lingering signs of infection before attempting to conceive.

Otherwise, prevention is the best approach to controlling PID. Any woman who is not in a mutually monogamous sexual relationship should take the same precautions against PID that are recommended to protect against AIDS; namely, always insist on the use of a condom as well as spermicides, which also have an antibacterial effect.

Other Causes of Pelvic Infections

Abortion, miscarriage, and complications resulting from childbirth or pelvic surgery cause a small number of pelvic infections. Also, a ruptured appendix or perforated colon can mimic the symptoms of PID.

fallopian tube

uterus

ovary

331

Phlebitis/Venous Thrombosis

(Acute venous occlusion; superficial thrombophlebitis)

The veins of the leg are vulnerable to two types of blockage caused by clots: phlebitis, in which a superficial vein becomes blocked and inflamed, and acute deep venous thrombosis, in which a clot occludes an inner vein. The latter is the more serious of the two because it can lead to a pulmonary embolism, stroke, or heart attack, if a piece of the clot breaks away and enters the circulation.

The cause of superficial phlebitis is unknown, although it generally develops in older people, often after an injury or prolonged period of inactivity. Varicose veins also increase the likelihood of phlebitis. The symptoms are usually unmistakable: The blocked vein becomes swollen, inflamed, and very painful. There may also be a fever.

In contrast, a deep venous thrombosis often does not produce any obvious symptoms until the person suffers a pulmonary embolism or another life-threatening consequence. Being bedridden for a time is a common precipitating factor because inactivity reduces blood flow in the legs, giving clots a chance to form. Other causes include the use of birth control pills or other products containing estrogen, recent childbirth or miscarriage, paralysis, a clotting disorder, and cancer. Smoking also increases the risk of deep venous thrombosis.

Diagnostic Studies and Procedures

To diagnose superficial phlebitis, a doctor will look at the area and feel the vein. Doppler ultrasonography, in

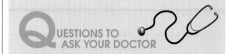

QUESTIONS TO ASK YOUR DOCTOR

▶ What preventive measures can I take against future episodes of phlebitis?
▶ Will support stockings help? If so, should I invest in the more expensive prescription type?

which high-frequency sound waves are used to study blood flow, may be ordered to confirm the diagnosis.

A deep venous thrombosis is more difficult to diagnose, but Doppler ultrasound and venography, special X-rays taken following the injection of a dye into a vein, can detect most blockages.

Medical Treatments

Treatment depends upon whether the clot is in a superficial or a deep vein. Superficial phlebitis can usually be managed with self-treatment (see below) and an anti-inflammatory drug such as indomethacin (Indocin).

If a deep vein is blocked, one large intravenous dose of heparin, an anti-clotting drug, will be given, followed by periodic injections of smaller doses over several days. In some cases, streptokinase (Streptase and others) or urokinase (Abbokinase), which dissolve blood clots, may be administered also.

As the condition improves, the patient will usually be started on warfarin (Coumadin), an oral anticlotting agent, and tapered off heparin. Depending upon the site of the thrombosis, warfarin will be continued for one to six months, then reduced gradually.

In complicated cases, surgery may be necessary to remove the clot or insert a graft to bypass the occluded vein. Recurrent phlebitis also may be treated surgically by tying off and stripping the affected veins.

Rather than wait for a deep thrombosis to develop, some doctors will advocate preventive measures, such as long-term

or even life-long anticoagulant therapy, for their high-risk patients.

Another preventive strategy calls for a low dose of heparin to be administered prior to any operation and continued for several days afterwards. Bedridden patients should also wear special elastic surgical stockings.

High-risk patients, such as those who have developed a pulmonary embolism despite anticoagulant therapy, may have an umbrella-like device implanted in the lower vena cava—the large vein that carries blood from the lower extremities back to the heart—in order to prevent the passage of clots.

Alternative Therapies

Physical Therapy. A physical therapist might be engaged to make sure that an immobilized patient moves his legs periodically. Passive exercises, in which a therapist exercises the patient's limbs, are used for persons who are unable to move on their own. The patient is encouraged to move about as soon as possible, at first simply by moving the legs in bed, then sitting up with legs dangling over the edge, and finally, by walking around.

Self-Treatment

Superficial phlebitis usually can be self-treated as follows:

▶ Keep the affected leg elevated a few feet above the floor when possible.
▶ Apply warm wet compresses to the area several times a day.
▶ Wear surgical or prescription elastic stockings to promote blood flow.
▶ If your doctor approves, take aspirin, ibuprofen, or other nonsteroidal anti-inflammatory medication.

To prevent future attacks, exercise every day to promote leg circulation. A brisk walk is ideal, but if this is not feasible, try an exercise cycle or low-impact aerobics. During long trips and long hours seated at work, stretch your legs every hour. Also ask your doctor about long-term use of surgical stockings and low-dose aspirin therapy.

Anyone who suffers from phlebitis should refrain from smoking, and women with this or other clotting problems should not take oral contraceptives or estrogen replacement therapy.

Other Causes of Phlebitis Symptoms

Bacterial cellulitis, inflammation and infection of the connective tissue, can produce symptoms similar to those of phlebitis, as can lymphangitis, an inflammation of the lymph channels.

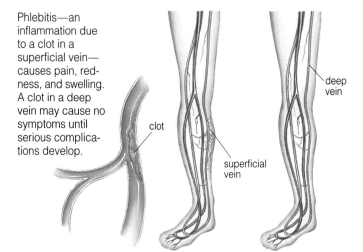

Phlebitis—an inflammation due to a clot in a superficial vein—causes pain, redness, and swelling. A clot in a deep vein may cause no symptoms until serious complications develop.

clot

deep vein

superficial vein

Pica

Pica is the abnormal desire to eat such inedible substances as clay, plaster, dirt, and paint. This compulsion is most common in children of both sexes between the ages of one and six. Although it gradually diminishes with age, it can sometimes do irreversible damage.

The consequences of pica are well known, especially among economically deprived urban children who may eat paint chips from a flaking tenement wall. These chips invariably contain old lead-based paint, and their consumption is our most common cause of childhood lead poisoning. On the other hand, a rural child with pica may eat earth and animal feces, and acquire intestinal parasites such as pinworms.

(Pica should be distinguished from the normal tendency of a toddler to explore and experience the environment orally. Especially between ages one and three, practically everything goes into the mouth, and it takes a vigilant parent to prevent a child from ingesting dangerous or poisonous substances.)

The cause of childhood pica is unknown, but some experts theorize that a neglectful or otherwise inadequate parent-child relationship which results in ungratified oral needs is responsible. In unusual cases, pica may point to a dietary lack of a specific nutrient such as iron.

Pica is rarely seen in adults, except in individuals who are mentally retarded. People who are severely deficient in iron and zinc commonly resort to eating large amounts of ice, but this behavior, as well as the pica that sometimes develops in persons suffering from schizophrenia, autism, and other severe mental disorders, is viewed as a manifestation of an underlying illness rather than a true eating disorder.

Diagnostic Studies and Procedures

Pica may come to the attention of a doctor or other health professional because a family member or some other caregiver sees the child repeatedly eating some bizarre substance. A doctor may also uncover the problem after diagnosing lead poisoning or another serious consequence. In other instances, the disorder may go undetected until the child enters nursery school or kindergarten and teachers note that she eats crayons, clay, paste, sand, and other possibly harmful substances.

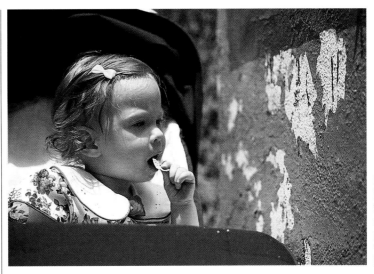

Lead poisoning is a major threat to toddlers who eat paint chips peeling from the walls of older buildings.

A child who has pica will be given a complete physical examination, and blood samples will be obtained for laboratory analysis to measure lead levels as well as to look for iron and other nutritional deficiencies.

Medical Treatments

There is no specific medical treatment for pica. If a dietary deficiency of iron is detected, supplements of the mineral will be prescribed. Lead poisoning resulting from pica is treated with drugs that bind to the metal and promote its excretion in the urine (see page 268).

Alternative Therapies

Nutrition Therapy. Adults who eat inedible substances may benefit from nutrition counseling. This is especially important for pregnant women who eat clay, starch, and soil (see below) because these substances can reduce the body's absorption of nutrients that are needed by both the mother and infant. Nutrition counseling is sometimes combined with psychotherapy in order to explore the underlying causes of the compulsion.

Psychotherapy. When the inadequacy of parental attention and nurturing seem to be contributing to pica, some guidance by a family counselor may prove beneficial. Behavior modification techniques might be employed to help older children or mentally retarded adults overcome persistent pica. Methods that have been successful include giving rewards for resisting the urge to eat a favored inedible substance, sometimes coupled with aversion therapy in which engaging in pica results in a mild electric shock or some other unpleasant consequence.

Self-Treatment

Experts emphasize that the likelihood of pica can be minimized by fulfilling a child's emotional needs through loving care and concern. Providing a balanced, wholesome diet and interesting play materials also helps to counteract abnormal cravings. Another practical preventive measure includes repainting or papering over crumbling surfaces that may contain lead-based paint.

Other Causes of Abnormal Cravings

Pregnant women in the rural South sometimes engage in a type of cultural pica in which they eat clay, soil, or laundry starch. Among African-Americans, this practice is believed to stem from the African folk tradition of eating soil during pregnancy in the belief that it makes childbirth easier. Other women engage in eating soil in the mistaken belief that it adds iron to the diet. (In fact, soil eating actually interferes with the body's ability to utilize iron and other essential nutrients and increases the risk of malnutrition.) These forms of pica, which cease with childbirth, should not be confused with the sometimes eccentric food cravings that occur during pregnancy.

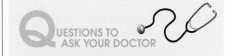

QUESTIONS TO ASK YOUR DOCTOR

▶ What is the best way to discourage a toddler from putting harmful things in his mouth without squelching his normal need to explore and learn?

Pigment Disorders

(Albinism; hyper- and hypopigmentation, melanocytic or pigmented nevi, melasma, moles)

Pigment disorders are discolorations of the epidermis, the outermost layer of the skin, which gets its color from melanin, a chemical produced by a specific type of skin cells called melanocytes. The affected skin may appear bleached—hypopigmented—from insufficient melanin; or it may have become abnormally dark—hyperpigmented—due to excessive melanin.

A lack of melanin may be hereditary; the most extreme example of it is albinism, a genetic disorder in which

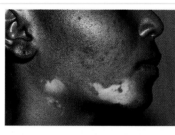
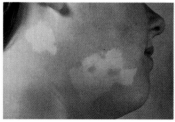

Vitiligo is especially obvious on African-Americans and other dark-skinned people, who are more commonly affected than Caucasians. In these people, dark cosmetics will usually mask the blemish. Small patches of vitiligo on light skin (lower photograph) can be camouflaged by bleaching the surrounding skin.

melanocytes are present but do not produce melanin. People with albinism have white hair, pale skin, and pink eyes that are extraordinarily sensitive to light. They sunburn easily and are very susceptible to skin cancers.

When melanocytes are damaged, areas of hypopigmentation develop, ranging from small patches to large segments that cover most of the body. This condition, known as vitiligo, sometimes affects light-skinned people, but is more prevalent among those who are dark skinned. Between 2 and 5 percent of all African-Americans are affected. (The pop star Michael Jackson is one of the most famous examples.)

More commonly, bleached skin develops at the site of a healed injury such as a cut, burn, abrasion, or infection—a condition called postinflammatory hypopigmentation. Sometimes the opposite occurs and the skin darkens

instead. This tends to happen to black people who have had severe acne.

A temporary loss of pigmentation, pityriasis alba, is a benign disorder in which small, smooth white patches appear, usually on the cheeks and arms. Though not painful, the spots may itch. They commonly occur in children and adolescents, and often come and go for years, generally disappearing entirely between ages 20 and 30.

By far the most common examples of hyperpigmentation are pigmented moles, the vast majority of which are harmless (see box, opposite page). Also, with age, most people develop so-called liver spots, or senile lentigines. These pigmented areas have nothing to do with the liver, but are caused by excessive exposure to sun. They too are generally benign. More serious is the widespread skin darkening that may result from the hormonal changes in Addison's disease (page 68), a life-threatening endocrine disorder.

Another harmless form of pigmentation is melasma gravidarum, or the mask of pregnancy, a manifestation of hormonal changes. Women with melasma develop patches of darkened skin, usually on the forehead, temples, or cheekbones, especially after exposure to sun. The patches generally disappear following childbirth, although the process may take several months.

Diagnostic Studies and Procedures

Abnormalities in pigmentation are readily apparent; a dermatologist can usually determine the condition simply by inspecting affected skin. To confirm a diagnosis, however, skin scrapings may be examined under a microscope.

Finding the underlying cause may require various tests, especially if it involves an organic disorder. Blood tests and hormonal studies will be ordered if Addison's disease or some other hormonal disorder is suspected.

Medical Treatments

Treatments vary according to the underlying problem, and for some, such as albinism, there is no medical treatment other than frequent checkups for skin cancer.

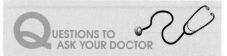
For treatable disorders, the goal is to make the discolorations less noticeable. Vitiligo, for example, may be treated either by repigmentation (restoring of the normal pigment) or depigmentation (destroying the remaining pigment). Neither of these approaches is totally satisfactory, and the degree of success varies from one person to another. Some dermatologists treat senile lentigines cosmetically with Retin A, a cream containing the vitamin A derivative tretinoin, which is said to have antiaging properties.

The most frequently used approach for repigmentation is a combination of drug and light therapy. First, a psoralen drug, the type used to treat psoriasis, is taken internally. This is followed by exposure to ultraviolet light, either by sitting in the sun or under artificial lamps. When this drug is activated by the light, it stimulates repigmentation by increasing the availability of color-producing cells at the skin's surface. Treatment may go on for months, with a rest period usually taken during the winter. Protective sunglasses must be worn during exposure to the sun and throughout the day on which the psoralen drug is taken.

If vitiligo consists only of small, scattered patches, drugs to stimulate pigmentation may be applied directly to the affected skin. These areas are then exposed to sunlight, taking care to avoid overexposure, because the treatment makes a person highly susceptible to severe sunburn and blistering.

Anyone who has vitiligo covering more than half the body is not considered a good candidate for repigmentation. Instead, the person may try depigmentation, aimed at making the patches less noticeable by bleaching the rest of the skin. Bleaching agents such as hydroquinone (Solaquin Forte 4%)

may be prescribed. A sunblock must be used because exposure to ultraviolet rays will cause repigmentation. Allergic reactions to the drug also are common.

Pityriasis alba is usually treated with hydrocortisone creams, which may be applied to the affected patches of skin once or twice a day.

When melasma gravidarum persists after childbirth, the condition may be treated with hydroquinone to decrease the pigmentation, provided there is no allergic reaction when the substance is tested on a small patch of skin. Some doctors may prescribe hydroquinone combined with Retin-A to enhance its effects. These drugs should never be used during pregnancy.

Alternative Therapies

No effective alternative therapies exist for stimulating pigmentation, but there are numerous remedies for hyperpigmented areas, especially those that develop with age.

Herbal Medicine. Aloe vera gel is said to bleach age spots. Many herbalists advocate rubbing them with a fresh piece of aloe, rather than using commercial preparations, which often contain very little aloe vera. An alternative remedy calls for rubbing a spot for a few minutes twice a day with the milky sap from crushed dandelion stems. A paste made of dried comfrey root is also said to bleach pigmented spots. Leave the paste on for 20 minutes, and then rinse off with lemon juice.

Nutrition Therapy. Vitamins A, C, D, and E are believed to help protect the skin from damage and perhaps hyperpigmentation caused by ultraviolet radiation. Use vitamin A supplements with caution; too much can damage the liver. High doses of vitamin A can also cause serious birth defects; supplements and drugs containing vitamin A or its derivatives should not be used during pregnancy and should be stopped at least three months before attempting to conceive a child.

Self-Treatment

Avoiding sunburn is fundamental to self-treatment of most pigment disorders, especially albinism. People with this condition—as well as those with vitiligo—should stay out of the sun as much as possible and always wear protective clothing and use a sunscreen with a sun protection factor of 15 or more on skin that is exposed to sunlight. People with albinism should also wear sunglasses that screen out 100 percent of ultraviolet rays. In fact, many are so sensitive to light that they must wear dark glasses even indoors.

The right combination of cosmetics can be very effective in concealing or deemphasizing affected patches of skin for both hyperpigmentation and hypopigmentation disorders. However, anyone with sensitive skin should use hypoallergenic products to minimize the risk of allergic reactions.

To avoid or reduce post-inflammatory hyperpigmentation from acne, treat the skin gently during eruptions. Avoid picking, harsh scrubbing, and abrasive products unless they are prescribed by a physician. In general, washing with soap and water is sufficient to cleanse skin affected by acne (see page 65).

A word of caution: Most over-the-counter bleaching creams and lotions that are advertised as freckle and spot removers are not effective and may irritate the skin, causing an allergic reaction. Anyone interested in commercial bleaching products, dyes, and stains should consult a dermatologist for the names of suitable products.

Other Causes of Pigment Disorders

In addition to Addison's disease, darkening of the skin may be caused by high-estrogen birth control pills and other hormonal preparations. Light skin spots may be due to tinea versicolor, a fungal infection that starts as small spots scattered over the upper arms, chest, and back. The spots expand slowly and are more noticeable on dark skin where they appear as white to pale tan. On light skin they may not be recognized or may appear as tan to pink spots. This disorder is treated with antifungal creams or pills.

PIGMENTED MOLES AND BIRTHMARKS

These two types of skin blemishes are exceedingly common and, in most instances, are harmless, although some are disfiguring.

Pigmented moles, or melanocytic nevi, develop from a benign proliferation of melanocytes before birth, but most don't become apparent until sometime during childhood or adolescence. (The exception, congenital nevi, are obvious at birth.) Typically, they begin to disappear during middle age and are rare in the elderly.

Moles vary greatly in size and coloration; for example, some are large and hairy, while others are tiny and flat, and still others form in raised wart-like clusters. One type—halo nevi—is surrounded by a patch of vitiligo that eventually eliminates the mole. Normal repigmentation of the skin follows.

Despite a widespread belief that pigmented moles may give rise to malignant melanoma, the most deadly form of skin cancer, this association is relatively rare. Only one uncommon type of mole, the congenital giant hairy pigmented nevi, does carry an increased risk of cancer. Otherwise, about 80 percent of melanomas arise from previously normal skin. Still, moles should be inspected regularly for any suspicious changes, such as accelerated growth, altered color, development of uneven margins, and crusting or bleeding. If such changes do develop, a dermatologist should be consulted. In some cases, the moles will be removed as a preventive measure; in others, a biopsy might be necessary to rule out the possibility of cancer.

Moles that are unsightly or situated in a place where they are easily irritated can be removed either with a scalpel, laser surgery, by freezing (cryosurgery), or burning them off using an electric needle.

Birthmarks, or vascular nevi, are actually benign vascular tumors rather than collections of melanocytes. Superficial birthmarks such as strawberry nevi, purplish dome-shaped growths that appear shortly after birth, usually disappear by age six or seven. In contrast, the flat, deep red or purple nevi known as port-wine stain birthmarks are permanent. Large ones, especially on the face, can be quite disfiguring, but special cosmetics make it possible to camouflage them. Also, many now can be removed with laser surgery (see photos at right).

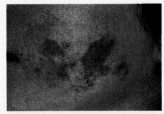

Before treatment, this extensive port-wine birthmark was prominent and disfiguring.

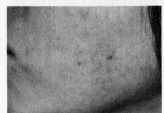

Now, most discoloration has been removed by laser surgery; the remainder can be hidden by cosmetics.

Pityriasis Rosea

Pityriasis rosea is a common, relatively short-lived skin disorder exhibiting a scaly rash of symmetrical pink patches. The underlying cause is unknown, but an unidentified virus is believed to be the culprit. Even so, it is not contagious.

Pityriasis typically occurs during the spring and autumn months and affects mostly adolescents or young adults. It begins with a large pink spot—called a herald or mother patch—on the chest or back. (This initial patch is often mistaken for ringworm or an insect bite.) Within a week or two, other, smaller pink spots appear over the trunk, upper arms, and legs. The spots may also occur on the neck, but they rarely spread to the face. The rash on the trunk sometimes resembles an evergreen tree with drooping branches. On individuals who are suntanned, the rash may be confined to unexposed areas of the body, such as the breasts, armpits, buttocks, and pubic area.

Racial differences among pityriasis patients have been noted. In African-Americans, for example, the rash often covers the lower arms and legs in addition to the usual distribution, and the pink spots may give way to dark, hyperpigmented spots that persist for months after the rash disappears.

In about 50 percent of cases, the rash causes itching, which can be quite intense, especially if the person becomes overheated. In some instances, there is a more severe inflammatory skin reaction, often accompanied by other symptoms such as fatigue and achiness.

The rash usually fades and disappears within six weeks after reaching its peak, but there have been cases in

The lesions of pityriasis rosea are usually concentrated on the trunk, sometimes in a distribution that resembles a Christmas tree.

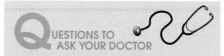
which it lasted much longer. Sometimes the patches show up in two or more waves, with subsequent waves appearing at intervals of up to several weeks after the first one. Occasionally, additional outbreaks occur after many months, and certain environmental or physical factors, such as overheating or developing some other type of skin irritation, can cause a worsening or even reappearance of the rash.

Diagnostic Studies and Procedures

A dermatologist usually can diagnose the condition by examining the skin for the characteristic herald patch. She will also check the appearance of individual lesions—the lesions of pityriasis rosea typically have raised borders where scaling is most prominent—and closely examine the distribution of the rash. If it has an unusual appearance, skin scrapings may be sent to a laboratory for analysis to rule out a fungal infection. Blood tests also may be ordered.

Medical Treatments

Pityriasis rosea is a self-limiting condition and will eventually clear up without treatment. If the itchiness interferes with sleep or other activities, steroids may be prescribed. Medicated lotions and lubricants may also be given to help alleviate itching. In severe cases, ultraviolet light treatments may help. Such treatments should always be supervised by an experienced health professional.

Alternative Therapies

Herbal Medicine. Compresses soaked in witch hazel or an infusion of geranium, chamomile, lavender, or juniper berry are recommended to help ease the itching and skin inflammation. Ointments or salves that contain arnica, calendula, chickweed, or elder have been found effective too. A cucumber poultice is yet another method for relieving itchiness.

Hydrotherapy. A time-honored way to alleviate itchiness is to add two cups of apple cider vinegar to tepid bathwater. Alternatively, a cup of baking soda or a pint of thyme tea may help. Avoid hot baths and saunas, as heat often worsens the itchiness of pityriasis.

Hypnotherapy and Visualization. These techniques may be helpful in coping with itching. For example, by using self-hypnosis, an individual may be able to create a sensation of numbness in the itchy spots.

Self-Treatment

Resist the urge to scratch, which actually worsens the condition by setting in motion an itch-scratch-itch cycle. Scratching also can lead to infection. Nonprescription products such as hydrocortisone creams and calamine lotion applied to the rashy areas will usually ease the itching. Bath preparations containing colloidal oatmeal may also be soothing, but be sure the water is tepid rather than hot or cold.

Over-the-counter antihistamines such as Benadryl may also relieve itching, but they often cause drowsiness, which may make it difficult to use these medications for long periods.

Because physical exertion and overheating sometimes worsen the disorder, try to avoid vigorous exercise that is likely to produce sweating. And don't use strong soaps and cosmetics, as they may increase the irritation.

Exposing the rash to sunlight may hasten healing, but should be limited to a few minutes in the morning or late afternoon when you are less likely to become sunburned.

Other Causes of Itchy Rashes

Eczema and dermatitis cause itchy rashes, but unlike pityriasis, these conditions tend to be chronic. Psoriasis is also characterized by scaly lesions, but they are usually larger and thicker. Among infectious disorders, ringworm and other forms of tinea can produce an itchy, scaly rash that may be confused with pityriasis rosea, as may a reaction to penicillin and other medications.

Syphilis causes a red, scaly, bumpy rash during its second stage, usually about six weeks after the infection is contracted. Thus, a laboratory test to check out the possibility of syphilis is in order if such a rash is accompanied by a fever or enlarged lymph nodes in the neck, armpit, or groin.

Pleurisy

(Pleural effusion; pleural inflammation)
Pleurisy is an inflammation of the pleura, the thin, double membrane that covers the lungs and lines the chest cavity. Sometimes fluid accumulates in the space between the layers of the pleural membrane, a condition called pleural effusion.

Pleurisy and plural effusion are not disease entities; instead, they are complications of other disorders, such as pneumonia, a collapsed lung (pneumothorax), a pulmonary embolism, tuberculosis, or cancer. Certain connective tissue disorders, such as lupus, can also cause pleural pain. A fractured rib or other chest injury may damage the pleura, causing inflammation and producing pleural effusion. Other possibilities include congestive heart failure, kidney disorders, and liver disease.

Typically, pleurisy comes on suddenly, and breathing produces a sharp pain when the two inflamed pleural layers rub against the lungs as they expand and contract. Coughing, sneezing, or other abrupt movement worsens the pain, which may be alleviated by holding the breath or pressing on the chest. Depending upon the cause, there may also be a fever and other symptoms.

Shortness of breath is the major symptom of pleural effusion, which is not as painful as pleurisy. In fact, a lessening of pleural pain accompanied by increasing shortness of breath is a possible sign that pleural effusion is developing, and prompt medical attention is required.

Diagnostic Studies and Procedures

Pleurisy usually can be diagnosed on the basis of symptoms and a chest examination. When a doctor listens to the chest sounds with a stethoscope, she can hear a characteristic rubbing sound.

A chest X-ray will be ordered to look for possible causes such as pneumonia. If plural effusion is present, a hollow needle may be inserted between two ribs to withdraw a fluid sample for laboratory analysis. Sputum analysis and a biopsy also may be done. Blood studies and other tests may be needed to determine the underlying cause.

Medical Treatments

Treating the underlying cause of the pleurisy is essential to achieving a cure. Antibiotics are prescribed if bacterial pneumonia or some other infection is responsible. Drainage usually alleviates any pleural effusion, although repeat drainage may be necessary. If the fluid contains pus, antibiotics may be administered through a tube inserted directly into the chest cavity.

Acetaminophen will usually control the pain, which also may be relieved by wrapping the entire chest firmly with two or three wide elastic bandages; these should be loosened and reapplied once or twice a day.

Alternative Therapies

Because pleurisy may indicate a serious underlying disease, treatment should always be overseen by a medical doctor, with alternative therapies used as adjuncts to alleviate symptoms.

Aromatherapy. A massage using camphor oil may help ease the discomfort. It should be given once a day for about three weeks. However, the chest area itself should not be massaged if the action causes any pain.

Herbal Medicine. Western herbalists may prescribe drinking an infusion of *Asclepias tuberosa,* also known as pleurisy root, two or three times a day, or boneset, which may be taken as an infusion or decoction. Garlic—either fresh or in capsules—is recommended sometimes for its anti-infective properties. Chinese herbalists most often use a formula called Pu-Chung-I-Chi-Tang, made up of ginseng root, Chinese angelica, licorice root, mandarin orange peel, paichu, ginger rhizome, bupleurum, cimicifuga, and astragalus.

Homeopathy. Aconitum may be prescribed in the earliest stages of pleurisy, to be taken as often as three times an hour. When movement is painful, sulphur may be taken every two hours. Apis is used to treat pleural effusion, and hepar sulphuris may be used when pleurisy is chronic and a large amount of mucus is present.

Self-Treatment

Rest until pain and fever disappear, then gradually resume your normal activities. If coughing causes pain, use a cool-mist humidifier to help loosen bronchial secretions and make them easier to cough up. Holding a pillow firmly against the chest wall when coughing can also help limit the pain. Do not take a cough suppressant, however, because coughing is essential to clearing the lungs and bronchial tubes. Try to breathe deeply and cough after taking a painkiller.

Exposure to any form of tobacco smoke can aggravate pleurisy; refrain from smoking, and also stay away from secondhand smoke.

Other Causes of Painful Breathing

Pericarditis, an inflammation of the heart covering, can produce pain and a rubbing sound similar to those of pleurisy. Various lung disorders, including pneumonia and a collapsed lung, also may be mistaken for pleurisy.

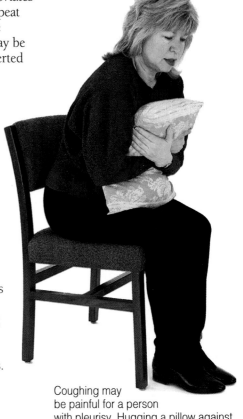

Coughing may be painful for a person with pleurisy. Hugging a pillow against the chest can help reduce the pain.

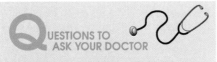

QUESTIONS TO ASK YOUR DOCTOR

► Do I have a condition that predisposes me to pleurisy? If so, what can I do to prevent a recurrence?
► What is the best sleeping position?
► Should I take an expectorant to make it easier to cough up phlegm?
► How long should I wrap my chest with an elastic bandage? How can I tell if it's too tight?

Pneumonia

(Bacterial and viral pneumonitis;
Pneumocystis carinii *pneumonia)*
Pneumonia is an acute infection of the lungs that can be caused by bacteria, viruses, fungi, or parasites. About 2 million Americans contract it each year. Up to 70,000 die, making it our most lethal infectious disease.

Many types of bacteria cause the disease, but pneumococcus is the most common. Viral pneumonia is often caused by flu viruses, whereas fungal pneumonias are frequently contracted by inhaling dust or air that harbors spores of *Coccidioides, Histoplasma, Cryptococcus, Aspergillus,* and others. It is uncertain whether *Pneumocystis carinii,* the organism responsible for AIDS-related pneumonia, is a fungus or parasite, but research favors the former.

PNEUMONIA IMMUNIZATION

Two common forms of pneumonia can be prevented by immunization. Preventive shots for pneumococcal pneumonia are advocated for everyone over age 65 and for anyone over the age of two who has a chronic disease that increases their risk for pneumonia. Immunization against *Haemophilus influenzae B* (HIB) is recommended for all babies, beginning at two months of age.

Aspiration pneumonia, in which stomach contents are inhaled into the lungs, can occur after surgery.

Regardless of the cause, pneumonia is most serious in young children, the elderly, or anyone whose immunity is low or whose health is poor. Symptoms vary somewhat according to the cause and site of the infection in the lung, but all pneumonias result in breathing problems, such as pain when inhaling and shortness of breath. Coughing may produce thick, greenish or yellow sputum. There may also be a high fever and chills, which come on suddenly.

Diagnostic Studies and Procedures

A doctor begins by examining the lungs with a stethoscope to listen for characteristic crackling sounds, or rales, that occur when the patient takes a deep breath. He will also place the fingers of one hand over a rib and thump with a finger of the other hand, listening for a normal, resonant sound. A dull sound

may indicate a patch of pneumonia. A chest X-ray and laboratory examination of blood and sputum samples are needed to confirm the diagnosis.

Medical Treatments

To fight bacterial pneumonia, broad-spectrum antibiotics, such as penicillin, a cephalosporin, or erythromycin, are usually prescribed.

Pneumocystis pneumonia is treated with trimethoprim/sulfamethoxazole (Bactrim and Septra) and pentamidine (NebuPent, which is inhaled, and Pentam 300, given by injection). Antifungal drugs are administered to treat pneumonia caused by a fungus.

Antiviral drugs, such as amantadine (Symmetrel) and acyclovir (Zovirax), may be given to prevent or shorten the course of viral pneumonia, but this treatment is generally reserved for patients with a chronic disease that increases the risk of complications.

Other treatments are aimed at alleviating symptoms; an expectorant, for example, may be prescribed to make the mucus easier to cough up.

Alternative Therapies

Herbal Medicine. Western herbalists may prescribe an expectorant decoction consisting of licorice root, wild cherry bark, coltsfoot, anise, and horehound. Practitioners also recommend drinking infusions of hyssop or marsh mallow or taking diluted tinctures or extracts of echinacea several times a day. Chinese herbalists may use the combination of pueraria, ma-huang, cinnamon, peony, jujube, licorice, and ginger to treat pneumonia.

Homeopathy. In acute cases, a homeopath may prescribe aconitum, to be taken hourly, or the ABC formula every one to two hours. Bacillinum may be taken once but should not be repeated if it has no effect. If pus-filled mucus is being coughed up, hepar every three to four hours may be recommended.

Naturopathy and Nutrition Therapy. Extra vitamin C with bioflavonoids and vitamin A or its precursor, beta

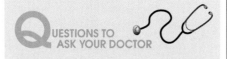
▶ Should I be immunized against pneumonia? (See box, left.)
▶ If I have pneumonia, what can I do to keep from infecting others?

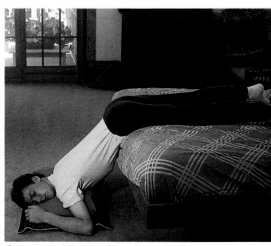

Coughing while lying face down with the upper body hanging downward promotes drainage of mucus from the lungs.

carotene, are advocated to hasten recovery, and zinc lozenges to help bring up phlegm. During the acute phase, the diet should be mainly fruits, vegetables, and chicken broth and other clear soups. The patient should abstain from alcohol and caffeine. Any individual being treated with antibiotics should also take acidophilus capsules in order to prevent an overgrowth of yeast.

Self-Treatment

Bed rest is necessary until any fever disappears, and even then, normal activities must be resumed gradually. Viral pneumonia may require a convalescence of four to six weeks; recovery from other pneumonias varies depending upon the causes.

Placing a heating pad on the chest helps to relieve pain, but it should not be left on while sleeping. You can use a cool-mist humidifier to increase air moisture. Refrain from taking cough suppressants, especially if you are coughing up sputum, because coughing helps eliminate lung secretions.

Practicing postural drainage for 5 to 15 minutes several times a day also helps clear the lungs. To do this, lie face down across a bed with the upper part of your body hanging over the edge; and then cough up as much sputum as you can (see photo, above). If someone is available to help you, have him gently tap your back to loosen the mucus.

Other Causes of Lung Symptoms

Flu, bronchitis, emphysema, and various occupational lung disorders are among the many respiratory conditions that produce symptoms similar to those of pneumonia.

Poisoning Emergencies

Most poisoning emergencies result from ingesting a toxic substance; less common are poisonings caused by inhaling gases, such as exhaust fumes; absorbing chemicals through the skin; or injecting drugs into the body.

More than 75 percent of poisonings reported in the United States each year are of children under age five who have swallowed toxic substances ranging from excessive doses of vitamins and medications to household cleaners. Another high-risk group is the elderly, who accidentally (or intentionally) take an overdose of a drug or other toxic substance.

Symptoms of poisoning vary. Some substances produce vomiting, cramps, abdominal pain, and other intestinal

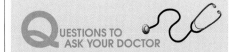

QUESTIONS TO ASK YOUR DOCTOR

► Should vomiting be induced or should the poison be diluted with milk?

problems; others primarily affect the central nervous system, causing an altered state of consciousness, blurred vision, or paralysis, for example. Certain poisons work almost instantly; others may not produce symptoms for a number of hours or even days.

Diagnostic Studies and Procedures

At a hospital or emergency room, blood tests may be performed to determine how much poison is circulating in the body. Depending on the substance, blood and urine tests and X-rays may

be needed to evaluate its impact on various organs, especially the liver, kidneys, and lungs. If a caustic substance has been ingested, endoscopy may be done to assess the extent of damage to the esophagus and stomach.

Medical Treatments

Depending on the poison ingested, medical personnel may be able to give an antidote, such as atropine for an organic phosphate or acetylcysteine for an overdose of acetaminophen. Metal poisoning, including an overdose of iron pills—one of the most common childhood poisoning episodes—may respond to administration of a chelating agent that binds to the metal and facilitates its elimination from the body.

In other cases, vomiting may be induced with medication and/or a pump device might be used to empty the stomach. In addition, activated

AVOIDING POISONOUS HERBS AND OTHER PLANTS

The increased use of herbal medicine has led to a growing number of poisonings and serious health problems from ingesting toxic herbs. Commercial herbal products are generally safe, provided they are used according to instructions. Most poisonings occur when herbs meant for external use are ingested or when people preparing their own remedies mistake a poisonous plant for a medicinal herb. Some older herbal books list plants that have subsequently been found unsafe. The following list is a sampling of dangerous herbs.

Herb	Uses	Dangers
Aconite	Liniments; Chinese and homeopathic remedies.	Contains dangerous alkaloids and other substances that slow the heartbeat, lower blood pressure, and can cause death. Is absorbed through the skin and should not be used in any form.
Bloodroot	Used by Native Americans to treat breast cancer and other disorders.	Contains alkaloids that can cause paralysis, GI upset, vertigo, and collapse.
Broom	Induce menstruation.	Causes reaction similar to nicotine poisoning, with rapid heartbeat, nausea, vertigo, convulsions, respiratory collapse, and death.
Chaparral	General tonic, blood builder.	Overuse can cause hepatitis and liver failure.
Deadly nightshade (atropa belladonna)	Atropine extracts are used in many drugs and homeopathic remedies.	Overdose causes dilated pupils, thirst, nausea, hallucinations, and rapid, weak pulse. Sap causes dermatitis.
Foxglove (digitalis)	Cardiac stimulant; used in many heart drugs.	Overdose causes nausea, diarrhea, arrhythmias, convulsions, possible death.
Goldenseal	Native Americans and some herbal texts recommend it to induce labor and to treat infections and inflammation.	Safety is disputed, but some studies show direct contact can cause severe ulcerations; ingestion may produce nausea.
Hellebore (both American and black)	Older herbal books recommend it for warts, amenorrhea, tumors, and other disorders.	Taken internally, it can be a lethal sedative and narcotic agent; used topically it causes intense hives. Poisoning usually occurs as a result of confusion with other herbs.
Jimson weed	Hallucinogen.	Irregular heartbeat, convulsions, elevated blood pressure, dimness of vision, dilated pupils, giddiness, and delirium.
Lobelia	Weight-loss aid, respiratory problems.	Overdose can cause low blood pressure, rapid heartbeat, respiratory collapse, coma, and even death.
Mayapple	Purgative and laxative.	Causes severe nausea and intestinal disorders; overdose can be fatal.
Pokeweed	Native Americans used it externally and internally for rheumatism.	Powerful narcotic; overdose can be fatal.
St. John's wort	Older herbal books recommend it for indigestion, ulcers, diarrhea, nausea, and pain. Topical forms used to treat bruises and hemorrhoids.	May cause extreme sun sensitivity, swelling, and bleeding disorders.
Tansy	Used by Native Americans to induce abortion; older herbal books recommend it for external treatment of sprains, headaches, and rheumatism.	Oil is highly toxic; overdose causes gastritis, convulsions, and death.
Yohimbe	Africans use it as a male aphrodisiac; also used for impotence and male fertility problems.	Lowers blood pressure; can cause severe anxiety.

FIRST AID FOR POISONING EMERGENCIES

The majority of poisoning victims can be saved if appropriate procedures are followed quickly. The most important steps are to discern what poison has been ingested and to call your local poison control center or emergency room for instructions.

In general:

1. Don't panic.

2. If the person is conscious, try to find out what substance was taken and observe the nature of any symptoms.

3. If the person is unconscious, but does not appear to be in immediate danger, look for an open or empty container or other clue as to what might have been ingested, such as a drinking glass or food remnants. Smell the person's breath, which may reveal a characteristic odor, such as that of alcohol or kerosene. Look for any burns on the lips or mouth that could come from a caustic substance such as lye.

4. Call your local poison control center or hospital emergency room for instructions. Be prepared to report the age of the victim, the substance that was ingested if it is known, symptoms, any first aid being administered, and your location and phone number.

5. Never give any drugs, beverages, or foods to a poisoning victim, except as described here or as directed by health care personnel.

6. After administering first aid, preferably as directed by health professionals, get the victim to the nearest hospital emergency room. Take with you a sample of the toxic substance or its container and a sample of any vomit.

For caustic substances:

(Lye, bleach, benzene, paint thinner, gasoline or kerosene, or drain, oven, or toilet bowl cleaners)

1. If the victim is conscious, try to dilute the poison by giving him milk or water— 1 to 2 cups for children, 2 to 3 cups for a teenager or adult. Milk is better for acids and alkalis, such as lye; water is preferred for petroleum products such as gasoline.

For other poisons:

1. If the victim is conscious and is not experiencing pain or burning sensations in the throat, chest, or stomach, induce vomiting, preferably by administering 1 or 2 tablespoons of ipecac syrup followed by a glass of water. Repeat the process if vomiting does not occur within 20 minutes. If ipecac syrup is unavailable, insert a spoon or finger in the mouth and gently stroke the gag reflect center at the back of the throat.

2. Keep the victim's head lower than his chest during vomiting to prevent inhaling vomit into the lungs.

For unconscious victims:

1. Call an ambulance immediately.

2. Look for a heartbeat and signs of breathing. If these are absent, maintain an open airway and begin cardiopulmonary resuscitation (see page 217).

3. Do not induce vomiting or give fluids.

first aid kit. Post phone numbers of the local poison control center and hospital emergency room near your telephone.

Certain self-care measures formerly printed on product labels or in now-outdated first aid manuals, may do more harm than good for poisoning victims. These are things you should never do:

▶ Do not give vinegar or citrus fruit juice following ingestion of drain or oven cleaners and lye-containing products, based on the mistaken assumption that they will provide a neutralizing effect on these alkalis. These natural acids may increase gastrointestinal burning.

▶ Do not give butter, cooking oil, or other fatty substances to soothe the effects of lye and other caustic substances. Fats coat and conceal the amount of damage, interfering with medical diagnosis and treatment.

▶ Do not give sodium bicarbonate to anyone who has ingested an acidic substance, thinking that it will have a neutralizing effect. It could cause serious stomach damage instead.

▶ Do not induce vomiting with a salt and water solution at any time. It is usually ineffective and could cause fatal salt poisoning.

Other Causes of Poisoning

Food poisoning can result from eating something contaminated with bacteria or bacterial toxins produced by certain organisms. The most common offending bacteria are staphylococcus, clostridia, and salmonella. Rarer, but more severe, is botulism, caused by a toxin that is produced by a strain of *Clostridium* bacteria. Poisoning also may occur from the bites of insects, marine life, or snakes.

POISONING EMERGENCIES (CONTINUED)

charcoal may be left in the stomach to absorb any remaining poison.

A person who is unconscious or having trouble breathing will be given extra oxygen or will be placed on life-support equipment, and possibly given intravenous fluids and replacement electrolytes to treat dehydration.

If a caustic substance has burned the esophagus or damaged the airway, a tracheostomy will be performed to facilitate breathing.

Renal dialysis will be used if kidney function has been damaged or if the procedure will speed elimination of the poison from the bloodstream. Intravenous nutrition and medication also may be provided as needed.

Alternative Therapies

There are no alternative therapies for poisoning victims.

Self-Treatment

The best approach is prevention. Never take medication in the dark. Always store toxic substances (see box, right)

in their original containers and keep them out of the reach of small children, preferably on a high shelf in a cabinet that can be locked. When giving medication to youngsters, never present it as a treat. Keep syrup of ipecac, which induces vomiting, in your home and

SAFETY FIRST IN POISON PREVENTION

The following substances, commonly found in many households, pose a serious threat to life if ingested or taken in overdoses. These and other potentially toxic substances should always be kept out of the reach of children.

Alcohol	Dishwashing liquid	Lye	Rat poison and other pesticides
Ammonia	Drain cleaner	Lighter fluid	
Aspirin and acetaminophen	Fabric softener	Medications, both prescription and over-the-counter	Rubbing alcohol
	Floor wax		Scouring pads
Benzene	Furniture polish		Shoe polish
Bicarbonate of soda	Glue	Metal polish	Stain removers
	Grease remover	Mineral oil	Toilet cleaner
Bleach	Hair dyes, perms, and straighteners	Nail care products	Turpentine
Carpet cleaner		Oven cleaner	
Deodorants	Insecticide	Paint	Vitamin and iron pills
Depilatories	Laundry detergent	Paint thinner	Weedkiller

Polio/Postpolio Syndrome

(Infantile paralysis; poliomyelitis; postpolio syndrome)

Polio, a highly contagious disease, is caused by three different types of polio virus. Most infections are asymptomatic, with illness becoming evident in only about 5 in 100 cases, and then, usually limited to a low-grade fever, malaise, sore throat, and other flu-like symptoms. This manifestation is referred to as abortive polio.

A small percentage of people develop viral, or aseptic meningitis, characterized by severe headache, stiff neck, back and muscle pain, and sometimes muscle spasms or paralysis. Most recover completely, and only in the most severe cases is there permanent paralysis. (The most well-known case of this type was that of President Franklin Delano Roosevelt.)

Polio is now rare in the United States thanks to vaccines introduced in 1955 and 1963. Ironically, use of the live polio virus in an oral vaccine is now responsible for most of the cases in this country—an average of nine a year. The disease is, however, still common in some developing countries.

In recent years, postpolio syndrome, characterized by fatigue, muscle weakness, pain, and sometimes even paralysis, has been identified among people who decades earlier suffered polio. Of 250,000 polio survivors in the U.S., some 20 to 25 percent are expected to develop the syndrome. The cause is unknown, but some researchers have theorized that aging further depletes nerve cells originally damaged by polio. However, some patients experience atrophy and weakening even of muscles that were not affected earlier. Nor is there any correlation between the severity of the two attacks. Some patients

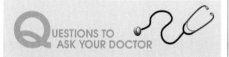

POLIO VACCINE

There are two types of polio vaccine—Sabin live oral and Salk inactivated; this last is given in a series of shots. The oral vaccine is recommended for most children, to be taken first between 2 and 4 months of age, again at 15 to 18 months, and before entering school between ages 4 and 6 years. Adults who have never been immunized and are traveling to parts of the world where polio is common should also be vaccinated. People with weakened immune systems should not receive the oral vaccine because they may contract the disease; instead, they should have the Salk injected vaccine.

whose initial bouts were mild suffer progressively severe symptoms.

Diagnostic Studies and Procedures

An initial diagnosis of polio can be based on symptoms, but laboratory tests will be ordered to rule out other possible causes. A person who may have postpolio syndrome will undergo electromyography and other muscle tests, as well as a chest X-ray and perhaps pulmonary function tests.

Medical Treatments

There is no effective antiviral treatment against polio; thus, therapy is aimed at relieving symptoms. If breathing is affected, long-term use of a respirator may be necessary. In less severe cases, postural drainage and suction are used to remove accumulations of mucus in bronchial tubes. Sometimes a tracheostomy, an opening in the trachea, is created to function as an airway.

Perhaps the most important aspect of treating polio is medically supervised physical therapy during convalescence. About half of patients with paralytic polio recover completely; 25 percent retain mild disabilities, and 25 percent remain severely handicapped.

Patients with postpolio syndrome are treated by experts in rehabilitation medicine, with the goal of helping them adapt to loss of muscle strength.

Alternative Therapies

Hydrotherapy. Swimming is the best exercise for polio patients. Water temperature should be warm to promote flexibility of muscles and joints. Range-of-motion and stretching exercises also can be done in the water.

Music Therapy. Music has long been part of the programs at New York's Goldwater Memorial Hospital and

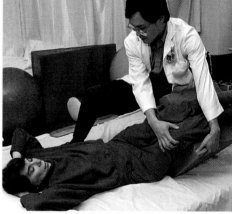

Patients with postpolio syndrome can benefit from physical therapy and exercises.

the Rusk Institute of Rehabilitation Medicine—leading treatment centers for polio patients—where it is used to encourage movement and control pain.

Physical and Occupational Therapy. As soon as the acute phase passes, physical and occupational therapists begin working with patients to increase muscle tone and strength. For those who suffer disability, occupational therapists can provide training in how to care for themselves independently even with limited strength and mobility.

Self-Treatment

Extra rest is important both during convalescence from polio and in dealing with postpolio syndrome. While exercise is significant, it is equally important not to overdo it.

Maintaining ideal weight is critical, because excess weight makes it more difficult to get about. When eating, a patient should chew slowly and swallow carefully to avoid choking, especially if respiratory muscles have become weakened. The best eating position is sitting up straight with the head leaning slightly forward. Alcohol should be avoided with meals, because it may further inhibit swallowing.

Anyone who has had polio should avoid sleeping pills and narcotic medications, because these can suppress breathing. Swollen feet and ankles are a common complication in partially or completely paralyzed legs. Support stockings might be considered.

Other Causes of Polio Symptoms

Guillain-Barré syndrome is sometimes confused with polio. Postpolio syndrome can be mistaken for multiple sclerosis and other disorders of the neuromuscular system.

Polycystic Kidney Disease

Polycystic kidney disease is a hereditary disorder in which fluid-filled sacs, called renal cysts, form in the kidneys. About 50,000 American adults have the disorder, which is responsible for about 5 percent of chronic kidney failure in the United States. There are two general types of this disease:

The adult, or autosomal dominant form, is more common and less severe. It generally does not appear until early adulthood, and when kidney failure occurs, it is usually after age 50.

The infantile, or autosomal recessive form, is relatively rare. It shows up at birth or shortly afterward and results in early kidney failure. A variation of the infantile form of this disease remains asymptomatic during the early years, and generally causes less severe renal impairment. However, it develops in association with a congenital liver disease that often proves fatal.

As they become increasingly filled with cysts, the kidneys may grow to three or four times their normal size. Early symptoms include flank pain, a mass that can be felt in the kidney area, blood and protein in the urine, recurrent bladder or kidney infections, and kidney stones. High blood pressure is common, and some patients develop anemia. Alongside this condition, cysts often form in other internal organs as well, especially the liver and, less commonly, the spleen, pancreas, lungs, ovaries, testes, thyroid, uterus, and bladder. A major danger of the disease is development of kidney cancer, which is far more common than in people with noncystic kidneys.

Diagnostic Studies and Procedures

A complete physical examination and blood and urine tests are standard. A definitive diagnosis of this disease is

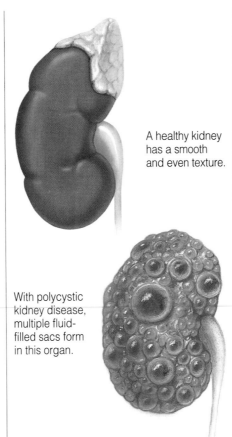

A healthy kidney has a smooth and even texture.

With polycystic kidney disease, multiple fluid-filled sacs form in this organ.

made with the additional help of X-rays, ultrasonography, CT scans, and other imaging studies that show the kidney cysts and enlargement.

Medical Treatments

Because there is no cure for polycystic kidneys, treatment is designed to help prevent or control its complications. Hypertension may be treated with one or more medications (see page 230), and antibiotics may be prescribed for bladder and kidney infections. Kidney stones may be treated with medication or pulverized with sound waves that make them easier to pass through the urinary system (see page 264).

Sometimes, large cysts are punctured surgically, especially if they are causing acute pain, bleeding, or urinary obstruction. In severe cases, one or both kidneys may be removed.

Chronic kidney failure, which occurs when more than 90 percent of kidney function has been lost, can be treated with dialysis (see page 262) or by transplanting a new kidney. If a transplant is feasible, the approach that has the greatest probability for success is to use a donor organ from a living relative who is a close genetic match with the

patient. Otherwise, a genetically compatible kidney taken from a recently deceased person may be used.

Alternative Therapies

There are no alternative therapies for treating polycystic kidneys, but some are helpful in preventing complications.

Herbal Therapy. To treat bladder and kidney infections, herbalists recommend uva-ursi (bearberry) in capsules or dried and mixed with warm water (1 tablespoon of herb to 8 ounces of water), which may be used as an adjunct to antibiotics.

Nutrition Therapy. Some research has suggested that a low-protein diet can ease the workload on the kidneys. A registered dietitian should be consulted for assistance in planning such a diet. If ample citrus fruits and juices are included, they will help acidify the urine, which may inhibit bacterial growth and reduce the risk of bladder infections. Blueberry and cranberry juices also inhibit bacterial growth within the bladder.

Self-Treatment

Because polycystic kidneys are hereditary, there is nothing you can do to prevent the disease. However, you may want to seek genetic counseling before starting a family. Because pregnancy puts extra strain on the kidneys, a woman with polycystic disease may be advised to forego having children.

Anyone with polycystic kidney disease must be especially cautious about using drugs, as there are many that affect the kidneys; do not take any medication, including over-the-counter painkillers, without checking first with a doctor.

In general, patients with polycystic kidneys should never restrict either water or salt intake, because this can lead to dehydration. It is important to drink adequate fluids—at least 8 to 10 glasses of water or other nonalcoholic beverages a day—and consume a moderate amount of salt, unless a doctor advises otherwise.

Moderate exercise is safe, but contact sports such as football should be avoided because a blow to the kidneys can cause severe bleeding and more damage.

Other Causes of Chronic Kidney Failure

Chronic kidney failure may also be caused by kidney diseases such as nephropathy and glomerulonephritis, as well as by diabetes, hypertension, lupus, and atherosclerosis.

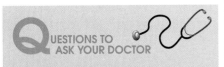

QUESTIONS TO ASK YOUR DOCTOR

► What type of polycystic disease do I have? Should other members of my family be evaluated?
► What possible signs of kidney failure should I watch for?

Post-Traumatic Stress Syndrome

Post-traumatic stress syndrome is a psychiatric disorder that arises from having endured an event that is outside the range of usual human experience. In the past, it was referred to as shell shock, and was associated mostly with war. Now, it is generally recognized that any devastating event—a flood, earthquake, plane crash, rape, assault, accident, or fire—can precipitate the syndrome in susceptible persons.

Post-traumatic stress disorder can occur at any age, but the very young and the aged appear to be the most vulnerable, presumably because they have less ability to cope and adjust to trauma. For example, one study found that 80 percent of young children who have suffered severe burns experience post-traumatic stress symptoms one to two years after the injury, compared with 30 percent of adults. Another survey

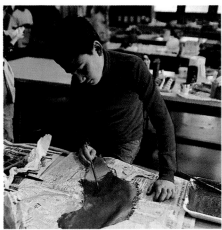

Survivors of natural disasters are prone to post-traumatic stress syndrome. Here, a victim of the devastating 1992 fires in Oakland expresses his feelings through art therapy.

indicated that 12 percent of women and 6 percent of men in the United States have experienced post-traumatic stress at some time in their lives. Among the women, half the cases resulted from having been raped or otherwise sexually molested, while combat duty was the major cause among men.

Persons suffering from post-traumatic stress repeatedly relive the event in disturbingly realistic dreams, hallucinations, or flashbacks. Often, these flashbacks are triggered by sights, sounds, or smells associated with the trauma. Many such persons maintain a constant state of vigilance to avoid stimuli that are likely to trigger a flashback. They are often irritable and given to outbursts of uncontrollable anger. They may have difficulty sleeping and be unable to concentrate. Any situation that resembles an aspect of the event can set off a fight or flight response. For example, a survivor of a plane crash may experience sudden sweating, rapid heartbeat, and mounting fear whenever a plane flies overhead.

Others may withdraw and appear unresponsive to their environment, taking little interest in important or pleasurable activities and feeling detached or estranged from loved ones and friends. Feelings of survivor guilt are not uncommon when the trauma involved the death of others.

It is not known why some people develop the syndrome while others who shared the same experience do not. One recent hypothesis holds that hormonal factors may be responsible; another attributes the symptoms to withdrawal from high levels of endorphins and other opium-like body chemicals that are released during the flashbacks.

Diagnostic Studies and Procedures

To diagnose the disorder, the American Psychiatric Association notes that, in addition to persistently reliving the event, at least three of the following must be present for at least one month:
► Avoidance of thoughts and feelings associated with the trauma.
► Avoidance of activities or situations likely to trigger recall of the event.
► Amnesia of the event.
► Lack of interest in normal activities.
► Feelings of detachment.
► Restricted range of feelings or emotions, such as an inability to love.
► Gloomy outlook for the future.
Two of the following conditions must also be present:
► Insomnia.
► Irritability or angry outbursts.
► Difficulty in concentrating.
► Excessive vigilance.
► Exaggerated startle response.

Medical Treatments

Treatment varies depending upon the symptoms and their severity, but a combination of medication and pschotherapy appears to work best.

Tricyclic antidepressant drugs such as amitriptyline (Elavil), imipramine

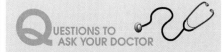

(Tofranil), and phenelzine (Nardil) may be prescribed to help reduce anxiety and depression. In severe cases marked by violent or agitated behavior, antipsychotic medications such as haloperidol (Haldol) or thiothixene (Navane) may be used for a brief time. If the patient is suicidal or self-destructive, hospitalization might be necessary.

Short-term cognitive psychotherapy may be advised for helping the patient develop effective coping techniques. Group and family therapy could also prove helpful, especially if the traumatic event is one that affected a large number of people, such as a flood.

Alternative Therapies

Art, Dance, and Drama Therapy. Under the guidance of a qualified therapist, these arts can be effective in helping post-traumatic stress patients come to grips with the devastating event and to express fears or thoughts they might not be able to verbalize. These modalities are especially helpful in the treatment of children.

Meditation. Relaxation therapies, especially meditation, self-hypnosis, and biofeedback training, can help ease anxiety.

Self-Treatment

It is important to acknowledge and discuss the experience, rather than trying to forget or ignore it. Sometimes spending time talking about it with a supportive family member or friends can help integrate the event effectively. It is also wise to try to resume normal activities as soon as possible.

Joining a support group of people who have survived a similar experience may also help. Such groups have proved especially beneficial for rape victims and Vietnam veterans.

Other Causes of Post-Traumatic Symptoms

Panic attacks and other manifestations of an anxiety disorder can cause symptoms similar to those of post-traumatic stress, as can certain phobias.

Postpartum Depression

Postpartum depression, or the baby blues, is a feeling of sadness and/or despair that appears shortly after giving birth. The symptoms range from mild to incapacitating, but are usually short-lived. The cause is probably a combination of factors. Sudden hormonal changes at the time of childbirth play a major role, as does the mother's realization that she is now responsible for a tiny, helpless person who requires 24-hour care. Fatigue is also involved. Childbirth itself is often painful and exhausting, and newborns demand to be fed every two hours or so. The result is that most new mothers fail to get adequate rest until the baby's routine stabilizes, which may not happen until six weeks to two months after birth.

A past history of depression or other preexisting psychological problems increases the likelihood of more severe postpartum depression. Still other contributing elements include the need to return to work before a woman feels physically and emotionally ready to leave the baby, and lack of support from one's partner, family, or friends.

In some cases, postpartum depression inhibits bonding between mother and baby, which can have serious consequences for both. In rare instances, serious and long-lasting depression may be accompanied by aggressive feelings toward the infant, loss of pride in appearance and home, lack of appetite or compulsive eating, withdrawal from others, and even suicidal tendencies.

Diagnostic Studies and Procedures

Most women manage to diagnose themselves and report the symptoms to a doctor if they last more than a few days. A doctor should perform a careful physical examination that includes blood and urine studies to make sure that an organic disorder is not contributing to the depression.

Medical Treatments

In a severe or persistent case, a doctor may prescribe an antidepressant drug to be taken for several weeks. Alternatively, he may advocate hormones to help speed the body's return to normal. If the mother is breast-feeding, however, careful consideration must be given to the effect on the baby of any medication she takes, as traces of most drugs that she ingests will pass into the milk.

Psychological counseling or therapy may be recommended if depression seems severe or other emotional difficulties are complicating it. Therapy is more likely to be considered for a woman who has previously experienced a psychological problem Hospitalization is extremely rare, but it might be needed in an acute situation, especially if the woman is potentially suicidal.

Alternative Therapies

Aromatherapy. To elevate mood, therapists recommend adding a few drops of clary sage, geranium, and ylang ylang oils to bathwater. A massage using lavender, geranium, or chamomile is also said to chase depression. For a quick uplift, one can sniff a handkerchief sprinkled with clary sage, rose, and/or sandlewood oils.

Exercise. Physical activity helps quell depression and promotes a sense of well-being by prompting the brain to increase production of endorphins, the body's natural painkiller and mood elevator. When you feel down, try putting the baby in a stroller or body sling and taking a half-hour walk. Not only will you and the baby benefit from an outing, but the exercise will also help get your body back in shape.

Meditation and Yoga. These and other relaxation therapies can help overcome stress and counter fatigue.

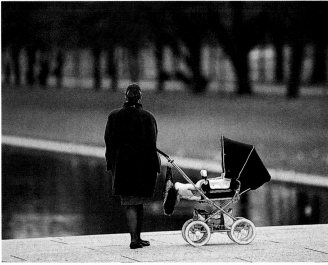

The responsibility of caring for a newborn can seem overwhelming, especially if the new mother has little opportunity for time to herself.

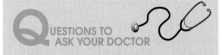

QUESTIONS TO ASK YOUR DOCTOR

▶ How can I convince my partner that my feelings are serious, when everyone says I'll feel better in a week or two?
▶ What effect will antidepressant drugs have on breast-feeding?
▶ Am I likely to experience similar feelings of depression after subsequent pregnancies?

Music Therapy. Music is an age-old remedy for depression. Research indicates that listening to music increases endorphin levels, which would explain how it improves mood.

Self-Treatment

There is a great deal you can do for yourself to overcome baby blues. Start by realizing that it's normal to have mixed feelings about the upheaval that a new baby brings to your life, even though you wanted the child very much. Give yourself time to adjust and bond with your baby rather than feeling upset and guilty.

If you are depressed, don't attempt to hide these feelings. Talking to someone you trust can be highly therapeutic; in fact, many women say that talking to other new mothers, the majority of whom share some of their feelings, helps them put postpartum depression and other problems in perspective.

It is also important to have time away from the baby. Ask for help from your family and friends to care for the child and give you some time alone.

Make sure you get as much rest as possible. Plan to nap when the baby is asleep to make up for getting up several times during the night.

If you find yourself sliding deeper into depression or harboring thoughts of suicide, call your doctor or mental health professional immediately. This is an emergency, especially if the arrival of the baby coincides with other major life changes such as a move, divorce, financial difficulties, a death in the immediate family, or a career change.

Posture Defects

(Kyphosis; lordosis)

The spinal column is made up of 33 bones, arranged in such a way that humans can maintain an upright posture while walking about on two legs instead of all four limbs. Normally, the spine has a slight S curve, which gives it extra strength and flexibility. Posture defects are exaggerations of the spine's natural curves, and they throw the normal body alignment out of kilter. For example, swayback, or lordosis, is an excessive curvature of the lower spine; a person with lordosis will have a protruding abdomen. A hunchback, or kyphosis, involves a curvature of the

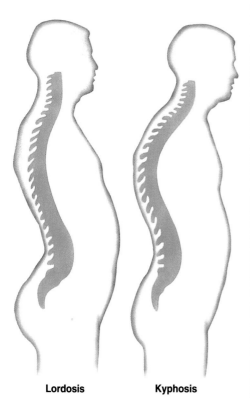

Lordosis   **Kyphosis**

A person with lordosis, or swayback, stands with the abdomen thrust forward. Someone with kyphosis, or hunchback, has rounded shoulders and the head pushed forward.

upper (thoracic) spine. It is often associated with scoliosis (page 370), a sideways curvature. Kyphosis results in a rounding of the shoulders and pitching forward of the head.

Our concept of what constitutes good posture has changed in recent decades. At one time, children were admonished to "straighten up," which meant holding themselves in an exaggerated military posture. We now know that this

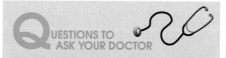

can lead to fatigue, back strain, and nerve pain. The ideal posture is more relaxed, with the head held high, the shoulders in a relaxed position that allows deep breathing, and the pelvis tucked in. A weighted line dropped from just in front of the ear should end just in front of the ankle bone.

Numerous structural defects and diseases can produce abnormal posture. Spinal arthritis and osteoporosis are common causes of kyphosis. Obesity and pregnancy can lead to lordosis. Chronic slouching and various muscle disorders can also cause rounded shoulders or a swayback. Whatever the cause, most posture defects are painless cosmetic deformities. In some cases, however, there may be backaches, impaired lung function, shortening of chest muscles, and loss of flexibility.

Diagnostic Studies and Procedures

Posture defects can usually be diagnosed visually while the patient walks, sits, and bends forward; this last position makes the spine stand out. A doctor will measure the shoulder and hip symmetry, or have X-rays taken from the back and the side, to explore the extent of the defect and try to trace its underlying cause.

In more serious cases, MRI may be ordered. Less commonly, a myelogram—a dye-enhanced X-ray study of nerves arising from the spinal cord—and a bone scan are done to look for a cause. If osteoporosis is suspected, bone density will be studied. Blood analyses, muscle and nerve studies, and other tests may be ordered to identify any underlying disease.

Medical Treatments

Some treatments focus on physically correcting the curvature, while others aim at treating an underlying disease. In the absence of a disease such as spinal arthritis or osteoporosis, treatment will be directed to correcting the posture. Often, corrective exercise is all that is needed. In more severe cases,

bracing or orthopedic surgery may be advised. Aspirin or stronger nonsteroidal anti-inflammatory drugs may be prescribed to treat back pain.

Alternative Therapies

Mild curvature usually can be corrected through alternative therapies that work to strengthen the supporting muscles and encourage proper posture.

Alexander Technique. A trained instructor analyzes your posture and movements while you perform various tasks, and then uses gentle physical and verbal instructions to improve body alignment. The technique is especially useful to correct postural problems stemming from bad habits.

Chiropractic. Chiropractors use spinal manipulation to alleviate back and neck pain. These adjustments do not correct posture defects, but when they ease pain, it is usually possible to hold the back in proper alignment.

Osteopathy. Osteopaths are licensed physicians who believe that proper postural alignment has a direct influence on a person's overall health. They often specialize in treating back problems, using gentle manipulation and teaching patients effective movements.

Physical Therapy. A physical therapist can recommend exercises that will help reduce back strain, strengthen supporting muscles, and correct any mild posture problems.

T'ai Chi and Yoga. These movement therapies promote strength, flexibility, alignment, and harmony between body and mind. In yoga, the body is placed in a series of poses, many of which involve isometric tension and stretching simultaneously. Many yogic poses can be performed only when one uses correct posture techniques. T'ai chi involves a set series of slow exercises.

Self-Treatment

All of the following can help you to avoid posture defects: Make a conscious effort to keep from slouching and to maintain good posture. Use a straight-backed chair or other type that provides lower back support, and sit with your thigh resting horizontally on the chair seat. Wear low-heeled shoes that provide good support. Sleep on a firm mattress. Exercise regularly, and strive to maintain normal weight.

Other Causes of Poor Posture

Scoliosis, congenital birth defects, chronic back pain, and various neuromuscular disorders can alter posture.

Pregnancy Complications

(Morning sickness; placenta abruptia; placenta previa; pre-eclampsia; toxemia of pregnancy)

From the moment of conception, a woman's body begins undergoing changes; some are scarcely noticeable, others are annoying or uncomfortable but not serious, and a few are signs of dangerous complications.

Even before pregnancy has been confirmed, a woman is likely to notice that her breasts are more swollen and tender than usual. This is due to rising levels of estrogen and progesterone, hormones essential to establishing and maintaining pregnancy. She may also experience the nausea and vomiting of morning sickness, actually a misnomer, as the queasiness can occur at any time of day, starting in about the sixth week of pregnancy and usually continuing until the tenth or eleventh week and, for some women, even longer.

As pregnancy progresses, certain other symptoms commonly develop, but they are generally no cause for concern and disappear shortly after childbirth. They include the following:

Heartburn, indigestion, and constipation, especially during the last trimester when the growing fetus crowds the stomach and intestines. Constipation may be due to pressure on the colon as well as to relaxation of muscles, including those that control the bowels' rhythmic action.

Fatigue, particularly in the early months when the woman's body uses much of its energy for the fetus.

Insomnia, which may develop because it is difficult to find a comfortable sleeping position. In addition, restful sleep may be interrupted by a need to urinate, a kicking baby, or leg cramps brought on by changes in the body's electrolyte balance.

Mildly swollen hands and feet, due to increased fluid retention, a normal change of advanced pregnancy. (If swelling is accompanied by high blood pressure, this could be a sign of pre-eclampsia; see hypertension, right.) As the blood supply expands and the uterus enlarges, blood tends to collect in the body's extremities. The pooling of blood in the legs can, however, cause dizziness and fainting.

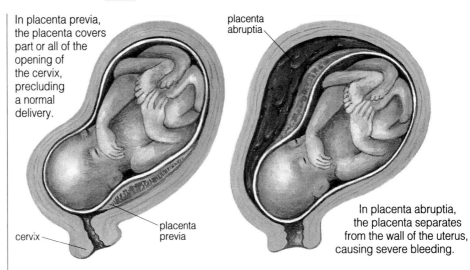

In placenta previa, the placenta covers part or all of the opening of the cervix, precluding a normal delivery.

cervix

placenta previa

placenta abruptia

In placenta abruptia, the placenta separates from the wall of the uterus, causing severe bleeding.

Varicose veins in the legs and hemorrhoids (varicose veins in the anus), brought on by increased abdominal weight, pressure, and other factors that resolve themselves after childbirth.

Bleeding teeth and gums, a result of higher levels of progesterone.

Pregnancy increases a woman's vulnerability to other conditions and itself can bring on complications that require medical attention. These include:

Vaginitis, an infection or inflammation of the vagina. Again, high levels of certain hormone are responsible; they alter the acidity of the vagina, creating an environment that favors overgrowth of yeast and bacteria. A higher body temperature during pregnancy is also a contributing factor.

Urinary tract infections, due to increasing pressure on the bladder by the uterus, which affects the normal flow of urine. Such infections can be dangerous to both the mother and baby if left untreated.

Hypertension, either preexisting or pregnancy-induced. This is potentially dangerous because it can lead to pre-eclampsia, a condition that is marked by a steep rise in blood pressure, generalized swelling, and kidney failure. If not brought under control, pre-eclampsia can evolve into eclampsia, or toxemia of pregnancy, in which uncontrollable seizures and coma occur.

A marked rise in blood pressure and swelling of the face, hands, and feet that is especially pronounced in the morning are the clearest early warning signs of pre-eclampsia. If untreated, these symptoms may worsen and soon be accompanied by headache, abdominal pain, and irritability. The next stage is true eclampsia, which can lead rapidly to death. Any indication of pre-eclampsia demands prompt treatment.

Bleeding from the uterus. This always calls for immediate attention. If it occurs in the first trimester, it may indicate a miscarriage (page 299). During late pregnancy, it could be a sign of one of two serious complications: placenta previa—in which the placenta has become implanted in the lower part of the uterus and is covering part or all of the opening into the cervix; or placenta abruptia—in which the placenta has become partially detached from the wall of the uterus (see illustrations, above). The resulting severe bleeding threatens both the mother and baby.

Premature labor and delivery. Pregnancy normally lasts 40 weeks, but very few babies are born on their exact due date and about 5 percent of deliveries are premature. Great strides in neonatal intensive care now enable doctors to save many premature babies that had little or no chance in the past. Even so, the longer a pregnancy can be maintained, the better it is for the baby.

Diagnostic Studies and Procedures

Throughout pregnancy, a woman should see a doctor or nurse-midwife for regular examinations that include urinalysis, blood glucose tests to detect gestational diabetes (page 203), and blood pressure measurement. At these checkups, she should discuss any problems, including seemingly minor ones. If an infection or other evolving complication is suspected, additional tests may include laboratory cultures, blood studies, an ultrasound examination, and fetal monitoring.

Medical Treatments

Most minor complications of pregnancy do not require medical treatment; more serious problems are treated according to the underlying cause.

Many pregnant women are reluctant to take any drug for fear that it will harm the fetus. Although this is an important concern, foregoing needed medical treatment can be even more dangerous. For example, high blood pressure should be treated with anti-hypertensive drugs, though the dosage and/or drug selection may have to be altered. Methyldopa (Aldomet) and hydralazine (Apresoline) have been used safely during pregnancy. Studies indicate that some beta blockers, such as labetalol (Normodyne), may also be safe. Diltiazem (Cardizem), verapamil (Calan or Isoptin), and other calcium channel blockers seem to be relatively safe, although they should be used during pregnancy only if clearly needed. In contrast, angiotensin converting enzyme (ACE) inhibitors such as captopril (Capoten) or enalapril (Vasotec) are not advisable because these medications have been linked with an increased risk of fetal death.

Pre-eclampsia may be treated with antihypertensive drugs to lower blood pressure and anticonvulsant drugs to prevent seizures. If toxemia develops, hospitalization will be required, and an early delivery may be advisable.

Urinary tract infections call for antibiotic treatment; again, any effects on the fetus must be taken into consideration when selecting a medication.

Premature labor can sometimes be stopped by bed rest and administration of ritodrine (Yutopar), a drug that halts uterine contractions.

Placenta previa and abruptia usually require hospitalization and strict bed rest until the bleeding stops. In some cases, an immediate Cesarean section will be performed.

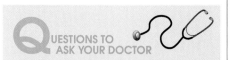

QUESTIONS TO ASK YOUR DOCTOR

▶ How often should I come in for a checkup during pregnancy?
▶ How much exercise is safe while I am pregnant?
▶ Should I monitor my blood pressure regularly at home?

AVERAGE WEIGHT GAIN IN PREGNANCY

The baby	Pounds
Fetus	7.5
Placenta	1
Amniotic fluid	2
The mother	
Fat and protein stores	4–6
Increased fluid volume	1–3
Uterus	2.5
Breast enlargement	2
Increased blood volume	4
TOTAL	**24 to 28**

Alternative Therapies

Alternative therapies and folk remedies must be approached with the same caution as medical treatments during pregnancy. Herbs or high-dose vitamins can be as dangerous as any drug, so it's a good idea to check with your doctor before taking any preparation or engaging in unusual activities.

Alexander Technique. Back pain is often due to poor posture, which is aggravated by increased abdominal weight during pregnancy. A practitioner of the Alexander technique can teach posture exercises to bring the spine into proper alignment and strengthen the supporting muscles.

Homeopathy. Practitioners claim that homeopathic remedies are safe during pregnancy because the doses are so low that they pose no threat to the fetus. Sepia is recommended for relief of morning sickness and vomiting.

Massage. A soothing massage can relax tense muscles, but the abdominal area should not be massaged vigorously. A gentle classic, or Swedish, massage, with the woman lying on her side, may be the most beneficial.

Nutrition Therapy. To give birth to a healthy, normal-size baby, a woman who enters pregnancy at or close to her desirable weight should gain 24 to 28 pounds by her due date. An underweight woman probably needs to gain more, and an overweight woman may be advised to gain no more than 20 pounds (see box, below).

Nutritionists generally advise that a pregnant woman eat ample amounts of skim milk and low-fat dairy products, vegetables, fruits, whole-grain cereals and breads, lean meats, and eggs. Vitamin and mineral needs increase during pregnancy but, except for iron

and folic acid, supplements are usually not necessary if the diet is properly balanced. High doses of vitamin A can cause severe birth defects.

Yoga and Meditation. These and other relaxation techniques are helpful in coping with the minor discomforts and stress of pregnancy. Any exercises that require abdominal straining or lying flat on the back during the last trimester should be avoided.

Self-Treatment

Self-care can keep annoying pregnancy complications in check. To alleviate nausea, try to get out into the fresh air as much as possible. Eat crackers or dry toast, keeping a supply by the bedside if you feel nauseous on awakening. Sucking on crushed ice can also help. Eat small, frequent meals and avoid fried and spicy dishes. Food odors can trigger nausea; meals served cold or at room temperature may be better tolerated because they have less odor.

To relieve heartburn, eat slowly and chew thoroughly. Try to identify and avoid foods that provoke indigestion. Chewing gum or sucking a lemon can help neutralize stomach acid. If the problem persists, ask your doctor about taking an antacid.

Constipation can be lessened if you drink plenty of liquids, exercise regularly, and eat foods that are high in fiber. To avoid hemorrhoids, try not to strain during a bowel movement.

If you have vaginitis, do not douche unless your doctor recommends it. Vaginitis often can be prevented by drying the genital area thoroughly after showering and wearing cotton panties. Never sit around in a wet bathing suit or damp clothing after exercise.

Moderate daily exercise enhances a sense of well-being and helps maintain muscle tone. Most women can continue their prepregnancy exercise program as long as it does not raise their heart rate above 110 to 140 beats per minute (depending upon fitness level). Excessive body heat can be harmful to a fetus; exercise should not be so vigorous or prolonged that it raises the core body temperature above 100.4°F (40.2°C), measured rectally. Pregnant women should also avoid hot tubs and saunas for the same reason.

Other Pregnancy Complications

Miscarriage and gestational diabetes—two very common complications of pregnancy—are covered separately.

Premenstrual Syndrome

(PMS)

Premenstrual syndrome, or PMS, is a collection of physical and emotional symptoms associated with the menstrual cycle. Symptoms typically appear in the week before menstruation begins and disappear as soon as it starts. Although most women experience some physical or emotional changes during their premenstrual phase, only about 40 percent have symptoms that require treatment, and in 10 percent, the problem is classified as severe.

More than a hundred symptoms are associated with PMS, but most women suffer only a small number (see box, opposite page), which may vary somewhat from month to month.

Until recently, PMS was regarded as a psychological problem, but it is now believed that many of the symptoms have organic causes that may be related to hormonal changes during the menstrual cycle. Exactly how these shifts affect women physically and emotionally is still a mystery, and researchers do not yet know why there are such differences in the ways that women are affected by their menstrual cycles.

Diagnostic Studies and Procedures

An accurate medical history is very important in diagnosing PMS, because the timing of symptoms is the key to

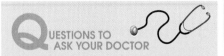

QUESTIONS TO ASK YOUR DOCTOR

▶ Will my PMS symptoms lessen as I grow older?
▶ Can you recommend a PMS clinic or self-help group?
▶ If I suffer from PMS, are my daughters likely to have the same problem?

distinguishing this condition from other disorders. A doctor may ask you to keep a diary for several months, noting any symptoms and indicating the dates on which your menstrual periods begin and end.

Blood and urine studies and additional tests may be done to rule out other possible causes. Hormone levels may be measured, perhaps at different phases in the menstrual cycle, to determine whether they fluctuate abnormally.

Medical Treatments

How best to treat PMS is still controversial. Because the cause is not completely understood, treatment is aimed at alleviating symptoms. It might be necessary to try a variety of approaches before finding an effective treatment or combination of treatments.

In severe cases, when anxiety, insomnia, and other psychological symptoms predominate, tranquilizers or sedatives may be prescribed, although long-term use of these drugs is discouraged

because of their addictive nature. Women who suffer from PMS-related migraines may be helped by a low dose of a beta blocking drug such as propranolol (Inderal), which prevents the vascular changes associated with these headaches. Similarly, taking a nonsteroidal anti-inflammatory drug such as ibuprofen may prevent or alleviate cramps, backache, joint pain, and other types of premenstrual achiness.

A mild diuretic is sometimes prescribed to alleviate fluid retention and swelling. Some doctors advocate treating PMS with progesterone and other hormones, but this approach appears to help only a few women.

Alternative Therapies

Aromatherapy. To ease anxiety and nervousness associated with PMS, some therapists recommend taking a soothing bath to which a few drops of any of the following oils have been added: chamomile, rosemary, lavender, rose, or lemon. A massage that includes the use of clary sage, lavender, and melissa or rose oil is said to balance emotions and lift spirits. A headache and/or emotional unrest may be eased by sprinkling two drops each of melissa, lavender, and chamomile oils on a tissue and inhaling the scent.

Herbal Medicine. A study conducted by the PMS clinic at St. Thomas Hospital in London found that evening primrose oil, long recommended as a remedy for PMS, alleviated symptoms

---

A CASE IN POINT

Since her early twenties, Christine Tanner had suffered from PMS severe enough to make life miserable for 7 to 10 days before each menstrual period. "I felt like I was on an emotional roller coaster," she explains. "I'd feel irritable and anxious one moment and depressed and withdrawn the next." She experienced insomnia, achiness, clumsiness, and a bloated feeling. Ibuprofen eased the achiness, but upset her stomach. Her doctor offered little concrete help.

Then one day, Tanner answered a small ad that was seeking volunteers for a PMS study at a nearby women's health clinic; it involved forming support groups, which would hold monthly meetings, to try out various nondrug self-help strategies

"At my first meeting, I found that most of the other women were experiencing similar

symptoms and feelings," she later recalled. "Just knowing I was not alone was reassuring." The doctor and nurse-practitioner conducting the study reviewed medical treatments for PMS, such as hormones, sleeping pills, diuretics, and tranquilizers, pointing out their potential benefits and risks. Members were then given brochures listing the many PMS symptoms and alternative and self-help strategies.

Tanner noted that evening primrose oil and vitamin E were recommended for achiness and joint pain; yoga, meditation, and vitamin B_6 for emotional swings; dietary changes for bloating; and exercise to counter depression.

"There were so many options, I didn't know where to start," Tanner recalls. She was advised to try a regimen for three cycles

to help the worst symptoms. "If you don't notice an improvement, devise a different regimen," the nurse-practitioner said. "That way, you can tell what helps."

Tanner was most troubled by emotional swings, so she began taking yoga. "I was amazed to notice an improvement after just one month," she says. "The support group sessions were also helpful."

Tanner also decided to try evening primrose oil. She then cut back on salt to help ease fluid retention. Her diet was short on dairy products, so she started taking a calcium supplement. After six months, she described her improvement at one of the group sessions. "I know I've adopted a healthier lifestyle, and maybe this accounts for my reduced PMS. The important thing is, what I'm doing seems to be working!"

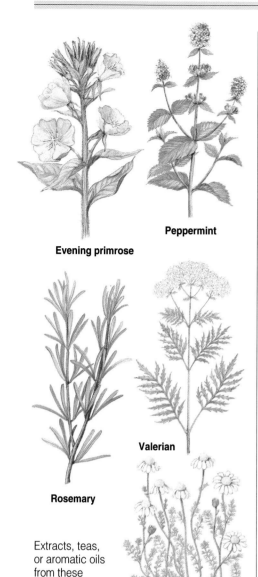

Peppermint

Evening primrose

Valerian

Rosemary

Extracts, teas, or aromatic oils from these herbs have been shown to help ease at least some PMS symptoms.

Chamomile

in more than 70 percent of patients. The recommended dosage is two 250-milligram tablets after breakfast and dinner beginning three days before the expected onset of symptoms and continuing until menstruation starts.

Women who are not helped by evening primrose oil may respond to dong quai capsules. This herb, sometimes called the female ginseng, is used by Chinese herbalists to treat various gynecologic disorders.

Teas or infusions of valerian, skullcap, raspberry leaves, sarsaparilla, and squaw vine, are also said to alleviate PMS. Drinking a cup of peppermint tea

after eating may help prevent digestive problems linked to the condition.
Homeopathy. Practitioners use sepia to treat PMS symptoms.
Hypnotherapy. Self-hypnosis can be helpful for controlling stress, fear, and pain, especially when practiced at the onset of symptoms.
Naturopathy and Nutrition Therapy. A common dietary approach calls for reducing intake of calories, caffeine, sugar, and salt for two weeks before menstruation. The suggested diet emphasizes fresh fruits and vegetables, whole-grain cereals and breads, beans, peas, lentils, nuts, and seeds. Red meat may be eliminated in favor of fish and skinless chicken or turkey. Small, frequent meals possibly help to reduce digestive problems. Likewise, cutting back on dietary fat may ease indigestion and reduce bloating.

Vitamin therapy is widely used in addition to dietary changes, but as with most approaches to PMS, its success varies from one woman to another. Vitamin B_6 supplements help some; others appear to benefit from extra vitamin E, calcium, or magnesium. Be cautious about using vitamin B_6. High doses may cause nerve damage, which is characterized by tingling in the fingers and toes.
Yoga. The corpse pose (lying on the back, legs apart, with arms at the side and palms up) may reduce the severity and duration of PMS symptoms when practiced at their onset .
Self-Treatment
Self-care entails trial and error to find out what works best. You can experiment with the alternative therapies outlined above. Often, simply recognizing that mood swings and other symptoms are a natural aspect of your menstrual cycle—and not a sign of mental illness—makes them easier to deal with.

You may be able to avoid crying spells and emotional swings by anticipating certain reactions and steering clear of stressful situations that invariably trigger negative feelings. Plan to do things that are calming and pleasurable during your premenstrual phase, saving more stressful activities for the early part of your cycle. If you suffer from PMS insomnia, set aside time for an afternoon nap. In general, make every effort to get plenty of rest during the two weeks before menstruation. Also, avoid alcohol during these two

weeks. Studies have shown that a number of women have a reduced tolerance for alcohol at this time.

Many women find that regular aerobic exercise relieves or reduces PMS symptoms. During exercise, the brain produces extra endorphins, which are natural mood elevators and painkillers; thus a good workout may alleviate both emotional and physical responses.

If the problem persists, consider joining a self-help group comprised of fellow PMS sufferers. Many medical centers and women's health clinics offer special PMS programs.
Other Causes of PMS Symptoms
Because symptoms are so numerous, one or another can be associated with virtually any medical condition. Some of the mood changes and other emotional symptoms mimic those of other psychological disorders. However, if these symptoms occur only during the premenstrual period they indicate PMS, not a mental disorder. The same can be said of physical symptoms. If one or more persists throughout the menstrual cycle, the cause is probably not PMS and should be evaluated by a physician.

COMMON MANIFESTATIONS OF PMS

Physical symptoms may include:
▶ Breast swelling and tenderness.
▶ Abdominal bloating, discomfort, and perhaps constipation.
▶ Headaches, especially migraines.
▶ Backache and cramps.
▶ Dizziness.
▶ Digestive disorders.
▶ Swelling of feet, ankles, and hands.
▶ Joint and muscle pain.
▶ Palpitations.
▶ Urinary frequency.
▶ Increased thirst.
▶ Reduced tolerance to alcohol.
▶ Flare-up of acne.

Psychological symptoms may include:
▶ Food cravings, especially for sweets and salt.
▶ Feelings of tension or anxiety.
▶ Mood swings.
▶ Crying spells.
▶ Irritability.
▶ Lethargy.
▶ Fatigue.
▶ Depression.
▶ Insomnia or increased sleepiness.
▶ Forgetfulness or mental confusion.
▶ Panic attacks.
▶ Aggressive or violent behavior.

Prostate Cancer

(Prostatic adenocarcinoma)

With about 244,000 new cases in the United States each year, prostate cancer is the most common type of malignancy in men and, with 44,000 deaths a year, second only to lung cancer in male cancer mortality. According to the American Cancer Society, about 1 in 11 men develops prostate cancer, usually after age 65, and the risk becomes greater with age. International studies link a high-fat diet to increased risk, but what triggers the cancer is unknown. It appears that certain population groups are more vulnerable than others. For example, the incidence of prostate cancer among African-American men is 32 percent higher than in Caucasions.

Early signs of prostate cancer include difficulty in starting urination, inability to empty the bladder fully, and frequent urination, especially at night. There may also be pain or burning during urination, blood in urine, and dull, chronic pain in the lower back, pelvis, or upper thighs.

Diagnostic Studies and Procedures

The American Cancer Society recommends that all men over the age of 40 undergo annual screening for prostate cancer, starting with a digital rectal examination. For this test, a doctor inserts a gloved finger into the rectum and then feels the gland for unusual hardness or lumps. The same group also advocates that a blood test to measure prostate specific antigen (PSA, a substance secreted by prostate cells) should be done annually in addition to the digital exam, beginning at the age of 50. An elevated PSA level indicates an enlarged prostate, which is a sign of possible cancer.

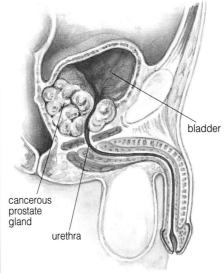

Prostate cancer produces hard lumps, or nodules, that can be felt by a doctor during a rectal examination.

labels: bladder / cancerous prostate gland / urethra

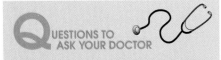

QUESTIONS TO ASK YOUR DOCTOR

▶ Will treatment with female hormones cause feminization? What body changes should I expect?
▶ If my testicles are removed, will I still be able to have sexual relations? Will I develop a high voice and other female characteristics?
▶ Should I arrange to store my sperm in a sperm bank so that I can father children if I become sterile as a result of surgery or radiation?

If either test produces suspicious results, a transrectal ultrasound examination, CT scan, or MRI may be ordered to detect any tumors. But none of these tests actually confirms prostate cancer; this requires a biopsy of tissue from suspicious areas of the gland. If cancer is detected, bone scans and other tests are necessary to determine whether or not it has spread.

Medical Treatments

Treatment varies, depending upon the type and stage of the cancer and the patient's age. Surgery to remove the prostate gland—a prostatectomy—can cure localized prostate cancer in more than 90 percent of cases. New surgical techniques usually make it possible to preserve the man's sexual function and urinary continence as well.

In some cases, surgery may be followed by radiation. Radiation therapy by itself is successful in men with certain early stages of prostate cancer.

Hormone treatment, using female hormones such as estrogen to suppress male hormones that the cancer cells need for growth, and chemotherapy with anticancer drugs, may control prostate cancer for long periods. Orchiectomy, removal of the testicles, may be performed to slow cancer growth spurred by testosterone.

Alternative Therapies

The following alternative therapies may be helpful adjuncts to medical treatment for controlling pain, maintaining a healthful nutritional status, and alleviating anxiety.

Acupuncture and Acupressure. These techniques are especially useful for controlling pain.

Hydrotherapy. To increase circulation in the prostate region and also alleviate pain, sitting in a hot tub is sometimes recommended. Yet another technique involves sitting in hot water while immersing the feet in cold water for three minutes, then reversing the process for three more minutes.

Imagery or Visualization. Practitioners teach patients to picture their bodies fighting and overcoming the disease.

Nutrition Therapy. Because studies have linked a high-fat diet to an increased risk of prostate cancer, a low-fat, mostly vegetarian diet may help prevent it. Fruits, vegetables, nuts and seeds, dried beans, peas, brown rice, and fresh juices should be emphasized. Some nutritionists advocate abstaining from coffee, tea, and alcohol, although a specific association of these beverages with prostate cancer has not been established. Eating an ounce of pumpkin seeds daily or taking pumpkin seed oil capsules is said to be helpful for all types of prostate problems. Pumpkin seeds are high in zinc, and deficiency of this mineral has been linked to prostate inflammation.

Self-Treatment

There is very little you can do to treat prostate cancer on your own. However, you can reduce your risk of developing it by adopting the low-fat diet described above and maintaining your ideal body weight.

If you are diagnosed with prostate cancer and are concerned about the effects of treatment on sexual function, discuss your options with your doctor. New methods of removing the prostate reduce the likelihood of impotence, but you may have to seek out a surgeon trained in the procedure.

Even when sexual function is preserved, a prostatectomy alters the route of ejaculation, sending the semen backward into the bladder instead of forward into the penis. This does not affect sexual pleasure for either party, but if conception is desired, artificial insemination will be necessary.

Other Causes of Prostate Symptoms

Prostate enlargement (benign prostatic hypertrophy) and prostatitis, an infection of the prostate, produce symptoms similar to those of prostate cancer.

Prostate Enlargement

(Benign prostatic hypertrophy; BPH)
About one-third of all men over age 50 experience noncancerous enlargement of the prostate gland, the result of a gradual process that can eventually cause severe obstruction of urinary flow. The prostate gland surrounds the neck of the male bladder and the urethra, the tube that carries urine from the bladder during voiding. Why it enlarges with age is not completely understood. Some theorize that chronic inflammation of the prostate may cause the enlargement; others suggest nutritional or metabolic factors play a role.

An enlarged prostate presses against the urethra and sometimes the bladder, preventing the bladder from emptying completely. Typically, an older man notices that he needs to urinate more often, the flow is slow to start, and the stream is weak, with dribbling at the end of voiding. There may also be pain and burning during urination, especially if the prostate is pressing against the urethral canal. If stagnant urine collects in the bladder, it increases the risk of urethritis (page 429) and bladder stones (page 100). More severe blockage can cause urine to back up to the kidneys, damaging those organs.

Diagnostic Studies and Procedures
Two tests are useful in diagnosing benign prostatic enlargement. One is a digital rectal examination, during which a doctor palpates the prostate with a gloved finger inserted into the rectum, feeling it for enlargement and unusual hardness or lumps that may suggest the presence of cancer.

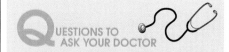

QUESTIONS TO ASK YOUR DOCTOR

▶ Am I a candidate for Proscar? If so, are there side effects I should watch for?
▶ If I have prostate surgery, am I likely to experience sexual problems? Will the operation prevent prostate cancer?

The other is a relatively new blood test that measures levels of prostate specific antigen (PSA), a substance normally produced by prostate tissue. In 30 to 50 percent of men with prostate enlargement, the PSA is elevated; the test is considered worthwhile because it can screen for prostate cancer. Blood for the test should be drawn before the digital rectal examination because palpating the prostate may produce a misleading temporary rise in PSA levels.

Other diagnostic studies may include placing a catheter in the bladder to measure the amount of urine remaining after voiding; an ultrasound examination; and cystoscopy, the insertion of a viewing tube into the bladder. A biopsy may be ordered to rule out cancer.

Medical Treatments
Initial therapy may involve medication to treat the urinary infections and kidney problems that frequently accompany an enlarged prostate. A bladder catheter may be necessary if the urinary flow is obstructed.

Until recently, the only treatment for the condition itself was surgery, usually transurethral resection of the prostate, or TURP. For this procedure, the surgeon uses a cytoscope (flexible tube) to reach the prostate through the urethra and then inserts a scalpel-like device through the tube to snip away overgrown prostate tissue. Most men who undergo this procedure remain in the hospital for about three days. The operation usually provides long-term relief from the symptoms of prostate enlargement, but there is about a 10 percent risk of impotence, and some 60 to 70 percent of patients lose the ability to ejaculate from the penis. Instead, they develop a retrograde

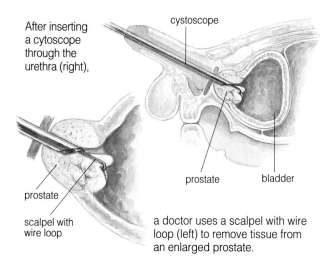

After inserting a cytoscope through the urethra (right), a doctor uses a scalpel with wire loop (left) to remove tissue from an enlarged prostate.

ejaculation, in which they ejaculate semen into the bladder. This does not affect the ability to have an orgasm, but it does impair fertility.

A new drug, finasteride (Proscar), that shrinks the overgrown prostate when taken long-term now offers an alternative to surgery for some men. Experimental treatments include dilation of the portion of the urethra surrounded by the prostate, a method similar to the balloon angioplasty used to open clogged arteries.

Alternative Therapies
Herbal Medicine. Parsley and corn silk teas are popular herbal remedies advocated for alleviating mild prostate problems. An extract of saw palmetto berry is said to inhibit production of dihydrotestosterone, a body chemical that may be instrumental in prostatic enlargement. Herbalists also claim that ginseng can shrink an enlarged prostate.
Hydrotherapy. Warm sitz baths taken for 3 to 10 minutes two or three times a day may relieve symptoms, at least temporarily. Water temperature should be 105° to 115°F (40.5° to 46°C).
Naturopathy and Nutrition Therapy. Because zinc deficiency has been linked to prostate inflammation and enlargement, supplements of zinc may be advocated both to prevent and alleviate an enlarged prostate. Some nutritionists also recommend taking 1 teaspoon of flax, evening primrose, or walnut oil a day. Drinking two to four ounces of coconut milk daily is also said to tone the prostate gland.

It's a good idea to drink at least 8 to 10 glasses of water or other clear fluids a day. You should, however, be sure to avoid alcohol and caffeine.

Self-Treatment
You cannot prevent the development of an enlarged prostate. You should, however, avoid certain drugs that worsen the problem, including cold and allergy pills, which can cause urinary retention. Some prescription drugs, including medications used to treat ulcers, irritable bowel syndrome, and depression, may have a similar effect.

Urinate when you first feel the urge, rather than delaying. Avoid sexual stimulation and arousal without ejaculation.

Other Causes of Prostate Symptoms
Prostate inflammation and prostate cancer produce symptoms similar to those of enlarged prostate; both should be ruled out in the diagnostic process.

Prostatitis

(Acute or chronic bacterial prostatitis; chronic nonbacterial prostatitis)

Prostatitis is an infection or inflammation of the prostate. This is the plum-shaped gland that surrounds the neck of the male bladder and urethra, the tube that transports urine during voiding.

Symptoms of prostatitis include low back pain and an urgent and frequent need to urinate, even during the night, with difficulty in starting the urine flow and in emptying the bladder completely. Urination and ejaculation often produce pain or burning; there also may be blood and bacteria in the urine. Acute bacterial prostatitis is often accompanied by chills, fever, and achy joints and muscles.

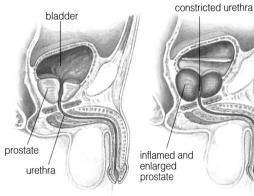

A normal prostate surrounds the urethra, but does not obstruct urinary flow.

An inflamed and enlarged prostate can constrict the urethra and trap urine.

Of the two basic types, chronic non-bacterial prostatitis is the more common; its cause is unknown. Bacterial prostatitis, which can be chronic or acute, is often due to organisms found in feces. These may reach the prostate through the bloodstream, the lymph system, or the urethra. Young men and those with urinary catheters are most often affected. There has been speculation that a vasectomy increases vulnerability to prostatitis, but this has not been established.

Diagnostic Studies and Procedures

Generally, several urine samples will be obtained—one from the beginning of the first voiding of the day, a second from urination at midstream, and a third following examination and massaging of the prostate. These will be studied for the presence of white blood cells and also cultured for bacteria.

A doctor will perform a digital rectal exam by inserting a gloved finger into the rectum to palpate the prostate. Pain experienced during this examination indicates that the prostate is inflamed. The gland itself may feel swollen and warm, and gently massaging it may force prostate secretions into the penis. A culture of these secretions can also determine whether or not the cause is bacterial and, if so, identify the infecting organism. An ultrasound examination and other diagnostic tests may be performed to rule out cancer.

Medical Treatments

Acute bacterial prostatitis is most often treated with antibiotics, usually trimethoprim and sulfamethoxazole (Bactrim, Septra, and others) or a cephalosporin. Treatment, which may include both the oral and intravenous forms, is sometimes continued for 30 days or longer in order to prevent chronic prostatitis.

If the prostate is so swollen that it blocks urinary flow, the bladder may be drained with a procedure called cystostomy, in which a surgical opening is made into the bladder just above the pubic bone. Cystostomy is preferred to catheterization (inserting of a tube), as the latter carries the risk of introducing bacteria into the urethra.

Hospitalization might be necessary in serious cases, especially if bacteria have invaded the bloodstream. Occasionally, surgery may be required to drain an abscess of the prostate or even to remove part of the gland.

Chronic bacterial prostatitis almost always involves recurring urinary tract infections. Antibiotics are usually prescribed, but even prolonged treatment often does not eradicate the source of the infection.

Chronic nonbacterial prostatitis is quite difficult to treat, although some patients do benefit from antibiotics. In such cases, researchers theorize that chlamydia or some other sexually transmitted organism may be responsible for the infection, but evidence for this is lacking. As a rule, treatment is aimed at alleviating symptoms with painkillers and anticholinergic drugs, agents that relax the muscles and block spasms that cause pain and retention of urine in the bladder.

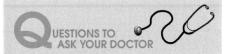

Alternative Therapies

Certain alternative therapies can ease symptoms of prostatitis and may help prevent recurrent attacks.

Herbal Medicine. The extract and flower pollens of saw palmetto are popular European herbal remedies for prostatitis and they are gaining popularity among American herbalists. A decoction made by simmering equal amounts of gravel root, sea holly, and hydrangea root is said to alleviate chronic prostatitis. Buchu, a diuretic herb, also may be beneficial. Goldenseal root, parsley, juniper berries, uva-ursi, slippery elm bark, and ginseng are all used by Western herbalists to help relieve the symptoms of prostate problems.

Hydrotherapy. Sitting in a hot tub, particularly a whirlpool bath, is helpful in alleviating the discomfort of nonbacterial prostatitis. The usual procedure is to sit in 6 to 8 inches of warm to hot water for about 15 minutes at least three times a day.

Naturopathy and Nutrition Therapy. It's best to avoid alcohol, caffeine, and spicy foods, which cause bladder and urethral irritation and can further aggravate prostatitis. Some nutritionists advise eliminating acidic foods such as tomatoes. They may also recommend zinc supplements or unsweetened cranberry juice, especially for chronic prostatitis accompanied by cystitis.

Self-Treatment

Drinking two to three quarts of water daily will stimulate urine flow and help prevent cystitis, inflammation of the urinary bladder. Bed rest is important during an acute attack. Aspirin, acetaminophen, or ibuprofen can be taken to alleviate pain.

Doctors generally advise abstaining from sexual intercourse until symptoms have disappeared completely.

Other Causes of Urinary Symptoms

An enlarged prostate and prostate cancer produce symptoms similar to those of prostatitis. Urethritis and cystitis also can cause difficult and painful urination.

Protozoal Infections

Caused by protozoa, a class of single-cell parasites, protozoal infections are common in rural areas of underdeveloped countries in Africa, Asia, and South America. They are relatively rare in the United States and other industrialized nations, but do occur among Western travelers to Third World countries. Such infections include:

Amebiasis, which can infect the skin, intestines, liver, lungs, and chest cavity; it is caused by *Entamoeba histolytica.*

Babesiosis, an infection of the red blood cells that can lead to hemolytic anemia; it is caused by *Babesia* organisms that are transmitted by ticks.

Cryptosporidiosis, an intestinal infection that is usually self limiting, but can be life-threatening to an AIDS patient; its cause is *Cryptosporidium.*

Giardiasis, an intestinal infection that often produces diarrhea; it is caused by *Giardia lamblia,* an organism contracted by drinking water contaminated with animal and human waste.

Leishmaniasis, an infection of the skin, mucous membranes, or internal organs, depending on the cause; it is brought on by any of several *Leishmania* protozoa carried by sand flies. Kala-Azar, which produces recurrent fever and severe weight loss, and cutaneous leishmaniasis, which causes boils and skin ulcers, are among the more common types of this illness.

Trypanosomiasis, or African sleeping sickness, an often fatal disease; its cause is *Trypanosoma,* which is spread by tsetse flies. A South American variation, called Chagas disease, is spread by assassin, or kissing reduviid, bugs and is generally milder.

Diagnostic Studies and Procedures

Characteristic symptoms and recent travel to a developing country may lead a doctor to suspect a protozoal infection, but identifying the organism is often difficult. Analyses of blood, urine, stool, and perhaps stomach juices and other body fluids are needed.

Medical Treatments

Treatment will depend on the infecting organism. Metronidazole (Flagyl) is usually the first choice for an uncomplicated case of amebiasis or giardiasis. This drug, which is given orally or by injection for 5 to 10 days, often causes nausea, loss of appetite, abdominal pain, and dark urine. It is important to abstain from alcohol while taking it.

Giardiasis may also be treated with quinacrine (Atabrine), a drug used to treat malaria (page 284). Babesiosis is usually treated with intravenous clindamycin, an antibiotic, and quinine, an antimalaria drug.

Cryptosporidiosis can be difficult to treat, especially if a patient's immune system is weakened by other diseases or drugs. Sometimes, strengthening the immune system by stopping immunosuppressive drugs and correcting any nutritional deficiencies aids healing.

African trypanosomiasis is treated with intravenous eflornithine (DFMO), an antiprotozoal drug. An alternative is melarsoprol, which is more potent but also more dangerous because it contains arsenic and can damage the kidneys. Suramin and pentamidine, an antiprotozoal drug, may be prescribed to treat leishmaniasis.

Other treatments are directed to controlling symptoms and manifestations of the disease, and may include blood transfusions and intravenous fluids.

Alternative Therapies

No alternative therapy can cure a protozoal infection, but when used alongside the appropriate medical treatment, some can alleviate symptoms.

Herbal Medicine. Meadowsweet is commonly recommended to control all types of diarrhea. For acute attacks, herbalists prescribe a tea made with a mixture of equal parts meadowsweet, American cranesbill, and bayberry, to be consumed hourly until the symptoms subside, and then before meals until the digestive system returns to normal. A glass of unsweetened black

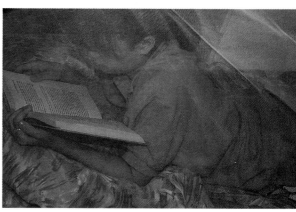
Covering sleeping areas with protective netting can help prevent protozoal infections carried by insects in endemic areas.

currant juice three times a day is an alternative remedy. Other herbs used to treat diarrhea include teas made from raspberry leaves or chamomile.

A poultice of echinacea root may be used to lower a fever. Other treatments for fever include a tea made from a mixture of hyssop, licorice root, thyme, and yarrow, and tea made with blackthorn, fenugreek seed, feverfew, ginger, poke root, or echinacea.

Homeopathy. Practitioners use podophyllum, several times a day, to treat severe chronic diarrhea.

Naturopathy and Nutrition Therapy. Extra fluids are advised, especially distilled water and vegetable juices, to protect against dehydration caused by diarrhea and fever. In severe cases, rehydration fluids (see page 161) or Gatorade may be needed to restore the electrolyte balance. As the diarrhea subsides, a patient can resume solid foods with the BRAT diet of bananas, rice, applesauce, and toast. Coffee, alcohol, milk, and spicy or fatty foods should be avoided.

Self-Treatment

Prevention is the best approach. If you are spending time outdoors or sleeping in infested places, wear clothing with long sleeves and pants legs, and cover your sleeping area with mosquito netting. Drink, cook with, and brush teeth with bottled or boiled water; wash your hands often, and always before meals.

Other Causes of Protozoal Infections

Other protozoal infections that occur in the United States include toxoplasmosis, which is transmitted by eating undercooked meat or by contact with cat feces; trichinosis, from eating infected pork; and trichomoniasis, a sexually transmitted disease.

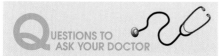
QUESTIONS TO ASK YOUR DOCTOR

▶ Can you contract giardia by swimming in contaminated lakes or rivers?
▶ Can protozoal infections be transmitted through intimate contact?

Psoriasis

Psoriasis is a recurrent disorder in which patches of skin become red and covered by dry, silvery scales. About 5 million Americans have the condition, which usually develops during young adulthood through late middle age. Although psoriasis is seldom serious medically, the unsightly lesions can lead to emotional problems.

Normally, the skin is in a constant state of renewal, with new cells forming in the dermis, or inner layer, and pushing upward into the epidermis, which sheds the old, dead cells. With psoriasis, the skin makes new cells so fast that they form silvery scales. Then, new blood vessels are created to nourish these immature cells, resulting in the typical reddening of the skin.

The initial patches typically form on the scalp, behind the ears, on the back of the neck, between the shoulders, and on elbows and knees or near fingernails and toenails. Some patients also develop psoriatic arthritis, a potentially crippling joint disorder that resembles rheumatoid arthritis. In unusual cases, the entire body is covered with red, scaly patches, a variation called exfoliative psoriasis. Another form, pustular psoriasis, is characterized by blisters, usually on the palms and soles.

The cause of psoriasis is unknown, but it is thought to be an autoimmune disorder, perhaps with an inherited predisposition. The condition tends to wax and wane, with symptoms often disappearing for months or even years at a time. Recurrences can be triggered by a severe sunburn, a reaction to a medication, an injury, or stress.

Diagnostic Studies and Procedures

Diagnosis is usually made by inspecting the skin for the typical layers of dry, silvery scales, but a skin biopsy may be ordered in some cases. If joints are painful and inflamed, X-rays and blood studies will be done. The absence of rheumatoid factor in the blood serum distinguishes psoriatic arthritis from rheumatoid arthritis.

Medical Treatments

If only small patches of skin are affected, self-treatment or application of a prescription-strength corticosteroid ointment may be effective. Calcipotriene (Dovonex), a topical drug derived from vitamin D, appears promising in slowing the growth of new skin cells.

Severe cases can benefit from photochemotherapy, a treatment in which the skin is exposed to ultraviolet A light rays following administration of psoralen, an oral medication that enhances the healing potential of the light. This approach is known as PUVA, an acronym for psoralen plus ultraviolet A.

Very severe conditions may be treated with anticancer drugs, such as methotrexate, which slow the production of new cells. Etretinate (Tegison), an antipsoriatic drug, or isotretinoin (Accutane), a derivative of vitamin A used to treat severe cystic acne, are effective against pustular psoriasis.

Alternative Therapies

Herbal Medicine. Herbalists and naturopaths recommend applications of a mixture of lavender and olive oils, or bergamot and comfrey oils, to the scaly patches. Yarrow oil added to bath water is also said to help reduce scaling. A combination of the tinctures of burdock, sarsaparilla, and cleavers in equal parts, taken in doses of 1 teaspoon three times a day, may also be helpful.

Hydrotherapy. Warm compresses applied to affected skin for several minutes each day may be soothing. Some people with severe psoriasis have traveled to the Dead Sea area in Israel for special water and sun treatment. Sunbathing in this locale is beneficial because of its unique geography, 1,300 feet below sea level. At this altitude, the concentration of ultraviolet A light rays is higher than anywhere else on earth. Salt and mud mixtures from this region are also sold as treatments for psoriasis.

Meditation. Because stress is known to provoke psoriasis, this and other relaxation techniques can be preventive.

Nutrition Therapy. Although it has not been proved that psoriasis is related to food allergies or sensitivities, some people appear to benefit from dietary changes. To identify possible offenders, eliminate a food or group of foods for a few weeks to see if there is any improvement. Then return the food to the

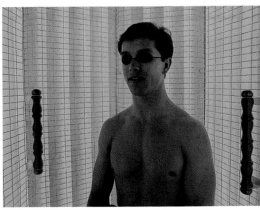
Protecting the eyes is essential during PUVA, the combination of psoralen drugs and exposure to ultraviolet A rays.

diet; if it produces a flare-up, it may well play a role in triggering psoriasis.

High doses of vitamin D have been found effective for treating psoriasis. Because this approach is still experimental, patients should not attempt to treat themselves with it.

Self-Treatment

Mild cases often can be controlled with diligent self-care that includes regular use of lubricants such as white petrolatum or a vegetable shortening. Using an oatmeal soap and adding a cup of sea salt to bath water may also help.

If scaling persists, nonprescription cortisone cream or coal tar ointments, creams, or shampoos, such as Pentrax lotion, P&S Plus gel, or Sebutone cream or solution, can be tried. Their use should be checked beforehand with a dermatologist, but a typical regimen calls for applying the cream or lotion at night, covering it with plastic wrap, washing it off in the morning, and then exposing the skin to the sun or artificial ultraviolet light.

Thick scalp plaques can be treated with overnight applications of a solution of mineral oil and 10 percent salicylic acid. To enhance the effectiveness and keep the preparation off bedding, wear a shower cap to bed.

Judicious exposure to the sun often helps, but care is needed because too much sun can worsen psoriasis.

Other Causes of Skin Scaling

Seborrheic dermatitis (dandruff), can cause scalp scaling, though the lesions are usually greasy and yellow. Other conditions that should be ruled out include squamous cell skin cancer, dermatitis, fungal infections, eczema, and lichen planus, a recurrent itchy rash.

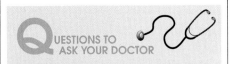
QUESTIONS TO ASK YOUR DOCTOR

▶ Could I benefit from PUVA treatments?
▶ Are my joint pains related to psoriasis? How should they be treated?

Pulmonary Embolism

(Thromboembolism)

A pulmonary embolism occurs when an artery in the lung becomes obstructed, usually by a clot, or embolus. Most often, the clot forms in a deep vein of the leg or pelvic area and a piece breaks away, traveling through the venous system and heart and into the lungs. Less commonly, the obstruction may be due to a globule of fat that enters the bloodstream following a fracture.

Symptoms and complications vary depending on the site of the obstruction and the extent of impaired lung function. Chest pain, breathlessness, and shallow breathing are typical early signs, combined sometimes with lightheadedness and agitation or restlessness. Life-threatening deterioration is signaled by worsening pain, especially when coughing or taking a deep breath; blood-streaked sputum; a rapid heartbeat; heavy perspiration; and the onset of shock.

Many conditions promote the development of a pulmonary embolism, including heart failure, stroke, obesity, thrombophlebitis, and leg or hip fractures. Prolonged bed rest, especially after surgery, increases the risk, as does use of birth control pills by women who smoke or have a history of phlebitis or other clotting disorders.

Pulmonary hypertension, increased blood pressure in the lung, is a potential complication, especially if the embolism blocks blood flow to 30 percent or more of a lung. A deadly complication is pulmonary infarction, in which part of the lung dies and is replaced with scar tissue. Fortunately, this does not happen often because clots begin to dissolve, or lyse, almost immediately after reaching the lungs.

About 500,000 Americans suffer pulmonary embolisms each year, with a mortality rate of about 10 percent. Before age 45, the condition is somewhat more common in women, but after that age, the incidence is about equally divided between the sexes.

Diagnostic Studies and Procedures

If a doctor suspects a pulmonary embolism, an immediate chest X-ray and lung scan will be ordered. A pulmonary angiogram, an X-ray of the lungs' blood vessels after injection of an opaque dye, will provide a definitive diagnosis. Doppler ultrasound, a test that uses high-frequency sound waves to study blood flow, also may be performed to locate the clot.

Medical Treatments

An individual experiencing a massive pulmonary embolism is hospitalized and immediately placed in an intensive care unit where procedures are started to improve heart and lung function. Supplemental oxygen will be given to compensate for temporary reduction in lung function, and analgesics offered if pain is severe. When medical measures appear to be inadequate, emergency surgery may be considered to remove the obstructed portion of the lung.

Treatment concentrates on dissolving the blood clot and preventing the formation of new ones. Unless there are complications such as bleeding or a stroke, clot-dissolving (thrombolytic) drugs, such as streptokinase or tissue plasminogen activator (TPA), may be administered. To prevent new clots from forming, anticoagulant drugs such as intravenous heparin, perhaps combined with warfarin, may be given.

Complications, such as pulmonary hypertension and cardiac arrhythmias, are also treated with drugs. Antibiotics are prescribed if the embolus has resulted in a bacterial infection.

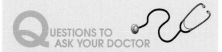
Alternative Therapies

Physical Therapy. Prolonged bed rest can lead to sluggish circulation and a pooling of blood in the legs, thus increasing the risk of clots. Early ambulation to increase circulation following surgery, a fracture, childbirth, or a serious illness is an important preventive measure. Even if a person cannot get up, a physical therapist can teach the patient ankle and leg movements and other exercises that can be done in bed. Patients who are unable to move themselves can benefit from passive exercises in which a caregiver physically moves their limbs.

Self-Treatment

As noted, regular exercise can help prevent clots from forming in the legs and elsewhere. Cycling is an especially good activity to promote leg circulation; so is walking. If your job involves sitting for long periods, get up and walk about every hour or so. Between walks, elevate your feet and legs by placing them on a stool under your desk. Interrupt long auto trips by stopping every hour or two for a brief walk, even if it means getting off a major highway. Similarly, during a long plane trip, take regular strolls in the aisle.

If you have varicose veins, talk to your doctor about prescription elastic stockings to help improve circulation.

If you have a history of thrombophlebitis or another condition that increases the risk of a pulmonary embolism, you may be instructed to take a daily aspirin to help prevent the formation of blood clots.

Other Causes of Lung Obstructions

An air bubble that enters the bloodstream during intravenous therapy or a transfusion can travel to the lungs and disrupt blood flow. Disorders to be ruled out in a diagnosis include septic shock, pericarditis, heart attack, congestive heart failure, and pneumonia, all of which produce symptoms similar to those of a pulmonary embolism.

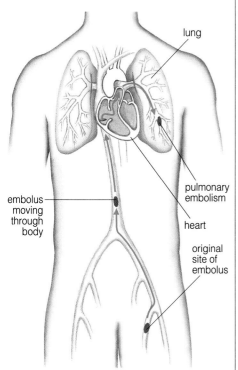

lung

embolus moving through body

pulmonary embolism

heart

original site of embolus

Most pulmonary emboli develop when a blood clot from the leg travels to the lungs.

Rabies

(Hydrophobia)

Rabies, or hydrophobia, is an acute, highly lethal viral disease that can affect the central nervous system of any warm-blooded animal, including humans. It is almost always transmitted through the bite of a rabid animal, although it can also be contracted if saliva containing the virus enters the body through an open sore, the eyes, or the mucous membranes of the mouth.

Once inside the body, the virus travels along nerves until it reaches the spinal cord and brain, where it multiplies, destroys tissue, and eventually causes paralysis and death. In humans, the average incubation period between exposure to the virus and onset of symptoms is 30 to 50 days, although it can range from 10 days to a year.

Typically, rabies begins with fever, headache, muscle aches, vomiting, and malaise, followed by uncontrollable agitation, drooling, and painful spasms of throat muscles, which prevent drinking despite tremendous thirst (hence the name hydrophobia). Death usually occurs from widespread paralysis that leads to suffocation.

The disease is found in all states except Hawaii; it also occurs in most other countries in both hemispheres. Worldwide, rabid dogs present the greatest risk, but in the United States, immunization has almost eradicated rabies in dogs and cats. The disease is widespread, however, among raccoons, skunks, foxes, and bats. Rabies has also been reported in squirrels, chipmunks, and other rodents. These animals rarely pose a threat to humans, but may infect an unimmunized pet.

RABIES IMMUNIZATION

Rabies immunization is recommended now for people at high risk. Included are veterinarians, animal handlers, cave explorers, and laboratory workers. Two types of vaccine are available for active immunization: human diploid cell rabies vaccine (HDCV) and rabies vaccine absorbed (RVA). HDCV is given in a series of three injections under the skin in the upper arm. RVA is administered as a single intramuscular injection. Testing for the antibodies is recommended every two years; a booster shot should be given to those with inadequate immunity.

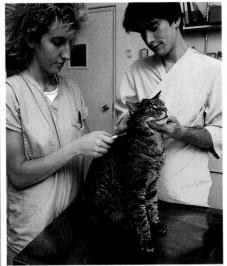

All domestic pets should have an annual rabies shot even if they don't go outdoors.

Diagnostic Studies and Procedures

Diagnosis centers on trying to determine whether or not a bite was inflicted by a rabid animal. If it came from a seemingly healthy cat, dog, or other pet, the animal should be given to a veterinarian or local health department for 10 days of observation and an antibody test. If the test is negative and the animal remains healthy, it can be assumed that the animal was not rabid and treatment is not necessary.

If the bite has been inflicted by a wild animal or a domestic animal that seems rabid or sick, the animal should be killed and its brain examined for signs of rabies. Only laboratory proof that the animal in question is not rabid justifies foregoing a course of preventive treatment for a person who has sustained a suspicious animal bite.

Medical Treatments

For Humans. Immediately wash the area several times with a strong antiseptic soap and warm water. Flush a deep puncture wound with soapy water. Then seek medical treatment, either in a hospital emergency room or from a private physician.

When a doctor has decided that preventive treatment is advisable, a series of shots will be given, usually beginning with rabies immune globulin or antirabies serum for passive immunization; this will be followed by active immunization with five or six injections, and then testing for immunity. The vaccine is usually injected into the arm muscle and may cause local swelling, itching, and other adverse reactions,

which can be minimized by taking antihistamines and other medications.

At one time, onset of rabies invariably ended in death. Recently, aggressive treatment to control symptoms that affect breathing, circulation, and the brain has resulted in a few survivals. *For Animals.* Wear protective gloves, wash the bite area thoroughly with soap and hot water, and take the animal to a veterinarian at once.

Alternative Therapies

There are no alternative therapies that can be used to prevent or treat rabies.

Self-Treatment

Health officials stress the importance of rabies immunization for all cats and dogs, as well as for horses and other domestic animals that might come in contact with a wild rabid animal. To further protect pets, keep cats indoors, and keep a dog on a leash or in a pen or fenced yard when outdoors.

In areas where rabies has been reported, try to avoid contact with stray cats and dogs and be alert for any wild animal that acts strangely. A rabid animal may be aggressive and attack people, animals, or objects. But sometimes the animal simply behaves strangely. For example, a bat, raccoon, or other normally nocturnal animal might come out during the day and appear friendly and unafraid of humans. It may have an unsteady gait and seem to be sick or disoriented; possibly, it will be drooling or foaming around the mouth, symptoms caused by jaw and throat paralysis.

If you suspect that an animal has rabies, do not attempt to catch it yourself. Instead, notify your local animal warden or health department so that the animal can be captured.

Other Causes of Rabies Symptoms

Hysteria following an animal bite can sometimes mimic rabies, but symptoms subside when the person is assured that the disease can be prevented.

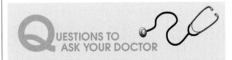

QUESTIONS TO ASK YOUR DOCTOR

▶ If my travel or work brings me in contact with rabid animals, what type of vaccine do you recommend?
▶ Why is it necessary to immunize my cats against rabies even though they never go outdoors?

Raynaud's Disease

(Secondary Raynaud's phenomenon)
Raynaud's (pronounced ray-nose) disease is a circulatory disorder characterized by spasms of the arteries that carry blood to the fingers and toes. Exposure to cold or emotional stress triggers the spasms; researchers theorize that the underlying mechanism may be similar to that of migraine headaches (page 298).

Typical symptoms are sensations of coldness, numbness, and tingling in the affected areas. There are also pronounced changes in color, ranging from pale pink or white due to reduced blood flow, to blue because of insufficient oxygen reaching the affected tissues, and finally, a deep red as extra blood rushes to the area. In about 10 percent of patients, the skin of affected fingers and toes becomes smooth, shiny, and tight due to a loss of underlying tissue. In severe cases, the blood vessels may thicken and become blocked by the formation of clots.

Raynaud's phenomenon was first described as a neurotic disorder in 1862 by the French physician for whom it is named. Doctors now recognize that there are two different forms of the disease. Primary, or idiopathic, Raynaud's, which has no identifiable cause, is comparatively mild and most common among young women. Secondary Raynaud's, which is potentially more serious, is always associated with some other ailment, such as a thyroid disorder, or is triggered by an identifiable circumstance, such as occupational hazards or the use of various drugs, including ergot medications.

Diagnostic Studies and Procedures

A doctor can usually diagnose Raynaud's disease and identify the type by asking detailed questions about the symptoms, the triggering circumstances, and other medical problems. A physical exam and blood and urine tests can help determine whether the condition is primary or secondary to some other disorder. The doctor will look for tissue damage, especially skin ulcers, and signs of arthritis or other connective tissue disease. He will also feel pulses in the hands and feet and note their response to cold.

In a diagnostic procedure called nailfold capillarioscopy, the skin at the base of the fingernails is viewed through a

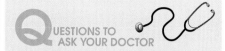

magnifying lens. The presence of abnormally large or deformed capillaries around the fingernails points to a connective tissue disease, such as scleroderma, a condition in which the skin thickens and hardens, or dermatomyositis, skin inflammation that can cause secondary Raynaud's.

Medical Treatments

Mild primary Raynaud's disease can usually be controlled with self-treatment or alternative therapies. If not, drugs that open, or dilate, the small arteries may be prescribed. Possible medications include prazosin (Minipress or Minizide) or nifedipine (Procardia or Adalat), agents more commonly used to treat high blood pressure. Promising results also have been reported from experimental use of pentoxifylline (Trental), a drug used to treat reduced blood flow to the legs.

Secondary Raynaud's usually can be alleviated by treating or removing the underlying cause. For example, if the spasms are due to ergot preparations, prescribed for migraine headaches, or beta blockers, often used to treat high blood pressure and angina, alternative medications can be substituted.

For severe cases, an operation called sympathectomy may be recommended. In this procedure, the small nerves serving the affected blood vessels are destroyed. Unfortunately, benefits are often temporary, and symptoms typically return in one to two years.

Alternative Therapies

Acupuncture. Studies at New York's Rusk Institute of Rehabilitation Medicine have demonstrated that acupuncture can increase blood flow and raise the temperature of hands and feet affected by Raynaud's disease. The symptoms may recur, however, and require repeated treatments.

Biofeedback Training. Most patients with primary Raynaud's disease can be taught to increase circulation to their extremities by using special electronic temperature sensors. The objective is

to learn to raise the temperature of the fingers and toes by increasing the flow of blood to these areas.

Meditation. Spasms triggered by stress can be alleviated by meditation and similar relaxation techniques.

Self-Treatment

Primary Raynaud's disease can usually be controlled by consistently protecting the hands and feet from cold. When the weather is even mildly chilly, wear woolen socks and mittens (or wool-lined gloves) and layers of garments for insulation and ease of movement. If your job or recreational pursuits require hours of outdoor exposure in cold weather, investigate battery-powered "hot" socks and chemical warmers that can be inserted into gloves and footwear. Wear cotton tights instead of nylon hose in cold weather, and make sure your shoes permit free movement of your toes. You may also need to wear mittens and warm socks to bed.

Handling cold objects often provokes spasms. Wear gloves to take items from a freezer or refrigerator, and cover a glass containing an iced drink with an insulator to protect your hands.

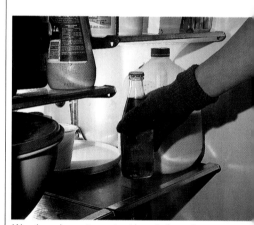

Wearing gloves to protect hands from the cold can prevent painful Raynaud's attacks.

If you smoke, make every effort to stop. Also, abstain from alcoholic beverages before going out into the cold.

Try this simple exercise to relieve circulatory spasms in your fingers: extend your arms straight out from the shoulders and swing them around energetically windmill fashion several times.

Other Causes of Cold Extremities

Secondary Raynaud's phenomenon may accompany scleroderma, carpal tunnel syndrome, rheumatoid arthritis, psoriasis, cancer, and lupus.

Renal Artery Disease

(Renal artery stenosis; renovascular hypertension)

In renal artery disease, one or both major arteries that supply blood to the kidneys become narrowed or obstructed, creating a progressive rise in blood pressure. If untreated, this condition can progress to such life-threatening problems as malignant hypertension, kidney failure, stroke, or heart attack. About 2 percent of all high blood pressure cases can be traced to this disease.

When arterial narrowing occurs in a child or young adult, it is usually due to a congenital defect or an overgrowth of fibrous muscle tissue, a condition referred to as fibromuscular dysplasia.

In older persons, atherosclerosis, a buildup of fatty deposits on the inner walls of the arteries, is the likely cause. Trauma or disorders such as sickle cell disease are responsible in some cases. Complete blockage may result from progression of untreated renal artery disease or a blood clot.

Generally, narrowing of the renal artery causes no symptoms other than a steady rise in blood pressure. If the artery becomes completely blocked, then there may be pain in the side or back, fever, nausea, vomiting, and blood in the urine.

Diagnostic Studies and Procedures

Because its early phase seldom produces symptoms, the condition is often found by chance when a doctor seeks a cause for an abrupt rise in blood pressure. Important clues are a particular kind of murmuring sound, or bruit,

heard through a stethoscope placed over the abdomen, and the presence of microscopic amounts of blood, protein, and white blood cells in the urine, indicating reduced kidney function. To confirm the diagnosis, imaging studies of the kidneys and related structures are needed, which may include:

Renal sonography, in which high-frequency sound waves provide images on the size and shape of the kidney. Doppler sonography is a variation that measures blood flow.

Intravenous pyelogram and renal angiography, in which X-rays of the renal circulation are taken after injection of a radioactive dye.

If renal artery disease is diagnosed, a captopril test may be performed to evaluate levels of renin, a chemical produced by the kidneys. Reduced blood flow to the kidneys increases its production, setting in motion a complex biochemical chain of events that raises blood pressure. The patient is given captopril, an antihypertensive agent that interrupts this process, and blood samples are taken repeatedly to measure changes in blood renin levels in response to the drug. The test helps doctors determine the best treatment.

Medical Treatments

Treatment varies according to the underlying problem. Balloon angioplasty may cure a congenital defect or fibromuscular dysplasia. In this procedure, a balloon-tipped catheter is inserted into the renal artery and the balloon inflated to widen the channel and increase blood flow. Angioplasty may be tried when atherosclerosis is causing the narrowing, but the success rate is not as high, especially if blockage is at or near the site where the renal artery branches off from the abdominal aorta.

Alternatively, a physician may recommend bypass surgery, in which a portion of healthy vein from a leg is used to bypass the narrowed artery and create a new passage for blood flowing from the heart to the kidney.

When a blood clot is occluding a renal artery, it may be

QUESTIONS TO ASK YOUR DOCTOR

▶ Can my renal artery disease be cured by angioplasty or surgery? If so, will my blood pressure return to normal?

removed surgically or dissolved with streptokinase or another fibrinolytic medication. Anticoagulants such as heparin, warfarin (Coumadin), or low-dose aspirin may be given to prevent new clots.

If these treatments are not feasible or fail to lower blood pressure, an angiotensin converting enzyme (ACE) inhibitor such as captopril (Capoten) will be prescribed (see page 230 for a discussion of these medications).

Alternative Therapies

Although the crisis of renal artery occlusion and rising blood pressure must be treated medically, alternative therapies can augment treatment by helping to reduce blood pressure.

Herbal Medicine. Garlic, fresh or in tablet form, can help prevent atherosclerosis by lowering blood cholesterol.

Meditation and Yoga. These can help lower blood pressure. Some therapists recommend assuming the yoga corpse pose (lying on the back, on a firm surface, with legs slightly spread and arms at the side) for 30 minutes each day. Avoid positions that require breath holding or isometric straining as they can raise blood pressure.

Nutrition Therapy. If renal artery disease has been caused by atherosclerosis, adopting a diet that restricts salt intake, is low in cholesterol and fat and high in soy protein, fiber, and starches can be very helpful. Studies indicate that vitamin E supplements reduce the risk of stroke, heart attack, and other complications of high blood pressure, probably by preventing clot formation.

Self-Treatment

There is no self-treatment for renal artery disease, but following a common-sense regimen that includes regular exercise and the diet recommendations described above can help prevent the type that results from atherosclerosis. Not smoking is important as well.

Other Causes of Renal Hypertension

Renal cancer and other tumors that press upon the renal artery can cause a rise in blood pressure.

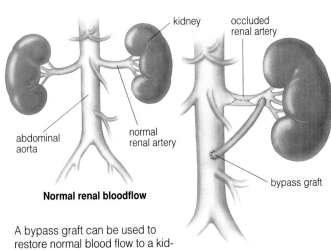

Normal renal bloodflow

A bypass graft can be used to restore normal blood flow to a kidney with a blocked renal artery. **Rerouted bloodflow**

Restless Leg Syndrome/ Leg Cramps

(Neurologic sleep disorder; muscle spasms)
When uncomfortable sensations prompt an irresistible urge to move one or both legs, the condition is known as restless leg syndrome. The feelings are centered usually in the calf, although the thighs and feet are sometimes affected as well. Symptoms occur when sitting or lying down, and are especially noticeable when trying to fall asleep. In fact, restless leg syndrome is medically classified as a neurological sleep disorder. A variation, myoclonic jerks, causes involuntary leg movements that disrupt sleep.

In most cases, the cause is unknown, but stress and heredity appear to be contributing factors. Neurologic conditions such as Parkinson's disease sometimes are associated with the syndrome.

A different type of discomfort is caused by leg cramps—painful, involuntary muscle contractions, or spasms, in the legs and feet. These occur when nerves send out excessive electrical charges and prompt a group of muscles to contract at the same time. As a rule, they last only a few minutes. Prolonged leg cramps, which occur mostly in the elderly or people with underlying neuromuscular disorders, can cause persistent muscle tenderness and even death (necrosis) of some muscle fibers.

Leg cramps can occur at any time, but are most common at night and sometimes interfere with sleep. Overexertion can bring them on; they are also linked often to pregnancy. Less common precipitating factors include nutritional deficiencies, dehydration, and electrolyte abnormalities, especially among patients who are on kidney dialysis.

Occasional leg cramps that abate within a few minutes are normal. Also normal is a sudden but painless jerk of the legs or body that occurs while falling asleep. Recurring or more troubling symptoms should be evaluated by a physician.

Diagnostic Studies and Procedures
Evaluations may include physical and neurological examinations, blood and urine studies, and electromyography, which measures the electrical activity of muscles. Patients may be advised to attend a sleep laboratory where they can be monitored by electronic devices and observed by sleep specialists.

Medical Treatments
Some physicians treat restless leg syndrome with clonazepam (Klonopin), a member of the benzodiazepine class of drugs that is usually prescribed for seizure disorders such as epilepsy. It is not fully understood how Klonopin alleviates restless legs, but all benzodiazepines subdue the central nervous system. They should never be used with tranquilizers, sleeping pills, or alcohol, however, because the combination might lead to an overdose. Long-term use of these medications can also result in mild drug dependence.

Quinine sulfate (Quinamm), was once recommended to alleviate leg cramps, but is no longer advocated by the FDA for this purpose, because it has produced severe adverse effects such as tinnitus, gastrointestinal bleeding, and even death.

Alternative Therapies
Acupressure. Firmly pinching the skin between the nose and the center of the upper lip for 30 seconds is reputed to dispel a leg cramp.
Biofeedback Training. Patients may use this technique to learn how to increase blood flow to the legs, thus alleviating both restless leg syndrome and recurrent cramps.
Meditation. The syndrome may be controlled by using this to reduce stress.
Nutrition Therapy. Some practitioners advise an increased intake of high-potassium foods such as bananas, tomatoes, citrus fruits, fresh vegetables, legumes, and whole grains. Studies have shown that daily supplements of 400 IU of vitamin E often reduce or eliminate nighttime leg cramps. Other supplements that may help are vitamins B_6 and C, calcium, and magnesium.

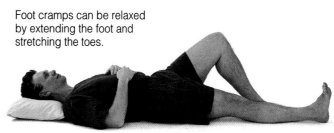

Foot cramps can be relaxed by extending the foot and stretching the toes.

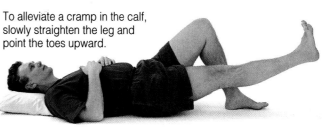

To alleviate a cramp in the calf, slowly straighten the leg and point the toes upward.

T'ai Chi and Yoga. These therapies improve muscle tone and ease restless leg syndrome and leg cramps.
Self-Treatment
Most leg cramps can be alleviated by massaging and stretching the muscle involved. If the cramp is in the calf, slowly straighten the leg and bend your foot upwards with toes pointing toward you. For a foot cramp, it usually helps to extend the foot and stretch the toes.

To avoid leg cramps brought on by post-exercise dehydration, drink a glass of water before working out and another 4 ounces every 20 minutes during vigorous activity. Try exercising early in the morning or in the evening to avoid becoming overheated.

If leg cramps awake you, try massaging the muscles before going to bed. Also, do the calf-stretch exercise shown on page 305. To ease leg cramps due to overexertion, sleep on your side with a pillow between your knees.

Taking a warm bath before bed can reduce the discomfort of restless legs.

Placing books or bricks under the foot of the bed to raise it a few inches can prevent restless legs by facilitating blood flow from the lower part of the body to the heart. If the weight of bed linens causes leg discomfort, fashion a frame to keep blankets off your legs.

To prevent leg cramps in the late stages of pregnancy, doctors advise sleeping on the left side with the knees drawn up to relieve nerve pressure.
Other Causes of Leg Cramps
Intermittent claudication, in which the arteries of the lower legs are blocked by fatty deposits, can cause cramps and leg pains during exercise. Diabetic neuropathy can cause sensations similar to those of restless leg syndrome.

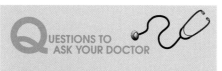

QUESTIONS TO ASK YOUR DOCTOR

▶ Would an evaluation in a sleep laboratory be helpful?
▶ Should I take vitamin supplements?

359

Retina Disorders

(Retinitis pigmentosa; retinopathy)

The retina, the thin membrane that lines the back of the eyeball, receives the images formed by the lens and transmits them to the optic nerve, an extension of the brain. Anything that interferes with the retina's ability to receive or transmit visual images can impair eyesight. A problem may originate in the membrane itself; examples are detached retina (page 157) and macular degeneration (page 282). It may also result from occlusion of blood flow to the retina due to glaucoma (page 205). The retinal disorders described below are either hereditary or are caused by other diseases.

Diabetic retinopathy. About half of the approximately 14 million Americans with diabetes have some degree of retinal impairment, with about 700,000 of them threatened by blindness. Diabetic retinopathy has two major manifestations: Macular edema, the most prevalent of the two, develops when the small retinal blood vessels leak fluid into the macula, the part of the retina responsible for clear vision. As the fluid accumulates, the macula swells and vision becomes blurred.

More serious, but much less common, is proliferative retinopathy, in which abnormal new blood vessels multiply on the surface of the retina. These vessels frequently rupture, forming scar tissue that blocks vision.

Retinitis pigmentosa. This inherited disorder leads to progressive destruction of the retina's rods and cones, the cells that send signals about light perception to the brain. The earliest symptom is a loss of normal nighttime vision. There is also a gradual loss of peripheral, or side, vision. Typically, the person has only tunnel vision by the age of 40 and may become blind within the following 20 years. Nearly 100,000 Americans and 1.5 million people worldwide have this disorder.

QUESTIONS TO ASK YOUR DOCTOR

- If I have diabetes, how often should I see my ophthalmologist?
- Is there a chance that laser treatments can damage the healthy parts of my eye?
- Could I benefit from high doses of vitamin A? If so, how long would I have to stay on this regimen?

Diagnostic Studies and Procedures

Retinal disorders are usually diagnosed by examining the eye with a lighted magnifying device, such as an ophthalmoscope. A doctor will first apply medicated eye drops to widen, or dilate, the pupil. By training the magnifying instrument through the enlarged pupil, he can inspect the retina and other eye structures for diabetes-related retinal changes, even before symptoms occur.

A doctor may also order fluorescein angiography, special X-rays of the eye's blood vessels taken after injecting dye into a vein to make them more visible.

Retinitis pigmentosa is often diagnosed early in life when a child complains of not being able to see clearly at night. Special tests are used to measure the eye's adaptation to the dark as well as any loss of the peripheral vision.

If a retinal problem is caused by a systemic disease, such as diabetes or high blood pressure, the patient will be referred to an internist or other primary-care physician for a complete physical examination that includes blood and urine studies. X-rays and a CT scan or MRI may also be ordered, especially if the patient recently suffered a head injury, a stroke, or a mini-stroke.

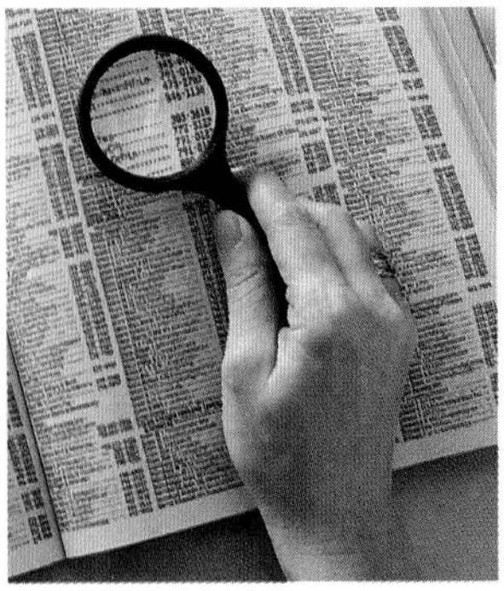

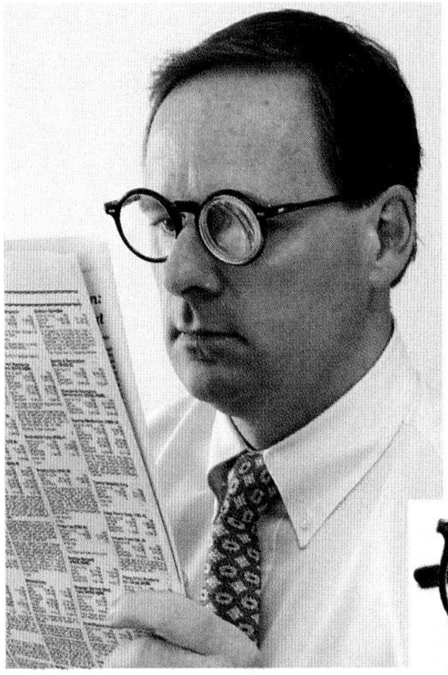

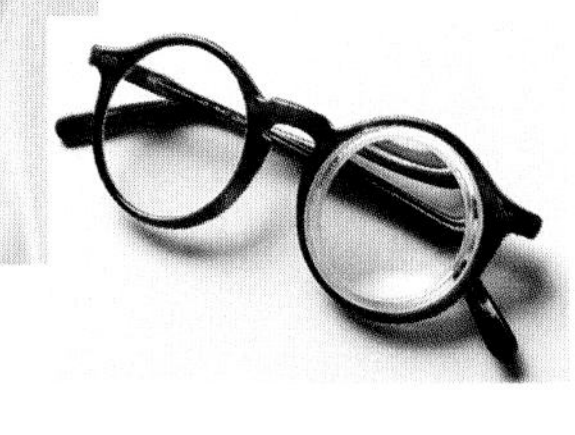

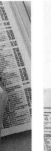

Special glasses and magnifying devices can help some patients with a damaged retina see well enough to read and carry out other daily activities. The glasses at the right have two distinctly different lenses, with one designed to compensate for retinal degeneration affecting the left eye.

Medical Treatments

Treatment varies according to the specific retinal disorder and its cause. Achieving good control of diabetes, high blood pressure, and other diseases that affect the eyes is essential.

Diabetic retinopathy can now be treated with laser surgery. Powerful light beams are directed into the eye to seal off leaking blood vessels, a procedure called photocoagulation. Laser photocoagulation also is used to stop proliferative retinopathy by destroying the diseased retinal tissue.

There is no specific treatment for retinitis pigmentosa, although nutrition therapy may slow its progress.

Alternative Therapies

Nutrition Therapy. A study published in 1993 in the Archives of Ophthalmology reported that a daily dose of 15,000 international units of vitamin A can slow the progress of retinitis pigmentosa. Because this dosage is four or five times the normal dietary intake, this treatment should not be undertaken without a doctor's supervision. A buildup of vitamin A in the body can cause liver disease and, if taken during pregnancy, can result in severe birth defects or even fetal death.

Self-Treatment

Self-care for retinal disorders centers on controlling any underlying disease, such as diabetes or high blood pressure. If diminished vision cannot be avoided, there are numerous optical devices that maximize partial sight, or low vision. Practical aids to daily living include large-print newspapers, magazines and books; special calculators and typewriters; television screen magnifiers; and voice-activated computers, clocks, and other devices.

Patients with retinitis pigmentosa are advised to plan for progressive vision loss by learning to read braille and use other aids for the visually impaired.

Other Causes of Retinal Damage

In addition to the disorders cited above, the retina may be damaged by sickle cell anemia, kidney disease, leukemia, syphilis, and toxicity from quinine drugs.

Rheumatic Fever

Rheumatic fever is an acute infection that can cause inflammation of the joints, eyes, nerves, and heart. Most often it is a complication of strep throat, or streptococcal pharyngitis. The usual symptoms are a high fever, rash, and joint and muscle pains that follow or accompany a sore throat. Chorea—jittery body movements and facial twitches—also may develop.

At one time, rheumatic fever was a widespread childhood disease in the United States, especially in crowded urban areas, and it was the most common cause of chronic heart disease. The arthritic pain and other aches associated with the disease were often dismissed as growing pains, allowing it to go unchecked until the heart had incurred permanent damage.

Due largely to the use of antibiotics to treat strep throat, the incidence of rheumatic fever has dropped by more than 90 percent in the United States over the last 50 years. However, there have been recent sporadic outbreaks. These cases have been ascribed to a new strain of streptococcus bacteria that produces a sore throat so mild and brief that it goes unnoticed.

Diagnostic Studies and Procedures

Although not all episodes of strep throat develop into rheumatic fever, any sore throat in a child that lasts for more than a couple of days should be seen by a physician. After inspecting the throat for characteristic inflammation and pus, a doctor will use a swab to collect a sample of secretions for a laboratory culture.

If there is no sore throat but other symptoms suggest the presence of rheumatic fever, blood tests will be ordered to look for strep antibodies, and an electrocardiogram done to check for heart damage. Some fluid may be aspirated from swollen joints to rule out other types of infectious arthritis.

Years after the initial infection, a cardiac examination may reveal a heart murmur, indicating possible damage to the mitral valve and perhaps other heart structures. Echocardiography, an ultrasound examination of the heart, can identify specific abnormalities.

Medical Treatments

Antibiotics are prescribed to eliminate any lingering strep organisms, followed by low-dose prophylactic antibiotics to prevent recurrent attacks. This preventive regimen varies, but may involve a monthly injection of penicillin or a daily oral dose of a sulfa drug or penicillin. Some doctors advocate lifelong prophylaxis with antibiotics, while others prescribe it for the first few years after a bout of rheumatic fever.

If prophylactic antibiotics have been stopped, they should be temporarily resumed before and after dental work or surgery. During such procedures, bacteria may enter the bloodstream and travel to the heart where they can multiply and cause endocarditis (page 178), a serious infection of the heart valves and lining.

Other treatments will vary according to symptoms. If mild arthritis is the only problem, aspirin or another painkiller may be all that is needed. More severe arthritis requires higher doses of aspirin or other nonsteroidal anti-inflammatory medications.

High doses of aspirin, plus prednisone or another corticosteroid drug, are prescribed for heart inflammation. Cardiac arrhythmias are treated with antiarrhythmic drugs; other heart medications are prescribed as needed.

Surgery to repair or replace damaged heart valves is sometimes necessary, but usually not until many years after the bout of rheumatic fever.

Alternative Therapies

Aromatherapy and Massage. A therapist may gently massage painful joints with eucalyptus, mint, thyme, or rosemary oils. However, the massaging or manipulating of badly inflamed joints should be avoided.

Herbal Medicine. Teas made of feverfew or a combination of dandelion and catnip are said to help reduce fever, and garlic and onions are recommended to strengthen the heart. To reduce joint pain and inflammation, herbalists sometimes prescribe white birch capsules, which contain salicylate, the

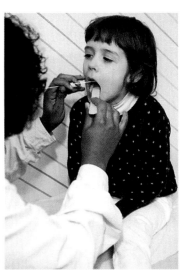

A throat culture is the surest way to diagnose a strep infection. Prompt antibiotic treatment can prevent rheumatic fever from developing as a complication of strep throat.

major ingredient in aspirin. A comfrey poultice may also help alleviate pain. *T'ai Chi.* These gentle range-of-motion exercises are especially suitable for people with arthritis, chorea, and reduced heart function. The routine also fosters a sense of well-being, an important factor in recovery.

Self-Treatment

The high doses of aspirin prescribed to treat the inflammation of rheumatic fever can cause severe stomach irritation. To minimize this effect, take aspirin and similar anti-inflammatory drugs with meals. If you still suffer stomach upset, ask your doctor about taking enteric (coated) aspirin, which does not dissolve until the pill reaches the small intestine. When taking aspirin, be alert for other adverse reactions, especially ringing in the ears (tinnitus), loss of hearing, palpitations, or easy bruising and bleeding.

Bed rest is imperative during the acute phase of rheumatic fever, when heart and joint inflammation are most severe. In the past, patients were advised to stay in bed for months after symptoms disappeared. Many doctors now believe that prolonged bed rest has no value, and may cause unnecessary psychological problems.

Other Causes of Rheumatic Symptoms

Juvenile rheumatoid arthritis can cause many of the same symptoms as rheumatic fever. Depending upon the patient's age and symptoms, other disorders that a doctor may consider include Lyme disease, rheumatoid arthritis, drug reactions, and complications of gonorrhea.

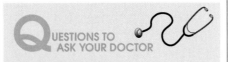

QUESTIONS TO ASK YOUR DOCTOR

▶ Should a child with rheumatic fever be isolated from siblings? And how long should he stay in bed?
▶ How long should antibiotic prophylaxis be continued?

Ringing in the Ears

(Tinnitus)

Ringing in the ears is a general term to describe a condition in which a person perceives sounds that have no acoustic origin. Although tinnitus, the medical name for the condition, comes from the Latin term "to ring," the noises can take many forms—whistling, buzzing, humming, or roaring—and range from a soft hum to a high-pitched squeak. Some people hear the sounds constantly in one or both ears, while others hear them only intermittently. Sometimes the sounds pulsate, synchronizing with the heartbeat.

At any given time, approximately 35 million people in the United States are affected by some degree of ringing in the ears, which may impair their hearing. For many, it is a minor nuisance that can be ignored or handled without medical intervention. For others, the condition can be eliminated or minimized when the underlying cause is discovered. For about 7 million people, however, the noises are distressing and distracting enough to interfere with normal activities.

Tinnitus has many causes. One of the most common is ear damage from exposure to very loud noise. Such damage may occur from a single event, such as an explosion, or develop over time

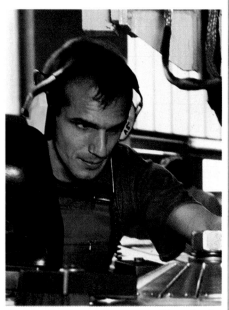

Any person whose jobs exposes him to loud noise should wear protective earmuffs to block out the sound.

from listening to superamplified rock music, operating noisy machinery, or living close to an airport.

The problem often originates in the ear itself; possibilities include infection, a blocked eustachian tube, obstruction by earwax, a tumor, or—especially in the elderly—the progressive growth of spongy bone in the middle ear, a condition called otosclerosis.

Ringing in the ears is frequently a side effect of medications, especially aspirin and other drugs that contain salicylates, quinine, aminoglycoside antibiotics, and certain diuretics. Alcohol abuse, carbon monoxide poisoning, or toxicity from lead, mercury, and other metals can also produce the ringing. Less commonly, systemic diseases, such as high blood pressure, thyroid disease, arteriosclerosis, and anemia, can cause tinnitus, as can meningitis, syphilis, and head injuries.

Diagnostic Studies and Procedures

Diagnosis begins with asking numerous questions about medications, work and recreational exposure to noise, and other illnesses. A physician will then examine the inside of the ear with an otoscope, looking for obvious causes such as an infection, a foreign object, or accumulation of earwax.

If the patient complains of pulsating tinnitus, a doctor will look for circulatory problems, a process that may require angiograms, dye-enhanced X-rays of the blood vessels. In some cases, a physical examination that includes blood and urine studies may reveal the cause. But if no obvious explanation is forthcoming, the patient may be referred to an ear specialist (otologist) or an ear, nose, and throat doctor (otorhinolaryngologist), who may order CT scans or MRI and conduct various hearing tests. The purpose of these procedures is to determine whether the problem originates in the ear itself, in the acoustic nerve, or in the brain.

Medical Treatments

There are no treatments for tinnitus as such; efforts are directed to eliminating the underlying cause. An easy one to remedy is tinnitus caused by medication; stopping the drug or substituting another usually solves the problem.

Certain devices can be helpful. For some patients, a hearing aid works. For others, especially people who cannot tolerate the noise, a tinnitus masker brings relief. This is a device that

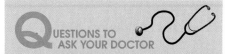

resembles a hearing aid and provides a sound that is more pleasant than the troubling noise. Deaf patients may be helped by having a device that provides electrical stimulation implanted in the cochlea portion of the inner ear.

Alternative Therapies

Hypnosis. Self-hypnosis techniques can help patients to ignore the noises or perceive them as pleasant sounds. For example, a buzzing sound may be imagined as flowing water or waves.
Meditation. Deep breathing and other meditation methods, perhaps combined with visualization, may make the tinnitus less intrusive and bothersome.
Music Therapy. Playing background music to mask tinnitus is a time-honored remedy that many ear specialists recommend. If headphones are used, the volume should be loud enough to mask the noise in the ears, but not so loud that it causes further damage.

Self-Treatment

In addition to the alternative therapies discussed above, you might investigate a white sound machine, a device that plays a monotonous yet pleasant masking sound, such as falling rain or waves. People who suffer from chronic tinnitus find these machines especially useful for helping them to fall asleep.

To prevent tinnitus from getting worse, wear earplugs when you find yourself in an excessively noisy environment. If your job exposes you to loud noise, wear protective earmuffs. Avoid listening to loud rock music, especially through a headset.

Other Causes of Ringing in the Ears

Ménière's disease and vertigo are often accompanied by ringing in the ears. People who suffer from motion sickness may also experience tinnitus along with the more common queasiness. Some persons have temporary ringing in the ears when riding in a fast elevator or during descent on a plane trip. In such cases, the problem is due to changes in atmospheric pressure.

Rosacea

Rosacea is a chronic disorder of the facial skin that produces skin swelling and inflammation, along with small blisters and telangiectasia, clusters of tiny blood vessels just under the skin surface. It usually appears after age 30 and affects women, especially those with light skin and fair hair, three times more often than men. The disease is more severe in males, however.

Often beginning as a prominent flushed appearance in the center of the face that gradually covers the cheeks and chin, rosacea develops over time. At first, it may be mistaken for a ten-

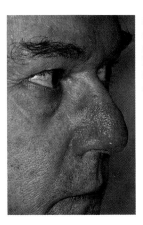

Severe rosacea can produce disfiguring facial inflammation and deformity of the nose.

dency to blush easily or an extreme sensitivity to cosmetics. As the disease progresses, the skin is persistently ruddy. Symptoms may come and go, but rarely disappear permanently. Also, the nose may become red and bulbous, a complication that is often mistakenly attributed to alcoholism. The use of alcohol may aggravate rosacea, but it does not cause the nasal deformity.

About half of all people with rosacea also have chronic conjunctivitis, an inflammation of the membrane covering the eye. In a few serious cases, the eyelids and mucous membranes of the eyes are also affected, and rosy patches may develop on trunk, arms, and legs.

The cause is unknown, but some researchers theorize that an infectious agent may play a role. Anything that increases the flow of blood to the surface may worsen the condition; for example, stress, menopausal hot flashes, spicy foods, alcohol, exposure to sun and warm temperatures, and vasodilating drugs, agents that cause small arteries to dilate, or open wider.

Diagnostic Studies and Procedures

Dermatologists can often diagnose rosacea on the basis of a skin examination and the patient's description of its onset. However, a physical examination, blood tests, and perhaps a skin biopsy may be needed.

Medical Treatments

Although rosacea is not known to be a bacterial disease, antibiotics are a mainstay in its treatment. Tetracycline is the preferred drug, because its long-term use normally does not produce serious side effects. Initially, the drug is taken three times a day, but after the symptoms improve, the dosage usually can be lowered.

Antibacterial skin cleansers or gels may also be prescribed, and in some cases, a topical antibiotic such as metronidazole gel (Flagyl). Topical agents can take up to two months to produce noticeable improvement.

In severe cases, oral isotretinoin (Accutane), a derivative of vitamin A that is used to treat cystic acne, may be recommended. Because this drug can cause severe birth defects, it should not be taken by any woman who might be pregnant. Doctors are instructed to do a pregnancy test before prescribing the drug for a woman of reproductive age, and to stop the drug at least three months before conception is attempted.

A deformed nose may require surgery to remove the excess tissue. Small growths can be taken off with a laser beam or electric needle; larger ones are excised with a scalpel. Dermabrasion, a skin-peeling technique using rapidly revolving abrasive brushes, may then be used to smooth the skin's surface.

Alternative Therapies

Naturopathy and Nutrition Therapy.
Hot or spicy foods that can cause facial flushing should be avoided, along with alcohol, caffeine, and other substances that have a vasodilating effect. Some practitioners recommend vitamin B supplements, but caution against high doses of niacin because it is a vaso-

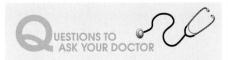

QUESTIONS TO ASK YOUR DOCTOR

▶ Will early treatment of rosacea prevent a deformed nose?
▶ How can I dispel the assumption that my skin condition stems from drinking?

dilator that can cause facial flushing and thus tends to worsen the condition.

Rosacea patients have been found to produce less gastric acid and lipase, a digestive enzyme. Therfore, some nutritionists prescribe hydrochloric acid capsules and enzyme supplements such as pancreatin. However, their effectiveness has not been proved.

Patients on antibiotic therapy are advised to eat yogurt with live cultures or to take acidophilus tablets to prevent an overgrowth of yeast.

Self-Treatment

Anyone with rosacea must be extremely careful to avoid irritating the facial skin. Stay away from all skin products that contain alcohol, including toners, moisturizers, cosmetics, sunscreens, and aftershave lotions. Even herbal and hypoallergenic products may create problems, especially if they contain yeast, mint, camphor, or other ingredients that bring blood to the surface.

Medicated cosmetics formulated for acne or some other skin problem are not effective for treating rosacea and might even worsen the problem. Similarly, DO NOT apply fluorinated cortisone or other corticosteroid creams or ointments to the skin.

Accutane greatly increases the skin's sensitivity to sun; if you are taking this drug, be sure to wear a sunblock such as titanium dioxide outdoors.

As much as possible, avoid activities that increase surface blood flow, especially to the face. For example, try not to stand over a hot stove or steamy food. Exercise is important to maintain health, but pick activities such as walking or swimming that are unlikely to result in overheating and perspiring. Do not use saunas or hot tubs, and don't apply hot towels or ice-cold compresses to the face. You can use a cool compress, however, to reduce redness and alleviate irritation temporarily. Try a combination of 1 tablespoon of oatmeal and ½ cup of cool water, soaking a smooth, soft cloth such as a man's handkerchief in the mixture, and patting it gently onto the skin.

Other Causes of Skin Inflammation

Similar symptoms may be caused by an allergic reaction to medications, or by discoid lupus, which affects only the skin. Perioral dermatitis produces redness and papules around the mouth and on the chin. Granulomas, benign skin tumors, have a similar look.

Runner's Knee

(Patellofemoral stress syndrome)

Runner's knee, a pain in the knee joint, is a very common sports injury. In many cases, no cause can be found; in others, overpronation, a tendency for the feet to roll too far inward, plays an important role. In a normal running gait, the heel lands first, and as the foot moves forward, body weight is transferred to its outside edge. The foot then rolls inward, transferring weight to the inside. This part of the cycle is pronation, which distributes the force of each foot strike throughout the entire foot and leg and protects against injuries.

Excessive pronation results in an exaggerated inward twisting of the lower leg, which causes the kneecap (patella) to rub against the thigh bone (femur). In time, this action produces pain behind the kneecap, especially when running downhill. If the condition is not corrected, walking will eventually become painful.

Weak ankles are often responsible for excessive inward rotation of the foot, and wearing the wrong running shoes can worsen the problem.

Diagnostic Studies and Procedures

A doctor will examine the feet and ankles and observe how the patient stands and walks barefooted. A foot

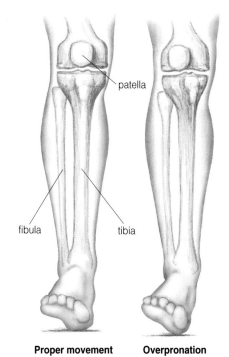

Proper movement   **Overpronation**

Overpronation (rolling too far inward on the feet) is often a factor in runner's knee.

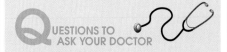
that appears flat signals overpronation. A doctor may also examine a patient's shoes, particularly a pair worn for running. People who overpronate wear down the outside back of the heel first.

X-rays may be ordered to rule out arthritis and other joint conditions. Sometimes, the interior of the knee will be examined with an arthroscope, a flexible viewing tube with a lighted tip and magnifying devices. However, this procedure usually is not necessary for a case of runner's knee when there have been no previous problems.

Medical Treatments

Aspirin or a stronger nonsteroidal anti-inflammatory drug may be prescribed to relieve pain and reduce inflammation. Successful treatment mandates not running until the knee pain has disappeared, and undergoing physical rehabilitation (see Alternative Therapies) before gradually starting again.

Alternative Therapies

Acupressure. Pressing on pressure points on both sides of the knee joint may provide temporary relief.

Alexander Technique. An instructor can analyze your gait and teach you the correct posture and motions to minimize stress on your knees.

Hydrotherapy. Applying ice reduces swelling and inflammation and provides temporary relief from pain.

After a few days of cold packs, some people find that switching to hot compresses, warm water soaks, or a whirlpool bath provides more relief than ice. During rehabilitation, exercising in water may be advisable, because its buoyancy and cushioning effect minimize stress on the knee joint.

Physical Therapy. Ideally, rehabilitation should be directed by a physical therapist who specializes in sports injuries and will have a variety of techniques to reduce pain. The therapist can design an exercise program that will strengthen the quadriceps muscles, which support and protect the knee,

and utilize proper running gait and warm-up and cool-down exercises. (See box, below, for two helpful exercises.)

Self-Treatment

If knee pain strikes, stop running immediately and refrain from exercises that place extra demands on your knees until you are free of all pain. When you do return to running, try wearing an elastic bandage or a knee sleeve for compression and support. Ankle supports also may be advisable.

Wear the right shoes; the wrong ones could be the root of the problem. Certain models are designed specifically for people who overpronate; among their features are a special arch support and a flared heel for stability. Some runners with knee problems may be helped by additional arch supports designed for running shoes; others may need orthotics, custom-made shoe inserts that can be obtained through a podiatrist or orthopedist. Orthotic devices may be rigid or flexible and usually have posts under the heel to prevent the foot from rolling too far inward.

Other Causes of Knee Pain

Various types of arthritis can cause knee pain. Runner's knee is sometimes confused with chondromalacia of the patella, a softening and inflammation of the cartilage that lines the inside of the kneecap. Running or any other sport that requires repeatedly bending the knee can cause this problem, which is treated with many of the techniques used for runner's knee.

KNEE EXERCISES

The most important muscles that support the knees are the quadriceps in the front of the thighs. A simple strengthening method is to sit on the floor with legs straight out in front of you. Press the backs of the knees into the floor, hold for 10 seconds and relax. Another strengthener for the quadriceps is to assume the same position with toes pointed, and then outline each letter of the alphabet in the air with one leg at a time.

To stretch the hamstring muscles in the backs of your thighs, assume the same position and slowly reach forward and tuck your hands under your thighs or your knees, depending on your flexibility. Then slowly and gently pull your chest toward your legs until the backs of your thighs feel stretched. Take care not to jerk or bounce; instead, strive for an easy, fluid motion.

Ruptured Disk

(Herniated or prolapsed vertebral disk)
The human spine has 33 vertebrae separated by disks made of cartilage and fibrous tissue that act as cushions. These disks have a tough outer portion, the annulus fibrosis, which holds the pulpy inner nucleus in place. If the annulus weakens or becomes stretched, the nucleus bulges out, resulting in a so-called slipped disk. Depending on the extent of the abnormality, more accurate medical terms are a bulging, herniated, extruded, ruptured, or prolapsed disk.

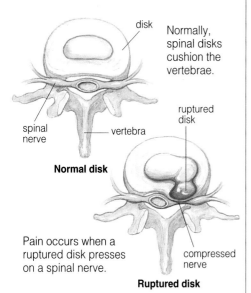

Normally, spinal disks cushion the vertebrae.

disk

spinal nerve — vertebra

Normal disk

ruptured disk

compressed nerve

Pain occurs when a ruptured disk presses on a spinal nerve.

Ruptured disk

Not all protruding disks produce symptoms, but if the herniated portion presses on a nerve root, it can cause mild to severe back pain, sciatica (a pain shooting down one leg), or arm pain. The pain often subsides during rest, only to return as soon as the patient moves around. There may also be numbness, tingling, or even paralysis and loss of bladder control.

Diagnostic Studies and Procedures
A doctor will observe the patient's posture while standing and walking, test muscle strength in the arms and legs, and stimulate certain nerves to detect any loss of sensation.

X-rays are usually made, as well as a CT scan or MRI. Myelography may also be used to identify more precisely whether a disk is bulging or ruptured. In this procedure, a dye is injected into the spinal column while the patient lies on a special table that can be tilted as a series of X-rays are taken.

Medical Treatments
In most cases, nonsurgical treatment is tried first. This usually consists of a few days of bed rest, followed by a gradual return to normal activities. Aspirin or a stronger nonsteroidal anti-inflammatory drug (NSAID) may be prescribed for pain and inflammation. If this fails to provide adequate relief, a short course of a narcotic painkiller, such as meperidine (Demerol) or propoxyphene (Darvon), may be justified. In some cases, diazepam (Valium) or another drug that relaxes muscles is prescribed to stop the spasms that often contribute to back pain. Hydrocortisone and other steroid drugs are occasionally used for a short period to relieve acute pain and inflammation. Traction may also be employed to relieve pain and, depending on the disk's location, a neck collar or back brace may be recommended.

Surgery is considered if symptoms persist after four to six weeks of rest and drug therapy. It may be done sooner if there is numbness or loss of bowel and bladder function.

The operation usually involves removing part or all of the ruptured disk and possibly some of the lamina, the bone that makes up the back wall of the spine. Increasingly, disks are being removed by microsurgery, which requires only small puncture openings (see photograph above). There is very little bleeding and the patient usually can go home within a day or two.

Alternative Therapies
A word of caution: Alternative therapies should be tried only after a doctor has established the diagnosis.
Acupuncture. This is now a widely accepted treatment for back pain that is caused by muscle spasms.
Alexander Technique. Correcting posture and learning more effective ways to carry out day-to-day activities can be useful in reducing back pain as well as preventing its recurrence.

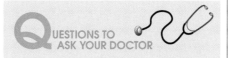

QUESTIONS TO ASK YOUR DOCTOR

▶ If surgery is indicated, what type of operation will I have? What are the risks? And how long will convalescence take?
▶ Is it safe to undergo chiropractic and other manipulative treatments?

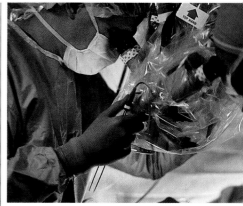

Microsurgery, using special cameras and tiny instruments, allows surgeons to remove a ruptured disk with minimal bleeding and scarring.

Chiropractic. Practitioners use manipulation to treat many neck and back problems. Caution is needed, however: Some manipulative methods can worsen a ruptured disk; it is advisable to determine beforehand whether or not chiropractic treatments are likely to exacerbate the problem.
Massage. This approach is especially useful for relieving muscle spasms. Shiatsu, rolfing, and other vigorous types of massage should be approached with caution if a disk is ruptured.
Osteopathy. In addition to conventional treatment methods and surgery, osteopaths also use manipulative techniques to relieve muscle tension and improve body function.
Physical Therapy. Physical therapists often provide an alternative to surgery by supervising rehabilitative exercise, and using pain-relieving techniques, including application of heat or cold, massage, and electrical stimulation.

Self-Treatment
Although a ruptured disk needs medical care, self-care may prevent its occurrence. A doctor or physical therapist can recommend exercises to help strengthen the abdominal muscles and support the back. (See pages 90–91 for a few examples of back exercises.) A Scandinavian study also found that regular aerobic exercises may reduce the incidence of ruptured disks.

Other Causes of Back Pain
Various types of arthritis or spondylosis can cause back pain, as can osteoporosis (the thinning of bones), and scoliosis, an abnormal curvature of the spine. Cancer that has originated in the spine or metastasized to the bones is still another possible source of back pain.

Scabies

(Sarcoptes scabiei infection)

Scabies is an intensely itchy, highly infectious parasitic skin disease caused by the *Sarcoptes scabiei* itch mite. The mite is usually transferred from one person to another by direct skin contact, especially during sexual activity or while sharing a bed. Far less often it is spread by indirect contact, such as sharing a towel or clothing. This is not typical because the mites do not survive long when not on a human body.

To reproduce, the tiny female mite searches for places where the skin is thickest—especially the palms and soles. She then burrows tunnels under the skin into which she deposits her eggs, about two a day for two months. The larvae hatch in two to four days, leave their mother's tunnel, and cluster around hair follicles. The nymphs will mature within two weeks and begin a new life cycle.

Hypersensitivity to the eggs, and perhaps to the waste products of the mites and larvae, causes the characteristic itchy rash, which usually begins on the thighs and spreads to most parts of the body, particularly the trunk, hands, feet, armpits, and genital region, but not the face. Itching is intermittent and can be quite severe.

Diagnostic Studies and Procedures

It is difficult to diagnose scabies by visual inspection of the rash because it resembles many other skin conditions. Instead, a doctor will look for burrows on the palms or soles, and scrape away the overlying skin. The female mite clings to the top of her burrow and may be visible to the naked eye. Placing the scrapings under a microscope will clearly show the mite. Even if mites cannot be found, a diagnosis may be based on symptoms and recent contact with someone who had scabies.

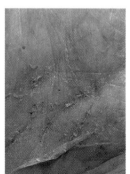

The female scabies mite (above) lays her eggs in burrows under the skin (left).

Medical Treatments

To destroy the mites and their eggs, doctors have traditionally prescribed very potent parasite-killing medications, such as gamma benzene hexachloride, malathion (Ovide), and lindane (Kwell), available as prescription creams or lotions. Because these can cause skin irritation and nerve damage, especially in infants and children, milder but equally effective nonprescription drugs such as permethrin (Nix, Elimite) are now preferred. In children under the age of two, a 5 percent permethrin cream or a 5 or 10 percent sulfur ointment might be used.

Whichever drug is prescribed, it should be applied to the entire body, completely covering the skin from the neck down. It must be left on for at least 12 hours, or preferably 24 hours, before being washed off. Household members and others who have been in physical contact with the patient should be treated at the same time. All recently used clothing, towels, and bed linens should be laundered in hot water.

In most cases, one treatment will kill the mites and their eggs, but a follow-up doctor's visit in a week or two is advisable to see if retreatment is necessary. Itching may persist for a week or two. If it is severe, a doctor can prescribe a topical corticosteroid ointment to be applied twice daily.

Alternative Therapies

While waiting for medical therapy to destroy the parasites, alternative methods can help to ease the itching.

Herbal Therapy. Capsules of a freeze-dried extract of the stinging nettle plant, with one or two taken every two to four hours, might alleviate the itch.

Hydrotherapy. Topical poultices or bath additives often ease itching. Try cornstarch or colloidal oatmeal, available at your pharmacy or health food store. Alternating cold and hot water sprays may also relieve itching.

Meditation and Self-Hypnosis. Because the skin is highly responsive to hypnotic suggestion, meditative practices may help ease itching.

Self-Treatment

Make every effort not to scratch—this may temporarily relieve itching, but it sets in motion an itch-stratch-itch cycle that results in increasingly intense itchiness. Also, scratching may open the skin to a secondary bacterial infection.

In addition to the alternative therapies suggested above, a nonprescription antihistamine cream may also ease mild to moderate itching.

To prevent spreading the infection, avoid physical contact or sharing a bed, towels, linens, or other personal items with anyone until the scabies is completely eliminated.

Other Causes of Itchy Skin Rashes

Itchy skin rashes may be caused by chickenpox, insect bites, eczema, allergies, and contact dermatitis.

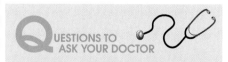

QUESTIONS TO ASK YOUR DOCTOR

► What is the safest, most effective drug for treating scabies?
► What should I do if I have an allergic reaction to the medicine?

Scarlet Fever

(Scarlatina)

Scarlet fever, a contagious childhood disease, usually begins with an acutely sore throat that is caused by a particular strain of streptococci bacteria. If allowed to progress, the bacteria produce a toxin that quickly spreads throughout the body and causes the symptoms that give scarlet fever its name: a high temperature accompanied by a red speckled rash and strawberry colored tongue.

In typical cases, the rash extends from the chest and arms to the lower abdomen and the legs, increasing in redness in the skin folds of the groin,

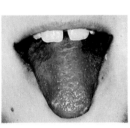
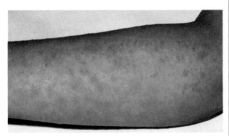

A strawberry colored tongue and speckled red rash (below) are hallmarks of scarlet fever.

armpits, and inner elbow. The reddened area turns pale when pressure is applied, and the skin itself, which has the rough texture of sandpaper, peels. The skin may continue to flake or peel for several weeks after the infection has been controlled.

At one time, scarlet fever was quite common, but today it is relatively rare because of the widespread use of antibiotics to treat strep infections. The disease is contagious from about 24 hours before any symptoms appear until two weeks after the rash disappears, especially if there are lingering complications, such as a middle ear infection or a sinus infection.

Diagnostic Studies and Procedures

A doctor can diagnose scarlet fever on the basis of the characteristic rash and strawberry colored tongue and by inspecting the inflamed throat and tonsils. It may be necessary to have a throat culture done to verify the presence of streptococcal infection. When a child is known to have been exposed to a strep infection from other family members or close associates, a throat culture is considered advisable, even if symptoms have not yet developed. If the result is positive, prompt antibiotic treatment at this point can prevent the onset of scarlet fever.

Medical Treatments

Penicillin is the antibiotic of first choice for treating scarlet fever, but if the patient is allergic to it, erythromycin or a similar broad-spectrum antibiotic is an effective alternative. To prevent ear infections and other potentially serious complications, the full course of medication—usually 10 days—must be completed. Sometimes, a single large dose of the antibiotic is given by injection instead of having the patient take daily pills. If severe complications such as pneumonia or meningitis develop, hospitalization and intravenous antibiotics are usually necessary.

Alternative Therapies

Alternative therapies cannot substitute for antibiotic treatment of a strep infection, but they are useful for reinforcing medical treatment or reducing the risk of its side effects.

Herbal Medicine. To ease the discomfort of a sore throat, herbalists often recommend gargles and teas made of eucalyptus, red sage, fenugreek, or horehound. Vervain or feverfew tea is said to reduce fever. Garlic and goldenseal have mild antibacterial properties, and may be advised to augment therapy with antibiotics. Both are available either as capsules or powders, but some herbalists recommend chewing a fresh clove of garlic.

Naturopathy and Nutrition Therapy. Sucking on zinc lozenges alleviates a sore throat. Some nutritionists advocate supplements of vitamin C and beta carotene, a precursor of vitamin A, to build resistance against further infection. Others feel that including ample foods in the diet that are high in these nutrients, especially fresh fruits and vegetables, is preferable to supplements.

Self-Treatment

The child should be kept in bed until the rash and sore throat abate. Ask your doctor about giving acetaminophen to lower the fever and reduce the pain of swallowing. (Aspirin is a safe medication when a child has a bacterial

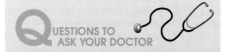

QUESTIONS TO ASK YOUR DOCTOR

▶ How long after the rash disappears should I wait before sending my child back to school or day care?
▶ What precautions should I take to protect my other children from scarlet fever?

infection, but when given for a viral infection, it has been associated with Reye's syndrome, a life-threatening condition affecting the brain and liver (see box, page 437). Many doctors advise not giving aspirin to anyone under age 18 unless there is a compelling reason, such as the presence of juvenile rheumatoid arthritis, to use it.

Sponge baths with lukewarm water also help lower a high temperature. Do not use rubbing alcohol, however, because its fumes are potentially harmful and some of the substance can be absorbed through the skin.

Gargling with warm salt water is a time-honored home remedy for a sore throat. Chicken soup and other broths can ease a sore throat and help prevent dehydration from a high fever as well. Sorbet, gelatin, and similar smooth, cold foods are also soothing to a sore, inflamed throat. In general, bland, soft foods are recommended.

When a child's temperature returns to normal, bed rest is not necessary, but quiet activities should be encouraged until she recovers completely. A doctor should be consulted about when the child can return to school without spreading the infection to others.

It is possible to contract scarlet fever and other strep infections more than once, so children should always be monitored for sore throat, rash, and other signs of illness after contact with someone who has the infection.

Other Causes of Scarlet Fever Symptoms

Rheumatic fever, also a complication of strep throat, can cause inflammation of the joints, nerves, and heart. Measles and rubella produce red rashes and perhaps a sore throat, but these are viral infections that a doctor can easily distinguish from scarlet fever. Juvenile rheumatoid arthritis sometimes starts with a rash, sore throat, and fever, but the tongue is not bright red.

Scars and Keloids

(Fibroblastic cutaneous overgrowth; hypertrophic scars)

Whenever skin is damaged—due to an accidental cut, surgery, burn, or other trauma—scar tissue forms as part of the healing process. Such tissue is composed of special cells called fibroblasts, which make the affected area stronger, thicker, and tougher than usual and cause it to stand out from surrounding skin. Usually, such scars tend to shrink slightly with age, becoming less noticeable or even invisible.

Sometimes, however, a scar continues to grow even after an injury has healed. It forms a keloid, a growth composed of connective tissue, which is raised, shiny, and pink or red in color. In some cases, keloids resemble small tumors; in others, they have claw-like extensions around the growth. The keloid itself may be tender or itchy.

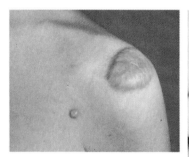

Keloids, such as the one pictured above, often continue to grow, even after wound healing is complete. Laser surgery (right) is sometimes successful in removing small keloids without provoking further scar formation.

It is not known why some people develop keloids, but genetic factors are probably involved. For example, keloids are far more common among people of African descent than Caucasians. Repeated injuries or stretching of a wound during healing can promote keloid growth. They may result also from ear piercing, burns, severe acne, or ingrown hairs. The earlobes, chin, neck, shoulders, breastbone area, and upper trunk are especially vulnerable to keloid development. While some keloids stop growing or even disappear on their own, others continue to enlarge and may eventually require treatment.

Diagnostic Studies and Procedures

Scars and keloids are diagnosed by a physician based on their characteristic physical appearance.

Medical Treatments

Treatment depends on the extent of the disfigurement, including the size and location of the blemish.

Corticosteroids, such as prednisone, are the primary medications for treating keloids. A doctor may inject them directly into the keloid and also prescribe topical steroid salves for home use. Sometimes, a dermatologist will freeze a keloid with nitrogen before such an injection. These treatments are likely to be repeated at monthly intervals for six months or longer to flatten and lighten the coloration of a keloid.

In general, surgical removal of keloids is not advised because it may result in an even larger growth. In some cases, however, surgical removal followed by steroid injections can reduce the visible

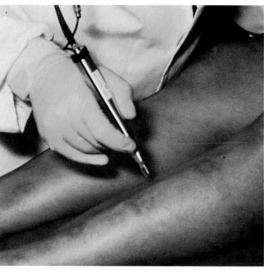

scar. Other techniques include laser surgery or freezing (cryosurgery) to remove small keloids, and radiation therapy for larger, more severe ones. Topical applications of tretinoin (Retin-A), a derivative of vitamin A used to treat acne, also may be helpful.

Plastic surgery can often minimize disfiguring scars that have not formed keloids. In such cases, the surgeon reduces the blemish by cutting out the scar tissue and realigning the surrounding skin. Although this surgery will also leave a scar, it is likely to be a far smaller and less visible one when healing is complete.

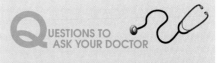

QUESTIONS TO
ASK YOUR DOCTOR

▶ Is this scar or keloid likely to fade or to worsen?
▶ If I must have surgery, what can be done to minimize scaring and keloids?

Scars that form following a severe burn may require skin grafts, in which patches of healthy skin are removed from one place and transplanted to the burned area.

Alternative Therapies

Nutrition Therapy. Appropriate nutrition is essential to assure that the body repairs itself after injury. In particular, you may need extra protein, vitamins A and C, and zinc to support skin repair. Vitamin C is vital for the synthesis of collagen, a major supportive protein in the skin, and daily supplements of 100 to 300 milligrams may be recommended. For their anti-inflammatory effects, vitamin E supplements may also be helpful. In addition, vitamin E oil applied directly to the skin may speed healing and minimize scarring.

Self-Treatment

Avoid exposing any skin area that has recently been cut or otherwise damaged to sunlight, which may impair normal scar formation. Use sunscreens that contain titanium dioxide, which forms a mechanical barrier against the sun's rays. To avoid irritation, do not apply any cosmetics to a scar until it is completely healed.

If you have a tendency to develop keloids, be careful not to scratch or squeeze pimples. Avoid all unnecessary surgery, including chemical facial peels or dermabrasion. If surgery is needed, ask your doctor about preventive steps that may minimize keloid formation, such as a pressure bandage or steroid applications during the healing process.

If the appearance of a scar or keloid is upsetting even after treatment and healing are complete, consult a cosmetologist, preferably one recommended by a plastic surgeon. Such experts are knowledgable about products and techniques that can be quite effective in hiding scars.

Other Causes of Scars

Acne and rashes that have become infected can leave scars.

Schizophrenia

Schizophrenia is a mental disorder that is characterized by severe disturbances of thought, perception, feeling, and behavior. Mental health professionals classify it as a psychotic disorder, defined as being out of touch with reality and unable to separate real from imaginary experiences.

Acute schizophrenia is marked by severe psychotic symptoms, which may include hallucinations, delusions, irrational acts, and bizarre behavior. Some people have only one such episode, while others have experienced many throughout their lives, sometimes interspersed with relatively normal periods. Still others suffer chronic recurrences without ongoing treatment.

About 200,000 new cases are diagnosed in the United States each year. The disease affects about 1 percent of the population from all economic, racial, and cultural groups, with men and women affected equally. Its cause is unknown, but researchers believe that a combination of inherited and environmental factors are involved.

Diagnostic Studies and Procedures

Since many patients with schizophrenia think, feel, and act quite normal much of the time, it is often hard to establish a diagnosis. In the active phase of the disease, at least two of the following symptoms must be present for most of the time for at least one month: delusions, hallucinations, disorganized speech or behavior, catatonic behavior, and a flat or abnormal facial expression.

A medical history is important in determining if the patient has become withdrawn and dysfunctional suddenly or over a period of time. Tests might include psychological and neurological studies, a blood workup, and CT scans or MRI to rule out a brain tumor.

Medical Treatments

Hospitalization is often needed for an initial episode or severe relapse. Long-term hospitalization is uncommon, but a few patients may require it.

The mainstays of treatment are antipsychotic medications, or neuroleptics. These drugs, which include chlorpromazine (Thorazine), haloperidol (Haldol), thiothixene (Navane), prochlorperazine (Compazine), loxapine (Loxitane), and clozapine (Clozaril), do not cure the condition, but they do enable most patients to think more

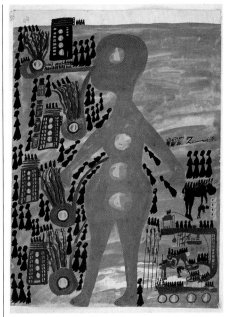

This painting by Carlo Zinelli, an Italian artist and a severe schizophrenic, reflects the hallucinations that plagued his life.

clearly and rationally. Antipsychotic drugs unfortunately have a number of adverse side effects, some of which can be eliminated by lowering the dosage. If this is not possible, some of the side effects can be controlled with other medications. Long-term use, however, can lead to tardive dyskinesia, a disorder in which involuntary movements occur, most often of the mouth, lips, and tongue.

Electroconvulsive therapy (page 29) is rarely used to treat schizophrenia but may be helpful if a severe depression accompanies or triggers a psychotic episode. Lobotomy, a brain operation once used for severe chronic schizophrenia, is no longer advocated.

Alternative Therapies

Art Therapy. This modality encourages patients to express thoughts they cannot verbalize. The art also gives some insights into a patient's mental turmoil.

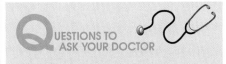

QUESTIONS TO ASK YOUR DOCTOR

▶ What type of continuing care and medication are needed to prevent a relapse?
▶ How long will it take for antipsychotic medication to work? What are the side effects and how can they be minimized?
▶ Do you recommend counseling for other family members?

Behavior Modification. During hospital treatment this therapy is often used to encourage patients to adopt more socially acceptable behavior. A typical approach calls for praising and rewarding tolerable conduct while ignoring or punishing unacceptable behavior.

Music Therapy. Music not only has a soothing effect, but it also encourages movement, social interactions, and emotional expression.

Naturopathy and Nutrition Therapy. Although there is no scientific proof that diet helps control schizophrenia, some nutritionists recommend a high-fiber diet that also includes foods rich in niacin, such as poultry, seafood, seeds and nuts, potatoes, and fortified or whole-grain breads and cereals. They also advise against refined foods such as white flour, instant rice, sugar, and soft drinks.

Psychosocial Treatment. This is an essential adjunct to medical treatment, since antipsychotic drugs do not relieve all symptoms of schizophrenia. Even when schizophrenic patients are not suffering from psychotic symptoms, many still have trouble establishing and maintaining relationships. Therefore, psychosocial treatment usually includes one or more forms of psychotherapy, such as group and family therapy, as well as rehabilitation programs. The latter are often in group homes with other patients and emphasize social skills and lessons in daily living.

Self-Treatment

Self-treatment is not effective, although participation in self-help groups is often valuable both for patients and their families. Such groups provide continuing mutual support as well as comfort in letting individuals know that others have similar problems.

Because many patients with schizophrenia relapse when they stop taking medication, supervision is essential to make sure that they comply with their drug regimens. Following a routine that emphasizes regular meals, daily exercise, and adequate rest also helps.

Other Causes of Psychotic Symptoms

Organic brain disorders, mental retardation, severe depression, or paranoid disorders may produce some of the same symptoms as schizophrenia. Brain tumors, certain medications, and alcohol or drug abuse also can lead to psychotic behavior.

Scoliosis

Scoliosis, an exaggerated sideways, or lateral, curvature of the spine, comes from the Greek term for curved or askew. Very few people have perfectly straight spines, but to qualify as scoliosis, the curvature must be more than 10 degrees. The abnormality often affects the symmetry of the shoulders, hips, or rib cage, but in some cases, double curves may balance each other without affecting the shoulders or hips.

This structural defect most often becomes apparent during an adolescent growth spurt, and girls are affected more often than boys. Possible early signs include a shoulder blade or hip that is more prominent than the other, uneven hip and shoulder levels, and clothes that hang unevenly.

In 80 to 90 percent of all cases, the cause is unknown, although the condition appears to run in families. Complications of severe scoliosis depend upon the site of the curvature. For example, if the upper spine is involved, heart and lungs may be compressed.

Diagnostic Studies and Procedures

A home test (see box, right) can help detect scoliosis, but a medical evaluation, preferably by an orthopedist, is needed to assess the severity. It begins with a careful physical examination that includes studying the symmetry of shoulders, arms, and hips, and measuring the length of each leg. X-rays are taken, and the degree of spinal rotation, is determined. A curvature of 20 degrees or less is considered mild, more than 25 degrees, moderate to severe.

Medical Treatments

Only 2 to 3 percent of scoliosis cases require treatment, but all should be checked periodically to monitor any progression, which occurs mostly during periods of growth. Instead of taking X-rays each time, a doctor may use an OSI Scoliometer to measure any significant changes in the curve.

When treatment is necessary, it usually entails wearing a rigid brace that exerts pressure on the apex of the curve to achieve a more normal alignment. Typically, a brace is worn 18 hours a day, but at the end of treatment, it may be needed only at night.

In about one case in a thousand, surgical correction will be needed. The operation may involve insertion of metal rods to hold the vertebrae in

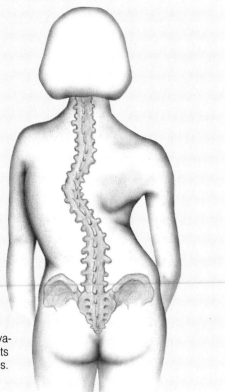

The exaggerated spinal curvature of severe scoliosis results in uneven shoulders and hips.

proper alignment. Usually, some of the vertebrae are fused in order to prevent further progression of the curvature.

Although the chances of arresting or even reversing scoliosis are greatest with early treatment, braces or surgery also may be recommended for an adult, especially someone who suffers from chronic back pain or spinal arthritis, or is experiencing breathing or heart problems related to scoliosis.

Alternative Therapies

Alexander Technique. Practitioners believe they can help mild scoliosis by analyzing body movements and then increasing the person's awareness of how to achieve better posture.

Chiropractic. Manipulation is advocated by some chiropractors as the way to prevent mild curvature from becoming more pronounced. Orthopedists discount its benefits.

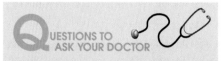

Electro-Stimulation. This approach, which uses low-voltage electrical stimulation, was once hailed as a promising new treatment. However, studies indicate that it is of little or no value.

Physical Therapy. A therapist can design an exercise program suitable for the person's age and extent of curvature to help maintain good muscle tone and strength while the torso is immobilized in a brace. Patients who do not require a brace are encouraged to pursue activities such as swimming or horseback riding that strengthen muscles and encourage good posture.

Self-Treatment

Scoliosis can be difficult for adolescents because it comes at a time when they want to be like their peers. Fortunately, there are braces that can be worn under clothing, and those patients who must have surgery usually do not require the bulky body casts used in the past. Still, joining a scoliosis support group may be helpful in dealing with emotional problems related to the condition.

Other Causes of Spinal Curvatures

Congenital anomalies, cerebral palsy, muscular dystrophy, spinal fracture, or advanced osteoporosis are among the disorders that can cause spinal curvatures. Degenerative scoliosis may be caused by osteoarthritis.

Seborrhea

(Inflammatory dandruff; seborrheic dermatitis; seborrheic eczema)

Seborrhea, a common chronic skin disorder, is characterized by rough, dry, inflamed skin that gives off yellowish scales. There may be itching, and when it develops in skin folds, these areas are often red and sore. The term seborrhea is misleading because the scaling has little or nothing to do with the production of sebum, the waxy substance secreted by the skin's sebaceous glands; instead, the scales are dead cells shed by the epidermis layer. Seborrhea can develop at any age, but occurs most often in young adults. (An infant form, cradle cap, is discussed on page 148.)

The areas generally affected are the scalp; the face, especially the eyebrows, eyelids, moustache area, around the nose, and behind the ears; the torso,

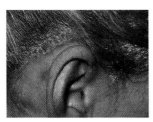

The inflammation and scaling of seborrhea is especially evident when the scalp is involved.

usually the central chest and upper back; and the skin folds of the armpit and groin and under the breasts.

The cause is unknown, but stress and climate may be factors. For example, many people find that their skin clears up when they are on vacation, especially if the locale is warm and sunny, only to have the problem recur when they return to work or when winter arrives.

In older people, seborrhea is sometimes associated with Parkinson's disease or other neurological disorders. The condition tends to run in families, so there may be an inherited predisposition, but it is not a genetic disease.

Diagnostic Studies and Procedures

Dermatologists can diagnose seborrhea simply by inspecting the skin. In unusual cases, a skin biopsy may be ordered to rule out other conditions.

Medical Treatments

Treatment varies according to the part of the body affected. A physician may recommend a mild, 1 percent hydrocortisone cream, available without a prescription, for facial seborrhea. If this does not help, a prescription of a 2.5 percent strength solution may be tried.

Seborrhea on the trunk is harder to treat, and often recurs. Topical hydrocortisone usually doesn't help, although oral or injected steroids may bring it under control. Stubborn cases may respond to overnight tar preparations.

Mild seborrhea in skin folds generally responds to a topical prescription-strength steroids. For severe cases, 10-minute, twice-daily applications of compresses soaked in aluminum acetate or potassium permanganate may be prescribed, along with steroids and antibiotics. In these areas, seborrhea is often accompanied by secondary bacterial or *Candida* infections; thus, antibacterial or antifungal medications may be added to the regimen.

Scalp seborrhea is treated with special shampoos containing tar, zinc pyrithione, selenium sulfide, or sulfur and salicylic acid or tar.

Alternative Therapies

Aromatherapy. Practitioners recommend bathing the affected skin with 2 percent essence of geranium in a base of distilled water. This should be done three times a week before bedtime. The scalp, chest, and skin folds may be treated twice a week with 10 percent essence of sage in an olive oil base, which is massaged into the affected areas and washed out in two hours.

Herbal Medicine. Compresses soaked in dandelion, goldenseal, or red clover teas may help seborrhea. Some herbalists also recommend a chaparral tea rinse following a shampoo.

Meditation. Because stress appears to be a precipitating factor, meditation and other relaxation techniques may prevent flare-ups.

Nutrition Therapy. Some naturopathic practitioners believe seborrhea could be due to vitamin A deficiency and recommend a daily supplement, although

QUESTIONS TO ASK YOUR DOCTOR

▶ Could I benefit from ultraviolet light therapy during the winter months? If so, are tanning parlor lights okay?
▶ Should I try compresses or soaks of aluminum acetate or potassium permanganate? What precautions are needed when using these substances?

A CASE IN POINT

When Anne Johnson, a 46-year-old legal secretary, developed a red, scaling rash in her genital area, she assumed that it was an allergic reaction. But wearing only white cotton next to her skin and eliminating other possible allergens failed to help. In fact, the rash was spreading when Johnson consulted her gynecologist.

"I don't think it's anything serious," the doctor assured her, but he referred her to a dermatologist for a more expert opinion. The specialist quickly diagnosed seborrheic intertrigo; this is a form of seborrhea that typically develops in the genital area or other major skin folds.

A more careful inspection of the rash revealed a secondary yeast, or *Candida*, infection, as well as a couple of crusted sores that were infected with bacteria. The doctor explained that it's not unusual to find such infections when seborrhea develops in the genital area, but they also made treatment more difficult. He prescribed a 1 percent hydrocortisone cream with miconazole, a drug that is effective against both bacteria and yeast. Within a month, all the conditions had cleared up.

Because recurrences are common, Johnson was told to treat any recurring rash with the 1 percent hydrocortisone cream, and to see a doctor if it persisted for more than a week.

other medical specialists disagree. Vitamin B complex and zinc supplements may also be recommended.

Self-Treatment

Mild seborrhea can usually be self-treated with nonprescription hydrocortisone creams and antidandruff shampoos. Judicious exposure to sun may also help, but care must be taken not to burn, which can worsen the condition.

Other Causes of Skin Scaling

Ordinary dandruff may resemble scalp seborrhea without the inflammation. Psoriasis may be mistaken for seborrhea, but its scales are thicker and the skin is likely to be redder. Tinea versicolor, a superficial fungal infection, sometimes resembles seborrhea, as do several other fungal infections, especially those affecting the skin folds.

Seizures

(Convulsive disorders; epilepsy)

When the brain's normal electrical activity is disrupted, seizures, or convulsions, can occur. They are classified as generalized or partial, with variations in each category. Generalized seizures include the following:

Tonic-clonic, or grand mal. The person abruptly halts all activity and loses consciousness briefly. This tonic phase lasts for only a few seconds and is characterized by a sustained contraction of muscles. The subsequent clonic phase may last for five minutes, during which time muscles spontaneously relax and contract, creating convulsive twitching. If only one phase occurs, it is called either clonic or tonic.

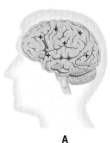

A

A certain amount of electrical activity (denoted by + in these drawings) is needed to transmit messages within the brain. A surge in electrical impulses can produce a seizure (B), which can be prevented by a neutralizing anticonvulsant drug (C).

electrical charge

B

C

Atonic, or drop attack. The person suddenly loses muscle tone, goes limp, and is unconscious for several minutes.
Myoclonic. The person usually remains conscious, but exhibits brief, random contractions and twitching of a muscle.
Absence, or petit mal. The person, usually a child, has a brief episode of altered awareness, in which he stares blankly ahead.

Partial seizures may involve muscles, sensory organs, or mental function, but do not result in generalized convulsions. In some occurrences, muscles may twitch in a specific area, such as a leg, or there may be localized tingling. Others involve brief mental lapses that are similar to absence seizures. A common partial seizure is characterized by repetitive motions that are a continuation of an activity but lacking in

purpose. For example, a child might continue a writing motion without actually forming letters.

Epilepsy, the most common seizure disorder, is characterized by recurrent seizures that follow a specific pattern.

Diagnostic Studies and Procedures

Seizures can be diagnosed from symptoms and an eyewitness account of an attack, but determining the cause is often difficult, sometimes impossible. Tests include blood studies, an electroencephalogram (EEG) to measure the brain's electrical activity, X-rays, and perhaps a CT scan or MRI.

Medical Treatments

Medication with anticonvulsant drugs can prevent seizures or reduce their frequency. Commonly used anticonvulsant medications are phenytoin (Dilantin), phenobarbital, primidone (Mysoline), carbamazepine (Tegretol), ethosuximide (Zarontin), clonazepam (Klonopin), and valproic acid (Depakene). The side effects vary, but may include lethargy, drowsiness, dizziness, nausea and vomiting, gait problems, and mental changes.

Finding the right drug or combination of drugs usually involves a period of trial and error. Once a regimen is found to work however, the patient should stay on it. This is one instance in which a generic drug should not be substituted for a brand-name product. Even though the active ingredients may be the same, the two drugs may react differently in the body. Some patients are eventually able to discontinue their medication, while others must remain on it for life.

Surgery may be tried if seizures cannot be controlled by drugs.

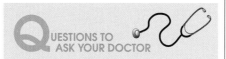

QUESTIONS TO
ASK YOUR DOCTOR

▶ Is it safe for me to drive if I have a seizure disorder? What about sports?
▶ If I must take anticonvulsant drugs, what side effects might I expect?
▶ Might a ketogenic diet eliminate my seizures?

Alternative Therapies
Nutrition Therapy. Fasting has been known to eliminate seizures, but this was hardly a feasible treatment for epilepsy until neurologists at Johns Hopkins devised a diet that mimics fasting metabolism. The regimen calls for a high intake of fats, only enough protein for growth, and little or no carbohydrates. This ketogenic diet is recommended mostly for children whose epilepsy cannot be controlled by drugs or who suffer severe side effects from anticonvulsants. It must be tailored individually and followed carefully; after two years, most children can resume a normal diet without recurrence of seizures.
Meditation. This and other relaxation techniques may be helpful for seizures that are triggered by stress.

Self-Treatment
Some people can modify their tendency to have seizures by identifying and then avoiding triggering factors. An orderly, moderate lifestyle, adequate rest, and a nutritious diet help most patients. Others with severe seizures may benefit from the Johns Hopkins ketogenic diet (see Resources Directory, page 467).

Anyone who has a seizure disorder should wear a medical identification bracelet or necklace that lists the illness and an emergency phone number.

Other Causes of Seizures
A rapidly rising temperature can produce febrile seizures, especially in babies. A brain injury, certain drugs, poisons, lack of oxygen, and either high or low blood sugar can cause seizures.

Sexual Dysfunction

Sexual dysfunction is the inability to achieve an orgasm as the culmination of sexual activity with one's partner. Such achievement depends on an unbroken chain of events, involving both the body and the mind. Beginning with desire and an expectation of pleasure, this mental state proceeds to physical arousal, during which the man has an erection and the woman's vagina becomes lubricated to ease penetration. Intercourse can then take place, ideally continuing to orgasm for both partners.

In a woman, orgasm takes the form of pleasurable contractions of muscles within the vaginal walls; in the male, orgasm is immediately followed by the ejaculation of semen. After orgasm, both partners experience a feeling of total relaxation and well-being. Sexual dysfunction exists if emotional and physical responses at any point in this continuum prevent a satisfying outcome for both partners.

It is only in recent decades that the medical profession has gained a better understanding of the many reasons for sexual dysfunction and how to deal with them. The 1966 publication of *Human Sexual Response*, a landmark study by Dr. William H. Masters and Virginia E. Johnson, is viewed as a major turning point. Following this study, medical schools began offering courses in human sexuality, and sex therapy clinics were established in leading medical centers. Ongoing research into the physiology, not just the psychology, of sex has helped health professionals to identify the source of a problem and offer effective treatment.

One factor in sexual dysfunction of women may be painful intercourse (page 326). In men, the most common problems are impotence (the inability to have or maintain an erection sufficient for sexual intercourse) and premature ejaculation (the inability to delay orgasm). Two additional difficulties are common to both sexes: deficiency or absence of sexual fantasies and desire, and sexual aversion disorder, which takes the form of avoiding any genital contact with a sexual partner.

Psychological factors, such as guilt, anxiety, anger, and fear, may play a role in sexual dysfunction, but doctors are

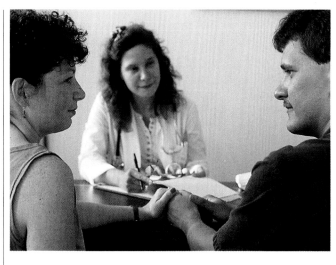

Sex therapy is more likely to work if both partners participate in counseling sessions.

increasingly aware that many cases have an organic origin. For example, diabetes is a relatively common cause of male impotence. Certain medications, especially those used to treat high blood pressure, produce sexual dysfunction in both men and women. Long-term alcohol abuse can cause male impotence, and may also lower sexual desire in women.

Many women who have had a hysterectomy report diminished sexual response, but the reasons for this are not entirely clear.

Diagnostic Studies and Procedures

Correct diagnosis of a particular aspect of sexual dysfunction begins with a doctor who asks the right questions, takes the time to listen, and understands the relationship between various health problems, medications, and lifestyle on the one hand, and sexual fulfillment on the other. Information gathered from the physical examination and laboratory tests is then evaluated against this background.

When there is no obvious cause for the dysfunction, specific tests may be ordered. In a man, this may include nocturnal penile tumescence testing. During the rapid eye movement (REM)

Q UESTIONS TO ASK YOUR DOCTOR

► Could one of my medications account for my sexual problems? If so, is there an alternative drug that will work as well but won't have the same side effect?
► Can you recommend a reliable sex therapist or program?

phase of sleep, men have as many as five erections of varying duration. If a snap gauge device attached to the penis is open in the morning, it is assumed that at least one erection occurred, indicating that impotence while awake is probably due to psychological rather than physical causes. Other procedures include testing nerve reflexes and evaluating circulatory problems that might reduce blood flow to the penis.

Identifying the cause of sexual dysfunction in a woman can be more difficult. If she is able to achieve orgasm through self-stimulation but not during intercourse, a doctor might assume that the problem is psychological. However, a gynecological examination may reveal an infection, a tumor, or other abnormality that inhibits orgasm during sexual intercourse.

Medical Treatments

When a situation calls for it, a primary-care doctor will refer patients to other specialists: a man to a urologist or an endocrinologist, a woman to a gynecologist. Either might need the expertise of a sex therapist or psychiatrist.

Because an estimated 25 percent of all cases of sexual dysfunction are related to the use of various medications, the first aspect of treatment may be to review all drugs being taken for other conditions. Otherwise, treatment is determined by the person's gender and the nature of the problem.

Male Impotence. Increasingly, male impotence is treated with drugs or devices that help achieve or maintain an erection.

One strategy, developed in France in the 1980s and now the most popular impotence treatment worldwide, involves injecting medication into the side of the penis a few minutes before intercourse to increase blood flow and achieve an erection.

Another regimen entails taking two drugs, papaverine, an artificial opium alkaloid, and phentolamine (Regitine), a drug normally used to treat high blood pressure. The drugs work by relaxing the smooth muscles in the walls of the blood vessels, allowing them to open wider and let more blood flow into the penis. Sometimes a synthetic form of prostaglandin E-1 is taken to achieve a similar effect.

In yet another approach, a medicated patch containing nitroglycerin is placed directly on the penis. The medication, which is more often used to treat angina, promotes a rush of blood to the penis and results in an erection.

Still in the testing stage are several creams that dilate blood vessels: one is a topical form of minoxidil, the antihypertensive drug that is also marketed as a treatment for baldness; another is a drug that is massaged into the penis to induce erection and heighten arousal in the female by increasing blood flow to the vagina; a third type is inserted into the tip of the penis with a plunger.

A number of mechanical implements are also used to treat male impotence. One is a vacuum apparatus that applies a negative pressure to achieve an erection, which is then maintained by a tight rubber ring placed at the base of the penis. Another, made of semirigid material, is placed over the penis like a condom. A vacuum device then draws out the penis to fill the covering, which is left in place during intercourse.

Surgical penile implants are now considered the treatment of last resort because of their inherent risk of infection and tissue damage. The simplest are those that hold the penis in a semirigid position all the time; the more complex have devices that allow a man to make the penis rigid during intercourse and relax it at other times.

Female Sexual Dysfunction. The cause of sexual problems in women is not always apparent, so self-treatment, counseling, or alternative therapies may take precedence over medical approaches. An estrogen cream or hormone replacement therapy can usually solve the problem of postmenopausal dryness and thinning of the vaginal tissue, a common cause of sexual dys-

SEX THERAPY

Before beginning sex therapy, it is critical to make sure that the therapist is reputable and has undergone proper training. Sex therapists associated with the human sexuality programs of medical schools and many major medical centers are usually reliable, but it's still advisable to check credentials.

To overcome anxieties about sexual performance, a typical treatment program might guide a couple through sensate exercises, in which different parts of the body are stimulated to achieve arousal without proceeding to actual intercourse. These exercises are practiced at home until mutually satisfying levels of arousal have been achieved. At that time, intercourse can be attempted.

Treatment for premature ejaculation might consist of teaching a man to concentrate on aspects of sexual activity without aiming for intercourse. The goal is to help him identify the pre-ejaculatory phase, and then learn how to control it.

Couples counseling and one-on-one psychotherapy can be effective treatment for lack of desire that originates in boredom, anger, anxiety, or depression. Through cognitive therapy, a man or woman whose sex drive has been suppressed since childhood because of guilt, fear, or sexual abuse can arrive at the insights necessary for seeing the past in a new light. Women who have been raped or battered also may benefit from counseling by a qualified therapist.

function in older women. Surgery may be advised to correct a condition such as endometriosis (page 179) if it causes painful intercourse.

Alternative Therapies

Acupuncture. Practitioners claim to have achieved positive results in treating impotence and orgasmic difficulties. A series of five or six sessions is usually required.

Herbal Medicine. Ginseng root, available fresh, powdered, or as a tea, is widely prescribed as an aphrodisiac by Asian herbalists. Some herbalists also recommend infusions made from licorice root or from damiana, a desert plant. Various fungi and yeast are also believed to contain chemicals similar to the human sex hormones. Yohimbine, an African plant said to stimulate blood flow to the genitals, should be avoided because of its toxicity.

Massage. Mutual massage using aromatic oils can be a relaxing and enjoyable prelude to sex.

Meditation and Visualization. Stress and anxiety, which often cause sexual dysfunction, can be overcome through breathing exercises and meditation skills. Using the technique of guided imagery, individuals can visualize themselves in relaxed and erotic settings to enhance arousal.

Yoga. For centuries, teachers have recommended specific exercises that reportedly liberate sexual energy by inducing relaxation and increasing blood flow. Once learned, they can be a form of self-treatment.

Self-Treatment

Bookstores and libraries can provide enlightened how-to books for over coming nonorganic sexual dysfunction. The most useful ones are graphic and detailed, and include information about massage, erotic gadgets, and ways to stimulate the mind and body through the use of aromatic oils, music, lighting, and verbalizing one's fantasies.

Take the time to communicate to your sexual partner what you find pleasurable and what you don't like.

Occasionally watch a sex video together. According to Dr. Stephen B. Levine, professor of psychiatry at Case Western Reserve University and a sex researcher, the two most potent aphrodisiacs are "psychological intimacy and voyeurism—looking at pictures or movies of people engaged in genital or romantic interplay."

Sometimes, arthritis, a bad back, heart disease, and other chronic health problems interfere with sexual enjoyment. Experimenting with different positions may help, especially if pain is a factor. Talking with a doctor can also provide important insight. For example, many heart patients and their partners are afraid to engage in sex, fearing that it will provoke a heart attack. In general, if a person has enough cardiac stamina to walk up one flight of stairs, sexual intercourse should be safe. Prophylactic use of nitroglycerin can prevent an attack of angina brought on by sexual excitement.

Other Causes of Sexual Dysfunction

In addition to conditions cited earlier, disorders that can cause sexual problems include arteriosclerosis and other circulatory problems, spinal cord injuries and other neurological disorders, obesity, and thyroid disease or other hormonal imbalances.

Shin Splints

(Anterolateral shin splints)

The term shin splints is often used to describe any persistent pain in the front part of the lower leg, but medically, the condition involves an injury to the muscles that attach to the tibia, or shin bone. The direct cause is scarring from small tears in the shin muscles, especially where they attach to the bone.

The underlying problem often stems from an imbalance in muscle strength; the shin muscles, which pull the forefoot upward, typically are weaker than the calf muscles, which pull the forefoot down. As calf muscles become disproportionately stronger, running or jogging increases wear and tear on the weaker shin muscles.

Pain, ranging from mild tenderness to progressively severe achiness that is centered in the outer side of the shin's bony ridge is the major symptom. It is usually felt in both legs and in mild cases, occurs only when running or walking. Sometimes, the shin muscles become inflamed and swollen, causing chronic pain because they are encased in a tight-fitting sheath, or compartment, that allows little room for swelling. In unusual cases, the inflammation may spread to the membrane surrounding the shin bone, a condition referred to as periostitis.

Diagnostic Studies and Procedures

A principal diagnostic clue is the location, nature, and duration of the pain. A medical history that includes the patient's daily activities helps pinpoint the source of discomfort. A physical examination might reveal swelling and tenderness. X-rays or a bone scan may be ordered to rule out a stress fracture or other bone problem.

Medical Treatments

Mild shin splints generally can be handled by self-treatment and physical therapy (see below). Aspirin, ibuprofen, or other anti-inflammatory medication might be prescribed. More severe swelling and inflammation may require a cortisone injection. Surgery is sometimes needed if swelling within the muscle compartment threatens to block the flow of blood.

Alternative Therapies

Herbal Medicine. Although it cannot cure the problem, a soothing poultice may alleviate pain. One combination said to relieve muscle pain consists of

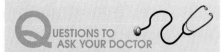

comfrey, echinacea, goldenseal, mullein leaves, poke root, turmeric, and yellow dock. To prepare a poultice, mix the herbs and add lukewarm water to make a thick paste. Cover the painful area with a clean cloth and spread the paste over it. Cover with another cloth and elevate your legs with the poultice in place for 30 minutes.

Hydrotherapy. Ice packs help relieve pain, swelling, and inflammation, but ice should never be placed directly on the skin; put it in a plastic bag and cover it with a clean cloth. Remove the pack after 20 minutes and wait 10 to 15 minutes before applying it again.

Physical Therapy. A therapist who specializes in sports medicine can design a program of rehabilitation for a specific type of shin splint, the extent of inflammation, and the patient's athletic goals. One basic strategy involves strengthening the shin muscles and lengthening the calf muscles. Exercises might include running up stairs to exercise the shin muscles and doing wall push-ups to stretch the calf muscles.

Tai Chi. The gentle exercises and stretching of this movement therapy can help retain muscle tone and

strength while waiting for your muscles to heal. It also fosters a sense of well-being to compensate for the frustration that comes with inactivity.

Self-Treatment

Rest is an essential element in self-care. Because most shin splints result from too much exercise, they will become progressively worse unless the legs are rested and the muscles given a chance to heal—a process that may take up to six weeks. If pain persists after that time or if it recurs with the gradual resumption of exercise, check with a doctor. It could be due to a stress fracture or some other problem.

Recurrent shin splints may indicate a need for physical therapy or a change in your exercise program. Perhaps you can run on a softer surface, or less often. Swimming, bicycling, and using a stair-climber or a cross-country skiing machine all provide aerobic benefits and are unlikely to cause a recurrence. Devise a cross-training program in which you alternate among these forms of exercise and keep your running to a minimum. A personal trainer can help you find the type and level of exercise that provide health benefits without creating new problems.

Other Causes of Shin Pain

Tingling shin pain that lasts several hours after exercising may be caused by swelling within the compartments that encase the lower leg muscles. This condition, known as anterior compartment syndrome, often results from muscle enlargement due to overtraining or frequent uphill running. A stress fracture of the tibia can also produce shin pain.

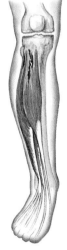

Normal leg muscles   **Overdeveloped calf muscles**

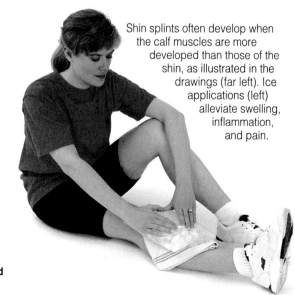

Shin splints often develop when the calf muscles are more developed than those of the shin, as illustrated in the drawings (far left). Ice applications (left) alleviate swelling, inflammation, and pain.

Shingles

(Herpes zoster; postherpetic neuralgia)
Shingles is almost always an adulthood recurrence of chickenpox, but differs from the original disease in that it involves inflammation of a peripheral sensory nerve that originates in the spinal cord.

The varicella zoster virus, which causes chickenpox and shingles, is related to herpes simplex, the virus that produces cold sores and genital herpes. As with these herpes infections, the varicella virus remains in the body after chickenpox clears up, taking refuge in certain nerve cells. Thus, shingles is characterized by nerve pain and the eruption of painful blisters along the pathway of a root nerve. (The varicella virus can be transmitted from someone who has shingles and become the cause of chickenpox.)

A typical case of shingles begins with general discomfort, gastrointestinal upset, fever, and pain in the part of the body that is supplied by the affected root nerve, most often the upper torso. In a few days, the skin becomes red and slightly swollen, and a spotted rash appears. The red spots turn into small blisters that dry up and crust over

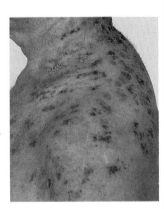

The rash of shingles follows a peripheral nerve on one side of the body, usually the upper torso.

within a week. Permanent scarring is rare, and for many people recovery is complete in two weeks. Sometimes, however, an attack of shingles will be followed by persistent and intractable pain, or neuralgia, along the nerve pathway, a complication known as postherpetic neuralgia.

Another complication is ophthalmic herpes zoster, also called zoster keratitis, which can occur if shingles affects the face. Blisters break out along the forehead, the eyelids swell, and, in the most serious cases, the cornea becomes inflamed and ulcerated. Since ulceration may lead to scarring and irreversible damage to vision, a physician should be consulted without delay at the first sign of facial shingles.

What triggers shingles is not known, but the incidence increases with advancing age. Stress and reduced immunity also appear to play a role. For example, widespread shingles that lasts for more than two weeks is sometimes associated with Hodgkin's disease, a cancer of the lymph system. Patients undergoing cancer chemotherapy, long-term treatment with steroids, or immunosuppressive therapy also have an increased incidence.

Diagnostic Studies and Procedures

A diagnosis of shingles is usually based on the characteristic distribution of blisters along the path of a nerve on one side of the body. If there is any doubt, a laboratory culture may be ordered. Because shingles sometimes develops in people with Hodgkin's disease or other conditions marked by reduced immunity, blood studies and other tests may be ordered.

Medical Treatments

Although there is no medical cure for shingles and its consequences, treatments can reduce discomfort and prevent some of the complications. If the condition is diagnosed early, acyclovir (Zovirax), an antiviral drug, may be prescribed to hasten healing of blisters and perhaps lower the likelihood of postherpetic neuralgia. Early use of acyclovir is especially critical if the eyes are involved or if the patient has a condition that lowers immunity.

Dexamethasone, a cortisone-like drug, may be prescribed as an eye ointment and/or a salve to speed the healing of blisters.

Drugs that can diminish the pain of postherpetic neuralgia include codeine combined with aspirin or acetaminophen; carbamazepine (Tegretol), an antiseizure medication; and amitriptyline (Elavil), antidepressant medication. Also under study is Zostrix, a cream that contains capsaicin, a substance in hot peppers. When rubbed on the blisters, capsaicin produces a stinging sensation that appears to reduce the discomfort of shingles.

Some doctors advocate injections of a corticosteroid medication, but this is a controversial treatment.

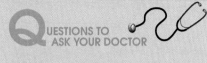
Alternative Therapies

Acupuncture. This has been shown to alleviate postherpetic neuralgia. Six sessions over a one- or two-month period are usual. Practitioners stress that prompt treatment contributes to the likelihood of success.

Herbal Medicine. Herbalists recommend applications of aloe vera gel, fresh leek juice, or compresses soaked in goldenseal, mugwort, or peppermint tea to soothe the shingles blisters.

Meditation. This relaxation technique, perhaps combined with self-hypnosis or biofeedback training, may be helpful in coping with the pain of shingles or postherpetic neuralgia.

Nutrition Therapy. Vitamin E supplements are said to reduce the likelihood of postherpetic pain. Some nutritionists also recommend high-dose vitamin C to help heal the blisters.

Self-Treatment

Self-care is directed to bolstering immunity by eating balanced, nutritious meals and getting adequate rest. If pain interrupts sleep at night, compensate by taking naps during the day.

Discomfort from blisters can be reduced by applying cool wet compresses or soaking in a tepid bath containing a cup of colloidal oatmeal or a cup of baking soda. Another home remedy calls for mixing a crushed aspirin with a tablespoon of unscented skin lotion and applying it to the blisters. To reduce the likelihood of scarring, apply vitamin E oil or cream to the blisters as they begin to dry up.

Lingering nerve pain may be controlled by TENS, or transcutaneous electrical nerve stimulation produced by a pocket-sized device. After an accredited physical therapist provides instruction in its use, it is a convenient form of self-treatment.

Other Causes of Herpetic Blisters

Herpes simplex can cause blisters similar to those of shingles, but they do not follow a nerve pattern.

Shock

(Hypovolemic shock; traumatic hemorrhagic shock)

Shock is a life-threatening emergency in which insufficient oxygenated blood reaches vital body organs and tissues because of extremely low blood pressure. One type, traumatic hemorrhagic, or hypovolemic, shock, results from a severe loss of blood. Typical causes range from a major accident to a ruptured tubal pregnancy, a perforated intestinal ulcer, or ruptured aneurysm. Other types of shock may be due to serious illnesses (see Other Causes). For example, septic shock occurs when bacteria multiply in the bloodstream and then release toxins. Whatever the type of shock, emergency first aid calls for similar procedures (see box, right).

When blood pressure falls, the body compensates by rerouting blood away from the skin and muscles to the more vital organs, such as the heart, lungs, and brain. The skin then becomes pale, cool, and clammy and the individual feels weak. As the heart and lungs struggle to function, the pulse becomes very rapid, although weak, and the rate of breathing increases but the person feels short of breath, and perhaps also extremely anxious and restless.

As shock progresses, other symptoms may include unusual thirst, vomiting, blotched or streaked skin, dilated pupils, and disorientation and confusion. A delay in treatment can lead to permanent damage of the intestines, kidneys, and other vital organs; failure to treat shock may result in death.

Diagnostic Studies and Procedures

Shock should be suspected in any situation in which a person has suffered severe internal or external bleeding. Blood pressure may be so low that it cannot be measured. A physical examination and certain blood tests can confirm the presence of shock. After the emergency medical needs of the victim have been met, further tests may be necessary to help determine the cause.

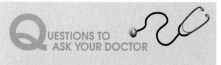

QUESTIONS TO ASK YOUR DOCTOR

▶ Do I have any medical condition that increases my risk of shock?

FIRST AID FOR SHOCK

If you suspect shock, take the victim to the nearest hospital emergency room. If this is not possible, call for an ambulance immediately. While awaiting medical help, start these first aid measures:

1. Keep the victim lying down and covered with a blanket or coat to maintain warmth.
2. Do not move the person if injury to the head, neck, or spine may have occurred. Movement can cause further damage and should be done only by trained medical personnel.
3. In the absence of such injuries, elevate the feet 8 to 10 inches to increase blood flow to the trunk. You can prop the feet on pillows, books, or other such items. If nothing is available, simply hold them up with your hands.
4. If the person shows signs of heart attack—chest pain, difficulty in breathing, profuse sweating—do not elevate the feet. Instead, raise the head and shoulders 8 to 10 inches.
5. If an arm or leg is bleeding severely, apply direct pressure to the wound. Bright red blood that is gushing or spurting indicates an injured artery. If pressing on the wound does not stop the bleeding, apply pressure to the appropriate point along the artery (see page 103 for pressure points).
6. Do not give the victim anything to drink or eat, except as discussed below.
7. If nausea occurs, turn the person's head to one side so that vomiting won't cause choking.
8. If the victim falls unconscious and is not breathing, maintain an open airway and begin cardiopulmonary resuscitation immediately (page 217).

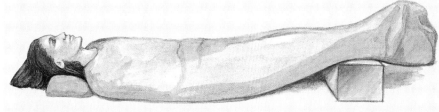

A shock victim should be warmly covered, with the legs elevated 8 to 10 inches.

Medical Treatments

When a shock victim is brought to the hospital, emergency treatments may include the following:

▶ Blood transfusions to restore blood lost from severe injuries.

▶ Intravenous fluids to help restore the body's fluid volume.

▶ Medications to help raise and maintain the blood pressure.

In addition, steps will be taken to treat the underlying cause of the shock. For example, surgery may be necessary to halt internal bleeding due to tearing of blood vessels in an accident, a ruptured aneurysm, or a tubal pregnancy.

Alternative Therapies

No alternative therapy can replace medical treatment for shock. However, if medical attention cannot be obtained immediately and is not likely to be available for several hours, steps may be taken to help the patient retain body fluid, but only if she is conscious and has not suffered convulsions, a stomach wound, or bleeding from the mouth or rectum. If these conditions apply, the patient may be given a weak saline solution made with ½ teaspoon of salt added to 4 ounces (½ cup) of water. Children under 12 should be given only 2 ounces of such a solution and infants 1 ounce. The liquid should be sipped very slowly over a period of 15 minutes or more.

Self-Treatment

If you have any medical condition that increases your risk of shock, follow your doctor's recommended self-care regimen scrupulously. Keep the phone numbers of your nearest hospital emergency room posted near your telephone and wear a medical ID bracelet.

Other Causes of Shock

A heart attack, cardiac arrhythmias, pericarditis, or a pulmonary embolism can cause cardiogenic shock. Severe blood poisoning or infections such as toxic shock syndrome can lead to septic shock. Extensive burns, prolonged diarrhea or vomiting, or other conditions that upset the body's fluid and electrolyte balance can cause shock. Still other possible causes of shock include uncontrolled diabetes or an overdose of insulin, poisons, and a severe allergic reaction that results in anaphylactic shock.

Sickle Cell Disease

(Hemoglobin S; sickle cell anemia)
Sickle cell disease is the general term for a group of inherited blood disorders characterized by abnormal hemoglobin, the pigment in red blood cells that contains iron and carries oxygen throughout the body. Sickle cell disorders derive their name from the abnormal crescent shape of the red blood cells, which are also easily destroyed.

The disease varies greatly in severity, but it invariably causes anemia. Thus, fatigue, shortness of breath, delayed growth, and rapid heartbeat—common components of anemia—generally occur. The anemia, however, is not the most serious aspect of the disorder. From time to time, a person with sickle cell disease develops an aplastic crisis in which the circulation is flooded with sickled cells that clog small blood vessels and may block blood flow to vital organs. In time, the kidneys, lungs, heart, and joints may suffer permanent damage. In severe cases, early death from kidney failure, respiratory failure, or stroke is common.

Sickle cell disease occurs in most racial and ethnic groups, but is most widespread among people of African origin. In the United States, it affects about 150 in every 100,000 African-Americans, or a total of 60,000 to 80,000 people. To develop sickle cell disease, a child normally must inherit the gene from both parents. Those who inherit only one gene become carriers of the sickle cell trait and can pass the gene to the next generation.

Although a person with the sickle cell trait may have deformed blood cells, he usually has no symptoms. However, travel to a high altitude may actually precipitate symptoms because reduced

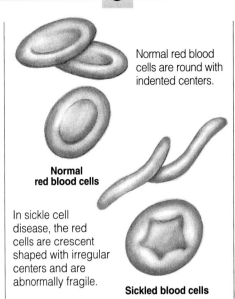

Normal red blood cells are round with indented centers.

Normal red blood cells

In sickle cell disease, the red cells are crescent shaped with irregular centers and are abnormally fragile.

Sickled blood cells

availability of oxygen can accelerate breakdown of the fragile red blood cells.

A rare type of sickle cell disease, called hemoglobin S-C, develops when a child inherits the sickle cell trait from one parent and a variant called hemoglobin C from the other. The disorder causes mild to moderate anemia, but does not shorten life expectancy.

Diagnostic Studies and Procedures
Sickle cell disease is diagnosed by taking a family history and by hemoglobin electrophoresis, a blood test that can detect the abnormal red cells.

Medical Treatments
Anyone diagnosed as having sickle cell disease should be referred to a specialist in genetic blood diseases for future monitoring and treatment.

Experimental drugs that prevent sickling of the red blood cells are being tested; in the meantime, guarding against infection is a major focus of treatment. Specialists generally recommend that all babies diagnosed with sickle cell disease receive prophylactic antibiotics. Before this preventive treatment was instituted, 20 percent of children with this disease died before the age of three; now the mortality rate is less than 3 percent among children who are on long-term antibiotic therapy.

Immunization is also critical; in addition to the usual vaccines, pneumonia, influenza, and hepatitis immunizations are recommended.

Aplastic crises and their complications are treated as they arise. Blood transfusions are sometimes necessary to treat severe anemia. Supplemental oxygen may also be needed.

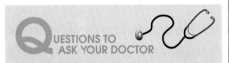
TESTING FOR SICKLE CELL DISEASE
Sickle cell disease can now be diagnosed in a prenatal procedure called a fetoscopy. Early in pregnancy, blood samples are taken from the fetus through a long, narrow tube and needle inserted into the mother's uterus through a small abdominal incision.

Federal health experts recommend that all newborns be screened for sickle cell disease. More than half the states nationwide conform to this recommendation, screening for sickle cell disease at the same time that they conduct other neonatal blood tests. Ten states provide sickle cell screening only for high-risk groups, and the rest have no screening programs at all.

Alternative Therapies
Nutrition Therapy. Supplements of folic acid are often prescribed, but should be taken only under the supervision of a qualified nutritionist.
T'ai Chi. Running and other vigorous activities usually are precluded because sickle cell disease often damages large, weight-bearing joints. T'ai chi, with its gentle exercises, helps maintain muscle tone and fosters well-being.

Self-Treatment
If you have sickle cell trait, exercise caution when flying. Travel in a plane with a pressurized passenger cabin and make sure that supplemental oxygen is available if you need it.

About 2.5 million African-Americans carry the sickle cell gene, or trait. Couples who are contemplating parenthood and are at risk for transmitting the disease may want guidance from a genetic counselor. For example, if both partners carry the gene, there is a 50 percent chance that any child they have will inherit one gene and also become a carrier. In each pregnancy, there is a 25 percent chance that the child will inherit two genes, and develop the disease, and also a 25 percent chance that the baby will have two normal genes and be free of the trait.

Other Causes of Abnormal Hemoglobin
More than 400 different hemoglobin disorders interfere with the blood's ability to transport oxygen. Thalassemia, a genetic disease that is most common among people of Mediterranean origin, has some of the same characteristics of sickle cell disease.

Sinusitis

Sinusitis, or inflammation of the sinuses, is an exceedingly common problem, affecting millions of Americans of all ages. The nasal sinuses consist of eight air pockets in the bones around the nose, cheeks, and eyes. These cavities are lined with mucous glands, which keep the passages moist. Sinusitis develops when these passages become inflamed and swollen, usually due to an infection or allergic response.

Most sufferers complain of a feeling of congestion accompanied by a headache and perhaps a runny nose. The nature of the headache varies according to which sinuses are affected. Inflammation of the maxillary sinuses, those situated below the eyes and on either side of the nose, can cause facial

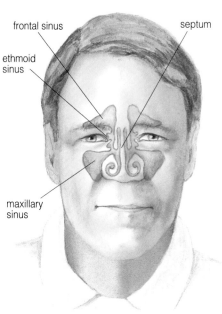

Sinusitis typically causes a feeling of nasal congestion and a frontal headache.

pain, toothache, and a frontal headache. A blockage in the frontal sinuses, located in the forehead, also produces a headache in that area. A so-called splitting headache and pain behind the eyes point to inflammation of the ethmoid sinuses, which are located on either side of the eyes and just over the nose. In addition to a headache, there might be visible swelling in the area over the affected sinus.

Sinusitis may be acute or chronic; acute attacks are more likely to be due to an upper respiratory infection, while chronic sinusitis is often caused by

allergies, although many people who have it do not suffer from them. Dental abscesses or infections are responsible for about 25 percent of chronic maxillary sinusitis. Infectious agents that can cause acute sinusitis include strains of streptococci, pneumococci, staphylococci, and *Haemophilus influenzae* bacteria as well as some viruses.

Diagnostic Studies and Procedures

Diagnosis is usually based on the patient's description of the symptoms and a physical examination of the sinus areas. The mucous membranes of the nose may also be red and swollen and nasal discharge may be greenish-yellow or tinged with blood. X-rays are sometimes ordered, but they often fail to find any abnormality because swollen mucous membranes usually are not visible on film. A CT scan may produce better results, but is not necessary as a rule. In a few cases, dental X-rays will be taken if an abscess is suspected of causing the sinusitis. A laboratory culture of the nasal discharge may also be ordered. This facilitates identification of any infecting organism.

Medical Treatments

Antibiotics are used to fight the underlying infection. They will probably be prescribed for 10 to 12 days; it is important to complete the full course of antibiotics, even if symptoms of sinusitis have already disappeared. Otherwise, the infection may recur.

Chronic sinusitis is most often treated with ampicillin or tetracycline, which may be needed for four to six weeks to eradicate the underlying infection. Nasal sprays may be prescribed to shrink swollen membranes and ease congestion, but should not be used for more than a week. In severe cases or when some deformity of the sinus passages is contributing to the problem, surgery to correct the abnormality, drain the sinuses, and remove infected material may be necessary.

Alternative Therapies

Aromatherapy. Therapists recommend inhalation of eucalyptus, peppermint, basil, or lavender oils to help clear blocked sinuses. This can be done by putting about 10 drops of the oil on a handkerchief and inhaling from it. A more effective means is to bring a pot of water to a boil, add a few drops of the aromatic oil after removing the water from the heat, and then inhale the steamy vapors that rise from it.

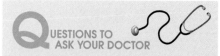
Herbal Medicine. A capsule containing a mixture of echinacea, goldenrod, goldenseal, and marsh mallow leaf may be prescribed. Herbalists also recommend taking garlic, which is considered a natural antibiotic, and drinking teas or infusions made of mullein, fenugreek, red clover, rose hips, or a combination of anise and horehound.

Homeopathy. A wide variety of homeopathic remedies may be used, with kali bi, pulsatilla, ignatia, and thuya often suggested.

Self-Treatment

Over-the-counter decongestants are sometimes helpful, but they should not be taken for longer than a week. Use them only as directed; these drugs should be avoided if you have high blood pressure, glaucoma, diabetes, heart disease, and certain other chronic conditions. Also, do not take cold or allergy pills containing antihistamines, since they dry up the sinus mucus and interfere with drainage.

Blow your nose gently; blowing too hard can worsen the problem by forcing mucus into the sinus cavities. To help clear nasal and sinus passages, some doctors recommend a daily nasal wash. This can be done by filling a nasal syringe with warm, salty water and drawing it into one nostril at a time.

Placing a warm compress over your forehead or taking a hot, steamy shower can provide temporary relief. Keep air moist by using a misting vaporizer.

Drink plenty of fluids, especially steamy bullion and other hot liquids, to help thin mucus. Eating hot, spicy food such as chilies or horseradish also may help clear congested sinuses.

Other Causes of Sinus Symptoms

A cold or other upper respiratory infection can cause congestion, headache, and other symptoms similar to those of sinusitis. Head pain from muscle tension and other causes should also be ruled out when making a diagnosis.

Skin Cancer

(Basal cell and squamous cell carcinomas)
Skin cancer is by far the most prevalent
malignancy in the United States, with
more than 800,000 cases a year. The
two most common forms are basal cell
carcinoma, which arises in the lowest
part of the epidermis, or surface layer
of the skin, and squamous cell carcinoma, which originates in the cells that
make up the skin's outer surface. Both
types are readily curable if detected
early and treated properly.

These two cancers are heralded by
growths or skin sores that do not heal.
A basal cell cancer is typically an irregular shape. It may appear as a flat spot
or a firm lump that is scaly and crusty
or smooth and shiny. A squamous cell
cancer also appears as a scaly or crusty
patch that may bleed occasionally.
Squamous cell cancers develop most
often on the rim of the ear, the mouth,
and scalps of bald men. People with
fair skin, red hair, and blue eyes are
most vulnerable to both cancer types.

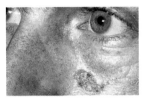

Basal cell
carcinoma is
the most com-
mon form of
skin cancer.

Excessive exposure to the sun's ultraviolet rays is the most common cause of
skin cancer. Occupational exposure to
coal tar, pitch, creosote, arsenic, and
radium also increase the risk.

Diagnostic Studies and Procedures
A dermatologist often suspects skin
cancer from the appearance of a sore or
other lesion, but a skin biopsy is essential to make a definitive diagnosis and
to determine the type.

These skin cancers rarely metastasize
to distant parts of the body, but the
squamous cell type may invade nearby
organs. Thus, MRI or a CT scan may be
ordered if the cancer is near the eyes or
other pathway to the brain.

Medical Treatments
Removal is the usual treatment for
skin cancer, although radiation is
sometimes used when surgery is not
possible. Chemotherapy with topical
5-fluorouracil may also be considered.

There are several different surgical
methods; the choice depends on the

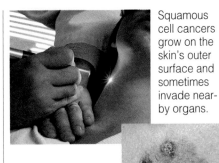

Squamous
cell cancers
grow on the
skin's outer
surface and
sometimes
invade near-
by organs.

cancer's appear-
ance, size, loca-
tion, and type. A
small surface can-
cer can be treated with curettage—the
scraping away of the cancerous tissue
with a sharp surgical instrument.
Bleeding is stopped with electrodesic-
cation, the use of an electric needle that
also cauterizes a zone of normal tissue
surrounding the lesion, reducing the
likelihood of recurrence.

Cryosurgery is the use of liquid
nitrogen spray or a device called a
cryoprobe to freeze the cancerous tissue and destroy the malignant cells
with minimal scarring. Laser surgery
can also be used to pinpoint and kill
certain types of skin cancer cells.

Surgical excision involves removing
the growth along with a margin of normal tissue, then closing the wound
with stitches or skin clips. A skin graft
and plastic surgery may be needed.

In the Mohs procedure, layers of tissue are cut away in an expanding circle
around the cancer, and each layer is
examined microscopically to determine
the extent of malignant cells. Successive
layers are removed until only normal
tissue is found. Plastic surgery may be
needed as a follow-up procedure.

Alternative Therapies
Meditation, hypnosis, and visualization
can be helpful in controlling pain and
promoting healing.

A diet that includes foods rich in
antioxidants—vitamins C, E, and A (or
beta carotene, its precursor), can help
protect against cancer. Vitamin E oil
applied to the excised areas may hasten
healing and reduce scarring, but check
with your doctor before applying this
(or anything else) to the wound.

Self-Treatment
While self-treatment cannot cure skin
cancer, it is the key to prevention and
avoiding recurrences. Because most
skin cancers are related to damage from
the sun's ultraviolet rays, you should

SKIN SELF-EXAMINATION
Know the warning signs of skin cancer
and examine your skin thoroughly and
regularly in a brightly lit room. Examine
your body front and back, then the right
and left sides with the arms raised.
Check your forearms, upper underarms,
and palms carefully. Examine the feet,
including the spaces between toes and
the soles. Look at the back of the neck
and the scalp. Part the hair and lift it for
a closer look. Check the lower back and
buttocks. See a doctor promptly if you
note the appearance of:
▶ Any new skin growth that does not disappear in four to six weeks.
▶ Any lesion that grows and turns translucent, brown, black, or multicolored.
▶ Any mole, birthmark, or beauty mark
that increases in size, changes color or
texture, or develops an irregular outline.
▶ Any open sore or wound that does not
heal for more than four weeks, or heals
and then recurs.
▶ Any skin spot or growth that continues
to itch, hurt, crust over, form a scab,
erode, or bleed for several weeks.

minimize your exposure. Avoid being
outside during the peak sunlight hours
from 10 A.M. to 2 P.M. If you must be
out then, wear a hat with a wide brim
and loose-fitting but tightly woven
clothing that covers most exposed skin.
Use a sunscreen with a sun protection
factor (SPF) of at least 15 on remaining
exposed skin; reapply it often. For a
baby, ask your doctor to recommend a
safe sunscreen, and make sure that she
wears a sun hat and protective clothing.

Remember that sand, snow, and
water reflect the sun's rays and thus
magnify their potential harm to skin.
Tanning booths and sun lamps can also
give off harmful ultraviolet rays.

Other Causes of Skin Lesions
Moles, warts, and other benign skin
growths and discolorations sometimes
resemble skin cancer. Skin disorders
such as psoriasis and dermatitis can be
confused with malignant lesions.

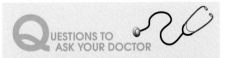

QUESTIONS TO
ASK YOUR DOCTOR

▶ If I have dark skin, do I need to worry
about skin cancer?
▶ What sunscreen can you recommend
for extremely sensitive skin? For babies
and young children?

Sleep Apnea

(Central, mixed, or obstructive apnea)
While breathing is an automatic function that most people take for granted, persons who have sleep apnea stop breathing repeatedly for anywhere from 10 seconds to 2 or 3 minutes during sleep. The majority of these persons are unaware of such episodes, although their bed partners may complain of their loud snoring and fitfulness.

Overweight middle-aged or older men are the ones most commonly afflicted, but sleep apnea can occur at any age and in either sex. Adults with the disorder have an increased risk of sudden death from a heart attack while sleeping. Infants who have experienced sleep apnea account for about 5 percent of all cases of crib death, or sudden infant death syndrome (page 397).

In obstructive apnea, the most common form, the upper air passages in the nose and mouth are temporarily blocked. Also referred to as the Pickwickian syndrome, this type occurs most often in obese people. Typically, the person is sleeping on his back and snoring loudly. The snoring and breathing suddenly stop briefly, then resume as the person thrashes about or gasps for breath. During the day, the sufferer may be inordinately drowsy, and will often nod off, only to awaken feeling starved for air. The restless sleep and reduced oxygen intake can lead to personality changes.

A variation called central apnea is caused by a malfunction in the brain's respiratory center. The airway is open, but the respiratory structures in the

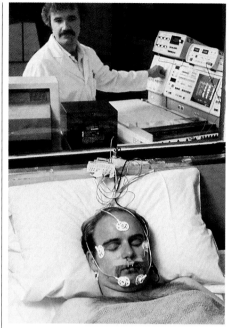

Monitoring in a sleep clinic is the best way to diagnose sleep apnea.

chest and abdomen do not receive the proper messages from the brain.

Diagnostic Studies and Procedures

Diagnosing sleep apnea in an awake individual is difficult because breathing usually appears to be normal in this state. A physical examination may reveal a deviated septum or polyps in the nose, enlarged tonsils, large adenoids, or some other predisposing abnormality, but many people with apnea do not have such anomalies. A diagnosis may require a night being monitored in a sleep laboratory. As sleep apnea is often associated with arrhythmias and other cardiac complications, a cardiovascular workup may also be ordered.

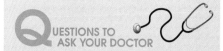

Medical Treatments

A positive air flow machine, which blows air into the nose during the night, can help keep the upper airways open.

Surgery to widen the air passages in the throat can cure apnea in some persons. In others, a tracheostomy may be necessary. This is a surgical procedure in which a small hole is made in the trachea, or windpipe, at the base of the neck. A tube is inserted into the hole and at bedtime, a valve is opened so that air can flow directly through the tracheostomy to the lungs. When the patient is awake, the valve is closed, allowing normal speech and breathing.

Alternative Therapies

There are no alternative therapies for sleep apnea itself. If the problem is related to obesity, a nutritionist can help devise a weight-loss plan.

Self-Treatment

Mild cases can be treated with the self-care remedies for snoring that prevent sleeping on the back (page 384).

A baby who has frequent bouts of sleep apnea may be fitted with a monitor that sounds if breathing stops.

Other Causes of Apnea Symptoms

Nasal infections, allergies, and obstructions in the nose, mouth, or throat can cause snoring and fitful sleeping.

A CASE IN POINT

For years, Sally Kline had complained about her husband Larry's loud snoring. He had tried various devices and home remedies, but nothing had helped. Sally finally resorted to wearing earplugs to block the noise. This worked until Larry developed a new sleep habit—a fitful thrashing about during which he unintentionally hit or kicked her, sometimes even leaving bruises.

Although Larry seemed to get a full night's sleep, however restless, he invariably woke up tired, and often dozed off during the day.

"I was exhausted by being wakened several times every night," Sally recalled. "Twin beds or even separate bedrooms seemed to be the only solution."

But then she came across a magazine article about sleep apnea, which described her husband's snoring pattern and fitfulness exactly. The article stressed the association of sleep apnea with sudden death, so Sally urged her husband to see their family doctor.

Aside from the fact that Larry was markedly overweight, the doctor could not find any physical abnormalities. He

then referred Larry to a sleep disorders clinic, where a night in the sleep laboratory confirmed that he had obstructive sleep apnea. The clinic doctor urged Larry to see a nutritionist for some help in getting his weight down. She also prescribed a positive air flow machine, which he could use at home.

"It took a bit of getting used to," Larry said later in describing what it was like to sleep with a nasal tube that blew air into his nostrils. But the device also ended the episodes of apnea, so both Klines could again enjoy a full night of restful sleep.

Sleep Disorders

(Cataplexy; hypersomnia; insomnia; narcolepsy; nightmares; somnambulism)
Sleep needs vary: some people feel alert and rested after only four or five hours of sleep, while others require eight or nine hours. On average, a healthy person feels best with seven to eight hours of sleep per night.

A sleep disorder can affect almost every aspect of daily life—mood, alertness, and the ability to concentrate. The more common sleep disorders include:
Insomnia, defined as difficulty in getting to sleep, or experiencing disturbed sleep patterns that result in the perception of insufficient sleep. Some people with insomnia fall asleep easily, then awaken during the night and cannot return to sleep. Others are convinced they cannot get to sleep, when in fact, studies in sleep laboratories show that they sleep a normal amount of time.

With rare exceptions, everyone has an occasional sleepless night. If the problem lasts a few days, it is termed transient insomnia, and is usually triggered by stress or travel that upsets the body's normal wake-sleep cycle.

If the difficulty continues for up to three weeks, it is classified as short-term insomnia. Typical causes include worries about money or a job, the death of a loved one, marital problems, or serious concerns about health.

Long-term insomnia, which lasts more than three weeks, has many possible causes—noise, night-shift work, chronic pain or disease, drug or alcohol abuse, depression or other psychological problems, overuse of caffeine, or abuse of sleeping pills. It may also be due to another sleep disorder, such as sleep apnea (page 381) or restless legs syndrome (page 359).
Narcolepsy, characterized by sleep attacks and abnormal patterns of REM, or rapid eye movement, sleep. The person cannot resist falling asleep and almost immediately enters the REM dream stage. If undisturbed, the person may sleep a few minutes or an hour or more. The frequency of attacks is unrelated to the amount of sleep.
Cataplexy, a sudden loss of muscle tension that causes weakness or even brief paralysis. The individual may experience weak knees or a drop of the head, or might even collapse. Such an attack is usually triggered by an intense emotional reaction. It may last for just seconds or for a minute or two. During a brief episode, the person is awake, but a longer attack may merge with a period of narcolepsy and REM sleep.
Sleep paralysis, manifested as brief episodes of being unable to move when falling asleep or upon awakening. These incidents often accompany narcolepsy and cataplexy, but also occur in people who have no sleep disorders.
Hypersomnia, an increase of 25 percent or more in the hours an individual normally sleeps. It is often a manifestation of depression, but is also caused by a brain disorder or abuse of hypnotic drugs, or downers.
Sleepwalking, or somnambulism, which is more common in children than adults. About 15 percent of children walk in their sleep at least once between ages 5 and 12. The cause is unknown, but some researchers believe it is due to a minor neurological abnormality. It usually occurs in the early part of the night. Typically, the sleepwalker has a blank, staring expression, but may perform various tasks. The episode usually ends with the person waking in confusion and then falling asleep with no memory of it.
Nightmares and night terrors, characterized by intense feelings of fear. Most people experience an occasional nightmare or vivid dream, but children are affected more frequently by night terrors, which occur during a nondreaming stage of sleep. Typically, the child sits up in bed, screams, and perspires profusely. Night terrors usually occur between the ages of 4 and 12 and are more common in boys than girls.

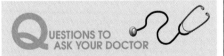

Q UESTIONS TO ASK YOUR DOCTOR

▶ How can I determine whether I'm getting enough or too much sleep?
▶ Is it true that older people need less sleep? How much sleep is enough for a person over age 60?
▶ If I make my child go to bed on time, he says he can't sleep for hours. Do some children need less sleep and should they be allowed to stay up later?
▶ How can I tell whether my child's nightmares, sleepwalking, or night terrors are related to an emotional problem?
▶ Could I benefit from spending a night or two in a sleep laboratory?

Diagnostic Studies and Procedures
Initial diagnosis is usually based on the patient's description of symptoms. A medical history may provide clues about habits and other health problems that could prompt a sleep disorder. A physical examination provides further clues, and blood tests and other laboratory studies may be ordered.

Sometimes patients are referred for evaluation to a clinic for sleep disorders. There, they are examined by neurologists, psychologists, psychiatrists, and other specialists, and then electronically monitored while they sleep.

Medical Treatments
Treatment depends on the nature of the problem and its underlying cause. Therapy for insomnia may include, for example, psychotherapy for an emotional problem, such as depression, or medical treatment for an organic disorder. Sleep-inducing barbiturates and other hypnotic drugs may be given for a short time, but doctors are prescribing such medications less because their misuse can be addictive and even fatal. Benzodiazepines such as diazepam (Valium) are more likely to be used because they are less addictive. Still, caution is needed; these medications can be dangerous if used in combination with alcohol, or if taken by someone with a respiratory problem.

Narcolepsy is treated with a stimulant such as ephedrine or an amphetamine. Patients who also have cataplexy are given a second drug, usually imipramine (Tofranil). Anyone taking both stimulants and imipramine is at risk of developing hypertension (high blood pressure) and must be monitored.

Hypersomnia is dealt with by finding and treating the cause. Sleepwalking, night terrors, and nightmares in children rarely require medical treatment, although psychotherapy may reveal whether emotional problems are at fault.

Alternative Therapies
Aromatherapy. Therapists suggest taking a warm bath to which lavender, ylang ylang, and chamomile oils are added, or having a massage with the same combination of oils. Sprinkling these oils on the bed sheets is also said to promote sound sleep. A massage or bath using marjoram, pennyroyal, or peppermint oils is recommended to counter excessive drowsiness.
Herbal Medicine. For insomnia, Western herbalists suggest pouring

Reflexologists treat insomnia by pressing certain pressure points, including one just below the ankle bone on each side of the foot.

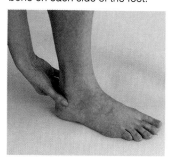

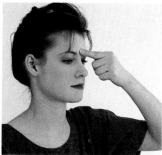

Two other sleep-inducing pressure points can be found behind each side of the jaw, just below the ear lobe.

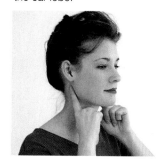

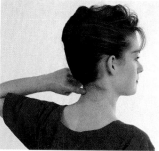

Another insomnia pressure point is located above the bridge of the nose between the eyebrows.

One other point is at the center of the nape of the neck. Select any two points and press on each for 30 seconds at a time.

1 quart of boiling water over a cup of dried valerian root, letting it steep for 25 minutes, then adding the strained liquid to a warm bath, taken just before bedtime. Two capsules or an infusion of California poppy or passion flower or a cup of chamomile tea consumed just before going to bed are also thought to combat insomnia. Drinking thyme tea is said to protect against nightmares.

Homeopathy. To prevent awakening in the middle of the night, nux vomica is taken before bed. Passion flower is used to combat restless sleep.

Hydrotherapy. A warm bath just before bedtime is soothing and relaxing. Sipping warm milk and listening to soft music while soaking enhances the effect.

Hypnosis. Self-hypnosis—a variation of the age-old counting sheep remedy—is a relaxation technique that may help people with stress-related insomnia. Some hypnotherapists teach patients to give themselves mental clues to induce relaxation and drowsiness.

Light Therapy. People who travel frequently or work swing shifts may develop sleep problems related to disturbed circadian rhythms, the internal clock that controls sleep cycles. Studies show that exposure to very bright light can help reset these internal clocks. Thus, a person who works a night shift and has trouble sleeping during the day should make sure that the bedroom is dark and then, before going to work in the late afternoon or evening, spend two hours exposed to lights.

Massage. A gentle massage is extremely relaxing, especially if oils are used, and can be a fine antidote to overcoming stress-related sleeplessness.

Meditation and Visualization. Any form of meditation can be useful in coping with sleep problems. Regular deep breathing combined with progressive muscular relaxation produces a relaxed state that promotes sleep.

Music Therapy. Some people find that soft, relaxing music helps them to fall asleep. In contrast, more lively music can combat daytime sleepiness.

Naturopathy and Nutrition Therapy. Supplements of melatonin, a hormone secreted by the pineal gland, are promoted as a safe natural therapy for insomnia. Studies show 2.5 to 10 milligrams of melatonin, which is sold in health food stores or in vitamin sections, restore normal sleep patterns in chronic insomniacs. As an added benefit, melatonin is said to slow the aging process and bolster immunity. Researchers caution that much remains to be learned about the hormone, but early studies appear promising.

Eating a light bedtime snack of foods high in tryptophan, an amino acid, can combat insomnia. Such foods include milk, yogurt, turkey, bananas, dates, figs, tuna, whole-grain crackers, and nut butter. In the evening, avoid foods that contain tyramine, such as cheese, sugar, chocolate, bacon, ham, sausage, eggplant, spinach, and tomatoes, as well as wine and other alcoholic beverages.

Psychotherapy. Counseling may help sleep disorders linked to anxiety, depression, or other psychological problems.

Reflexology. Pressure points that are said to promote sleep are illustrated above. The outside edge of the nail of the second toe is also a sleep inducer. Reflexologists suggest pressing on two points for about 30 seconds.

Self-Treatment

A few common sense measures may be all that is needed to overcome common sleep problems. Avoid caffeine for at least four hours before going to bed. People who are very sensitive to caffeine should eliminate it completely.

Don't go to bed hungry, but also avoid eating a heavy meal late in the evening. Have a moderate dinner and a low-fat snack an hour before bedtime.

Exercise regularly, but not within the few hours before bedtime.

Invest in a truly comfortable bed that suits your needs. Make the bedroom as soundproof as possible. If it's still noisy, try earplugs or a white noise machine that plays soothing sounds to mask outside noise. Use dark drapes to block out light, and set the temperature at a comfortable level. Wear comfortable bed clothes and use a blanket or comforter that is neither too hot nor heavy.

Don't go to bed until you are sleepy. If you can't fall asleep, get up and engage in some relaxing activity, such as taking a warm bath. If you have slept poorly one night, a nap the next day may or may not be helpful. Experiment to find what works for you.

Keep to a regular sleeping schedule, picking a time when you are usually sleepy and going to bed at about the same time each night. Set your alarm clock for about the same time every morning, regardless of how much sleep you have had. Force yourself out of bed even if you slept poorly, and if you awaken before the alarm goes off, get up then. Sleep researchers say most insomniacs stay in bed too long.

Never punish or tease a child who sleepwalks or has night terrors and nightmares. Sleepwalkers usually avoid obstacles, but may stumble against furniture or lose their balance and tumble down stairs or out a window. If your child sleepwalks, make sure to protect against these possibilities.

Anyone with narcolepsy should not operate hazardous machinery or drive a car unless the disorder is effectively controlled with medication.

Snoring

Snoring, a very common occurence, affects some 100 million Americans, mostly older adults. Why so many snore is unknown, but the source of the noise is clear. When these people sleep, their throat muscles relax, and as air passes over the uvula (the pendant of flesh that hangs down at the back of the mouth), it causes vibrations similar to those produced when someone plays a woodwind instrument. Instead of musical tones, however, snoring creates harsh, rasping noises. These sounds are more disturbing to sleeping partners than to the snorers themselves, who are usually unaware of the problem until someone complains of the noise.

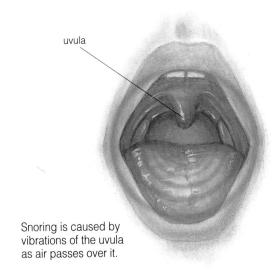

uvula

Snoring is caused by vibrations of the uvula as air passes over it.

Males who snore greatly outnumber women, and the likelihood that a person of either sex will snore increases with age. Among people in their thirties, about 5 percent of women and 20 percent of men have the problem, compared with 40 percent of women and 60 percent of men at age 60.

Snoring can occur at any stage of sleep, but it seems to be most pronounced during the REM, or dreaming stages. Sleeping on one's back often contributes to the problem, and having the mouth open might also be a factor. However, some people snore no matter what sleeping position they assume and whether their mouth is open or closed. The use of alcohol, tranquilizers, sleeping pills, and antihistamines and other medications that relax the muscles of

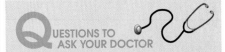

QUESTIONS TO ASK YOUR DOCTOR

▶ Should I consider wearing a mouth guard to prevent snoring?
▶ Would I benefit from spending a night in a sleep laboratory?

the throat and dry the mucous membranes can promote snoring. Smoking can have a similar effect.

Certain physical characteristics promote snoring. People who are markedly overweight are three times more likely to snore than those who are thin. Blockage of nasal passages accounts for some cases of snoring, especially in children with overgrown adenoids and adults who have a deviated septum.

Diagnostic Studies and Procedures

A person who consults a doctor because snoring is interfering with sleep (or threatening to destroy a relationship) will be given a physical examination to look for possible airway obstructions in the nose, throat, and palate. If no physical abnormality is found, the physician will investigate other possible causes, including the use of medications and alcohol.

Spending a night in a diagnostic sleep laboratory for observation may be recommended, especially if sleep apnea (page 381) is suspected. This potentially dangerous condition is marked by loud snoring and fitful sleep, interrupted by brief periods during which the person stops breathing altogether.

Medical Treatments

There are no medical treatments for snoring itself, but a doctor may advise self-help strategies or seek ways to eliminate the underlying cause. For example, if the use of certain medications is contributing to the problem, a physician may suggest alternative drugs. Taking a decongestant before going to bed may help if nasal congestion is causing snoring.

Some patients are helped by wearing a mouth guard, a device that fits inside the mouth to hold the upper and lower

teeth together while sleeping. Ask your dentist about using such a device and where to have one made.

Surgery may be suggested for overgrown adenoids or a deviated septum, especially if the abnormality is linked to other problems such as breathing abnormalities or an increased number of sinus infections. A surgical procedure in which a laser is used to remove or reshape the uvula and nearby structures may be recommended. However, this operation does not always solve the underlying problem, and experts advise seeking a second or even a third opinion before undergoing it.

Alternative Therapies

These are directed to remedying possible underlying causes. If you are overweight, consult a nutritionist for help in working out a sensible weight-loss program that emphasizes adopting new eating habits and increasing exercise. If alcohol abuse is the underlying problem, participating in a support group such as Alcoholics Anonymous may bring about a desired change in lifestyle habits.

Self-Treatment

The problem of snoring is frequently solved through the process of trial and error. For example:

▶ If you snore mainly on your back, make every effort to sleep on your side or stomach. Some people find it helpful to sew a pocket on the back of pajamas and insert a tennis ball into it to discourage rolling over while sleeping.

▶ To make breathing easier, try elevating your head by putting a bolster under the mattress or a brick or piece of two-by-four lumber under each leg at the head of the bed.

▶ Make sure that your bedroom is as free of dust and other allergens as possible. A cool-mist humidifier will keep the air moist and prevent the drying of nasal passages. Washing your nasal passages with a saline solution before going to bed will also ease any nasal congestion.

▶ Instead of taking a sleeping pill or an alcoholic nightcap to help you fall asleep, have a glass of warm milk and honey before going to bed.

If all else fails, the person being disturbed by the noise might consider wearing earplugs at night.

Other Causes of Snoring

Hay fever and other allergies that affect the nasal passages may contribute to a snoring problem.

Sore Throat

(Pharyngitis)

In the United States, sore throats account for 40 million visits to medical facilities each year. Although many factors and circumstances promote them, the pain usually indicates inflammation of the pharynx, which extends from the back of the mouth to the esophagus. Common types of sore throats include:

Viral infections, especially colds and flu. The most prevalent sore throats, these are self-limited and may be accompanied by fever, muscle aches, and a runny nose. Less commonly, a sore throat may result from mononucleosis or viral pneumonia.

Bacterial infections, especially streptococcal bacteria. A strep throat typically comes on suddenly, is acutely painful, and is accompanied by fever. Such an infection usually occurs between the ages of 5 and 25 and if not treated promptly with antibiotics, it can spread to other organs and may cause irreversible heart and kidney damage.

Tonsillitis, usually due to infection and inflammation of the tonsils. Quinsy is a severe infection of the tonsils themselves or bits of tonsillar tissue left behind after a tonsillectomy.

Diagnostic Studies and Procedures

A doctor will ask about other symptoms, feel for swollen glands under the jaw and in the neck, and then inspect the throat using a bright light and magnifying devices. A sample of pus or other secretions may be taken for microscopic examination and a culture to identify any infecting organism.

Medical Treatments

If strep or another bacterial infection is suspected, a broad-spectrum antibiotic will probably be prescribed even before results of the culture are known. The medication may be changed later, depending upon the causative organism. For strep throat, the first choice of treatment is 10 days of penicillin. Erythromycin may be used instead for persons who are allergic to penicillin.

A chlamydial throat infection is treated with a seven-day course of oral tetracycline or doxycycline. Gonococcal pharyngitis is typically treated with a single dose of ceftriaxone and seven days of oral doxycycline.

It is critical to complete the full prescribed course of antibiotics to fully eradicate the bacteria, even if symptoms

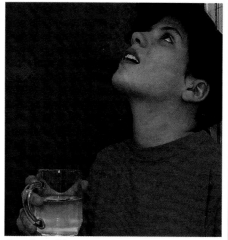

Gargling with warm salt water is a time-honored measure to alleviate a sore throat. Herbal brews also may be used.

disappear after two or three days. Otherwise, any surviving bacteria can cause a relapse or smoldering infection, which can damage vital organs.

Alternative Therapies

Aromatherapy. Therapists recommend oils of eucalyptus, geranium, lavender, and sage to alleviate discomfort. The oils can be massaged into the skin, from under the chin to the base of the throat, or they may be inhaled after placing them in a steam humidifier.

Herbal Medicine. Gargling with a sage preparation is said to alleviate a sore throat. Make an infusion of 1 cup of sage tea, and add a teaspoon each of honey and cider vinegar. Use as a gargle four times a day. Gargling with warm chamomile tea as often as needed may help. A Russian herbal remedy calls for drinking a mixture of a tablespoon of horseradish and a teaspoon each of honey and ground cloves added to a glass of warm water.

Naturopathy. Practitioners advise taking garlic capsules three times a day for their antibiotic properties, and sucking on a zinc lozenge every two hours for a week. Some also suggest high doses of vitamin C to hasten recovery or act as a

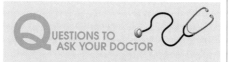

QUESTIONS TO **ASK YOUR DOCTOR**

▶ Will a tonsillectomy help prevent my recurrent sore throats?
▶ If the cause of my sore throat is a chlamydia infection, should my sexual partner be treated with antibiotics too?

WHEN TO SEE A DOCTOR

Although most sore throats are not serious health threats, some indicate a more serious underlying condition. Any throat inflammation that causes swelling and difficulty in breathing is potentially fatal. In such a case, call an ambulance or go to the nearest emergency room. Otherwise, a doctor's assessment is needed if a sore throat lasts for more than four days of self-treatment. See one sooner if strep throat is suspected or the pain is accompanied by:

▶ A high fever (over 103°F or 39.5°C) or any temperature that lasts more than three days.
▶ A skin rash.
▶ Very painful swallowing.
▶ The spitting up of bloody phlegm.

preventive, but this remains unproven. In any event, these should not substitute for antibiotics to treat strep throat.

Self-Treatment

The body gets rid of most sore throats by itself in a few days, but to ease discomfort, you can:

▶ Add ½ teaspoon of salt to ½ cup of warm water and gargle with it every few hours. Or try gargling with 3-percent hydrogen peroxide (1 part to 4 parts of water).

▶ Drink extra fluids, especially warm broth, herbal teas, and fruit juices. A time-tested home remedy calls for sipping a mixture of 1 tablespoon each of honey and cider vinegar or lemon juice in 1 cup of warm water.

▶ Suck on honey, eucalyptus, or other lozenges. A throat spray containing phenol helps temporarily, but ask a doctor before using it on children.

▶ Use a humidifier to keep air moist.

▶ Take aspirin, acetaminophen, or ibuprofen to lower a fever and alleviate pain. However, do not give aspirin to anyone under the age of 18 who has a viral infection. In this situation, aspirin is linked to an increased risk of Reye's syndrome (see box, page 437).

Other Causes of Sore Throats

Excessive shouting or singing, allergies, environmental irritants, tobacco use, polyps, and oral or throat cancer are among the many noninfectious causes of sore throats. The infectious causes include chickenpox, mumps, diphtheria, and herpes. Bacterial sore throats also can be caused by sexually transmitted diseases such as chlamydia and gonorrhea when contracted through oral-genital sex.

Speech Defects

(Aphasia; dysphonia; stuttering)

Because speech is essential to human communication, anything that interferes with it can be isolating and emotionally distressing. Primary mutism, in which a person cannot speak due to absent vocal cords or another structural defect, is rare. More commonly, difficulty speaking is secondary to other conditions, including paralysis, deafness, retardation or other mental disorders, and larynx cancer. In certain cases, a person knows how to speak but has difficulty forming words. Three often encountered disorders are:

Aphasia (from the Greek, meaning "without speech"), in which brain damage impairs a person's ability to speak and/or understand spoken or written words. Sudden aphasia usually is due to a stroke or a head injury, whereas the likely cause of slowly developing aphasia is a brain tumor or progressive dementia.

Stuttering, in which speech is disrupted by the involuntary repetition or prolongation of certain sounds. About 2.5 million Americans stutter. The problem usually begins between ages two and five, with male stutterers outnumbering females threefold. Many youngsters outgrow stuttering by the time they reach adolescence, but for others it remains a lifelong problem. Until recently, stuttering was attributed mostly to anxiety or other emotional problems. Although these may be contributing factors, research implicates subtle brain abnormalities as the major cause.

Spastic dysphonia (from the Greek, meaning "faulty sound"), a neuromuscular disorder in which unpredictable spasms compress the vocal cords, causing irregular speech that may sound choked or whispered. The problem, which originates in the nerve cells at the base of the brain that control the laryngeal muscles, usually begins between ages 40 and 50 and affects more women than men. In some cases, the condition seems to be hereditary; in others, it is triggered by an injury, stroke, or exposure to certain chemicals. Stress intensifies the symptoms but does not cause them.

Diagnostic Studies and Procedures

The nature of the speech problem is usually obvious; hence, diagnostic studies are directed to finding a possible

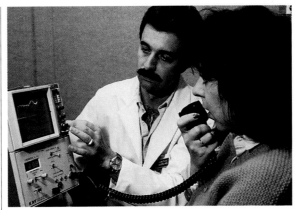

In helping patients who have stuttering or aphasia problems overcome them, speech therapists sometimes use a computer technique that analyzes different speech patterns.

underlying cause. In the case of aphasia, tests generally include X-rays and CT scans or MRI to assess a stroke or look for a tumor. An evaluation by a psychologist or psychiatrist may be recommended if the aphasia is associated with Alzheimer's disease or other forms of dementia.

An ear-nose-throat specialist (ENT physician or otolaryngologist) is able to diagnose dysphonia by inserting a flexible viewing tube into the larynx and observing the structure and functioning of the vocal cords.

Medical Treatments

The underlying causes of aphasia and dysphonia may be treated with drugs, surgery, or a combination of the two.

A promising experimental treatment for dysphonia involves injecting very small amounts of botulinum toxin, the substance that causes botulism, into the muscles that control the vocal cords. Preliminary studies show that this can restore normal or near-normal speech for up to four months, after which the injection is repeated. The injections are administered through the neck under local anesthesia.

Stuttering is best treated with a combination of the speech therapy and self-help techniques described below.

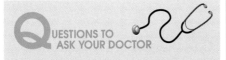

Alternative Therapies

Biofeedback. This technique may help some persons overcome stuttering and mild dysphonia.

Music Therapy. Stutterers and people with aphasia can often sing without difficulty. A form of music therapy called melodic intonation can improve the ability to communicate.

Speech Therapy. Trained therapists use a combination of physical therapy, speech techniques, computer aids, tape recordings, and other devices to help patients overcome aphasia or stuttering. Patients are taught special techniques for talking on the telephone and public speaking. An experimental method of communication called computerized visual communication employs pictures on a computer screen to represent the various parts of speech.

Visualization and Meditation. These and other relaxation techniques can help a person overcome some speech problems, especially those that are worsened by stress.

Self-Treatment

Speech therapists usually prescribe fluency exercises, which should be done daily. A tape recorder can be helpful in measuring progress.

The National Aphasia Association suggests the following to help those with speech problems:

▶ Reduce background noise and give the speaker your full attention. Be patient; refrain from finishing sentences or speaking for the person unless it is absolutely necessary.
▶ Try not to ask questions that require complicated answers. Give the person time to answer or to backtrack and correct a mistake.
▶ Speak simply, slowly, and use a normal tone of voice. If the person has suffered brain damage and reacts with incomprehension, repeat what you said, perhaps using simpler key words.

Other Causes of Speech Problems

In addition to the disorders listed earlier, speech problems may be caused by cerebral palsy and other birth defects, Parkinson's disease, multiple sclerosis, and autism. Laryngitis causes temporary loss of voice. Rarely, a type of hysterical neurosis can produce mutism.

Spinal Arthritis

(Ankylosing spondylitis; Marie-Strümpell disease)

Spinal arthritis is a chronic, progressive joint disease that affects mostly men. The condition's medical name, ankylosing spondylitis, comes from Greek words that describe what happens as the disease progresses: The spine (spondyl) becomes inflamed (itis) and the vertebrae fuse together (ankylosing). An estimated 300,000 Americans have been diagnosed with spinal arthritis, but the actual incidence may be much higher, because a large number of cases are so mild that they go undetected for decades.

The cause of spinal arthritis is unknown, but there is probably a hereditary predisposition In many cases, a specific genetic marker, designated as HLA-B27, shows up in blood tests.

Although the disease process may begin in childhood, the first symptoms typically show up between ages 15 and 30. Early indications include severe pain and stiffness in the affected joints, which may be accompanied by fatigue, loss of appetite, and perhaps an intermittent low-grade fever. The spinal inflammation typically begins around the sacroiliac joints, where the lowermost spine (the sacrum) connects with the pelvic bone (ilium). The disease usually progresses up the spine, sometimes as high as the neck. It also affects

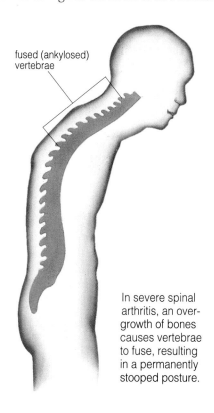

fused (ankylosed) vertebrae

In severe spinal arthritis, an overgrowth of bones causes vertebrae to fuse, resulting in a permanently stooped posture.

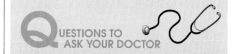
QUESTIONS TO ASK YOUR DOCTOR

▶ What are the best exercises to keep my back strong and straight?
▶ Should I wear a back brace? If so, what kind do you suggest?

other joints, including the shoulders, knees, or ankles. The inflammation causes overgrowth of the bones. As the spinal column becomes more rigid, the vertebrae may fuse so that the person has a permanently stooped posture, a major characteristic of the disease.

Some patients also suffer inflammatory bowel diseases, such as ulcerative colitis or Crohn's disease; heart-valve abnormalities; and/or related eye inflammation.

Diagnostic Studies and Procedures

Spinal arthritis is diagnosed on the basis of family history, a physical examination, X-rays, and blood tests. The presence of the genetic marker helps confirm the diagnosis, but its absence does not rule out the disease.

Medical Treatments

Although no medical cure exists for spinal arthritis, drugs play an essential role in reducing inflammation and pain. The condition appears to be less responsive to aspirin than most other inflammatory joint disorders, but some patients find they can manage with over-the-counter nonsteroidal anti-inflammatory drugs (NSAIDs) in the ibuprofen category (Advil, Motrin, Nuprin, and others). The most effective prescription drug for spinal arthritis is indomethacin (Indocin), one of the more potent NSAIDs.

A corticosteroid shot can alleviate a sudden flare-up. However, steroids are not a part of long-term treatment because of their serious side effects, which include lowered immunity, bleeding problems, and bone loss.

Various braces may be used to hold the back straight and prevent fusing of the spinal column in a stooped position. Surgery is sometimes recommended in advanced cases to remove some of the bone overgrowth and improve posture.

Alternative Therapies

Acupuncture. For some people, occasional treatments by an acupuncturist reduce the amount of pain-killing medication they need to do their exercises.

Alexander Technique. Patients with severe spinal arthritis tend to stoop

because this posture is less painful than standing erect. After analyzing the individual's way of standing, sitting, and performing daily tasks, a therapist of the Alexander technique can recommend special preventive exercises that will help retain as much spinal flexibility as possible. If fusing is inevitable, it is preferable to have the spine in a rigid upright position rather than one that is bent forward.

Hydrotherapy. Swimming and exercising in warm water helps maintain muscle tone and strength without putting undue stress on weight-bearing joints. Whirlpool baths and water massage can alleviate joint pain.

Occupational Therapy. An occupational therapist can provide suggestions on how best to perform daily tasks.

Physical Therapy. Daily exercise is a critical aspect of managing spinal arthritis. A physical therapist can help devise a suitable regimen that will stretch and strengthen the muscles surrounding the affected joints so that they remain flexible. The therapist may also teach deep-breathing exercises, especially if the rib cage is deformed.

Psychotherapy. Spinal arthritis can take a heavy emotional toll, especially if it produces disability and deformity. Counseling may be helpful in coping with the problems of living with a progressive chronic disease. Joining a support group may also prove beneficial.

T'ai Chi. The gentle range-of-motion exercises of t'ai chi can help maintain strength and flexibility, even if a person is unable to perform all of the prescribed movements.

Self-Treatment

To keep the spine as straight as possible, even during the night, doctors advise sleeping on your back on a hard mattress, with your body stretched out full-length and without pillows under your head. Always avoid slouching. If your job entails sitting, make sure your chair provides proper back support.

When driving, always wear your seat belt and adjust your head rest for maximum support. A pillow behind the small of your back eases strain. You may need to wear neck and back braces for additional support; discuss this with your doctor or physical therapist.

Other Causes of Back Symptoms

Back pain may result from muscle spasms, a ruptured disk, an injury, an infection, spinal stenosis, and other forms of arthritis.

Sprains and Dislocations

A stretching or tearing of ligaments, the fibrous bands that bind bones together at a joint, is referred to as a sprain. Typically, the surrounding blood vessels are also injured, resulting in bruising.

Although ligaments are very strong, almost any fall or misstep that twists a joint into an unnatural position can result in a sprain; in fact, a sprained ankle is the most common of all sports injuries. The knees are also vulnerable to severe sprains, especially among skiers. Improved bindings and inflexible boots have resulted in a 90-percent decrease in broken legs and ankles, but knee sprains have increased threefold.

Some sprains are accompanied by a dislocation, in which the end of the bone is displaced from its joint. Most dislocations result from a fall, a blow, or a movement that forces the joint beyond its normal range of motion, such as may occur in wrestling, football, and gymnastics.

The finger joints are especially susceptible to dislocation; in fact, some people with lax finger joints can dislocate them at will. Of larger joints, the shoulder is the most commonly dislocated, because of the ball-and-socket construction that gives it a 360-degree range of motion. When swung by their arms, young children may suffer dislocated shoulders. The wrists, knees, ankles, and toes are other joints that are frequently dislocated.

Both sprains and dislocations cause swelling, pain, and eventual discoloration at the affected site. An obvious deformity with the bones at odd angles to each other indicates a dislocation.

Diagnostic Studies and Procedures

X-rays are taken to determine the extent of damage and whether there are any fractures. A dislocation is always X-rayed before any attempt at correction. Severely torn ligaments may also be studied by MRI scanning. In some cases, arthroscopy, a procedure in which a lighted viewing instrument is inserted into a joint, may be ordered.

Medical Treatments

Treatments of sprains vary according to their classification (see box, Degrees of Sprain) and which joint is involved. Grades 1 and 2 sprains can usually be handled with self-care, although physical therapy may be needed (see facing page), especially if the knee or another major weight-bearing joint is injured.

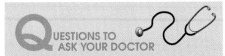
Aspirin, ibuprofen, or other nonsteroidal anti-inflammmatory drugs are recommended to control pain and inflammation. If a stronger painkiller is necessary, codeine or another morphine derivative may be prescribed.

Usually, a doctor can successfully manipulate a dislocated bone back into its socket after administering a local anesthetic. In some cases, however, surgery is necessary.

Torn ligaments, especially of the knee and shoulder, often require surgical repair. This can now be done through arthroscopic surgery, in which surgeons use tiny instruments and a surgical microscope to work through a lighted viewing tube, or arthroscope, inserted into the joint. Arthroscopic surgery requires only small puncture openings instead of a long, open incision, thereby minimizing bleeding and scarring. Thanks to this development, shoulders and knees can be stabilized with much less loss of strength and mobility than was previously possible.

Alternative Therapies

Herbal Medicine. A liniment made by boiling 1 tablespoon of cayenne pepper in 1 pint of cider vinegar and applied as a cool compress is said to reduce swelling of a simple grade 1 sprain. Rubbing marjoram oil or tincture of arnica into the area is also suggested.

Physical Therapy. Patients who have severe sprains involving the knees and perhaps other weight-bearing joints frequently require physical therapy. The objective is to strengthen the surrounding muscles in order to give the joint more stability. Physical therapy is also necessary following surgery to repair torn ligaments.

Self-Treatment

RICE—an acronym for **r**est, **i**ce, **c**ompression, and **e**levation—is the basic self-treatment for sprains (see page 306). It's best to refrain from using the injured joint for the first 24 hours. To reduce swelling, rest the injured part

FIRST AID FOR A BAD SPRAIN

1. Do not allow the person to walk if the knee or ankle is injured. Keep the limb elevated until transport is available.
2. If ice is available, apply a plastic bag packed with crushed ice wrapped in cloth to the injured area for 30 minutes. This reduces blood flow and swelling.
3. To immobilize a sprained ankle, use a roll of three-inch wide cotton gauze. Start by making two turns around the foot (A), then begin wrapping upwards using figure-eight turns (B). Bandage until the foot, ankle, and lower leg are wrapped (C); anchor with a safety pin.

FIRST AID FOR A DISLOCATION

1. DO NOT ATTEMPT TO RESTORE THE BONE TO ITS JOINT. Instead, make the person comfortable and immobilize and splint the joint in the position in which it is found. You can immobilize a dislocated finger or toe simply by taping or wrapping it firmly between its two adjacent members. To improvise a splint, use a rolled newspaper, piece of wood, or other firm object.
2. Apply a sling if appropriate. If the jaw is dislocated, loop an improvised bandage under the chin and tie at the top of the head.
3. Apply cold packs, if available, and seek emergency medical help.

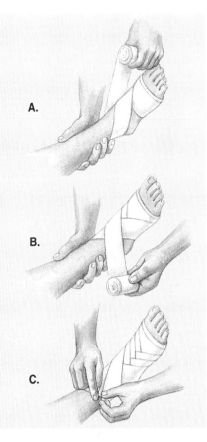

A.

B.

C.

REHABILITATING A SPRAINED ANKLE

These exercises can prevent repeated injuries by strengthening supporting muscles.
1. Stand with your feet comfortably apart and rise up on the balls of your feet as high as you can without losing your balance (A). Then lower your heels. Repeat this 20 times.
2. Stand on your heels by raising your toes off the ground (B). Walk around the room on your heels for several minutes. Then walk on the insides of your feet for a while; follow this exercise by walking on the outsides (C).

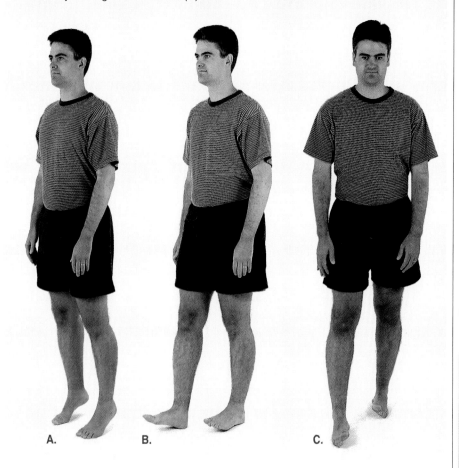

A.   B.   C.

and place an ice bag wrapped in a cloth over the area. A typical regimen calls for applying ice 15 minutes of every hour for the first 12 to 24 hours.

To further minimize swelling, wrap the area with an elastic bandage and elevate the joint so that it is higher than the heart. Take care not to make the bandage too tight; loosen it if swelling increases or there is any numbness, tingling, or loss of feeling in the area below the bandage.

After the first 24 to 48 hours, heat may be substituted for the ice packs.

DEGREES OF SPRAINS

Doctors classify sprains as follows:

Grade 1: The ligament is stretched, and any tearing is visible only under a microscope.
Grade 2: The ligament is partly torn apart.
Grade 3: The ligament is completely torn.

At this stage of healing, the application of heat, in the form of a heating pad or other warm compress, increases blood flow to the area and may speed healing.

Follow your doctor's guidelines for resuming use of the joint. He may encourage some movement of the joint early in the healing process to prevent stiffness, but this advice varies according to the site and extent of injury.

To reduce the risk of recurrent sprains and dislocations, follow these commonsense precautions:
▶ Use elastic supports, taping, wrapping, and bracing for protection of ankles, knees, wrists, or elbows during active sports.
▶ Pay special attention to footwear, making sure that your shoes are suitable for your particular activity.

Other Causes of Joint Swelling
A fracture can produce many of the symptoms of a sprain or dislocation.

David Roberts suffered his first dislocated shoulder while skiing at the age of 17. "I was sure I had broken something," he recalls, "but the resort doctor immediately saw that my shoulder was dislocated." X-rays were taken, which confirmed the injury and the absence of any broken bones. The doctor then used simple traction to ease the joint back into place. Roberts was placed prone on an examination table with his arm dangling over the edge and a five-pound weight attached to his wrist. Within 15 minutes, the shoulder had eased back into proper alignment. The doctor instructed Roberts to lay off skiing for at least four weeks, and recommended he see a physical therapist.

But Roberts wasn't going to let such a simple injury keep him down for long. He skipped the physical therapy and was back on the slopes before the month was up. He finished that ski season without further mishap, but the following summer, he suffered a second dislocation while playing golf with his father. Again, the doctor was able to manipulate his shoulder into place, and suggested that Roberts take up running or cycling to give his shoulder a chance to mend. This time Roberts heeded the doctor's advice, but even so, he suffered four more incidents of shoulder dislocation during the next two years.

"It was reaching the point where I couldn't ski, play tennis, or golf without having my shoulder pop out of place," Roberts said. This is a common story—up to 80 percent of persons who experience a dislocated shoulder at an early age suffer recurrences. Roberts was referred to a center for sports medicine and a surgeon who specializes in shoulder repair. In Roberts' case, tears in the shoulder's anterior capsule were contributing to the joint instability.

The objective of the operation was to limit the external rotation of the shoulder enough to prevent dislocation, but not enough to restrict the range of motion needed for sports like tennis and golf. After an overnight hospital stay, Roberts was sent home with his shoulder in an immobilizing brace for three weeks. This was followed by six months of physical therapy, which included relearning tennis and golf swings.

Stomach Cancer

(Gastric adenocarcinoma)

Most stomach cancers are adenocarcinomas, malignancies that arise in the glandular cells that line the stomach and produce various hormones and mucus. Less common types are gastric lymphomas, tumors that form in the stomach's lymph tissue, and gastric sarcomas, which develop in connective tissue.

Although stomach cancer is now a relatively rare form of intestinal cancer —with about 24,000 new cases and 14,000 deaths a year—only 50 years ago it was the leading cause of cancer mortality in American men and third for women. Dietary changes appear to be a factor in this decline; in particular, less consumption of nitrates. (In Japan, which leads the world in stomach cancer, studies implicate nitrates—preservatives in pickled vegetables, salty sauces, and dried salted fish—all staples in the Japanese diet.) Some cases of stomach cancer have been linked to drinking water that is naturally high in nitrates.

The risk of stomach cancer increases with digestive disorders that reduce stomach acidity; for example, chronic bile reflux and atrophic gastritis. Pernicious anemia, which is marked by reduced production of a substance called intrinsic factor, is also linked to an increased risk of stomach cancer. People who have had part of their stomach removed sometimes develop gastric cancer 15 to 20 years later.

In its early stages, stomach cancer is often easy to overlook because its symptoms—persistent heartburn, bloating and discomfort after eating, nausea, loss of appetite, and sometimes mild abdominal pain—are vague and similar to those of other digestive disorders. Later, additional symptoms may include weight loss, fatigue, vomiting, blood in stools, and more severe pain.

Diagnostic Studies and Procedures

Iron deficiency anemia (in men) and blood in the stools should alert a doctor

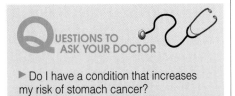

A small stomach cancer is treated by removing part of the stomach. tumor

Before surgery   **After surgery**

to possible intestinal cancer. When the stomach appears the likely site, tests will include an upper GI series—X-rays taken after swallowing barium, a chalky substance that coats the upper GI tract to make it more visible on film.

Any abnormality calls for gastroscopy, a procedure in which a viewing tube is inserted through the mouth and esophagus into the stomach, allowing a doctor to inspect its lining and collect biopsy samples from any suspicious area. Cells shed from the stomach lining can also be collected by using a washing technique, called gastric lavage, or by scraping the lining. These cells are then studied microscopically for cancer. If cancer is diagnosed, CT scans, MRI, and ultrasonography may determine whether it has spread.

Medical Treatments

Treatment depends on the stage of the cancer and such considerations as age, overall health, and previous history of cancer. The usual treatment involves surgical removal of the malignant tumor, which may entail taking out all or part of the stomach and possibly portions of other digestive organs if the cancer has spread to them.

Surgery is usually followed by chemotherapy with a combination of anticancer drugs, especially if the cancer has spread beyond the stomach. Some cancer specialists advocate adjuvant chemotherapy even if it appears that the cancer has not spread, because more than two-thirds of these patients eventually develop metastases.

Radiation is generally of little value as a primary treatment for stomach cancer, as the dosage needed would

cause extensive internal damage. Under study, however, is a technique called intraoperative radiotherapy, in which a single large dose of radiation is beamed directly into the tumor site at the time of surgery. In advanced cases, low-dose palliative radiation therapy may be used to alleviate pain.

Alternative Therapies

These may relieve pain and minimize the adverse effects of chemotherapy and other medical treatments. Effective pain control techniques may include meditation, guided imagery, hypnosis, and biofeedback. Other, more controversial therapies include the following:

Herbal Medicine. Western herbalists use Siberian ginseng, sarsaparilla, and wild Oregon grape, in capsule or extract forms, to minimize the side effects of chemotherapy.

Homeopathy. Euphorbium is prescribed every two hours for pain.

Nutrition Therapy. For the first few days after removal of all or part of the stomach, nutrients are given intravenously or via a feeding tube inserted directly into the remaining portion of the stomach through a small incision. Normal eating begins with a liquid diet for a few days, followed by gradual reintroduction of solid foods. Before leaving the hospital, the patient will be given a detailed eating plan and may also be advised to take supplements.

Good nutrition also plays a role in preventing stomach cancer. A diet made up mostly of fruits, vegetables, legumes, and grains probably helps prevent all types of intestinal cancers. These foods are high in fiber, vitamin C and other antioxidants, and other natural chemicals that are believed to protect against cancer.

Self-Treatment

Patients can still eat many of their favorite foods, even after removal of the stomach. However, a different meal pattern will be necessary to prevent too much food from entering the small intestine at once; this condition, referred to as dumping syndrome, can produce weakness, dizziness, sweating, nausea, vomiting, and palpitations. The best approach is to eat six to eight small meals a day, emphasizing foods high in protein and low in sugar and fat.

Other Causes of Stomach Symptoms

Digestive disorders that produce symptoms similar to those of stomach cancer include ulcers, gastritis, pancreatitis, diverticulosis, and gallstones.

QUESTIONS TO ASK YOUR DOCTOR

▶ Do I have a condition that increases my risk of stomach cancer?
▶ Would changing my diet reduce my risk?

Strep A

(Invasive streptococcus A)

Outbreaks of a deadly streptococcal infection that results in toxic shock and the rapid destruction of muscle and flesh have raised concern among scientists that a strain of strep A, the bacterium involved, is reemerging as a major health threat. According to the Centers for Disease Control and Prevention, the current wave of invasive strep A infections began in the late 1980s, and by 1990, about 10,000 to 15,000 cases were being reported in the United States each year. Although this is less common than other bacterial infections, it is of concern because of the rapidity with which strep A can maim and kill.

The strep organism multiplies rapidly, dividing every 45 minutes and producing progressively worse symptoms that include a rising fever and rash. By the third day, the patient's temperature may soar above 102°F (39°C). By the fourth day, 25 to 50 percent of patients begin to suffer tissue destruction

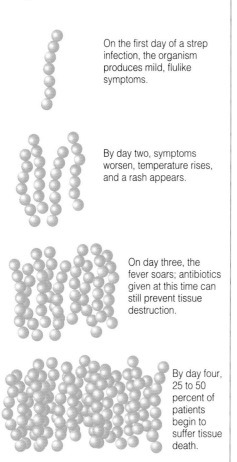

On the first day of a strep infection, the organism produces mild, flulike symptoms.

By day two, symptoms worsen, temperature rises, and a rash appears.

On day three, the fever soars; antibiotics given at this time can still prevent tissue destruction.

By day four, 25 to 50 percent of patients begin to suffer tissue death.

The rapid proliferation of the strep A organism and mounting toxin production can cause gangrene and even death.

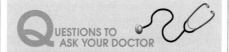

QUESTIONS TO ASK YOUR DOCTOR

▶ What is the likelihood that a strep throat might be caused by the invasive strep A strain?
▶ Is there any danger in traveling to an area where strep A has been reported?

because the bacterium, through a complex genetic process, produces toxin that rapidly kills muscle and other tissue. There may also be a severe drop in blood pressure and impaired circulation that causes further tissue death and gangrene. Although popularly dubbed "the flesh-eating" bacterium, tissue-killing is a more accurate description of what it does.

Sufferers have included Jim Henson, creator of the Muppets, who died within days of falling ill, despite massive antibiotic therapy. Survivors are often left disfigured or severely handicapped.

Contrary to media reports, strep A is not new, nor is it resistant to penicillin and other antibiotics. Populations of bacteria, like viruses and many other organisms, tend to wax and wane. The last major upsurge of invasive strep A was during World War II, but it seemed to die out, probably due to its natural life cycle. Researchers in the United States and abroad reported clusters of infections caused by "flesh-eating bacteria" in the 1980s. Since then, the number of cases has increased worldwide.

Strep A can be a complication of a skin rash, especially in children. During an epidemic of chickenpox in California in the early 1990s, 28 children developed invasive strep A when their skin blisters became infected with the organism. Five of these children died.

Fortunately, the infection does not appear to be as contagious as the more common strep strain that causes a strep throat. The invasive strep A bacterium typically infects the body through a minor cut and, rarely, via a sore throat. Initially, the patient may experience flulike symptoms—muscle aches, a sore throat, fever, and swollen lymph nodes. The skin wound becomes increasingly painful and inflamed.

Diagnostic Studies and Procedures

A rapid rise in temperature occurring in the presence of even a trivial wound or sore throat should raise a suspicion of invasive strep A, which can be identified by a laboratory culture.

Medical Treatments

Penicillin or another broad-spectrum antibiotic administered during the first three days of a strep A infection cures most cases. Even if treatment is delayed until the toxin has already begun its tissue destruction, antibiotics are still the mainstay of therapy. In this situation, clindamycin may be the most effective antibiotic, because it appears to prevent the bacteria from producing toxin. Antibiotics may be given by injection or intravenously, along with intravenous fluids, electrolytes, and other medications used to raise and maintain blood pressure.

All dead flesh must be removed surgically. In severe cases, amputation of infected limbs or other body parts may be necessary. Otherwise, the dead tissue becomes an ideal refuge for the bacteria, providing a haven that cannot be reached by antibiotics.

Alternative Therapies

There is no effective alternative to the immediate use of antibiotics for overcoming a strep A infection; medical treatment is of primary importance. But alternative therapies may play a role in rehabilitation, especially after amputation or extensive muscle loss.

Physical and Occupational Therapy. These therapists can teach exercises to help the patient regain muscle strength and can provide practical pointers in overcoming physical handicaps to retain independence.

T'ai Chi. This structured regimen of gentle exercises can improve muscle tone and function while fostering an enhanced sense of well-being.

Self-Treatment

Prevention is the best approach for dealing with this deadly disease. You should always take care to treat even the most minor cut immediately by washing the wound thoroughly with soap and water, flushing it with an antiseptic solution such as hydrogen peroxide or alcohol, and then applying an antibiotic cream.

See a doctor right away should you develop such symptoms as fever, swollen lymph nodes, or other signs of an infection.

Other Causes of Tissue Death

Staphylococcal toxic shock syndrome can cause a drop in blood pressure, tissue destruction, gangrene, and death.

Stress

Increasingly, doctors are recognizing that too much stress, or an inability to cope with it, is a serious health threat. Although many people think of stress as a modern phenomenon, humans have never lived in a stress-free environment. Indeed, many experts contend that our prehistoric ancestors, in their quest for food, shelter, and safety, faced stressors much worse than those of the 20th century. Still, the way in which our bodies respond to stress is a holdover from our earliest forebears.

When confronted with any stress, the body automatically goes into high gear, preparing either to defend itself or escape, the so-called fight or flight response. Here's what happens:

▶ Acting on the brain's command, the adrenal glands immediately pump out adrenaline, cortisol, and other hormones that travel through the body and prepare various organs to go into action to either flee or fight.

▶ Digestion slows to divert blood from the intestines to the muscles and brain. This sudden diversion and halt of digestion produce the stomach knotting or fluttering sensations, and perhaps nausea, associated with fear.

▶ Breathing speeds up to draw more oxygen into the body.

▶ The heart beats faster and blood pressure rises to ensure that muscles and the brain get enough blood.

▶ The liver pours extra sugar (glucose) into the bloodstream, and the pancreas supplies the insulin needed to metabolize it quickly.

▶ Sweating increases to cool the body, allowing it to burn extra energy.

▶ Muscles tense, getting ready to move.

▶ Chemicals that increase formation of blood clots are released in case the ensuing danger results in a wound.

If faced with a real emergency, the body remains in a state of preparedness until the danger is past or the person becomes exhausted. But the body responds in a similar fashion to such minor stresses as running late for an appointment or standing in a long line. We are so accustomed to facing scores, even hundreds, of such stressors each day that we barely notice our physical reactions. The effects add up, however. Frequent rises in blood pressure can eventually take a toll on the heart and blood vessels. Repeated shunting of

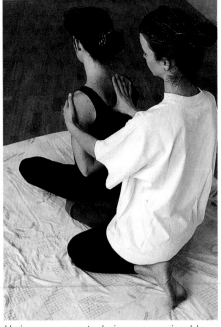

Various massage techniques are enjoyable and effective ways of countering stress.

blood from the intestines can promote digestive problems. Formation of a clot in a key artery of the heart or brain can precipitate a heart attack or stroke. Tensed muscles can trigger headaches, back pain, and other discomforts.

Not all stress is detrimental. Without some, life would be impossibly boring. In fact, many people seem to thrive on stress; they need a deadline or confrontation to get going. Others, however, fall apart when faced with even minor stress. Experts say that it's not necessarily the degree of stress that is harmful, but rather the way in which the individual copes with it.

Diagnostic Studies and Procedures

Before concluding that symptoms are stress-induced, a doctor must investigate and rule out organic causes. A person experiencing chest pains could be having a heart attack, suffering a bout of indigestion, or overreacting to stress. In this situation, an ECG and other heart studies are needed to eliminate the possibility of a heart attack. Only after a careful physical examination and appropriate tests fail to find a physical cause can a doctor safely conclude that stress is the problem.

Medical Treatments

Stress can generally be controlled with a combination of alternative therapies and self-care (see below). But in some instances, short-term medication may be needed to get through a particularly

STRESS-RELATED DISORDERS

Following are some of the many medical and psychological conditions caused or worsened by stress:

▶ Alcoholism
▶ Angina and other forms of heart disease
▶ Asthma and allergies
▶ Backache and other pain syndromes
▶ Chronic fatigue syndrome
▶ Diabetes
▶ Eating disorders
▶ Headaches, both migraine and tension
▶ High blood pressure
▶ Irritable bowel syndrome and other intestinal disorders
▶ Lupus and other autoimmune disorders
▶ Menstrual irregularities
▶ Obesity
▶ Rheumatoid arthritis
▶ Sexual dysfunction
▶ Ulcers

trying period, especially if tension is contributing to a serious medical condition, such as angina or an intestinal disorder.

If stress is interfering with sleep and thereby contributing to a worsening cycle of stress and insomnia, a doctor may prescribe a sedative for a few weeks. Severe anxiety or panic attacks may be treated with a benzodiazepine tranquilizer, such as diazepam (Valium). Because illness contributes to stress, treating an underlying medical condition may also help.

Alternative Therapies

Aromatherapy. Relaxing in a bath scented with chamomile, sandalwood, lavender, geranium, cypress, juniper, rose, or clary sage can be helpful in alleviating stress. Alternatively, a few drops of one of these oils can be placed on a handkerchief and its scent inhaled when stress is felt.

Biofeedback Training. This technique can help lessen the body's response to stress by fostering relaxation and also by allowing the patient to control, at least for short periods, blood pressure, heart rate, breathing, and other body functions that are normally automatic.

Massage. Few activities are more relaxing than a massage, especially one that uses the aromatic oils listed above. When a full body massage is impractical, shoes and socks can be removed and the feet massaged.

Meditation. Deep breathing, progressive relaxation, visualization, and other techniques are the key to finding effective ways of coping with stress.

Music Therapy. Playing some of your favorite music can help relieve stress. It doesn't have to be slow or boring to be relaxing; listening to music you enjoy is more important than its tempo.

Yoga and T'ai Chi. These movement therapies foster relaxation and enhance well-being—important factors in effective stress management.

Self-Treatment

Stress is especially detrimental when you feel that you have no control over the situation. When faced with a seemingly impossible task, try breaking it into manageable segments and then tackle them one at a time.

Learn to set priorities. If you have so much to do that you don't know where to start, list the various tasks. Assign each a number signifying its priority; for example, *1* might designate what needs to be accomplished today, *2* what

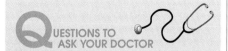

can wait until tomorrow, and *3* what can be postponed until later. Then look at today's list, arrange the tasks in order of importance, and tackle them one at a time. As you finish each task, cross it off your list, reflect on what has been accomplished, take a 10-minute break, and then continue. If you don't get through the entire list by quitting time, shift what's left to tomorrow, and try to make that day's list more realistic.

No matter how rushed you feel, leave some time each day for pleasurable activities—reading a good book, visiting a friend, or simply enjoying a sunset or pleasant scenery. Regular exercise

is also a good means of combatting stress. DO NOT turn to alcohol or recreational drugs as a means of relaxation; such escapes only create new problems, leading to further stress.

Finally, learn to share your stress and ask for help. Confiding in a relative or good friend can help put a problem into proper perspective. If you feel you cannot turn to a friend or family member, consider participating in group therapy or a self-help group of others who are experiencing similar problems. Just knowing that you are not alone can help alleviate stress.

Other Causes of Stress

Pheochromocytoma, an adrenal tumor that produces adrenaline and other hormones, can cause body responses that mimic those related to stress, as can other hormonal disorders. Many women going through menopause or those experiencing premenstrual syndrome develop unexplained periods of anxiety. Grief, illness, and traumatic experiences can also bring about significant stress.

A CASE IN POINT

Kate Arnold had always had absolutely normal blood pressure, so the 56-year-old editor was understandably upset and puzzled when a routine checkup turned up a pressure reading of 140/105. Her doctor explained that the stress of being in a doctor's office often raises blood pressure temporarily. He asked her to sit quietly for 15 minutes before he took a second reading. This one was 142/103.

"I'm not overly concerned about a systolic reading in the 140s in people in their fifties," the doctor said, "but any diastolic reading over 95 needs follow-up." Arnold was instructed to buy an automated blood pressure machine and to test herself once or twice a day for the next few weeks. "Be sure to write down your pressure, time of day, and any recent activities."

Arnold followed these instructions, and after three weeks, she noted an interesting pattern. When she took her blood pressure in the morning, it ranged from 120-135/78-85—normal readings. But when she took a reading after coming home from work, it was invariably 135-145/90-105. When Arnold showed the doctor her blood

pressure diary, he immediately sensed what the problem might be.

"What's going on at work?" he asked, explaining that normally, blood pressure is at its highest in the early morning, and lower in the late afternoon and evening. Arnold's opposite pattern pointed to on-the-job stress as a possible explanation for her high blood pressure.

"I don't know how much longer I'll even have my job," Arnold said, explaining that her publishing house was consolidating three divisions, which would eliminate a large number of positions. Further probing revealed that Arnold was also worried about her husband's health. On top of her other stresses, she was planning her daughter's wedding. "Sometimes I don't know whether I'm coming or going," she confessed, "and now I have my blood pressure to worry about!"

Under other circumstances, the doctor might have started the patient on antihypertensive medication, but in Arnold's case, he felt that an alternative course was worth a try.

"I think stress is driving up your blood pressure," he explained. "If I'm

right, relaxation therapy and exercise should bring it down." He taught Arnold a simple, 10-minute progressive relaxation routine. "Just close your door, take off your shoes, and do this routine twice a day."

The doctor also instructed Arnold to exercise for 20 to 30 minutes each day. "I know you don't think you have time, but regular exercise is one of the best ways to overcome stress and to lower blood pressure. Try leaving for work a half-hour earlier and walking for a couple of miles on your way to the office. Or take a long walk on your way home in the evening."

Arnold was instructed to follow this regimen for six weeks while continuing to monitor her blood pressure. After only four weeks of religiously practicing the progressive relaxation routine and walking two miles a day, her blood pressure was again stabilized in the normal range. In addition, she survived the job cuts at her office. But even with life on a more even keel, she was determined to continue her relaxation therapy and exercise, simply because she enjoyed a renewed sense of well-being.

Strokes

(Cerebral embolism, hemorrhage, or thrombosis; cerebrovascular accident; subarachnoid hemorrhage)

A stroke occurs when a portion of the brain is deprived of blood, resulting in ischemia or even tissue death. More than 500,000 Americans suffer a stroke each year, about one every minute. Although the stroke death rate has been cut in half over the last 25 years, the affliction still claims 144,000 lives annually, making it the third leading cause of death in the United States (after heart attacks and cancer). Strokes are also a major cause of serious disabilities, which include varying degrees of paralysis, speech problems, visual disturbances, and impaired memory.

Men suffer a slightly greater number of strokes than women, but women account for 60 percent of the deaths. Strokes are more widespread, more severe, and twice as likely to be fatal for African-Americans of both sexes than for Caucasians.

Most strokes fall into one of the following categories:

Cerebral thrombosis, the most common type. It occurs when a blood clot, or thrombus, forms in an artery supplying blood to the brain and is often preceded by mini-strokes, also called transient ischemic attacks or TIAs (see Warning Signs on facing page).

Cerebral embolism, which accounts for 5 to 14 percent of strokes. It occurs when an embolus (wandering clot) forms in the body, travels through the bloodstream, and lodges in the brain.

Cerebral hemorrhage, which accounts for 10 percent of strokes. It is caused by the rupture of a weakened blood vessel, or aneurysm, in the brain.

Subarachnoid hemorrhage, which is responsible for 7 percent of strokes. Often the result of an injury, a burst blood vessel bleeds into a space between the brain and skull, rather than inside the brain itself.

Although strokes appear to strike out of the blue, contributing factors are well-known. Poorly controlled high blood pressure greatly increases the risk, as does atherosclerosis, narrowing of blood vessels by fatty deposits. Heart disease, diabetes, excessive red blood cells, obesity, and high blood cholesterol all raise susceptibility to stroke. Other risk factors include such habits

as smoking and moderate-to-heavy alcohol use (defined as two or more drinks a day). Women who both smoke and take birth control pills also suffer a higher incidence of strokes. In addition to race, risk factors beyond one's control include advancing age and a family history of strokes.

Diagnostic Studies and Procedures

A doctor will immediately assess vital signs—blood pressure, heart rate, respiration—and listen for turbulent sounds, or bruits, in the neck's carotid arteries and in other key blood vessels. A suspected stroke calls for immediate neurological evaluation, including assessment of consciousness, orientation, memory, coordination, and vision, hearing, and other sensory responses. Blood studies will be ordered and an electrocardiogram taken, especially if a disturbed heart rhythm is suspected.

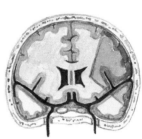

Cerebral thrombosis

When a clot forms in one of the brain's arteries and cuts off blood flow, that portion of brain becomes damaged.

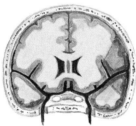

Cerebral embolism

A clot that forms elsewhere and travels to the brain can also block crucial blood flow and cause brain damage.

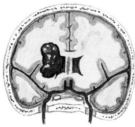

Cerebral hemorrhage

Bleeding from a burst blood vessel inside the brain injures the surrounding tissue.

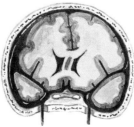

Subarachnoid hemorrhage

Bleeding into the subarachnoid space between the skull and brain can cause damage by encroaching on brain tissue.

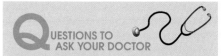

QUESTIONS TO ASK YOUR DOCTOR

► Am I in a high-risk group for stroke? If so, what can I do to lower that risk?
► After a stroke, at what point should I assume that a loss of function is going to be permanent?

The most important diagnostic study, however, is MRI or a CT brain scan to look for cerebral bleeding or blockage. Angiography can pinpoint blocked vessels and reveal damaged areas of the brain. In this procedure, radioactive dye is injected into a vein in the arm and then followed with a camera as it flows through the brain.

Other possible tests include Doppler ultrasound, for studying blood flow through the carotid arteries and other vessels; and carotid phonoangiography, in which a sensitive microphone is used to listen for bruits. An echocardiogram may be ordered if a doctor suspects the stroke is due to a clot that has traveled from the heart to the brain.

Medical Treatments

Intensive treatment within the first six hours after the onset of symptoms is critical in limiting the damage of a stroke. If stroke is due to a thrombus or embolus, clot-dissolving drugs may be administered, as well as heparin or similar medications to prevent more clots from forming. Other drugs may be given to lower blood pressure, steady the heartbeat, and prevent brain swelling.

In some cases, surgery is performed to remove accumulated blood or to repair a ruptured artery or aneurysm.

As soon as the patient's condition is stabilized, attention turns to rehabilitation, which involves a combination of medical and alternative therapies. The sooner rehabilitation begins, the greater the chance of a good recovery.

After a TIA, the goal of treatment is to prevent a full-blown stroke. Aspirin or other drugs that inhibit clot formation will be given. If the carotid artery is severely clogged, an endarterectomy—a surgical procedure is which an occluded carotid artery is cleared of fatty deposits—may be considered.

There is increasing emphasis on stroke prevention. For example, control of high blood pressure can reduce stroke risk by 50 percent or more. Treatment of atrial fibrillation, a type of cardiac arrhythmia often ignored because it usually produces only minor symptoms, also lowers the risk of a stroke.

Numerous studies have shown that a regimen of low-dose aspirin—typically, a baby aspirin or one regular aspirin a day—cuts the incidence of stroke. A doctor should be consulted first, however, because aspirin can increase the risk of hemorrhagic stroke, especially if a person has high blood pressure.

Alternative Therapies

Rehabilitation is a team effort that usually involves a neurologist, a physiatrist (a physician who specializes in rehabilitative treatment), and numerous therapists. Increasingly, a combination of conventional and alternative therapies is used to help patients regain lost function. New York University's renowned Rusk Institute of Rehabilitative Medicine employs the following alternative modalities in addition to conventional medicine.

Acupuncture. Doctors are studying the value of this ancient Chinese practice as a means of stimulating nerve pathways and restoring lost function.

Music Therapy. Therapists use music to improve mood, encourage movement, and help patients regain memory. Because the brain programs and remembers music differently than it processes language, a patient who has difficulty speaking or is suffering memory loss may be able to hum a melody or recall an incident associated with a particular song. As rehabilitation progresses, dance therapy may be added to improve coordination.

Physical and Occupational Therapy. As noted earlier, physical therapy should begin as soon as the immediate crisis is past. Initially, passive range-of-motion exercises, in which a therapist moves the patient's limbs, are used to keep muscles limber and help prevent clots from forming. As nerve function returns, the patient assumes a more active role in these exercises. In some cases, rehabilitation exercises are performed in water, especially if the patient is unable to walk.

Occupational therapy also begins as soon as possible. Partially paralyzed patients learn new approaches to self-care, which may entail using special eating utensils and grooming devices. Patients also learn how to use a cane or, if unable to walk, a wheelchair.

Stroke rehabilitation often takes years; therefore, patients (and family members) should expect to continue working with various therapists.

Speech Therapy. These therapists can help patients relearn speech and improve memory, often by using tape recorders, computers, and other devices.

Self-Treatment

Stroke recovery varies considerably; some patients who initially are totally paralyzed recover fully, while others become increasingly helpless. Experts stress that all family members play an indispensable role in helping the patient recover. Optimism, patience, and understanding are vital, but it is also important to resist the temptation to help too much; instead, encourage the patient to be as independent as possible.

A stroke often alters behavior and personality, but the nature of change depends upon the side of the brain that is damaged. Left-brain injury usually results in speech problems and a more cautious, less organized, and slower behavior style. Because they have difficulty in communicating, these patients often appear to be more handicapped than they actually are. However, if a task, such as relearning speech, is broken down into simple steps, they are often able to make great progress.

In contrast, a person who suffers right-brain damage may be able to speak, understand, and respond more quickly, but may have difficulty with tasks requiring spatial and perceptual skills. These patients, as well as their caregivers, tend to overestimate their capabilities, resulting in frustration when they fail. It is important to provide cues and encouragement, but it's also necessary to protect the patient from falls or self-injury.

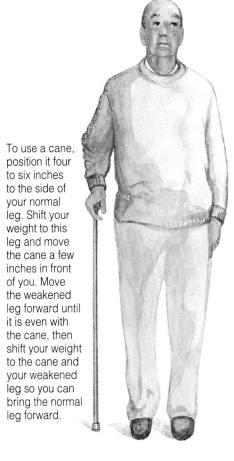

To use a cane, position it four to six inches to the side of your normal leg. Shift your weight to this leg and move the cane a few inches in front of you. Move the weakened leg forward until it is even with the cane, then shift your weight to the cane and your weakened leg so you can bring the normal leg forward.

Emotional ups and downs are to be expected after a stroke. Crying is especially common, but it may not reflect sadness—brain damage may be responsible. If the person stops crying immediately when you call his name or snap your fingers, the crying probably stems from organic causes rather than sadness. Similarly, do not assume that bursts of laughter signal happiness; they also may reflect brain damage.

To cope with these and other aspects of stroke recovery, specialists recommend joining a stroke survivors support group, which can be as beneficial for family members as for the patient (see Health Resources, page 466).

Other Causes of Stroke Symptoms

Head injuries can cause paralysis, disorientation, and other symptoms that characterize stroke. Memory loss, visual disturbances, and gait abnormalities can be caused by alcohol or drug abuse, as well as some medications. Other disorders that can mimic symptoms like those of a stroke include complicated migraine headaches, seizures, multiple sclerosis, and encephalitis, an inflammation of the brain.

WARNING SIGNS OF A STROKE

Seek immediate medical attention if any of these symptoms develop, even if they then disappear. Temporary symptoms may be due to a mini-stroke, or a transient ischemic attack (TIA), a common precursor to a full-blown stroke.

▶ Sudden weakness or numbness of the face, arm, or leg on one side of the body.

▶ Sudden dimness or loss of vision, especially in one eye.

▶ Loss of speech or difficulty understanding speech.

▶ Unexplained dizziness, a sudden fall, or loss of coordination.

▶ Confusion and unusual behavior.

▶ Sudden severe headache unlike any previous one.

Sty

(Hordeolum)

A sty develops when a pimple-like abscess forms in one or more of the specialized oil glands that line the eyelid. The term sty (or stye, as it is sometimes spelled) derives from the old English word *stigend,* which means "to rise." Hordeolum, the medical term for a sty, is Latin for "a small grain of barley," which describes its appearance.

Most sties develop at the base of an eyelash on the outside of an eyelid, but some, called internal hordeola, form on the inner edge. Regardless of where they appear, sties are usually caused by staphylococcal bacteria, organisms that normally live on the skin and in the nasal passages without causing harm.

Sties occur equally in women and men of all ages, but for reasons that are unknown, some people, especially children, seem to be particularly vulnerable to recurrent episodes. Exposure to chemical and environmental irritants, including tobacco smoke, is thought to increase the risk of sties.

An external sty typically begins as a red, itchy or sore spot that swells and eventually forms a pink or yellow head, similar to that of a pimple or small boil. The entire eyelid and surrounding area may be red and painful. The eye may feel as if something is in it and be more sensitive to light. In most cases, the sty comes to a head and ruptures in a few days and then heals itself.

An internal sty is more painful, but is not as readily apparent as an external one. Lifting the eyelid reveals the yellowish head, which is not as likely to rupture as that of an external sty. Instead, an internal sty may gradually subside

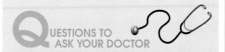

QUESTIONS TO ASK YOUR DOCTOR

▸ What measures should I take to prevent sties from recurring?
▸ If I have an internal sty, what is the best way to protect the eye from becoming infected?

in three or four days. Recurrence is more common than with external sties.

Diagnostic Studies and Procedures

Most sties can be diagnosed on the basis of their symptoms and appearance. In unusual cases, a doctor may order a laboratory culture of discharge from the sty to identify the infecting organism and prescribe an antibiotic.

Medical Treatments

Most sties can be handled with self-treatment, but medical care is warranted if a sty fails to rupture or does not drain spontaneously after it bursts. When a sty does not burst or drain, it may be opened with a fine-tipped lance, allowing a doctor to express its contents. To hasten healing and help prevent recurrence, an antibiotic ointment or cream may be applied to the edge of the eyelid several times a day. Antibiotic eyedrops also may be prescribed, especially for internal sties, to protect the eye itself from infection. In such cases, the drops should be applied to both eyes as a precaution.

Alternative Therapies

Herbal Medicine. Herbalists recommend washing the eyes with a cool tea made from raspberry leaves to alleviate pain. Parsley compresses are said to hasten healing of external sties. To prepare a compress, pour a cup of boiling water over a handful of fresh parsley and let it steep for 10 minutes. Soak a clean cloth in the hot tea and place it on the closed eyelid for 15 minutes. Continue with this procedure twice a day until the sty heals. A topical lotion made from eyebright is thought to help alleviate the pain and inflammation of sties.

Hydrotherapy. Warm, moist compresses applied to the eye for

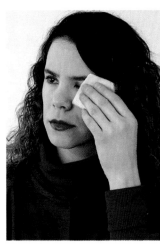

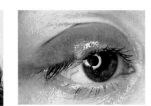

Typically, a sty forms near an eyelash on the upper lid. Holding a warm compress to the area eases pain and helps bring the sty to a head.

10 minutes three or four times a day help bring a sty to a head. They also relieve pain and inflammation.

Naturopathy. Some practitioners attribute the recurrence of sties to an inadequate intake of vitamin A or beta carotene, its precursor. Thus, increased consumption of orange, yellow, and dark-green leafy vegetables and yellow and orange fruits—all good sources of beta carotene—may be recommended to help prevent sties from forming.

Self-Treatment

See a doctor if a sty does not improve after two days of treatment with warm compresses or if several sties develop simultaneously or recur in rapid succession. Don't try to open a sty yourself. Squeezing or pressing it can spread the infection and make it worse. Always wash your hands with soap and water before and after touching a sty, and use boiled water and sterile gauze or cloth for compresses.

After a sty has come to a head and burst, you can help release the pus by gently easing the tip of the involved eyelash out of the infected area. Use a dilute solution of baby shampoo to bathe the eyelid and remove pus and any crusts that may have formed around the sty. Afterward, wash your hands again, and apply a thin layer of an antibacterial ointment.

To help prevent sties, avoid dust and other substances that can irritate the eye. If you work in an environment with irritants, be sure to wear protective goggles at all times.

If you wear removable contact lenses, be sure to clean and disinfect them daily. Never put a lens in your mouth to moisten it before putting it into your eye, as this transports germs from the mouth into the eye. Mascara and other eye cosmetics can also harbor bacteria. Replace them approximately every two or three months, and never share these items with others.

Other Causes of Eyelid Symptoms

A sty may easily be confused with a condition called chalazion, an inflammation of sebaceous glands in the eyelid. Instead of coming to a head, a chalazion forms a slowly expanding, grainy mass in the eyelid, which usually disappears on its own in a month. Sties are also similar to blepharitis, a chronic inflammation of the margins of the eyelid that can cause redness, discomfort, and sometimes ulcerations.

Sudden Infant Death Syndrome

(Crib death; SIDS)

When an apparently healthy infant dies and a medical investigation fails to uncover an explanation, cause of death is attributed to sudden infant death syndrome (SIDS). This syndrome, or crib death, claims about 8,000 infants in the United States each year, making it one of the most common causes of death in babies under one year.

The cause of SIDS is unknown, but researchers believe that it probably involves abnormalities in the mechanisms that control breathing and heart rate. Specific contributing factors may include a narrowed and inflamed airway, chronic oxygen deficiency, and irregular breathing, all of which may predispose an infant to spasm of the trachea, or windpipe, and death.

About 5 percent of babies who die of SIDS have had prior episodes of apnea, a condition in which breathing stops, usually during sleep. In most instances, the apnea is brief and the baby resumes breathing without incident. During a prolonged breathing lapse, however, the brain and heart become starved for oxygen, and this situation may result in a life-threatening cardiac arrhythmia. Death usually occurs rapidly, and most babies do not cry or struggle. Even a person in the same room may hear nothing. There have been cases in which an apparently healthy baby died silently in a car seat or a parent's arms.

Babies born to women who smoke have a markedly increased risk of SIDS, as do those who had a sibling die unexpectedly. Other possible predisposing factors include prematurity, low birth weight, and slower than normal growth. Racial, social, and economic factors may also play a role; SIDS occurs most

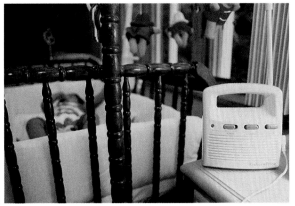
A crib monitor sounds an alarm when the baby's breathing stops for more than a few seconds.

often among Native Americans, followed in order by African-Americans, Caucasians, and Asian-Americans.

SIDS is most common during the winter and sometimes follows a cold. However, most SIDS babies were completely well before they died. They may even have seen a doctor recently and been pronounced healthy.

Diagnostic Studies and Procedures

In most cases, there are no symptoms before SIDS occurs to give any indication that the baby is in any danger. Therefore, after a death, an autopsy should be performed immediately to look for a possible cause, such as an undiagnosed congenital defect.

Medical Treatments

There is no medical treatment for SIDS, but in some cases, a baby who has had repeated episodes of apnea may be hospitalized for monitoring.

Alternative Therapies

Nutrition Therapy. There are many theories about what to feed or not feed a baby to prevent SIDS. Although some nutritionists have attributed SIDS to food allergies and bottle-feeding, this has not been proven. While experts agree that breast-feeding provides the best nutrition for young babies, SIDS occurs with equal frequency among breast-fed and bottle-fed infants.

Psychotherapy. The sudden loss of a baby is one of life's hardest blows. Psychological counseling can be very beneficial to the surviving family members, who invariably need help in coming to terms with this death. Siblings, for example, may develop a fear of falling asleep, especially if they have been told that the dead baby has "gone to sleep." They may also feel guilty, thinking that the baby died because they secretly wished it would go

away. Parents, too, may feel guilty or blame each other, even when assured that they were not at fault.

Different forms of psychotherapy are available, including family counseling or individual sessions with a therapist, social worker, or another professional trained in helping people to cope with a death in the family. There are also support groups of parents who have lost children to SIDS (see Health Resources, page 468).

Self-Treatment

Electronic monitoring is sometimes recommended for a high-risk baby. Such a monitor, placed in the crib, will sound an alarm if the baby ceases breathing for more than a few seconds.

A baby's sleeping position may have something to do with the risk of SIDS. Several studies here and abroad have found an increased incidence of SIDS among babies who slept on their stomachs rather than their sides or backs. This has led many pediatricians to recommend that infants be placed on their backs, but this advice is somewhat controversial. Some doctors maintain that babies who are prone to spitting up should be placed on their stomachs to prevent possible choking. Increasingly, however, pediatricians are advising that infants be placed on their backs.

Regardless of his sleeping position, a child should be placed on a firm, smooth mattress that is covered with a tight-fitting sheet. Pillows should not be used, nor should the baby be swaddled snugly. Instead, loosely cover him with a light blanket. Also, avoid overheating the bedroom.

Parents and others should not smoke around infants, as secondhand smoke can damage their vulnerable respiratory systems and may contribute to SIDS.

Other Causes of Sudden Death in Babies

Autopsies sometimes reveal that sudden death is due to a brain hemorrhage, often the result of a fall or child abuse. Other causes of infant death may include myocarditis, an inflammation of the heart muscle; and meningitis, an infection of the membranes that cover the brain and spinal cord. Unlike SIDS, these usually produce prior symptoms.

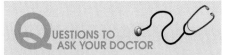

QUESTIONS TO ASK YOUR DOCTOR

▶ Should I use an electronic monitor for my baby during sleep?
▶ After losing one baby to SIDS, what are the chances that a future baby will suffer a similar fate?
▶ What is the best way to explain the baby's death to my other children?

Sunburn

Overexposure to the sun is by far the leading cause of skin damage, with consequences ranging from mild sunburn to premature aging and even skin cancer. Most sunburns are classified as first-degree, meaning they are limited to the epidermis, the top layer of the skin. More severe, second-degree burns extend into the dermis, the inner layer of skin. Although very painful, these burns eventually heal as the skin renews itself. Third-degree sunburns, which damage both layers of skin as well as the underlying nerves and subcutaneous tissue, are rare. They occur mainly in babies or young children, who have thin, delicate skin that is especially vulnerable to the sun.

Sun can harm skin the year-round in both bright and overcast weather, but the amount of damage depends upon the intensity of ultraviolet, or UV, radiation. In the northern hemisphere, UV radiation is highest in the summer between 10 A.M. and 2 P.M.

Ultraviolet radiation has two components: the shorter UVB rays, which are responsible for most sunburns, and the longer UVA rays, which are involved more in suntanning. Both types cause skin damage as well as promote skin cancer (page 380). Overexposure to UV rays also encourages actinic keratoses; these are scaly lesions that may be precancerous.

The tanning process is the body's way of protecting the skin from the sun's damage. Pigment-producing cells send an increasing amount of melanin to the skin's surface to block the harmful incoming rays. Thus, fair-skinned, blue-eyed people who do not readily tan are the most vulnerable to sunburn. Those with dark skin are also susceptible, but their heavier layer of melanin helps protect them against sunburn.

While an occasional mild sunburn may seem harmless, research indicates that any prolonged exposure to the sun causes irreversible damage and increas-

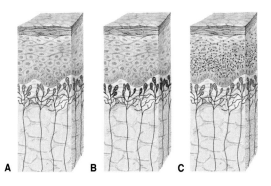

Sun exposure causes normal healthy skin (A) to redden and the capillaries beneath the surface to become dilated (B). More melanin is then sent to block out harmful rays, thus darkening the skin (C).

es the risk of cancer. Especially dangerous are blistering sunburns suffered in childhood; even one or two at an early age can more than double the risk of developing melanoma (page 287), the deadliest of the skin cancers.

Diagnostic Studies and Procedures

A sunburn is easily diagnosed simply by observing the characteristic skin reddening, blistering, and peeling.

Medical Treatments

A severe sunburn that covers a large area of the body or produces fever, chills, and nausea within 12 hours of exposure, should be treated by a doctor. Oral prednisone may be prescribed to alleviate inflammation and swelling, especially if a rash develops. Penicillin or another broad-spectrum antibiotic may be advisable to prevent or treat a secondary infection from blistering. Aspirin or ibuprofen can relieve pain and inflammation. A mild tranquilizer may be prescribed if loss of sleep and itching become a problem.

Alternative Therapies

Herbal Medicine. To ease the discomfort of mild sunburn, herbalists suggest applying a cool compress of apple cider vinegar. The juice of a freshly cut aloe plant may also alleviate pain and speed healing. However, do not apply this or any other preparation to severely blistered skin; to do so risks infection.
Meditation. Deep-breathing exercises can help overcome the desire to scratch itchy, peeling skin.

Self-Treatment

Mild sunburn may be relieved with a cool shower or cold-water compresses, or by sitting in a tub of cool water to which a cup of cornstarch has been added.

Doctors advise against self-care with ointments or lotions that contain the

anesthetic benzocaine. They recommend ice packs wrapped in cloth to alleviate severe pain or itching (applying ice directly to skin can increase damage), and staying out of the sun until skin is completely healed.

Of course, prevention is the best approach to sunburn. Dermatologists stress that there is no such thing as a "healthy" tan. Any time spent outdoors during the day, even if no tan results, exposes the skin to potentially harmful ultraviolet rays. This includes cloudy days, when 80 percent of UV radiation reaches the earth. Remember, too, that water and sand reflect the sun's rays, thus increasing exposure.

Many dermatologists now recommend daily use of protective clothing and a sunscreen on exposed skin all year round. Some makeups contain sunscreens, but most do not provide complete protection. Also, sunscreens vary in the amount of protection they provide. Look for one with a sun protection factor, or SPF, of at least 15 or more. Also look for a brand that protects against both UVA and UVB rays. Many sunscreens contain para-aminobenzoic acid (PABA), to which some people are allergic. They can substitute sunscreens that contain benzophenone.

If you are especially sun-sensitive, you may need a sunblock, which prevents any UV rays from penetrating the skin. The most familiar sunblock is zinc oxide, the opaque white salve that some lifeguards use to cover their noses and lips. Similar protection for all parts of the face and body is now available in less visible preparations made with micronized titanium dioxide.

Do not apply sunscreens to babies under six months; instead, shield them from the sun. After six months, an alcohol-free sunscreen may be used.

Other Causes of Sunburns

Artificial lights that emit ultraviolet rays can cause sunburns and other skin damage. This is especially true of equipment used in tanning parlors, which may give off 200 times more UVA than natural sunlight. Also, many drugs, including antihypertensives, antibiotics, steroids, acne medications, and anticancer drugs, make skin extra-sensitive to the sun, as does pregnancy and such diseases as lupus.

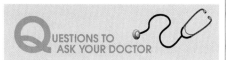

QUESTIONS TO ASK YOUR DOCTOR

▶ Am I taking a medication that increases my sensitivity to the sun?
▶ What are the best sunscreens for babies and young children?

Sweating Disorders

(Hyperhidrosis)

Sweating, or perspiring, helps remove some of the body's wastes through the pores of the skin. It also aids in regulating the body's temperature by cooling through evaporation, and it provides an acidic coating that controls the growth of skin bacteria.

Two types of glands—apocrine and eccrine—produce sweat, but their production differs. Apocrine glands, which enlarge as puberty approaches, are located in the armpits, where they are the most active, as well as selected areas of skin on the trunk, face, and scalp. They exude a scant amount of milky perspiration that contains proteins, carbohydrates, and lipids, which give it a somewhat unpleasant smell as these substances are broken down by bacteria. Apocrine sweat is thought to broadcast sexual signals through the odor of a group of chemicals known as pheromones. Nothing inhibits the production of this sweat, but deodorants diminish its smell.

The wetness associated with sweating is produced by the approximately three million eccrine glands, located all over the body except in the ear canal. Eccrine sweat is mostly water, plus small amounts of potassium, salt, urea, and a few other ingredients. It is sterile and odorless, except when transmitting the smells of onion, garlic, and similar foods.

Under normal circumstances, the eccrine glands produce about one quart of sweat every day, but this amount varies from person to person and depends on age, sex, race, and sensitivity to heat. From time to time, an individual may produce up to 10 quarts of sweat in a day, due to heat, heavy physical activity, or undue emotional turmoil; this is still considered normal.

A variety of circumstances, ranging from eating highly spiced food to having a heart attack, may produce abnormally heavy sweating, or hyperhidrosis, but stress is the most common cause. Technically referred to as emotional hyperhidrosis, this type of chronic sweating appears to run in families and is most obvious in the armpits or on the palms and soles. It begins during childhood and is more prevalent in men than in women.

Diagnostic Studies and Procedures

A doctor who is consulted about heavy sweating will take into account the individual's sex, age, and medical history. A diagnosis of emotional hyperhidrosis often entails a process of eliminating possible medical causes. A physical examination is conducted, and blood and urine studies, X-rays, and other tests may be ordered.

Medical Treatments

If excessive sweating is a manifestation of an underlying disorder, treatment of that condition often solves the problem.

For excessive underarm sweating, the most effective medication is Drysol, a 20 percent solution of aluminum chloride (hexahydrate) in ethyl alcohol. At bedtime, it is applied under the arms to completely dry skin and then covered with a thin layer of polyethylene (plastic wrap). In the morning, the wrap is removed and the area is bathed. After application on two or three consecutive nights, Drysol usually need not be used more than once or twice a week.

Medications with an anticholinergic action, for example, drugs prescribed to calm excessive bowel spasms, may be prescribed as a short-term solution for heavy sweating because of their drying effect. In especially troublesome cases, surgical removal of overactive sweat glands may be considered. This may entail removing a strip of underarm skin or severing some of the nerves that control areas rich in sweat glands. Such operations carry a risk of infection and loss of sensation and so are reserved for the most refractory cases.

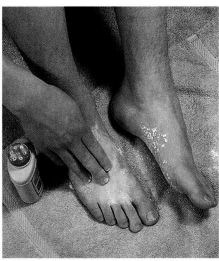

Daily application of a medicated foot powder can help control both the odor and moisture of sweaty feet.

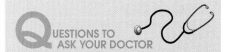

QUESTIONS TO ASK YOUR DOCTOR

▶ If I am allergic to commercial antiperspirants, would Drysol help? Can you recommend other alternatives?

Alternative Therapies

Biofeedback training. A person who sweats excessively when under stress may learn how to control the process by using electronic monitors to alter normally automatic body responses.

Relaxation techniques. The body's response to stress is controlled by the hypothalamus, a part of the brain that also regulates the sweating process. Thus, stress management through meditation and breathing exercises can help reduce heavy sweating.

Self-Treatment

Most sweating problems can be controlled through common sense and self-care. If you are especially sensitive to heat, wear light, layered clothing that is easy to remove as needed and use a small hand fan. To reduce night sweats, sleep in a cool room, use a light covering, and wear light, cotton nightclothes. (For additional suggestions, see Menopause, page 290.)

To control sweaty feet:

▶ Use a medicated foot powder to absorb moisture.

▶ Choose footwear made of leather or fabric. Wear sandals when possible.

▶ Wear white cotton socks and change them whenever necessary.

To reduce underarm sweating:

▶ Use a deodorant with antiperspirant action. Select a cream or roll-on product instead of an aerosol spray, which may contain harmful propellants.

▶ If your skin won't tolerate any antiperspirant or deodorant, try using a cream or ointment containing the antibiotic neosporin, or experiment with various antibacterial soaps.

Other Causes of Heavy Sweating

Recurring episodes of heavy sweating may signal an underlying medical condition; possibilities include certain cancers, AIDS, malaria and other infections, and an overactive thyroid and other hormonal disturbances. Transient heavy sweating may be prompted by fever, medications, and withdrawal from various addictive drugs, including alcohol and narcotics.

Syphilis

Until the 20th century, syphilis was a lethal disease, decimating entire populations. At the end of the 15th century, for example, a massive pandemic of the great pox, a name used to distinguish syphilis from smallpox, swept through Europe and Asia, causing thousands of deaths. At that time, syphilis became recognized as a sexually transmitted disease, but it was not until 1903 that the causative organism—*Treponema pallidum*, a spiral-shaped bacterium, or spirochete—was identified.

Because this spirochete can survive for only a brief time outside the body, primary syphilis is almost always contracted by means of direct sexual or oral contact with an infected person. Congenital syphilis is passed to an unborn baby by an infected woman during pregnancy.

After decades of decline, syphilis is again increasing in the United States, with about 50,000 new cases reported each year since 1987. The rise is attributed to changes in sexual behavior and declining public health services.

Untreated syphilis typically progresses in three stages:

Primary syphilis is characterized by the appearance of one or more painless ulcers, or chancres, two to three weeks after exposure. Chancres develop where the bacteria enter the body, usually on the penis, vagina, cervix, anus, mouth, or hands. If scraped, a chancre gives off a clear fluid that contains numerous *T. pallidum* organisms. Nearby lymph nodes may swell painlessly. Even without treatment, these symptoms disappear after three to eight weeks.

Syphilis is most contagious during this stage, because the bacteria can pass directly from a chancre to the skin or mucous membranes of a sexual partner.
Secondary syphilis appears 4 to 10 weeks after the initial lesions and is

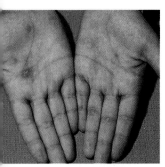

The rash of secondary syphilis sometimes appears as patches on the palms and other parts of the body.

marked by waves of a painless skin rash that usually covers the entire body. Less commonly, the rash appears in a few patches on palms, soles, genitalia, and mucous membranes. It may be accompanied by mild symptoms—sore throat, fever, fatigue, swollen lymph nodes, and perhaps headache. A few people will become acutely ill with syphilitic meningitis and others will experience deafness and other nerve problems. Without treatment, these symptoms typically disappear in 3 to 12 weeks, but in some cases, there may be relapses for up to one year.

At this stage, the disease is not as contagious as primary syphilis, but the organism can still be shed from the recurring skin lesions and passed to others during sexual activity.
Latent syphilis carries a risk of recurrent relapses of the rash and other symptoms. About a third of patients develop severe complications of late, or tertiary, syphilis, which may affect the skin, bones, nerves, brain, heart, and other internal organs. In the past, this stage brought blindness, deafness, heart problems, insanity, and death.

Latent syphilis is rarely contagious, but recurring complications can produce permanent damage.

About 25 percent of unborn babies who contract congenital syphilis are born dead or die within a few weeks of birth. Untreated survivors often become deaf. (Beethoven's deafness is attributed to congenital syphilis.) They may also develop anemia, growth problems, and other complications.

Diagnostic Studies and Procedures
In its primary stage, syphilis is diagnosed by finding the causative organism in a microscopic test. A sample of chancre fluid is placed on a slide, a bright light is shown through it, and the organism is then visible under a microscope. Blood studies that test for syphilis exist, but can be misleading. In secondary and latent syphilis, the spinal fluid may also be examined.

Anyone who has been diagnosed with syphilis is advised to be tested for HIV, the virus that causes AIDS. Studies have shown that people with syphilis are three to five times more likely to be HIV-positive than those in the general population.

Medical Treatments
Penicillin is the drug of choice for treating all stages of syphilis. Primary

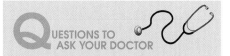
QUESTIONS TO ASK YOUR DOCTOR

▶ After treatment for syphilis, how often and for how long should I undergo follow-up testing? At what point should tests for HIV be performed?

syphilis can usually be cured with a single high-dose injection that remains effective for six to eight days. Secondary syphilis requires two high-dose injections, or 10 days of smaller injections. For patients who are allergic to penicillin, erythromycin or tetracycline, taken orally every 6 hours for 14 days, may serve as viable alternatives.

Penicillin is also given to treat late-stage complications. Other medications—for example, painkillers or antipsychotic drugs—may be added to the regimen to treat specific symptoms.

Penicillin and erythromycin are 98 percent effective in preventing congenital syphilis in the babies of pregnant women who have the disease.

Relapses are common in secondary and latent syphilis. Repeated blood studies are recommended at suitable intervals to confirm that the syphilis has been eradicated.

Alternative Therapies
Before the discovery of antibiotics, arsenic, mercury, and other toxins were used to treat syphilis. These dangerous agents have no place in modern treatment, and there is no alternative therapy that can cure the disease.

Self-Treatment
Prevention is the only possible self-care approach with syphilis. Use of a condom during sexual intercourse reduces, but does not eliminate, the risk of contracting it. A mutually monogamous sexual relationship is the only assurance against transmission.

If you are infected with syphilis, your doctor must notify public health officials, who will try to locate all of your sexual contacts so that they can be tested and treated.

Other Causes of Syphilis Symptoms
The chancre of primary syphilis and the later rashes are easily mistaken for other skin disorders. Later complications of tertiary syphilis might be confused with heart disease, psychosis, nerve disorders, and Alzheimer's disease or progressive dementia.

Taste and Smell Disorders

(Chemosensory loss)

The senses of taste and smell are so closely related physiologically that a disorder affecting one is likely to have an adverse effect on the other as well. An estimated 80 to 90 percent of the people who think they have lost their sense of taste have actually lost their ability to smell instead.

The sense of smell declines sharply with age; studies show that more than half of Americans aged 65 to 80, and three-fourths of those over 80, have serious problems in detecting or identifying odors. A significant number in both age groups cannot smell at all.

The sense of taste originates in the tongue's taste buds, which can differentiate among sweet, sour, bitter, and salty. When food is chewed and swallowed, its odors make their way from the back of the mouth to the upper nasal cavity where they stimulate specialized olfactory cells that send odor signals to the brain. This information enables a person to distinguish between foods that have the same texture but different flavors. Someone who cannot smell may find that an apple, onion, and peach all taste alike.

Research indicates that the brain's olfactory receptor cells can differentiate among thousands of odors, including pheromones, chemicals in sweat that appear to play an important role in sexual attraction. Still, our sense of smell lags behind that of most animals. For instance, each person emits a unique scent, yet we generally do not recognize each other by odor; your pet, however, can probably recognize you solely by sniffing.

While taste and smell disorders are rarely fatal, loss or distortion of these perceptions diminishes enjoyment of many of life's important pleasures, including the savoring of food. In some

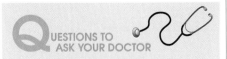

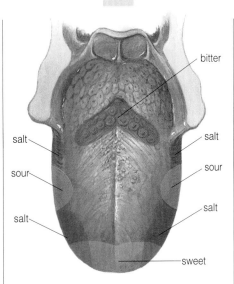

Taste buds in different parts of the tongue differentiate among the four basic flavors—sweet, sour, bitter, and salty.

instances, these disorders can have dangerous consequences, as may occur when a person does not smell an incipient kitchen fire or recognize the rancid taste of spoiled food.

Some disorders that affect taste and smell, such as the common cold and hay fever, are minor and self-limiting. Prolonged exposure to tobacco smoke and other environmental pollutants and toxic industrial chemicals can cause a gradual loss of smell sense, which is usually reversible if the irritant is removed.

Permanent destruction of the olfactory cells can result from a severe head injury or from radiation treatment for neck or head cancer. The loss of the ability to smell may accompany Alzheimer's or Parkinson's diseases. Tumors of the nose, mouth, or brain can also cause permanently impaired taste and smell.

Diagnostic Studies and Procedures

Diagnosis of taste and smell disorders may require a team effort involving a neurologist, psychologist, and nutritionist, as well as a doctor who specializes in this aspect of otolaryngology. A patient may be given a scratch-and-sniff test to determine whether or not she can identify familiar odors.

To identify the cause, additional procedures may include a careful inspection of the head and neck, including the tongue. Substances may be placed on the patient's tongue to see if he can differentiate among sweet, salty, sour, and bitter tastes. A CT scan may be used to check for anatomical defects or tumors that might affect taste and smell.

Medical Treatments

Treatments depend on the underlying cause of the disorder. Chronic nasal sinus blockage from allergies or the blockage of air flow by nasal polyps may be treated by hydrocortisone injections and/or surgery. Sinus infections will be treated with antibiotics. Surgery may also be recommended to correct a deviated septum or other defect causing nasal congestion and an impaired sense of smell.

Alternative Therapies

Herbal Medicine. Horseradish, cayenne pepper, and other hot herbs and spices can help clear sinuses and may restore a sense of smell due to nasal congestion. The spices can be sniffed or added to food.

Naturopathy. Some naturopaths attribute loss of taste perception to vitamin and mineral deficiencies; they may recommend supplements of vitamins A and B_{12}, zinc, and copper. However, be sure to consult a doctor before taking high doses of these nutrients.

Nutrition Therapy. A nutritionist can advise an older person who is inadequately nourished because "everything tastes the same" in ways of preparing more appealing and nutritionally balanced meals. Sometimes, using extra spices and herbs—for example, sage, garlic, cinnamon, nutmeg, and mint—give foods more flavor, even for those with an impaired sense of smell. Varying the texture and color of foods in a meal can also make it more appetizing.

Self-Treatment

If your loss of smell is due to allergies, ask a doctor about medication or allergy shots. If you smoke, make every effort to stop, and avoid secondhand smoke and other irritants.

Pay attention to good dental hygiene; tooth decay and gum disease can leave a bad taste in your mouth and interfere with your ability to taste food.

If you live alone and you have an impaired sense of taste and/or smell, label all perishable foods with the date of purchase and discard any for which freshness is in doubt.

Other Causes of Impaired Taste

Advanced cancer can alter taste perception, especially of meat. In addition to the disorders cited earlier, circumstances that can diminish senses of taste and smell include dry mouth, nose deformities, oral thrush, and disorders affecting the tongue.

QUESTIONS TO ASK YOUR DOCTOR

▶ Is it possible that one of the medications I'm taking has changed the way everything tastes?
▶ Can very spicy foods permanently damage taste buds?

Tendinitis

(Epicondylitis; tenosynovitis)
Tendons are the tough, fibrous bands of tissue that connect muscles to bones; tendinitis occurs when these tissues become inflamed. Athletes often suffer tendinitis, and the disorder may be identified with a particular sport or activity to indicate its location—for example, tennis elbow, golfer's shoulder, runner's ankle, or housemaid's knee.

Because tendons have only a limited ability to stretch and contract, they are also easily torn when subjected to excessive strain. A torn Achilles tendon, which connects to the heel, is common among athletes and dancers.

An even more frequent occupational complaint is tenosynovitis, inflammation of the synovium, the fibrous sheath that surrounds or lines the tendons. When the synovium becomes inflamed, the tendon is unable to move smoothly within its covering. This is a special problem for people whose jobs entail repetitive motions.

Tendinitis begins with weakness, stiffness, swelling, and tenderness in the area. Continued use of the inflamed tendons brings worsening pain until even the slightest demand becomes excruciating. The condition is often confused with, or accompanied by, bursitis (page 119), an inflammation of the bursa, the fluid-filled sac that reduces friction between tendons and bones.

With proper treatment, mild tendinitis usually heals completely after two or three weeks. However, continued use of the inflamed tendons can result in chronic tendinitis and, in turn, increasing disability.

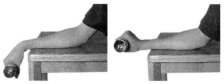

Working with weights can help prevent tennis elbow by strengthening forearm muscles. Do the exercises above for your backhand game.

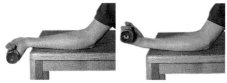

These exercises strengthen muscles for forehand shots. Extend and flex the wrist, repeating until your muscles tire. Do this twice a day.

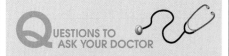

QUESTIONS TO ASK YOUR DOCTOR

▶ Do I need surgery to correct my chronic tendinitis?
▶ At what point is it safe for me to resume workouts and other activities?

Diagnostic Studies and Procedures

A doctor can usually diagnose tendinitis on the basis of symptoms and a physical examination. However, X-rays may be taken to rule out a fracture, arthritis, and other disorders that cause pain, swelling, and inflammation.

Doctors who specialize in sports medicine and performing-arts medicine may use electromyographic studies and videotapes to analyze movements of joints and their supporting structures. They can then identify specific movements that may induce tendinitis.

Medical Treatments

Most tendinitis can be managed with self-care (see below), but in chronic cases, injections of a steroid, such as hydrocortisone, directly into the inflamed area may be recommended. These injections do not cause as many side effects as steroids taken systemically; even so, excessive shots can weaken the tendon and lead to its rupture.

In some cases, such as so-called baseball, or mallet, finger, splinting may be necessary to immobilize the finger and allow the tendon to repair itself.

A ruptured tendon that fails to reattach itself may require surgical repair.

Alternative Therapies

Alexander Technique. By analyzing the faulty postural habits that strain the joints and supporting tissues, a practitioner of this technique can help an individual relearn postures and body movements to prevent tendinitis.
Herbal Medicine. Compresses soaked in comfrey, arnica, or witch hazel are said to alleviate inflammation and speed up healing of tendinitis. To prepare a comfrey or arnica compress, brew a strong tea of the herb, allow it to cool, soak a clean cloth in it, and apply it to the painful area. These herbs can also be used to make a poultice for the same purpose (see page 45).
Hydrotherapy. Whirlpool baths, hot and cold soaks, and exercising in water may alleviate pain and help restore the function of the injured area.

Massage. Gentle kneading and massaging of the area surrounding the inflammation can ease discomfort and may hasten healing by increasing circulation in the area. However, avoid direct massage of the inflamed portion, as this may exacerbate the injury.
Physical Therapy. A physical therapist who specializes in sports injuries can provide exercises that gradually restore function without causing a recurrence of the tendinitis. Such a therapist may use whirlpool baths and devise a rehabilitation program to restore normal joint movement by strengthening the affected muscles. Follow-up visits are scheduled to monitor progress and add to the exercise regimen. A physical therapist can also give advice on support bandages to prevent future flare-ups.

Self-Treatment

Rest is the key to prompt recovery from tendinitis. If necessary, immobilize the injured area with a splint or sling. In the early stages of inflammation, apply ice packs. As healing progresses, switch to heat, or alternate hot and cold packs.

To avoid a recurrence and the risk of chronic tendinitis, it may be wise to consult an exercise physiologist or a professional trainer. An improper grip on a tennis racket or a faulty golf swing may be responsible for tennis elbow or golfer's shoulder.

Consider asking a pro to check your equipment. Using a racket that is too heavy or too tightly strung can cause tennis elbow; wearing improper or poorly fitted running shoes can result in Achilles tendinitis.

Overuse is responsible for many cases of chronic tendinitis, especially among youngsters. Budding baseball pitchers have had their careers cut short by little leaguer's elbow, a traction injury affecting the cartilage caused by throwing too much at an early age.

Weight training to strengthen certain muscles can help prevent tendinitis. If you are plagued with tennis elbow, for example, work on strengthening your forearm muscles by exercising with small (three- to five-pound) weights; flex and extend your wrists with your forearms resting on a flat surface (see photographs, left).

Other Causes of Tendon Pain

Symptoms similar to those of tendinitis can result from muscle strain, frozen shoulder, shin splints, stress fractures, runner's knee, and other sports injuries.

Testicular Cancer

(Testis carcinoma)

Each year, about 7,000 men in the United States are diagnosed with testicular cancer and 370 die it. While this accounts for only about 1 percent of malignancies in all men, it is 19 percent of cancer in those aged 15 to 34. There is another, though lesser, peak risk period among men in their seventies. Caucasians with the disease outnumber African-Americans four to one.

Testicular cancer typically appears as a firm, painless lump or swelling in the front part of a testicle. Some men have also described a dull aching or heavy sensation located in the lower abdomen, groin, or scrotum, and swollen lymph nodes in the groin.

About 95 percent of testicular cancers arise in the sperm-making germ cells. The cause is unknown, but men who have an undescended testicle (page 428) have about a fivefold increase in risk for developing the disease. There has been a marked increase in both undescended testes, or cryptorchidism, and testicular cancer in the last 40 years, especially among white males. Some researchers attribute this rise to mothers using hormones just before or during pregnancy. Studies have found a twofold increase in undescended testes among males born to women who took oral contraceptives in the month before

TESTICULAR SELF-EXAMINATION
Start by taking a warm bath or shower to relax the scrotum and make any lumps or abnormalities easier to feel. While standing, roll one testicle at a time between the thumb and fingers. Feel for lumps, swelling, or any other changes in consistency. A normal testicle is egg-shaped and feels smooth and fairly firm.

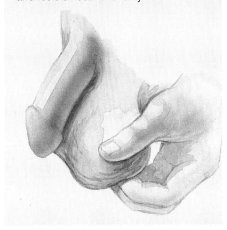

STAGES OF TESTICULAR CANCER
Cancer specialists use a complicated system of cell type and cancer spread to determine the stage of testicular cancer. A simplified version identifies the following five stages:

Stage A: Tumor is confined to the testicle.

Stage B1: Cancer has spread to fewer than six nearby lymph nodes, and none are larger than two centimeters, or three-fourths of an inch.

Stage B2: Cancer has spread to more than six nearby nodes and/or some are larger than two centimeters.

Stage B3: Nearby lymph nodes are larger than six centimeters, but there is no evidence of metastases to other organs.

Stage C: Cancer has spread to the liver, lungs, bones, brain, or other organs.

conception. Risk was also increased by the use of DES, an artificial estrogen given to women until the late 1960s to prevent a threatened miscarriage.

Possible risk factors for testicular cancer include exposure to cadmium and other industrial chemicals or metals.

Diagnostic Studies and Procedures
Any lump, swelling, or change in the way a testicle feels calls for prompt medical investigation. An ultrasound examination of the scrotum can locate the lesion and differentiate it from other conditions, such as epididymitis, an inflammation of a cordlike structure on the back of the testicle. A biopsy confirms the presence of cancer.

If cancer is diagnosed, X-rays, CT scans, and other imaging studies of the abdomen and chest will be ordered to determine whether it has spread. Additional tests may include a urine-flow study, or urogram, to detect any obstruction of the urinary tract; blood tests for various tumor or genetic markers; lymphography, X-ray depiction of the lymph system; and possible scans of the liver, brain, and bones.

Medical Treatments
Treatment usually begins with surgical removal of the entire testicle through inguinal orchiectomy, an incision in the groin. However, in some cases, radiation or chemotherapy alone is sufficient.

Depending upon the cancer type and extent of any spread, surgery may be followed by radiation, chemotherapy, or a combination of the two.

Even after treatment is complete, frequent checkups are important to spot any recurrence as early as possible. Testicular cancer is highly curable when detected and treated early.

Alternative Therapies
There is no substitute for medical treatment in dealing with testicular cancer, although such alternative therapies as meditation, self-hypnosis, and visualization can help control pain and foster a sense of well-being.

Nutrition Therapy. Some naturopaths recommend zinc supplements for men who have testicular tumors, based on laboratory findings that zinc injections sometimes shrink these cancers in animals. However, this treatment has not been studied scientifically in humans; indeed, there is some evidence that excessive exposure to zinc may actually promote testicular tumors.

Self-Treatment
Early detection is the key to curing testicular cancer, and monthly self-examination is the best means of early detection (see illustrated box, left).

Men who find an abnormality often delay seeing a doctor, perhaps because they believe that removal of one or both testicles will prevent normal sexual intercourse. This fear is unfounded; a man can still achieve a normal erection following removal of one or both testicles. However, the cancer treatment may result in infertility; thus, he may want to have some of his sperm frozen for future use.

Another important preventive step involves early treatment of an undescended testicle. Even after treatment, anyone born with an undescended testicle should be particularly conscientious about regular self-examination.

Other Causes of Testicular Abnormalities
An injury to the scrotal area, a hernia, and epididymitis are among the benign conditions that can cause testicular swelling or lumps.

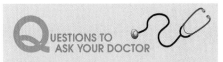

QUESTIONS TO ASK YOUR DOCTOR

▶ Should a man who had an undescended testicle as a baby have more frequent medical checkups?
▶ What effect will cancer treatment have on my sexual function? Fertility?

Testicular Pain and Swelling

(Epididymitis; testicular torsion)
Many conditions produce testicular pain, but the two most common are epididymitis, inflammation of the spaghetti-like tubules at the back of each testicle, and torsion, the twisting of the testicle on its own cord.

A bacterial infection, often a sexually transmitted disease such as chlamydia, usually causes epididymitis. Any bacteria, including those responsible for urinary infections, can travel through the genitourinary passageway and reach the epididymis, where sperm from the testes is stored until transported to the vas deferens in preparation for discharge from the body.

In a typical case of epididymitis, only one testicle is affected. If both become infected and are not treated, infertility may result. In addition to local pain, symptoms include swelling of the entire testicle and the spermatic cord, which may feel hot. There may also be abdominal pain, fever, discharge from the penis, and difficulty in urinating.

Sometimes epididymitis recurs frequently or becomes chronic. When this happens, it is usually secondary to chronic prostatitis (page 352) or urethritis or due to an indwelling urethral catheter to remove urine.

Testicular torsion is unpredictable and can occur at any age, but is most common in adolescents and young adults. Sometimes it is triggered by strenuous activity, but may also develop spontaneously, often during sleep. As the testicle turns or rotates on its cord, the twisting blocks blood flow. The lack of oxygen produces sudden excruciating pain, and the twisted testicle may appear swollen, inflamed, and higher in the scrotal sac than the other one. The pain may produce nausea and vomiting. Unless blood flow to the testicle is restored promptly, the organ dies and gangrene develops.

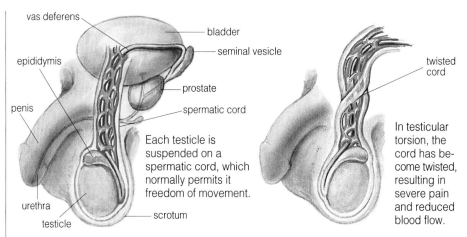

Each testicle is suspended on a spermatic cord, which normally permits it freedom of movement.

In testicular torsion, the cord has become twisted, resulting in severe pain and reduced blood flow.

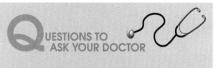

QUESTIONS TO ASK YOUR DOCTOR

▶ When will it be safe for me to resume my exercise routine, which includes weightlifting?
▶ Could my recurrent epididymitis be related to another underlying disease?

Diagnostic Studies and Procedures

A doctor can usually distinguish between epididymitis and torsion by observing whether the twisted cord and displacement characteristic of torsion has taken place. If there is any doubt, he will study blood flow to differentiate between the two conditions: in torsion, it is decreased, whereas it usually is increased in epididymitis.

If epididymitis is diagnosed, additional studies are needed to identify the cause. These may include blood and urine analyses and cultures of any penile discharge and secretions from the prostate gland. In some cases, ultrasound or a CT scan may be ordered to rule out testicular cancer.

Following treatment, repeat cultures may be ordered to make sure that the bacteria have been eradicated.

Medical Treatments

Epididymitis. Antibiotics are the mainstay of treatment, but the choice of drug depends upon the infecting organism. Chlamydia is treated with a prolonged regimen of tetracycline. Because many strains of gonococci are now resistant to penicillin and tetracycline, the current antibiotic therapy consists of one injection of ceftriaxone followed by seven days of doxycycline (see Gonorrhea, page 206). If epididymitis stems from a sexually transmitted disease, the patient's sexual partner should be treated also. Aspirin may be recommended to reduce fever and pain. Persistent inflammation may require a short course of steroids.

Recurrent or chronic epididymitis is difficult to treat, especially when due to treatment-resistant urethritis or prostatitis. A vasectomy may be considered to prevent infectious organisms from invading the epididymis via the vas deferens.

Recurrences linked to an indwelling urethral catheter may be cured by finding an alternative method of urine removal, such as creating an opening (stoma) in the pubic area. Surgical removal of the epididymis is a treatment of last resort.

Testicular torsion. This is a medical emergency, because the cord rarely straightens on its own. Prompt surgery is critical to prevent tissue death. The operation, which can be done on an outpatient basis under local anesthesia, involves unwinding the testicle and stitching it and its partner to the inside of the scrotum to prevent recurrence.

Alternative Therapies

Hydrotherapy. To relieve inflammation and pain from epididymitis, apply an ice pack for a few minutes and then recline in a warm bath. Avoid excessive heat, which can inhibit sperm production.

Self-Treatment

Wearing a scrotal support during treatment and recovery from a bout of epididymitis can ease discomfort. Doctors also advise avoiding strenuous activity until the inflammation disappears.

Because epididymitis often results from a sexually transmitted disease, practicing safe sex is essential to prevention. Always use a condom during sexual intercourse unless you are in a mutually monogamous relationship.

After treatment for either epididymitis or testicular torsion, follow your doctor's instructions concerning resumption of sexual activity.

Other Causes of Testicular Pain

Testicular cancer can cause swelling and other symptoms similar to those of epididymitis. Mumps in an adolescent or adult can also cause testicular pain and swelling. Other possible causes include prostatitis, bladder infections, hernias, hydrocele, and varicocele.

Tetanus

(Lockjaw)

Tetanus is an acute infectious disease of the nervous system caused by a microorganism that usually enters the body through an open wound or cut. The infectious agent, *Clostridium tetani*, is a type of bacterium, or bacillus, that reproduces by forming spores. These spores are found almost everywhere, but especially in soil, dust, and the manure of cows, horses, and other plant-eating animals.

Anyone who sustains a severe burn or deep puncture wound is vulnerable to tetanus; so too are intravenous drug users. Farmers, gardeners, and others who work with the soil are especially susceptible. In underdeveloped countries, newborns sometimes contract a form of the disease called tetanus neonatorum, when the spores enter the umbilicus. The practice of covering a cut umbilicus with mud increases the risk of this type of tetanus.

As tetanus bacilli invade the bloodstream, they produce a toxin that causes intermittent spasms of the voluntary muscles. An early symptom is jaw stiffness, quickly followed by headache, restlessness, and irritability. The facial expression may freeze and the muscles of the arms, legs, and neck go into spasms. Opening the mouth or moving the jaw may become difficult or impossible, hence the well-known name of lockjaw.

As the infection advances, throat-muscle spasms may interfere with speech and swallowing, and sphincter spasms may cause urine retention. When the breathing muscles are affected, tetanus becomes life threatening.

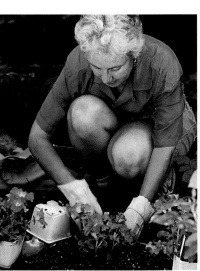

Wearing gloves when gardening helps safeguard against tetanus, but even so, you should have a tetanus booster shot every 10 years.

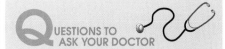

QUESTIONS TO ASK YOUR DOCTOR

▶ Do you have a record of when I had my last tetanus booster shot?
▶ After a puncture wound, am I likely to need a tetanus shot even if I am not due for a booster?

Diagnostic Studies and Procedures

Tetanus can usually be diagnosed solely on the basis of symptoms, especially if they follow a recent injury or wound. However, blood tests and analyses of cerebral spinal fluid may be ordered to rule out the possibility of other diseases, such as meningitis (inflammation of the membranes covering the brain and spinal cord) and encephalitis (inflammation of the brain).

Medical Treatments

Prevention is the best medical approach to tetanus. All infants should be immunized against the disease (see box, right). If an injured person has never been immunized or has not received a tetanus booster shot in the last five years, an injection of tetanus immune globulin is given as a preventive measure. Depending upon previous immunizations, tetanus toxoid may also be given in three doses.

Immediate and thorough cleansing of a deep puncture wound is critical. This should be followed by a 10-day course of penicillin or tetracycline, which kills *C. tetani* and also helps prevent or cure other infections.

If tetanus develops, hospitalization is necessary. Serum antitoxin may be administered and diazepam (Valium) or similar medications may be given to control seizures and muscle spasms. An antibiotic, either penicillin or tetracycline, is also administered.

The patient should be kept in a quiet room with vigilant nursing care to watch for breathing difficulty and other complications. In severe cases, a tracheotomy—an opening into the windpipe, or trachea—is made and a breathing tube inserted to prevent suffocation. The patient must be turned frequently and forced to cough to clear the lungs and prevent pneumonia. Intravenous feeding, a rectal tube, and a bladder catheter may be necessary.

Even with treatment, tetanus has a high mortality rate—about 50 percent worldwide and somewhat lower in the United States, provided that intensive treatment has been started promptly.

Alternative Therapies

Tetanus always demands prompt and intensive medical treatment. During recovery, physical therapy and various types of massage may aid in the rehabilitation process.

Self-Treatment

To prevent tetanus, make sure that you have a tetanus booster every 10 years. Seek immediate medical attention for any deep puncture or dirt-contaminated wound. Even if it seems relatively minor, you may not be able to remove all the dirt yourself.

Wear sturdy-soled shoes when walking in a barn or an open pasture where contaminated animal dung presents a potential source of infection. Also, be sure to wear protective gloves when gardening or working with soil.

Although tetanus is rare in the United States, when it occurs, the victim is often a middle-aged or older gardener who has not had booster shots.

Other Causes of Tetanus Symptoms

Acute meningitis, encephalitis, and other central nervous system infections can produce muscle spasms, seizures, and stiffness similar to those of tetanus. However, these conditions also alter mental alertness, which is not a characteristic of tetanus.

TETANUS IMMUNIZATION

Primary immunization. The tetanus vaccine is usually given together with diphtheria and pertussis (whooping cough) vaccines in a shot called DPT. The American Academy of Pediatrics recommends that DPT shots be given at 2, 4, 6, and 15-to-18 months, with a fifth dose between ages 4 and 6 years or before entering school.

Booster shots. Adult tetanus toxoid should be given between ages 14 and 16, and repeated every 10 years thereafter. This vaccine is usually combined with an adult dosage of diphtheria toxoid.

After an accident. Antitoxin blood levels may fall below the minimum protective level before 10 years have elapsed. Therefore, to prevent possible tetanus following a deep puncture or dirt-contaminated wound, a tetanus toxoid shot is recommended if more than five years have elapsed since the last booster.

Following tetanus. Having the disease does not confer immunity; therefore, regular immunization is necessary after recovery from tetanus.

Thalassemia

(Cooley's anemia; Mediterranean anemia; thalassemia major and minor)
Thalassemia refers to a group of inherited blood disorders in which the body's bone marrow is unable to form normal amounts of hemoglobin, the oxygen-carrying pigment in red blood cells. People of Mediterranean, African, and Southeast Asian origin are most commonly affected.

Thalassemia is classified as alpha or beta, with each type displaying varying degrees of severity depending upon the number of genes that are inherited. In the most severe form—beta thalassemia major, or Cooley's anemia—a child inherits the causative gene from both parents. At birth, such an infant appears normal, but severe anemia develops during the first few months of life. These babies grow slowly and are thin and jaundiced. They are likely to develop a variety of skeletal abnormalities and enlargement of the heart, liver, and spleen. Most will die before reaching adulthood, although advances in treatment are extending survival.

Children who inherit only one of the beta thalassemia genes become carriers. They usually do not develop anemia even though their blood cell counts and hemoglobin may be slightly atypical.

Normally, a person inherits four alpha globin genes, two from each parent. If one is missing, the child will be an asymptomatic carrier of alpha thalassemia. Two missing genes result in

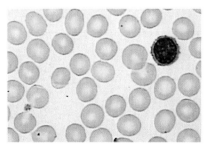

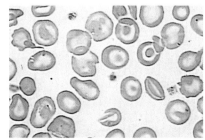

Normal red blood cells (top photo) are round and fairly uniform, compared to the misshapen cells (bottom) that characterize thalassemia.

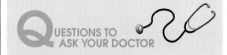

some blood abnormalities, but anemia and other health consequences are unlikely. Someone with only one alpha gene has more pronounced abnormalities; a complete absence results in a fatal syndrome called hydrops fetalis.

Diagnostic Studies and Procedures
The primary diagnostic test is a blood smear to look for abnormal red blood cells. Other blood tests may be ordered, as well as X-rays to see if there are skeletal abnormalities indicating bone thinning and overactive bone marrow.

People who have a family history of thalassemia can be tested for the genetic trait. Problems generally occur only if both parents are carriers, in which case genetic counseling may be advisable when planning a family. Beta thalassemia can often be diagnosed before birth through amniocentesis or chorionic villi sampling (CVS)—tests in which the DNA in cells shed from the fetus is analyzed. If the results indicate possible thalassemia, analysis of a sample of fetal blood can confirm it.

Medical Treatments
Genetic carriers and people with asymptomatic thalassemia minor do not need treatment, but children with the major form require periodic transfusions of red blood cells. Frequency varies according to the severity of the disease and local medical practice. In most areas, moderate transfusions are given every three to four weeks. As a child grows, more red blood cells must be given with each transfusion.

Although transfusions control the anemia and allow for more normal growth and development, they create new problems for thalassemia patients. Even with proper screening and tests, transfusions carry a slight risk of transmission of hepatitis, HIV, and other blood-borne diseases. Also, repeated transfusions produce a buildup of excess iron in the body, which can damage the heart, liver, and other organs. Therefore, thalassemia patients must usually undergo treatment with

deferoxamine (Desferal), a chelating drug that binds to excess iron and is then excreted. The drug is dripped into the body by way of a special pump for 8 to 12 hours, usually during sleep.

Researchers are working on oral chelating drugs that can eliminate the need for desferoxamine treatment. Another drug under study is phenylbutyrate, commonly used for rare metabolic disorders, which appears to increase hemoglobin production.

An enlarged spleen, which destroys excessive numbers of red blood cells, lessens the effectiveness of transfusions. In such cases, it may be best to remove the spleen. Because spleen removal lowers immunity, doctors recommend immunization against pneumonia beforehand. Some also prescribe preventive antibiotics for patients who have had a splenectomy.

Alternative Therapies
Nutrition Therapy. People with thalassemia should avoid foods that are rich in iron or fortified with the mineral; they may need folic-acid supplements to aid in making red blood cells. Those being treated with deferoxamine may require extra vitamin C. However, no supplements of any kind should be taken without a doctor's supervision.

Self-Treatment
Children with thalassemia should be encouraged to attend school regularly, engage in suitable activities, and live as normal a life as possible. If transfusions are given on weekends or in the late afternoon or evening, then treatment will not interfere with the youngster's normal school day.

Barring a serious problem, thalassemic children can usually participate in sports, but they should avoid overexertion. As these children enter their teens and come to realize their high risk of premature death, psychological counseling or a self-help group may enhance their ability to cope.

Traveling to high altitudes can cause problems for people with thalassemia. They should either avoid altitudes above 11,000 feet or have a transfusion immediately before ascending. In such cases, the stay should not last more than a week.

Other Causes of Anemia
Iron deficiency is the most common cause of anemia. Other nutritional deficiencies, autoimmune diseases, genetic disorders, and bleeding disorders can also produce anemia.

Throat/Oral Cancers

(Buccal cavity carcinoma; esophageal cancer; head and neck cancer; upper aerodigestive tract carcinoma)

Cancers of the upper aerodigestive tract, which extends from the mouth and nasal passages to the stomach, are relatively rare, especially when compared with malignancies of the colon and other lower digestive organs. But cancers arising anywhere in the mouth and throat are especially devastating because of their effect on appearance and the ability to eat.

Pharynx and Esophageal Cancers. The pharynx, the muscular structure that begins in the back of the mouth, and the esophagus, the tube that receives food from the pharynx and transports it to the stomach, are two common sites of cancer in the throat portion of the upper digestive tract. Each year, more than 9,000 cases of pharynx cancer and 12,000 cases of esophageal cancer are diagnosed, resulting in about 4,000 and 11,000 annual deaths respectively. (The larynx, another throat structure, is the site of about 12,000 new cancers a year; see page 267 for a more detailed discussion.)

Men with esophageal or pharynx cancer greatly outnumber women, but this situation is changing with the growing number of women who smoke—the major cause of these cancers. The combination of smoking and heavy alcohol use seems to compound the risk. Less commonly, esophageal cancer is associated with iron deficiency anemia. Tylosis, a hereditary disease characterized by thickening of the palms and soles, is also linked to an increased incidence of esophageal cancer.

Difficulty in swallowing is the most common symptom suggesting throat cancer. Initially, the problem is confined mostly to solid foods, but eventually, swallowing even puréed foods or fluids may be difficult. Often, the person describes a feeling of a chronic lump in the throat, frequent spitting up of undigested food, and choking. There may also be a sore throat and possible voice changes as the tumor grows.

Oral Cancers. Each year, more than 19,000 Americans are diagnosed with oral cancer, which can develop in any of the structures in and around the

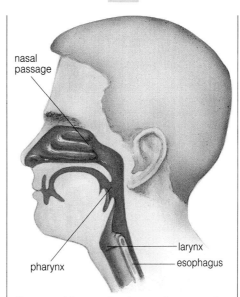

Cancers of the mouth, pharynx, larynx, and esophagus are most prevalent among heavy users of tobacco and alcohol.

mouth—the tongue, cheeks, gums, lips, soft and hard palate, and other oral tissues. In recent years, a marked increase of oral cancer has occurred among young people, especially those who use chewing tobacco or snuff. Overall, tobacco users have 15 times more oral cancer than nonsmokers, but the risk rises to more than 50-fold among those who use chewing tobacco and snuff. As with esophageal and throat cancers, the combination of alcohol and tobacco further increases risk. Pipe and cigar smokers have a higher-than-normal incidence of lip cancers.

Other contributing factors include nutritional deficiencies, which are rare in the United States; chronic mouth infections and poor dental hygiene may also contribute to the development of oral cancer. Excessive sun exposure carries a risk of lip cancer.

Oral cancers are easier to detect in an early stage than those that develop in the pharynx and esophagus. Any persistent sore on the lips, tongue, or soft tissue inside the mouth raises a suspicion of oral cancer. The development of white or red patches that don't go away and bleed easily calls for prompt medical investigation. There also may be painless swelling of the lymph nodes located in the neck.

Lip cancer may appear first as a growth, most often on the lower lip, that forms a dry crust which bleeds when removed and then crusts over again. Cancer of the hard palate usually manifests itself as a

persistent sore, which may ulcerate. All of the oral cancers can produce mild irritation and pain, which worsen as the cancer progresses. These pains may be felt eventually in or around the ear as well.

Diagnostic Studies and Procedures

A dentist is often the first to notice signs of oral cancer, especially patches of leukoplakia, a whitish lesion that is often precancerous, or erythroplakia, similar patches that are red.

A doctor begins the diagnostic process with a physical examination that includes careful examination of the inside of the mouth and throat and palpating of the lymph nodes in the neck to check for swelling or a change in consistency. To diagnose oral cancer, however, a biopsy is necessary.

If esophageal cancer is suspected, X-rays will be taken, usually after the patient first swallows a liquid containing barium, a chalky substance that enhances the organs on film. Using a fluoroscope, a doctor can observe the motion and outline of the esophagus as the barium passes through it. Additional X-rays, taken once the esophagus is coated with barium, will reveal any abnormalities in its outline.

Esophagoscopy—an examination in which a lighted tube with magnifying devices is inserted into the esophagus—and a biopsy of suspicious tissue provide a definitive diagnosis.

After a doctor confirms the presence of cancer, additional tests are needed to determine the extent of the disease, a procedure called staging that is used to decide the most effective treatment approach. Staging usually requires additional X-rays and CT scans, blood tests, and perhaps ultrasound examination or other imaging studies of the liver, lungs, bones, and other organs.

Medical Treatments

Pharynx and Esophageal Cancers. Early pharynx cancer is highly curable by surgical removal of the tumor and a surrounding margin of healthy tissue, usually followed by radiation therapy. Depending upon the location of the cancer, this may require extensive neck surgery that affects both appearance and function. In some cases, the larynx must also be removed, even if the cancer has not spread to it.

Esophageal cancer is more difficult to treat because it is often quite advanced at the time of diagnosis. Surgery offers the best possibility of a cure, especially if the cancer is in the middle to lower segment of the esophagus. When all or most of the esophagus must be taken out, the uppermost portion of the stomach can be fashioned into a replacement food tube. If this is not feasible, a portion of the colon may be used.

In some cases, radiation is the primary treatment; in others, it is used as an adjunct to surgery or as a means of controlling pain and other symptoms when a cure is unlikely. Radiation must be administered carefully to avoid damaging the heart, spinal cord, and other vital structures.

Chemotherapy may be used, either alone or with radiation, to shrink a tumor before surgery.

Oral Cancers. Most oral cancers are treated surgically. Depending on the location of the cancer and its size, the operation can result in changes in appearance and difficulty in chewing, swallowing, and speaking, especially if the tongue is involved.

Fortunately, great strides in reconstructive plastic surgery have helped minimize the disfigurement and functional disabilities associated with oral cancer. Following treatment, skin, bone, and cartilage grafts may all be necessary. Internal prostheses can restore the teeth, palate, jawbone, and other structures inside the mouth. These devices are made by maxillofacial orthodontists, dentists who have special training in oral reconstruction.

Radiation is also used to treat oral cancers and is particularly effective in those detected at an early stage. It may be given either by external beam or by implanting radioactive seeds at the site of the tumor. In either approach, the overall objective is the same: to direct the cancer-killing radiation towards the tumor while sparing as much of the surrounding healthy tissue as possible.

Chemotherapy can be an effective method in reducing the size and density of certain types of tumors.

Alternative Therapies

Although alternative therapy cannot cure these cancers, some are useful in managing pain and in mitigating the symptoms and side effects of treatment. In particular, imaging, visualization, meditation, and other relaxation therapies are often employed.

Acupressure. You may be able to alleviate nausea associated with chemotherapy and radiation treatments by pressing on the middle of your inner wrists either manually or by wearing acupressure bracelets (see page 260) designed to prevent motion sickness.

Herbal Medicine. Gingerroot is highly effective in preventing or minimizing nausea, a common complication of radiation treatments and chemotherapy. For some people, sipping flat ginger ale helps; others may respond to ginger capsules or tablets. Avoid chewing raw or candied ginger, however; these forms can further irritate and damage the lining of the mouth and esophagus among patients undergoing cancer therapy.

Nutrition Therapy. Oral and throat cancers often interfere with normal eating. A clinical nutritionist trained in treating patients with these cancers can devise a balanced diet of soft or liquid foods. Enriched liquid supplements may be needed; if treatment makes it impossible to swallow, feeding can be accomplished via a gastric tube inserted directly into the stomach through a small abdominal incision. Small, frequent meals of nutrient-rich liquids are poured into this tube. Medication can be given intravenously or in a liquid added to the gastric feedings.

Physical, Occupational, and Speech Therapy. Rehabilitation is essential after extensive head and neck surgery, especially when normal eating and speaking have become impaired. Rehabilitation usually involves a team of therapists who are trained in teaching patients new ways to eat, swallow, and speak. The team may also include a dentist and plastic surgeon.

Psychotherapy. A potentially disfiguring oral cancer or an incurable esophageal cancer is likely to cause a patient great psychological distress. Some form of counseling or therapy is often recommended as part of the rehabilitation process. Support groups of people with similar problems are of special value because they usually provide both emotional support and practical tips for coping with the condition.

Self-Treatment

Oral and throat cancers develop slowly, and some experts believe that early preventive action may stop precancerous lesions from developing into invasive cancer. If you use tobacco in any form and notice white or red patches in your mouth, it is imperative that you stop the habit. Treatment at this stage, along with giving up tobacco, may prevent further progression.

If you've had surgical treatment for for oral or throat cancer, it can hinder your ability to eat normally. Consult a qualified nutritionist (see Nutrition Therapy) for guidance and eat frequent, small meals; puréed foods served cold or at room temperature are less likely to provoke nausea than warm foods.

Radiation therapy to the head and neck can reduce or even halt the flow of saliva, adding to eating problems. Drink extra fluids and ask your doctor to recommend an artificial saliva product. This therapy can also cause hair loss and increase the skin's sensitivity to sunlight. Although the hair loss is usually temporary, it can be devastating, especially if surgery has already caused disfigurement. Investing in an attractive wig can boost morale; many insurance policies cover wigs, which are also tax deductible for people undergoing cancer treatment. To prevent sunburn, use a sunblock or wear protective clothing.

Maintaining oral hygiene during treatment is extremely important. Have a complete dental checkup before radiation therapy begins, and get instructions on caring for your teeth and gums. Radiation treatments can increase the likelihood of developing cavities, so you should see a dentist regularly and follow instructions on oral care.

Other Causes of Throat and Mouth Symptoms

Dental disease, recurrent canker sores, and irritation from a broken tooth, jagged filling, or ill-fitting dentures can produce symptoms that could be mistaken for those of oral cancer. Esophageal outpouches, or diverticula, as well as esophageal webs and chronic throat irritation or infections can cause swallowing problems and other symptoms that resemble those of pharynx or esophageal cancer.

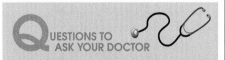

QUESTIONS TO ASK YOUR DOCTOR

▶ Will surgical treatment of my cancer cause disfigurement? If so, can it be minimized with reconstructive surgery?
▶ Will I be able to eat and speak normally after treatment?
▶ What other side effects are likely? Are these temporary or permanent?

Thrush

(Oral candidiasis)

Thrush, or oral candidiasis, is a common yeast infection that develops in and around the mouth. It usually appears as a heavy, whitish coating on the tongue and as creamy patches that resemble milk curds on the mucous membranes of the mouth. The patches may spread to the gums, lips, throat, and skin. In severe cases, thrush may progress to the esophagus, which results in pain and difficulty swallowing. In rare instances, it enters the bloodstream and may affect various organs throughout the body; this serious complication develops mostly in patients with AIDS, cancer, or other disorders marked by reduced immunity.

Although thrush is generally painless, it can cause mouth soreness, especially in babies. Sometimes painful fissures

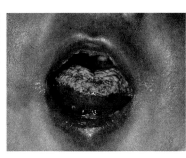

Babies often develop oral thrush, which may spread to the lips, throat, and other tissues.

develop on the corners of the mouth, and trying to wipe away the creamy patches may cause small, painful ulcers.

Thrush is caused by the common fungus called *Candida albicans,* which is also responsible for vaginal yeast infections. Small numbers of the fungus normally reside in the mouth without creating problems. But if an illness or some other circumstance upsets the body's normal balance of these microorganisms, the yeast can overgrow and result in thrush.

Oral thrush occurs most commonly in newborns, who may pick up the yeast organism during birth or in a hospital nursery. Babies are especially vulnerable because their immune systems are not yet fully developed. It is also a frequent problem for AIDS patients, and may develop as well among people with diabetes and those taking antibiotics, corticosteroids, anticancer drugs, or other medications that suppress the immune system.

Diagnostic Studies and Procedures

An initial diagnosis can be made on the basis of the appearance and location of the creamy patches, but to confirm thrush, a doctor uses a swab to remove a small sample for study under a microscope. In most cases, the reason for the yeast overgrowth is obvious, but in some, tests may be necessary to determine the underlying cause. The testing procedures may include blood, urine, and bone-marrow studies, endoscopy, and testing for HIV, the virus that causes AIDS.

Medical Treatments

Nystatin, an antifungal drug that is available in pill, liquid, cream, ointment, lozenge, and powdered form, is the mainstay for treating oral thrush. A cream or ointment is applied directly to the patches. The oral solution is held in the mouth as long as possible and then swallowed. Lozenges should be allowed to dissolve slowly.

Clotrimazole (Mycelex Troche) lozenges are an alternative to nystatin. If neither of these drugs is effective, a doctor may prescribe a stronger antifungal medication such as ketoconazole (Nizoral). Systemic candidiasis is usually treated with an intravenous antifungal drug such as fluconazole (Diflucan). The complete course of antifungal medication should always be taken, rather than stopped when the symptoms disappear. Even when this procedure is followed, recurrences are common. In such cases, the treatment—perhaps with a different drug regimen—will be repeated.

Alternative Therapies

Herbal Medicine. Herbalists recommend alternating pau d'arco and clove tea, drinking three to six cups a day. Taking garlic pills or chewing a clove of raw garlic may also help.

Naturopathy and Nutrition Therapy. Because yeast thrives on sugar, naturopaths stress omitting it from the diet until the thrush subsides. This means avoiding fruit, milk and other dairy products, and the hidden sugar in many foods. The exception to the ban on dairy foods is yogurt made with live lactobacillus cultures. Lactobacillus acidophilus pills also help control yeast.

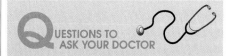
Self-Treatment

Thrush often results when a person is run-down and thus resistance is low. In general, getting enough sleep, exercising regularly, and maintaining a nutritious, balanced diet helps to prevent thrush and minimize the risk of other health problems that increase vulnerability. If you have a disease or are taking a drug that increases the risk of thrush, be especially scrupulous about dental hygiene. Brush your teeth after each meal and rinse your mouth with a solution of 1 tablespoon of hydrogen peroxide (3 percent strength) in ½ cup of warm water.

If you have thrush, you should take care to protect others from contracting it by sterilizing shared household items. Boiling all your eating utensils or using disposable items until the condition is completely cured will help keep the infection from spreading. After treatment, replace your toothbrush to prevent reinfection. To promote healing, rinse your mouth several times a day with a solution of 1 teaspoon of salt in ½ cup of water.

A baby who develops thrush should be given ½ ounce of cool, boiled water after each feeding to help rinse away any milk remnants, which may promote yeast growth. A woman who has a vaginal yeast infection during pregnancy should have it treated before giving birth. A newborn with thrush should be isolated from other babies in a hospital nursery. His bottle nipples should be boiled separately for 20 minutes before the final sterilization.

Other Causes of Mouth Ulcers

Early oral cancer and a mouth condition called leukoplakia, which is often precancerous, can cause flat, white patches that resemble thrush on the tongue and oral mucous membranes. In children, scarlet fever produces a strawberry-colored tongue sometimes with overlying white patches.

Thyroid Cancer

Thyroid cancer is by far the most common malignancy affecting the endocrine, or hormone-producing, system. Even so, it is relatively rare, with about 13,000 new cases and 1,000 deaths a year.

Hormones secreted by the thyroid, a butterfly-shaped gland whose two lobes rest over the front of the trachea (windpipe) in the lower neck, regulate metabolism (see Thyroid Disorders, opposite page). The thyroid gland is highly sensitive to radiation, especially when exposure occurs in a person under age 21. This became evident when studies found a greatly increased incidence of thyroid cancer among people who underwent radiation treatment as children for such disorders as an enlarged thymus, chronic tonsillitis, and even acne, a practice that has been abandoned. About 10 percent of those receiving such treatments later developed thyroid cancer. Similarly, people accidentally exposed to radiation, such as the Marshall Island inhabitants who were under the fallout of an atomic bomb detonated on the atoll Bikini in 1954, also have an increased incidence of thyroid cancer.

For unknown reasons, the course of thyroid cancers varies dramatically according to age. When the malignancy develops before the age of 40 in men and 50 in women, it is rarely fatal, even if it is quite advanced. In contrast, the outlook is poor after the age of 50, with the disease progressing rapidly and resisting treatment.

Thyroid cancer typically starts as a small lump, or nodule, that a doctor can feel when palpating the gland. Sometimes the first obvious sign is an enlarged lymph node in the neck. As

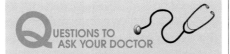

the primary thyroid tumor grows, it may encroach on surrounding organs, resulting in possible voice changes, paralysis of the vocal cords, and swallowing problems due to a narrowing of the esophagus.

Diagnostic Studies and Procedures

Most thyroid nodules are benign, but these can be hard to distinguish from those that are cancerous. A thyroid scan using radioactive iodine can make the distinction, however, because benign, or hot, nodules produce hormones and tend to absorb more of the iodine than nodules that do not make hormones. These so-called cool nodules are more likely to be cancerous, but in either instance, a biopsy is needed to rule out malignancy.

Sometimes what feels like a nodule is actually a cyst, in which case an ultrasound examination may verify that it is. However, some cysts are mixtures of solid and cystic tissue, which can produce misleading results. Thus, only a biopsy can determine whether a thyroid lump is cancerous. This can be done by withdrawing tissue samples from the nodule using a hollow needle.

If cancer is confirmed, a CT scan or MRI may be ordered to detect any spread to nearby organs. A lung X-ray may also be needed, as some thyroid cancers spread to the lungs.

Medical Treatments

Thyroid cancer is generally treated surgically, but the extent of the operation depends upon the patient's age and type of cancer. Removal of the suspicious nodules, perhaps along with treatment using radioactive iodine, may be enough in a young person. Most experts, however, advise removing half or all of the affected thyroid lobe, especially if the patient is over 50 or the tumor is large and has invaded nearby tissue. Some or all of the opposite lobe may also be removed. When all of the thyroid is removed—a total thyroidectomy—lifelong hormone replacement therapy will be needed.

In advanced cases, radiation treatments, either alone or combined with chemotherapy, can alleviate pain and other symptoms. A tracheostomy, an opening in the trachea, or windpipe, may be necessary to allow breathing if the cancer threatens to close the airway.

Occasionally, during surgery to remove the thyroid cancer, the parathyroid glands—small clusters of tissue in the thyroid that produce hormones for controlling calcium metabolism—are inadvertently destroyed. If this happens, additional hormone replacement is needed, although an experimental treatment to implant salvaged parathyroid tissue appears promising. Other possible complications of thyroid surgery include damage to the nerves that control the opening of the airway, making a permanent tracheostomy necessary, and speech problems that result from larynx nerve damage.

Alternative Therapies

No effective alternative therapies for thyroid cancer exist, other than meditation, imaging, deep breathing, and other relaxation therapies to control pain and stress.

Self-Treatment

Thyroid cancer itself cannot be self-treated, but preventive measures can be taken. As much as possible, avoid exposing the head and neck to radiation, especially during childhood. Because people with Hashimoto's disease, a disorder in which the thyroid is chronically inflamed and gradually destroyed, have an increased risk of thyroid cancer, they should be diligent about having regular examinations.

Other Causes of Thyroid Symptoms

A goiter due to an over- or underactive thyroid can cause swelling of the gland.

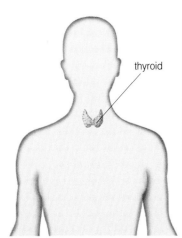

thyroid

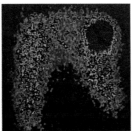
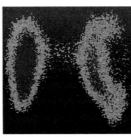

"Hot" thyroid nodules (see photo, above left) are less likely to be cancerous, whereas nonfunctional or "cold" nodules (photo, above right), tend to be cancerous. Ultimately though, only a biopsy can confirm whether or not a malignancy is present.

Thyroid Disorders

(Goiter; Graves' disease; Hashimoto's disease; hyperthyroidism; hypothyroidism; myxedema)

The thyroid, a butterfly-shaped gland that rests over the windpipe at the base of the neck, produces hormones that regulate metabolism and many other body processes. Both an overproduction (hyperthyroidism) or an underproduction (hypothyroidism) of these hormones can have a profound effect on almost all body functions.

The thyroid is regulated by the pituitary, a gland in the brain that produces thyroid-stimulating hormone, or TSH. A rise in TSH levels signals the thyroid to extract iodide from the bloodstream, convert it to iodine, and create the hormones known as thyroxine (T_4) and triiodothyronine (T_3). (The numbers refer to how many iodine molecules each hormone contains.)

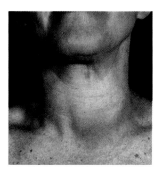

A goiter, an enlargement of the thyroid, often points to an iodine deficiency.

The thyroid gland appears to be the only tissue in the body that uses iodine. Although the thyroid needs only a very small amount to create the T_3 and T_4 hormones, an iodine deficiency can cause a goiter, an overgrowth of thyroid tissue produced as the gland enlarges itself to increase its ability to extract and process iodine. Goiters have become increasingly rare in the United States, thanks to the widespread use of iodized salt and the consumption of iodine-rich seafood.

An estimated 10 million Americans have some sort of thyroid disorder, with women outnumbering men five to one. Some of the disorders are triggered by female sex hormones and by pregnancy; they may also be a response to excessive stress, to a disturbance in the immune system, and to occupational hazards, especially exposure to radiation and certain industrial chemicals.

Thyroid disorders can occur at any age, but are sometimes hard to detect because their symptoms are easily ascribed to other conditions, especially in older people. These disorders fall into two main categories: hyperthyroidism, in which the gland produces excessive hormones; and hypothyroidism, which is characterized by too little.

Approximately 2 million Americans have some form of hyperthyroidism, which tends to run in families. The most common type is Graves' disease, one of many autoimmune disorders in which the body's defense system attacks its own tissues. Antibodies in the blood stimulate an overproduction of the thyroid hormones, which in turn speed up metabolism.

A person with Graves' disease feels on edge all the time; other symptoms include weight loss (even with an increased appetite), nervousness, irritability, insomnia, fatigue, muscle weakness, hand tremors, undue heat intolerance, excessive sweating, and frequent, loose stools. The heart rate speeds up, causing palpitations and potentially dangerous cardiac arrhythmias. An increase in bulk of the muscular tissue behind the eyes causes the eyeballs to bulge, and in some cases, to become inflamed.

Hyperthyroidism may be caused by excessive production of TSH because of a pituitary tumor, an inflammation of the thyroid gland (thyroiditis), or development of thyroid nodules. Less commonly, abuse of thyroid pills to control weight is responsible.

An acute form of hyperthyroidism, thyroid storm, may be triggered by a severe infection, surgery, pregnancy, or the sudden withdrawal of antithyroid medications. This condition is indicated by a rapid rise in body temperature, a fast heartbeat, and mental changes that may lead to delirium and coma. Thyroid storm is always a life-threatening emergency calling for medical attention.

Hypothyroidism (thyroid deficiency), also known as myxedema, affects about 5 million Americans. Babies born with such a deficiency are at great risk for developing cretinism, a devastating form of mental retardation and abnormal growth, unless treatment begins within the first few weeks of life. Consequently, all babies born in hospitals in the United States are tested for thyroid deficiency.

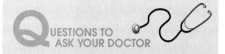
An autoimmune disorder called Hashimoto's disease is the most common form of hypothyroidism. Named for the Japanese doctor who first described it, the disease is characterized by chronic inflammation of the thyroid, causing it to enlarge and impairing its ability to produce hormones. The cause is unknown, but there appears to be a hereditary disposition to develop it and it is more prevalent in women than men.

Hypothyroidism can sometimes result from treatment for hyperthyroidism (see page 412). Secondary hypothyroidism is attributed to failure of the pituitary gland to produce the essential supply of thyroid-stimulating hormone.

The typical symptoms of hypothyroidism—weight gain, lethargy, fatigue, and constipation—emerge slowly and initially may be ascribed to other disorders. In time, the skin changes, becoming thicker, dry, and scaly; it may feel cold and clammy, and sweating diminishes. Nails also thicken and grow more slowly. The hair becomes coarse and sparse, and in young women, it may gray prematurely. Speech becomes thick and slow, and the voice turns husky. Younger women experience unusually heavy menstrual flow; older women often feel uncomfortably cold, even in a warm room. Personality changes, memory loss, and other signs of intellectual impairment approaching psychosis (myxedema madness) may be incorrectly diagnosed as a form of senile dementia.

Diagnostic Studies and Procedures

Symptoms and the patient's appearance usually raise the suspicion of a thyroid disorder. A doctor will feel the thyroid gland for any nodules or enlargement. A referral may then be made to an endocrinologist for more specific tests to evaluate thyroid function. Various blood tests will be ordered to measure levels of thyroid hormones and antibodies. One of the most sensitive tests

A CASE IN POINT

When Carolyn Kent, a 36-year-old real estate agent, first experienced symptoms of a thyroid disorder—lack of energy, hair loss, a thickening of her skin, and constipation—she misinterpreted them as a nutritional problem. But self-care with high-dose vitamin and mineral supplements failed to help; instead, her list of symptoms grew. Her hands and feet always felt cold and her family kept complaining that she "seemed a different person."

When Kent finally saw her doctor, a careful physical examination turned up an enlarged, rubbery feeling thyroid gland. Blood tests showed high levels of thyroid-stimulating hormone (TSH) and low levels of the T_4 thyroid hormone—a classic picture of autoimmune hypothyroidism, or Hashimoto's disease. To confirm the diagnosis, additional tests were ordered to look for antibodies against thyroid tissue. In Hashimoto's disease, the immune system attacks the thyroid gland and causes chronic inflammation. As the disease progresses, parts of the thyroid gland are replaced by lymphatic or fibrous tissue.

Kent was started on T_4 replacement therapy. It took several weeks to arrive at the proper dosage; after that, her symptoms began to abate gradually. After 18 months of treatment, however, she began to experience alarming palpitations in which her heartbeat was fast and irregular. She also felt nervous and had difficulty sleeping. Blood tests ordered by her doctor showed that she had abnormal levels of T_4 hormone.

"Have you been following your medication schedule?" the doctor asked. Kent insisted that she had. Further questioning revealed that Kent had recently joined a new insurance plan in which the use of generic drugs was mandated. Her doctor quickly determined that this switch was causing the problems. "Whenever you change T_4 preparations, you must be reevaluated to make sure that the dosage is correct," the doctor explained. "We had established your dosage under a brand-name drug. A different preparation may be chemically the same, but your body may react differently to it. So it's essential to stay with the same drug."

The doctor further explained that if Kent wanted to switch to a generic T_4 preparation, the dosage would have to be titrated again. "And after that, you must make sure you are getting the same preparation each time your prescription is filled," the doctor stressed. "In your case, it might be better to talk to your insurance company to find out if you can continue on your original brand-name drug, even if it is somewhat more expensive." This she did, and her insurance company agreed that the brand-name drug could be used.

THYROID DISORDERS (CONTINUED)

for hypothyroidism measures the amount of thyroid-stimulating hormone produced in the pituitary gland.

An ultrasound examination of the thyroid can detect nodules and other abnormalities. Sometimes tests using radioactive iodine—for example, thyroid scanning—are ordered. However, because they are costly, require hospitalization, and expose the patient to radiation, they are not done routinely. Nodules are usually biopsied.

Medical Treatments

In treating hyperthyroidism, the goal is to reduce the production of thyroid hormones, but the method used varies according to the age and general condition of the patient. Propranolol (Inderal), a beta-blocking drug normally used to treat high blood pressure and angina, is the first-choice emergency treatment of thyroid storm, because it slows the heart rate. Alternatively, iodine may be given, especially before surgery.

There are three approaches to treating Graves' disease:

Antithyroid drugs. These include methimazole (Tapazole) and propylthiouracil (PTU), which prevent the gland from making hormones. This is the first-choice treatment for pregnant or breast-feeding women.

Radioactive iodine. Because the thyroid is very sensitive to radiation, carried directly to it by the iodine, this drug destroys part of the gland, thereby decreasing its hormone-making capacity. It should not be used during pregnancy or breast-feeding due to the risk it poses for the fetus or infant.

Surgery. Removal of all or part of the thyroid is advised for hyperthyroid patients who should not receive radioactive iodine and cannot tolerate other antithyroid medications. It is also used to remove a large goiter and thyroid nodules. Following surgery, thyroid replacement drugs are necessary.

Hashimoto's disease and other forms of thyroid deficiency are treated with thyroid pills, preferably such T_4 preparations as Synthroid and Levothroid. Even though it is less expensive, T_3 made from animal thyroid glands is generally not recommended for use because of variability in products (see case, above) and an increased risk of cardiac arrhythmias.

Alternative Therapies

Naturopathy. Naturopaths recommend that the following foods be eliminated from the diet because they are reputed to stimulate goiter growth: soybeans, peanuts, pine nuts, turnips, cabbage, and mustard greens. In treating thyroid disorders, naturopathic practitioners prefer to use dried natural thyroid hormones rather than synthetic equivalents. However, it is best to follow the recommendations of an endocrinologist who is experienced in treating thyroid problems, and to clear any hormone preparation with this specialist.

Nutrition Therapy. An individual who has lost a great deal of weight before the diagnosis and treatment of Graves' disease may benefit from the guidance of a nutritionist, who can recommend a diet that provides extra calories without excessive fat.

Self-Treatment

People with thyroid disorders need to be especially diligent about taking their medication regularly and having checkups to make sure that the dosage is appropriate. Pregnancy poses a special risk to both mother and fetus. A baby born with thyroid deficiency must receive hormone therapy early to prevent retardation and growth problems.

Other Causes of Thyroid Symptoms

Thyroid cancer can induce enlargement of the gland and imbalance of thyroid hormones. Sometimes lithium, a medication used to treat manic-depression, causes hypothyroidism.

Tick Fever

(Human granulocytic ehrlichiosis; Rocky Mountain spotted fever; tick typhus)
Ticks are often carriers of organisms that can cause human disease. One of the most familiar is Rocky Mountain spotted fever, which is transmitted to humans by ticks carrying rickettsia, an organism that is classified as bacteria but which also has some characteristics of viruses. This particular form of tick fever is named for the part of the United States where it was discovered, but occurs in all of the states except Maine, Alaska, and Hawaii.

Various types of hard-shelled (Ixodidae) ticks, especially the wood, dog, and Lone-Star varieties, carry rickettsia organisms. In northern states, people are most likely to contract tick fever from May to September. In the South, where ticks are out the year around, they may be vulnerable during any month.

Symptoms develop 3 to 12 days after a tick bite. The fever comes on suddenly along with chills, a headache, and muscle pain. Body temperature may soar to 104°F (40°C) and remain high for up to three weeks if untreated.

The rash generally appears about the fourth day, quickly spreading to the neck, face, and trunk. At first, the rash is flat and pink, but it soon produces small bruises called petechia. The petechia eventually run together, forming large bruises. Brain inflammation, or encephalitis, may develop, causing agitation, delirium, and eventually coma. The gastrointestinal tract is often involved, with nausea, vomiting, and diarrhea. Other target organs for infection include the lungs, liver, spleen, heart, and kidneys. In severe cases, patients may suffer circulation failure and cardiac arrest.

Another deadly type of tick fever, human granulocytic ehrlichiosis (HGE) was identified in 1995. This disease is transmitted by the deer tick, which also carries Lyme disease (page 280). HGE is characterized by the sudden

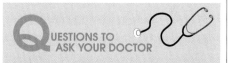

QUESTIONS TO ASK YOUR DOCTOR

▶ What tick repellents are safe to use on children?
▶ Can I contract tick fever when removing the insects from a pet?

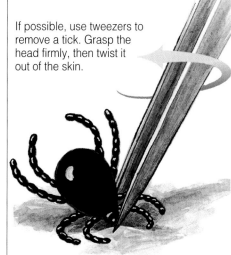

If possible, use tweezers to remove a tick. Grasp the head firmly, then twist it out of the skin.

onset of fever, chills, muscle and joint pain, and other flu-like symptoms.

Tick fever is always considered life threatening. Untreated, it carries a 20-percent mortality rate; early antibiotic therapy can cut this death toll.

Diagnostic Studies and Procedures

A recent tick bite and rapid onset of symptoms are key diagnosing factors. In some cases of spotted fever, however, the rash fails to appear or it develops late, making early diagnosis difficult. The rickettsia may be detected by using special staining techniques of tissue and blood samples. They can also be grown in a laboratory culture, but this should be done only in facilities with protective equipment; otherwise, technicians may be exposed to the disease.

Blood tests showing low white blood cell and platelet counts point to the possibility of HGE. There may be arthritis and other symptoms of Lyme disease also, because the two infections may occur simultaneously.

Medical Treatments

If spotted fever is suspected, antibiotic treatment with tetracycline and/or chloramphenicol in pill form will be started immediately, even before laboratory results are available. For a critically ill patient, drugs are given intravenously.

Doxycycline is the first-choice drug for HGE; tetracycline is also effective. Amoxicillin—used to treat Lyme disease—does not work against HGE.

Alternative Therapies

There are no alternative therapies that can cure tick fever.

Self-Treatment

Avoiding tick bites is the best approach. When outdoors in a tick-infested area,

wear protective clothing, such as high boots, long pants, and long-sleeved shirts that fit tightly at the ankles and wrists. Use an insect repellent that is specifically effective against ticks. Even then, after being outdoors, examine your entire body, including the scalp and body folds, for ticks.

Use special collars, sprays, and shampoos on pets during warm weather. Inspect their coats at least once a day and carefully remove any ticks.

If you do find a tick on your body, pull it out, preferably with a pair of sterilized tweezers (see illustration, left). If this is not possible, use clean fingers. Wash the wound with soap and water. Do not burn a tick out or kill it with kerosene or turpentine.

If you are diagnosed with tick fever, rest in bed until fever and other symptoms disappear; this should take only a few days if antibiotic treatment has been started promptly.

Other Tick-Borne Disorders

Lyme disease has become one of the most prevalent tick-borne disorders in the United States. Colorado tick fever is a mild viral disease spread by ticks in the Western states. In Africa and South America, ticks spread various forms of typhus, as well as rickettsial diseases similar to spotted fever.

In its early stages, the rash of tick fever can be easily confused with measles, but the spreading pattern is different. Measles starts on the face and trunk and spreads outward, whereas the tick-fever rash begins on the hands and feet and spreads inward.

RICKETTSIALPOX

This rickettsial disease is spread by bites of infected mouse mites. Like spotted fever, rickettsialpox produces a spotted rash that appears mostly on the face, trunk, and extremities. Other symptoms include fever, chills, headache, muscle aches, appetite loss, light sensitivity, and swollen lymph nodes. But unlike other tick fevers, rickettsialpox is mild and self-limiting, with symptoms usually disappearing in a week.

Tetracycline or chloramphenicol can hasten recovery, but even without treatment, serious complications are unlikely.

Rickettsial is now rare in the United States, but at one time, it was common among people who lived in mouse-infested tenements in New York City and other urban areas.

Tics

(Habit spasms; Tourette's syndrome)

Tics are rapid, involuntary movements that are usually jerky and repetitive. They commonly involve muscles of the face, shoulders, or arms, producing such motions as eye blinking, mouth twitching, forehead wrinkling, head shaking, and shoulder shrugging. Sometimes tics are accompanied by grunts or other involuntary noises or words.

Simple tics, or habit spasms, frequently begin during childhood or adolescence. Some researchers have theorized that they develop as nervous mannerisms to relieve tension. These habitual patterns usually disappear spontaneously, but in some people, they become ingrained behavior. Once a tic has been established, the person may be able to control it for a short period, but it soon returns and often is even more noticeable than before.

Simple tics are three times more common in males than females. Sometimes they are associated with an obsessive-compulsive behavior disorder, such as a need to wash every few minutes. A tendency to develop tics seems to run in some families. In a few instances, tics may be caused by an underlying neurological disorder.

With time, some people become totally unaware of their tics and lose any ability to control them. The mannerisms tend to intensify when these persons feel stressed, anxious, or self-conscious and lessen or even disappear during sleep or an absorbing activity, such as reading or watching television.

The most severe type of tic is called Gilles de la Tourette's syndrome, named for the French physician who first described it in 1885. This movement disorder, believed to be caused by a chemical imbalance in the brain, is characterized by a variety of facial and body tics and noises such as sniffing, throat clearing, grunting, or barking. Some people constantly repeat what is said to them, and others stutter or repeat their own words. An especially disturbing vocal aspect is coprolalia, the involuntary use of obscenities.

Tourette's syndrome usually begins between the ages of 2 and 15 and often lasts for a lifetime, although in some people it disappears by adulthood. In severe cases, the person is unable to hold a job or engage in social activities.

Diagnostic Studies and Procedures

Diagnosis begins with a doctor asking questions about the nature of the tics, such as when they began, how often they occur, and whether stress or specific activities bring them on. This questioning is followed by an examination that includes simple neurological tests. In some cases, a CT scan or MRI may be ordered, as well as EEG (electroencephalography), a study of the brain's electrical activity.

Medical Treatments

A decision as to the necessity of medical treatment is based on the type and severity of the tic, its underlying cause, and the degree to which it interferes with normal activities. Minor nervous tics in children are usually temporary and are best ignored.

Patients with simple anxiety-induced tics may be treated with a short course of a benzodiazepine tranquilizer, such as diazepam (Valium). While these drugs do not have a direct effect on a tic itself, they may alleviate anxiety while the patient undergoes psychotherapy to resolve the problem.

Haloperidol (Haldol), a drug that is normally used to treat psychotic disorders, helps up to 80 percent of patients who have Tourette's syndrome, with a 70- to 90-percent decrease in the symptoms. Unfortunately, symptoms are likely to return if the drug is stopped. Even so, only 20 to 30 percent of patients continue long-term use of Haldol because of its side effects, which include drowsiness, a dulling of mental function, and problems in muscle control that resemble Parkinson's disease. A safer drug is clonidine (Catapres), an antihypertensive drug that blocks certain nerve impulses. Some studies suggest that it helps 40 to 70 percent of Tourette's patients.

Patients who are not helped by Haldol or Catapres may be given pimozide (Orap), a new drug created specifically for Tourette's syndrome. It works by inhibiting the brain's receptors for

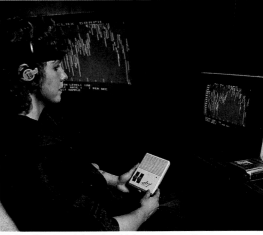

Biofeedback training, in which one learns how to control certain neuromuscular responses, helps people with simple tics overcome them.

dopamine, a chemical that transmits nerve messages. Its side effects are similar to those of Haldol, but unlike Haldol, Orap has not yet been studied for use in children under the age of 12.

Alternative Therapies

Biofeedback Training. Some patients are able to overcome simple tics by learning to control the responsible nerve and muscle responses.

Meditation. Deep breathing and other relaxation techniques associated with meditation can help alleviate stress and may reduce the frequency and severity of simple tics. Related techniques like self-hypnosis may also help.

Self-Treatment

Trying to control tics by voluntarily suppressing them does not work and may even worsen the problem. A better approach is to identify the stressors that seem to exacerbate a tic, and then avoid them or work on improving stress-coping techniques.

Tourette's syndrome can be difficult to live with, especially because many people have little or no understanding of the disease and assume that the afflicted person is mentally unbalanced. Joining a self-help group (see page 468) can help, as can psychological counseling for the patient and family members. Although Tourette's syndrome does not affect intelligence, it can disrupt the thought processes and learning.

Other Causes of Abnormal Movements

Tics and related abnormal movements may also be caused by Huntington's disease, dystonia, Parkinson's disease, and other neuromuscular disorders.

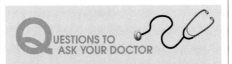

QUESTIONS TO **ASK YOUR DOCTOR**

► How can I prevent my child's nervous mannerisms from becoming ingrained?
► Could drugs help lessen my tic? If so, what are the likely side effects?

TMD Syndromes

(Temporomandibular joint; TMJ syndrome)
Temporomandibular disorders, or TMD, refers to syndromes that cause pain, clicking noises, locking, or stiffness when opening or moving the jaw. In the past, these disorders were referred to as temporomandibular joint (TMJ) dysfunction, but TMD is now the preferred term, because it also covers muscle problems. Research has shown that only 5 to 10 percent of TMD disorders result from structural problems in the joint itself. Facial pain, restricted motion, earaches, and clicking noises, which make up the majority of complaints previously attributed to structural abnormalities, are more likely to originate in muscles that control the lower jaw, or mandible.

Although the cause of most TMD problems is unknown, a number of predisposing factors have been identified, including overusing jaw muscles as a reaction to emotional stress. This may manifest itself as bruxism, the unconscious clenching or grinding of teeth, especially during sleep; gnashing the teeth in suppressed anger; and clenching the jaw or thrusting it forward in an unnatural position. In some few cases, jaw muscle fatigue may be

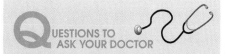

caused by poorly fitted dentures, a faulty bite (malocclusion), or teeth and fillings that are too high.

Ear pain is the TMD symptom that prompts most visits to a doctor. This pain is not necessarily restricted to the ear; it may radiate upward to the forehead or downward to the neck. Chewing sometimes intensifies the pain. Jaw motion may be limited, and in some cases, a crisis may occur when muscle spasms are so severe that the jaw locks and can be opened only by force. Contrary to popular belief, TMD problems seldom cause headaches.

Diagnostic Studies and Procedures

Diagnostic studies begin with a careful dental examination to look for poorly aligned teeth, high fillings, loose dentures or bridges, and other obvious causes. To detect possible dysfunction of the jaw joints, a doctor or dentist will observe the jaw to see if it moves symmetrically when the patient opens his mouth. The doctor may also position three fingers vertically between the patient's upper and lower incisors to find out if it causes pain (it should not). He might also place his fingers deep inside the patient's mouth to test the range of the muscles surrounding the temporomandibular joint.

X-rays can reveal if the problem is due to structural abnormalities of the bones—for example, severe arthritis or fusing (ankylosis) of the joints. However, X-rays may be normal despite the presence of TMD. If a tumor is suspected, a CT scan or MRI might be ordered, but in most cases, a diagnosis is based on the patient's description of symptoms and lifestyle factors, which

may reveal unusual stress or such habits as unconscious teeth-grinding.

Medical Treatments

Mild TMD can usually be treated with self-care or alternative therapies (see below). If muscle spasms are a problem, a muscle relaxant such as diazepam (Valium) may be prescribed. Arthritis and other inflammatory problems can be controlled with aspirin, ibuprofen, or other nonsteroidal anti-inflammatory drugs.

Special dental appliances to be worn at night can prevent teeth grinding, jaw clenching, and other unconscious habits. In addition, TMD problems related to a poor bite can be alleviated with orthodontics, the use of braces to realign teeth. In other cases, a dentist may recommend grinding down the teeth and crowning them to change their height and bite.

Corrective surgery should be done only after obtaining a second or even a third opinion. There are two surgical approaches: open temporomandibular-joint, which entails removing scar tissue and repositioning jaw structures through a large incision, and arthroscopic, in which a surgeon works through a viewing tube inserted via a small puncture over the joint. There is also orthognathic surgery to correct a faulty bite and jaw positioning with a combination of braces and jaw surgery.

Alternative Therapies

Biofeedback Training and Meditation. These and other stress-management techniques can help overcome bruxism, jaw clenching, and other stress-related habits contributing to TMD.

Physical Therapy. There are special exercises designed to retrain chewing muscles that go into spasm. Therapists can also suggest exercises to increase the jaw's range of motion.

Self-Treatment

Doctors generally recommend three months of alternative therapies and self-care before embarking on surgery, orthodontics, and other extensive treatments. For example, TMD muscle pain often can be alleviated by applying moist hot packs several times a day and massaging the painful areas. A soft, easy-to-chew diet is advisable until symptoms subside.

Other Causes of Facial Pain

Arthritis, a dental abscess, head injury, fracture, sprain, or dislocation are among the many conditions that can cause facial pain similar to that of TMD.

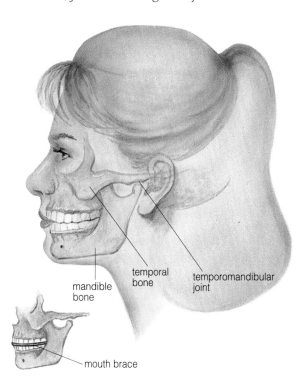

temporal bone
temporomandibular joint
mandible bone
mouth brace

Wearing a special mouth brace while sleeping can prevent the jaw clenching and teeth gnashing or grinding that are often the causes of TMD symptoms.

Tonsillitis

The tonsils, a pair of lymph nodes at the back of the throat, are part of the body's defense system against bacteria and other harmful organisms entering through the nose and throat. Sometimes the tonsils become enlarged and inflamed. This condition, called tonsillitis, is especially common in children.

Both viruses and bacteria can cause tonsillitis, with strains of streptococcus—the bacteria responsible for strep throat and other common infections—the most common culprit.

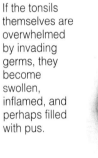

The tonsils' location at the back of the throat allows them to attract bacteria and viruses entering the body through the nose and mouth.

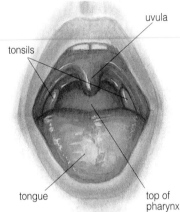

uvula
tonsils
tongue
top of pharynx

Normal

If the tonsils themselves are overwhelmed by invading germs, they become swollen, inflamed, and perhaps filled with pus.

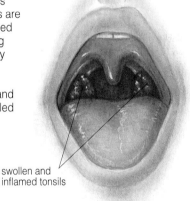

swollen and inflamed tonsils

Tonsillitis

Tonsillitis typically starts with a sore throat that comes on suddenly and is most painful when swallowing. The pain may radiate to the ears and be accompanied by fever, headache, vomiting, and a feeling of general malaise. Also, the lymph nodes on either side of the jaw often swell.

Sometimes tonsillitis sets the stage for more serious disorders. Strep tonsillitis, if left untreated, can develop into rheumatic fever or acute glomerulonephritis, a serious kidney disorder. Another

possible consequence is a peritonsillar abscess, or quinsy. This condition, rare in children but fairly common in young adults, usually develops when strep infects tissue between a tonsil and the pharyngeal muscle at the back of the throat. In severe cases, the swelling is so great that it may close off the airway, creating a medical emergency. As with tonsillitis, severe sore throat, difficulty swallowing, and fever are symptoms.

Diagnostic Studies and Procedures

A doctor can readily determine whether the tonsils are enlarged and reddened by depressing the tongue and looking into the mouth and throat with the aid of a lighted instrument. The tonsils may give off yellowish pus and be covered by a white membrane that can be peeled away without bleeding.

A sample of secretions from the tonsils may be cultured or examined under a microscope to identify the causative organism.

Medical Treatments

Streptococcal tonsillitis is treated with a 10-day course of oral penicillin. A week later, another smear will be collected from the throat and examined to determine if streptococci are still present. Other family members may also be asked for throat cultures and asymptomatic carriers should be treated with antibiotics to avoid passing the infection back and forth. Prophylactic antibiotics may be given to children who have had close contact with someone with a strep throat infection.

Viral tonsillitis does not respond to antibiotics, but it usually clears up on its own within a few days. Children may be given acetaminophen to relieve pain and lower a fever, but not aspirin, because of an increased risk of Reye's syndrome (see box, page 437). Adults can take either aspirin or ibuprofen, which will alleviate both the pain and inflammation.

Surgery to remove the tonsils may be recommended if tonsillitis recurs, becomes chronic, or if peritonsillar abscesses develop. The procedure, a tonsillectomy, was once performed on almost all children who had a bout of tonsillitis, but today doctors recommend it more selectively.

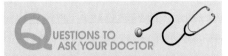
Alternative Therapies

These remedies are not a substitute for antibiotics in treating tonsillitis caused by strep or other bacteria. They may, however, alleviate the sore throat, fever, and other symptoms.

Aromatherapy. Therapists recommend inhaling essence of bergamot once a day for a week.

Herbal Medicine. Some herbal books advocate pokeroot to treat tonsillitis, but this herb should never be ingested, even in small amounts, because it is highly toxic. Safer herbal remedies include echinacea and chamomile, which can be taken in capsule form or brewed into a tea.

Homeopathy. To treat tonsillitis, homeopaths may use aconitum, baryta carb, a phytolacca gargle, or hepar sulphuris if there is pus or an abscess.

Naturopathy. Zinc lozenges are said to relieve the pain of a sore throat and stimulate the immune system to promote healing. Acidophilus capsules or yogurt with live cultures may be taken in conjunction with antibiotics in order to prevent a yeast overgrowth.

Self-Treatment

Gargling is an age-old method of alleviating the pain of sore throat temporarily. A teaspoon of salt in a cup of warm water is perhaps the best-known formula. Other gargle mixtures include 2 teaspoons of apple cider vinegar in a cup of warm water or 1 part of 3-percent hydrogen peroxide to 4 parts water.

Using a cool-mist humidifier in a room or inhaling the steam of hot vinegar are other popular home remedies; so too is drinking a mixture of lemon juice, hot water, and honey.

Other Causes of Throat Symptoms

Diphtheria and infectious mononucleosis can resemble tonsillitis, but there are differences. Diphtheria produces a gray, thick, membrane that bleeds if peeled away, and mononucleosis usually is accompanied by fatigue and other symptoms.

Toothaches

Although pain of a toothache originates in part of the tooth, the surrounding soft tissue, or underlying bone, it can radiate up and down and extend from the forehead to under the jaw.

Most toothaches result from caries, or dental decay, triggered by bacteria that live in the mouth. These bacteria give off acids that can erode tooth enamel, allowing organisms to invade the underlying dentin—the beginning of a cavity (page 125).

Initially, the person may experience minor twinges, especially when eating sweets or something hot or cold. But as the bacteria expand into the tooth's soft tissue, the pulp and tiny blood vessels that nourish the tooth become inflamed. Because the pulp is tightly encased by hard tissue, it cannot swell enough to make room for inflammation. The swelling also blocks the opening at the end of the root and reduces blood flow. Nerves become compressed and starved for oxygen, resulting in intense and relentless pain. Eventually, the pulp dies and the pain disappears. Pain may return, however, if an abscess forms at the root of the tooth, but it is likely to be duller and more localized.

A toothache may occur if a dental filling falls out or a tooth cracks or breaks, exposing the underlying dental tissue and nerves. Also, some people have otherwise healthy teeth that are supersensitive to hot or cold.

Diagnostic Studies and Procedures

Several approaches may be necessary to determine the cause of pain and the tooth responsible for the problem. These include tapping the teeth with a metal probe and observing your response, taking X-rays, applying a small amount of electrical stimulation to suspected teeth in a pulp vitality test, and exposing them to a jet of cold water or air. Drilling a small hole in a tooth can reveal infection under the enamel.

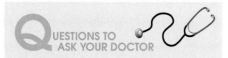

QUESTIONS TO ASK YOUR DOCTOR

▶ Does disappearance of a toothache mean that the tooth is dead? If so, does it still need treatment?
▶ Does root canal treatment mean I'll have no future pain in that tooth?

To alleviate tooth pain in the upper jaw, press firmly on the indentation just under the upper jaw bone (at the jaw joint) for one minute.

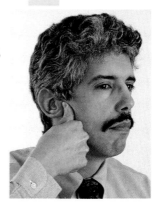

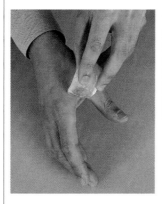

Try using ice to stimulate the acupressure point in the web between the thumb and index finger.

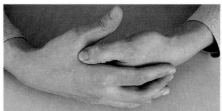

As an alternative to ice, use your other thumb and first finger to squeeze the area for a few seconds, repeating until pain eases.

Medical Treatments

A toothache due to dental caries requires drilling out the decayed area and filling the cavity. If decay is deep, the dentist may apply medicine to the underlying tissue before inserting the filling to help prevent sensitivity.

If an abscess is present, the dentist will drill a hole in the tooth to allow the pus to drain. Opening the tooth to relieve internal pressure usually provides immediate relief from pain. Depending on the extent of the infection, the tooth may be left open to drain for several days or it may be temporarily filled. The dentist will also prescribe antibiotics.

When the abscess affects a primary, or baby, tooth, the dentist may extract it. If a permanent tooth is affected, he will likely try root canal treatment, which involves cleaning out the canals, removing the nerve, and then filling and sealing the tooth.

If the nerve is dying, either extraction or root canal treatment will be recommended, depending on whether the tooth is primary or secondary.

Alternative Therapies

Dental care is essential for curing a toothache, but alternative therapies can help ease pain until you see the dentist. *Acupressure.* Rubbing an ice cube over the web of the hand between the thumb and forefinger, or massaging this same area, may help short circuit dental pain (see lower and middle photos, left).

For toothache in the lower jaw, use the thumb of one hand to massage the jawbone vigorously where it angles toward the front of the head. To ease a toothache in the upper jaw, place your thumb over the middle of the ear and slide it forward until it reaches the indentation under the bone about an inch in front of the ear; then press hard for one minute (see photo, top left). *Herbal Medicine.* Traditional herbal remedies for toothaches call for applying full-strength oil of cloves or cinnamon to the tooth. Dentists discourage this practice, however, because these oils can burn and irritate the gums and other oral tissue. Safer alternatives are oil of sassafras or fresh aloe vera gel, which can be applied around the tooth.

Self-Treatment

Over-the-counter analgesics, such as aspirin or acetaminophen, can provide temporary relief of mild to moderate toothache. Don't, however, resort to the old home remedy of pressing crushed aspirin against the tooth; this can burn gums and damage tooth enamel.

Moist heat or a heating pad applied over the aching area may help ease the aching. However, for throbbing pain that indicates a possible infection, apply instead an ice compress to the side of the face for 5 to 10 minutes every half-hour to an hour. It should help alleviate both pain and swelling.

If your teeth are sensitive, brush with baking soda or a toothpaste formulated for sensitive teeth. To protect your teeth from cold air in the winter, wear a ski mask or a scarf over your mouth.

Other Causes of Toothaches

Gingivitis can cause gums to recede, exposing parts of the tooth root and leading to dental pain. In addition, bruxism—grinding of the teeth when awake or asleep—can cause toothaches. An impacted molar or other tooth is another cause of dental pain.

Toxic Shock Syndrome

(Staphylococcal toxic shock; TSS)

Toxic shock syndrome, a type of blood poisoning, made headlines in the early 1980s when an outbreak of cases was linked to use of a new, highly absorbent tampon. The tampon was taken off the market and public concern waned. At the time, toxic shock syndrome was believed to be a new disease; scientists now realize that it has been in existence since the 1920s, but it was then regarded as a childhood disease called staphylococcal scarlet fever.

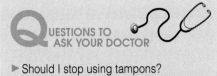

A painless red rash that often resembles a severe sunburn is an early sign of toxic shock syndrome. The rash typically starts on the trunk and quickly spreads to the legs, arms, soles, and palms. One to two weeks later, the skin begins to peel, especially on the soles and palms.

Although toxic shock syndrome no longer makes headlines, it is far from gone—researchers estimate that there are 5,000 to 10,000 cases every year. Even with treatment, 2 to 4 percent of patients die, compared with a 15 percent mortality rate among the untreated.

About 60 percent of those affected are women who use tampons, vaginal sponges, or diaphragms, but toxic shock can occur at any age and in both sexes. The usual cause is a toxin produced by a strain of *Staphylococcus aureus* bacteria, organisms commonly found in the mucous membranes of the nose, mouth, throat, and vagina. If the bacteria enter the bloodstream, they can produce life-threatening poisons. Doctors now believe that the bacteria can

invade the bloodstream through any cut or infection. Some cases of toxic shock have been associated with respiratory infections, including the flu.

Symptoms, which appear abruptly, include a fever above 102°F (38.9°C), vomiting, diarrhea, and a severe drop in blood pressure that can cause dizziness, fainting, and mental confusion. A red rash develops, followed a week or two later by peeling of the skin, especially on the palms and soles.

Diagnostic Studies and Procedures

Diagnosis of toxic shock syndrome is based on an evaluation of symptoms. The presence of fever, low blood pressure, and a peeling rash, as well as involvement of three or more organ systems—the liver, kidneys, and intestines, for example—points to the disorder. Blood studies and cultures may detect the *S. aureus* organism and help to confirm the diagnosis.

Medical Treatments

Time is essential in treating toxic shock syndrome. Immediate hospitalization, preferably in an intensive care unit, and administration of intravenous fluids and electrolytes, substances that maintain the body's chemical balance, are needed to counter the effects of shock and protect against kidney failure.

It is important to find the bacteria's point of entry. Tampons, contraceptive devices, wound packings, or other foreign objects have to be removed immediately; any wounds or abscesses must be cleaned and, if appropriate, drained. Although antibiotics cannot neutralize the toxins that are causing the symptoms, they will be administered to eradicate the bacteria in the hope of preventing a recurrence of the infection.

In some cases, blood pressure may be reduced severely enough to cause death. In others, there may be tissue death and gangrene, especially of fingers and toes, and amputation may be necessary.

Alternative Therapies

Any alternative therapy must be used as an adjunct to intensive medical treatment and should be undertaken only with a physician's approval.

Naturopathy and Nutrition Therapy. As soon as the patient is again able to eat and drink, large quantities of fluids—water, diluted juices, clear soups, and herbal teas—are recommended. Some practitioners also advocate zinc lozenges and supplements of vitamins C and A to strengthen the immune system and promote recovery.

Physical Therapy. Recovering from toxic shock syndrome can be arduous, especially if the infection has resulted in tissue death and amputation. In such cases, physical and occupational therapists can help patients learn new ways of performing everyday tasks.

Self-Treatment

Recurrence is a danger, particularly among patients whose infection is linked to menstruation. Some studies have revealed that up to two-thirds of women experiencing toxic shock have had subsequent bouts during their menstrual periods. To reduce this risk, doctors advise women who have had the syndrome to switch to sanitary napkins and not to use vaginal sponges or diaphragms for birth control. Others can protect themselves by:

▶ Changing tampons at least every four hours and not using the superabsorbent types.

▶ Using a sanitary napkin instead of a tampon overnight.

▶ Not leaving a vaginal sponge in place for more than 24 hours.

▶ Abstaining from sexual intercourse while menstruating.

Other Causes of Toxic Shock or Similar Symptoms

Blood poisoning from *Streptococcus A*, a bacterium related to the strain that causes strep throat, can produce a syndrome similar to that of toxic shock. Kawasaki syndrome, a serious childhood illness, produces early symptoms like those of toxic shock syndrome but does not cause shock. Other diseases with similar symptoms that a doctor should rule out, especially in children, include scarlet fever and Rocky Mountain spotted fever.

Toxoplasmosis

Toxoplasmosis, a parasitic disease, occurs worldwide in nearly all warm-blooded animals, including humans. It is caused by a single-celled (protozoan) parasite called *Toxoplasma gondii*, an organism usually contracted by eating undercooked meat from infected animals. Cats are often wrongly blamed as the major source of infection. Because the parasite produces eggs only in cats, they are the definitive *T. gondii* host. However, humans can acquire toxoplasmosis from them only by direct contact with cat feces containing *T. gondii* eggs. A cat may eat infected mice or raw meat containing cysts of *T. gondii*. The protozoan then reproduces sexually in the cat's small intestine, and one to four weeks later, its eggs are excreted.

When a human or another animal ingests the *T. gondii* organism or its eggs, the parasite makes its way to various tissues—usually the muscles, but also the brain, eyes, heart, and lungs—where it forms cysts. The body makes antibodies against the organism, though the *T. gondii* in the cysts remain viable for the lifetime of their host.

The vast majority of people are never aware that they have been infected. When symptoms do develop, they generally last for a few weeks and may include malaise, muscle aches, sore throat, and perhaps a fever and swollen lymph nodes. In a few cases, cysts form in the eyes, causing inflammation and sometimes vision problems. Otherwise, toxoplasmosis usually is not a serious disease, with two major exceptions:

Fulminating, disseminated infection, which can produce encephalitis, hepatitis, pneumonia, and inflammation of the heart. This form occurs mostly in AIDS patients and others who have weakened immune systems.

Congenital toxoplasmosis, in which a pregnant woman passes the infection to her fetus. Babies who contract toxoplasmosis may suffer such consequences as mental retardation, seizures, deafness, and blindness.

Diagnostic Studies and Procedures

In otherwise healthy people, a blood test shows a characteristic rise in toxoplasmosis antibodies. Some doctors recommend routine testing of newly pregnant women for the antibodies. An infection acquired during, but not before, pregnancy carries a high risk

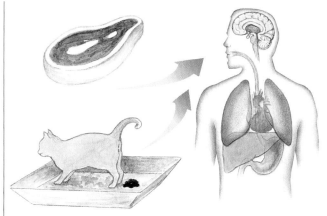

Undercooked meat is the most common source of toxoplasmosis. Cat feces containing *T. gondii* eggs is another possible source.

of fetal infection. If congenital toxoplasmosis is suspected in a newborn, confirmation is based on blood tests, analysis of cerebrospinal fluid, and inspection of the placenta for presence of *T. gondii*. The eyes may be examined for cysts and other abnormalities.

Antibody tests are of little value in detecting toxoplasmosis in AIDS patients and others with compromised immune systems. In these cases, diagnosis is based on symptoms and perhaps a culture.

Medical Treatments

Most cases are asymptomatic and self-limited, requiring no treatment. An acute infection, especially in an AIDS patient, is treated with oral sulfa drugs and an antiparasitic drug. One such combination is sulfadoxine plus pyrimethamine (Fansidar). Patients taking this should call their doctor immediately if they develop a skin rash, a sign of a potentially life-threatening adverse reaction.

Because of the high rate of relapses among AIDS patients, treatment is continued indefinitely. All patients receiving pyrimethamine need periodic blood tests to monitor for toxic effects and suppression of bone marrow function.

Treatment during pregnancy is somewhat problematic. Studies show that treating a woman who has an acute infection reduces the incidence and

severity of congenital toxoplasmosis, but the drugs used, especially pyrimethamine, are potentially hazardous to the fetus. In each case, a doctor considers the stage of pregnancy. Pyrimethamine and sulfa drugs are relatively safe after the first trimester and may prevent or reduce the severity of the disease. Spiramycin, a drug used in Europe and available from the Food and Drug Administration for special use in the United States, is safer during the first trimester.

Infants who have congenital toxoplasmosis usually are treated with pyrimethamine plus a steroid.

Chronic toxoplasmosis affecting the eyes may be treated with clindamycin, an antibiotic. In some cases, corticosteroids may reduce inflammation.

Alternative Therapies

Alternative therapies are not useful in treating toxoplasmosis.

Self-Treatment

Prevention is the best approach to self-treatment. The following are some practical guidelines:

▶ Make sure that all meat is cooked until well done, or to an internal temperature of 151° F (71° C).

▶ Wash your hands and utensils thoroughly after handling raw meat.

▶ To protect pet cats, feed them only commercially prepared food and prevent them from hunting in the wild.

▶ Use dry cat litter and dispose of the feces every day. Be sure to wash your hands afterwards. (To be extra safe, a pregnant woman or AIDS patient can ask someone else to change the cat's litter box.) The *T. gondii eggs* are not infective until 24 to 48 hours after passage. After that time, they remain infective for a year or more.

▶ Wear gloves when gardening or handling soil that may contain cat waste. If children play in a backyard sandbox, keep it covered when not in use.

Other Causes of Toxoplasmosis Symptoms

Mononucleosis, flu, and other viral infections can produce symptoms similar to those of toxoplasmosis.

QUESTIONS TO ASK YOUR DOCTOR

▶ Should I be tested for toxoplasmosis antibodies before becoming pregnant?
▶ Should I also have my cats tested?

Traveler's Diarrhea

(Infectious gastroenteritis; turista)
Traveler's diarrhea is characterized by the passage of four or five loose, watery stools a day, usually for two to four days. Studies show that 20 to 50 percent of travelers develop diarrhea, but the incidence varies greatly according to destination. For Americans, the developing countries of Latin America, Africa, the Middle East, and Asia pose the greatest risk. But travelers who go anyplace where their intestinal tracts encounter unfamiliar microorganisms can acquire diarrhea. For example, Mexicans often develop the problem when visiting the United States.

Numerous bacteria, viruses, and protozoa can cause traveler's diarrhea, but 40 percent of cases are caused by strains of *E. coli*. When these bacteria enter the small intestine, they produce a toxin that induces the intestinal wall to draw in large amounts of water and salt. Although the large intestine can absorb several quarts of liquid a day, it is quickly overwhelmed by the excessive water flowing in from the small intestine, resulting in diarrhea. Until the bacteria are washed out (about 48 hours), the person is likely to suffer abdominal cramps and may also experience nausea and vomiting.

Other organisms that commonly cause traveler's diarrhea include *Shigella, Salmonella*, various viruses, and protozoa such as *Giardia lamblia. Cryptosporidium*, an intestinal parasite that has been found in water here and abroad, is an increasingly common cause of a more serious form of diarrhea that may last 10 or more days.

Diagnostic Studies and Procedures
Traveler's diarrhea can usually be diagnosed on the basis of its symptoms. Blood tests and a stool culture may be ordered if the diarrhea persists for more than three or four days, or if it is

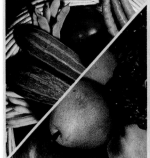
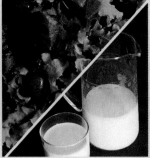
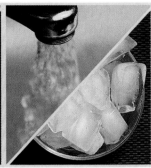

E. coli is usually ingested in food and liquids that have not been heated to a temperature high enough to kill it, such as raw vegetables, unpeeled fruit, unpasteurized milk, tap water, and ice.

accompanied by a high fever, blood in the stools, and other severe symptoms.

Medical Treatments
Most traveler's diarrhea is self-limiting and requires no care other than fluid replacement to prevent dehydration (see Self-Treatment). Most doctors advise against taking antidiarrheal medications, because they may slow recovery. However, if diarrhea is interfering with travel, some may prescribe an antibiotic such as trimethoprim with sulphamethoxazole (Bactrim or Septra) or ciprofloxacin (Cipro). Metronidazole (Flagyl) is used for giardiasis or other parasitic infections.

For situations in which it is difficult to get to a bathroom, loperamide (Imodium) or codeine, drugs that slow intestinal motility, may be recommended. Some doctors prescribe a combination of Bactrim and Imodium for two or three days for travelers who want relief from their symptoms.

Alternative Therapies
Herbal Medicine. Chamomile or ginger tea can help settle the stomach. Teas made of barberry, cayenne pepper, or summer savory are said to alleviate diarrhea. Caution is called for, however, because some of these may further irritate the intestinal tract.

Homeopathy. Practitioners recommend arsenicum, veratrum album, and belladonna to treat diarrhea.

Naturopathy. Naturopaths advocate switching to a liquid diet during the acute phase and reintroducing foods slowly (page 161). They also suggest drinking 3 cups of boiled rice water a day. This is made by boiling a cup of brown rice in 6 cups of water for 45 minutes, then straining it.

Self-Treatment
Prevention is the best approach. When traveling, eat at clean, long established restaurants. Select well-cooked foods; avoid raw vegetables, unpeeled fruits, and unpasteurized milk and milk products. Use only bottled or boiled water for drinking and brushing your teeth. Don't use ice cubes unless you know they were made with sterile water. Wash your hands frequently and always before eating or handling foods.

People who follow these precautions can still develop diarrhea, so it's wise to take preventive medicine with you. One study found that travelers to Mexico who took two bismuth tablets four times a day cut their risk of diarrhea from 63 to 21 percent. Alternatively, low-dose prophylactic antibiotics may be taken; ask your doctor about a prescription.

If diarrhea does develop, you will probably need a couple of days to recover. Bismuth tablets or nonprescription diarrhea products are generally safe, but may prolong the diarrhea.

Replacing lost fluids is essential, especially in young children and the elderly. It's wise to carry packets of a rehydration replacement product that you can reconstitute with sterile water.

REHYDRATION FORMULA
The Centers for Disease Control and Prevention recommends this fluid/electrolyte replacement drink:

Prepare two separate glasses. Fill one with 8 ounces of orange or apple juice (to replace potassium) and add ½ teaspoon of honey or corn syrup and a pinch of salt. Fill the second glass with 8 ounces of boiled or bottled water and add ¼ teaspoon of baking soda.

Take a sip from each glass every few minutes. When possible, supplement the rehydration formula with carbonated beverages, boiled or carbonated water, or tea made from sterile water.

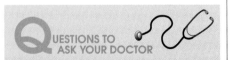

QUESTIONS TO
ASK YOUR DOCTOR

▶ Should I take medication to prevent traveler's diarrhea?
▶ Should I carry an antibiotic or an antidiarrheal drug with me just in case?

Trichinosis

Trichinosis, a parasitic infection, occurs worldwide and affects people of all ages. The parasite, *Trichinella spiralis*, forms cysts in the flesh of pigs, bears, some marine animals, and certain wild scavengers. In the United States, pigs fed garbage that contains raw meat scraps are the most common trichinosis carriers. Humans typically contract the disease by eating raw or undercooked pork, especially ready-to-eat sausages.

After a person ingests infected meat, the cyst wall surrounding the parasite is broken down in the digestive tract and the larvae penetrate the intestinal walls. Within two days, they mature and mate, and in another week the females begin to discharge larvae. These are carried by the lymph system into the bloodstream, where they are circulated to all parts of the body.

Symptoms vary according to the part of the body harboring the parasites. Early ones usually include abdominal pain, nausea, vomiting, and diarrhea. Fever develops as the larvae spread. Some of the parasites invade skeletal muscles, where they coil up and form cysts that can live for several years. Those that invade other types of muscle do not form cysts; they either reenter the bloodstream or are killed by the body.

Eye muscles are a favored target; in fact, swelling of the eyelid is a common early symptom, followed by eye pain, hemorrhages, light sensitivity, and impaired vision. The tongue is another common site of infection, resulting in swelling and difficulty in swallowing and speaking. Other symptoms include a persistent high fever (102°F, or 39°C), profuse sweating, chills, swollen and

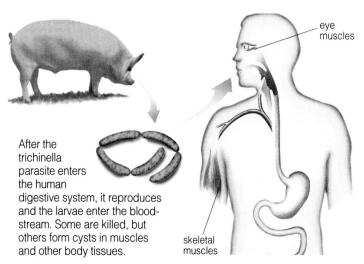

After the trichinella parasite enters the human digestive system, it reproduces and the larvae enter the blood-stream. Some are killed, but others form cysts in muscles and other body tissues.

eye muscles

skeletal muscles

painful lymph nodes, rash, coughing, itching, and muscle aches. Depending upon the site, later manifestations of the infection may include inflammation of the heart and lungs, meningitis, seizures, and impaired hearing.

Although death sometimes results, most patients recover in about three months, but some experience fatigue, diarrhea, and muscle pain for months.

Diagnostic Studies and Procedures

Early diagnosis is difficult, because there is no simple test for trichinosis until the larvae invade the muscles. However, an upset stomach, fever, facial swelling, and other symptoms after eating undercooked pork suggest trichinosis. Blood tests showing a rapid rise in eosinophils, a type of white blood cell, is another indicator. About three weeks after infection, antibody tests can confirm the diagnosis; so too can muscle biopsies for the larvae.

Medical Treatments

The trichinosis parasite can be killed by taking mebendazole (Vermox) or thiabendazole (Mintezol) for 5 to 10 days. A corticosteroid, usually prednisone, may be prescribed to control inflammation, especially of the heart, lungs, or brain. Aspirin or ibuprofen will usually alleviate muscle aches; if not, codeine or one of the more potent nonsteroidal anti-inflammatory drugs (NSAIDs), such as those that are used to treat arthritis, may be prescribed. NSAIDs, however, can cause further intestinal upset, and thus should not be taken when the person is suffering any gastric symptoms.

Alternative Therapies

No alternative therapies can cure trichinosis, but some can reduce symptoms.
Aromatherapy. To relieve intestinal symptoms, therapists recommend inhaling two drops of geranium or chamomile oil three times a day. Soaking in a hot tub to which you've added a few drops of juniper oil can alleviate muscle aches.
Herbal Medicine. Teas or capsules made of marsh mallow root and meadowsweet are used for gastric symptoms. Ginger tea often eases nausea and vomiting. Applying a poultice of juniper berries that have been simmered in olive oil may relieve muscle pain, as can a poultice made from crushed and boiled uva-ursi leaves.
Hydrotherapy. A whirlpool bath, a hot tub, or hot compresses can ease muscle aches that persist after other symptoms subside. Or try contrast bathing, sitting in a tub of hot water for 10 minutes, then taking a brief cold shower.

Self-Treatment

Bed rest is advised until a fever and other acute symptoms have subsided. Acetaminophen is usually the best choice to lower a fever if there are also intestinal symptoms.

Trichinosis is preventable simply by making sure that all pork, including ready-to-eat sausages, is well-cooked. The parasite also can be killed by freezing the meat at a very low temperature (-10°F, or -23°C) for 7 to 10 days. Even so, it's a good idea to cook it until well-done.

Home-raised pigs should not be fed scraps that contain raw meat waste. They should be given commercial feed or root vegetables, as is the custom in France, where trichinosis is rare.

Remember, too, that other meat or foods that come in contact with raw pork can become a source of trichinosis. For example, the disease has been traced to rare hamburger that was ground with the same machine used to make pork sausage. Always thoroughly wash all cutting boards, utensils, and other objects used in the preparation of pork.

Other Causes of Trichinosis Symptoms

The first stage of trichinosis may be mistaken for another type of food poisoning. In the later stages, muscle pain may be wrongly attributed to arthritis and other rheumatic disorders.

Tubal Pregnancy

(Ectopic pregnancy)

A tubal, or ectopic, pregnancy occurs when a fertilized egg becomes implanted in one of the fallopian tubes (or less commonly, elsewhere in the pelvic cavity) rather than in the uterus. Normally, an egg enters a fallopian tube after it is released from an ovary during ovulation. When conception takes place, it usually does so within the tube and the fertilized egg then proceeds to the uterus. If all goes well, pregnancy is established. In about 1 in 80 pregnancies in the United States, however, something goes wrong; the fertilized egg fails to reach the uterus and develops instead in the tube.

A tubal pregnancy is always a medical emergency and should be regarded as such. In fact, it is the leading cause of maternal death during the first trimester. As the embryo grows, it stretches the fallopian tube. When untreated, it can result in a rupture of the tube and sudden, massive bleeding.

The first signs of a tubal pregnancy may occur before a woman even knows she is pregnant. Soon after the first menstrual period is missed, spotting and abdominal cramping begin. If the tube ruptures, there is sudden sharp and intense abdominal pain. Severe bleeding can cause a drop in blood pressure, dizziness, or fainting. The woman also may go into shock; its symptoms include paleness, a rapid heartbeat, low blood pressure, and cold, clammy skin.

The frequency of tubal pregnancy varies greatly from country to country. In Jamaica, for example, the incidence is 1 for every 28 normal births. The rate in the United States has increased fourfold since the 1960s, paralleling the rise in pelvic inflammatory disease (PID, page 331), an infection of the female reproductive organs. PID often scars and damages the fallopian tubes, preventing the normal passage of eggs to the uterus. Other factors increasing the likelihood of a tubal pregnancy include use of an IUD (or, less commonly, a progestin-only oral contraceptive), multiple abortions, and a chromosomal abnormality in the embryo. Women whose mothers took DES, an artificial estrogen, during pregnancy have an increased risk of tubal pregnancy. A faulty tubal ligation can also result in tubal pregnancy.

Diagnostic Studies and Procedures

In some cases, an ectopic pregnancy can be diagnosed on the basis of the symptoms and a physical examination. More often, however, a number of tests are needed, starting with a positive pregnancy test and pelvic examination.

A blood test will be ordered to measure levels of hCG—a hormone that rises markedly early in a normal pregnancy. A lower than normal rise in hCG calls for further investigation using ultrasound to examine the uterus; if it appears empty, an ectopic pregnancy is highly likely. In such situations, a procedure called culdocentesis may be performed. This involves obtaining fluid from the pelvic cavity in order to determine whether abnormal bleeding is taking place. If doubt still remains, laparoscopy, the insertion of a viewing tube into the abdominal cavity through a small incision, will be ordered. The procedure, performed using general anesthesia, allows a doctor to examine the fallopian tubes, the uterus, and other pelvic organs.

Medical Treatments

Treatment depends upon the stage and location of the pregnancy. If the tube has ruptured, immediate surgery is essential to save the woman's life. In such cases, blood transfusions may be needed.

Sometimes, an ectopic pregnancy degenerates on its own, precluding the need for any treatment. In other cases, methotrexate—a drug normally used to treat cancer, severe arthritis, and psoriasis—is given to halt growth of the

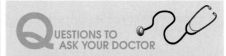

QUESTIONS TO ASK YOUR DOCTOR

▶ Is it safe for me to attempt another pregnancy?
▶ What is the likelihood of having another tubal pregnancy?

embryo, which is then gradually resorbed by the body. In such situations, a woman will remain in the hospital for a few days of careful monitoring to make sure that a crisis does not develop.

When medication does not work or a ruptured tube is likely, an operation must be performed to remove the developing embryo. If the problem is caught early enough, the doctor may be able to spare the tube. In more advanced cases, however, removal of part or all of the tube is usually necessary. If the remaining tube is normal, a future pregnancy is possible. Or if enough of the tube remains and a future pregnancy is desired, reconstructive surgery can be tried. In either instance, there is a high risk of another ectopic pregnancy. In vitro fertilization is a possible alternative when pregnancy cannot be achieved naturally.

Alternative Therapies

No alternative therapy is effective in treating a tubal pregnancy.

Self-Treatment

While resting in bed following surgery, move your legs often to prevent blood clots from forming. Your doctor may recommend specific leg exercises and also instruct you to wear surgical elastic stockings to improve blood flow.

After leaving the hospital, resume normal daily activities as soon as possible but avoid becoming overly fatigued. This helps to prevent postoperative depression. However, do not attempt vigorous exercise, heavy lifting, and straining for about six weeks or until your doctor approves such activities. Abstinence from sexual intercourse is essential until healing is complete.

Other Causes of Pelvic Symptoms

A threatened or incomplete miscarriage can produce symptoms similar to those of a tubal pregnancy; so too can a ruptured ovarian cyst, PID, and acute appendicitis. Some pain, bleeding, and other symptoms might be due to a normal pregnancy.

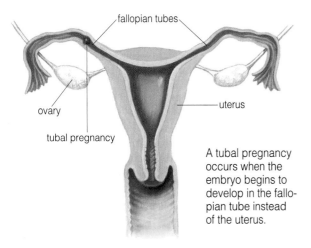

fallopian tubes

ovary

uterus

tubal pregnancy

A tubal pregnancy occurs when the embryo begins to develop in the fallopian tube instead of the uterus.

Tuberculosis

(Mycobacterium tuberculosis;TB)
Tuberculosis is an ancient disease that remains one of the leading causes of death. According to one estimate, about half of the world's population is infected with *Mycobacterium tuberculosis*, the major causative organism. Of these, 30 million have active tuberculosis, with 10 million new cases and 3 million deaths each year.

In the United States, tuberculosis is relatively rare, but there has been an alarming increase in recent years, especially among impoverished people who live in crowded, unsanitary conditions, persons with AIDS, and the elderly. The incidence of the disease among African-Americans in all age groups is twice that of Caucasians.

The disease spreads when a person inhales the *M. tuberculosis* bacilli expelled into the air from the lungs of someone who has an active infection. Typically, when the bacilli enter the lungs, they set off an inflammatory response. Attacking white blood cells, called macrophages, carry the bacilli to lymph nodes, where most are eventually destroyed. Those that escape into the bloodstream travel through the body, prompting the immune system to produce antibodies against them.

About 95 percent of patients in the United States with disseminated primary TB heal completely, and most are unaware that they have been exposed. Even so, these individuals still harbor the bacilli, which can be reactivated later.

The scenario is quite different for people who are malnourished or weakened by age or disease. In some, the bacilli quietly multiply for months or years before producing symptoms. Others may show signs of TB within a few weeks; weight loss, fatigue, a chronic fever, and night sweats are common. Pulmonary TB is the most frequent type, signaled by a chronic cough that may produce blood-streaked sputum. Less often, the infection attacks the kidneys, brain, heart, liver, spine, and other organs and bones.

Diagnostic Studies and Procedures

A positive reaction to a tuberculin skin test indicates the presence of TB antibodies, but it cannot diagnose an active infection. Skin tests also produce many false negative results, especially among AIDS patients and others who have

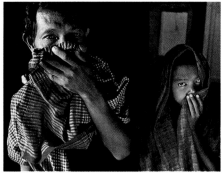

In developing countries, poverty, poor sanitation, and crowded living conditions promote the spread of tuberculosis.

weakened immune systems. A chest X-ray and other imaging studies can detect lesions typical of TB, but a diagnosis requires culturing the bacilli from the sputum and other fluids or tissue.

Medical Treatments

Treatment of an active or recurrent infection entails taking antituberculosis drugs, usually for at least six months. The most common are isoniazid (Nydrazid), rifampin (Rifadin and Rimactane), ethambutol (Myambutol), streptomycin, and pyrazinamide. Typically, two or more medications are prescribed.

Drugs must be taken in adequate doses for the entire duration of treatment. Because they can cause numerous side effects, including diarrhea, liver and kidney problems, and hearing loss, many patients stop taking their medication as soon as they begin to feel better. This can result in reactivation of surviving bacilli that have developed resistance to the drugs.

The emergence of TB strains that are resistant to multidrug regimens is a growing threat, especially among the homeless, prison populations, and other groups of people who lack diligent medical supervision. New York and other urban areas have stringent programs that include, when necessary, institutionalization to ensure that TB patients take their medication.

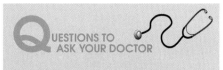

QUESTIONS TO ASK YOUR DOCTOR

▶ How can I protect myself and other household members from contracting TB while caring for someone who has it?
▶ How long must I continue drug therapy? What are the chances of recurrence?

Fulminating TB requires hospitalization for intensive drug therapy, usually in an isolation unit. After a few weeks of antibiotic treatment, most TB patients are no longer contagious. Even so, prophylactic isoniazid or rifampin may be prescribed for household members, such as young children, even though they may test negative for the disease. Antibiotics usually are recommended for asymptomatic persons who test positive for TB, to lower their risk for later activation of the bacilli. The BCG vaccine, which is made from a bovine strain of *Mycobacterium*, is safe and widely used in other countries, but its efficacy is doubtful.

Alternative Therapies

Alternative therapy must be approached as an adjunct to, not a substitute for, drug treatment.

Light Therapy. The *M. tuberculosis* bacilli are highly sensitive to ultraviolet light. Exposure to the sun or special sunlamps reduces transmission of the disease and may also promote healing.

Naturopathy and Nutrition Therapy. A balanced, nutritious diet emphasizing fresh fruits and vegetables, high-protein foods, and whole-grain products is critical. Also, extra calories are needed to counter the weight loss typical of TB. Naturopaths usually prescribe supplements of vitamins C and A, selenium, and zinc to boost immune function, but you should check with your doctor before taking any high-dose supplement. Garlic, either fresh or in capsule form, is said to boost immunity; it is also a natural antibiotic.

Self-Treatment

Most importantly, comply with your drug regimen, even if your symptoms improve. Get adequate rest and consume balanced, nutritious meals. Abstaining from smoking and avoiding secondhand smoke are also crucial, and the house should be aired frequently, even in cold weather. A dry, sunny climate has traditionally been recommended to help speed recovery.

To avoid spreading the disease, always cover your mouth and nose when coughing, and dispose of used tissues immediately.

Other Causes of TB Symptoms

Pneumonia and lung cancer sometimes resemble TB on lung X-rays, and flu, bronchitis, and emphysema can cause coughing, shortness of breath, and other symptoms similar to those of TB.

Tularemia

Although this infectious disease is commonly referred to as rabbit fever, it is carried by some 100 other species of wild animals as well as sheep, cattle, cats, and at least six other species of domestic animals. Tularemia is spread to humans by handling infected animals, eating their meat, drinking contaminated water, inhaling contaminated particles, or being bitten by ticks, deer flies, or other insects carrying the causative *Francisella tularensis* bacterium.

Until recently, tularemia was considered a rare disease, confined mostly to hunters, trappers, and fur handlers.

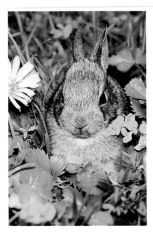

Many wild animals and even some domestic ones carry tularemia, but rabbits are especially identified with the disease; in fact, it is commonly called rabbit fever.

Doctors now think that some mild cases of illness attributed to flu are actually tularemia. Those at risk of contracting the disease include butchers, farmers, and campers and others who frequent tick-infested areas. In the United States, cases of tularemia are also reported among laboratory workers who have come in contact with the *F. tularensis* organism.

Symptoms appear suddenly a few days after exposure. Typically, a painful, ulcerative sore develops at the spot where the organism has entered the body—often the hands, mouth, or eyes, or the site of an insect bite—and lymph nodes become inflamed, swollen, and

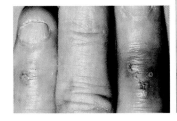

A sore typically points to the initial site of infection.

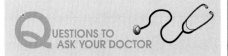

QUESTIONS TO ASK YOUR DOCTOR

▶ Can I be tested to find out if I am immune to tularemia?
▶ Should I be immunized against tularemia?

tender. A measles-like rash may appear. About 8 percent of cases are classified as typhoidal, in which the organism travels throughout the body, causing fever, abdominal pain, liver and spleen enlargement, and additional symptoms.

Other common forms of the disease include oculoglandular, characterized by severe conjunctivitis and swollen lymph nodes; oropharyngeal, marked by a severe sore throat and swollen nodes; and glandular, in which the lymph nodes become swollen without the usual skin ulceration.

Some patients develop pneumonia, either as the primary manifestation of the disease or in association with other symptoms. Most people recover completely, but about 6 percent of those who do not receive treatment for the disease die. After one attack, the person develops immunity against future tularemia infections.

Diagnostic Studies and Procedures

A doctor will suspect tularemia if a skin ulcer and swollen lymph nodes develop within a few days of contact with a rabbit or other rodent or after a tick bite. But diagnosis may be missed or delayed, especially if the disease was contracted from other animals or follows a different course. In these cases, a laboratory culture can establish the diagnosis. Blood tests can also detect tularemia antibodies, but not until about 10 days after infection.

Medical Treatments

Antibiotics can cure almost all cases of tularemia. One regimen calls for giving streptomycin by injection twice a day until the fever disappears, and then once a day for five days. Gentamicin is also effective against tularemia. In other cases, chloramphenicol or tetracycline are given, but a relapse may occur when using these treatment methods.

Severe cases require hospitalization. Although normally the disease is not passed from one human to another, an isolation unit may be advisable for patients with tularemic pneumonia.

Large abscesses in infected lymph nodes may require surgical drainage. Patients with tularemia of the eyes may benefit from atropine eye drops. Codeine is prescribed to alleviate a severe headache, which may accompany ocular tularemia.

Alternative Therapies

Hydrotherapy. Warm water soaks and compresses dipped in salt water can speed healing of skin ulcers and ease the pain of swollen lymph nodes.

Self-Treatment

Prevention is the best approach. You should always exercise special caution when handling wild animals and warn children about approaching them, especially if they appear sick. Hunters should wear rubber gloves and a protective face mask when butchering and skinning their kill. All wild game meat, especially rabbit, should be cooked until it is well-done. The tularemia organism is extremely hardy; studies show that it can survive for three years in frozen rabbit meat.

When venturing into areas with ticks or deer flies, wear protective clothing. An insect repellent containing DEET offers some protection against ticks. Inspect your body carefully for ticks and remove any carefully. Use tweezers to ensure that the entire insect is removed (see Tick Fever, page 413). If you live in an area where there are ticks, try to keep pets indoors; those that go outdoors should wear tick collars. Even so, comb them daily to remove any ticks. For people who have tularemia and experience fever, bed rest may be advisable until the fever subsides.

Other Causes of Tularemia Symptoms

Flu and other viral illnesses can cause fever, swollen lymph nodes, and other symptoms of mild tularemia. A strep throat resembles oropharyngeal tularemia; mononucleosis and numerous other infections can cause swollen and tender lymph nodes.

TULAREMIA IMMUNIZATION

Laboratory workers and others at high risk of exposure to tularemia can be immunized against the disease with a vaccine made from the weakened *F. tularensis* organism. The vaccine is available from the Centers for Disease Control and Prevention (CDC) in Atlanta.

424

Typhoid Fever

Typhoid fever, a serious intestinal infection, is now uncommon in the United States, with only about 500 cases a year, but it continues to thrive in areas lacking proper sanitation. The disease is caused by the *Salmonella typhi* bacterium and is considered the prototype of salmonella infections.

Infection is caused by ingesting food or water contaminated by the *S. typhi* organism, which is shed in the feces and urine of typhoid carriers, some of whom may be asymptomatic. Initially, the bacteria multiply in the small intestine for 24 to 72 hours before entering the bloodstream. Most are destroyed by the body's immune system, but those that survive continue to multiply. The surviving bacteria commonly infect the gallbladder and bile ducts; from there, they are able to return to the intestinal tract by way of the bile, allowing for reinfection.

As *S. typhi* bacteria enter the bloodstream, the person may develop fever, chills, generalized aches in the muscles and joints, abdominal pain, and a rose-colored rash. Unlike other salmonella infections, diarrhea and vomiting are minimal or absent.

The course of typhoid fever is unpredictable. In some mild cases, it is self-limiting. In others, fever disappears, only to return one or two weeks later. In still others, life-threatening complications, such as intestinal bleeding and perforation, pneumonia, and hepatitis develop.

Some people become asymptomatic typhoid carriers without knowing it. There are an estimated 2,000 such persons in the United States. In most of these individuals, *S. typhi* is harbored in the gallbladder. For unknown reasons, most carriers are women over the age of 50. When carriers are identified, they must be reported to local health authorities and are prohibited from handling commercially served food.

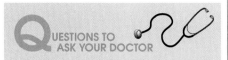

QUESTIONS TO ASK YOUR DOCTOR

▶ Should I be immunized against typhoid fever? If so, which type of vaccine do you recommend?
▶ What are the chances I will become a typhoid carrier?

TYPHOID IMMUNIZATION

Two vaccines are available to the public. The newer one is an oral type containing weakened strains of live *S. typhi* bacteria. A capsule is taken every other day until four have been consumed. Reactions, which occur rarely, may include nausea, vomiting, abdominal cramps, and skin rash. This immunization should be repeated every five years if the person is at continued risk.

The other vaccine consists of two shots spaced four weeks apart. Reactions may include discomfort at the site of injection for a few days, a low fever, headache, and malaise. A booster shot every three years provides continued protection. Neither vaccine offers more than 75 percent protection against typhoid fever, especially if a large number of bacteria are ingested.

Most Americans who contract typhoid fever do so during travel to Mexico, India, and other countries where the disease is endemic. Cases in the United States are usually traced to food handled by an asymptomatic carrier, although there have been instances of typhoid fever contracted by eating oysters and other shellfish from polluted waters.

Diagnostic Studies and Procedures
Diagnosis is based on the isolation of *S. typhi* organism from the blood, stools, or other tissues of an infected person.

Medical Treatments
Untreated typhoid fever has a mortality rate of more than 10 percent, but antibiotic therapy can cut this to less than 2 percent. In the past, chloramphenical was the drug of first choice, but in some parts of the world, *S. typhi* has developed resistance to this drug as well as to ampicillin. If chloramphenicol does not work, newer cephalosporin antibiotics, such as ceftriaxone (Rocephin) or cefoperazone (Cefobid), are given intravenously twice a day for one to two weeks. Other drugs that may be used include furazolidone (Furoxone), ciprofloxacin (Cipro), ofloxacin (Floxin), and trimethoprim with sulfamethoxazole (Bactrim or Septra).

Asymptomatic carriers are also treated with antibiotics. Typical regimens include trimethoprim with sulfamethoxazole or rifampin (Rimactane or Rifadin). To make sure the *S. typhi* organism has been destroyed, a series of three negative stool tests, taken at weekly intervals, are needed.

In individuals with gallbladder disease, its removal is often necessary to eradicate the *S. typhi*. Intestinal perforation usually requires emergency surgery. Transfusions are sometimes needed if there is hemorrhaging or chronic intestinal bleeding.

Alternative Therapies
Nutrition Therapy. Recovery may be faster with a suitable high-calorie, high-protein diet to restore energy and normal weight. Frequent, small meals are recommended. If diarrhea occurs, a clear liquid diet or intravenous fluids and feeding might be necessary. Iron supplements are needed if intestinal bleeding has caused anemia.

Self-Treatment
Bed rest is advisable, especially when there is a fever and other symptoms. Aspirin should be avoided because it increases the risk of intestinal bleeding and other complications. Laxatives and enemas pose similar dangers.

Anyone who has had typhoid fever can continue to shed the *S. typhi* organisms for up to six months, even after antibiotic treatment. Thus, they should not handle food served to others until stool tests are negative. Thorough hand washing and meticulous attention to personal hygiene can help protect others from contracting the disease.

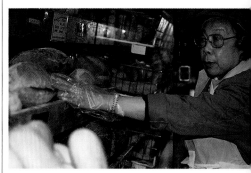

In many places, food handlers are required to wear protective gloves to avoid spreading typhoid and other diseases.

Immunization is advised for travelers to underdeveloped areas, laboratory workers, and others at high risk for exposure to typhoid fever. Because it is not 100 percent effective, immunized persons should be cautious about food and water in areas where typhoid is endemic.

Other Causes of Typhoid Symptoms
Some other salmonella infections can produce fever, prostration, and other symptoms similar to those of typhoid.

Ulcers

(Duodenal, esophageal, gastric, and peptic ulcers)

Small, open craters or sores that develop in the lining of the stomach or small intestine are commonly referred to as ulcers. (Less often, ulcers form in the esophagus, especially in the lower portion that may be exposed to stomach acids.) Technically, however, those that develop in the stomach are gastric ulcers, and those that form in the section of small intestine just below the stomach are duodenal ulcers. Doctors usually add the term peptic because such ulcers develop only in the areas of the digestive system that come in contact with pepsin, an enzyme that breaks down proteins.

At one time, researchers thought that an overabundance of pepsin and other digestive juices was the cause of ulcers, but studies have since shown that most ulcer patients do not have this problem. Indeed, many have lower than normal levels of stomach acid.

Doctors theorize that hereditary factors, such as a thin or overly fragile protective mucous membrane lining the stomach and duodenum, may be involved. In addition, research has linked the presence of a bacterium called *Helicobacter pylori* to the incidence of ulcers. Whatever the cause, ulcers can be exacerbated by poor dietary habits, excessive stress, caffeine, smoking, and heavy drinking. They are also worsened by aspirin and other nonsteroidal anti-inflammatory drugs.

Studies reveal that 1 in 10 persons will develop one or more ulcers at some point. They can occur at any age, but duodenal ulcers typically develop between ages 40 and 50, and gastric ulcers between ages 50 and 60. Many ulcers heal within a year, often without any special treatment or without even making their presence known.

Symptoms vary considerably. Some patients experience abdominal burning or a gnawing sensation, usually just under the breastbone. This type of ulcer pain typically occurs when the stomach is empty. Other sufferers complain of feeling bloated or nauseated after eating, and still others describe a feeling of persistent hunger.

Often, an acute episode of bleeding is the initial tip-off. This may manifest itself as vomiting fresh, bright red

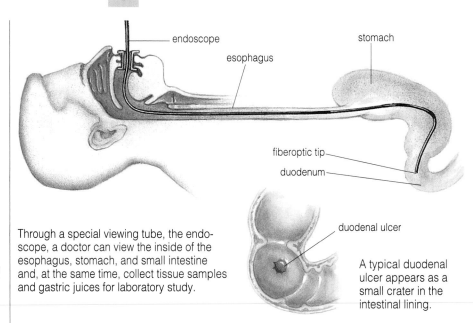

Through a special viewing tube, the endoscope, a doctor can view the inside of the esophagus, stomach, and small intestine and, at the same time, collect tissue samples and gastric juices for laboratory study.

A typical duodenal ulcer appears as a small crater in the intestinal lining.

blood or material that resembles coffee grounds. The stools may be bloody, maroon, or tarry and black, also indications of intestinal bleeding. Severe bleeding can lead to shock, a medical emergency characterized by a drop in blood pressure, rapid heartbeat, and cold, clammy skin. Chronic loss of small amounts of blood can result in anemia (page 77).

The ulcer may perforate the stomach or intestinal wall, allowing the contents to spill into the abdominal cavity. The first sign of a perforation is sudden, intense, unrelenting abdominal pain. This also is a medical emergency, as it can lead to peritonitis, a life-threatening inflammation of the abdominal lining.

Intestinal obstruction is still another complication of ulcers, usually the result of accumulated scar tissue that narrows the passage between the stomach and duodenum. Symptoms include distended stomach, intense pain, and vomiting of partially digested foods.

Diagnostic Studies and Procedures

Endoscopy, a procedure in which a long, thin, flexible viewing instrument is inserted into the stomach or duodenum by way of the mouth and esophagus, is the major diagnostic tool. This examination allows a doctor to view the lining of these organs, take pictures of suspicious areas, and collect samples of tissue and intestinal fluids.

An upper GI series is another diagnostic procedure. It entails taking X-rays after the patient has swallowed barium, a chalky substance that makes the intestines more visible on film.

Medical Treatments

Drug Therapy. A number of different medications are used to treat ulcers. *Antacids* reduce the acidity of digestive juices, alleviating pain and inflammation and promoting healing. Most antacids are available without prescription; common ingredients include aluminum hydroxide, calcium carbonate, magnesium hydroxide, and sodium bicarbonate. *Histamine (H₂) blockers* work by hindering the action of chemicals that can trigger inflammation and pain. Examples include cimetidine (Tagamet) and ranitidine (Zantac). *Antibiotics* clear up infection from harmful bacteria, especially *H. pylori,* sometimes found in the lining of the stomach or intestine. Antacids or other antiulcer drugs may be prescribed along with the antibiotics. *Coating agents* form a barrier over the ulcer to protect it from acid and allow it to heal; sucralfate (Carafate) is a coating agent. Certain antacids containing aluminum also perform this function. *Prostaglandin agents* such as misoprostol (Cytotec) protect the lining of the stomach from the side effects of

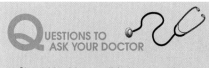

QUESTIONS TO ASK YOUR DOCTOR

▶ Should I add an antibiotic to my ulcer treatment regimen? If so, what are the possible side effects?
▶ What precautions should I take following ulcer surgery?

aspirin, ibuprofen, and other non-steroidal anti-inflammatory drugs.

Surgery. Most ulcers do not require surgery unless there are serious complications, such as obstruction, perforation, or hemorrhaging. The extent of the operation depends upon the complication. For a bleeding ulcer, perhaps only the blood vessel needs to be tied, although the ulcer may be taken out at the same time. In other cases, part of the stomach may be removed.

Alternative Therapies

Biofeedback Training. Biofeedback, in which machines are used to identify specific body responses and to learn ways to control or change them, may be useful in treating stress-related ulcers.

Herbal Medicine. Numerous herbs, including cayenne, catnip, chamomile, licorice, sage, and slippery elm, are said to alleviate ulcer symptoms. These herbs may be taken either as teas or in capsule form.

Meditation and Hypnosis. Although stress itself probably does not cause ulcers, it certainly aggravates them. Thus, many doctors who specialize in treating ulcers recommend meditation, yoga, self-hypnosis, deep breathing, and other relaxation techniques.

Naturopathy and Nutrition Therapy. In the past, diets for ulcer patients relied heavily on milk, rice, mashed potatoes, and other bland foods. Naturopaths now believe that milk has a rebound effect; while it neutralizes stomach acid, the calcium and protein it contains stimulate the production of

ACUTE STRESS ULCERS

Acute stress ulcers develop suddenly in response to surgery, extensive burns or other severe injuries, shock, organ failure, or other acute illnesses. The ulcers form in the stomach and often progress rapidly from small bleeding erosions to massive hemorrhaging, which is fatal in more than 60 percent of patients.

This type of ulcer can often be prevented by early intervention with histamine blockers, such as Tagamet or Zantac. These drugs are now given routinely before many operations and to patients with severe burns and other injuries.

more acid. Many now recommend drinking the juice of raw cabbage to dilute stomach acids. Small, frequent meals are advocated and, when symptoms are severe, soft foods, with a switch to baby foods if bleeding occurs. To prevent constipation, a nonirritating fiber such as psyllium seed or guar gum may be added to the regimen.

Iron supplements may be prescribed to overcome anemia caused by chronic or severe bleeding. Zinc is said to promote ulcer healing, and vitamin A emulsion or capsules are believed to protect the mucous membranes of the stomach and intestines.

Self-Treatment

Learn to slow down and be patient; ulcers often take a year or more to heal. In the meantime, strive for a healthy lifestyle that stresses regular exercise, a balanced diet, ample sleep, and time to relax and enjoy life.

Avoid aspirin and other nonsteroidal anti-inflammatory drugs unless you need them for arthritis or another medical problem. In such cases, ask your doctor about taking either an alternative medication or the drug in a coated (enteric) form that passes through the stomach without being broken down. If this is not feasible, investigate taking a protective medication, such as an antacid or coating agent.

If you smoke, make every effort to stop—there is a definite association between smoking and ulcers. Also, do not drink coffee, even decaffeinated types; coffee in all forms stimulates acid production. Abstain from alcohol as well; it irritates the intestinal lining and prevents healing. Spicy foods probably do not exacerbate ulcers, but you should avoid any that seem to provoke symptoms.

Some patients who undergo ulcer surgery develop a condition called dumping syndrome, which is marked by abdominal distress, lightheadedness, sweating, diarrhea, and sometimes vomiting an hour or so after eating. The symptoms are caused by an overly rapid emptying of the stomach contents into the duodenum. To avoid this problem, eat small, frequent meals, limit your intake of sweets, and avoid drinking fluids at mealtime.

Other Causes of Ulcer Symptoms

Stomach or intestinal pain may signify diverticular disease, gallstones, irritable bowel syndrome, inflammatory bowel disease, or even stomach cancer.

A CASE IN POINT

At the age of 62, Agnes Jackson—a Montana homemaker—suffered a severe episode of bleeding from a gastric ulcer that landed her in the emergency room. Until then, she had not experienced pain or other ulcer symptoms, but years of high-dose aspirin therapy for rheumatoid arthritis had put her in a high-risk group.

Doctors were unable to stop the bleeding, so emergency surgery was necessary to remove part of her stomach. She made a good recovery, but soon learned that she had to develop new eating habits as well as to take different drugs to control her arthritis. "I was used to eating three meals a

day," she explained. "Now my doctor told me to eat six or eight small ones." Heretofore, she had started her day with two cups of coffee, which was now on the list of forbidden foods and drinks. Various herbal teas became her coffee substitute; sticking to a schedule of a small meal every two hours or so was more difficult.

"I found myself snacking on crackers or cookies instead of consuming nutritious food," she related. "I simply didn't know how to spread my normal diet into so many little meals." A dietitian at the hospital showed her the way by making a list of the foods Jackson would normally eat in three

regular meals and then parceling them out in six to eight small ones. Jackson would start the day with a bowl of cereal and cup of herbal tea. Two hours later she might have two slices of toast and a piece of fruit. At noon, she'd have a bowl of vegetable soup and crackers; at 2 P.M., a slice each of roast chicken and bread; at 4 P.M., a cup of yogurt and crackers; at 6 P.M., salad, pasta, and cooked carrots; and before going to bed, a glass of milk and baked apple. On days when she would not be home, she packed a few small sandwiches, yogurts, a container of fresh vegetables, and a couple of pieces of fruit to eat at regular intervals.

Undescended Testicle

(Cryptorchidism)
The testicles are the two egg-shaped male sex glands suspended in the scrotal sac behind the penis. They normally develop inside the abdominal cavity and then descend through the inguinal canal into the scrotum shortly before birth or during the first few months of life. In about 3 percent of full-term and 30 percent of premature baby boys, however, one or both testicles fail to fully descend, a condition known medically as cryptorchidism.

There are varying degrees of the condition. With true cryptorchidism, a testicle is not visible nor can it be felt when the baby is in a supine, frog-legged position. The condition is due usually to mechanical or hormonal abnormalities. Maldescent, incomplete testicular descent, or arrested testis refers to a testicle that has descended only partially to the scrotum, the result of mechanical barriers to complete passage. When certain conditions cause a testicle to move off the normal course of descent and settle elsewhere, such as along the inner thigh or above the pubic bone, this is referred to as an ectopic or misplaced testis.

In cases of highly mobile or retractile testes, a testicle is positioned properly in the scrotum only at certain times

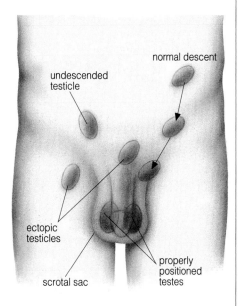

Normally, both testicles develop in the abdomen and then move through the inguinal canal to the scrotum just before birth, or within a few months afterward.

(such as during a hot bath); at other times it retracts up into the inguinal canal or abdomen, due to tightening and squeezing of the muscle that lines the scrotum. This usually harmless condition, sometimes called pseudo-cryptorchidism, eventually abates, leaving normal genital structure and sexual function. During a thorough examination of the baby in a warm tub it is possible to differentiate between a truly undescended and a retractile testicle.

Although some types of undescended testicles have no impact on sexual function or fertility, true cryptorchidism may result in a poorly developed testicle that cannot produce viable sperm. When both testicles are so affected, the condition results in sterility if left untreated.

Men with a problem in testicular descent have an increased incidence of testicular cancer, and therefore should be particularly careful about regularly doing self-examination of their testes and having medical checkups.

Diagnostic Studies and Procedures
Parents are likely to suspect an undescended testicle if the baby's scrotum is totally flat or flat on one side. A physical examination by the pediatrician can confirm the diagnosis. Depending on the nature of the problem, other tests may be ordered, including ultrasound and other imaging studies and hormonal and genetic evaluations.

Medical Treatments
No treatment is advised for retractile testes as a rule, because they rarely cause problems and tend to become normal by puberty. Otherwise, treatment will depend on the type of cryptorchidism and the doctor's approach.

In many instances, the recommendation will be to wait and see what happens, because about 80 percent of misplaced testes descend normally within the first year of life.

In some cases of true cryptorchidism, doctors will prescribe intramuscular injections of the hormone human chorionic gonadotropin (hCG), to be given several times a week for five weeks. Such hormonal therapy may promote normal testicular descent.

When hormonal treatment fails, surgery may be recommended. In one surgical approach, orchiopexy, the undescended testicle is repositioned into the scrotum. This is usually done before two years of age because any

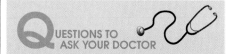

QUESTIONS TO ASK YOUR DOCTOR

► What type of testicular problem does my son have?
► Can hormone therapy help? What are the risks and benefits of the various treatment options?

delay, especially beyond the age of five, may impair the boy's normal sperm production.

If an abnormal testicle has not corrected itself by puberty, then removing it may be advised. An artificial implant can be placed in the scrotum so that the testicles appear normal. The decision to do so can be particularly important psychologically.

In the rare cases in which both testicles must be removed, the boy will be given injections of male sex hormones at puberty to ensure normal growth and development. Hormonal therapy will continue for life, making normal sexual function possible, even though the man will be infertile.

Alternative Therapies
No alternative therapy can aid promote descent of the testicles.

Self-Treatment
Parents should never try to reposition a baby's testicle manually; such maneuvering could cause serious damage.

A boy who has had a testicular descent problem should be taught the techniques of testicular self-examination at puberty and instructed to perform the simple, three-minute check once a month throughout life (for instructions, see page 403). Starting young is important because it may take several months for the boy to get to know his own body.

Any abnormality in sexual development can cause serious psychological problems. In those unusual cases in which sterility occurs, it is important that parents assure their son that he is normal in other respects, and that with proper hormone therapy, he can also function sexually, even though he will not be able to father children.

Other Causes of Absent or Abnormal Testicles
Various hormonal and genetic disorders can result in a baby with absent or incomplete sex organs, but these syndromes are very rare.

Urinary Obstruction

A urinary obstruction can result from any growth or narrowing that partially or totally blocks the normal passage of urine anywhere between the kidneys and its exit from the body through the urethra. In most cases, the obstruction is only partial, so that urine flow is restricted. For example, the flow may be reduced and marked by dribbling before or after normal urination. In some instances, attempting to urinate produces pain or burning. Though rare, total obstruction sometimes occurs, in which there is no urination; medical intervention must be immediate to prevent urine from backing up into the kidneys and damaging those vital organs.

Up to 15 percent of the population is born with urinary tract abnormalities, such as a muscle or nerve problem that affects the ureters or bladder. Most of these disorders never cause any difficulty, but the following can be serious:

▶ A marked narrowing of a ureter, either at the point where it meets the kidney (ureteropelvic junction obstruction) or where it meets the bladder (ureteral stenosis).

▶ A shortening of the outlet where urine leaves the bladder, a condition known as vesical neck contracture.

▶ Bands of fibrous tissue in the urethra that narrow it (urethral stricture).

Urinary tract obstructions can also be acquired; common causes include:

▶ Enlargement of the prostate gland, due to benign overgrowth (page 351) or cancer (page 350).

▶ Inflammatory conditions, including cystitis, or inflammation, of the bladder (page 152), and prostatitis, a disorder of the prostate gland (page 352).

▶ Genitourinary tumors, which may arise in the bladder, ureters, kidneys, or nearby organs, such as the prostate, uterus, or cervix.

▶ Sagging pelvic muscles that make the bladder shift position, a common condition among older women (page 100).

▶ Injury or scar tissue that is caused by infections, radiation treatments, surgery, or trauma.

▶ The use of cold pills and other drugs that interfere with urinary flow.

Diagnostic Studies and Procedures

Diagnosis typically begins with a physical examination and routine blood and urine studies. The lower urinary tract may be inspected by uroscopy, in which a viewing tube with lights and magnifying devices is inserted into the urethra and bladder.

Imaging procedures may include intravenous urography, X-rays taken after injection of a dye that outlines the kidney and ureter; retrograde pyelography, in which the dye is injected through the urethra into the bladder, ureters, and kidney; or anterograde pyelography, in which a catheter is inserted into a dilated ureter at a point

The flow of urine can be obstructed anywhere along the urinary tract. Common examples include narrowing of the ureters, tumors of the bladder and other urinary organs, and stricture of the urethra.

kidneys
ureter
narrowing of the ureter
tumor
urethra

above the obstruction and then dye is injected. Ultrasound and CT scans, which are less invasive, can often pinpoint the underlying problem as well.

Medical Treatments

Some ureteral obstructions can be resolved during anterograde pyelography; for others, a doctor may be able to provide immediate relief by inserting a catheter, a thin, flexible tube, through the urethra and into the bladder. If the obstruction is in the lower urinary tract, blocked urine may immediately flow out through the catheter.

Further treatment depends on the cause and location of the obstruction. Antibiotics will be prescribed for urinary tract infections. Tumors may be treated by surgical removal, chemotherapy, radiation, or a combination of these methods. Congenital problems often require surgery. Depending on the site of obstruction, surgery may be done using tiny instruments inserted through the urethra or an incision in the abdomen.

Alternative Therapies

Because a urinary tract obstruction potentially threatens the kidneys, a physician must diagnose the condition. Depending upon the cause, some alternative therapies may be useful adjuncts to medical treatment.

Herbal Medicine. Herbalists recommend tinctures or infusions of red clover, catnip, or bearberry (uvi-ursa) for a variety of urinary disorders. Herbal diuretics include juniper, saw palmetto, and gravelroot, which can be taken as tinctures or infusions.

Naturopathy. Drinking two or three glasses of cranberry juice, preferably in unsweetened form, every day acidifies urine and helps to prevent bladder inflammation. Some naturopaths recommend taking high doses of vitamin C, but many doctors discourage this practice because it can promote bladder stones and irritation.

Self-Treatment

Drink at least eight glasses of water, diluted juice, and other nonalcoholic beverages a day to help flush out the urinary tract. It is best to abstain from alcohol and caffeine, which can cause bladder irritation and urinary urgency. Also, do not take over-the-counter cold and allergy pills, as they can cause urinary retention.

Beyond these steps, urinary tract obstructions generally cannot be self-treated. However, if you are suddenly unable to pass urine but have no pain, take a warm bath. If the problem persists, you should call your physician.

Other Causes of Urinary Tract Obstruction

In addition to the conditions already listed, urinary obstructions may be the result of kidney or bladder stones, cancer and other tumors, and a variety of structural abnormalities.

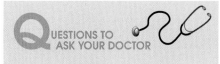

QUESTIONS TO ASK YOUR DOCTOR

▶ Could my problem be due to a medication I'm taking?
▶ What are the chances that the obstruction will recur?

Uterine Cancer

(Endometrial cancer; uterine sarcoma)
A malignancy anywhere in the uterus or its lining is referred to as uterine cancer. However, the major forms are distinguished from each other by their site of origin and types of malignant cells. Cancer arising in the endometrium, the lining of the uterus, is now the most common gynecologic cancer in the United States, with about 33,000 new cases and 6,000 deaths a year. (In the early 1900s, cervical cancer was the most prevalent form of cancer of the reproductive organs, but widespread use of the pap smear to detect precancerous changes has greatly diminished this malignancy.)

Most endometrial cancers are classified as adenocarcinomas, malignancies derived from glandular tissue. Many of these cancers are heralded by an overgrowth of endometrial tissue, a condition called hyperplasia (see opposite page). Much less common are uterine sarcomas, cancers made up of a type of connective tissue.

Typically, endometrial and other forms of uterine cancer develop following menopause; more than 75 percent of patients are over age 50 compared to 4 percent who are 40 or younger. The cause is unknown, but estrogen is thought to be an important factor, as it stimulates growth of the endometrium. Before menopause, the levels of estrogen, progesterone, and other hormones fluctuate during the menstrual cycle, resulting in shedding of the endometrium during menstruation. But if it is exposed only to estrogen, the endometrium grows unchecked. The resulting hyperplasia is believed to set the stage for cancer.

Studies conducted in the 1960s and 1970s found that postmenopausal women who took estrogen replacement alone had a greatly increased incidence of endometrial cancer, as did women who had entered menopause late, those who had never had a baby, and those with polycystic ovaries and hormonal disorders resulting in high estrogen production.

Obesity is another major risk factor; women who are 50 or more pounds overweight have a ninefold increase in uterine cancer, compared to women of normal weight. Here, too, estrogen is important, as it can be produced in fat

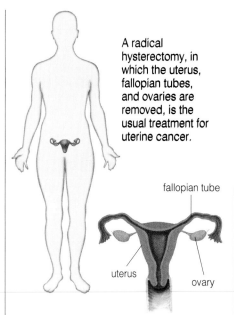

A radical hysterectomy, in which the uterus, fallopian tubes, and ovaries are removed, is the usual treatment for uterine cancer.

fallopian tube

uterus
ovary

tissue, even after menopause. Genetics also may play a role, because uterine cancer tends to run in families.

Early uterine cancer does not usually produce symptoms, but as the tumor grows, it may cause bleeding. Women with unexplained vaginal bleeding after menopause should be examined for possible endometrial or cervical cancer.

Diagnostic Studies and Procedures

An abnormal pap smear indicates the possibility of cancer, but it is more helpful in detecting cervical than endometrial cancers. A physician may use a long, slender cannula to collect cells from inside the uterus, but a definitive diagnosis usually requires a biopsy of tissue removed during a D&C (dilation and curettage). When cancer is diagnosed, blood tests, scans, and other tests will be ordered to determine whether it has spread to other organs.

Medical Treatments

Early uterine cancer has a very high cure rate. A radical hysterectomy, which entails removal of the uterus, fallopian tubes, and ovaries, is the standard procedure for uterine cancer.

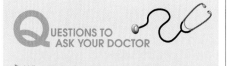

QUESTIONS TO
ASK YOUR DOCTOR

▶ When can I resume my regular activities following a hysterectomy?
▶ Has my cancer spread?
▶ Should I consider taking androgens to restore my sexual drive?

Also, a sampling of pelvic lymph nodes are tested for cancerous cells.

In all but very early, localized uterine cancer, a postoperative series of radiation treatments is recommended. External beam radiation is generally used, but in some instances, radioactive seeds may be implanted in the pelvic cavity temporarily.

Chemotherapy may be added to the regimen as well, especially if the cancer has spread. Progesterone is also used sometimes, particularly in cases of recurrent cancer.

Alternative Therapies

No alternative therapies can cure uterine cancer, but techniques such as meditation and self-hypnosis may help ease the pain of advanced cancer.

Self-Treatment

It takes four to six weeks to recover from a hysterectomy, although some women have reported that it took six months or longer to regain their former energy. Some feel depressed, especially if their surgery has abruptly brought on symptoms of menopause. If the cancer precludes hormone replacement therapy, a patient must find other means of controlling these symptoms (see Menopause, page 290).

Following a hysterectomy, some women experience reduced interest and pleasure in sexual activity. In the past, doctors rejected the notion that sexual function was affected, but a number of studies confirm that it can have a detrimental effect, especially for women who previously experienced deep, or internal, orgasms. Also, a hysterectomy that shortens the vagina may make intercourse uncomfortable, a problem that is compounded by vaginal dryness due to a lack of estrogen. Experimenting with different positions during lovemaking and using a water-based vaginal lubricant are usually helpful.

Androgens (male sex hormones) can help restore libido, but they can also produce side effects, such as growth of facial hair, deepening of the voice, and acne. To reduce these adverse results, European and Canadian doctors sometimes implant a pellet that releases small amounts of testosterone under the skin in the hip area, but this treatment is not used in the United States.

Other Causes of Uterine Symptoms

Abnormal vaginal bleeding may be due to fibroids and other benign uterine growths, infection, and trauma.

Uterine Disorders

(Benign fibroids; hyperplasia; polyps; prolapse)

The uterus, or womb, is a hollow, pear-shaped muscular organ whose main function is to house and nourish the fetus as it develops during pregnancy. Normally, the uterus is about the size of a medium pear, but it stretches to many times that size to accommodate the growing fetus. When fetal growth is complete, the uterine muscles begin the powerful contractions of labor and the birth process.

The uterus is divided into two parts—the uterine corpus, which is the upper portion; and the cervix, the narrow, lower part. The corpus is lined with soft, blood-enriched tissue called the endometrium, which is shed as part of menstruation if conception does not take place. When conception occurs, the embryo becomes embedded in this lining, where it develops into a fetus.

The cervix opens into the vagina to allow menstrual fluid and other uterine discharges to exit and sperm to gain entry. Both the cervix (page 127) and the endometrium (page 430) are relatively common sites of cancer, but far more common are a variety of benign conditions, which may develop in any part of the uterus.

Fibroids and other benign tumors. Doctors estimate that 20 to 25 percent of all women between the ages of 30 and 50 have one or more of these benign growths. Known medically as leiomyomas, these tumors are composed mostly of muscle tissue. Some

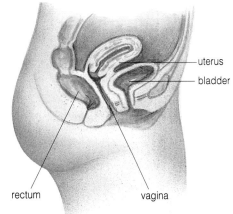

Normal uterus position

Under normal conditions, pelvic muscles and ligaments hold the uterus in its proper position above the bladder.

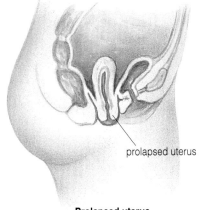

Prolapsed uterus

A weakening of supporting structures, usually as a result of several pregnancies, can allow the uterus to move downward into the vagina.

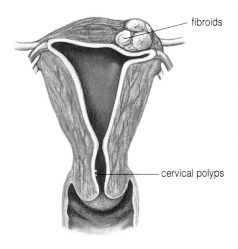

Fibroid tumors, or leiomyomas, may distort the shape of the uterus. Cervical polyps can cause abnormal bleeding.

are embedded in the uterine wall, while others resemble mushrooms growing into the hollow interior. They vary in size from less than an ounce to many pounds; the largest one on record weighed 147 pounds when it was finally removed. Most are asymptomatic, but larger tumors can produce abdominal swelling, miscarriage, fertility problems, discomfort, and excessive or prolonged menstrual bleeding that can cause anemia. If the distorted uterus presses on the bladder, urinary frequency may result. Other possible complications include constipation, chronic backache, and painful intercourse.

What causes fibroids is unknown, but estrogen appears to stimulate their growth. They tend to shrink and eventually disappear after menopause, but estrogen replacement therapy may stimulate their regrowth. Most of the time, fibroids do not become cancerous, but in some cases, they may mask a malignant growth.

Dysplasia/hyperplasia. Dysplasia is a general term for the abnormal overgrowth of tissue. In some instances, cervical dysplasia represents an early stage of cancer. Cervical hyperplasia is characterized by a proliferation of mucous and other glands, often as a consequence of taking birth control pills that contain estrogen. This type of hyperplasia often causes an increased vaginal discharge.

An overgrowth of the uterine lining, called endometrial hyperplasia, is often linked to high levels of estrogen that are not opposed or kept in check by progesterone and other hormones. This

commonly occurs in older women approaching menopause, resulting in heavier than normal menstrual bleeding. It also develops in women taking estrogen-only hormone replacement therapy, in which case it increases the risk of endometrial cancer.

Polyps. Polyps are smooth, tubelike growths that may project from the mucous membrane in any part of the body, including a portion of the uterus. Those that grow in the corpus may cause fertility problems and heavier than normal menstrual bleeding. Cervical polyps can cause abnormal bleeding or a heavy discharge, especially after sexual activity.

Prolapse. This refers to displacement of internal organs, usually due to weakness of the supporting muscles and ligaments. Prolapsed uterus—a condition in which the uterus protrudes downward into the vagina—is the most familiar. (This should not be confused with a tipped, or retroverted uterus, a variation of the organ's normal position.) Prolapse is most likely to occur after several pregnancies or after menopause, when supporting tissue becomes thin and weak. When the prolapse coincides with a weakening of the muscles supporting the bladder, as is often the case in older women, urinary incontinence (page 244) may result. A prolapsed uterus can also cause vaginal bleeding and backaches.

Diagnostic Studies and Procedures

Diagnosis starts with a doctor asking a woman detailed questions about her symptoms, menstrual pattern, and the use of oral contraceptives and other

UTERINE DISORDERS (CONTINUED)

hormonal preparations. This is followed by a physical examination that includes inspection of the genitalia and internal pelvic organs. If the pelvic examination is to be performed by a male doctor, he usually asks a female assistant to be present. A speculum, a plastic or metal device shaped like a duck's bill, will be inserted into the vaginal opening. When the device is expanded, it keeps the walls of the vagina open so that the cervix can be inspected. At this time, a swab is used to collect cell samples for a routine pap smear test, a laboratory analysis that looks for abnormal cells.

The next step is a bimanual examination. The doctor removes the speculum and inserts two fingers of one hand into the vagina and presses down on the abdomen with the other hand to locate the uterus and assess its size, shape, and hardness. A prolapsed uterus, for example, is easily diagnosed in this way. An enlarged, hard, or irregularly shaped uterus may indicate the presence of fibroids.

Colposcopy, an examination of the cervix using a lighted magnifying device, may be performed as a next step to look for cervical polyps, as well as abnormalities in the cells lining the cervix. The doctor may also perform a hysteroscopy, a procedure in which a lighted viewing tube is inserted through the cervix into the uterus to look for polyps, fibroids, and other abnormalities. Tissue samples of the endometrium can be collected at this time as well.

A more extensive diagnostic procedure is a D&C (dilation and curettage), in which the cervix is dilated and a small spoon-shaped instrument called a curette is used to scrape away part of the endometrium. The removed tissue will later be analyzed for possible cancer. The D&C by inself may suffice in treating the excessive bleeding from endometrial hyperplasia.

Other possible diagnostic studies include X-rays, ultrasonography, and a CT scan or MRI. Laparoscopy, a procedure usually done under general anesthesia, involves insertion of a lighted viewing tube into the abdomen through a small incision in order to view the uterus and other pelvic organs.

Medical Treatments
Once it is established that the patient's condition is noncancerous, treatment may range from watchful waiting to

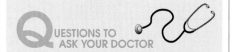

surgery. For example, asymptomatic fibroids usually do not require treatment, especially if menopause is only a few years away. If, however, the tumors are causing pain and heavy bleeding, several options can be considered, depending on the woman's age and her future pregnancy plans.

Hormonal manipulation may be tried to see if the tumors will regress. If not, endometrial ablation may be an option. In this procedure, the uterine lining and the fibroids are destroyed by electric current transmitted by a probe inserted through the cervix into the uterus. While this technique is less costly and simpler than surgical removal, it also results in infertility because the uterine lining no longer has the ability to support a fetus.

When an operation is necessary, a doctor may try to remove only the tumors—a procedure called a myomectomy—especially if a future pregnancy is desired. The success of this procedure depends upon the size, type, and location of the tumors. Sometimes trying to remove a fibroid that is deeply embedded in the uterine wall causes severe bleeding. If this happens, a hysterectomy, removal of the entire uterus, may be necessary. In other cases, hysterectomy is the best option, especially if fibroids are large and causing excessive bleeding and anemia.

A D&C is usually all that is needed to treat endometrial polyps and hyperplasia. Cervical polyps can be removed during outpatient surgery, often with a laser or an electric needle.

Treatment of a prolapsed uterus varies according to the degree of displacement. Frequently, it can be controlled by wearing a pessary—a donut-shaped rubber device inserted into the

vagina to support the uterus and keep it in place. If this procedure is unsuccessful, reconstructive surgery may be attempted to shorten and strengthen the ligaments that hold the uterus in place. In extreme cases, a hysterectomy may be necessary.

Alternative Therapies
In general, alternative therapies are of little use in treating uterine disorders. If heavy bleeding causes anemia, a doctor is likely to recommend iron supplements as well as a diet that includes iron-rich foods—red meat, liver and other organ meats, and seafood—along with abundant servings of leafy green vegetables, citrus fruits, and other foods high in vitamin C to help increase iron absorption.

Self-Treatment
Most uterine disorders cannot be self-treated, although some of the consequences can be alleviated. For example, if a prolapsed uterus or other condition causes painful intercourse, experimentation with positions that do not entail deep penetration may help to resolve this problem. A pessary usually must be removed before intercourse; it also requires careful cleaning on a regular basis to prevent infections.

After a D&C for endometrial hyperplasia, a woman may experience bleeding and discomfort for a few days. Sexual intercourse should be avoided until bleeding stops or a doctor says it is safe. Also, heavy menstrual bleeding may persist for one or two cycles, so don't immediately assume that the procedure did not help.

A hysterectomy generally requires four to six weeks for recovery, although most women leave the hospital after four or five days. You should avoid straining and heavy lifting for at least six weeks, and take care to prevent infection; for example, shower instead of taking a tub bath. It is usually safe to resume sexual intercourse after four or five weeks; check with your doctor first.

Other Causes of Uterine Symptoms
Cervical and uterine cancer can produce symptoms similar to those of benign conditions. A rapidly growing fibroid tumor, for instance, may be mistaken for pregnancy. Pelvic inflammatory disease, endometriosis, and other inflammatory conditions can cause pelvic discomfort, vaginal discharge and bleeding, and other symptoms similar to those of other uterine conditions.

Vaginitis

Vaginitis is an inflammation of the vagina and often the vulva as well. The most common symptoms are intense itching and a vaginal discharge that varies in color, consistency, and odor depending on the cause. Pain and a burning sensation may occur during urination and intercourse.

A number of infectious agents can cause vaginitis; one of the most common is the protozan parasite *Tricho-monas vaginalis*. Vaginitis also results from an overgrowth of organisms that normally inhabit the vagina or intestinal tract; for example, the *Gardnerella vaginalis* bacterium or *Candida albicans*, a yeast-like fungus. The nature of the discharge usually provides clues to the cause. *Trichomonas* causes a profuse, frothy discharge with an unpleasant odor. *Gardnerella* may produce a blood-streaked, white or yellow discharge with a fishy odor, whereas a cheesy discharge with a yeast-like odor points to *Candida*.

In some cases, the problem is due to a sexually transmitted disease, such as herpes, gonorrhea, or chlamydia.

The hormonal changes of puberty, pregnancy, and menopause sometimes predisposes a woman to vaginitis, as does sexual intercourse without adequate lubrication, and sensitivity to soaps, deodorants, douches, and spermicides. Sometimes careless personal hygiene, including failure to remove a tampon or contraceptive device, is responsible. Diabetes can increase vulnerability to vaginitis as can impaired immunity or the use of antibiotics or steroid medications.

Diagnostic Studies and Procedures

A doctor can often diagnose vaginitis and its cause by examining the vulva and vagina, but to make sure, she will take a sample of the vaginal discharge and send it for microscopic examination. If trichomoniasis or a sexually transmitted disease is responsible,

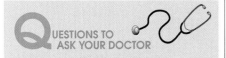

▶ Could my vaginitis be secondary to diabetes or some other disease?
▶ Is it safe for me to use a nonprescription drug or douche for self-treatment?

sexual partners should also be examined and treated to prevent reinfection. Additional tests may include blood and urine studies and a biopsy.

Medical Treatments

Candida, or yeast, infections are treated with antifungal suppositories, creams, or ointments; these products include butoconazole (Femstat), nystatin (Mycostatin), terconazole (Terazol), tioconazole (Vagistat-1), clotrimazole (Gyne-Lotrimin, Mycelex, and Femcare), and miconazole (Monistat), which are available in both prescription and over-the-counter forms.

Gardnerella infections may be treated with oral antibiotics, usually metronidazole (Flagyl or Protostat). Ampicillin or a cephalosporin are sometimes used, but they are not as effective. Topical antibiotic creams such as clindamycin (Cleocin) or vaginal creams and tablets that contain a combination of sulfa drugs, such as Sultrin, may also be used, but are not as effective as the systemic drugs. Trichomoniasis can be treated with oral metronidazole.

Estrogen replacement alleviates postmenopausal vaginitis (page 290).

Alternative Therapies

Natural remedies for vaginitis abound; but a doctor should be seen first for a proper diagnosis.

Herbal Medicine. Some books advocate a goldenseal-myrrh douche, but this should be avoided because it can irritate delicate mucous membranes. Herbalists recommend douching with yellow dock tea two or three times a week for yeast infections or a chickweed douche for trichomoniasis. (Boil 3 tablespoons of dried chickweed in 3 cups of water for two minutes, let stand for five minutes, strain, and cool.)

Naturopathy and Nutrition Therapy. Acidophilus pills or yogurt made with live cultures is a popular remedy for yeast infections (see A Case in Point, above). Drinking unsweetened cranberry juice to acidify vaginal secretions may also help. Another natural remedy for yeast infections entails inserting boric acid capsules into the vagina daily for two weeks. For trichomoniasis, naturopaths (and many doctors) recommend vinegar douches. Iodine (Betadine) may eliminate bacterial vaginitis.

Self-Treatment

In attempting to self-treat vaginitis, make sure you know what type you have. If you recognize a yeast infection

A CASE IN POINT

When Darlene Adams was put on a 10-day course of antibiotics to treat a strep throat, she had no idea that this would create a new set of problems; namely, a vaginal yeast infection. The persistent itching and profuse discharge prompted a quick visit to her gynecologist. The doctor explained that the drug had killed not only the harmful strep germ, but also the beneficial bacteria that help keep in check the yeast that normally live in the vagina and elsewhere in the body.

In Adams' case, the culprit was *Candida albicans,* a common yeast organism that is readily brought under control by antifungal agents. The gynecologist recommended a nonprescription miconazole product.

As a further measure to hasten a return of the body's natural balance between yeast and bacteria, the doctor suggested that each day she eat two or three cups of yogurt containing live cultures and also insert a few tablespoons of plain yogurt directly into the vagina.

"To do this," she instructed, "fill the kind of applicator that is used for contraceptive foam with plain yogurt and then wear a tampon to keep it from leaking out."

Adams was dubious about the yogurt treatment, but was pleased to report that her vaginitis cleared up within three days.

from a prior diagnosis, you can try an over-the-counter antiyeast product or an alternative remedy.

If you douche, don't overdo it, as this in itself can cause inflammation.

Future bouts can often be prevented by following these measures:
▶ Keep the genital area as dry as possible. Wear loose-fitting cotton underclothes and don't stay in a wet bathing suit any longer than necessary.
▶ Use a mild, unscented soap; avoid vaginal deodorants, perfumed bubble baths, scented tampons, and other potentially irritating products.
▶ Use a water-based lubricating jelly during sexual intercourse.

Other Causes of Vaginal Irritation

Cervicitis, pelvic inflammatory disease, herpes, and other genital infections can result in vaginal symptoms.

Varicose Veins

(Varicosities)

Varicose veins—which are widened and twisted—develop when the tiny one-way valves within the vessels malfunction and allow some blood to seep backwards. The most familiar are those in the lower legs, which appear bluish and bulging, but they also form in the anal area (see hemorrhoids, page 225). Less often, veins in the esophagus become varicosed; this condition, usually linked to liver disease, can cause serious intestinal bleeding.

In general, varicose veins are more of a cosmetic problem than a health threat. In some instances, however, they cause pain and ulcers; they also increase the risk of phlebitis, an inflammation of the veins (page 332).

A predisposition for varicose veins is often inherited. Obesity and straining during bowel movements also contribute to the condition. The hormonal changes of pregnancy that promote relaxation and stretching of connective tissue can cause varicose veins, which often disappear within a few months of giving birth. About 10 percent of men and 25 percent of women are affected by the disorder. Occupations that require standing in one place for long periods do not cause varicose veins, but can worsen them once they develop.

Diagnostic Studies and Procedures

A doctor can detect superficial varicose veins by sight and by palpating, or feeling, for swollen vessels while the patient stands. Other signs may include a brownish-gray discoloration of the skin

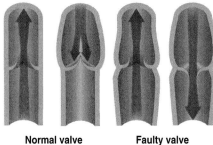

Normal valve   **Faulty valve**

One-way valves keep blood flowing through veins. A faulty valve allows a back flow and pooling of blood.

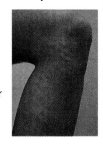

The saphenous and other superficial leg veins are especially susceptible to varicosities.

and skin ulcers in the lower legs. To pinpoint the faulty valves, the doctor elevates the leg to empty the saphenous vein there and then, while applying pressure to this same vein in the upper thigh, asks the patient to stand, which will cause bulges to form over the diseased vessels. Doppler ultrasound, using high-frequency sound waves, can detect less obvious abnormalities, as can venography, X-ray studies of the vessels taken after injection of a dye.

Medical Treatments

Normally, varicose veins do not require treatment unless their appearance is troublesome or they are causing pain, skin changes, or ulcers. For mild cases, sclerotherapy may suffice. In this procedure, an irritating solution, such as sodium tetradecyl sulfate, is injected into the vein, foam pads are placed over it, and the leg is wrapped with a compression bandage. The solution collapses the treated veins and blood is diverted to other veins, causing the discolored bulges to disappear. The patient can resume normal activities almost immediately, although the leg will remain bandaged for three weeks or longer.

Less than 10 percent of patients require surgical stripping, or removal, of the saphenous vein. In this procedure, done under general anesthesia, at least two incisions are made, one in the ankle and the other in the groin. Other incisions may be made along the vein and its branches tied off. The surgeon passes a plastic stripper up the length of the vein, which is removed through the incision in the groin. The operation takes about 30 minutes. A week later, the stitches are removed and moderate activities resumed. However, vigorous exercise must be avoided until healing is complete, which usually takes two weeks. The operation leaves a few scars, and other veins may develop varicosities. Some 2 to 5 percent of patients experience ankle numbness due to damage of nerves in the skin.

Alternative Therapies

Herbal Medicine. Herbalists recommend covering the diseased veins with compresses soaked in a solution of horse chestnut extract and witch hazel, herbs that are said to improve the tone of venous muscles. Applying lotion containing butcher's broom to the bulging veins is also reputed to help. Garlic, taken fresh or in capsules, is recommended to prevent clots.

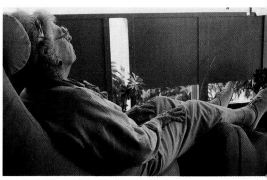

Resting with the leg elevated promotes blood flow and eases pressure on varicose veins.

Nutrition Therapy. People in developing countries who eat a high-fiber diet rarely have varicose veins. Consuming a diet that provides plenty of fruits, vegetables, and whole grains may prevent the problem. Losing excess weight is also important.

Self-Treatment

Elastic stockings promote blood flow by compressing varicose veins. They are most effective if you put them on before getting out of bed in the morning and wear them throughout the day.

Daily exercise is a critical aspect of self-treatment. Cycling, walking, and swimming are good choices. Avoid standing in one place for any length of time; if your job requires standing, walk in place every few minutes, and if possible, alternate standing on each foot with the other supported on a low stool. When resting, elevate your legs so they are higher than your heart, a position that uses gravity to increase blood flow from the legs.

Hot tubs, heating pads, and saunas may worsen varicose veins; instead, apply cold compresses or ice packs.

Other Causes of Leg Pain

Phlebitis causes inflammation, pain, and swelling in leg veins. Reduced blood flow through the leg arteries can also result in pain, especially during exercise. Nerve disorders, including the neuropathy associated with diabetes, frequently produce leg pain.

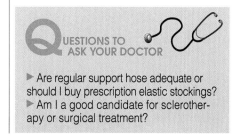

QUESTIONS TO ASK YOUR DOCTOR

▶ Are regular support hose adequate or should I buy prescription elastic stockings?
▶ Am I a good candidate for sclerotherapy or surgical treatment?

Vascular Bleeding

(Petechia; purpura)

Any condition in which blood leaks out of the vessels that normally contain it constitutes vascular bleeding. If the leaking blood invades skin tissue, it shows up as bruises, ranging from tiny reddish-brown or purple dots, called petechiae, to larger patches, referred to as purpura.

Of the various types of vascular bleeding, two of the most common are purpura simplex, a condition marked by easy bruising, and senile purpura, which occurs among older people. Easy bruising appears to run in families, and is often seen in women of childbearing age who develop discolored patches on their upper arms, thighs, and buttocks without sustaining any injury. In the past, these patches were sometimes referred to as devil's pinches and interpreted as a sign of witchcraft. They may develop during the night or immediately before a menstrual period. As a rule, they are not painful and vanish as unaccountably as they appeared.

Senile purpura takes the form of irregular, deep purple splotches that appear on the forearms and hands of older people. These patches usually disappear within a week or two, but sometimes they last for months or even years, often evolving into permanent brown areas on the skin.

Allergic purpura, also called anaphylactoid purpura, shows up as a skin rash that appears suddenly, most commonly on the arms, legs, buttock, and feet. Although it occasionally occurs in adults, more frequently it affects children, often following an infection such as strep throat. It might also be a reaction to a drug, during which the body's immune response causes an inflammation that weakens the vessel walls. The bleeding may be accompanied by fever, kidney damage, and joint pain and swelling, especially of the knees, hips, wrists, and elbows.

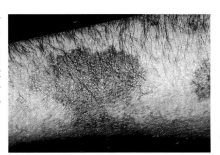

Some elderly people develop senile purpura, large purplish splotches that resemble bruises, on their arms and hands.

Another childhood bleeding disorder is called acute idiopathic thrombocytopenic purpura (ITP). It typically follows a viral infection that has reduced the number of platelets, which are blood cells instrumental in clotting. Chronic ITP, which occurs mostly in women aged 20 to 40, is an autoimmune disorder that causes accelerated destruction of platelets.

Most types of vascular bleeding are the result of a temporary change in blood composition (especially the condition or supply of platelets) or the deterioration of the tissue making up the blood vessel walls, causing them to rupture easily. This deterioration is presumed to be the underlying cause of

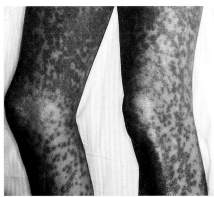

The rash of Rocky Mountain spotted fever can cause severe purpura, especially on the legs, soles, and palms.

senile purpura, which may also be triggered by excessive exposure to the sun.

Other possible causes of purpura include rare hereditary disorders of connective tissue and autoimmune diseases that reduce the level of platelets in the blood. Rocky Mountain spotted fever can also cause a type of purpura.

Diagnostic Studies and Procedures
Vascular bleeding can easily be detected by examining the skin, but finding the underlying cause generally requires blood studies to determine the platelet count and clotting function.

Medical Treatments
Easy bruising is not serious and no drug can prevent its occurrence. Individuals who are afflicted with this condition may be advised to avoid aspirin and other medications containing salicylates, although no

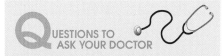

compelling evidence has shown that these drugs contribute to this type of bleeding. Similarly, there is no treatment for senile purpura.

If a particular drug appears to trigger allergic purpura, an alternative medication should be sought. When the kidneys are involved, steroids may be given, but caution is needed because these drugs themselves can also cause easy bruising.

ITP is usually treated with steroids and sometimes removal of the spleen. Researchers are hopeful that the hormone thrombopoietin, which speeds up the production and regrowth of blood platelets, may prove to be an effective treatment for ITP and other types of vascular bleeding.

Alternative Therapies
Naturopaths and nutrition therapists often advocate high doses of vitamin C for vascular bleeding. Although this vitamin is essential to maintain the walls of blood vessels, there is no evidence that vascular bleeding is a deficiency disease. A well-balanced diet that provides ample citrus fruits and other fresh fruits and vegetables should supply all the vitamin C that the body needs.

Self-Treatment
Aside from avoiding drugs or other substances that provoke allergic purpura, there is not much you can do to self-treat vascular bleeding. If you have thin skin and tend to bruise easily, minimize your time in the sun. Unsightly bruises that appear on the arms and legs can be covered with an opaque cosmetic.

Other Causes of Vascular Bleeding
Scurvy, a rare disease caused by severe vitamin C deficiency, can result in bruising and bleeding gums. Other possible causes of vascular bleeding include leukemia, hemophilia, and clotting disorders. Heavy alcohol consumption and frequent use of aspirin can also cause bleeding.

Viral Infections

Viruses, the smallest of all parasites, can live, grow, and reproduce only within the living cells of a host organism, which may be any plant or animal, including human beings. The world is populated by many billions of viruses; most are harmless, but others are the sources of our most persistent and even deadly diseases—everything from the common cold to AIDS.

In recent years, viral illnesses have gained new attention from researchers because viruses undergo genetic changes, or mutations, and new viral diseases keep cropping up. Researchers are especially concerned by the rapidly increasing global range and speed with which disease-bearing viruses can spread, due, at least in part, to wars, population density, human migration, deforestation, and air travel. Epidemiologists are attempting to establish an international warning system to spot newly evolving viral diseases quickly, so that they can be contained and treated when possible. These efforts were spurred by the 1995 outbreak in Zaire of the deadly Ebola virus, which causes widespread internal hemorrhaging.

There is mounting evidence that certain viruses may trigger a number of chronic diseases, including multiple sclerosis, Alzheimer's disease, and juvenile onset, or Type I, diabetes. Viruses are also implicated in some malignancies. Cervical cancer, for example, is associated with the papilloma virus, which causes genital warts. Hepatitis C increases the risk of liver cancer; HIV appears to cause AIDS-related lymphoma in some AIDS patients and the herpes virus is implicated in Kaposi's sarcoma, another AIDS-related cancer. New insight into the possible viral origins of such diseases may ultimately lead to new vaccines and treatments.

In humans, viral infections are spread mainly by blood and respiratory and intestinal secretions. They may also be

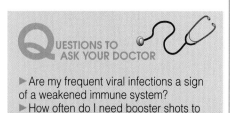

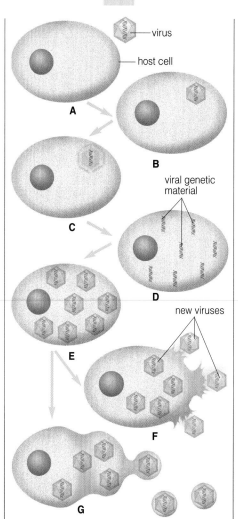

To reproduce, a virus must enter a host cell (B), where its own shell is shed (C), releasing its genetic material when it then replicates itself (D) to form new viruses (E). Some types of viruses destroy the host cell as they enter the body (F); others encapsule themselves in membranes of the host cell but leave without killing it (G).

sexually transmitted (as in genital herpes and HIV infection) or carried from one person to another by a biting insect. (Two examples: epidemics of dengue, or breakbone fever, have been traced to a mosquito originating in Hawaii; the Asian tiger mosquito, which entered the United States in 1986, is responsible for spreading the Eastern equine encephalitis virus.)

Although viral diseases differ greatly in severity and duration, they follow similar patterns of infection and replication. Once a virus invades the body, it enters its host's target cells. Some attach themselves to receptors on the cell's surface; others have proteins that allow them to penetrate the cell. Once inside, the virus sheds its coat or

undergoes other changes that allow it to insert its genetic material into that of the host cell and then reproduce many times. Eventually, the new viruses escape from the host cell and travel through the body seeking new target cells. Depending upon the virus, they may travel through the bloodstream, the lymph system, or along nerve pathways until reaching their target organ.

Much remains to be learned about viral infections and their consequences. With so-called slow viruses, such as HIV, for example, there are no symptoms until months or years after infection. Other viruses cause acute, but self-limiting illnesses; colds, flu, and measles are common examples. Still others, such as the varicella-zoster virus, which causes chickenpox and shingles, seem to disappear, but may reemerge months or years later in somewhat different manifestations.

Fortunately, the body has many defenses against viruses, beginning with the skin. Those that enter through the respiratory or gastrointestinal tract face attack from the body's immune defenses as well as chemical and structural barriers. As soon as a virus enters the body, the immune system begins to make antibodies against it. This response does not always halt infection, but it may result in immunity against future attacks. A bout of rubella or measles, for example, confers lifelong immunity against these diseases.

Diagnostic Studies and Procedures
Specific viral infections are usually diagnosed on the basis of the symptoms they produce. Epidemics of viral infections are tracked by state health authorities, laboratory reports, and the Centers for Disease Control and Prevention (CDC). Tissue and blood samples are examined for antibodies.

Medical Treatments
Many viral illnesses are short-lived and do not require treatment. Others, such as colds and flu, have no remedies, but there are medications that alleviate symptoms. Still others, such as AIDS, are incurable, but various treatments can slow the progress of the virus. Specific antiviral treatments include:
Immune globulins. These are substances derived from blood plasma taken from a large number of adults who have antibodies against the infecting virus. A few diseases that can be prevented by prompt administration of

INFECTIOUS VIRAL DISORDERS

Hundreds of different viruses can cause human disease. The following table lists some of the more common; not included are those commonly prevented by childhood immunization.

VIRUS	CAUSES	PREVENTION
Adenoviruses	Pneumonia, conjunctivities, diarrhea	Vaccine*
Coxsackie	Respiratory symptoms, meningitis, pericarditis, numerous other disorders	None
Cytomegalovirus	Pneumonia, congenital defects, other disorders	None
Echoviruses	Meningitis, paralysis, respiratory disease, other disorders	None
Epstein-Barr	Mononucleosis	None
Gastroenteritis virus	Nausea, vomiting	None
Hepatitis (A, B, C, and D)	Liver disease	Immune globulin (types A and B); vaccine (type B)
Herpes	Cold sores, genital herpes, conjunctivitis, encephalitis	None
Influenza	Respiratory symptoms	Vaccine; amantadine
Papillomavirus	Warts, possible genital cancer	None
Parvovirus	Rash, skin infections	None
Reoviruses	Respiratory symptoms	None
Rhinoviruses	Common cold	None

*Available only for military use.

immune globulins following exposure to a specific virus are hepatitis A and B, chickenpox, and rabies.

Antiviral drugs. Although not as effective as antibiotics in treating bacterial infections, antiviral drugs can halt or lessen a viral infection if they are given early enough. Acyclovir (Zovirax), the first effective antiviral drug, is prescribed mostly for herpes infections, especially genital herpes and herpes encephalitis. It is also used to treat shingles in patients who have lowered immunity. Ribavirin (Virazole) is given as an inhalant for severe viral respiratory infections. Amantadine (Symmetrel) or rimantadine (Flumadine) is given to prevent or reduce the severity of influenza A, and vidarabine (Vira-A) to treat viral eye infections. There are also several new drugs used against HIV (page 69) and its complications.

Interferon. This protective protein, which the body makes in response to a viral infection, is produced artificially by cloning techniques and is used to treat several diseases, including AIDS and other viral disorders.

Immunization. Effective virus vaccines include those for measles, mumps, rubella (German measles), influenza, hepatitis B, and rabies. A chickenpox vaccine is also now available.

Alternative Therapies
Some alternative therapies are directed toward boosting immunity and countering factors that increase susceptibility to viral infections. Others are used to alleviate symptoms.

Herbal Medicine. Garlic, taken fresh or in capsule form, is said to fight infections of all kinds. Herbs recommended to boost immunity include huang qu, available as a tincture or decoction, and purple coneflower (echinacea), taken as a powder or tincture.

Meditation and Visualization. Stress increases vulnerability to viral and other infections; meditation and other relaxation techniques can help offset its harmful effects on the immune system. Visualization, in which a person creates a mental image of the body fighting viruses, is also said to bolster immunity.

Nutrition Therapy. A healthy immune system requires a balanced diet that daily provides adequate protein, 5 to 9 servings of fresh fruits and vegetables, and 6 to 11 servings of starchy foods. Some nutritionists also recommend supplements of vitamins C and A and zinc to help prevent infection, but others feel these are unnecessary for people who consume a proper diet.

Self-Treatment
A healthful lifestyle—a balanced diet, adequate sleep, regular exercise, abstinence from smoking, safe sex practices, and prudent use of alcohol—is perhaps your best defense against viral illnesses. In addition, make sure you are immunized against the more common viral infections and that you have your scheduled booster shots. In planning a trip abroad, have any necessary immunizations before departure.

Remember that most viral infections are self-limiting and some of your symptoms represent your body's way of fighting off an invading virus. For example, viruses are sensitive to heat; thus, a fever is actually part of the healing process and is best left alone unless it rises to 104°F (40°C) in a child or 102°F (39°C) in an adult or lasts for more than two days. However, it's necessary to drink extra fluids to prevent dehydration from a fever.

During a mild illness, eat small meals of light, easy-to-digest foods—soups, gelatin, rice, toast. Switch to a liquid diet if diarrhea occurs. Try to stay in bed; extra sleep helps speed recovery.

Other Causes of Infections
Bacteria, fungi, and a variety of parasites can produce infections.

CHILDREN, ASPIRIN, AND REYE'S SYNDROME

Children under the age of 18 should never be given aspirin if they have the flu, a cold, chickenpox, or other viral illness. In this situation, aspirin increases the risk of developing Reye's syndrome, a rare, potentially fatal disorder that causes brain inflammation and swelling and severe liver damage. Typically, Reye's comes on during recovery from a viral illness, and initially can be mistaken for many other disorders. The child may be cranky, lethargic, or confused. As these symptoms worsen, protracted vomiting develops. The child may fall into a coma and, if untreated, could die.

What causes Reye's syndrome is unknown, but the incidence has dropped dramatically with the decreased use of aspirin during childhood. Although aspirin may be safe under most circumstances, doctors urge parents not to use it, unless directed to do so by their pediatrician to treat a specific illness such as juvenile rheumatoid arthritis. Otherwise, acetaminophen is the recommended aspirin substitute for children.

Vision Disorders

(Astigmatism; color blindness; near- and farsightedness; presbyopia)

Vision is a complex and delicate process that can be affected by injuries, aging, and various diseases. Vision problems are due mainly to errors of refraction—the way in which the lens of the eye focuses light on the retina at the rear of the eye. The most familiar are:

Astigmatism, in which the cornea, the transparent membrane at the front of the eye, is misshapen. Light rays fail to focus on a single point of the retina, resulting in distorted images.

Farsightedness, or hyperopia, in which light rays focus at a point just beyond the retina, blurring near objects.

Nearsightedness, or myopia, in which light rays focus just before the retina, making far objects difficult to see.

Presbyopia, a condition that develops with age, in which the lens loses some elasticity, resulting in farsightedness.

Color blindness, in which the cone cells of the retina are unable to distinguish the full spectrum of colors. Most color blindness is hereditary, affecting men 10 times more often than women. Other forms may develop with age or be secondary to diabetes, glaucoma, medications, or accidental poisoning.

Diagnostic Studies and Procedures

Most vision problems are readily diagnosed by an ophthalmologist or optometrist. These eye specialists test visual acuity with a Snellen test, a chart with rows of letters or numbers in different sizes. (Special picture charts are used to test young children.) Typically, the patient reads the chart, first using the naked eye and then with special lenses or instruments. Peripheral vision may be tested by a device that blinks lights on and off while the person looks into it. If a color vision problem is suspected, the patient will be shown patterns of colored dots and asked to identify objects traced in different colors. Eye drops may be given to dilate the pupils, in order to inspect the inside of the eye.

Medical Treatments

Vision problems involving refraction errors are usually treated successfully with corrective glasses or contact lenses that refocus the light rays on the retina. Because vision changes over time, a prescription for corrective lenses must also be changed periodically. With advancing age, more than one lens strength may be needed, which can be combined into bifocal glasses.

Color vision abnormalities are sometimes treated with colored contact lenses, but these reduce visual acuity, distort three-dimensional perception, and offer little help with light shades, generally the major problem area.

Nearsightedness can be corrected with radial keratotomy. This outpatient surgical technique, developed in Russia, involves making a series of tiny radial incisions in the cornea. Each eye is done separately, with several days between operations. An eye patch or dark glasses are worn for several days. The full effects may not be felt for several months.

In one long-term follow-up study, more than half of the patients reported fully corrected vision, and another one-fourth said their eyesight was improved. Anyone contemplating radial keratotomy should make sure that the surgeon has a high success rate.

Alternative Therapies

Exercises. In the Bates method, exercises are used to improve poor or weak eyesight. Ophthalmologists discount their value, but others contend that the exercises balance the optic muscles, nerve, and other eye structures.

Nutrition Therapy. High doses of vitamin A are reputed to improve faulty color vision, but this has not been proven. However, vitamin A is essential for night vision; good sources include yellow and dark green vegetables.

Self-Treatment

To test yourself for a possible refractive error, make a pinhole in a piece of paper and look through the hole at a well-lit object. If the object is clearer this way, you probably need corrective lenses. If not, your blurred vision may be due to another disorder. In either case, seek professional care.

Other Causes of Vision Disorders

Glaucoma, cataracts, and certain retinal disorders are some conditions that impair vision. Amblyopia, or lazy eye syndrome, is common in children and may occur with strabismus, or crossed eyes. Diabetes and untreated high blood pressure can also affect the eyes, as can many drugs.

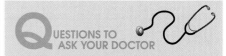

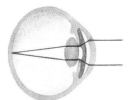

Normally, the lens focuses light at a precise point on the retina.

Normal

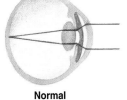

Nearsightedness

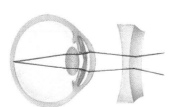

Nearsightedness is corrected with a concave lens to lengthen the focus.

Concave lens

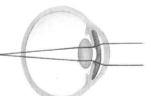

Farsightedness

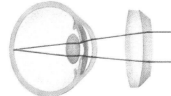

A convex lens shortens the focus, correcting the refraction problem of farsightedness.

Convex lens

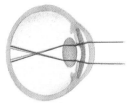

Astigmatism

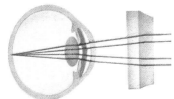

A cylindrical lens corrects astigmatism by bringing the light rays into a single focal point.

Cylindrical lens

Warts

(Papilloma; verrucae)

At least 50 different skin growths are classified as warts. All are caused by strains of the human papillomavirus (HPV), which infect the skin's epithelial cells, prompting them to multiply abnormally fast. The virus can be passed readily from person to person by direct contact.

The most prevalent are verrucae vulgaris, also called common warts. From time to time, almost everyone has one or more of these benign growths, which are easily identified by their appearance. They usually develop on the fingers, elbows, knees, or face. Other types of warts include:

Filiform warts, long, narrow growths on the face, neck, or eyelids.

Flat warts, usually multiple, which tend to develop on the face, back of the hands, neck, or chest. They are often spread by scratching or shaving.

Laryngeal papillomas, which develop on the larynx in infants following vaginal birth or in adults due to oral sex.

Pedunculated warts, which resemble a cauliflower and usually appear on the head or neck.

Periungual warts, which develop around the nails.

Plantar warts, which form on the soles of the feet, and mosaic warts, which are clusters of small plantar warts.

Venereal, or *moist, warts,* which develop in the genital area (page 201) and are sexually transmitted.

The majority of warts are benign, but there are exceptions. For example, genital warts and laryngeal papillomas may become cancerous, and in people with lowered immunity, malignancies may develop in preexisting warts.

Diagnostic Studies and Procedures

Most warts are diagnosed on the basis of appearance and location. Any that are potentially malignant are biopsied.

Medical Treatments

While common warts usually disappear on their own, it may take months or years. These warts are not dangerous, but treatment may be advisable if they are on the hands or other areas where they spread easily. A doctor can quickly remove them by freezing with liquid nitrogen, burning with an electric needle, or performing laser surgery. These methods, however, may result in scarring, and about one-third will recur.

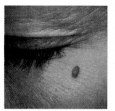

Filiform warts appear mostly on the neck and face, especially near the eyes and on the lids.

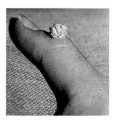

A pedunculated wart looks like a tiny cauliflower; the fingers and neck are favored sites.

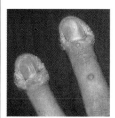

Periungual warts, which grow on the fingers, can distort the area around the nails.

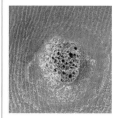

Plantar warts grow on the soles of the feet and can make walking very painful.

Chemical treatment may be preferable. One approach calls for applying a potent acid, cantharidin (Cantharone), two or three times, then covering the area for seven hours with tape. The wart should come off when the tape is removed; if not, the treatment can be repeated in one or two weeks.

Flat warts are sometimes treated with daily applications of tretinoin (Retin-A), which promotes skin peeling. In stubborn cases, other peeling agents, such as benzoyl peroxide or salicylic acid, are added to the regimen.

Plantar warts are notoriously difficult to get rid of. One treatment calls for wearing tape containing 40-percent salicylic acid for several days; when the wart is soft enough, a doctor can usually pare it away. Several treatments may be needed, however, and these warts also have a tendency to recur. Another approach entails injecting the wart with bleomycin, an anticancer drug. The wart may also be removed surgically.

Alternative Therapies

Folk and home remedies abound. Some work, but none are foolproof.

Herbal Medicine. Daily applications of aloe vera plant juice are said to make a wart disappear in a few weeks. Rubbing the wart with a clove of garlic is another popular herbal remedy.

Naturopathy. Naturopaths advocate placing some mashed fresh fig on the wart for half an hour daily, for two or three weeks. If this doesn't work, other suggested remedies are: Make a paste of grated carrots and olive oil and apply it to the wart for half an hour twice a day. Or dab lemon juice on the wart and cover it with raw chopped onion for half an hour. Do this daily for two or three weeks. Rubbing the contents of a capsule of vitamin E on the wart daily has worked for some people.

Self-Hypnosis and Visualization. These techniques have been credited with removing warts, but proof is lacking.

Self-Treatment

Various nonprescription wart-removal products are available at pharmacies. One is salicylic acid, available in a gel, liquid, or medicated plaster. To remove a common wart with it, soak the wart in warm water for 5 to 10 minutes, dry, apply the acid, and cover with tape for 8 to 10 hours. Remove the tape and gently rub or scrape the wart. Repeat the process until the wart disappears.

If you try to remove a plantar wart yourself, use extra care not to damage surrounding tissue. First soak the affected foot for 10 minutes in ½ gallon of warm water to which 2 tablespoons of a mild dishwashing or laundry detergent have been added. Then apply a 40-percent salicylic acid plaster directly over the wart and cover it with tape or a bandage for 48 hours. While the wart is still soft, scrub it vigorously with a toothbrush to peel away the upper layers. Repeat until the wart is gone, which typically takes two weeks. If your feet sweat heavily, wear absorbent cotton socks.

Other Causes of Skin Growths

Moles sometimes resemble warts. Skin cancers may also be mistaken for warts.

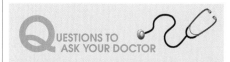

Q UESTIONS TO ASK YOUR DOCTOR

▶ What precautions can I take to prevent my child from spreading warts on his hands to other parts of his body?
▶ How long might it take for Retin-A to get rid of flat facial warts?

Whooping Cough

(Pertussis)

Whooping cough, or pertussis, is a contagious childhood disease that is now rare in industrialized countries, thanks to immunization during infancy. The causative bacterium, *Bordetella pertussis*, is far from extinct, however; outbreaks still occur among unimmunized children. Half of all cases occur before age two, and children under 12 months are the most severely affected, with a mortality rate of 1 to 2 percent.

About 7 to 14 days after exposure to the bacterium, the child develops what appears to be a lingering cold with a

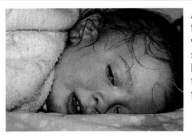

A young child may find it easier to cough while lying on her stomach with the head lowered and turned to one side to drain the lungs.

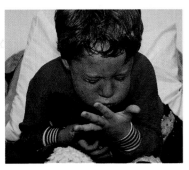

An older child can clear sputum from the lungs by coughing while sitting up and leaning forward.

cough. This catarrhal stage lasts for 7 to 10 days. Next follows the paroxysmal stage, marked by increasing production of sputum and frequent spells of violent coughing that end with a high-pitched whooping sound while the child gasps for breath. Large amounts of thick mucus are brought up, and vomiting often follows a coughing attack. This stage lasts for two to four weeks, with the cough gradually diminishing as the child enters convalescence. Full recovery takes another three or four weeks. In some cases, however, the illness takes up to three months to run its course. Paroxysms of coughing may, in fact, recur for months, especially if the child catches a cold.

Whooping cough carries a risk of serious complications, including ear infections, pneumonia, and convulsions.

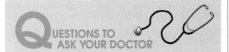

QUESTIONS TO ASK YOUR DOCTOR

▶ What preventive measures should I take for other household members?
▶ How should a baby who has not yet completed his DPT immunization schedule be protected?

Diagnostic Studies and Procedures

Early on, whooping cough is difficult to distinguish from other respiratory infections, but a laboratory culture can detect the causative bacterium. Fluorescent antibody testing of the sputum samples may also be performed to look for antibodies against *B. pertussis*.

Medical Treatments

Babies under six months old will usually be hospitalized; so, too, will older children who have severe symptoms. Choking is a major danger; infants may need suction to remove excess mucus, and some will require artificial respiration as well. Young babies may also require intravenous fluids and nutritional support. Otherwise, at the very least, bed rest is necessary, except for older children with mild cases.

Antibiotics prescribed during the catarrhal stage may help shorten the course of the disease and lower the potential for passing it to others, but these drugs are of little or no benefit in the paroxysmal stage. Complications such as pneumonia and ear infections are also treated with antibiotics.

Alternative Therapies

These can help during the convulsive stage, when coughing diminishes.

Herbal Medicine. Thyme tea and baths are recommended for treating whooping cough. To prepare a thyme bath, add 5 or 6 tablespoons of dry thyme to a quart of boiling water. Let it stand for about 20 minutes, and then add it to the bathwater. Some herbalists prescribe a tea made from a combination of coltsfoot, mullein, and licorice, to be drunk three times a day.

Self-Treatment

If the child is cared for at home, he will require close observation, especially during the paroxysmal stage. Keep him in bed in a quiet, darkened room; activity tends to provoke coughing.

Give plenty of fluids to help thin mucus and then offer warm broth and steamy chicken soup to loosen it. Do not give over-the-counter remedies without checking with a doctor. Use a cool-mist humidifier to help loosen sputum, and prepare small, frequent meals to help decrease vomiting.

During a coughing bout, have a baby or young child lie on her stomach with the head lowered and turned to one side to help drain the lungs. It is crucial to keep a close watch and remove expelled secretions and vomit. Older children usually do better if they sit up and lean forward during paroxysmal coughing.

Talk to your doctor about immunization of family members or children exposed to whooping cough. Prophylactic erythromycin is recommended for household members and other close contacts, such as day-care workers. Immunization or booster shots may be given to children, including those who have been immunized earlier.

Other Causes of Coughing

Many upper respiratory infections, including colds and flu, begin with symptoms similar to those of whooping cough. Bronchitis produces thick mucus but without paroxysmal coughing. Croup causes a barking, dry cough.

IMMUNIZATION

Immunization against whooping cough is included in the DPT (diphtheria, pertussis, and tetanus) shots administered routinely at 2, 4, and 6 months, again at some point between 15 and 18 months, and finally, before a child enters kindergarten or elementary school, or between 4 and 6 years of age.

The pertussis vaccine is generally safe, but some babies do suffer adverse reactions that may preclude further pertussis immunization with the current vaccine. These include seizures, allergic reactions, altered consciousness, a high fever (104°F, or 40.5°C), and inconsolable crying for more than three hours. Call your doctor immediately if your baby suffers any of these reactions. A new pertussis vaccine is being tested that appears to eliminate these problems.

Worms

(Hookworms; pinworms; roundworms; tapeworms; threadworms)

Infestation with parasitic worms is a common occurrence worldwide, but climate and other factors determine which are the most prevalent in any region. Most worms that infect humans reside in the intestinal tract, spreading through poor sanitation or food or water contaminated with worm eggs.

In the United States, pinworms are the most common, afflicting an estimated 5 to 15 percent of the population (mostly children) at any given time. These parasites, which look like tiny straight pins, mature in the human intestinal tract. While the host sleeps, the female worm emerges from the anus to lay thousands of eggs, causing skin irritation and severe anal itching. Scratching transfers some of the eggs to the hands and fingernails; if they are carried to the mouth and swallowed, the cycle of infestation begins again. The eggs can also be picked up from toilet seats, bedding, clothing, and other objects; some become airborne and can be inhaled and swallowed.

Hookworms infect about 25 percent of the world's population, but they are relatively uncommon in the United States, occurring mostly in the rural South. The eggs are discharged in the stool and hatch a day or two later in the soil. The larvae then enter the human body through the skin, usually on the soles of children or others who go barefoot. They migrate to the lungs, are coughed up, and swallowed. They then take up residence in the small intestine, where they attach themselves to its wall and feed on the person's blood. Left untreated, a large infestation of hookworms can cause iron-deficiency anemia and abdominal pain.

Threadworms, which have a life cycle similar to that of hookworms, can cause coughing, shortness of breath, and even pneumonia when lodged in the lungs. In the small intestine, they

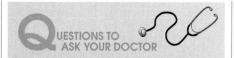

QUESTIONS TO ASK YOUR DOCTOR

▶ Are there any adverse effects from antiworm medications?
▶ How can we tell if one dose of medicine has eradicated all the worms?

can produce abdominal pain, severe diarrhea, and other GI symptoms.

Roundworms enter the body as eggs carried in contaminated water, food, or soil-contaminated hands. The adults resemble earthworms, and are sometimes found in the stool or vomit.

Tapeworms are rare in the United States but common in the developing countries of Africa, the Middle East, Asia, and Eastern Europe. Humans become infected by eating undercooked pork, beef, or fish that contain cysts of larvae. When these cysts reach the intestinal tract, the worms develop into their adult stage and may grow up to 30 feet in length. The body is made up of hundreds of segments called proglottids, which contain eggs. These break off and are passed in the stool, beginning a new life cycle. Many tapeworm infections are asymptomatic; others may cause anemia, diarrhea, and pain.

Diagnostic Studies and Procedures

The diagnostic procedure varies according to the type of worm. Pinworms can sometimes be seen by inspecting the anal area a few hours after a child has gone to bed. Otherwise, the eggs can be detected by patting the anal skin with a piece of transparent tape, sticky side down, and then examining the tape under a microscope. This should be done when the child first awakens in the morning. In other infestations, a doctor may order a stool analysis to look for eggs or worm parts. Repeated tests may be needed, as eggs may be discharged only sporadically.

Blood tests may be ordered to check for possible iron-deficiency anemia, especially if hookworms are found.

Medical Treatments

Worms are treated primarily with medications called antihelminthics, with specific drugs used depending on the type of worm. Pinworms, hookworms, and roundworms are usually eradicated with pyrantel pamoate (Antiminth) or mebendazole (Vermox). A single dose is usually effective, but a follow-up dose may be needed to eliminate all eggs and larvae. If one child in a family has pinworms, any siblings between ages 2 and 10 should also be treated. In some instances, adult family members may also be advised to take the medication.

Tapeworms are generally eliminated with niclosamide (Niclocide) or praziquantel (Biltricide).

Alternative Therapies

A number of folk remedies are said to eliminate worms, and some may actually work. However, antihelminthic drugs are the fastest and surest treatment; any alternative approaches should be considered adjuncts to a doctor's prescribed treatment.

Herbal Medicine. Garlic, taken fresh or in capsule form, is believed to help eliminate worms.

Nutrition Therapy. Worms can cause anemia and other nutritional deficiencies; maintaining a well-balanced diet is important. If you are anemic, iron supplements may be recommended, but you should consult a doctor before taking iron pills.

Self-Treatment

Self-care is focused on preventing reinfestation. To avoid resurgence of pinworms, clean the entire house on the same day that medication is taken. Wash towels, bed linens, pajamas, and underclothes in hot water, using a strong detergent and bleach. Clean the bathroom with a disinfectant and sterilize objects that might go into a child's mouth by washing them also with disinfectant, then rinsing thoroughly.

Trim children's fingernails and make sure that they wash their hands after going to the toilet and before eating.

To avoid hookworms or threadworms, do not go barefoot outdoors and use proper sanitary measures. To prevent tapeworm infestations, cook beef, pork, and fish until they are well-done.

Other Causes of Worm Symptoms

Hemorrhoids or an anal fissure can cause anal itching. Intestinal disorders, such as appendicitis, colitis, and irritable bowel syndrome can produce abdominal discomfort, and diarrhea.

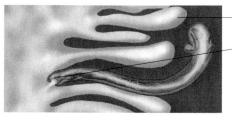

intestine

hookworm head

Hookworms attach themselves to the villa lining the small intestine where they feed on the host's blood.

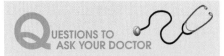
Wryneck/ Torticollis

(Focal dystonia; spasmodic torticollis)
Wryneck and torticollis are character-ized by painful spasms in the neck. A wryneck usually occurs suddenly and is self-limited, often vanishing mys-teriously. In contrast, torticollis comes on gradually; at first it is intermittent, but it keeps worsening until affected muscles are chronically contracted and the neck posture remains abnormal more or less permanently. Wryneck and torticollis are relatively common, affect-ing about 1 in 10,000 people, with women slightly outnumbering men.

What causes the muscle spasms is often unclear. In some acute cases, entrapment of a nerve arising from the upper (cervical) spinal cord is respon-sible. Infection, inflammation, disloca-tion of a joint in the neck, a thyroid disorder, and a tumor are other possi-ble causes. Heredity is also a possible factor. In congenital torticollis, a baby is born with an injured or malformed neck muscle. Many patients have other involuntary muscle tics and spasms, or spasmodic dystonia, as well.

Doctors are frequently unable to identify any single reason for wryneck or torticollis. In the past, cases were often attributed to hysteria and treated as a mental disorder. Physicians now agree that although torticollis can lead to emotional problems, those problems are rarely, if ever, the underlying cause of the affliction.

Diagnostic Studies and Procedures
Newborns should be carefully exam-ined for signs of muscular asymmetry affecting the neck. Adults will be ques-tioned about past nerve and muscle disorders, and recent accidents involv-ing the head and neck. Tests will include a neurological examination, X-rays, CT scans, or MRI, and possibly electromyography, which are studies of the muscles' electrical impulses.

Medical Treatments
Most patients benefit from a combina-tion of medical and alternative thera-pies. Regardless of treatment, 10 to 20 percent recover spontaneously within five years. The outlook, however, is best for patients whose problem stems from an identifiable orthopedic disorder.
Drug Therapy. Prescribed drugs usu-ally include such painkillers as aspirin

or stronger nonsteroidal anti-inflamma-tory agents; anticholinergic drugs such as trihexyphenidyl (Artane) to block cer-tain nerve impulses; and muscle relax-ants, such as diazepam (Valium). In some cases, haloperidol (Haldol) or per-phenazine (Etrafon or Triavil) are pre-scribed, but side effects such as lethargy and movement disorders limit their use.

Studies indicate that injections of botulinum toxin type A (BOTOX) into neck muscles reduce painful spasms and normalize head positions for up to three months in most patients. How-ever, this treatment has not yet been approved by the FDA for neck problems.
Surgery. When other approaches have been unsuccessful, neurosurgery to sever some of the nerves that control the neck muscles may help.

Alternative Therapies
A combination of physical therapy and massage sometimes provides temporary relief, and if started in the first year of life, can cure congenital torticollis. The daily regimen includes stretching the shortened neck muscle that holds the head at an abnormal angle. Other alternative therapies include:
Acupuncture and Acupressure. Six sessions with a qualified acupuncturist may provide relief and halt the muscle spasms. Applying pressure to the jaw may give temporary relief.
Biofeedback Training. This technique, which helps a patient control and relax neck muscles, is now a standard treatment.
Chiropractic. Many chiroprac-tors specialize in the treatment of neck pain, including wry-neck, using manipulation and electrical stimulation.
Hydrotherapy. Whirlpool baths, alternating hot and cold needle show-ers, and underwater massage are used by some physical therapists to alleviate muscle spasms and neck pain.
Massage Therapies. Traditional mas-sage, perhaps combined with physical

therapy, can be helpful. Others find the more vigorous massage of rolfing or shiatsu beneficial.
Meditation. People who have tension-induced wryneck might benefit from meditation and breathing exercises.

Self-Treatment
Application of heat can sometimes ease simple wryneck. A battery-operated vibrating neck massager that can be worn like a scarf while you read, work at a desk, or do chores may also help.

If you work at a computer or use the telephone often, take frequent breaks. Change positions, shrug your shoul-ders, and gently move your head from side to side. Don't cradle the phone between shoulder and neck; instead, try a speakerphone or headphone. Maintain good posture, keep your shoulders down, and avoid sudden head movements.

Try to sleep on your back, using a rolled neck pillow. If you suffer chronic neck pain, use a special pillow that pro-vides hot and cold therapy. Sold at med-ical supply stores, these have a gel pack that can be cooled in the freezer or heated in the microwave and then inserted into a sleeve that fits under the neck. On a long car or plane trip, rest your head on a traveler's neck pillow.

If a spasm develops, rub it with an ice cube wrapped in a plastic bag using a circular motion. If this doesn't help, take a hot shower. A pulsating shower mas-sage on the tensed muscle may relax it.

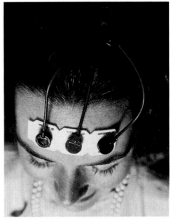

Some types of wryneck can be alleviated through biofeedback training, in which a person uses special sensors to learn how to control certain nerve impulses.

Other Causes of Neck Spasms
Whiplash and other neck injuries can cause muscle spasms and pain. In some cases, tardive dyskinesia, a move-ment disorder caused by potent antipsychotic drugs, affects the neck.

Yellow Fever

Yellow fever is an acute viral infection transmitted by the *Aedes aegypti* mosquito. These insects become yellow fever carriers, or vectors, by feeding on a person who has the virus.

Yellow fever, which gained notoriety when it felled thousands of workers during the building of the Panama Canal, is now rare in the United States, but there are still widespread epidemics every few years in Africa and in Central and South America. Fortunately, a better understanding of the spread and treatment of yellow fever has greatly reduced its mortality rate.

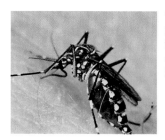

Yellow fever is spread by the *Aedes aegypti* mosquito.

Fever and jaundice are two hallmarks of the disease. The fever, which ranges from 102° to 104°F (39° to 40°C), comes on suddenly three to six days after a person is bitten by an infected mosquito. In this first stage, other symptoms include constipation, headache, a flushed face, nausea, vomiting, muscle aches, and a slow heartbeat. Bleeding from the gums and nose also may occur. The patient is likely to be restless and irritable. These symptoms last for two or three days, and in mild cases, the patient recovers without further symptoms and may not even be aware that he had yellow fever.

In moderate to severe episodes however, the symptoms subside only temporarily. After a period that lasts from several hours to a few days, the fever and other symptoms return, this time accompanied by jaundice, a yellowing of the skin and eyes that give the disease its name. The jaundice indicates liver damage, one of the more serious manifestations of yellow fever. The tongue turns a bright red at the edges and tip, and bleeding from the nose, mouth, and intestinal tract develops.

In the most severe incidences of yellow fever, the patient vomits black blood and becomes confused and lethargic. In life-threatening cases of the disease, this stage is usually followed by delirium and then coma.

Yellow fever that is severe enough to be diagnosed has a 10 to 20 percent mortality rate. However, because many mild cases are attributed to flu or other illnesses, the overall mortality rate is probably much smaller.

Diagnostic Studies and Procedures

The disease is suspected when typical symptoms develop in someone who has traveled recently to an area where yellow fever is endemic. Urine studies usually find a high level of protein; blood tests show clotting abnormalities and reduced liver function.

Medical Treatments

Because yellow fever is a viral disease, no specific drug or treatment can cure it. Instead, treatment focuses on relieving the symptoms, with an emphasis on total bed rest and nursing care. Because hemorrhaging is often a factor in severe cases, intravenous medications to reduce the risk of bleeding may be administered. If hemorrhaging does occur, blood transfusions may be needed. In other instances, widespread clotting is a potentially fatal complication. Therefore, this possibility must be treated early with preventive drugs.

Alternative Therapies

As with medical treatments, these are directed to lowering the fever and alleviating other symptoms.

Herbal Medicine. Ginger or chamomile tea may relieve nausea and vomiting. A tea brewed with hyssop, licorice root, thyme, and yarrow is reputed to help lower a high fever.

Homeopathy. Homeopaths use many different remedies to treat fevers. Belladonna is sometimes suggested for a fever of rapid onset, and sulphur for fever that returns after partial recovery. Belladonna is also prescribed for headaches that come on suddenly. Muscle aches and prostration may be treated with arnica.

Nutrition Therapy. A high-fiber diet and extra fluids can help overcome the constipation. Fresh fruits, dried prunes, brown rice, raw green leafy vegetables, and bran all add fiber to the diet. Two to three tablespoons of rapeseed oil taken once a day will help soften stools. Vitamin K supplements can promote proper clotting to help deal with bleeding gums, but these should be taken only under a doctor's supervision.

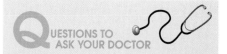

Self-Treatment

The best self-treatment for yellow fever is prevention. Vaccination confers immunity for up to 10 years. Anyone planning to travel in central Africa or certain areas of South and Central America where the disease is endemic should be immunized against yellow fever. Consult your doctor, local health department, or the Centers for Disease Control and Prevention (CDC) in Atlanta for immunization information.

Mosquito control is also an important aspect of prevention. If you are visiting or working in an area where yellow fever is prevalent, make certain that your accommodations are screened, and sleep under a mosquito net. Use insect repellent and wear long-sleeved shirts and pants when outdoors. Also, eliminate any standing pools of water that might attract mosquitoes and other undesirable insects.

Anyone who has yellow fever should be isolated in a well-screened room to protect against further mosquito bites. A bout of yellow fever will confer lifelong immunity.

Mild yellow fever is self-limiting and may be treated at home. Even so, a doctor should be consulted when the symptoms first appear; any worsening or recurrence of the symptoms may necessitate hospitalization.

Complete bed rest is essential. Tepid sponge baths can help lower a fever. In order to alleviate nausea, try sucking on cracked ice.

Other Causes of Yellow Fever Symptoms

Fever is associated with many other disorders, ranging from flu to malaria. Likewise, headaches, muscle pain, and other symptoms of yellow fever can have numerous other causes. It is the specific combination of symptoms, plus their rapid onset and the brief period of remission, that is characteristic of the yellow fever virus.

Drugs and Medications

The Proper Use of Medications

At the turn of the century, the typical pharmacy offered only a handful of patent medicines and preparations mixed by the pharmacist. Few were truly effective and many were addictive or dangerous. In contrast, today's pharmacies stock thousands of different prescription and over-the-counter (OTC) medications. Many also offer homeopathic, herbal, and other natural preparations. Faced with such an array of choices, it's understandable that the average patient is often confused as to when and how drugs should be used, often with serious consequences; more than 50,000 Americans are hospitalized each year with medication-induced illness.

Thus, it is essential for anyone taking a medication to be as knowledgeable as possible about how it should be used. This includes not only reading any written material provided by a doctor and pharmacist, but also being aware of the drug's proper dosage, possible side effects, adverse reactions, and interactions with other drugs.

How Drugs Work

Drugs work in many ways; in some cases, even medical scientists do not fully understand the precise mechanism of action. For example, lithium is highly effective in treating the manic phase of manic-depression, but how and why this medication affects the brain is unknown. For the most part, however, most drugs work in one of three ways:

▶ By *replacing or augmenting natural body chemicals*. The body is a complex biological structure made up of thousands of different chemicals and compounds; many diseases are a consequence of chemical deficiencies or imbalances. Diabetes, for example, results from a deficiency of insulin; an imbalance of brain chemicals can cause a variety of disorders, ranging from seizures to depression and Parkinson's disease. Drugs used to treat such diseases are designed to restore normal body chemistry.

▶ By *attacking harmful organisms or abnormal cells*. Numerous diseases are caused by the invasion of infectious organisms or the development of abnormal cells within the body. Drugs in this category work by destroying the source of such diseases, either by killing it directly or by preventing it from multiplying. Antibiotics and cancer chemotherapy are the most familiar examples of such medications.

▶ By *interfering with cell function*. Cells function as a system, directed by various chemical and electrical signals, or neurotransmitters. Millions of such messages are constantly being sent out from one part of the body to another; when some of these messages go awry, cells cease to function normally. Depending upon what organ is affected, drugs may be given to either speed up or slow down the cellular activity. For example, lupus and other autoimmune diseases are generally treated with drugs that reduce actions of the immune system. Ulcers and other digestive disorders are treated with drugs that slow down the production of digestive juices.

Adverse Side Effects

All medications can cause unwanted effects because it is impossible to design a drug that acts only on its target organ or cells. Unwanted responses vary from person to person and from one drug to another; some may cause nausea and constipation, others may produce drowsiness or insomnia, and still others may provoke rashes and other allergic responses. Some

DRUG ALLERGIES

Caution is critical in dealing with drug allergies. The first use of a medication cannot produce an allergic reaction, but it may prompt the body to create antibodies against the drug. If so, any future exposure to it could result in an allergic reaction.

Symptoms during the first reaction are likely to be mild, and may include fever, nausea, headache, a rash, or localized hives. Future responses may be more severe, producing widespread or intense itchiness, flushed skin, vomiting, muscle weakness, bleeding, impaired vision and hearing, and extensive swelling, which can interfere with breathing. These are the signs of possible anaphylaxis, a life-threatening medical emergency (see Allergies, page 71, for more details). You should report any allergic drug reaction to your doctor immediately, and avoid that drug, as well as any chemically related agents, in the future.

side effects appear immediately; others show up years later. In many instances, adverse effects lessen with time or can be eliminated by altering the dosage or trying an alternate drug.

Before taking a medication, ask the prescribing doctor and the pharmacist to list the most common side effects, also the more dangerous ones, and what to do if they should occur. Prior to using it, inform your doctor and pharmacist if you have ever had either an allergic or severe reaction to a particular drug, food, or any other substance, such as food dyes or sulfites. In addition, be sure to make a note of all reactions you have when you begin taking a new medication and relate them to your physician when you have a follow-up visit.

Some people face an increased risk of adverse side effects because they fall into one of the following groups:

Children. In regard to taking medications, anyone under the age of 12 should be considered a child. Usually, infants and children are given lower dosages of drugs than adults to compensate for their smaller size and lower body weight. Also, some medications that are safe for adults may be hazardous for a child. For example, aspirin given to a child who has a viral infection increases the risk of Reye's syndrome (page 437), a potentially fatal disease. Liquid cough medicines and other over-the-counter drugs may contain alcohol; read ingredient labels and look for nonalcoholic versions. Some OTC medications are specifically designed for children; others may have alternative instructions for children on the package. In most cases, a doctor or pharmacist should be consulted before giving a baby or young child any medication.

The elderly. As people age, the liver becomes less efficient at breaking down drugs, and the kidneys may take longer to excrete toxic remnants. As a result, even a regular dosage may produce severe side effects. This risk is compounded by the fact that many elderly people take different drugs simultaneously. Problems usually can be prevented by prescribing a reduced dosage and paying attention to potential drug interactions.

Pregnant and breast-feeding women. Almost any medication taken by a pregnant woman travels through her bloodstream and into that of the fetus. Some drugs are known to cause birth defects; others retard growth and some cause fetal death. Therefore, any over-the-counter or prescription drug should be taken during pregnancy only after consulting a doctor. Similarly, most drugs taken by a nursing mother can pass into her breast milk and may harm her infant. Consult a doctor beforehand about the safety of a medication.

FORMS OF MEDICATION

This table summarizes the different forms in which drugs are administered in order of the most to least frequently used types:

FORM — HOW IT'S TAKEN	VARIATIONS
Tablets Orally, usually with fluid	Sustained release or slow acting. Enteric-coated to prevent absorption in the stomach.
Capsules Orally, usually with fluid	Controlled-release.
Liquids Orally, or in some cases, as drops	Elixir, a solution of the drug, usually dissolved in alcohol and flavored with sugar. Emulsion, in which the drug is dispersed in oil and water. Syrup, in which the drug is dissolved in sugar and water. Mixture, one or more drugs suspended in a liquid (usually water) Drops, sterile solutions or suspensions, administered in the eyes, the ears, or the nose using a dropper.
Topical Skin Preparations Applied to the skin to treat local infections	Cream. Ointment. Lotion.
Injections Liquid solution is inserted into the body using a sterilized syringe	Intramuscular (IM), in which the drug is injected into a muscle. Intravenous (IV), in which the drug is placed directly into the bloodstream by being injected into a vein. Thus, IV drugs act more quickly in the body than other drugs. Subcutaneous (SQ), in which the drug is injected directly under the skin's surface.
Powders Usually orally, after being dissolved in either food or mixed in liquid	None.
Transdermal Patch Medicated patch, time-released, applied to skin	None.
Inhalants Inhaled into the lungs or nasal passages	Aerosol, a suspension or solution of a drug in air under pressure. Used for respiratory conditions such as asthma, aerosols are available in fixed doses, in which each squirt holds a measured dose of the drug, and non-fixed doses, in which the amount of the drug per squirt varies.
Suppositories Insertion of solid bullet-shaped tablet, either in the rectum or vagina, which melts at body temperature	Rectal. Vaginal.
Implants Inserted under the skin, releases the drug incrementally into the body over an extended period of time	Time-released capsules. Devices that dissolve in time. Devices that must be removed.

Drug Interactions

Many drugs interact with each other to produce effects not seen with the individual medications. This problem has been growing because more patients are taking multiple drugs, often to treat different problems—for example, a medication for blood pressure, an anti-inflammatory for arthritis, vitamin and mineral supplements, and perhaps an OTC allergy or cold preparation. Not only can each individual medication produce side effects, but any particular combination can also interact to create additional adverse reactions. In some cases, a combination may enhance the effects of one or all of the drugs being used; in others, the medications may cancel each other out, rendering them all ineffective.

Similarly, interactions may occur when drugs are combined with alcohol or certain of types of food. Taking aspirin with orange juice or other acidic foods, for instance, increases stomach irritation; taking certain antibiotics with food reduces or delays the drug's impact; the combination of alcohol with sleeping pills, tranquilizers, or even some cold pills can be deadly.

To minimize the risk of a dangerous drug interaction, always inform both your doctor and pharmacist of all other medications, including nonprescription drugs and vitamin and mineral supplements you are taking, as well as any herbal preparations, some of which have strong pharmacologic effects. Also, be sure to ask about any restrictions on alcohol or diet.

Taking Medication

Read all instructions before taking a medication and follow them precisely. When in doubt, ask your doctor or pharmacist to clarify any uncertainties. If, for example, the directions say "take three times a day," find out if this means morning, noon, and evening, or every eight hours. Also ask whether the drug should be taken with food or on an empty stomach.

Follow the doctor's instructions with regard to how long the drug should be taken. Certain medications, particularly over-the-counter remedies used to treat pain and other symptoms, are used only as needed. For instance, a person might

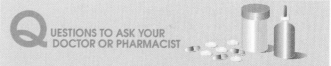

QUESTIONS TO ASK YOUR DOCTOR OR PHARMACIST

Use this list of questions as a checklist before starting any medication.

▶ What is the name of the drug? (Be sure to ask about both the brand name(s) and the generic name and write them down so you can be certain to remember them.)

▶ What exactly is the drug supposed to do?

▶ How long will it take for the effects of the drug to become apparent?

▶ Should the drug be taken with food or on an empty stomach? Are there any foods I should avoid while taking the drug? Or any foods I should add to my diet?

▶ What are the drug's most common side effects? Which are the most serious? What should be done if they appear?

▶ How much medication should I take? How often? For how long?

▶ Should I abstain from alcohol while taking this drug?

▶ Is there an expiration date on the medication's label? How should I store the drug? Should I discard any that is left over? If so, how should this be done?

▶ What should I do if I miss a scheduled dose?

▶ Are there any activities to avoid while using this medication?

▶ How much does the drug cost? Is there an equivalent generic form that is less expensive?

▶ Is the drug available in other, perhaps more convenient, forms?

▶ What written information is available on this drug and where can it be found?

▶ Are there any alternatives to drug therapy for the ailment, such as exercise, nutrition therapy, or alternative treatments?

WHAT TO DO IN CASE OF AN OVERDOSE

Many people mistakenly assume that a drug overdose implies drug abuse or attempted suicide. While this may apply sometimes, the fact is that most overdoses are unintentional. A patient may exceed the recommended dosage when he forgets he has already taken his medication—an especially common problem among the elderly. Or circumstances may increase a drug's effect. In most situations, one extra dose of a drug is not harmful, but in other cases, the consequences can be disastrous. The overdose threshold varies from drug to drug, so it is important to follow all dosage instructions carefully.

If you suspect that someone has overdosed, try to determine exactly how much was ingested. Review any package instructions on what to do in case of overdose. Symptoms vary from one drug to another; some resolve themselves, but medical treatment is often necessary, especially for drugs that affect the brain and nervous system. The first step is to call right away the doctor who prescribed the medication and follow her instructions. If the doctor cannot be reached, call the local poison control center and emergency medical services.

take aspirin, acetaminophen, or ibuprofen when a headache develops, and stop when the pain subsides. In contrast, some drugs, such as antihypertensives and insulin, are taken for a lifetime. In other cases, medications must be taken for the full duration of time instructed by a doctor or pharmacist for it to be effective. Many patients who have been prescribed an antibiotic regimen for 7 to 10 days stop taking the drugs as soon as their symptoms disappear, assuming they have been cured. However, while symptoms may have abated, some of the infecting organism may still be present, and can cause a recurrence of the infection. This time, the situation may be more serious, because the surviving organisms may have developed resistance to the first antibiotic, necessitating a switch to a different, more potent drug.

If you need a particular medication in the event of a medical emergency—such as insulin for diabetes or nitroglycerin for an attack of angina—carrying the drug on your person at all times is an important precautionary measure. Similarly, always carry this medical information on your person, written either on a card in your wallet or on a special MedicAlert bracelet. This will insure that any individuals assisting you in a medical emergency can aid you effectively and safely. Any drug allergies also should be noted.

Medication Labels

All medications—both OTC and prescription—should bear a label and additional written information regarding proper use and administration. Every prescription drug should come in a container with a label that includes all of the following information:

► Patient's name
► Pharmacy name, address, and phone number
► Physician's name
► Drug name and dosage
► Instructions for usage (when and how often to take the drug)
► Any special instructions for preparation or storage
► Date the prescription was filled
► Whether or not the prescription can be refilled

Check to make sure that the label information is written clearly and remember to question the pharmacist about how you should take the drug (see box on previous page). If you

have any questions after you get home, don't hesitate to call your doctor or pharmacist. It is in everyone's best interest to see that you take a medication properly.

Choosing Between Generic and Brand-Name Drugs

Check with your doctor and pharmacist to find out if a generic version of a particular medication is available and appropriate for your needs. Typically, generic forms are less expensive than their brand-name counterparts. In many cases, the only difference will be the price, and the generic drug will have the same effect as its brand-name version. In a few instances, however, the active ingredients of the two drugs may be the same, but the inert ingredients (binders, fillers, and other substances) may alter the absorption, or bioavailability, of the drug. Therefore, it is unsafe to assume that two versions of the same medication will produce the same effects during the same amount of time. These differences are especially critical in some heart medications and thyroid drugs and other hormone products; always check with your doctor about the advisability of switching to a generic product.

Storing Drugs

How drugs are stored determines whether they remain fresh, safe, and effective for as long as possible. To avoid confusion, keep all drugs in their original labeled containers. If a drug must be put into another container, affix to it the exact information as on the original label.

BASICS FOR YOUR MEDICINE CABINET

While many drugs should be purchased only as the need for them arises, certain medications, usually those used for common minor ailments, should be kept on hand:

Analgesics. Some kind of analgesic, such as aspirin, ibuprofen, or acetaminophen, should be on hand for relieving headaches, minor muscle aches, cramps, and other types pain.

Antacids. It is wise to have an antacid in the house to treat indigestion or heartburn. Since the ingredients of different antacids vary—for example, some products have a high salt content—be sure to talk to your doctor or pharmacist about which one would best suit your needs.

Allergy and Cold Medications. A number of these drugs contain antihistamines; others have decongestants that can ease nasal stuffiness. Before taking these medications, read the warning labels carefully. Many cause drowsiness and should not be used when driving or operating machinery. Some contain ingredients that interact with other medications or that can worsen certain medical conditions, especially high blood pressure, glaucoma, diabetes, and urinary tract problems. If you have doubts, check with your doctor or pharmacist before making the purchase to make sure that the product is safe for you to use.

Antipruritics. Calamine lotion is usually all that is needed to alleviate a bout of itching due to mosquito bites or poison ivy. In more severe cases, use of an over-the-counter low-dose corticosteroid cream or ointment may be more effective.

Antidiarrheals. For occasional episodes of diarrhea, an antidiarrheal medication is good to have on hand. You can ask your doctor or pharmacist to recommend the best available over-the-counter remedy. If an episode persists for more than a few days, make an appointment for a checkup with your physician.

Antiseptics. Always keep a product such as rubbing alcohol or 3 percent hydrogen peroxide with your medical supplies to use as a cleanser for minor scrapes and cuts. Application of an antiseptic to a small wound after it has been washed with soap and water helps to prevent infection.

Most drugs should be kept in a dry place away from direct sunlight. A bedroom or hallway cabinet may be the best choice, as drugs placed in a bathroom or kitchen cabinet may be adversely affected by heat and moisture. If the household includes children, store all medications either in a locked cabinet or in a place inaccessible to them. Follow the same precautions when other children visit. Also, you may want to ask your pharmacist to use child-proof safety bottles as an extra precaution.

Some medications must be refrigerated, but room temperature is fine for most of them. Keep containers away from all heat sources and always close the cap tightly after each usage. Remember, too, that drugs deteriorate over time.They should be labeled with a manufacturer's expiration date. Review all your medications every few months and discard those whose expiration dates have expired.

Never keep more than one drug on a bedside table; even then, get up and turn on the light before taking it. It is not uncommon for people to overdose inadvertently or take the wrong drug in the dark while half asleep.

Nonprescription Drugs

Over-the-counter (OTC) medications can be purchased at a pharmacy, supermarket, or other outlet without a physician's prescription. However, their widespread availability should not be interpreted as a sign that they are risk-free; while many drugs are appropriate and safe for self-treatment, they still have potential adverse side effects. Also, many former prescription drugs, such as ibuprofen and certain allergy and antifungal preparations, are now sold OTC. Although the dosage may be smaller than their prescription counterparts, they have a similar potential for side effects.

Most nonprescription drugs are designed to treat minor medical problems, such as coughs, colds, and minor infections. Regardless of the nature of the ailment, carefully follow all instructions for use, paying particular attention to dosage. This is especially important if you are taking medication for coexisting medical problems. Many OTC cold and allergy medications, for example, can exacerbate high blood pressure and glaucoma; others interact with medication to alter their effectiveness. If in doubt, ask your pharmacist. He can outline various options, and may suggest seeing a doctor if self-treatment is ill-advised or prolonged treatment with an OTC drug is unwise. Be especially cautious about administering OTC medication to children; in such cases, it is always best to check with a doctor beforehand.

Drug Dependency

Some drugs are potentially habit-forming, or addictive, meaning the user can become physically or psychologically dependent on them. Physical dependence is manifested by withdrawal symptoms when the user attempts to abstain from the drug. At the same time, increasing amounts are needed to forestall withdrawal symptoms. Psychological dependence is marked by constant craving for the drug and its effects. Physical and psychological dependence often co-exist, making it even more difficult to stop taking the drug.

The amount of time it takes to develop drug dependency varies according to the drug, its dosage, and frequency and duration of use. People who are already addicted to nicotine, alcohol, or other substances are especially vulnerable to dependency on a habit-forming medication. Fortunately, only a few groups of medications result in physical dependence;

examples include morphine and other opium derivatives, narcotics, antidepressants and antianxiety drugs, sleeping pills, and stimulants. (For more details, see Addictions, page 66). Although many of these medications have important medical uses, they also have a high potential for abuse as so-called recreational drugs. To differentiate among their potential risks, addictive drugs have been placed in the following controlled substance categories:

C-I, which has a high risk for physical and psychological abuse. Prescriptions are strictly limited and may not be refilled. Examples of drugs falling into this group include some opiates (derivatives of opium) and hallucinogens.

C-II, which has a high risk of both physical and psychological dependence. Prescriptions must be written and signed by a physician and cannot be refilled. Some examples include narcotics, amphetamines, and some barbiturates.

C-III, which may result in a high psychological dependence and a low-to-moderate physical dependence. Prescriptions for these drugs may be written or issued verbally by a doctor to a pharmacist. Up to five refills are allowed during a six-month period. Examples include certain antianxiety drugs, sleeping pills, and many other psychotropic drugs.

C-IV, which has a low potential for physical and psychological dependence. Physician prescriptions may be written or verbal. Up to five refills of the prescription may be filled during a six-month period. Examples include some barbiturates, propoxyphene, and benzodiazepines.

C-V, which has a low potential for physical and psychological dependence but may be subject to regulations in some states. A prescription may not always be needed, and there is no limit on refills. Examples include antidiarrheal agents and cough medicines containing mild narcotics.

Drug Directory

On the following pages, you will find tables of the most commonly used drugs, arranged by categories of use. Specific information for each drug includes its generic and brand names; whether it requires a prescription (indicated by an Rx), is sold over the counter, or both; a listing of its uses; its major side effects; and finally, any special precautions.

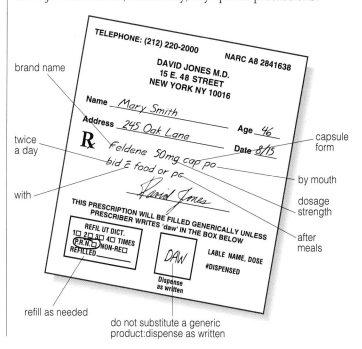

brand name
twice a day
with
refill as needed

TELEPHONE: (212) 220-2000
NARC A8 2841638
DAVID JONES M.D.
15 E. 48 STREET
NEW YORK NY 10016
Name Mary Smith
Address 245 Oak Lane   Age 46
Rx Feldene 50mg cap po   Date 8/15
bid c̄ food or pc
David Jones
THIS PRESCRIPTION WILL BE FILLED GENERICALLY UNLESS PRESCRIBER WRITES 'daw' IN THE BOX BELOW
REFIL UT DICT.
1☐ 2☐ 3☐ 4☐ TIMES
(P.R.N.☐) NON-REC☐
REFILLED.
DAW
LABLE NAME, DOSE #DISPENSED
Dispense as written

capsule form
by mouth
dosage strength
after meals
do not substitute a generic product:dispense as written

Generic (Brand-Name Examples)	OTC Rx	Used for	Major side effects	Special precautions
ANALGESICS/ANTI-INFLAMMATORY/ARTHRITIS **WARNING: DO NOT TAKE ANY of these drugs with alcohol, which increases the potential for intestinal, liver, and kidney damage.**				
acetaminophen (Aspirin-Free Anacin, Panadol, Tylenol)	OTC	Relieving pain and fever.	Few side effects, but large doses or prolonged use damage the liver and kidneys.	Take with milk or food to reduce stomach irritation.
aspirin (Bayer, Bufferin, Empirin) (Easprin, Zorprin)	OTC Rx	Relieving pain, fever, arthritis, and other inflammatory disorders; in a low dose for preventing stroke and heart attack.	Stomach upset, bleeding; prolonged use can cause ringing in the ears and hearing loss.	Take with milk or food to reduce stomach irritation. Do not give to children under 18 without consulting a doctor. Avoid if you have asthma, ulcers, nasal polyps.
aspirin/caffeine (Anacin)	OTC	Relieving pain, fever, migraine and other headaches.	Same as aspirin plus wakefulness.	Same as for aspirin.
aspirin/acetaminophen/caffeine (Excedrin)	OTC	Same as aspirin and acetaminophen.	Same as aspirin and acetaminophen, plus wakefulness. Stomach upset, bleeding; prolonged use can cause ringing in the ears and hearing loss.	Prolonged use increases risk of kidney damage. Take with milk or food to reduce stomach irritation. Do not give to children under 18 without consulting a doctor. Avoid if you have asthma, ulcers, nasal polyps.
ibuprofen (Advil, Nuprin) (Motrin) (Rufen)	OTC OTC Rx Rx	Relieving pain, arthritis, inflammation, and menstrual cramps.	Diarrhea, nausea, stomach upset, headache, dizziness.	Take with food or milk to reduce stomach irritation.
Stronger Nonsteroidal Anti-inflammatory Drugs (NSAIDs)				
diclofenac (Voltaren)	Rx	Relieving pain of arthritis and other conditions.	Stomach irritation, nausea, headache, ulcers, internal bleeding.	Take with food or milk and consult your doctor before combining this with aspirin, diuretics, warfarin, or oral diabetes drugs and other medications. Avoid driving and other hazardous activities if drowsiness occurs.
diflunisal (Dolobid)	Rx	Same as diclofenac.	Same as diclofenac.	Same as diclofenac.
etodolac (Lodine)	Rx	Same as diclofenac.	Same as diclofenac, plus increased urination and blurred vision. Prolonged use may cause kidney and liver inflammation.	Same as diclofenac.
fenoprofen calcium (Nalfon)	Rx	Same as diclofenac.	Same as etodolac.	Same as diclofenac.
flurbiprofen (Ansaid)	Rx	Same as diclofenac.	Same as etodolac.	Same as diclofenac.
indomethacin (Indocin, Indocin SR)	Rx	Same as diclofenac.	Stomach upset, headache, dizziness, drowsiness. Prolonged use may cause bleeding ulcers.	Same as diclofenac.
ketoprofen (Orudis, Oruvail)	Rx	Same as diclofenac.	Stomach upset, headache, dizziness, rash.	Same as diclofenac.
mefenamic acid (Ponstel)	Rx	Same as diclofenac.	Same as indomethacin, plus rash; also may cause bleeding ulcers.	Same as diclofenac.
nabumetone (Relafen)	Rx	Same as diclofenac.	Stomach upset, fluid retention, gas, ringing in the ears.	Same as diclofenac.
naproxen (Anaprox, Naprosyn) (Aleve)	Rx OTC	Relieving pain of arthritis, menstrual cramps, and other conditions.	Stomach upset, constipation, labored breathing, drowsiness, hearing and visual changes, fluid retention.	Same as diclofenac.
oxaprozin (Daypro)	Rx	Same as diclofenac.	Stomach upset, nausea, constipation, rash.	Same as diclofenac, plus prolonged use can cause anemia; regular blood tests are recommended.
piroxicam (Feldene)	Rx	Same as diclofenac.	Stomach upset, dizziness, itching and rash, drowsiness, ringing in the ears.	Same as diclofenac.
sulindac (Clinoral)	Rx	Same as diclofenac.	Stomach upset, dizziness, itching and rash, drowsiness, ringing in the ears.	Same as diclofenac.

Generic (Brand-Name Examples)	OTC Rx	Used for	Major side effects	Special precautions
tolmetin (Tolectin)	Rx	Same as diclofenac.	Stomach upset, nausea, constipation, diarrhea, vomiting, dizziness, headache, high blood pressure, edema, weight gain or loss. Prolonged use may cause bleeding ulcers.	Same as diclofenac.

Other Arthritis Drugs

Generic (Brand-Name Examples)	OTC Rx	Used for	Major side effects	Special precautions
auranofin (Ridaura)	Rx	Treating rheumatoid arthritis.	Stomach upset, diarrhea, nausea, vomiting, constipation, anorexia, stomatitis, conjunctivitis, rash.	Tell your doctor about other medications you are taking.
aurothioglucose (Solganal)	Rx	Same as auranofin.	Stomach upset, nausea, vomiting, stomatitis, weakness, fatigue, dizziness, sweating, rash, ulcers; may result in gold toxicity.	For intramuscular injection only. Use should be supervised cautiously in patients with skin rash, a history of kidney or liver disease, and cardiovascular or cerebral circulation problems. Tell your doctor about other medications you are taking.
azathioprine (Imuran)	Rx	Treating rheumatoid arthritis and as an adjunct for preventing rejection of kidney transplants.	Nausea, vomiting, diarrhea, rash, mouth sores.	Use should be supervised cautiously in patients with skin rash, a history of kidney or liver disease, and cardiovascular or cerebral circulation problems. Consult your doctor about combining with other drugs.
gold sodium thiomalate (Myochrisine)	Rx	Treating rheumatoid arthritis.	Same as aurothioglucose.	Same as aurothioglucose.
methotrexate (Rheumatrex)	Rx	Treating rheumatoid arthritis and psoriasis.	Nausea, vomiting, mouth sores, rash, dizziness. Prolonged use may damage liver or kidneys.	Use may potentially result in serious toxicity. Tell your doctor about other medications you are taking.
penicillamine (Cuprimine, Depen)	Rx	Treating severe, active rheumatoid arthritis, Wilson's disease, and cystinuria.	Stomach upset, nausea, vomiting, diarrhea, rash, decreased taste perception, serious liver or kidney adverse reactions.	Close medical supervision is necessary. Use is associated with a high incidence of potentially fatal reactions. Tell your doctor about other medications you are taking.
salsalate (Disalcid, Salflex)	Rx	Treating arthritis.	Nausea, rash, ringing in the ears, vertigo, reversible hearing impairment.	To avoid toxicity, do not combine with other salicylates. Use should be supervised cautiously in patients with chronic kidney insufficiency or peptic ulcer disease. Tell your doctor about other medications you are taking.

Narcotic Analgesics
Note: Prolonged use and/or high doses of these drugs may result in psychological and/or physical dependence.

Generic (Brand-Name Examples)	OTC Rx	Used for	Major side effects	Special precautions
hydromorphone (Dilaudid)	Rx	Relieving intractable or severe pain.	Dizziness, impaired mental function, slowed physical reflexes, anxiety, mood swings, labored breathing, constipation.	Use should be supervised if you have liver or kidney disease, heart arrhythmias, thyroid or adrenal gland disorders, or preexisting respiratory problems. Consult your doctor about combining with other drugs. Avoid alcohol. Suspend activities requiring alert reponses.
meperidine (Demerol)	Rx	Same as hydromorphone.	Drowsiness, nausea, vomiting, sweating, sedation.	Same as hydromorphone.
oxycodone/acetaminophen (Percocet)	Rx	Relieving severe pain and reducing fever.	Nausea, dizziness, lightheadedness.	Same as hydromorphone.
propoxyphene napsylate/acetaminophen (Darvocet-N)	Rx	Relieving pain, with or without fever.	Drowsiness, nausea, vomiting, sedation.	Same as hydromorphone.
propoxyphene/aspirin/caffeine (Darvon Compound-65)	Rx	Same as hydromorphone.	Same as hydromorphone, plus the side effects produced by aspirin.	Children under age 18 should not be given this drug unless approved by a doctor. If you have liver or kidney ailments, or have recurrent asthma problems, prolonged use is inadvisable.

Generic (Brand-Name Examples)	OTC Rx	Used for	Major side effects	Special precautions
Antimigraine agents				
ergotamine tartrate/caffeine (Cafergot)	Rx	Preventing vascular headaches, especially migraine and cluster types.	Digestive disturbances, nausea, muscle stiffness.	Regular use is inadvisable because of negative effects on circulation. If you have asthma, high blood pressure, heart problems, or have had a recent stroke, proceed with caution.
isometheptene mucate/dichloralphenazone/acetaminophen (Midrin)	Rx	Preventing tension headaches and migraines.	Dizziness, rash.	Same as ergotamine tartrate.
sumatriptan succinate (Imitrex Injection)	Rx	Aborting migraine and other vascular headaches.	Cardiac arrhythmias; feeling of tightness in chest, jaw, or neck; tingling or burning sensation; flushing; altered vision; muscle weakness, pain, or cramping; dizziness; drowsiness; anxiety; sweating.	Should not be used by persons with coronary artery disease, angina, or uncontrolled high blood pressure. Should not be used with ergotamine drugs or MAO inhibitors.
ANTI-INFECTIVES				
Antibiotics				
Aminoglycosides				
gentamicin (Garamycin)	Rx	Controlling complicated and serious infections.	Nausea, vomiting, itching, cloudy urine.	Do not use if you have kidney disease, myasthenia gravis, or hearing disability. Tell your doctor about other medications you are taking.
netilmicin (Netromycin)	Rx	Same as gentamicin.	Same as gentamicin.	Same as gentamicin, plus avoidance by those with Parkinson's disease.
streptomycin No brand names	Rx	Treating serious infections, especially tuberculosis.	Numbness in the face and hands, vertigo, hearing impairment.	Same as tobramycin. Use of this drug should be closely monitored.
tobramycin (Tobrex, Nebcin)	Rx	Same as gentamicin.	Dizziness, impaired hearing, rash, urine changes.	Report these side effects to your doctor without delay.
Cephalosporins				
cefaclor (Ceclor)	Rx	Treating a wide variety of bacterial infections, especially those resistant to penicillin.	Mild diarrhea, possible allergic reactions.	Do not use if you are allergic to penicillin, have impaired kidney function, or bleeding disorders.
cefadroxil (Duricef)	Rx	Treating specific bacterial infections, especially strep, staph, and *E.coli.*	Diarrhea, vomiting, allergic skin reactions.	Should not be used where there is a history of colitis or other bowel disease. Inform your doctor about allergies to other antibiotics.
cefazolin (Ancef, Kefzol)	Rx	Treating endocarditis, septicemia, and respiratory, urinary, genital, skin, bone, and joint infections resistant to other antibiotics. Also used to prevent postoperative infection in patients who have undergone surgery.	Diarrhea, stomach cramps, oral candidiasis, skin rash, itching and other allergic responses.	Do not use if you have impaired kidney function or a history of gastrointestinal disease (especially colitis). Inform your doctor if you have had previous allergic reactions to drugs, particularly penicillin.
cefmetazole (Zefazone)	Rx	Treating respiratory, urinary, genital, and skin infections, gonorrhea, and uncomplicated rectal infections. Also used to prevent infection in patients undergoing certain surgery.	Diarrhea, nausea, rash, localized pain, tenderness, or bruising following intramuscular injection, itching, and other allergic responses.	Same as cefazolin, plus this drug should be avoided if you have had previous allergic responses to cefmetazole or other cephalosporins.
cefoperazone (Cefobid)	Rx	Treating serious respiratory, urinary, and skin infections resistant to other antibiotics.	Diarrhea, nausea, vomiting.	Do not take this drug with alcohol. Consult your doctor about combining with other medications.
cefoxitin (Mefoxin)	Rx	Preventing infection during major surgery, also for treating blood poisoning, peritonitis, and other serious infections.	Diarrhea, nausea, vomiting.	Do not use if you have impaired kidney function. Tell your doctor about other medications.
cephalexin (Keflex)	Rx	Treating mild infections, such as cystitis and bronchitis.	Mild diarrhea, possible allergic response.	Inform your doctor about previous allergic response to penicillin. Avoid use if you have a kidney or bleeding disorder.

Generic (Brand-Name Examples)	OTC Rx	Used for	Major side effects	Special precautions
Erythromycins				
erythromycin (E-Mycin, Ery-Tab, EryPed, Eryc, Ilosone)	Rx	Treating some types of pneumonia, sexually transmitted diseases, and ear and throat infections. It is also an effective alternative to penicillins and tetracyclines.	Nausea and vomiting.	Do not use if you have liver or kidney disease, or if it caused a previous allergic response.
Lincosamides				
clindamycin (Cleocin)	Rx	Treating major lung, skin, and gynecological infections.	Mild diarrhea.	Inform your doctor if you have liver or kidney malfunction, a bowel disorder, or myasthenia gravis. Check combination with other drugs.
lincomycin (Lincocin)	Rx	Treating serious infections that are resistant to penicillin.	Same as clindamycin.	Same as clindamycin.
Penicillins				
amoxicillin (Amoxil) amoxicillin trihydrate (Augmentin, Moxilin, Trimox, Wymox)	Rx	Treating ear nose, throat, respiratory, and other infections.	Patchy skin rash, breathing difficulties, other allergic responses.	Advise your doctor about previous allergic reactions. Do not use if you have kidney disease or ulcerative colitis.
ampicillin (Ampicillin, Omnipen)	Rx	Same as amoxicillin; in large doses, for treating meningitis and typhoid fever.	Same as amoxicillin.	Same as amoxicillin.
cloxacillin (Cloxapen, Tegopen)	Rx	Treating staph infections.	Diarrhea, allergic responses.	Same as amoxicillin.
penicillin V (Ledercillin VK, Pen•Vee K)	Rx	Treating respiratory tract infections and certain uncommon strep infections such as scarlet fever.	Same as amoxicillin.	Same as amoxicillin.
Sulfa Drugs				
sulfacetamide (Bleph-10)	Rx	Treating eye infections.	Few if any when used as directed.	Do not use if you wear contact lenses or if you have had a previous history or allergic reaction to sulfa drugs.
sulfasalazine (Azulfidine)	Rx	Treating inflammatory bowel disorders and rheumatoid arthritis.	Gastrointestinal upset, allergic responses to large doses.	Do not use if you have kidney or liver disease, or a blood disorder such as porphyria, or are sensitive to aspirin.
sulfisoxazole (Gantrisin)	Rx	Treating urinary tract infections.	Gastrointestinal upsets.	Same as sulfasalazine.
Tetracyclines				
doxycycline (Doryx, Vibramycin)	Rx	Treating chronic bronchitis, chronic prostatitis, and pelvic inflammatory disease.	Nausea.	Take with food to reduce stomach upset. Do not give to young children or pregnant women because it may stain developing teeth.
tetracycline (Achromycin V, Panmycin, Sumycin)	Rx	Treating various pneumonias and sexually transmitted diseases.	Gastrointestinal upset, rash.	Do not take if you have kidney malfunction. Do not give to young children or pregnant women, because it may stain developing teeth.
General anti-infectives				
colistin (Coly-Mycin S)	Rx	Preventing and treating eye, ear, and skin infections, usually as ointment or drops.	Few if any when used in low doses.	Rarely given by injection because of potential damage to kidneys and nerves.
nitrofurantoin (Macrobid, Macrodantin)	Rx	Treating urinary tract infections.	Respiratory distress, loss of appetite, nausea.	Long-term use should be carefully monitored, especially because of effect on liver function and kidneys. Blood tests should be scheduled to rule out anemia.
Topical anti-infectives				
acyclovir (Zovirax)	Rx	Treating all types of herpes; may also be effective against the Epstein-Barr virus.	Itching, stinging; rash.	Should not be used in or near eyes.
amphotericin B (Fungizone)	Rx	Treating serious fungal infections, both systemic and local.	Possible allergic skin reactions.	Advise your doctor about previous allergic reaction.
bacitracin zinc (Cortisporin) (Neosporin, Polysporin)	Rx OTC	Treating skin infections.	Few if any when used in ointment form.	Stop if allergic reaction occurs.

Generic (Brand-Name Examples)	OTC Rx	Used for	Major side effects	Special precautions
mupirocin (Bactroban)	Rx	Treating the bacterial skin infection, impetigo.	Pain, itching.	Avoid use near the eyes.
nystatin (Mycostatin)	Rx	Treating candidiasis of the skin and mucous membranes.	None when used as directed.	Avoid use near eyes.
tetracycline (Achromycin 3% Ointment)	OTC	Treating cuts, burns, abrasions.	None when used as directed.	Best used as a first aid preparation.

Also: Lotrimin, Micatin, Mycelex, Mycitracin, and Tinactin.

Antifungals: Systemic

Generic (Brand-Name Examples)	OTC Rx	Used for	Major side effects	Special precautions
amphotericin B (Fungizone)	Rx	Treating potentially life-threatening systemic fungal infections.	Nausea, vomiting, bleeding.	Careful monitoring is essential if you have impaired kidney function and are taking other medications.
fluconazole (Diflucan)	Rx	Treating fungal and yeast infections of the genitourinary tract, as well as pneumonia and meningitis in people with AIDS.	Nausea, diarrhea.	Consult your doctor about the advisability of combining this drug with other medications.
griseofulvin (Fulvicin P/G, Grisactin Ultra, Gris-Peg)	Rx	Treating ringworm and fungal infections of the scalp, feet, fingernails, and toenails.	Dry mouth, impaired sense of taste, headache.	Inform your doctor about previous allergy to penicillin, any liver malfunction, and other drugs being used.
itraconazole (Sporanox)	Rx	Treating fungal infections such as histoplasmosis, aspergillosis, and blastomycosis.	Nausea, rash, headache, vomiting, diarrhea.	Do not use in conjunction with terfenadine or astemizole. Avoid this drug if you are hypersensitive to it or its inert ingredients. Do not breast-feed while taking this drug.
ketoconazole (Nizoral)	Rx	Treating fungal infections of the brain, kidneys, lungs, and lymph nodes (by injection).	Nausea, headache, constipation.	A history of ulcers or liver or kidney malfunction should be discussed with your doctor.
miconazole (Micatin, Monistat)	Rx	Same as ketoconazole.	Nausea, vomiting, fever.	Same as ketoconazole.

NOTE: Most prescription and OTC antifungals are also available for topical use in the form of creams and ointments. Brand-name preparations include: Exelderm, Lamisil, Loprox, Monistat-Derm, Mycelex, Mycostatin, Naftin, Nizoral, Oxistat, and Spectazole.

Antiparasitics

Generic (Brand-Name Examples)	OTC Rx	Used for	Major side effects	Special precautions
mebendazole (Vermox)	Rx	Treating hookworm, pinworm, and whipworm infestations.	Abdominal pain, diarrhea.	Inform your doctor about impaired liver function or any bowel disorder.
praziquantel (Biltricide)	Rx	Treating tapeworm and blood fluke (Bilharzia) infestations.	Dizziness and drowsiness.	Onset of severe diarrhea should be reported to your doctor without delay.
pyrantel (Antiminth)	Rx	Treating intestinal worm infestations.	Gastrointestinal discomfort.	Inform your doctor if you have impaired liver function, and provide information about other medications you are taking.

Antivirals

Generic (Brand-Name Examples)	OTC Rx	Used for	Major side effects	Special precautions
acyclovir (Zovirax)	Rx	Treating stubborn cases of genital herpes (by injection or by mouth).	From capsules—nausea, dizziness, headache; from injection—confusion.	Ask your doctor about adverse effects of combining with other medications.
amantadine (Symmetrel)	Rx	Preventing and treating influenza A in absence of flu vaccine.	Dizziness, insomnia, nausea, dry mouth, fluid retention, headache.	Do not combine with alcohol. Possibility of blurred vision and agitation makes driving hazardous.

Vaginal anti-infectives

Generic (Brand-Name Examples)	OTC Rx	Used for	Major side effects	Special precautions
butoconazole (Femstat)	Rx	Treating yeast-like infections of the vulva or vagina.	Soreness, swelling, itching, vaginal discharge.	Discuss the use of this drug with your doctor if you are pregnant or breast-feeding.
clindamycin (Cleocin Vaginal Cream)	Rx	Treating bacterial vaginosis.	Cervical and vaginal inflammation.	Do not use if you have a history of Crohn's disease or inflammatory bowel disease.
miconazole (Monistat-Derm)	Rx	Treating vaginal yeast infections.	Possible vaginal burning and irritation.	Do not use in combination with latex condoms or latex vaginal diaphragm because the mineral oil in this drug may reduce their effectiveness. Do not use during the first trimester of pregnancy.

Generic (Brand-Name Examples)	OTC Rx	Used for	Major side effects	Special precautions
sulfanilamide (AVC)	Rx	Treating yeast infections caused by the fungus *Candida albicans*.	Vaginal burning.	If you are pregnant or breast-feeding, ask your doctor about the safety of using this sulfa drug.
tioconazole (Vagistat-1)	Rx	Treating vaginal candidiasis.	Vaginal discharge, burning sensation during urination.	If you have diabetes, ask your doctor whether you can safely take this medication.

OTC: Femcare, Gyne-Lotrimin, Monistat 7, Mycelex.

ASTHMA/ALLERGY

Antianaphylactic Agents

epinephrine (Adrenalin, EpiPen)	Rx	Counteracting anaphylaxis and severe allergic responses to insect stings, shellfish, medications, and other allergens; severe asthma attack.	Restlessness, dry mouth, heart arrhythmias.	Used mostly in emergency situations. May exacerbate heart disease, high blood pressure, hyperthyroidism, or diabetes.

Bronchodilators

albuterol (Proventil, Ventolin)	Rx	Treating asthma, chronic bronchitis, emphysema.	Restlessness, anxiety, tremor, headache.	Must be used as directed to prevent worsening of asthma.
metaproterenol (Alupent)	Rx	Dilating the airways and to stop asthma attack.	Same as epinephrine.	Same as albuterol.
terbutaline (Brethaire, Brethine, Bricanyl)	Rx	Dilating the small airways to stop or prevent asthma attack.	Same as epinephrine.	Same as albuterol.

OTC: Primatene and others

Antihistamines/Antipruritics

astemizole (Hismanal)	Rx	Relieving allergic response known as "hay fever." Also for treating hives.	Headache, dry mouth, drowsiness, weight gain.	Take on an empty stomach (one hour before or two hours after eating). Consult your doctor if you are being treated for asthma or liver or kidney disease.
cyproheptadine (Periactin)	Rx	Relieving nasal congestion and other allergy symptoms. May also be prescribed to relieve cluster headaches.	Drowsiness, confusion.	Do not drive while taking this drug. A different antihistamine is advisable for the elderly and those who are taking antidepressant drugs or are breast-feeding.
loratadine (Claritin)	Rx	Treating runny nose and other hay fever symptoms.	Sleepiness, headache, drowsiness, dry mouth.	Dose should be adjusted if you have liver or kidney disease.
promethazine (Phenergan)	Rx	Treating allergies, hives, and inner ear disturbances that produce vertigo and vomiting (motion sickness and Ménière's disease).	Same as loratadine.	Same as loratadine; also your doctor should be informed of all other medications you are taking.
terfenadine (Seldane)	Rx	Treating allergic responses involving sneezing, runny nose, itching eyes, etc.	Diminished appetite, headache. (Unlike other antihistamines, it does not produce drowsiness.)	Consult your physician if you have liver or kidney disease, glaucoma, or epilepsy.

OTC: Benadryl, Caladryl, Chlor-Trimeton, Dimetane, Nolahist, Teldrin.

Topical Steroids

alclometasone dipropionate (Aclovate)	Rx	Relieving itching rashes, including psoriasis.	Excessive hair growth, pimples, increased inflammation.	For external use only; keep away from eyes. Watch out for changes in appearance that indicate excessive absorption.
betamethasone (Diprolene)	Rx	Treating skin problems.	High doses or prolonged use may aggravate symptoms.	Same as alclometasone.
hydrocortisone (Anusol HC, Bactine, Caldecort Cream)	Rx	Treating inflammatory skin problems.	Same as alclometasone.	Keep affected areas uncovered to reduce possibility of absorption.
triamcinolone (Aristocort, Aristospan, Mytrex)	Rx	Treating dermatitis, eczema, psoriasis.	Rare when used in topical form.	Same as alclometasone.

Inhaled Steroids

beclomethasone (Beclovent, Beconase, Vanceril, Vancenase)	Rx	Reducing asthma symptoms.	Nasal irritation, dry throat.	Inform your doctor about previous nasal surgery or nasal ulcers, or any respiratory diseases.

Generic (Brand-Name Examples)	OTC Rx	Used for	Major side effects	Special precautions
triamcinolone (Azmacort, Nasacort)	Rx	Controlling attacks of bronchial asthma and reducing nasal polyps.	Throat irritation, dry mouth.	Use should be monitored closely if you have a viral or bacterial infection and for possible development of fungal infections.
Xanthines				
oxtriphylline (Choledyl)	Rx	Expanding the airways to the lungs to stop or prevent asthma attacks.	Dizziness, nausea, agitation.	Inform your doctor if you have impaired liver function, coronary problems, or ulcers, or if you smoke.
theophylline (Slo-bid, Quibron, Theo-Dur)	Rx	Same as oxtriphylline.	Same as oxtriphylline.	Same as oxtriphylline.
CARDIOVASCULAR/ANTIHYPERTENSIVES				
ACE Inhibitors				
captopril (Capoten)	Rx	Lowering blood pressure, treating heart failure.	Loss of appetite, dizziness, cough.	Inform your doctor if you have liver, kidney, or coronary artery disease, and if you take other medications.
enalapril (Vasotec)	Rx	Same as captopril.	Dizziness, headache, cough.	Same as captopril.
Alpha Blockers				
prazosin (Minipress)	Rx	Treating high blood pressure.	Fainting, cardiac arrhythmias, dizziness, edema, headache, lassitude, depression, rash, impotence, visual problems, dry mouth, urinary frequency, GI upset.	May cause fainting if initial dosage is too high.
Anticoagulant Agents				
heparin No brand names	Rx	Preventing blood clots.	Bleeding, bruising.	Inform your doctor about allergies, high blood pressure, impaired liver or kidney function, and other medications you are taking.
streptokinase (Kabikinase, Streptase)	Rx	Same as heparin.	Excessive bleeding.	This is an emergency medication requiring close monitoring.
warfarin (Coumadin)	Rx	Same as heparin.	Nausea, loss of appetite, bleeding.	Same as heparin.
Beta Blockers				
acebutolol (Sectral)	Rx	Lowering blood pressure, treating angina and arrhythmias.	Lack of energy, slow heartbeat, cold extremities, depression, lassitude, impotence, headache, vivid dreams.	Inform your doctor if you have a respiratory or circulatory disorder or diabetes. Provide information about other medications you take.
metoprolol (Lopressor)	Rx	Same as acebutolol.	Same as acebutolol.	Same as acebutolol.
nadolol (Corgard)	Rx	Same as acebutolol; preventing migraine.	Same as acebutolol.	Same as acebutolol.
propranolol (Inderal, Inderal LA)	Rx	Same as acebutolol; preventing migraine.	Same as acebutolol.	Same as acebutolol.
timolol (Blocadren)	Rx	Treating high blood pressure, preventing migraine.	Same as acebutolol.	Same as acebutolol.
Calcium-Channel Blockers				
diltiazem (Cardizem CD, Cardizem SR)	Rx	Treating angina, cardiac arrhythmias, high blood pressure.	Headache, loss of energy, loss of appetite, swollen ankles.	Inform your doctor about impaired liver, kidney, or heart function. Provide information about other medications you are taking.
nifedipine (Procardia)	Rx	Same as diltiazem.	Headache, fatigue, dizziness.	Same as diltiazem.
verapamil (Calan, Isoptin)	Rx	Same as diltiazem.	Nausea, constipation, headache, swollen ankles.	Inform your doctor about impaired kidney or liver function, and other medications you are taking.
Digitalis Drugs (Cardiac Glycosides)				
digitoxin (Crystodigin)	Rx	Treating heart failure and arrhythmias.	Gastrointestinal upsets, fatigue.	Inform your doctor about impaired liver or thyroid function, and other medications you are taking.
digoxin (Lanoxicaps, Lanoxin)	Rx	Same as digitoxin.	Fatigue, loss of appetite, impaired vision.	Same as digitoxin.
Lanoxin injection	Rx	Same as digitoxin.	Same as digitoxin.	Same as digitoxin.

Generic (Brand-Name Examples)	OTC Rx	Used for	Major side effects	Special precautions
Diuretics				
chlorothiazide (Diuril)	Rx	Reducing fluid retention, lowering high blood pressure.	Leg cramps, weakness, possible electrolyte imbalance.	Inform your doctor if you have diabetes, impaired liver or kidney function, or a history of gout, and about other medications you are taking.
furosemide (Lasix)	Rx	Same as chlorothiazide, especially in persons with heart failure, kidney disease, and cirrhosis.	Same as chlorothiazide.	Same as chlorothiazide; also provide information about prostate problems.
hydrochlorothiazide (Esidrix, HydroDIURIL, Inderide, Moduretic, Oretic)	Rx	Same as chlorothiazide; relief of PMS.	Same as chlorothiazide.	Same as chlorothiazide.
Indolines				
indapamide (Lozol)	Rx	Lowering blood pressure and treatment of edema associated with congestive heart failure.	Headache, back pain, muscle cramps, dizziness, fatigue, anxiety, infection, and rhinitis.	Do not use if you have impaired kidney function or a history of hypersensitivity to indapamide or other sulfonamide derivatives.
Nitrates				
isosorbide dinitrate (Dilatrate-SR, Isordil, Sorbitrate)	Rx	Relieving the pain of angina.	Headache, dizziness.	Inform your doctor if you are anemic or are being treated for glaucoma or thyroid malfunction.
isosorbide mononitrate (Imdur)	Rx	Preventing angina attacks.	Same as isosorbide dinitrate.	Not a suitable drug following a heart attack. Blood pressure and heart function should be closely monitored.
nitroglycerin (Nitro-Bid, Nitro-Dur, Nitrolingual Spray)	Rx	Preventing and treating angina.	Dizziness, blurred vision, headache.	Doses should be carefully monitored so that side effects do not interfere with normal functioning.
DIABETES DRUGS				
Insulins (Human and Animal, all OTC)				
insulin (Humulin, Iletin, Novolin, NPH)	OTC	Replacing or supplementing natural insulin by injection.	Sweating, weakness.	A prescribed diet is essential. Tell your doctor about your other medicines. Always carry an ID that explains your diabetic condition.
Sulfonylureas				
chlorpropamide (Diabinese)	Rx	Treating adult-onset (non-insulin-dependent) diabetes mellitus.	Sweating, weakness, confusion.	Inform your doctor about liver or kidney problems, allergy to sulfa drugs, and current medications.
glipizide (Glucotrol)	Rx	Same as chlorpropamide.	Same as chlorpropamide.	Same as chlorpropamide.
glyburide (Diaßeta, Glynase, Micronase)	Rx	Same as chlorpropamide.	Same as chlorpropamide.	Same as chlorpropamide.
tolazamide (Tolinase)	Rx	Same as chlorpropamide.	Same as chlorpropamide.	Same as chlorpropamide.
tolbutamide (Orinase)	Rx	Same as chlorpropamide.	Heartburn, nausea.	Urine and blood should be monitored regularly. To decrease the risk of hypoglycemia, eat regular meals and avoid alcohol.
EYE DRUGS				
Antiglaucoma Agents				
acetazolamide (Diamox)	Rx	Maintaining normal eye pressure to treat glaucoma.	Nausea, diarrhea, loss of appetite.	Inform your doctor if you have liver or kidney disease or emphysema. Also, if you are taking high doses of aspirin, find out whether this drug is suitable.
betaxolol (Betoptic)	Rx	Same as acetazolamide.	Stinging in the eye.	Inform your doctor about asthma, heart disease, or diabetes.

Generic (Brand-Name Examples)	OTC Rx	Used for	Major side effects	Special precautions
dipivefrin (Propine)	Rx	Treating wide-angle glaucoma.	Same as betaxolol.	Use of this drug should be limited to wide-angle glaucoma.
levobunolol (Betagan)	Rx	Same as acetazolamide.	Stinging in the eye.	Same as betaxolol.
metipranolol (Optipranolol)	Rx	Same as acetazolamide.	Nausea, headache, eye irritation, rash, coughing, dizziness, anxiety.	Do not use if you have diabetes, hyperthyroidism, or a history of bronchial asthma, cardiac failure, or anaphylaxis.
timolol (Timoptic)	Rx	Same as acetazolamide.	Eye irritation and tearing.	Inform your doctor if you have asthma or a heart disorder, and provide information about other medications you are taking.

Ophthalmic anti-infective combinations

Generic (Brand-Name Examples)	OTC Rx	Used for	Major side effects	Special precautions
dexamethasone/neomycin (Neodecadron)	Rx	A steroid/antibiotic combination for treating inflammatory/bacterial eye infections.	Allergic skin reactions, increase in eye pressure.	Notify your doctor at once if you are exposed to measles or chickenpox while using these eye drops.
gentamicin (Garamycin, Genoptic)	Rx	Aminoglycoside drops to treat eye infections.	Stinging.	Discuss with your doctor other medications you are taking.
sulfacetamide (Bleph-10, Sodium Sulamyd)	Rx	An antibacterial sulfa drug for treating bacterial conjunctivitis.	Stinging.	Tell your doctor if you wear contact lenses and if you have a history of allergic response to sulfa drugs.
tobramycin (Tobrex)	Rx	An aminoglycoside antibiotic for treating conjunctivitis and inflammation of the eyelids.	Stinging.	Tell your doctor if you have had an allergic reaction to this drug category.

Ophthalmic decongestant/antiallergy agents

Generic (Brand-Name Examples)	OTC Rx	Used for	Major side effects	Special precautions
naphazoline/pheniramine (Naphcon-A)	Rx	Relieving eye irritation due to allergic response.	Drowsiness, high blood pressure.	Do not use if you have glaucoma. Do not give to young children. Tell your doctor if you have diabetes or heart disease, and about other medications you are taking.
oxymetazoline (Afrin, Dristan, Neo-Synephrine)	OTC	Same as above.	Nasal congestion.	Check with your doctor first if you have high blood pressure.

Ophthalmic steroids

Generic (Brand-Name Examples)	OTC Rx	Used for	Major side effects	Special precautions
dexamethasone (Dalalone, Decadron)	Rx	Treating eye inflammation.	Serious eye damage but only with long-term use.	Do not take if you have glaucoma or a herpes infection.
prednisolone (Hydeltra-T.B.A., Inflamase Mild, Inflamase Forte, Pred-G)	Rx	Treating conjunctivitis, iritis.	Rare with short-term use.	Same as dexamethasone.

GASTROINTESTINAL

Antacids (OTC)
Note: Habitual use of these products as a treatment for chronic heartburn or "acid indigestion" should not be considered a substitute for a doctor's diagnosis of the underlying cause.

Generic (Brand-Name Examples)	OTC Rx	Used for	Major side effects	Special precautions
aluminum hydroxide/magnesium hydroxide/simethicone (Di-Gel, Gaviscon, Gelusil, Maalox, and Mylanta)	OTC	Treating heartburn and flatulence.	Aluminum hydroxide can cause constipation and nausea; magnesium hydroxide can cause nausea and diarrhea.	Tell your doctor about other medications you are taking. Do not use at the same time as tetracycline drugs.
aspirin/sodium bicarbonate/citric acid (Alka-Seltzer)	OTC	Same as aluminum hydroxide/magnesium hydroxide/simethicone.	None with short-term use.	Not recommended if you have a negative reaction to aspirin.
magnesium hydroxide (Phillips' Milk of Magnesia)	OTC	Same as aluminum hydroxide/magnesium hydroxide/simethicone.	Nausea, diarrhea.	Overuse can lead to magnesium poisoning, which can be fatal.
simethicone/calcium carbonate/magnesium hydroxide (Di-Gel)	OTC	Same as aluminum hydroxide/magnesium hydroxide/simethicone.	Same as aluminum hydroxide/magnesium hydroxide/simethicone.	Same as aluminum hydroxide/magnesium hydroxide/simethicone.
sodium bicarbonate/sodium citrate (Citrocarbonate)	OTC	Same as aluminum hydroxide/magnesium hydroxide/simethicone.	Belching.	Tell your doctor if you have liver, kidney, or heart problems or high blood pressure. Provide information about other medications you are taking.

Generic (Brand-Name Examples)	OTC Rx	Used for	Major side effects	Special precautions
Antidiarrheal agents				
bismuth subsalicylate (Pepto-Bismol)	OTC	Treating diarrhea, stomach upset, indigestion.	Constipation, darkening of stools.	Should not be given to anyone under 18 with a viral infection.
dipenoxylate/atropine (Lomotil)	Rx	Treating diarrhea.	Drowsiness, constipation.	Not suitable for treating diarrhea caused by antibiotics, infection, or ingested poisons. Inform your doctor if you have urinary, liver, or kidney problems, or glaucoma, or if you have recently taken antibiotics.
loperamide (Imodium, Kaopectate II, Pepto Diarrhea Control)	OTC	Treating diarrhea.	Constipation.	Tell your doctor if you have impaired kidney or liver function, or if you have had recent abdominal surgery.
Antinauseants/antiemetics				
dimenhydrinate (Dramamine)	OTC	Treating vertigo, motion sickness, and Ménière's disease.	Dry mouth, drowsiness, blurred vision.	Tell your doctor if you have impaired liver, kidney, or prostate function, or a history of glaucoma.
diphenhydramine (Benadryl)	OTC	Treating motion sickness and vertigo, and relieving "morning sickness" in the early months of pregnancy.	Dry mouth, drowsiness.	Tell your doctor if you have urinary problems, kidney malfunction, or a history of seizures. Also provide list of other medications you are taking.
meclizine (Antivert) (Bonine)	Rx OTC	Treating vertigo and nausea produced by motion sickness, inner ear disturbances, etc.	Dry mouth, drowsiness.	Same as diphenhydramine.
ondansetron (Zofran)	Rx	Preventing nausea and vomiting resulting from anticancer chemotherapy.	Headache, constipation.	Inform your doctor of previous allergic reactions to this drug.
prochlorperazine (Compazine)	Rx	Reducing the side effects of certain medications or anesthesia. (It is not suitable for treating motion sickness or vertigo.)	Drowsiness, dry mouth, blurred vision, dizziness.	Tell your doctor if you have liver, kidney, heart, respiratory, or thyroid problems; also if you have a history of seizures or parkinsonism. Do not combine with alcohol or narcotics. Avoid exposure to the sun. Use of this drug must be closely monitored.
trimethobenzamide (Tigan)	Rx	Suppressing nausea and vomiting, especially after gastrointestinal surgery or radiation therapy.	Drowsiness.	Tell your doctor if you have parkinsonism, glaucoma, or prostate trouble, or if you have had a recent illness accompanied by a high fever.
Antispasmodics				
belladonna/ergotamine/ phenobarbital (Bellergal-S)	Rx	Treating irritable bowel syndrome, parkinsonism, and migraine.	Blurred vision, drowsiness, dizziness.	Tell your doctor if you have liver, kidney, or heart problems; high blood pressure, asthma, or glaucoma. Provide information about other medications you are taking.
dicyclomine (Bentyl)	Rx	Treating stomach cramps, infant colic, and incontinence.	Dry mouth.	Avoid alcohol. Tell your doctor if you have impaired liver or kidney function, ulcerative colitis, or glaucoma. Provide information about other medications you are taking.
hyoscyamine/atropine/ scopalamine/phenobarbital (Donnatal)	Rx	Treating cramps associated with ulcerative colitis, irritable bowel syndrome, and duodenal ulcers.	Blurred vision, drowsiness, constipation.	Tell your doctor if you have high blood pressure, hyperthyroidism; heart, liver, or kidney disease. Provide information about all meditions you are taking. Avoid alcohol.
Antiulcer/antireflux agents				
cimetidine (Tagamet) (Tagamet HB)	Rx OTC	Treating duodenal and stomach ulcers.	Diarrhea, headaches, breast enlargement in men, rash, rare instances of cardiac arrhythmias.	Tell your doctor if you have impaired kidney or liver function. Provide information about all other medications. Avoid alcohol. Inform your doctor if you are planning a pregnancy or are breast-feeding.

Generic (Brand-Name Examples)	OTC Rx	Used for	Major side effects	Special precautions
cisapride (Propulsid)	Rx	Treating duodenal and stomach ulcers, gastric reflux, esophagitis, and heartburn.	Headache, gastrointestinal upset.	Do not use if you have stomach bleeding. Tell your doctor about all medications you are using. Inform your doctor if you are pregnant or are planning a pregnancy; this drug also appears in breast milk.
famotidine (Pepcid)	Rx	Same as cisapride.	Headache.	Tell your doctor about the other drugs you are taking and whether you are pregnant or are planning a pregnancy; this drug also may appear in your breast milk.
misoprostol (Cytotec)	Rx	Same as cisapride.	Gastrointestinal upsets, cramps.	Because this drug causes uterine contractions, do not use during pregnancy. (Note: this drug is especially useful for long-term combination with NSAIDs to prevent stomach ulcers.)
nizatidine (Axid)	Rx	Same as cisapride.	Dizziness, headache, diarrhea.	Tell your doctor about kidney disease and all medications you are. taking. Combining this drug with heavy aspirin doses should be closely monitored.
omeprazole (Prilosec)	Rx	Same as cisapride.	Same as nizatidine.	This drug is not intended for long-term use. Take with an antacid before meals. Tell your doctor about other medications you are taking.
ranitidine (Zantac)	Rx	Same as cisapride.	Headache.	Tell your doctor about impaired kidney or liver function. Provide information about other medications. you are taking. Let the doctor know if you are pregnant, are planning a pregnancy, or are breast-feeding.
sucralfate (Carafate)	Rx	Same as cisapride.	Constipation.	Tell your doctor if you have impaired kidney function or a history of epileptic seizures.

Laxatives
Note: Most laxatives should not be used for more than one week. Excessive use of the chocolatelike laxatives containing phenolphthalein can irritate the lining of the bowel. Habitual dependence on laxatives weakens bowel muscles, producing "lazy bowel syndrome" thereby perpetuating rather than curing the problem.

Bulk producers

lactulose (Chronulac)	Rx	Softening stools.	Belching, flatulence, nausea.	Tell your doctor if you have high blood pressure, diabetes, or heart or kidney disease. Provide information about all medications you are taking.
psyllium (Metamucil, Syllact)	OTC	Same as lactulose.	Flatulence when used in high doses. As a beneficial effect, it lowes blood cholesterol levels.	Tell your doctor if you have rectal bleeding or acute constipation. Provide information about all medications you are taking.

Laxative Salts

calcium polycarbophil (Mitrolan)	OTC	Treating occasional constipation.	Diarrhea, bowel urgency.	Use for only a few days; long-term use can permanently disrupt bowel function.
magnesium hydroxide (Phillips' Milk of Magnesia)	OTC	Same as calcium polycarbophil.	Diarrhea, bowel urgency; excessive use can cause magnesium poisoning.	Same as calcium polycarbophil.

Lubricants

mineral oil	OTC	Same as magnesium hydroxide.	Diarrhea, bowel leakage.	Overuse can interfere with absorption of fat-soluble vitamins and other nutrients.
castor oil	OTC	Same as mineral oil.	Same as mineral oil.	Same as mineral oil.

Stimulant Laxatives

senna concentrates (Dosaflex, Fletcher's Castoria, Senokot)	OTC	Same as magnesium hydroxide.	Diarrhea, bowel irritation.	Same as magnesium hydroxide.

Generic (Brand-Name Examples)	OTC Rx	Used for	Major side effects	Special precautions
yellow phenolphthalein (Ex-Lax); (with docusate sodium) (Correctol, Dialose Plus)	OTC	Treating occasional constipation.	Diarrhea, bowel irritation.	Same as magnesium hydroxide.

Stool softeners

docusate sodium (Colace, Surfak); (with casanthranol) (Peri-Colace)	OTC	Treating occasional or chronic constipation.	Bowel urgency.	Safer than most laxatives for long-term use.

HORMONE PREPARATIONS

Growth Hormones

somatrem (Protropin)	Rx	Promoting normal growth in children with a hormone deficiency.	May reduce thyroid function and promote insulin resistance.	Tell the doctor if the child has diabetes or thyroid malfunction.

Hormone Replacement: Androgens

danazol (Danocrine)	Rx	Treating endometriosis, fibrocystic breasts	Unusual growth of hair, deepening of voice and other signs of masculinization; increased risk of stroke due to abnormal clotting.	Tell your doctor if you have liver, kidney, or heart disease, or a history of epileptic seizures or unexplained vaginal bleeding. Pregnancy should be postponed for three months after discontinuing use of this drug.
testosterone (Testoderm, DEPO-Testosterone)	Rx	Stimulating bone and muscle growth; stimulating sexual development in men.	(in women) Unusual hair growth; voice change, masculinization.	Tell your doctor if you have diabetes, liver, heart, or prostate problems. Provide information about other medications you are taking.

Hormone Replacement: Estrogens

estradiol (Delestrogen, Depo-Estradiol, Estrace)	Rx	Relieving hot flashes, vaginal dryness, and other menopausal symptoms; postmenopausal estrogen replacement to prevent osteoporosis and heart disease.	Nausea, breast tenderness, weight gain, bloating, fluid retention.	Tell your doctor if you have impaired liver or kidney function, high blood pressure, diabetes, if you smoke, or have had a stroke or repeated migraines or epileptic seizures. Do not use if you have breast cancer. Should have pap smear and pelvic exam every 6 to 12 months.
estropipate (Ogen)	Rx	Same as estradiol.	Same as estradiol.	Same as estradiol.
conjugated estrogens (Premarin)	Rx	Same as estradiol.	Same as estradiol.	Same as estradiol.

Hormone Replacement: Progestins

medroxyprogesterone (Cycrin, Provera)	Rx	Treating menstrual disorders and endometriosis, also with estrogen replacement therapy to prevent overgrowth of uterine lining (endometrium).	Swollen ankles, weight gain, vaginal bleeding.	Tell your doctor if you have diabetes, high blood pressure, impaired kidney or liver function, or have had a stroke. Provide information about all medications you are taking.

Other Hormonal Agonists/Antagonists

finasteride (Proscar)	Rx	Treating symptomatic benign prostatic hyperplasia (BPH).	Genitourinary problems such as impotence, decreased libido, and decreased volume of ejaculate.	Do not use if you are hypersensitive to any component of the drug. If your partner is pregnant, either avoid exposing her to your semen or stop using the drug during the pregnancy. Use caution if you have impaired liver function.

NEUROLOGICAL DRUGS

Anticonvulsants
Note: driving is inadvisable when taking these drugs.

carbamazepine (Tegretol)	Rx	Treating epilepsy/seizure disorders.	Drowsiness, dizziness, nausea.	Tell your doctor about liver or kidney malfunction; coronary, circulatory, or prostate problems, sensitivity to tricyclic antidepressants, and other medications you are taking.
clonazepam (Klonopin)	Rx	Same as carbamazepine.	Drowsiness, dizziness, behavioral changes.	Tell your doctor about liver or kidney malfunction, glaucoma, a history of respiratory diseases or substance abuse, and other medications you are taking. This drug usually is not prescribed during pregnancy.

Generic (Brand-Name Examples)	OTC Rx	Used for	Major side effects	Special precautions
ethosuximide (Zarontin)	Rx	Same as carbamazepine.	Drowsiness, dizziness, loss of appetite.	Tell your doctor if you have liver or kidney malfunction, diabetes or porphyria. Provide information about all medications. This drug is not usually prescribed during pregnancy.
felbamate (Felbatol)	Rx	Same as carbamazepine.	Acne, blurred vision, gastrointestinal upset.	Do not discontinue use without consulting your doctor. Inform your doctor if you are pregnant or planning a pregnancy.
phenytoin (Dilantin)	Rx	Same as carbamazepine.	Dizziness, blurred speech, increased body hair.	Tell your doctor if you have diabetes or impaired liver or kidney function. Provide information about all medications. Do not use this drug during pregnancy or breast-feeding.
primidone (Mysoline)	Rx	Same as carbamazepine.	Drowsiness, dizziness, confusion, irritability, appetite loss.	Tell your doctor about coronary, circulatory, or respiratory problems; liver or kidney malfunction, or chronic pain. Provide information about other medications. Do not use this drug during pregnancy or breast-feeding.
valproic acid (Depakene)	Rx	Same as carbamazepine.	Has caused fatal liver damage, especially when given to young children. Also may cause drowsiness, confusion, and abnormal clotting.	Tell your doctor about impaired liver or kidney function and provide information about all medications. Do not use this drug during pregnancy.

Antiparkinsonism Agents

Generic (Brand-Name Examples)	OTC Rx	Used for	Major side effects	Special precautions
amantadine (Symmetrel)	Rx	Treating Parkinson's disease and drug-induced movement disorders.	Fluid retention, low blood pressure, headache, dizziness, insomnia, mood changes, nausea and other GI symptoms, dry nose and mouth.	Tell your doctor about impaired liver or kidney function or a history of epileptic seizures. Provide information about other medications.
benztropine (Cogentin)	Rx	Same as amantadine.	Blurred vision, dry mouth and eyes, constipation, difficult urination, confusion, psychotic symptoms, and GI disturbances.	Tell your doctor if you have impaired liver or kidney function, high blood pressure, peptic ulcers, urinary problems, glaucoma, or a history of depression. Inform your doctor about other medications you are taking.
bromocriptine (Parlodel)	Rx	Same as amantadine, plus acromegaly; stop breast milk production.	Nausea, vomiting, dizziness, headache, drowsiness, fatigue, low blood pressure, fluid retention, shortness of breath.	Take with meals to reduce side effects. Tell your doctor if you have a stomach ulcer, inner ear disorder, or cold extremities. Inform your doctor about other medications.
levodopa (Larodopa); levodopa with carbidopa (Sinemet)	Rx	Treating Parkinson's disease.	Gastrointestinal disturbances, agitation, abnormal movements, cardiac arrhythmias, mental changes.	Tell your doctor about kidney and liver problems; heart, respiratory, or thyroid conditions, or glaucoma, also other medications you are taking.
selegiline hydrochloride (Eldepryl)	Rx	Treating Parkinson's disease (only in combination with other drugs).	May affect numerous body symptoms to produce side effects similar to those of amantadine.	Increasing the prescribed dose may result in a dangerous rise in blood pressure. Notify your doctor at once if you develop a severe headache.
trihexyphenidyl (Artane)	Rx	Same as amantadine.	Dry mouth and eyes, blurred vision, constipation, abnormal movements, cardiac arrhythmias, weakness.	Tell your doctor about impaired kidney, liver, or prostate function, high blood pressure, or glaucoma; also other medications you are taking.

Muscle Relaxants

Generic (Brand-Name Examples)	OTC Rx	Used for	Major side effects	Special precautions
chlorzoxazone (Paraflex)	Rx	Relaxing muscle spasms and relieving pain caused by injury.	Headache, drowsiness.	Tell your doctor about impaired liver or kidney function, allergies, and other medications you are taking.
cyclobenzaprine (Flexeril)	Rx	Same as chlorzoxazone.	Dry mouth, dizziness, drowsiness.	Tell your doctor about coronary, urinary, or thyroid problems or glaucoma, also other medications you are taking.

Generic (Brand-Name Examples)	OTC	Rx	Used for	Major side effects	Special precautions
methocarbamol (Robaxin)		Rx	Relaxing muscle spasms, treating tetanus.	Dizziness, headache, itchy rash.	Tell your doctor if you have impaired liver or kidney function and about other medications you are taking.
orphenadrine (Norflex)		Rx	Same as methocarbamol; also relief of muscular rigidity in parkinsonism.	Same as methocarbamol.	Same as methocarbamol, plus blurred vision.

PSYCHOTROPIC/MOOD ALTERING DRUGS
Note: Most of these drugs can become habit-forming if taken over a long period. Driving is inadvisable when taking drugs that induce drowsiness.

Antianxiety Agents

Generic (Brand-Name Examples)	OTC	Rx	Used for	Major side effects	Special precautions
alprazolam (Xanax)		Rx	Treating panic attacks and anxiety.	Dizziness, dry mouth, constipation, drowsiness; prolonged used may cause drug dependence.	Tell your doctor if you have impaired kidney or liver function, or a history of substance abuse, and about other medications you are taking.
chlordiazepoxide (Libritabs, Librium)		Rx	Treating anxiety; reducing symptoms of withdrawal from alcohol.	Same as alprazolam.	Same as alprazolam.
clorazepate (Tranxene)		Rx	Same as alprazolam.	Same as alprazolam.	Same as alprazolam.
diazepam (Valium, Valrelease)		Rx	Relieving psychological and physical tension and inducing sleep.	Same as alprazolam.	Same as alprazolam, plus information about respiratory disease.
lorazepam (Ativan)		Rx	Treating anxiety and insomnia.	Same as alprazolam.	Tell your doctor if you have impaired liver or kidney function, severe respiratory problems, or a history of substance abuse, and about other medications you are taking.
meprobamate (Equanil, Miltown)		Rx	Anxiety, stress, and (with aspirin) reducing pain.	Same as alprazolam.	Same as alprazolam.
oxazepam (Serax)		Rx	Reducing tension and inducing sleep.	Same as alprazolam.	Same as alprazolam.

Antidepressants

Generic (Brand-Name Examples)	OTC	Rx	Used for	Major side effects	Special precautions
amitriptyline (Elavil, Endep)		Rx	Treating clinical depression.	Drowsiness, dizziness, blurred vision, sweating, dry mouth, low blood pressure, breast growth in men, mental changes.	Tell your doctor if you have heart or prostate problems, glaucoma, or a history of epileptic seizures. Provide information about other medications.
amoxapine (Asendin)		Rx	Treating all types of depression, plus depression with anxiety and agitation.	Anxiety, tremors, confusion, palpitations, dizziness, sweating, increased appetite.	Same as amitriptyline.
bupropion (Wellbutrin)		Rx	Treating major depressive disorders.	Mental changes and instability, risk of suicide, weight loss, insomnia.	Do not combine with any other drug that might trigger seizures. Tell your doctor if you have an eating disorder. Provide your doctor with information about other medications.
doxepin (Adapin, Sinequan)		Rx	Same as amoxapine.	Dizziness, drowsiness, dry mouth, blurred vision, low blood pressure, GI upset, altered libido, male breast growth, weight gain.	Tell your doctor if you have heart or prostate problems, glaucoma, or a history of epileptic seizures, also about other medications you take.
fluoxetine (Prozac)		Rx	Treating uncomplicated depression.	Anxiety, agitation, dizziness, sweating, weight loss.	Do not take this drug if you are using an MAO inhibitor. Tell your doctor about liver or kidney malfunction, diabetes, or a recent heart attack; also other medications you are taking.
imipramine (Tofranil)		Rx	Treating simple depression.	Similar to doxepin.	Dizziness, dry mouth, sweating, blurred vision.
maprotiline (Ludiomil)		Rx	Treating depressive neurosis, manic-depression, anxiety with depression.	Drowsiness, rash, nervousness, dizziness, dry mouth, constipation, nausea and other GI upsets.	Same as imipramine; also tell your doctor if you are breast-feeding or taking other medications.
phenelzine (Nardil)		Rx	Treating atypical depression or when other drugs fail.	Dizziness, headache, drowsiness, constipation, low blood pressure, edema, sexual problems, blurred vision, nervousness and other mental changes, weight gain.	Same as maprotiline; also tell your doctor if you have celiac disease.

Generic (Brand-Name Examples)	OTC Rx	Used for	Major side effects	Special precautions
sertraline (Zoloft)	Rx	Treating simple depression.	Same as maprotiline, plus gastro-intestinal upset and difficulty with ejaculation.	Tell your doctor if you have liver or kidney malfunction, and about other medications you are taking. Do not drink alcoholic beverages.
trazodone (Desyrel)	Rx	Treating depression, with or without anxiety.	Drowsiness, dizziness, dry mouth, confusion, fatigue, head-ache, insomnia, nausea, muscle aches.	Tell your doctor if you have impaired liver or kidney function, have had a recent heart attack or a history of epileptic seizures. Be alert to possible erection abnormality (priapism).
Antimanic Agents				
lithium (Eskalith, LITHONATE, LITHOTABS)	Rx	Treating manic phase of manic-depression.	Gastrointestinal upsets, tremor, lithium toxicity.	Tell your doctor if you have liver, kid-ney, or thyroid malfunction; diabetes, or heart or circulation disorders, or a history of epileptic seizures. See your doctor frequently for blood tests to make sure dosage is appropriate.
Antipsychotic Agents				
chlorpromazine (Thorazine)	Rx	Treating severe psychotic dis-orders, including schizophrenia, manic episodes; severe nausea and vomiting, intractable hiccups.	Dizziness, drowsiness, blurred vision, tremor, drooling, difficulty controlling certain movements, rapid heartbeat, urinary problems, increased sun sensitivity, dry mouth, breast enlargement in men, milk production in women.	Tell your doctor if you have impaired liver or kidney function, glaucoma; heart, thyroid, or Parkinson's disease, or a history of epileptic seizures; also about other medications you take.
clozapine (Clozaril)	Rx	Severe schizophrenia.	Same as chlorpromazine, plus possible high fever.	Since in a few cases, this drug may cause a life-threatening drop in certain white cells, a weekly blood test is advisable. Do not take other medications of any kind, including OTC products, without your doctor's approval. Tell your doctor if you have glaucoma, an enlarged prostate, or liver or kidney disease.
fluphenazine (Permitil, Prolixin)	Rx	Severe psychotic disorders.	Same as chlorpromazine.	Tell your doctor if you have kidney or liver disease; prostate, thyroid, or heart problems; glaucoma or a history of epileptic seizures; also about other medications you take.
haloperidol (Haldol)	Rx	Treating psychotic disorders, Tourette's syndrome, severe hyperactivity, and severe compulsive behavior disorder.	Same as chlorpromazine.	Tell your doctor if you have impaired liver or kidney function, glaucoma, heart, circulation, or respiratory problems; parkinsonism or epileptic seizures; also about other medica-tions you are taking.
perphenazine (Trilafon)	Rx	Same as haloperidol.	Same as chlorpromazine.	Same as haloperidol.
thioridazine (Mellaril)	Rx	Treating psychotic disorders; also short-term use for treating severe depression with anxiety, agitation, or severe behavior disorders; short-term use for severe hyperactivity.	Same as chlorpromazine.	Same as haloperidol.
thiothixene (Navane)	Rx	Treating psychotic disorders.	Same as chlorpromazine, but usually not as pronounced.	This drug must be closely monitored if you have or have had a brain tumor, breast cancer, glaucoma, or are recovering from drug or alcohol addiction. Provide information about other medications you are taking.

Generic (Brand-Name Examples)	OTC Rx	Used for	Major side effects	Special precautions
trifluoperazine (Stelazine)	Rx	Treating psychotic disorders and generalized anxiety disorder.	Same as chlorpromazine.	This drug should not be used if you have abnormal liver, blood, or bone marrow conditions. Do not discontinue this drug without consulting your doctor. Provide information about medications you are taking.

Behavior Modifiers

Generic (Brand-Name Examples)	OTC Rx	Used for	Major side effects	Special precautions
disulfiram (Antabuse)	Rx	Helping to abstain from alcohol.	Drowsiness, headache.	Tell your doctor if you have kidney, liver, thyroid, or heart disease, diabetes, or a history of epileptic seizures. Since drinking even a small amount of alcohol when taking this medication may result in unconsciousness, you should carry a card with information about whom to notify in an emergency.
nicotine patches (Habitrol, Nicoderm, Nicotrol, Prostep)	Rx	Helping to gradually overcome addiction to nicotine.	Rash, itching, rapid heartbeat, diarrhea, insomnia, nervousness.	Watch for severe and unpleasant allergic skin reactions. Do not smoke while wearing the patch or for at least several hours after removing it. Tell your doctor about all your physical disorders and other medications you are taking.
nicotine polacrilex (Nicorette)	Rx	Same as nicotine patches.	Indigestion, nausea, mouth sores, bleeding gums, sweating, burning or tingling sensations.	Generally not recommended for persons with heart disease, high blood pressure, overactive thyroid, and peptic ulcers. Gum may stick to dentures or bridges. Should not chew more than 30 2-milligram (or 20 4-milligram) pieces day.

Sleep-Inducing (Sedative) Agents
NOTE: These drugs are potentially addictive. Alcohol should not be used when taking these drugs.

Generic (Brand-Name Examples)	OTC Rx	Used for	Major side effects	Special precautions
estazolam (ProSom)	Rx	Treating short-term insomnia.	Dizziness, impaired coordination, lack of energy and weakness.	Tell your doctor if you have had a recent serious illness, chronic respiratory problems, or kidney or liver malfunction, and about other medications you are taking. Do not take this drug if you are pregnant since it may result in birth defects.
flurazepam (Dalmane)	Rx	Same as estazolam.	Daytime drowsiness, dizziness, palpitations, drooling, stomach upset, urinary problems, generalized achiness.	Tell your doctor if you have impaired liver or kidney function, acute respiratory disease, or a history of substance abuse, and about other medications you are taking.
quazepam (Doral)	Rx	Same as estazolam.	Daytime drowsiness, headache, dizziness, indigestion.	Do not take this drug if you have sleep apnea, if you are suffering from depression, or if you are pregnant. A history of substance abuse increases the risk of addiction to this drug.
temazepam (Restoril)	Rx	Same as estazolam.	Daytime drowsiness, dizziness, headache, lethargy, confusion, nausea, dry mouth.	Tell your doctor if you have impaired liver or kidney function, respiratory disease, or a history of substance abuse. Provide information about other medications you are taking.
triazolam (Halcion)	Rx	Same as estazolam.	Daytime drowsiness, dizziness, coordination problems, nausea, lightheadedness.	Tell your doctor if you have impaired liver or kidney function or a history of substance abuse, and about other medications you are taking.
zolpidem (Ambien)	Rx	Same as estazolam.	Same as flurazepam plus lethargy, diarrhea or constipation, sore throat, sinusitis, coughing, and other respiratory symptoms.	Tell your doctor if you have kidney or liver disorders. Do not discontinue use of this drug without consulting your doctor.

ADDICTION

Alcoholism
Al-Anon Family Group
Headquarters
1372 Broadway
New York, NY 10018
(212) 302-7240
Mailing address:
P.O. Box 862
Midtown Station
New York, NY 10018-0862

American Council on Alcoholism
2522 St. Paul Street
Baltimore, MD 21218
(410) 889-0100
(800) 527-5344

Association of Halfway House
Alcoholism Programs of
North America
680 Stuart Avenue
St. Paul, MN 55102
(612) 227-7818

National Association of Children of
Alcoholics Inc.
11426 Rockville Pike, Suite 100
Rockville, MD 20852
(301) 468-0985

National Clearinghouse for Alcohol
and Drug Information
Box 2345
Rockville, MD 29847
(301) 468-2600 (800) 729-6686

National Council on Alcoholism and
Drug Dependence
12 West 21st Street
New York, NY 10010
(212) 206-6770 (800) NCA-CALL

Cocaine
Cocaine Abuse Hotline
P.O. Box 878
Port Hueneme, CA 93041
(800) 568-3303

Drug and Alcohol Helpline
(800) 787-7505

The Helpline
(800) 676-7574

Smoking
Action on Smoking and Health
(ASH)
2013 H Street NW
Washington, DC 20006
(202) 659-4310

Office on Smoking & Health,
Centers for Disease Control
Public Information Branch
Mail Stop K50
4770 Buford Highway
Atlanta, GA 30333
(404) 488-5705

Smokenders
4455 East Camelback Road,
Suite D150
Phoenix, AZ 85018
(800) 828-4357

Smoke Stoppers Program
National Center for Health
Promotion
3920 Varsity Drive
Ann Arbor, MI 48108
(313) 971-6077

Stop Teenage Addiction to Tobacco
511 East Columbus Avenue
Springfield, MA 01105
(413) 732-STAT

AGING
American Association of Retired
Persons
601 E Street NW
Washington, DC 20049
(202) 434-2277

Children of Aging Parents (CAPS)
1609 Woodbourne Road,
Suite 302A
Levittown, PA 19057-1511
(215) 945-6900

National Caucus & Center on Black
Aged Inc.
1424 K Street NW, Suite 500
Washington, DC 20005
(202) 637-8400

National Council on the Aging
409 Third Street SW
Washington, DC 20024
(202) 479-1200

National Council of Senior Citizens
1331 F Street NW
Washington, DC 20004
(202) 347-8800

ALLERGIES
American Allergy Association
P.O. Box 7273
Menlo Park, CA 94026
(415) 322-1663

National Allergy and Asthma
Network
3554 Chainbridge Road, Suite 200
Fairfax, VA 22030
(703) 385-4403

ALTERNATIVE THERAPIES

Acupuncture
American Academy of Medical
Acupuncture
5820 Wilshire Boulevard, Suite 500
Los Angeles, CA 90036
(213) 937-5514

American Acupuncture Society
1021 Park Avenue
New York, NY 10028
(718) 886-4431

American Association of Acupuncture
and Oriental Medicine
433 Front Street
Catasauqua, PA 18032
(610) 433-2448

American Oriental Acupuncture
Center
52 East Broadway
New York, NY 10002
(212) 343-2511

National Commission for the
Certification of Acupuncturists
1424 16th Street NW
Washington, DC 20036
(202) 232-1404

STATE REQUIREMENTS FOR ACUPUNCTURISTS

States that license, certify, or
register acupuncturists:
Alaska
California
Colorado
District of Columbia
Florida
Hawaii
Iowa
Maine
Massachusetts
Montana
Nevada
New Jersey
New Mexico
North Carolina
Oregon
Rhode Island
Texas
Utah
Vermont
Virginia
Washington
Wisconsin

Practice limited to physicians or
osteopaths:
Arizona
Georgia
Indiana
Kentucky
Louisiana
Minnesota
Mississippi
Nebraska
New Hampshire
North Dakota
Ohio
West Virginia

Practice limited to physicians,
osteopaths, or chiropractors:
Alabama
Illinois

Practice allowed under medical
supervision:
Connecticut
Delaware
Kansas
Michigan
Missouri
New York
Pennsylvania
South Carolina

No regulations:
Arkansas
Idaho
Maryland
Oklahoma
South Dakota
Tennessee
Wyoming

Alexander Technique
American Center for the Alexander
Technique
129 West 67th Street
New York, NY 10023
(212) 799-0468

North American Society of Teachers
of Alexander Technique
Box 517, Urbana, IL 61801
(217) 367-6956

Aromatherapy
National Association for
Holistic Aromatherapy
P.O. Box 4996
Boulder, CO 80306

Art Therapy
American Art Therapy Association
1202 Allanson Road
Mundelein, IL 60060
(708) 949-6064

Biofeedback
Association for Applied Psycho-
physiology and Biofeedback
Biofeedback Certification Institute
of America
10200 West 44th Avenue, Suite 304
Wheat Ridge, CO 80033
(303) 422-8436

Center for Applied Psychophysi-
ology and Biofeedback
Menninger Clinic, P.O. Box 829
Topeka, KA 66601
(913) 273-7500

Chiropractic
American Chiropractic Association
1701 Claredon Boulevard
Arlington, VA 22209
(703) 276-8800

Dance Therapy
American Dance Therapy
Association
2000 Century Plaza, Suite 108
Columbia, MD 21044
(410) 997-4040

Herbal Medicine
Herb Research Foundation
1007 Pearl Street, Suite 200
Boulder, CO 80302
(303) 449-2265

The American Botanical Council
Box 201660
Austin, TX 78720
(512) 331-8868

Homeopathy
American Institute of Homeopathy
(303) 898-5477 (answering service)

Foundation for Homeopathic
Education & Research
2036 Blake Street
Berkeley, CA 94704
(510) 649-8930

The National Center for
Homeopathy
801 North Fairfax, Suite 306
Alexandria, VA 22314
(703) 548-7790

Hypnosis

American Council of Clinical
  Hypnosis
2200 East Devon Avenue, Suite 291
Des Plaines, IL 60018
(708) 297-3317

American Guild of Hypnotherapists
7117 Farnam Street, Room 31
Omaha, NE 68132
(402) 397-1500

Hypnosis Consultation Center
1 Lincoln Street, Box 452
North Haven, CT 06473
(203) 239-7046

Light Therapy

Light Therapy Unit
Michael Terman, Ph.D., Director,
Columbia Presbyterian
  Medical Center
N.Y. State Psychiatric Institute
722 West 168 Street
New York, NY 10032
(212) 960-5712

Society for Light Treatment
10200 West 44th Avenue, Suite 304
Wheat Ridge, CO 80033
 (303) 424-3697

Massage and Manipulation

American Massage Therapy
  Association
820 Davis Street, Suite 100
Evanston, IL 60201-4444
(312) 761-AMTA

American Oriental Body Work
  Therapy Association
6801 Jericho Turnpike
Syosset, NY 11791
(516) 364-5533

Rolfing Institute
205 Canyon Boulevard
Boulder, CO 80302
(303) 449-5903

Meditation

American Association of Ayurvedic
  Medicine
P.O. Box 49667
Colorado Springs, CO 80949-9667
(719) 260-5500

Stress Reduction Clinic
Jon Kabat-Zinn, Ph.D., Director,
University of Massachusetts
  Medical Center
Worcester, MA 01655
(508) 856-0011

Movement Therapies

American Yoga Association
513 South Orange Avenue
Sarasota, FL 34236
(813) 953-5859
(800) 226-5859

Himalayan International Institute of
  Yoga Science & Philosophy
RR1, Box 400
Honesdale, PA 18431
(717) 253-5551

Music Therapy

American Association for Music
  Therapy
Box 80012
Valley Forge, PA 19484
(610) 265-4006

National Association for
  Music Therapy
8455 Colesville Road, Suite 930
Silver Spring, MD 20910
(301) 589-3300

Naturopathy

American Association of
  Naturopathic Physicians (referral
  and information request line)
2366 Eastlake Avenue East,
  Suite 322
Seattle, Washington 98102
(206) 323-7610
(206) 323-7612 FAX

Bastyr University
144 NE 54th Street
Seattle, Washington 98105
(206) 323-9585

Bastyr University Natural Health
  Clinic
1307 North 45th Street, Suite 200
Seattle, Washington 98105
(206) 632-0354

National College of Naturopathic
  Medicine
11231 SE Market Street
Portland, OR 97216
(503) 255-4860

Nutrition Therapy

American Dietetic Association
216 West Jackson Boulevard,
  Suite 800
Chicago, IL 60606-6995
(312) 899-0040

Nutrition Institute of America
200 West 86th Street, Suite 17A
New York, NY 10024
(212) 799-2234

Pet Therapy

People - Animals - Love
c/o MacArthur Animal Hospital
4832 MacArthur Boulevard NW
Washington, DC 20007
(202) 337-0120

Therapy Dogs International
6 Hilltop Road
Mendhan, NJ 07945
(201) 543-0888

Visualization

Academy for Guided Imagery
P.O. Box 2070
Mill Valley, CA 94942
(415) 389-9324

BIRTH DEFECTS

Association of Birth Defect Children
827 Irma Avenue
Orlando, FL 32803
(407) 245-7035

Spina Bifida

Spina Bifida Association of America
4590 MacArthur Boulevard,
  Suite 250
Washington, DC 20007
(202) 944-3285
(800) 621-3141

BLOOD DISORDERS

Cooley's Anemia

Cooley's Anemia Foundation
129-09 26th Avenue
Flushing, NY 11354
(718) 321-2873
(800) 522-7222

Hemochromatosis

Hemochromatosis Foundation
Box 8569
Albany, NY 12208
(518) 489-0972

Iron Overload Diseases Association
433 Westwind Drive
North Palm Beach, FL 33408
(407) 840-8512

Hemophilia

National Hemophilia Foundation
The Soho Building
110 Greene Street, Room 303
New York, NY 10012
(212) 219-8180

Leukemia

Leukemia Society of America
600 Third Avenue
New York, NY 10016
(212) 573-8484

BONE DISEASES

Osteoporosis

National Osteoporosis Foundation
1150 17th Street NW, Suite 500
Washington, DC 20036-4603
(202) 223-2226

Paget's Disease

Foundation for Paget's Disease of
  Bone & Related Disorders
200 Varick Street, Suite 1004
New York, NY 10014-4810
(212) 229-1582

Scoliosis

Scoliosis Association Inc.
Box 811705
Boca Raton, FL 33481-1705
(407) 994-4435
(800) 800-0669

CANCER

American Cancer Society Inc.
1599 Clifton Road NE
Atlanta, GA 30329
(404) 320-3333
American Cancer Society Response
  Line: (800) ACS-2345

Cancer Care
1180 Avenue of the Americas
New York, NY 10036
(212) 221-3300

Cancer Hotline
R. A. Bloch Foundation
(816) 932-8453
(For advice on seeking treatment.)

Cancer Information Clearinghouse,
  National Cancer Institute
1275 York Avenue, Box 166
New York, NY 10021
(800) 4-CANCER
In Hawaii:
University of Hawaii,
1236 Lauhala, Room 406
Honolulu, HI 96813
(808) 524-1234

National Bone Marrow Donor
  Program
3433 Broadway Street NE,
  Suite 400
Minneapolis, MN 55413
(800) 654-1247

The Candlelighters Childhood
  Cancer Foundation
7910 Woodmount Avenue,
  Suite 460
Bethesda, MD 20814
(301) 657-8401
(800) 366-2223

Breast Cancer

Susan J. Komen Breast Cancer
  Foundation
5005 LBJ Freeway, Suite 370
Dallas, TX 75244
(214) 450-1777
(800) 462-9273

National Alliance of Breast Cancer
  Organizations
9 East 37th Street, 10th Floor
New York, NY 10016
(212) 719-0154

Y-ME Breast Cancer
  Support Program
212 West Van Buren, 4th Floor
Chicago, IL 60607
(312) 986-8338
(800) 221-2141

Colorectal Cancer

United Ostomy Association
36 Executive Park, Suite 120
Irvine, CA 92714
(714) 660-8624
(800) 826-0826

Kaposi's Sarcoma

Gay Men's Health Crisis
  (for experimental treatments)
Department of Treatment,
  Education, and Advocacy
129 West 20th Street
New York, NY 10011
(212) 337-3505

Leukemia and Lymphoma

Leukemia Society of America
600 3rd Avenue
New York, NY 10016
(212) 573-8484

Prostate Cancer

US-TOO International
930 North York Road, Suite 50
Hinsdale, IL 60521-2993
(708) 323-1002
(800) 808-7866

CARDIOVASCULAR DISEASE AND STROKE

Heart Disorders

American Heart Association
1615 Stemmons Freeway
Dallas, TX 75207-8808
(214) 748-7212

American Heart Association's
   National Office of the Mended
   Hearts Club
7272 Greenville Avenue
Dallas, TX 75231
(214) 373-6300

Heartline
9500 Euclid Avenue, Room EE-37
Cleveland, OH 44195
(216) 444-3690
(800) 478-4255

National Heart, Lung, and Blood
   Institute Information Center
P.O. Box 30105
Bethesda, MD 20824-0105
(301) 251-1222

Stroke

American Paralysis Association
Box 187
Short Hills, NJ 07078
or 500 Morris Avenue
Springfield, NJ 07081
(201) 379-2690

Courage Center Stroke Network
3915 Golden Valley Road
Golden Valley, MN 55422
(612) 588-0811

National Stroke Association
8480 East Orchard Road,
Suite 1000
Englewood, CO 80111
(303) 771-1700
(800) STROKES
(800) 367-1990

The Stroke Foundation
898 Park Avenue
New York, NY 10021
(212) 734-3461

DIGESTIVE DISORDERS

Crohn's Disease & Colitis
   Foundation of America
386 Park Avenue South, 17th Floor
New York, NY 10016
(212) 685-3440
(800) 932-2423 (information)
(800) 343-3637 (literature)

National Digestive Diseases
   Information Clearinghouse
2 Information Way
Bethesda, MD 20892-3570
(301) 654-3810

GENETIC DISEASES

Alliance of Genetic Support Groups
35 Wisconsin Circle, Suite 440
Chevy Chase, MD 20815
(800) 336-4363

American Genetic Association
P.O. Box 39
Buckeyetown, MD 21717
(301) 695-9292

March of Dimes/Birth Defects
   Foundation
1275 Mamaroneck Avenue
White Plains, NY 10605
(914) 428-7100

National Foundation for Jewish
   Genetic Diseases
250 Park Avenue, Suite 1000
New York, NY 10017
(212) 371-1030

Cystic Fibrosis

Cystic Fibrosis Association
2250 North Druid Hills Road,
Suite 275
Atlanta, GA 30329
(404) 325-6973

Cystic Fibrosis Foundation
6931 Arlington Road
Bethesda, MD 20814
(301) 951-4422
(800) FIGHT CF

Sickle Cell Disease

National Sickle Cell Disease
   Program
National Heart, Lung, Blood Institute
Federal Building, Room 508
7550 Wisconsin Avenue
Bethesda, MD 20892
(301) 496-6931

Sickle Cell Disease Association of
   America
200 Corporate Point, Suite 495
Culver City, CA 90230
(310) 216-6363
(800) 421-8453

HEARING IMPAIRMENT

Alexander Graham Bell Association
   for the Deaf
3417 Volta Place NW
Washington, DC 20007-2778
(202) 337-5220

American Speech-Language-
   Hearing Association
Consumer Affairs Division
10801 Rockville Pike
Rockville, MD 20852
(301) 897-5700
(800) 638-8255

American Tinnitus Association
Box 5
Portland, OR 97207
(503) 248-9985

Better Hearing Institute
Box 1840
Washington, DC 20013
(703) 642-0582
(703) 642-0580
(800) 327-9355

Deafness Research Foundation
9 East 38th Street
New York, NY 10016
(212) 684-6556
(800) 535-3323
(212) 684-6559 TDD

Dogs for the Deaf
10175 Wheeler Road
Central Point, OR 97502
(503) 826-9220

Ear Foundation
2000 Church Street, Box 111
Nashville, TN 37236
(615) 327-7807
(800) 545-4327

Hear Now
9745 East Hampden Avenue,
Suite 300
Denver, CO 80231-4923
(303) 695-7797
(800) 648-4327 voice/TDD

National Association of the Deaf
814 Thayer Avenue
Silver Spring, MD 20910
Headquarters:
(301) 587-1788 voice
(301) 587-1789 TTD
(301) 587-1791 FAX
Bookstore:
(301) 587-6282 voice
(301) 587-6283 TTD
(301) 587-4873 FAX

National Information Center on
   Deafness
Gallaudet University
800 Florida Avenue NE
Washington, DC 20002
(202) 651-5051
(202) 651-5052 TDD

Self-Help for Hard of Hearing
   People Inc.
7910 Woodmont Avenue,
Suite 1200
Bethesda, MD 20814
(301) 657-2248
(301) 657-2249 TDD

INFECTIOUS DISEASES

National Institute of Allergies and
   Infectious Diseases
NIH Building 31, Room 7A50
9000 Rockville Pike
Bethesda, MD 20892-2522
(301) 496-5717

AIDS (Acquired Immune Deficiency Syndrome)

AIDS Clinical Trials Information
   Service
1600 Research Boulevard
Rockville, MD 20850
(800) 874-2572
(800) 243-7012 TDD

American Foundation for AIDS
   Research (AFAR)
733 Third Avenue, 12th Floor
New York, NY 10017-3204
(212) 682-7440

CDC National AIDS Clearinghouse
P.O. Box 6003
Rockville, MD 20849-6003
(800) 458-5231
The Centers for Disease Control

and Prevention (CDC) maintains a
24-hour hotline that provides confidential information and referral:
(800) 342-2437.
The hot line for deaf callers (M-F
10A.M.-10P.M.) is (800) 243-7889.
For Spanish speaking callers 8A.M.-
2A.M. daily): (800) 344-7432.
Hotline Director Mailing address for
   questions or problems:
CDC National AIDS Hotline
Box 13827
Research Triangle Park, NC 27709

HIV Center for Clinical and
   Behavioral Studies
722 West 168th Street, P.I. Unit
New York, NY 10032
(212) 740-0046
(212) 740-1774 FAX

People with AIDS Coalition
50 West 17th Street
New York, NY 10011
(212) 647-1415
Outside of NYC: (800) 828-3280

Sexually Transmitted Diseases

CDC's National STD Hotline
American Social Health Association
Box 13827
Research Park Triangle, NC 27709
(800) 227-8922

MENTAL HEALTH AND MENTAL ILLNESS

American Mental Health Foundation
2 East 86th Street
New York, NY 10028
(212) 737-9027

National Alliance for the Mentally Ill
200 North Glebe Road
Arlington, VA 22203-3754
(703) 524-7600
(800) 950-6264

National Association of State Mental
   Health Directors
66 Canal Center Plaza, Suite 302
Alexandria, VA 22314
(703) 739-9333

National Institute of Mental Health
Public Inquiries Section
5600 Fishers Lane, Room 7 C-02
Rockville, MD 20857
(301) 443-4513

National Mental Health Association
   Information Center
1021 Prince Street
Alexandria, VA 22314
(703) 684-7722
(800) 433-5959
(800) 969-6642

Anxiety Disorders

Council on Anxiety Disorders
P.O. Box 17011
Winston-Salem, NC 27116
(910) 722-7760

Autism

National Autism Services Hotline
Prichard Building
605 Ninth Street, Box 507
Huntington, WV 25710-0507
(304) 525-8014

Chronic Fatigue Syndrome
American Association for Chronic
   Fatigue Syndrome
Box 895
Olney, MD 20830

Chronic Fatigue and Immune
   Dysfunction Syndrome
   Association of America Inc.
Box 220398
Charlotte, NC 28222-0398
(800) 442-3437
CFIDS information line:
(900) 896-2343 $2/first minute and
   $1/each additional minute

CFS-News Electronic Newsletter
   Internet address:
cfs-news@list.nih.gov

Consumer Health Information
   Research Institute
300 East Pink Hill Road
Independence, MO 64057
(816) 228-4595

Depression
Depression Awareness
c/o National Institute of Mental
   Health
Public Inquiries Section
5600 Fishers Lane, Room 7 C-02
Rockville, MD 20857
(800) 421-4211

Foundation for Depression and
   Manic Depression
24 East 81st Street, Suite 2B
New York, NY 10028
(212) 772-3400

National Foundation for Depressive
   Illness
P.O. Box 2257
New York, NY 10116
(800) 248-4344

Eating Disorders
Anorexia Nervosa & Associated
   Disorders
Box 7
Highland Park, IL 60035
(708) 831-3438

Mental Retardation
American Association on Mental
   Retardation
444 North Capital Street NW,
Suite 846
Washington, DC 20001
(202) 387-1968

Association for Retarded Citizens
500 East Border Street, Suite 300
Arlington, TX 76010
(817) 261-6003

Kennedy Child Study Center
151 East 67th Street
New York, NY 10021
(212) 988-9500

National Down Syndrome Congress
1605 Chantilly Drive, Suite 250
Atlanta, GA 30324
(800) 232-6372

National Down Syndrome Society
   Hotline
666 Broadway, 8th Floor
New York, NY 10012
(800) 221-4602

Schizophrenia
American Schizophrenia
   Association
2401 Le Conte Avenue
Berkeley, CA 94709

National Alliance for Research on
   Schizophrenia and Depression
60 Cutter Mill Road, Suite 200
Great Neck, NY 11021
(516) 829-0091

METABOLIC AND HORMONAL DISORDERS
Diabetes
American Diabetes Association
National Center
P.O. Box 2575,
1660 Duke Street
Alexandria, VA 22314
(703) 549-1500
(800) 232-3472

Juvenile Diabetes Foundation
International Hotline
432 Park Avenue South
New York, NY 10016
(212) 889-7575
(800) 223-1138

National Diabetes Information
   Clearinghouse
7 Information Way
Bethesda, MD 20892-3560
(301) 654-3327

Thyroid Disorders
Thyroid Foundation of America
40 Parkman Street, RSL-350
Boston, MA 02114
(617) 726-8500

NEUROLOGICAL DISORDERS
Alzheimer's Disease
Alzheimer's Disease Education and
   Referral Center
P.O. Box 8250
Silver Spring, MD 20907-8250
(301) 495-3311
(800) 438-4380

Association for Alzheimer's &
   Related Disorders
919 North Michigan Avenue,
Suite 1000
Chicago, IL 60611
(800) 272-3900

Cerebral Palsy
United Cerebral Palsy
   Associations Inc.
1660 L Street, Suite 700
Washington, DC 20036
(202) 842-1266

Epilepsy
Epilepsy Foundation of America
4351 Garden City Drive
Landover, MD 20785-2267
(301) 459-3700
(800) EFA-1000

Pediatric Epilepsy Center
The Johns Hopkins Medical
   Institutions
Meyer 2-147
600 North Wolfe Street
Baltimore, MD 21287
(for information on ketogenic diet
   therapy)

Guillain-Barré Syndrome
GBS Foundation International
Box 262
Wynnewood, PA 19096
(610) 667-0131

Headaches
National Headache Foundation
5252 North Western Avenue
Chicago, IL 60625
(312) 878-7715
(800) 843-2256

Head Injuries
National Head Injury Foundation
1776 Massachusetts Avenue NW,
Suite 100
Washington, DC 20036-1904
(202) 296-6443
(800) 444-NHIF

Huntington's Disease
Huntington's Disease Society of
   America
140 West 22nd Street
New York, NY 10011
(212) 242-1968
(800) 345-4372

Hydrocephalus
National Hydrocephalus Foundation
400 North Michigan Avenue,
Suite 1102
Chicago, IL 60611
(815) 467-6548

Learning Disabilities
Challenge (Attention Deficit
   Disorder information service)
42 Way to the River Road West
Newbury, MA 01985
(508) 462-0495

Children with Attention Deficit
   Disorder (CHADD)
499 NW 70th Avenue, Suite 109
Plantation, FL 33317
(305) 587-3700

Learning Disabilities Association
4156 Library Road
Pittsburgh, PA 15234
(412) 341-1515

National Information Center for
   Children & Youth with Learning
   Disabilities
Box 1492
Washington, DC 20013-1492
(800) 695-0285

Orton Dyslexia Society
P.O. Box 9888
Baltimore, MD 21284
(410) 296-0232
(800) 222-3123

Lou Gehrig's Disease
Amyotrophic Lateral Sclerosis
Association
21021 Ventura Boulevard, Suite 321
Woodland Hills, CA 91364
(818) 340-7500

Multiple Sclerosis
National Multiple Sclerosis Society
733 Third Avenue
New York, NY 10017
(212) 986-3240
(800) 344-4867
(212) 986-7981 FAX

Muscular Dystrophy
Muscular Dystrophy Association of
   America Inc.
3300 East Sunrise Drive
Tucson, AZ 85718
(602) 529-2000

Myasthenia Gravis
Myasthenia Gravis Foundation of
   America Inc.
222 South Riverside Plaza,
Room 1540
Chicago, IL 60606
(800) 541-5454

Myasthenia Gravis Foundation of
   Greater New York Inc.
61 Gramercy Park North, Room 605
New York, NY 10010
(212) 533-7005
(800) MGF-0808

Parkinson's Disease
American Parkinson's Disease
   Association
60 Bay Street, Suite 401
Staten Island, NY 10301
(718) 981-8001
(800) 223-2732

National Parkinson's Foundation
1501 NW Ninth Avenue
Miami, FL 33136
(305) 547-6666
(800) 327-4545
(800) 433-7022 in FL

Parkinson's Disease Foundation
710 West 168th Street
New York, NY 10032
(212) 923-4700

Parkinson's Education Program
3900 Birch Street, Room 105
Newport Beach, CA 92660
(714) 250-2975 voice
(800) 344-7872

Parkinson Support Group of America
11376 Cherry Hill Road, Suite 204
Beltsville, MD 20705
(301) 937-1545

United Parkinson's Foundation
833 West Washington Boulevard
Chicago, IL 60607
(312) 733-1893

Polio
Polio Society
Box 106273
Washington, DC 20016
(301) 897-8180

Smell and Taste Disorders
Smell and Taste Center
Hospital of the University of
  Pennsylvania
5 Ravdin Building
3400 Spruce Street
Philadelphia, PA 19104
(215) 662-6580

Tourette's Syndrome
Tourette's Syndrome Association
42-40 Bell Boulevard
Bayside, NY 11361
(718) 224-2999
(800) 237-0717

OBSTETRICS AND GYNECOLOGY
Childbearing and Birth
American Fertility Society
1209 Montgomery Highway
Birmingham, AL 35216-2809
(205) 978-5000

International Childbirth Education
  Association Inc.
Box 20048
Minneapolis, MN 55420
(612) 854-8660

Planned Parenthood Federation of
  America
810 Seventh Avenue
New York, NY 10019
(212) 541-7800

The Compassionate Friends Inc.
P.O. Box 3696
Oakbrook, IL 60522
(708) 990-0010

Gynecological Concerns
American College of Obstetricians &
  Gynecologists (Resource Center)
409 12th Street SW
Washington, DC 20024-2188

Endometriosis Association
8585 North 76th Place
Milwaukee, WI 53223
(414) 355-2200
(800) 992-3636

Hysterectomy Educational
  Resources & Services (HERS)
422 Bryn Mawr Avenue
Bala Cynwyd, PA 19004
(610) 667-7757

PMS Access
P.O. Box 9326
Madison, WI 53715
(800) 222-4767

PAIN SYNDROMES
American Chronic Pain Association
Box 850
Rocklin, CA 95677
(916) 632-0922

American Pain Society
5700 Old Orchard Road
Skokie, IL 60077
(708) 966-5595

Committee on Pain Therapy
American Society of
  Anesthesiologists
520 North Northwest Highway
Park Ridge, IL 60068
(708) 825-5586

National Chronic Pain Outreach
  Association
7979 Old Georgetown Road,
  Suite 100
Bethesda, MD 20814
(301) 652-4948

Pain Treatment Program of Lenox
  Hill Hospital
130 East 77th Street
New York, NY 10021
(212) 249-2200

The Pain Center of the Hospital for
  Joint Diseases
301 East 17th Street
New York, NY 10003
(212) 598-6606

PARALYSIS AND SPINAL CORD INJURIES
American Paralysis Association
500 Morris Avenue
Springfield, NJ 07081
(800) 225-0292

National Spinal Cord Injury
  Association
545 Concord Avenue, Suite 29
Cambridge, MA 02138
(800) 962-9629

RARE AND MISCELLANEOUS DISEASES
National Organization for
  Rare Disorders
Box 8923
New Fairfield, CT 06812-8923
(203) 746-6518
(800) 999-NORD

Ménière's Disease
Ménière's Network
200 Church Street, Box 111
Nashville, TN 37236
(800) 545-4327

Reye's Syndrome
National Reye's Syndrome
  Foundation
P.O. Box 829
Bryan, OH 53506
(419) 636-2679

Sudden Infant Death Syndrome (SIDS)
American SIDS Institute
6065 Roswell Road, Suite 876
Atlanta, GA 30328
(800) 232-7437
(800) 847-7437 in Georgia

SIDS Alliance
1314 Bedford Avenue, Suite 120
Baltimore, MD 21208
(800) 221-7437

SIDS New York City Program
520 First Avenue, Room 506
New York, NY 10016
(212) 686-8854

SIDS Resource Center
8201 Greensboro Drive, Suite 600
McLean, VA 22102
(703) 821-8955

RESPIRATORY DISORDERS
American Lung Association
1740 Broadway
New York, NY 10019-4374
(212) 315-8700

International Society for
  Respiratory Protection
Box 158
Jonesborough, TN 37659
(615) 753-1388

Asthma
Allergy Information Referral Line
611 Wells Street
Milwaukee, WI 53202
(800) 822-2762

Asthma and Allergy Foundation of
  America
1125 15th Street NW, Suite 502
Washington DC 20005
(202) 466-7643

National Allergy and Asthma
  Network
3554 Chain Bridge Road, Suite 200
Fairfax, VA 22030
(703) 385-4403

National Institute of Allergies
  and Infectious Diseases
NIH Building 31, Room 7A50
9000 Rockville Pike
Bethesda, MD 20892-2522
(301) 496-5717

Emphysema
New York Lung Association
432 Park Avenue South
New York, NY 10016
(212) 315-8700
(800) LUNG-USA

RHEUMATIC DISEASES
Arthritis
Arthritis Foundation Information Line
1314 Spring Street NW
Atlanta, GA 30309
(404) 872-7100
(800) 283-7800

National Arthritis & Musculoskeletal
  & Skin Diseases
Information Clearinghouse
1 AMS Circle
Bethesda, MD 20892-3675
(301) 495-4484

Lupus
American Lupus Society
260 Maple Court, Suite 123
Ventura, CA 93003
(805) 339-0443
(800) 331-1802

Lupus Foundation of America
4 Research Place, Suite 180
Rockville, MD 20850-3226
(301) 670-9292
(800) 558-0121

Lupus Network
455 Main Street
West Hartford, CT 06107
(203) 521-9151
(203) 242-2684

Lyme Disease
Lyme Disease Information Hotline
1 Financial Plaza, 18th Floor
Hartford, CT 06103-2610
(800)-886-LYME

Spinal Arthritis
Ankylosing Spondylitis Association
Box 5872
Sherman Oaks, CA 91413
(818) 981-1616
(800) 777-8189

SEXUALITY AND SEXUAL DYSFUNCTION
General Information
Alan Gutmacher Institute
120 Wall Street
New York, NY 10005
(212) 248-1111

American Association of Sex
  Education, Counselors &
  Therapists
435 North Michigan Avenue,
  Room 1717
Chicago, IL 60611-4067
(312) 644-0828

Sexual Behaviors Consultation Unit
  of Johns Hopkins Medical Center
550 North Broadway, Suite 114
Baltimore, MD 21205
(410) 955-6318

Impotence
Impotence Information Center
P.O. Box 9
Minneapolis, MN 55440
(impotence information)
(800) 843-4315
(prostate information)
(800) 543-9632

Impotence Institute of America
8201 Corporate Drive, Suite 320
Landover, MD 20785
(301) 577-0650
(800) 669-1603

SKIN AND HAIR PROBLEMS
American Academy of Dermatology
P.O. Box 4014
Schaumburg, Il 60168
(708) 330-0230

Hirsutism
Electrolysis Society
122 Syosset Circle
Syosset, NY 11791
(516) 364-9706
(800) 656-ESNY

International Guild of Professional
  Electrologists
202 Boulevard, Suite B
High Point, NC 27262
(910) 841-6631
(800) 837-3247

Psoriasis
National Psoriasis Foundation
6600 SW 92nd Avenue, Suite 300
Portland, OR 97223
(503) 244-7404

SLEEP DISORDERS

American Sleep Disorders
Association
1610 14th Street NW, Suite 300
Rochester, MN 55901
(507) 287-6006

National Sleep Foundation
1357 Connecticut Avenue NW
Washington, DC 20036
(202) 785-2300

Sleep Apnea
American Sleep Apnea Association
P.O. Box 66
Belmont, MA 02178-0001
(617) 489-4441
(617) 489-4761 FAX

SPEECH PROBLEMS

Aphasia
National Aphasia Association
Box 1887, Murray Hill Station
New York, NY 10156-0611
(800) 922-4622

Dysphonia
National Spasmodic Dysphonia
Association
P.O. Box 203
Atwood, CA 92601-0203
(800) 714-NSDA

Stuttering
National Center for Stuttering
200 East 33rd Street, Suite 17C
New York, NY 10016
(212) 532-1460

National Council on Stuttering
Box 3093
Skokie, IL 60077
(708) 677-8200

National Stuttering Project
2151 Irving Street, Suite 208
San Francisco, CA 94122-1609
(415) 566-5324
(800) 364-1677

URINARY TRACT DISORDERS

American Association of Kidney
Patients
100 South Ashley Drive, Suite 280
Tampa, FL 33602
(813) 223-7099

American Foundation for Urologic
Diseases
300 West Pratt Street, Suite 401
Baltimore, MD 21201
(800) 242-AFUD

National Kidney Foundation Inc.
30 East 33rd Street, 11th Floor
New York, NY 10016
(212) 889-2210
(800) 622-9010

National Kidney & Urologic Disease
Clearinghouse
3 Information Way
Bethesda, MD 20892-3580
(301) 654-4415

Incontinence
Continence Restored Inc.
785 Park Avenue
New York NY, 10021
(212) 879-3131

Help for Incontinent People (HIP)
Box 544
Union, SC 29379
(803) 579-7900
(800) BLADDER

Simon Foundation for Continence
Awareness
Box 835
Wilmette, IL 60091
(708) 864-3913
(800) 23-SIMON

Interstitial Cystitis
Interstitial Cystitis Association
P.O. Box 1553
Madison Square Station
New York, NY 10159
(212) 979-6057

VISION IMPAIRMENT

National Eye Health Education
Program
Box 20/20 Vision Place
Bethesda, MD 20892-3055

National Eye Insitute
Building 31, Room 6A32
Bethesda, MD 20892
(301) 496-5248

The Lighthouse Inc.
111 East 59th Street
New York, NY 10022
(212) 821-9200
(800) 334-5497

Blindness
American Council of the Blind
1155 15th Street NW, Suite 720
Washington, DC 20005
(202) 467-5081
(800) 424-8666

American Foundation for the Blind
11 Penn Plaza
New York, NY 10001
(212) 502-7600
(800) 232-5463

Association for the Education &
Rehabilitation of the Blind
and Visually Impaired
206 North Washington Street,
Suite 320
Alexandria, VA 22314
(703) 548-1884

Foundation Fighting Blindness
1401 Mount Royal Avenue,
4th Floor
Baltimore, MD 21217
(410) 225-9400

National Association for Parents of
the Visually Impaired
P.O. Box 317
Watertown, MA 02272-0317
(617) 362-4945
(800) 562-6265

National Association for the Visually
Handicapped
3201 Balboa Street
San Francisco, CA 94121
(415) 221-3201

National Library Service for the
Blind & Physically Handicapped
Library of Congress
1291 Taylor Street NW
Washington, DC 20542
(202) 707-5100

Glaucoma
Foundation for Glaucoma Research
490 Post Street, Suite 830
San Francisco, CA 94102
(415) 986-3162
(800) 826-6693

Guide Dogs
Guiding Eyes for the Blind Inc.
611 Granite Springs Road
Yorktown Heights, NY 10598
(914) 245-4024
(800) 942-0149

Pilot Dogs
625 West Town Street
Columbus, OH 43215
(614) 221-6367

Macular Degeneration
Association for Macular Diseases Inc.
(at Manhattan Eye, Ear, and Throat
Hospital)
210 East 64th Street
New York, NY 10021
(212) 605-3719

WOMEN'S HEALTH ISSUES

International Women's Health
Coalition
24 East 21st Street, 5th Floor
New York, NY 10010
(212) 979-8500
(212) 979-9009 FAX

Jacobs Institute of Women's Health
409 12th Street SW
Washington, DC 20024
(202) 863-4990

National Women's Health Network
514 10th Street NW, Suite 400
Washington, DC 20004
(202) 347-1140

National Women's Health Resource
Center
2440 M Street NW, Suite 325
Washington, DC 20037
(202) 293-6045

Women's Sports Foundation
Eisenhower Park
East Meadow, NY 11554
(800) 227-3988

Breast-Feeding and Parenting
La Leche League International
1400 North Meacham Road
Schaumburg, IL 60173-4840
(708) 519-7730
(800) LA-LECHE

National Healthy Mothers, Healthy
Babies Coalition
409 12th Street SW
Washington, DC 20024-2188
(202) 863-2458

Domestic Violence
National Clearinghouse for the
Defense of Battered Women
125 South 9th Street, Suite 302
Philadelphia, PA 19107
(215) 351-0010

National Coalition Against
Domestic Violence
P.O. Box 18749
Denver CO 80218
(303) 839-1852

National Domestic Violence Hotline
(800) 333-SAFE

National Organization for
Victim Assistance
1757 Park Road NW
Washington, DC 20002
(202) 232-6682

Menopause
North American Menopause Society
University Hospitals of Cleveland
Department of OB/GYN
2074 Abington Road
Cleveland, OH 44016
(216) 844-3334

MISCELLANEOUS RESOURCES

Disease Prevention
Office of Disease Prevention and
Health Promotion
National Health Information Center
Box 1133
Washington, DC 20013-1133
(800) 336-4797

MedicAlert
MedicAlert Foundation International
Box 1009
Turlock, CA 95381-1009
(209) 668-3333
(800) 344-3226

Medical Specialists
American Board of Medical
Specialists
180 Allen Road, Suite 302
Atlanta, GA 30328
(800) 776-2378
(To check certification status of
individual physicians)

Osteopathy
American Osteopathic Association
142 East Ontario Street
Chicago, IL 60611
(312) 280-5800

Poison Control Centers
American Association of Poison
Control Centers
3201 New Mexico Avenue,
Suite 310
Washington, DC 20016
(202) 362-7217

Rehabilitation
Commission on Accreditation of
Rehabilitation Facilities
101 North Wilmot Road
Tucson, AZ 85711

Self-Help Groups
National Self-Help Clearinghouse
25 West 34th Street
New York, NY 10037
(212) 354-8525

CREDITS

PHOTOGRAPHS

20 *top* © Francis Leroy, Biocosmos / SPL / Photo Researchers, Inc.; *bottom left* © NIBSC/ SPL/Photo Researchers,Inc.; *bottom right* © Professor P. Motta / Dept. of Anatomy/ University "La Sapienza,"Rome/SPL/Photo Researchers,Inc. ***21*** *top left* E. Gueho-CNRI/ SPL/Photo Researchers,Inc.; *bottom left* Tektoff/Rhone-Merieux/ CNRI/SPL/ Photo Researchers, Inc.; *top middle and middle* © CNRI/SPL/Photo Researchers, Inc.; *bottom middle* © Professor P. Motta / Dept. of Anatomy/ University "La Sapienza", Rome/SPL/Photo Researchers, Inc.; *right* CNRI / SPL/ Photo Researchers, Inc. ***22*** FPG International. ***23*** *top left* © H. Sochurek/ The Stock Shop, Inc./ Medichrome; *bottom left* © Richard Shock/Gamma Liaison International; *top right* © Paul Shambroom/ Science Source / Photo Researchers, Inc.; *bottom right* © C.C. Duncan/Medical Images,Inc. ***24*** *top* © Thomas Braise / Tony Stone Worldwide; *bottom* © Ken Fisher / Tony Stone Worldwide. ***25*** *top* © Florence Durand/Sipa Press; *bottom* © Stevie Grand/SPL/Photo Researchers, Inc. ***26*** *left* © Bachmann / Photo Researchers, Inc.; *right* © Dan McCoy/Rainbow. ***27*** *top left* © SIU/Visuals Unlimited; *bottom left* © Yoav Levy/Phototake NYC; *top right* © Jon Riley/The Stock Shop, Inc./Medichrome. ***28*** *left* © James Wilson/Woodfin Camp & Associates; *right* © Joe Lynch/Medical Images, Inc. ***29*** © Will McIntyre / Photo Researchers, Inc. ***30*** *top* © Lester Lefkowitz/ Tony Stone Worldwide; *bottom* © Hank Morgan/ Rainbow. ***31*** © Chuck O'Rear/ Woodfin Camp & Associates. ***32*** © Alon Reininger/Woodfin Camp & Associates. ***33*** © Chris Maynard/Gamma Liaison International. ***34*** *left and right* Photo: Charles Lamb, courtesy Joan Arnold. ***36*** *left* © Fran Heyl Associates; *right* Irene Rosner David, M.A., A.T.R., Bellevue Hospital Center. ***37*** © Alon Reininger/Contact Press Images. ***38*** © Dan McCoy/ Rainbow. ***39*** *top* © Art Stein/Photo Researchers, Inc.; *bottom* Parker Chiropractic Resource Foundation. ***40*** © Paul Biddle & Tim Malyon/SPL/ Photo Researchers, Inc. ***41*** © Jeffrey Hamilton/Stock Boston. ***42*** *top* © Will & Deni McIntyre/ Photo Researchers, Inc.; *bottom* © Dilip Mehta/Contact Press Images. ***43*** © Francois Perri/Gamma Liaison International. ***46*** © Florence Durand / Sipa Press. ***47*** © Stan Levy/Photo Researchers, Inc. ***48*** Courtesy Dr. George Roston, D.D.S. ***49*** *left* © John Griffin/The Stock Shop, Inc./ Medichrome; *right* © 1991 C. Arthur Tilley/ FPG International. ***50*** © L. Steinmark /Custom Medical Stock Photo. ***51*** *top left* © Dan McCoy/ Rainbow; *top right* © Dan & Will McCoy/Rainbow; *bottom* © Florence Durand/Sipa Press. ***52*** © Yoav Levy/Phototake NYC. ***53*** © Andy Cox/Tony Stone Worldwide. ***54*** *left and right* © Leo Sorel, Courtesy Nordoff-Robbins Music Therapy Clinic, New York University. ***55*** © Greg Vaughn/Tom Stack & Associates. ***58*** *left* © S. Bamberg/Sipa Press; *right* © J.B. Diederich/ Contact Press Images. ***59*** *left* © Frank Fournier/ Contact Press Images; *right* © Kal Muller/ Woodfin Camp & Associates. ***60*** © Catherine Smith/Impact Visuals. ***61*** © Trippett / Sipa Press. ***62*** © Yoav Levy/Phototake NYC. ***67*** © TJ Florian/ Rainbow. ***68*** © NMSB / Custom Medical Stock Photo. ***69*** *left* © Hank Morgan / Photo Researchers, Inc.; *right* © Custom Medical Stock Photo. ***70*** © Porter Gifford / Gamma Liaison International. ***71*** *left* © CNRI / SPL/ Photo Researchers, Inc.; *right* © David Scharf/Peter Arnold, Inc. ***72*** *left* © SIU / Visuals Unlimited; *right* © Fran Heyl Associates. ***74*** © Bill Aron / Photo Researchers, Inc. ***75*** © Annebicque / Sygma. ***77*** © David M. Phillips/ Visuals Unlimited. ***81*** *top and bottom* © Ed Kashi. ***82*** © Fran Heyl Associates. ***85*** © SPL/Photo Researchers, Inc. ***86*** © Acupressure Institute of America, Inc. ***89*** © Leo Sorel, Courtesy Nordoff-Robbins Music Therapy Clinic, New York University. ***95*** © Lawrence Fried / Magnum. ***96*** *top* © J.P.Jackson/Photo Researchers, Inc.; *middle* © G. C. Kelley/ Photo Researchers, Inc.; *bottom* © C. K. Lorenz/Photo Researchers, Inc. ***97*** *left* © Jeff Lepore / Photo Researchers, Inc.; *middle left* © William J. Weber / Visuals Unlimited; *middle right* © M. P. Kahl / Photo Researchers, Inc; *right* R. Andrew Odum / Peter Arnold, Inc. ***98*** *left* © Bill Curt-singer / Photo Researchers, Inc.; *right* © Tom McHugh / Photo Researchers, Inc. ***104*** © David Stoecklein / The Stock Market. ***106*** *top* © Simon Fraser / SPL / Photo Researchers, Inc.; *bottom* © Bill Nation / Sygma. ***107*** © Biophoto Associates /Science Source / Photo Researchers, Inc. ***108*** *left* © Dan McCoy / Rainbow; *right* © Scott Camazine / Photo Researchers, Inc. ***114*** © Luis Castañeda / The Image Bank. ***115*** © Richard Trump / Photo Researchers, Inc. ***117*** © Dan McCoy / Rainbow. ***119*** © Patti McConville / The Image Bank. ***121*** *left* © Adam Hart-Davis / SPL/ Photo Researchers, Inc.; *right* © Andrew McClenaghan / SPL / Photo Researchers, Inc. ***124*** © Bob Masini/ Phototake NYC. ***126*** © Will & Deni McIntyre / Photo Researchers, Inc. ***128*** © Herb Charles Ohlmeyer/Fran Heyl Associates. ***130*** © Kit King/Gamma Liaison International. ***131*** *top* Biophoto Associates / Photo Researchers, Inc.; *bottom left* © Lannen / Kelly Photography; *bottom right* © Michael Molkenthin ***133*** © Frank Fournier / Contact Press Images. ***134*** © Brownie Harris/The Stock Market. ***135*** © Jim Stevenson / SPL / Photo Researchers, Inc. ***137*** *left* © Martin Rotker / Phototake NYC. ***138*** © Kathryn Abbe. ***143*** © Mauritius GMBH/ Phototake NYC. ***144*** *left* © Custom Medical Stock Photo; *right* © G. DeGrazia/ Custom Medical Stock Photo. ***146*** © Jennifer Watson-Holton / Custom Medical Stock Photo. ***148*** *top* © Caroline Brown / Fran Heyl Associates; *bottom* © Martin / Custom Medical Stock Photo. ***150*** *left* © John Watney / Science Source/ Photo Researchers, Inc.; *right* © Fran Heyl Associates. ***153*** *left and right* © Michael Newman / Photo Edit. ***154*** © Alan Oddie / Photo Edit. ***155*** © David Madison / Duomo. ***156*** © Dr. Michael Kramer/ Fran Heyl Associates. ***158*** © Michael Tamborrino /The Stock Shop, Inc./Medichrome. ***160*** © Fran Heyl Associates. ***161*** *top* © Charles Gupton / Tony Stone Worldwide. ***162*** © Andy Levin / Photo Researchers, Inc. ***164*** © Tony Freeman/ Photo Edit. ***166*** © David Young-Wolff / Photo Edit. ***167*** © Fran Heyl Associates. ***168*** © J.S. Reid / Custom Medical Stock Photo. ***170*** Dave Black. ***171*** © Tony Freeman / Photo Edit. ***172*** *left* © SPL / Photo Researchers, Inc.; *right* © Larry Voigt/Photo Researchers, Inc. ***173*** © Deborah Davis / Photo Edit. ***175*** © Tony Freeman / Photo Edit. ***181*** © Michael Furman/The Stock Market. ***182*** © Myrleen Ferguson / Photo Edit. ***184*** © Caroline Brown / Fran Heyl Associates. ***185*** © Ed Pritchard /Tony Stone Worldwide. ***186*** *all* © Fran Heyl Associates. ***189*** © Doug Plummer / Photo Researchers, Inc. ***190*** © Charles Gupton/ Stock Boston. ***194*** © 1991 B.S.I.P./ Custom Medical Stock Photo. ***195*** *top and bottom left* © Dr.Michael Kramer / Fran Heyl Associates; *right* Copyright © 1995, Carroll H. Weiss. All rights reserved. ***196*** © Tony Freeman / Photo Edit. ***198*** © Pix*Elation / Fran Heyl Associates. ***199*** © 1991 SPL / Custom Medical Stock Photo. ***202*** © 1992 NMSB / Custom Medical Stock Photo. ***203*** © Grapes / Michaud / Science Source/ Photo Researchers, Inc. ***205*** © Custom Medical Stock Photo. ***207*** *top* © Margaret Cubberly/ Phototake NYC; *bottom* © L.V. Bergman / Fran Heyl Associates. ***213*** © 1991 B.S.I.P./ Custom Medical Stock Photo. ***215*** *top* © Yoav Levy / Phototake NYC. ***216*** *top left* Photo © Herb Charles Ohlmeyer / Fran Heyl Associates, taken at Department of Cardiology, St. Joseph's Hospital, NJ; *top and bottom right* © SPL/Photo Researchers, Inc.; *bottom* © Charles Gupton / Stock Boston. ***218*** *left and right* © SIU/Peter Arnold, Inc. ***223*** Copyright © 1995, Carroll H. Weiss. All rights reserved. ***226*** © Custom Medical Stock Photo. ***230*** © Mauritius GMBH/ Phototake NYC. ***231*** © Barbara Alper / Stock Boston. ***232*** © David Young-Wolff / Photo Edit. ***234*** *left* © Dr. Jeremy Burgess / SPL / Photo Researchers, Inc.; *right* © Fran Heyl Associates. ***237*** © Fran Heyl Associates. ***238*** *left* © Fran Heyl Associates; *right* © Clive Robbins, Courtesy Nordoff-Robbins Music Therapy Clinic, New York University. ***239*** © Arthur Tress / Science Source/Photo Researchers, Inc. ***240*** © Fran Heyl Associates. ***241*** © Tom McCarthy 1992, The Picture Cube. ***243*** Copyright © 1995, Carroll H. Weiss. All rights reserved. ***247*** © Hank Morgan / Science Source / Photo Researchers, Inc. ***251*** *left* © Jean Claude Revy / Phototake NYC; *right* © Henley & Savage / The Stock Market. ***253*** © Varian Associates, Inc. / Fran Heyl Associates. ***255*** © David Young-Wolff / Photo Edit. ***258*** *top* Copyright © 1995, Carroll H. Weiss. All rights reserved.; *bottom* © Tom Raymond / The Stock Shop, Inc. / Medichrome. ***259*** © John Moss / Photo Researchers, Inc. ***260*** *left* © Dr. Libby Edwards / Fran Heyl Associates. ***262*** © Hank Morgan/ Rainbow. ***264*** © Mary Kate Denny / Photo Edit. ***265*** © Herb Charles Ohlmeyer / Fran Heyl Associates. ***267*** *left and right* INHEALTH Technologies, Carpinteria, CA. ***269*** © Laura Dwight. ***271*** © Herb Charles Ohlmeyer/ Fran Heyl Associates. ***272*** © Ettore Malanca / Sipa Press. ***274*** *left* © Fran Heyl Associates; *right* © Jean Claude Revy/ Phototake NYC. ***276*** © W. Bokelberg / The Image Bank. ***277*** © Melchior DiGiacomo / The Image Bank. ***280*** *right* © Bernard Furnival / Fran Heyl Associates. ***284*** © Dr. Leonard E. Munstermann / Fran Heyl Associates. ***285*** © A.Sieveking / Petit Format / Photo Researchers, Inc. ***286*** *top* © Biophoto Associates / Science Source / Photo Researchers, Inc.; *bottom* © Custom Medical Stock Photo. ***287*** © James Stevenson / SPL / Photo Researchers, Inc. ***290*** © Bill Bachman / Photo Researchers, Inc. ***292*** © Walter Bibikow / The Image Bank. ***297*** © Gary Parker/SPL/ Photo Researchers, Inc. ***298*** © Dan McCoy/ Rainbow. ***301*** © Willie L. Hill, Jr./ Stock Boston. ***302*** © Randy Brandon / Fran Heyl Associates. ***303*** © Joe Traver / Gamma Liaison International. ***304*** © C.James Webb / Phototake NYC. ***307*** © Yoav Levy / Phototake NYC. ***308*** Copyright © 1995, Carroll H. Weiss. All rights reserved. ***313*** Photo: Charles Lamb, courtesy Joan Arnold. ***314*** © Jack Reznicki. ***315*** *left* © David Young-Wolff / Photo Edit; *right* © Fran Heyl Associates. ***318*** © Frank Siteman / Stock Boston. ***324*** *left and right* © Dan McCoy / Rainbow. ***328*** © Yoav Levy /Phototake NYC. ***329*** © Ed Kashi/ Phototake NYC. ***333*** © Fran Heyl Associates. ***334*** *top* © J.F. Wilson/ Photo Researchers, Inc.; *bottom* © Biophoto Associates/Photo Researchers, Inc. ***335*** *top and bottom* © Dr. Bernard Cohen / Fran Heyl Associates. ***336*** *left* © 1993 NMSB/ Custom Medical Stock Photo; *right* © 1993 SPL/ Custom Medical Stock Photo. ***341*** © Kenneth Hayden / Black Star. ***343*** © Marvin Collins/ Fran Heyl Associates. ***344*** © Tim Bieber/The Image Bank. ***353*** © Fran Heyl Associates. ***354*** © Custom Medical Stock Photos. ***356*** © Blair Seitz / Photo Researchers, Inc. ***357*** © Herb Charles Ohlmeyer / Fran Heyl Associates. ***361*** © Caroline Brown / Fran Heyl Associates. ***362*** © Comstock, Inc. ***363*** Copyright © 1995, Carroll H. Weiss. All rights reserved. ***365*** © Erik Hildebrandt / Photo Researchers, Inc. ***366*** *left* © Custom Medical Stock Photo; *right* © Phototake NYC. ***367*** *top* © SIU / Visuals Unlimited; *bottom* © Custom Medical Stock Photo. ***368*** *left* © Biophoto Associates / Photo Researchers, Inc.; *right* © Herb Charles Ohlmeyer at Advanced Dermatology Associates, NY/ Fran Heyl Associates. ***369*** Collection: Phyllis Kind Gallery; Photo courtesy of Phyllis Kind Gallery, New York / Chicago. ***371*** Copyright © 1995. Carroll H. Weiss. All rights reserved. ***373*** © Custom Medical Stock Photo. ***376*** © Custom Medical Stock Photo. ***380*** *top left* © Andrew Popper / Phototake NYC; *top right* © Dr. Libby Edwards / Fran Heyl Associates; *bottom* Copyright © 1995. Carroll H. Weiss. All rights reserved. ***381*** © Custom Medical Stock Photo. ***385*** © Fran Heyl Associates. ***386*** © Yoav Levy / Phototake NYC. ***392*** © Dorothy Tanous Photography / Fran Heyl Associates. ***396*** © Western Ophthalmic Hospital / SPL/ Custom Medical Stock Photo. ***397*** © Rebecca C. Heyl / Fran Heyl Associates. ***400*** © SIU / Photo Researchers, Inc. ***405*** © David W. Hamilton / The Image Bank. ***406*** © Janice Godwin / Fran Heyl Associates. ***409*** © Dr. P. Marazzi / SPL/Custom Medical Stock Photo. ***410*** *left and right* © Dr. Lawrence Swayne, computer enhanced by © Pix*Elation / Fran Heyl Associates. ***411*** © SIU/ Visuals Unlimited. ***414*** © Ed Kashi / Phototake NYC. ***418*** *top* © Dr. Jeffrey P. Callen / Fran Heyl Associates; *bottom* © Dr. Anthony du Vivier / Fran Heyl Associates. ***423*** © Frank Spooner / Gamma Liaison International. ***424*** *top* © Scott Camazine / Photo Researchers, Inc.; *bottom* © Ken Greer / Visuals Unlimited. ***425*** © Fran Heyl Associates. ***434*** *top* © Bill Aron / Photo Edit; *bottom* © Rebecca C. Heyl / Fran Heyl Associates. ***435*** *top* © Dr. Fred Pereira / Fran Heyl Associates; *bottom* © Dr. Libby Edwards / Fran Heyl Associates. ***439*** *top* © J.F. Wilson / Photo Re-searchers, Inc.; *middle top* © Dr. Libby Edwards / Fran Heyl Associates; *middle bottom* © Biophoto Associates / Science Source/ Photo Researchers, Inc.; *bottom* © David Parker / Science Photo Library / Photo Researchers, Inc. ***440*** *top and bottom* © Fran Heyl Associates. ***442*** © Will & Deni McIntyre / Science Source / Photo Researchers, Inc. ***443*** © Leonard E. Munstermann, PhD. / Fran Heyl Associates.

Grateful acknowledgment is made for permission to excerpt featured material from the following works:

American Psychiatric Press, Inc. *DSM-III-R Case Book* edited by Robert Spitzer et al. Copyright ©1989 by American Psychiatric Press, Inc. Used by permission. **Atheneum.** *Hormones: The Woman's Answerbook* by Lois Jovanovic and Genell J. Subak-Sharpe. Copyright © 1987 by Lois Jovanovic and Genell Subak-Sharpe. **Oriental Healing Arts Institue of USA.** *Chinese Herb Medicine and Therapy, Revised Edition* by Hong-yen Hsu and William G. Peacher. Copyright © 1982 by Oriental Healing Arts Institute. Used by permission. **St. Martin's Press.** *Total Nutrition: The Only Guide You'll Ever Need* edited by Victor Herbert and Genell Subak-Sharpe. Copyright ©1995 by Mount Sinai School of Medicine.